THE
WRIST
AND ITS DISORDERS

THE
WRIST
AND ITS DISORDERS

SECOND EDITION

David M. Lichtman, MD
John S. Dunn Professor of Orthopaedic Surgery of the Hand
Department of Orthopaedic Surgery
Baylor College of Medicine
Houston, Texas

A. Herbert Alexander, MD
Professor of Surgery
Uniformed Services University of the Health Sciences
Bethesda, MD

W.B. SAUNDERS COMPANY
A Division of Harcourt Brace & Company
Philadelphia ▪ London ▪ Toronto ▪ Montreal ▪ Sydney ▪ Tokyo

W.B. SAUNDERS COMPANY
A Division of Harcourt Brace & Company

The Curtis Center
Independence Square West
Philadelphia, Pennsylvania 19106

Library of Congress Cataloging-in-Publication Data

The wrist and its disorders / [edited by] David M. Lichtman,
A. Herbert Alexander.—2nd ed.

p.   cm.

Includes bibliographical references and index.

ISBN 0–7216–4774–X

1. Wrist—Wounds and injuries.   2. Wrist—Pathophysiology.
 I. Lichtman, David M.   II. Alexander, A. H.
 [DNLM: 1. Wrist Injuries. 2. Carpal Bones—injuries.
 WE 830 W955   1997]

RD 559.W75   1997   617.5′74 — dc20

DNLM/DLC   96-7415

THE WRIST AND ITS DISORDERS   ISBN 0–7216–4774–X

Printed in the United States of America.

Last digit is the print number: 9   8   7   6   5   4   3   2   1

To Harry and Frances Lichtman, my parents, for their love and support.
To Frankie, my wife, for being my best friend.
To Elisa, Jamie, and Jenni, for being successful and independent children.
To Spencer and Miranda, for being everything we wanted in grandchildren.

DML

To my wife, Charlotte E. Alexander, for keeping me directed and for looking after the family.
To my daughters, Amy and Mandy, who brighten our lives daily with their enthusiasm and zeal.
To my mother, Mildred Alexander, for encouraging me to be everything I wanted to be.

AHA

CONTRIBUTORS

Charlotte E. Alexander, MD
Professor of Surgery, Uniformed Services University
of the Health Sciences, Bethesda, Maryland
 Triquetrolunate Instability; Kienböck's Disease and
 Idiopathic Necrosis of Carpal Bones

H. Herbert Alexander, MD
Professor of Surgery, Uniformed Services University
of the Health Sciences, Bethesda, Maryland
 Kienböck's Disease and Idiopathic Necrosis of Carpal
 Bones; Treatment of Acute Injuries of the Distal
 Radioulnar Joint

Gregory I. Bain, MBBS
Division of Orthopaedic Surgery, University of
Western Ontario Faculty of Medicine, London,
Ontario, Canada
 Wrist Arthroscopy

Robert D. Beckenbaugh, MD
Professor of Orthopaedic Surgery, Mayo Medical
School; Consultant, Department of Orthopaedics
and Division of Hand Surgery, Mayo Clinic,
Rochester, Minnesota
 Total Wrist Arthroplasty

Gerald Blatt, MD, FACS
Associate Clinical Professor, Orthopaedic Surgery,
University of California, Los Angeles, UCLA School
of Medicine; Hand Surgery Service, Harbor-UCLA
Medical Center; Consultant, Arthritis Center and
Children's Hospital of L.A., Los Angeles; Long Beach
Memorial Medical Center, Long Beach, California
 Scapholunate Injuries

George P. Bogumill, PhD, MD
Professor of Orthopaedic Surgery, Georgetown
University School of Medicine; Clinical Professor of
Orthopaedic Surgery, Uniformed Services University
of Health Sciences, Washington, DC
 Anatomy of the Wrist; Tumors of the Wrist

Michael J. Botte, MD
Professor of Orthopaedic Surgery and Chief,
Division of Hand and Foot Surgery, Department of
Orthopaedics, University of California, San Diego,
School of Medicine, San Diego, California
 Vascularity of the Carpus

William H. Bowers, MD
Chief, Children's Upper Extremity Service,
Children's Hospital, Richmond, Virginia
 Treatment of Acute Injuries of the Triangular
 Fibrocartilage Complex; Treatment of Chronic Disorders
 of the Distal Radioulnar Joint

Gordon A. Brody, MD
Clinical Associate Professor of Rheumatology and
Orthopaedic Surgery, Stanford University School of
Medicine; Hand Consultant, San Francisco Forty-
niners (National Football League), Stanford; Chief,
Hand and Wrist Surgery, Sports, Orthopaedics, and
Rehabilitation Associates, Menlo Park, California
 Advanced Imaging of the Carpus

David E. Brown, MD
Clinical Assistant Professor of Surgery, University of
Nebraska College of Medicine; Staff Orthopaedic
Surgeon, Sports Medicine Center, Omaha, Nebraska
 Physical Examination of the Wrist

Alvin H. Crawford, MD, FACS
Professor of Pediatrics and Orthopaedic Surgery,
University of Cincinnati College of Medicine;
Director of Pediatric Orthopaedic Surgery, Children's
Hospital Medical Center, Cincinnati, Ohio
 Congenital and Developmental Wrist Disorders in
 Children; Traumatic and Acquired Wrist Disorders in
 Children

David J. Curtis, MD
Clinical Assistant Professor, Duke University School
of Medicine; Staff Radiologist, Veterans
Administration Hospital (Durham), Durham, North
Carolina
 Soft Tissue Radiography of the Wrist

Gregory G. Degnan, MD
Assistant Professor of Orthopaedic Surgery,
University of Virginia School of Medicine,
Charlottesville, Virginia; Assistant Professor of
Surgery, Uniformed Services University of Health
Sciences, Bethesda, Maryland
 Soft Tissue Arthroplasty About the Wrist; Assessment;
 Conservative Rehabilitation

Edward F. Downey, Jr., DO
Clinical Associate Professor, Department of
Radiology, West Virginia University School of
Medicine; Chief, Department of Imaging Services,
Monongalia General Hospital, Morgantown, West
Virginia
 Soft Tissue Radiography of the Wrist

Paul W. Esposito, MD
Associate Professor of Pediatrics and Orthopaedic Surgery, University of Nebraska College of Medicine; Associate Professor, Pediatric Orthopaedic Surgery, University of Nebraska Medical Center, Omaha, Nebraska
   Congenital and Developmental Wrist Disorders in Children; Traumatic and Acquired Wrist Disorders in Children

Paul G. Feldon, MD
Clinical Associate Professor of Orthopaedic Surgery, Tufts University School of Medicine, Boston; Chief, Hand Service, St. Elizabeth's Medical Center of Boston, Brighton, Massachusetts
   Partial Wrist Fusions: Intercarpal and Radiocarpal; Arthrodesis of the Wrist: Indications and Surgical Technique

Donald C. Ferlic, MD
Associate Clinical Professor, University of Colorado School of Medicine; President, Denver Orthopaedic Specialists, Denver, Colorado
   Inflammatory and Rheumatoid Arthritis

Geoffrey R. Fisk, MB, BS, FRCSEng, FRCSEdin
Hunterian Professor, Royal College of Surgeons, London; Honorary Orthopaedic Surgeon, Princess Alexandra Hospital, Harlow and St. Margaret's Hospital, Epping, England
   The Development of Wrist Surgery: A Historical Review

Eric S. Gaenslen, MD
Milwaukee, Wisconsin
   Midcarpal and Proximal Carpal Instabilities

Richard H. Gelberman, MD
Professor of Orthopaedic Surgery, Washington University School of Medicine, Saint Louis, Missouri
   Vascularity of the Carpus

Louis A. Gilula, MD
Professor of Radiology, Washington University School of Medicine, Saint Louis, Missouri
   Post-Traumatic Wrist Pain and Instability: A Radiographic Approach to Diagnosis

Stephen Flack Gunther, MD
Professor, Department of Orthopaedic Surgery, George Washington University School of Medicine and Health Sciences, Washington, DC; Clinical Professor, Department of Surgery, Uniformed Services University of Health Sciences, Bethesda, Maryland; Chairman, Department of Orthopaedic Surgery, The Washington Hospital Center, Washington, DC
   Carpometacarpal Joint of the Thumb; The Medial Four Carpometacarpal Joints

Emily Jeter, OTR/L
Hand Rehabilitation Specialist, NRH Center for Spine, Sports and Occupational Rehabilitation, Bethesda, Maryland
   Assessment; Conservative Rehabilitation; Postoperative Wrist Rehabilitation

Samuel D. Kao, MD
Hand Fellow, Connecticut Combined Hand Surgery Service, Hartford, Connecticut
   Degenerative Disorders of the Carpus

Jon Pembroke Kelly, MD
Attending Orthopaedic Surgeon, Palomar Medical Center, Escondido, and Pomerado Hospital, Poway, California
   Scaphoid Non-Union

David M. Lichtman, MD
John S. Dunn Professor of Orthopaedic Surgery of the Hand, Department of Orthopaedic Surgery, Baylor College of Medicine, Houston, Texas
   Introduction to the Carpal Instabilities; Scaphoid Non-Union; Scapholunate Injuries; Triquetrolunate Instability; Midcarpal and Proximal Carpal Instabilities; Kienböck's Disease and Idiopathic Necrosis of Carpal Bones; Distal Radius Malunion; Treatment of Acute Injuries of the Distal Radioulnar Joint; Occupational and Sports Injuries of the Wrist; Soft Tissue Arthroplasty About the Wrist; Amputations About the Wrist; Assessment; Conservative Rehabilitation; Postoperative Wrist Rehabilitation

Jon B. Loftus, MD
Department of Orthopaedic Surgery, State University of New York Health Science Center at Syracuse College of Medicine, Syracuse, New York
   Disorders of the Distal Radioulnar Joint and Triangular Fibrocartilage Complex: An Overview

Gregory R. Mack, MD
Associate Clinical Professor, University of California, San Diego, School of Medicine; Chairman, Department of Orthopaedic Surgery, Naval Medical Center, San Diego, California
   Scaphoid Non-Union

Frederick A. Mann, MD
Professor of Radiology and Associate Professor of Orthopaedics, University of Washington School of Medicine, Seattle, Washington
   Post-Traumatic Wrist Pain and Instability: A Radiographic Approach to Diagnosis

Andrew D. Markiewitz, MD, BSChemEng
Associate Clinical Professor of Surgery, Uniformed Services University of the Health Sciences; Orthopaedic Surgeon, Hand Specialist, and Deputy, Element Leader, Keesler Medical Center, Keesler Air Force Base, Mississippi
   Carpal Fractures and Dislocations

Jack K. Mayfield, MD
Adjunct Professor, Department of Biologic, Chemical, and Materials Engineering, Arizona State University; Attending Orthopaedic Surgery Staff, St. Luke's Medical Center, Phoenix, Arizona
    Pathogenesis and Pathokinetics of Perilunate Wrist Instability

H. Relton McCarroll, Jr., MD
Associate Clinical Professor of Orthopaedic Surgery, University of California, San Francisco, School of Medicine; Chairman, Division of Hand Surgery, California Pacific Medical Center, San Francisco, California
    Nerve Injuries Associated with Wrist Trauma

Robert H. Meier, III, MD
Director of Medical Rehabilitation, O'Hara Regional Center for Rehabilitation, Denver, Colorado
    Amputations About the Wrist

Charles P. Melone, Jr., MD
Clinical Professor of Orthopaedic Surgery, New York University School of Medicine; Director of Orthopaedic Hand Surgery, New York University Medical Center, New York, New York
    Fractures of the Distal Radius

Edward A. Nalebuff, MD
Clinical Professor of Orthopaedic Surgery, Tufts University School of Medicine; Chief of Hand Surgery, New England Baptist Hospital, Boston, Massachusetts
    Partial Wrist Fusions: Intercarpal and Radiocarpal; Arthrodesis of the Wrist: Indications and Surgical Technique

Steven R. Novotny, MD
Hand and Microvascular Surgeon and Orthopaedic Surgeon, Arnett Clinic, Lafayette, Indiana
    Distal Radius Malunion; Occupational and Sports Injuries of the Wrist

Eugene T. O'Brien, MD
Division of Orthopaedic Surgery, Tufts University School of Medicine, Boston, Massachusetts
    Carpal Fractures and Dislocations

Andrew K. Palmer, MD
Professor of Orthopaedic Surgery and Director, Hand Surgery Section, State University of New York Health Science Center at Syracuse, Syracuse, New York
    Disorders of the Distal Radioulnar Joint and Triangular Fibrocartilage Complex: An Overview

Garry R. Pollock, MD, PharmD
Active Staff, Methodist Children's Hospital, St. Mary's of the Plains Hospital, South Park Hospital & Medical Center, Lubbock, Texas
    Midcarpal and Proximal Carpal Instabilities; Amputations About the Wrist

Sudhir B. Rao, MD
Private Practice, Big Rapids Orthopaedics PC, Big Rapids, Michigan
    Congenital and Developmental Wrist Disorders in Children; Traumatic and Acquired Wrist Disorders in Children

Keith B. Raskin, MD
Clinical Associate Professor, New York University School of Medicine; Attending Surgeon, New York University Medical Center, New York, New York
    Fractures of the Distal Radius

Michael E. Rettig, MD
Assistant Professor, Department of Orthopaedic Surgery, New York University School of Medicine, New York, New York
    Fractures of the Distal Radius

Robert S. Richards, MD
Division of Orthopaedic Surgery, University of Western Ontario Faculty of Medicine, London, Ontario, Canada
    Wrist Arthroscopy

James H. Roth, MD, FRCSC
Professor, Division of Orthopaedic Surgery, University of Western Ontario Faculty of Medicine; Director, Hand and Upper Limb Centre, Chief of Orthopaedics, St. Joseph's Hospital, London, Ontario, Canada
    Wrist Arthroscopy

Leonard K. Ruby, MD
Professor of Orthopedic Surgery, Tufts University School of Medicine; Director, Division Hand Surgery, New England Medical Center Hospitals, Boston, Massachusetts
    Carpal Fractures and Dislocations

Terri Skirven, OTR, CHT
Sports Medicine Center, Omaha, Nebraska
    Physical Examination of the Wrist

David W. Stoller, MD
Assistant Clinical Professor of Radiology, University of California, San Francisco, School of Medicine, Director, California Advanced Imaging; Director, Marin Radiology and National Orthopedic Imaging Associates; San Francisco, California
    Advanced Imaging of the Carpus

Alfred B. Swanson, MD, FACS
Professor of Surgery, Michigan State University College of Human Medicine, East Lansing; Director of Orthopaedic Surgery, Residency Training Program of The Grand Rapids Hospitals; Director of Hand Surgery Fellowship and Orthopaedic Research, Blodgett Memorial Medical Center, Grand Rapids, Michigan
    Implant Arthroplasty in the Carpal and Radiocarpal Joints

Geneviève de Groot Swanson, MD
Assistant Clinical Professor of Surgery, Michigan State University College of Human Medicine, East Lansing; Coordinator, Orthopaedic Research Department, Blodgett Memorial Medical Center, Grand Rapids, Michigan
   Implant Arthroplasty in the Carpal and Radiocarpal Joints

Andrew L. Terrono, MD
Clinical Assistant Professor of Orthopaedic Surgery, Tufts University School of Medicine; Hand Surgeon, New England Baptist Hospital, Boston, Massachusetts
   Partial Wrist Fusions: Intercarpal and Radiocarpal; Arthrodesis of the Wrist; Indications and Surgical Technique

Brian Tobias, DO
Clinical Assistant Professor, Department of Orthopaedics, Institute of Hand and Upper Extremity Disorders, Baylor College of Medicine; Clinical Assistant Professor, The Methodist Hospital, St. Luke's Episcopal Hospital, and Texas Children's Hospital, Houston, Texas
   Scapholunate Injuries

Craig M. Torosian, MD
Attending Staff Physician, Fox Valley Orthopaedic Institute, Geneva, Illinois
   Physical Examination of the Wrist

H. Kirk Watson, MD
Clinical Professor, University of Connecticut School of Medicine, Farmington, Connecticut; Assistant Clinical Professor, Yale University School of Medicine, New Haven, Connecticut; Associate Professor, University of Massachusetts Medical School, Worcester, Massachusetts; Director, Connecticut Combined Hand Surgery Fellowship, Hartford, Connecticut; Chief, Hand Surgery, Connecticut Children's Medical Center, and Senior Staff, Hartford Hospital, Hartford, Connecticut
   Degenerative Disorders of the Carpus

Edward R. Weber, MD
Associate Professor, Department of Orthopaedic Surgery, University of Arkansas College of Medicine, Little Rock, Arkansas
   Physiologic Bases for Wrist Function

Terry L. Whipple, MD
Clinical Professor of Orthopaedic Surgery, Bowman Gray School of Medicine at Wake Forest University, Winston-Salem, North Carolina; Clinical Associate Professor in Orthopaedic Surgery, Department of Surgery, Virginia Commonwealth University Medical College of Virginia, Richmond; Clinical Associate Professor of Orthopaedics and Rehabilitation, University of Virginia School of Medicine, Charlottesville, Virginia
   Clinical Applications of Wrist Arthroscopy

Ellison H. Wittels, MD
Associate Professor of Medicine, Baylor College of Medicine; Attending Physician, The Methodist Hospital, Houston, Texas
   Occupational and Sports Injuries of the Wrist

David S. Zelouf, MD
Assistant Clinical Professor, Virginia Commonwealth University Medical College of Virginia School of Medicine, Richmond, Virginia
   Treatment of Acute Injuries of the Triangular Fibrocartilage Complex; Treatment of Chronic Disorders of the Distal Radioulnar Joint

Preface

The first edition of *The Wrist and Its Disorders* was written to synthesize a vast amount of disparate information about the wrist into a well-organized and cohesive study of the carpus. It was also intended to be practical and very informative.

To accomplish these goals, the efforts of 38 different authors, all major contributors to the understanding of wrist disorders, were enlisted. The result was a 500-page text with 30 chapters divided into five sections. Judging by its widespread use and favorable reviews, the first edition met its objectives.

Now, 10 years later, there is once again a large accumulation of data and information pertaining to the wrist. And, again, there is a need to organize and synthesize this material. The object of the second edition therefore, is, to incorporate the discoveries of the past 10 years, keeping the text well-organized, profusely illustrated, and very practical. Given the magnitude of the effort, the founding editor (DML) was joined by a long-time colleague (AHA).

As a result, *The Wrist and Its Disorders*, second edition, has been expanded from five to nine general sections. Because of escalating interest in occupational disorders and sports medicine, this related material is placed into its own section—which also incorporates nerve injuries about the wrist. The section on trauma is reorganized into three sections based on anatomic location: the carpometacarpal joints, the carpus, and the distal radius and ulna. The latter contains new chapters on distal radius malunions and acute injuries of the distal radioulnar joint. It also examines injuries of selected levels of the forearm and elbow, as they are related to dysfunction of the distal radioulnar joint. A new section devoted to physical and occupational therapy of the wrist has been added. It is divided into chapters on therapeutic evaluation and assessment, conservative therapy, and postoperative rehabilitation.

Several other new chapters have been incorporated into the five pre-existing sections making a total of 42 chapters. Because of the complexity and increasing use of advanced imaging of the wrist, we included a chapter covering this topic, emphasizing magnetic resonance. Pediatric wrist disorders are expanded to two chapters—the first devoted to congenital and developmental disorders and the second to traumatic and acquired conditions in children. A new chapter on amputations, part of the surgical options section, reviews amputations at multiple levels about the wrist and discusses comparative indications and unique psychosocial implications.

The majority of the remaining chapters from the first edition are greatly expanded to keep abreast of the information explosion of the past 10 years. For example, *Scapholunate Injuries* contains more than 250 additional references and a new classification system based upon our newly developed treatment algorithm. The chapters on physical examination, wrist arthroscopy, carpal fractures and dislocations, scaphoid non-unions, and disorders of the distal radioulnar joint and triangular fibrocartilage complex have also undergone significant revision and expansion. Of particular interest is the introductory chapter—*The Development of Wrist Surgery: A Historical Review*—written by Professor Geoffrey R. Fisk. Drs. Novotny and Lichtman have taken great care to preserve Mr. Fisk's unique contribution. Extensive updates are included, but the reader can still identify and enjoy Mr. Fisk's original chapter. The updates also reflect Dr. Lichtman's personal opinion about which of the newer contributions will eventually join the "classics."

In summary, we are very pleased with the results of this effort. The size of the text greatly expands the original volume. It was more work than we expected for a "simple" revision, but collaborating for the second time with such a talented group of contributors was extremely rewarding. *The Wrist and Its Disorders*, second edition, is unique among a growing list of textbooks on the wrist. It still relies mainly upon the personal input of a wide variety of original researchers and contributors to the field, yet their efforts are bound with a common terminology and a systematic approach to the wrist—its anatomy, its biomechanics, and its disorders.

DAVID M. LICHTMAN, M.D.
A. HERBERT ALEXANDER, M.D.

Contents

PART I

Basic Science

CHAPTER 1

The Development of Wrist Surgery: A Historical Review

Geoffrey R. Fisk, MB, BS*

Surgery of the wrist and hand is no doubt as old as civilization itself, since the arm is the part of the body most exposed to injury, whether from falls, hunting accidents, or in battle (Fig. 1–1). The endeavors by the Egyptians, Greeks, and Romans to heal and minimize the baleful effects of the crippled hand have continued unabated by their successors to the present day. Amputation of part or the whole of the hand for ceremonial or penal purposes was practiced by early humans and illustrated on the walls of the caves in La Tene and Lascaux at least 30,000 years ago.[1]

A visit to the museum at Epidaurus in Greece, where the first asclepion was established in the fifth century BC, reveals surgical instruments that are instantly recognizable. Hippocrates (460–356 BC) wrote 28 books that contained all contemporary medical knowledge and included one section entitled "Fractures and Reduction of Dislocations." It would seem, however, that at the time amputation of the hand was the only life-saving measure available, and the provision of an artificial hand has an ancient lineage. On July 19, 1965, an account was written in the London *Times* of an operation to remove an artificial hand from an Egyptian mummy. Pliny the Elder (23–79 AD) described a similar case with an artificial hand.[2] Indeed, Johannes Scultatus wrote a learned treatise on the techniques of amputation of the upper extremity, entitled *Armamentarium Chirurgicum Bipartum*, that was published in Frankfurt in 1666. Ambroise Paré, the founder of French surgery, also described an artificial hand in a work entitled *Of the Means and Manner to Repair or Supply the Natural or Accidental Defects or Wants in Man's Bodie* (*Oeuvres*, 1664). He was also an early pioneer in the excision and resection of joints.

Paul of Aegina (256–290 AD) first described a "ganglion" as a swelling formed around joints, particularly the wrist, but he described this as a "round tumour of tendon." He did not recommend any treatment for such a swelling, but there is little doubt that

hitting or squashing it would have occurred to those early surgeons.

Jean Louis Petit (1674–1750) described congenital anomalies and dislocations of the hand and wrist. Jules Desault (1738–1795)[3] also wrote on dislocations of the carpus, and Pierre Brasdor described disarticulation of the hand at the level of the wrist. By the latter part of the eighteenth century, attempts were made to deal with the ravages of infection, particularly tuberculosis, and in 1805, Moreau (father and son) published in Paris *Resection of Articulations Affected by Caries*.

Vesalius (1543) first described and illustrated the wrist joint in his fundamental anatomy textbook, *De humani corporis fabrica* (Fig. 1–2),[107] and these illustrations were copied by Spigelius.[108] The ligamentous structures binding these bones together have also been fully described, but until relatively recently the physiology of the wrist has been neglected. In 1833, Sir Charles Bell regarded the wrist joint as a composite ball-and-socket articulation.[109] Bryce, through his work in 1896, has been credited with the notion that all carpal movements take place through a single axis that passes through the neck of the capitate bone.[110] In 1925, Destot referred to the bell-like movement of the scaphoid in normal carpal movements,[111] and in 1919, Wood-Jones drew attention to the different ranges of movement that occur at two levels of the carpus.[112] MacConaill also referred to the anatomy of the carpus in his general study of joint movement.[113]

FRACTURES OF THE FOREARM, WRIST, AND HAND

In the nineteenth century, long before the advent of x-rays, surgeons were describing fractures and their treatment. Much of this is anecdotal, with fulsome descriptions of physical signs, techniques of reduction, and the results in single cases. Nevertheless, remarkable clinical acumen was displayed, considering the limited resources available to the diagnostician. Indeed, an anatomist, G. W. Hind, wrote an

---

*Updates by Steven R. Novotny, MD, and David M. Lichtman, MD.

1

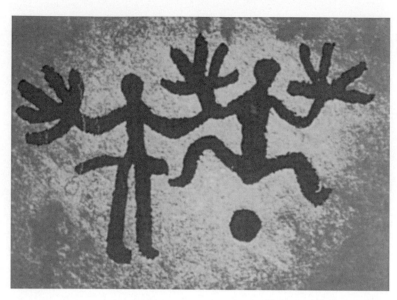

Figure 1–1. Rock carving of Bohuslän, about 3000 years old.

illustrated manual in 1836, entitled *Fractures of the Extremities*, showing from anatomic dissection of the forearm and hand how fractures might occur.[4] He was able to describe the expected deformity from the muscle attachments and their actions. Astley Cooper of Guy's Hospital in London (Fig. 1–3) gave a course of lectures and later wrote *A Treatise on Dislocations and Fractures of the Joints* in 1822,[119] and he did in

fact describe contracture of the palmar fascia before Dupuytren.[5]

Fractures of the lower radius were described in some detail in writings of this period. Colles' fracture recalls Abraham Colles (1773–1843) (Fig. 1–4). He qualified in Dublin, worked at Dr. Steeven's Hospital, obtained his MD degree at Edinburgh, and was Professor of Anatomy and Surgery at the Royal College of Surgeons of Ireland. In 1814, he described fracture of the wrist.[6] He prefaced his description by the note that it had not been "described by any other author," and it is doubtful, therefore, that he knew of the work of Petit (1723) and Pouteau (1783). Colles did, however, differentiate the fracture from a dislocation, and he observed the abnormal mobility of the ulna,

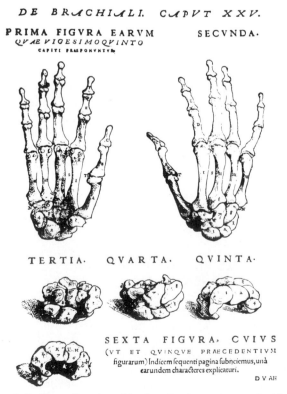

Figure 1–2. Illustrations from Vesalius: De humani corporis fabrica. Liber 1, 115, 1543.

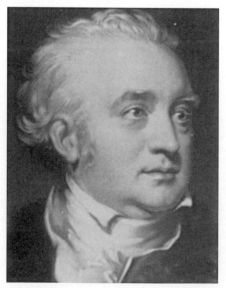

Figure 1–3. Astley Paston Cooper, 1768–1841. (From the Royal College of Surgeons of England.)

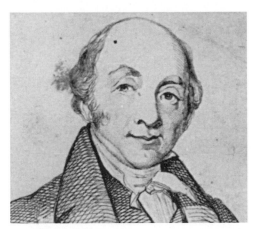

Figure 1–4. Abraham Colles, 1773–1843. (From the Royal College of Surgeons of England.)

but it was not until 1932 that this associated condition was described in some detail by Lippman.[7] In France at this time there were four surgeons quoted by Buxton[8]—Goyrand (1832), Diday (1837), Nelaton (1844), and Malgaigne (1850)[9]—who were all treating forearm and wrist injuries. Another Irish surgeon, Robert William Smith (1807–1873), in 1847 described the separation of the lower radial epiphysis and the less common forward displacement.[10]

Barton (1794–1871), an American surgeon working in Pennsylvania, described anteroposterior fracture-dislocations of the wrist, particularly those in which the carpus was displaced forward upon fragments broken from the anterior articular surface of the lower end of the radius.[11] Thomas, in 1957,[12] classified this fracture into three types: (1) an oblique fracture in which the carpus is displaced forward and proximally upon a triangular fragment of the radius, (2) a comminuted fracture of the radial articular surface that carries the carpus anteriorly, and (3) forward angulation of the lower part of the radius with or without comminution. Barton's fracture has proved difficult to hold in a reduced position; in 1965, Ellis described his buttress plate,[13] and there have been many other methods of fixation suggested.

In 1875, Alexander Gordon wrote a book on fractures of the radius, and in 1878, Lewis Pilcher, practicing in Brooklyn, taught the methods of reducing fractures of the wrist. In 1879, Alonzo Ferdinand Carr (1817–1887), who worked in Goff's Town, New Hampshire, described a wooden splint in which the forearm rested on a gutter with a dowel attaching to the distal end and then passing obliquely across the palm. It is remarkable how this universal splint has been the standard fixation procedure for wrist fractures for nearly a century and within the living memory of many surgeons alive today; indeed, in many parts of the world, this splint may still continue to be used.

Crushing of the lower radial epiphysis, like other injuries in growing bones, may result in premature fusion, which inevitably causes disproportion of the radius and ulna at the wrist joint. Compère drew attention to this in 1935,[14] as did Aitken (1935), writing on fractures of the distal radial epiphysis.[15] The inevitable cessation of growth in the radius leads to severe disproportion and an ugly deformity of the lower forearm, with loss of radioulnar movement. Correction is possible only by shortening the ulna. Excision of the ulnar head was described by William Darrach (1876–1948). Darrach was born in Germantown, Pennsylvania, and graduated from Yale University. His surgical life was spent at the Presbyterian Hospital in Philadelphia, and he described his operation in 1912,[16, 17] although it had first been suggested by Moore in 1880,[18] Tillmanns in 1911,[19] and van Lennep in 1897.[20] However, the operation has the disadvantage of altering the appearance of the wrist joint and disturbing the ulnar aspect of the carpus, particularly its support on the medial side, with later resorption of the ulnar shaft or regrowth of bone fragments if the ulnar head is removed subperiosteally. If an excessive amount of the ulna is removed, the remaining proximal portion becomes hypermobile, and pain and instability result.

However, an account of an operation that preserves the appearance of the wrist, appropriately shortens the ulna, and depends on the development of a pseudarthrosis at the neck of the ulna was published by Baldwin in 1921.[21] Baldwin described his procedure shortly after the 1914–1918 war, while he was still a colonel in the US Army. He practiced in San Francisco and was Bunnell's predecessor.[22] The operation has not enjoyed the popularity it deserves.

A variation of Baldwin's operation has been attributed to Lauenstein.[115] This procedure involves excision of the neck of the ulna, with fusion of the ulnar head to the lower end of the radius by a transversely placed transfixion screw. The transfixion screw will undergo fatigue fracture if persistent movement is allowed. Later attempts were made to realign the inferior radioulnar joint by careful recession of the ulna and internal fixation (Linscheid)[23]; but this presupposes normal articular surfaces.

Madelung (1845–1926) practiced in Bonn and drew attention to the dislocation of the inferior radioulnar joint from either congenital or traumatic causes,[24] but this had been previously described by Dupuytren[5] and R. W. Smith.[10] In 1791, Desault also wrote on the dislocation of the inferior radioulnar joint and rightly pointed to the fact that it is the radius that dislocates on the ulna.[3] Dameron classified the types and treatment of traumatic dislocation of the distal radioulnar joint.[25]

Milan, Italy, has the distinction of being the home of two surgeons, Monteggia and Galeazzi, who described fracture-dislocations of the forearm. Monteggia (1762–1815) wrote about the fracture of the upper third of the ulna associated with dislocation of the radial head at the elbow joint,[26] and Galeazzi (1866–1962) concentrated on fracture of the lower third of the radius with disruption of the inferior radioulnar joint.[27] Essex-Lopresti also described an injury affecting forearm function—fracture of the head of the radius associated with subluxation of the inferior radioulnar joint.[28]

Many innovations were introduced by Sir Robert Jones (Fig. 1–5) and R. W. Lovat in the textbook on *Orthopaedic Surgery*, published in 1929.[29]

In 1966, Buxton[8] reviewed the history of fractures of the lower radius in the *Annals of the Royal College of Surgeons*.

CARPAL TUNNEL SYNDROME

Sir James Paget[30] (1814–1899) (Fig. 1–6) of St. Bartholomew's Hospital, London, one of the great surgeons of the later nineteenth century, in 1853 described a case of median nerve compression following a fracture of the lower end of the radius complicated by "ulceration of the thumb, fore and middle fingers" which he was able to alleviate by bandaging the hand in flexion. In 1883, Ormerod accurately described the symptoms of tingling and numbness in the thumb, index, and middle fingers brought on in women at night and exacerbated by "ordinary work of housewives." He made no attempt to postulate the cause, and he attempted treatment by medication only. In 1913, Marie et Foix[31] demonstrated at autopsy bilateral thenar atrophy where the median nerve passed through the carpal tunnel. Indeed, medical students continued to be instructed in the occasional postmortem appearance of "median nerve

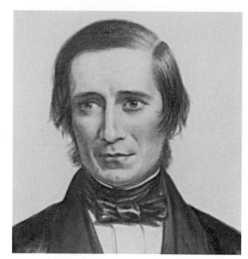

Figure 1–6. Sir James Paget, 1814–1899. (From the Royal College of Surgeons of England.)

neuroma" as an anatomic variant, even after its pathology had been appreciated.

Woltman[37] is credited with the first reported case of carpal tunnel syndrome (CTS) treated surgically in 1941, but sporadic cases of relief of symptoms in the hand by incision around the front of the wrist were reported in the first half of the twentieth century. Learmonth[33] of Edinburgh had reported surgical relief of such symptoms in 1933. Brain and colleagues,[34] writing in *The Lancet* in 1947, accurately described compression of the median nerve in the carpal tunnel and reported six cases treated surgically. As soon as the condition had been described, it rapidly became universally diagnosed, and its repair has become one of the most common operations in hand surgery. Indeed, in 1966, Phalen[35] was able to report the diagnosis and treatment of 654 hands with the syndrome. Carroll and Green[36] drew attention in 1972 to the risk of damage to the palmar cutaneous branch of the median nerve at the wrist with unwisely placed incisions of the carpal tunnel.

EXCISION, PSEUDARTHROSIS, AND ARTHROPLASTY OF THE WRIST

With the advent of listerian antisepsis, followed by asepsis, surgeons in the latter half of the nineteenth century embarked on wide excision of part or the whole of the carpus in an attempt to eradicate the ravages of infection and to overcome deformity and the complications of fractures and dislocations. This particularly applied to the treatment of tuberculosis of the joints, and pioneer work was performed by Ollier[37] in 1885 in Paris. Many such attempts to retain a mobile useful joint with cure of the disease resulted either unhappily in a flail joint and a useless hand or more happily in spontaneous ankylosis of the remaining bony elements. Steindler[38] stated that the

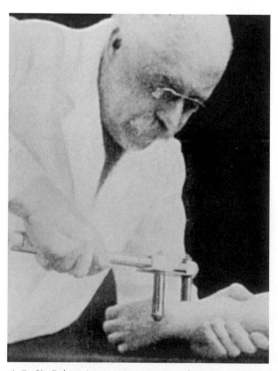

Figure 1–5. Sir Robert Jones (1858–1933) reducing a Colles' fracture using a wrench.

Malgaigne[120] is reported to be the first to apply an external fixation device to immobilize a fracture of the lower extremity. Parkhill[121] used half-pins connected by plates to a central clamp to hold long bones, including the forearm. Lambotte,[122] in Belgium, was the first to employ percutaneous half-pins to a rigid external bar in 1902. Though applied only after the fracture was reduced, the device provided satisfactory immobilization and was the prototype for many subsequent modifications.

In 1934, Anderson[123] provided the first suitable examples of adjustable clamps that allowed fracture manipulation after the frame had been applied. Otto Stader[124] modified Anderson's device to provide adjustments for distraction and compression. By 1938, Hoffmann[125] had used his carpentry skills to devise the ball-joint clamps to hold multiple pins. It allowed changing position of the fracture in three planes. Very few modifications of the equipment that bears his name have occurred to date. Anderson and O'Neil[126] describe their technique and early results for external fixation of comminuted and unstable distal radius fractures.

Clinically, the unilateral frame seemed not to provide significant rigidity. In 1969, Vidal and associates[127] studied the biomechanics of the Hoffmann device. They showed the quadrilateral or double upright frame to be the most stable with intact bone or in the compressive mode. If segmental bone loss exists, or in an unstable fracture, a supplemental anterior frame is required.

Though Rigaud[128] reported on an olecranon fracture immobilized by transfixing bolts surrounded by a plaster cast in 1870, Böhler[129, 130] is recognized to be the father of the pins-and-plaster technique. His technique for management of distal radius fractures has not been significantly altered or improved upon, as evidenced by Green's[131] review. During the 1970s and 1980s, reduction and maintenance of Colles' fractures via the principle of "ligamentotaxis" became highly popular, and the pins-and-plaster technique was the most widely utilized.

In the 1950s and 1960s, many authorities developed a very complacent attitude about displaced distal radius fractures. However, a more critical look showed that not all fractures of the distal radius uniformly did well. Bacorn and Kurtzke[132] reviewed 2000 workers' compensation cases involving Colles' fractures and showed a direct correlation between residual angulation or limited motion and disability. Gartland and Werley[133] reported a 31 percent rate of unsatisfactory outcome with reduction and plaster immobilization alone.

Their three-part classification system progressed from nondisplaced diaphyseal fracture to displaced intra-articular fracture. In 40 percent of cases with intra-articular displacement, arthritis developed. DePalma[134] in 1952 described a percutaneous pinning technique from ulna to distal radius with improved outcome. Max Scheck[135] in 1962 coined the term "die-punch fragment" to describe the dorsomedial radius fragment caused by impaction of the lunate.

Cole and Obletz[136] reviewed their pins-and-plaster technique and concluded that up to 8 weeks of treatment could be needed to prevent fracture settling after pin removal. In 1975, Green[131] reported on his series and modifications of the pins-and-plaster technique. Though reporting 86 percent overall good results, Green[131] did comment on the inability to restore volar tilt in all patients and to prevent subsidence in 50 percent. Patients who did poorly were young with high-energy injuries and articular comminution. He suggested that these more significant injuries are not true Colles' fractures and thus may necessitate different treatment.

Melone[137] in 1984 defined the four-part intra-articular comminuted distal radius fracture and its predictable components. He reaffirmed that anatomic reduction of the volar and dorsal medial radial fragments is required to restore both distal radioulnar joint (DRUJ) and radiocarpal congruity, which is essential for good outcome.

Cooney,[138] Nakata,[139] and Vaughan[140] reported outcomes for external fixation of unstable fractures. They showed that cast complications can be eliminated, complex soft tissue injuries can be aggressively treated, and results are better than for plaster treatment alone. As reported previously, an association of poor outcomes with intra-articular involvement and joint incongruity is noted. In 1986, Knirk and Jupiter[141] showed a 91 percent rate of arthritic complications in young adults if radiocarpal incongruity remained, and the die-punch lesion could be reduced by ligamentotaxis in only 49 percent of cases.

In 1990, Bartosh and Saldana[142] showed in cadaveric models that ligamentotaxis could not always restore radiocarpal alignment to preinjury status, especially for palmar articular fragments. This report provided scientific confirmation of the common clinical observation that certain distal radius fractures could not be reduced by ligamentotaxis alone. Thus, today most authorities recommend a wide array of open and closed techniques to achieve acceptable reduction of distal radius fractures.

Issues related to carpal tunnel syndrome have again assumed a prominent role in the medical literature. In 1988, Stevens and colleagues[143] reported a gradual increase in the incidence of CTS from 88 to 125 per 100,000 over the period 1961 through 1980. They believed that it was partly due to a greater appreciation of the disease process and diagnostic capability. But as part of the cumulative trauma disorders (CTD), the incidence of CTS doubled from 1.9 percent to 3.7 percent over the 4-year period 1987–1991.[144] Claims costs have reached almost $10,000 per case. The dramatic increase in CTS claims led Browne and coworkers[145] to proclaim it the new industrial epidemic.

In 1989, Okutso and associates[146] and Chow[147] reported on endoscopic techniques of transverse carpal ligament release. Both incorporated direct visualization of the transverse carpal ligament and its release during the operative procedure. Chow[148] reported on 149 carpal tunnel decompressions and showed dramatic resolution of symptoms and rapid return of function without significant complications; 85.9 percent of his patients returned to work or to normal activity within 4 weeks. Though a significant proportion of those not returning to work early were involved in workers' compensation cases, most had concurrent disease that precluded return to work. Agee and colleagues[149] reported a multicenter preoperative study of endoscopic versus open carpal tunnel release. No

significant complications were encountered. Dramatic resolution of symptoms and return to previous activity were achieved except in the workers' compensation cases. The mode of treatment did not influence the interval before returning to work in worker compensation patients.

Brown and coworkers,[150] in a prospective randomized multicenter study, reported four complications using endoscopic techniques, consisting of an injury to a superficial arch requiring repair, two resolving neurapraxias, and one resolving hematoma. They tempered their enthusiasm for endoscopic carpal tunnel release because of two digital nerve transections and a partial median nerve laceration during the learning curve period before the study. Agee and colleagues[151] reviewed 1049 endoscopic procedures without vascular or permanent neurologic injury.

Because of case reports of significant vascular and neurologic injury during endoscopic procedures, and high complication rates in smaller series, some physicians are using modified open techniques and are reporting good results. Bromley[152] and Wilson[153] reported excellent results with open carpal tunnel release using minimal incisions and subcutaneous tissue-sparing techniques. Achieving excellent patient recovery while retaining a reduction in incidence of pillar symptoms similar to that reported for endoscopic procedures is reported.

capitate was the bone most commonly affected by infection in the wrist. In fact, tuberculosis of the wrist was very rare, and Hodgson and Smith,[39] writing from Hong Kong, reported an incidence of only 0.7 percent.

Synovectomy was used in preantibiotic days in early cases and was often successful in the rarer forms of tuberculosis in which the onset of bone infection was late. Hodgson and Smith[39] believed that synovectomy was very effective, but in those cases in which suppression of the disease could not be safely achieved by drug therapy, panarthrodesis of the wrist extending from the radius to the third metacarpal gave the best results. They advocated Brittain's arthrodesis.[40]

However, until the advent of antibiotics, surgery of the hand remained limited and was almost totally devoted to overcoming and minimizing the dreadful effects of acute suppurative infections of the wrist and hand. Kanavel[41] (1874–1938) of Chicago was a pioneer in this respect, and his book on infections of the hand became a classic. Indeed, in his publication, coverage of surgery for nonsuppurative conditions is relegated to a few pages.

PARTIAL EXCISION OF THE CARPUS

Partial excision of the carpus or its unreduced elements has long been practiced and in fact can produce improved function. Certainly, excision of the lunate after persistent dislocation or Kienböck's disease is often acceptable. Excision of part or all of the scaphoid for non-union of a fracture, avascular necrosis, persistent dislocation, or Preiser's disease[42] had its advocates, although there is no unanimity about the wisdom or end results of such practice. In 1964, Crabbe[43] was able to report a series of excisions of the proximal row of the carpus in 24 patients who were followed up over a long period. He advocated this procedure, and although it resulted in the retention of a comfortable and useful wrist, inevitably some residual loss of power and movement occurred. In 1949, Dornan[44] reviewed the results of excision of the lunate in Kienböck's disease, and he recorded two thirds of patients as having a good or excellent result and being able to return to full-time work. This has been the general impression among previous generations of orthopedic surgeons, but the advent of prosthetic or soft tissue replacement has superseded simple excision, and Swanson[45] has popularized the use of silicon rubber for this and many other conditions in the wrist and hand. In the same way, excision of the trapezium for painful degenerative arthritis was reported by Gervis[46] and Murley.[47] Lasting, satisfactory results were reported for both series. Here again, the insertion of foreign materials of varying

Kienböck's Disease

In 1843, Peste[210] described through anatomic specimens the collapse of the lunate bone, which he attributed to trauma. Kienböck[211] in 1910 described the radiographic changes of lunatomalacia. He also believed this condition to be of traumatic etiology, related through repetitive injury to a precarious blood supply. Baum[212] in 1913 viewed surgical specimens and showed that necrosis of the lamellae and the marrow constituted the pathoanatomy of the disease. Hultén[213] in 1928 noted the relationship between the ulna minus variant and Kienböck's lunatomalacia; 78 percent of the patients with lunatomalacia had an ulna minus variant, and only 23 percent of the general population showed this discrepancy. Persson[214] in 1945 reported on a new procedure for joint leveling. He remarked on Hultén's previous reports of radial shortening procedures and discussed ulnar lengthening as an alternative and superior procedure. Stahl[215] reviewed 184 patients with Kienböck's disease, though only 142 were followed. He wrote that "every case of lunatomalacia may be interpreted as a stage in the development of a non-healing compression fracture" and further noted that cast immobilization must be used for a minimum of 2 months to significantly affect the outcome. Excision of the lunate was to be condemned as a crippling operation.

Lee,[216] using arterial injection techniques, showed the intraosseous vascular pattern of the lunate in 1963. He explained avascular necrosis in terms of the vascular anatomy and attributed the proximal origin of Kienböck's disease to a transverse compression fracture with disruption of the intraosseous blood supply. Gelberman and associates[217] in their 1980 study of the lunate, showed that vascular anastomosis occurred between the dorsal and volar nutrient vessels but that terminal vessels coursed to the subchondral area. They believed that their work supports repeated trauma with subsequent compression fracture leading to segmental interruption of the intraosseous blood supply as the most likely cause of Kienböck's disease.

Lichtman and colleagues[218] in 1977 produced a classification system that has withstood the test of time, though a minor complementary modification has been made. They emphasized the progressive nature of the disease and the common failure of immobilization and suggested an algorithmic treatment protocol based on stage and ulnar variance. In 1979, Hori and coworkers[219] repopularized the concept of direct revascularization of the small bones of the carpus, especially the lunate. Later studies have emphasized biomechanical means to decompress the lunate by radial osteotomy and or intercarpal arthrodesis, thus enhancing the possibility of indirect revascularization.

design has required stabilization by tendon or fascial grafts, which is the present fashion.

ARTHRODESIS

In contrast to natural ankylosis, surgical stiffening of the wrist has certainly been practiced for the last hundred years. Albert of Vienna recommended this operation in 1878. At the turn of the century, Tubby[48] advocated arthrodesis of the wrist for paralysis of the hand. Colonna[49] reviewed the methods of fusion of the wrist in 1944. In 1946, Steindler[50] discussed the advantages of fusion. These writers all recommended fusion of the wrist from the base of the second or third metacarpals to the radius without involvement of the inferior radioulnar joint, and most have suggested that a small degree of dorsiflexion assists function of the hand, but it has been agreed more recently that fusion is better performed with a little ulnar flexion and with the wrist in a neutral position. This is particularly important in patients with bilateral disease, for whom attendance to personal hygiene is facilitated. Brittain[40] described his operation of fusing the carpus from the dorsum using a "bail" graft taken from the tibia or iliac crest, i.e., a graft chamfered at either end and slotted into the radius proximally and the third metacarpal distally. Other methods have been recommended by Seddon,[51] in which an exposure from the radial aspect protects the dorsal tendons from adherence to the operation site; in 1940, Smith-Petersen[52] advocated the ulnar approach to the wrist using the lower end of the ulna as a free graft. Abbott and colleagues[53] advocated panarthrodesis of the wrist using multiple iliac crest grafts.

In 1919, Steindler[54] recommended partial arthrodesis (in reality, radiocarpal fusion) by scooping out part of the radius and the scaphoid to produce limited movement in preparation for tendon transfers in cases of paralytic or spastic dropped wrist.

Wedge resection of the carpus from the dorsum in order to overcome fixed flexion deformity has been practiced since the turn of the century, and attempts have been made to correct the deformity of malunited fractures around the wrist; these were reviewed by Durman.[55] Steindler[56] advocated this corrective osteotomy in 1918.

In 1943, White and Stubbins[57] recommended total carpectomy for intractable flexion deformities of the wrist; this induced a pseudarthrosis between the

Particulate Synovitis

Silicone elastomer implants were developed in the 1960s and have experienced widespread use that has continued to the present. Early application of these implants was heralded, but problems of implant failure, deformity, inability to regain function, and particulate synovitis were encountered with increasing frequency. Aptekar and colleagues[194] reported a case of metacarpophalangeal joint (MCP) synovitis with shards of silicone surrounded by foreign body reaction. Ferlic and associates[195] reviewed their experience in MCP surgery and found a 10 percent complication rate, though only one implant was removed for foreign body reaction. Worsing and coworkers[196] reported on reactive synovitis from a radial head implant and showed experimentally in laboratory animals that intra-articular injection of silicone elastomer particles caused an identical synovitis.

Manes[197] in 1984 described a foreign body granuloma forming in the distal radius articular surface with a silicone scaphoid implant. Smith and associates[198] in 1985 reviewed 9 cases of wrist particulate synovitis involving lunate, scaphoid, trapezium, and wrist implants. They believed that prolonged intermittent compression gradually caused fibrillation of the implant. Peimer and colleagues[199] in 1986 reviewed 18 cases of particulate synovitis. They concluded that cyclic loading, shear, and compression stresses cause surface deterioration of the prosthesis. The results deteriorate with time, and the severity of changes correlates with elapsed time. Surgery is required to arrest the process. Carter and associates[200] demonstrated lytic lesions adjacent to carpal implants in 75 percent of scaphoid implants, 53 percent of lunate implants, and 75 percent of scapholunate implants. Fifty-six percent of these patients complained of pain. Alexander and Lichtman,[201] after re-reviewing their patients with silicone lunate prostheses and finding significant deterioration of results over time, no longer recommend silicone implants for Kienböck's disease.

bases of the metacarpals and the radius, although the procedure appears to have been confined to adolescents. They particularly advocated this procedure in congenital contractures and after Volkmann's ischemia.

Partial Arthrodesis

In 1953, O'Rahilly[58] did a comprehensive review of carpal and tarsal anomalies from an anatomic point of view, and he described the incidence and variety of congenital fusion of carpal bones. Clinical observation has indicated a high degree of carpal function in the presence of such anomalies, and this encouraged surgeons in the past to carry out limited fusions in the wrist joint, where degenerative changes, infection, hypermobility, or non-united fractures appeared to have benefited from limited arthrodesis. However, it has not been sufficiently appreciated that congenital anomalies in the carpus can lead to premature degenerative changes in the remaining joints. It is postulated that partial arthrodesis may achieve only temporary amelioration and that in the long term, further arthrodeses may become necessary.

Not infrequently, infections and injuries have brought about spontaneous radiocarpal or midcarpal ankylosis. These have resulted in the patient's retaining a useful range of movement, usually about half that of normal, and a variable loss of ulnar or radial flexion. Indeed, it has been suggested in the past that the function of the hand is improved if panarthrodesis of the wrist has not been fully achieved!

Campbell and Keokarn[154] described an inlay technique for total wrist arthrodesis in 1964, utilizing en bloc resection of the radiocarpal joint and fusion with a cortical cancellous bone graft. Haddad and Riordan[155] described a radial approach to the wrist utilizing an intramedullary slotted bone graft. This approach avoided interference with dorsal tendon gliding. Carroll and Dick[156] refined the dorsal inlay technique and used a "rabbit ear"–shaped graft to bridge the radius to the second and third metacarpal bases. Though described for rheumatic wrists, the technique could be applied to osteoarthritis conditions. For rheumatoid arthritis, Clayton[157] in 1965 described an intramedullary pin technique stabilizing an iliac crest graft mortised into the radiocarpal articulation. The pin was intramedullary in the third metacarpal. Millender and Nalebuff[158] in 1973 described a variation wherein the pin exits between the metacarpals and morcellated bone graft is placed in the interspaces. Ryu and colleagues[159] believed that successful results could be achieved with a fibrous union, and that a fibrous ankylosis might be more desirable.

Larsson[160] in 1974 described a technique of wrist arthrodesis using a 3.5-mm dynamic compression plate. To eliminate irritation, Richards and associates[161] tested a tapering plate using 3.5-mm screws on the radius and 2.7-mm screws on the metacarpal. Hastings[162] has popularized this technique using low-profile precontoured plates.

Localized fusion of the wrist joint was reviewed by Schwartz[59] in 1967. He described localized radioscaphoid fusion of the wrist for old scaphoid fractures, osteoarthritis, and rheumatoid arthritis, especially with ulnar translocation, but this is admittedly difficult to achieve and has no advantage over inclusion of the lunate.

Scapholunate fusion has been advocated in cases of carpal instability or non-union of the proximal pole of the scaphoid when this fragment has already been excised. In 1960, Maguire[60] advocated this operation for all forms of carpal instability and avascular necrosis of the proximal pole of the scaphoid, but unfortunately, the scapholunate joint is essential to normal carpal movement.

Scaphotrapezial-trapezoid arthrodesis has likewise been advocated for scaphoid translocation within the carpus, and Watson and associates[61] have described its indications.

Instability of the ulnar column of the carpus has been similarly treated by triquetrohamate fusion.[62]

THE FRACTURED CARPAL SCAPHOID

Recognition of carpal scaphoid fracture and its subsequent treatment have gyrated wildly from studied neglect through prolonged immobilization to internal fixation with or without bone grafting. The fracture was certainly recognized before the advent of Roentgen's discovery of x-rays. Callender[63] described the fracture in 1866, and Codman and Chase[64] discussed the diagnosis and treatment of the fracture of the carpal scaphoid in 1905. Destot[65] also described the treatment of this fracture in 1921. It had been appreciated quite early that fracture of the carpal scaphoid could be found incidentally without any definite history of injury and that the patient would often be symptom free. In other patients, however, symptoms arose and persisted while the fracture remained non-united, and the condition might well have been followed by a periscaphoid degenerative arthritis. It was also agreed that this fracture would not normally unite unless it were immobilized, and during the first half of the twentieth century, many papers appeared describing the method of fixation, the position, and the extent of the splintage and its duration, most notably by Adams and Leonard[66] and Berlin.[67]

In 1961, London[68] reviewed the many attempts to immobilize the wrist effectively in many different positions. Snodgrass[69] used the flat palmar splint, Speed[116] slight flexion, and Hosford[70] hyperextension. Others, including Berlin,[67] advocated extension and radial deviation, whereas Watson-Jones[74] and Bunnell[22] (Fig. 1–7) advocated slight extension and ulnar flexion. Some authorities, such as Soto-Hall and Haldeman,[72] advocated fixation of the thumb in extension, but others advised a more physiologic position. Still others, including London[68] himself, following

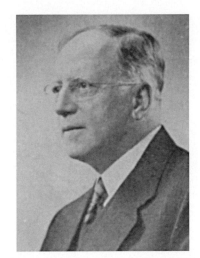

Figure 1–7. Sterling Bunnell, 1882–1957.

Bohler's example, left the thumb free. Yet others, such as Verdan,[9] advocated immobilizing the elbow or at least preventing rotation of the forearm. In 1959, Squire[73] advocated immobilization of the forearm fully supinated and in ulnar flexion.

London asserted that, using the criterion of clinical symptoms rather than radiologic appearance, immobilization was not necessary for more than 6 to 8 weeks and that some 90 percent or more of these fractures united at that stage. Those that were non-united on radiologic examination showed only an increased vulnerability to symptoms after heavy use or further injury to the wrist. The present author's experience, gained over some 20 years of wedge grafting non-united fractures of the scaphoid, shows three striking features.[117] First, all the patients seen were male; second, the original injury occurred early in the third decade of life; and third, the fractures had not been treated previously either because the patient had not attended hospital, the wrist had not been radiographed, or these young men would not tolerate prolonged immobilization.

Largely under the influence of Watson-Jones (Fig. 1–8),[74] it became fashionable to immobilize the wrist until union had been achieved as seen on radiographs, even if this meant plaster fixation for many months. This teaching was maintained during World War II, when fracture of the scaphoid was a relatively common injury and a considerable number of servicemen were withdrawn from active service during treatment while the wrist was immobilized in plaster. In the 1930s, several methods were advocated to obtain union of the fracture by longitudinal peg grafts, and Murray[75, 76] published a report of his first series in 1934 and then later a report of a series of 100 cases.

In 1939, Matti[118] described inserting a cancellous graft into the anterior aspect of the scaphoid. This operation was developed by Russe[77] in 1960 and remains the most popular method of treatment. However, these writers did not appreciate that in many

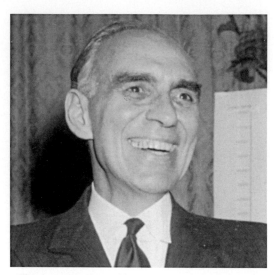

Figure 1–8. Sir Reginald Watson-Jones, 1902–1972.

cases of non-union, the anterolateral aspect of the fracture surfaces had resorbed, leaving a pyramidal defect with primary or secondary instability of the carpus. The present author has described a wedge graft that not only restores stability to the wrist but also results in union of the fracture without hump-back deformity.[78]

In 1954, McLaughlin[79] introduced the Vitallium lag screw, which was inserted at open operation. This was refined by Maudsley and Chen[80] in 1972, when they cannulated the screw so that it could be fitted over a Kirschner wire inserted under fluoroscopy through a small puncture wound. In 1984, Herbert and Fisher[81] introduced a new principle in internal fixation by means of a screw with a recessed head and a screw thread of different pitch at either end.

Removal of the radial styloid in the presence of painful localized scaphostyloid arthritis was studied by Barnard and Stubbins[114] in 1947. These authorities particularly recommended the operation of removing the styloid in the presence of non-union of the scaphoid, but they did not distinguish between fractures that occurred in stable versus unstable wrist joints. They recommended peg grafting of the scaphoid using the bone from the excised radial styloid. Styloidectomy is not approved of by many European writers, who claim that it destroys the ligamentous support on the radial aspect of the carpus, but Barnard and Stubbins[114] reported that there was no appreciable instability of the wrist joint in their cases, and the present author can confirm that this complication is theoretical only and is never seen purely as a result of removing the styloid. The operation is contraindicated, however, when there is an unstable pseudarthrosis of the scaphoid with an unstable carpus.

Other fractures of carpal bones with or without dislocation have been described at least since the days of Astley Cooper,[119] and there has been increas-ing emphasis not only on early diagnosis and reduction but on internal fixation of the scaphoid by screw or wire if it were involved, and stabilization of the rest of the carpus by impaled Kirschner wires. Destot,[88] one of the pioneers in the investigation of carpal movement, recommended manipulative reduction. Other writers include Conwell[89] in 1925, Schnek[90] in 1930, Watson-Jones[91] in 1928, and Johannson[92] in 1926, who discussed dislocation of the hamate bone.

Watson-Jones[93] classified carpal dislocation and fracture-dislocations in his textbook. He recommended manipulative reduction and, if necessary, excision of the displaced carpal bone, and he advocated prolonged immobilization of the wrist when a fractured scaphoid was involved. However, he did not differentiate between the first stage of dislocation of the carpus, leaving one or more bones in position, and the second stage, in which the carpus and hand spring back into position, dislocating those bones that originally were undisplaced. In 1949, Russell[94] reviewed wrist injuries treated in the Royal Air Force during World War II.

CARPAL INSTABILITY

In 1943, Lambrinudi[82] first expounded the principle of zigzag buckling, which he saw as taking place in the human body where there occurs a chain of three elements in which the central link could become unstable. Such an arrangement is seen not only in the fingers and toes but also in the carpus (Fig. 1–9). Guildford and associates,[83] in a fundamental paper, illustrated this concept in *Guy's Hospital Reports* in 1943. In 1961, Landsmeer[84] further developed the concept. In 1968, the present author set out to show that unpredictability of the fractured scaphoid depended upon the associated ligamentous injury, and that if this were recognized early, the treatment of the fractured carpal scaphoid could be logically planned.[85] In 1972, Linscheid and colleagues[86] further classified traumatic instability of the wrist in a fundamental paper in the *Journal of Bone and Joint Surgery*. Rotational subluxation of the scaphoid within the carpus has long been recognized,[87] but the exact pathologic process is not yet fully understood, and its treatment is insufficiently elaborated. Writers in the past have referred to "sprained wrist" with little attempt to analyze or specifically treat the effects of the injury. Attempts to stabilize the carpus by soft tissue repair are a later innovation.

TRIANGULAR FIBROCARTILAGE AND DISTAL RADIOULNAR JOINT

It has long been thought that triangular fibrocartilage lying between the radius and ulna and contributing to the smooth proximal carpal joint is subject to injury and responsible for pain, clicking, and locking of the wrist. Indeed, many surgeons have regarded

In 1970, Fisk[85] reported his observations that if the scaphoid fracture is associated with carpal instability, non-union may be expected with "humpback" deformity and subsequent degenerative arthritis. He devised a volar wedge bone graft technique to correct the deformity. Fernandez[163] expounded upon this idea by using preoperative templating and Kirschner (K) wire internal fixation to improve the results and expand the indications. Mack and associates[164] and Ruby and colleagues[165] demonstrated the long-term problems associated with scaphoid non-union and recommended bone graft and internal fixation when a non-union is identified. In 1989, Amadio and coworkers[166] reported an 83 percent satisfactory outcome if normal scaphoid anatomy was present at union. If the lateral intrascaphoid angle was greater than 45°, the results lessened to a 27 percent satisfactory outcome clinically with a 54 percent incidence of posttraumatic arthritis. Nakamura and associates[167] in 1991 reported on symptoms of 10 patients with scaphoid malunion, 7 of whom subsequently underwent corrective osteotomies with good results. These studies have encouraged most surgeons to treat displaced acute scaphoid fractures aggressively with open reduction and internal fixation. In addition, more attention is being given to proper alignment of non-unions at the time of grafting to avoid subsequent healing in the flexed or humpback position. The use of the Herbert screw and its modifications has been popular for stabilizing displaced acute scaphoid fractures and scaphoid non-unions.

In 1985, Green[168] reported his experience with Russe bone grafting. His paper included personal communication on technique modifications by Russe, and Russe's admonition that a completely necrotic proximal fragment excludes a good result. Green used direct inspection for punctate bleeding points in the proximal fragment to determine vascularity. None of the 5 patients with a totally avascular proximal fragment achieved successful union. Seventy-one percent (10 of 14) of patients with spotty vascularity and 92 percent (24 of 26) with good vascularity achieved union. Stark and associates[169] added K-wire fixation to all their Russe bone grafts; 21 of 25 patients with radiographic evidence of avascular necrosis (AVN) healed over periods ranging from 12 to 28 weeks. However, the 4 with AVN that did not unite were the only failures in the study, and the AVN group as a whole showed a tendency toward delayed union compared with those with normal osseous vascularity.

Reinus and colleagues[170] showed the value of magnetic resonance (MR) imaging in diagnosing AVN of carpal bones in 1986. Perlik and Guilford[171] confirmed the superiority of MR imaging in assessing vascularity over plain radiographs, tomograms, and intraoperative evaluations. Thus, definite preoperative determination of scaphoid vascularity and its healing potential is possible. This may direct the surgeon to a different procedure (e.g., vascularized bone grafts) than would otherwise be undertaken.

Braum[172] in 1982 reported his early good experience with the pronator pedicle vascularized bone graft from the distal radius. Eight patients had Kienböck's disease, 1 had Preiser's disease, and 5 had delayed scaphoid union. Kawai and Yamamoto[173] in 1988 reported on 8 patients with scaphoid non-union treated with this technique, all with good results. Hori and colleagues[174] in 1979 reviewed their experimental protocol of blood vessel transplantation to bone. They demonstrated the technique's applicability and early satisfactory clinical results for the treatment of carpal AVN, including scaphoid fractures with an avascular proximal fragment. Pechlaner and associates[175] in 1987 reported 25 patients treated with a free vascularized iliac crest graft. In 1991, Zaidemberg and colleagues[176] reported on a vascularized bone graft taken from the distal dorsal radius with successful results in treating long-standing scaphoid non-unions in 11 patients. The arterial branch that formed the vascular pedicle was present in all their cadaver and clinical specimens. Sheetz and coworkers[177] in 1995 detailed the vascular anatomy of the distal radius, providing other potential pedicles for vascularized bone grafts.

Pulsed electromagnetic fields (PEMFs) have been utilized for the treatment of delayed union and non-union of fractures in most parts of the body. Beckenbaugh[178] reported his experience with PEMFs on scaphoid non-unions. The overall union rate was 67 percent, which improved to 87 percent if long-arm casting was used. Frykman and colleagues[179] in 1986 reported a success rate of 80 percent. Adams and coworkers[180] presented a continuation of the Frykman study.[179] The overall success rate decreased from 80 percent to 69 percent. Only 50 percent of the proximal third non-unions healed, whereas 73 percent of the middle and distal third fractures united; 73 percent of fractures with AVN went on to union. Initiating treatment with a 6-week period of long-arm casting improved successful union to 83 percent, compared with 59 percent if short-arm casting was utilized. Patients who began treatment after 60 months from injury had only a 29 percent chance of healing.

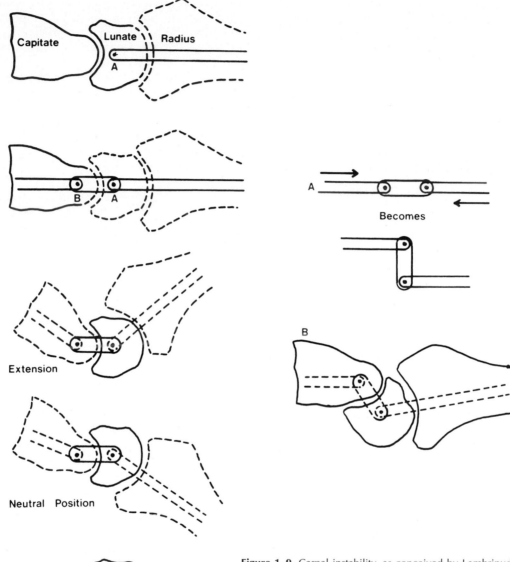

Figure 1–9. Carpal instability, as conceived by Lambrinudi. (After Guildford WW, Bolton RH, Lambrinudi C: Mechanism of the wrist joint with special reference to fractures of the scaphoid. Guy's Hospital Reports 92:52, 1943.)

Classification systems are usually developed to define and treat a related group of pathologic conditions. For this reason, Linscheid and colleagues coined the terms *dorsiflexion intercalary segment instability* and *volarflexion intercalary segment instability*, which have evolved into the popular acronyms *DISI* and *VISI*. Although the DISI pattern was seen with scaphoid fractures and scapholunate ligament instability, the exact pathokinetics of these disorders remained elusive. Palmer and associates[181] in 1978 demonstrated good results with open reduction and repair of scapholunate dissociation within 4 weeks of injury but poor results with immobilization alone after 4 weeks. Along with Linscheid and Dobyns, Palmer described a ligament repair for chronic scapholunate injuries.

Mayfield and coworkers[182, 183] experimentally demonstrated and defined the stages of progressive perilunar instability. Stage I corresponded to scapholunate dissociation. Stages II to IV described the progressive ligament disruptions and instability that resulted in perilunate and lunate dislocations. In 1981, Lichtman and colleagues[62] observed a different type of carpal instability. Clinically and experimentally, they defined ulnar mid carpal instability as a form of midcarpal instability (MCI) secondary to attenuation of the triquetrohamate ligaments and ulnar limb of the volar arcuate ligament. Louis and associates[184] defined a dynamic capitolunate instability pattern (CLIP) in 1984.

Johnson and Camera[185] reported on 12 patients with chronic capitolunate instability; 11 patients underwent tightening of the volar radiocapitate ligament, with 82% achieving good or excellent results.

An organizational framework to encompass present knowledge and future development was proposed by Dobyns and coworkers[186] in 1987. They introduced the term *carpal instability—dissociative (CID)*, which represents patterns of instability resulting from disruptions of ligaments within a carpal row. This is best represented by scapholunate dissociation with its attendant DISI deformity, and lunotriquetral ligament rupture with its attendant VISI deformity. *Carpal instability—nondissociative (CIND)* encompasses the entire spectrum of instabilities between carpal rows, rather than between individual bones in the same carpal row. This can be further subdivided into proximal carpal and midcarpal causes, as well as conditions intrinsic or extrinsic to the wrist. *Carpal instability—complex (CIC)* refers to patterns of deformity that include features of both CIN and CIND. In 1981, Lichtman and colleagues[62] introduced the "ring" concept that emphasizes the transverse row structure of carpal kinetics (see Chapter 12). The ring concept is compatible with observed carpal mechanics and is helpful in explaining the occurrence of interrelated wrist deformities secondary to specific ligament injuries.

this structure as analogous to the meniscus of the knee and have advised its excision. In 1960, Coleman[105] reported a series of 14 cases in which excision of the articular disk was performed, but it is likely that some patients with symptoms suggesting this injury in fact have instability of the medial column of the carpus. In addition, it is now realized that this structure is subject to degenerative change with age, and about half of patients in their middle years show perforation of the fibrocartilage with damage to or erosion of the lunate or the distal ulnar articular surface. In 1981, Palmer and Werner[106] estimated that in the neutral position of the forearm and wrist, some 40 percent of the load crosses the joint and is carried through the disk to the lower end of the ulna.

ARTHROPLASTY OF THE WRIST

Attempts to produce controlled movement of the carpus by the insertion of foreign material are of later origin and still in the early stages. Various types of pseudarthroses with limited but useful movement have been successfully employed over the last century, and the interposition of autogenous material has

been employed with varied success, using fascia lata, skin, and abdominal fat. Bourgeois[95] discussed wrist arthroplasty in 1925 and Albee[96] in more general terms in 1931. Foreign material, such as cellophane, has also been used, but the use of flexible material such as silicon rubber has allowed not only the replacement of individual carpal bones or parts of them but also the design of Swanson's prosthesis, giving rise to a "controlled pseudarthrosis."[97] Later attempts have been made to design a universal joint for the wrist in metal.[98–101]

Implant arthroplasty of carpal bones has also been advocated, including the scaphoid, the lunate, and the trapezium, but its durability remains unknown. However, replacement arthroplasty is no doubt the treatment of the future, although for the heavy manual laborer, arthrodesis is so satisfactory that replacement will require a very high standard of material and design to supersede it.

CONCLUSION

Although the development of wrist surgery stretches back into the mists of time, it is only over the last

Mikic[187] systematically studied 180 wrist joints from subjects ranging in age from fetus to 94 years. He concluded that the triangular fibrocartilage is very liable to degenerative alterations associated with aging. Degeneration begins in the third decade and progresses in frequency and severity. Changes are more common and more intense on the ulnar surface of the central part of the disk.

In their landmark article on the anatomy and function of the triangular fibrocartilage complex, Palmer and Werner[106] showed that the triangular fibrocartilage was not separable from the surrounding volar and dorsal radioulnar ligaments or extensor carpi ulnaris (ECU) sheath. They therefore introduced the term *triangular fibrocartilage complex* (TFCC). They showed that besides being a major stabilizer of the *distal radioulnar joint* (DRUJ), the TFCC bears significant load across the ulnocarpal joint. These loads were progressively decreased with incremental resection of the TFCC and distal ulna. Further, their specimens showed higher incidence of TFCC perforations with neutral or positive ulnar variance and demonstrated a corresponding area of ulnolunate chondromalacia consistent with an "abutment syndrome." Af Ekenstam and Hagert[188] contributed significantly to the understanding of DRUJ function and stability. They demonstrated that because of differing radii of curvature between the sigmoid notch and ulnar head, the radius not only rotates around the ulnar head but exhibits a translatory volar motion in pronation and a corresponding dorsal translation in supination. This helps explain the seemingly contradictory tightening of the volar radioulnar ligament in pronation and tightening of the dorsal radioulnar ligament in supination.

Palmer[189] classified TFCC injuries in 1989. The main categories are traumatic and degenerative disruptions. Traumatic lesions are further subdivided on the basis of the anatomic location of the tear, whereas degenerative lesions are subgrouped on a continuum of progressive degenerative changes in the TFCC and surrounding structures.

After failure of response to conservative measures, surgical unloading of the ulnocarpal joint should provide significant relief of symptoms. Darrow and colleagues[190] described a modern variant of the Milch ulnar cuff resection. The ulnar shortening provided significant relief of ulnar abutment symptoms. If significant DRUJ incongruity exists, then a matched ulnar resection[191] or hemiresection interposition arthroplasty[192] procedure may be a more desirable method of treating this combination of disorders. Feldon and associates[193] in 1992 reported the follow-up on 13 patients who underwent excision of a small "wafer" of distal ulna, all with good or excellent results.

Wrist Arthroscopy

Sporadic cases of wrist arthroscopy are mentioned mainly in the Japanese and North American literature until the late 1980s. Chen[202] reports on his center's experience in 1979. He remarks that at that time wrist arthroscopy was used for judging the intensity and extent of pathologic changes in the rheumatoid joint. It was also helpful in establishing the diagnosis of articular disc lesions, osteochondral fracture, and ligamentous pathology. Surgical intervention was not mentioned. With the advent of smaller arthroscopes and instruments, along with smaller motorized equipment, the feasibility of diagnostic and operative wrist arthroscopy increased.

In 1986, the techniques of wrist arthroscopy reported by Whipple and associates[203] were proven successful and reliable. Roth and Haddad[204] also demonstrated the superiority of arthroscopy to arthrography in diagnosing intra-articular pathology in undiagnosed ulnar wrist pain. Bora and colleagues[205] utilized arthroscopic techniques to successfully débride TFCC tears.

By 1990, Koman and associates[206] reported their evaluation of 54 consecutive arthroscopies for chronic wrist pain and made an arthroscopic diagnosis in 86 percent of patients; in 63 percent of patients, the lesions were incompletely diagnosed in preoperative studies. These researchers expanded the indications for wrist arthroscopy to TFCC tears, articular cartilage lesions, and undiagnosed wrist pain longer than 3 months' duration. Osterman[207] demonstrated the feasibility of TFCC débridement and early work on arthroscopic ulnocarpal decompression. In 1992 Wnorowski and colleagues[208] provided an experimental model and biomechanical analysis of arthroscopic distal ulnar resection. Pederzini and coworkers[209] compared MR imaging, arthrography, and arthroscopic evaluation. MR imaging and arthrography were 100 percent specific and 82 and 80 percent sensitive, respectively. Arthroscopy confirmed all the lesions and provided the benefit of diagnosing chondromalacia and ligament perforation not seen in the radiographic studies; arthroscopy permitted intervention when required.

100 years that it has become safe and effective. The post–World War II period has seen the greatest strides and advances, and the positive deluge of publications makes it impossible to provide a balanced assessment. No author can claim that he or she has presented an exhaustive review of this expansive topic, and the reader's indulgence is sought for any important omissions in this history.

The present author has relied heavily on Joseph Boyes' notable contribution *On the Shoulders of Giants*,[102] Mercer Rang's *Anthology of Orthopaedics*,[103] and the survey of European hand surgery by Verdan.[104]

References

1. Janssens PA: Medical views on prehistoric representations of human hands. Med Hist 1:318, 1957.
2. Lorthoir J: Essai sur l'histoire de la chirurgie de la main. Acta Orthop Belg Suppl 1, 24:15–27, 1958.
3. Desault J: . . . Sur la luxation de l'extrémité inférieure du radius. J Chir 1:78, 1791.
4. Hind GW: Fractures of the Extremities, ed 2. London, Taylor & Walton, 1836.
5. Dupuytren G: Leçons Orales de Clinique Chirurgicale. Paris, Ballière, 1832.
6. Colles A: On the fracture of the carpal extremity of the radius. Edinb Med Surg J 182, 1814.
7. Lippman RK: Laxity of the radio-ulnar joint following Colles' fracture. Arch Surg 35:772, 1932.
8. Buxton StJ D: Fractures of the forearm and wrist. Ann R Coll Surg 38:253, 1966.
9. Verdan C: Fractures of the scaphoid. Surg Clin North Am 40:461, 1960.
10. Smith RW: Treatise on Fracture in the Vicinity of Joints. Dublin, Hodges & Smith, 1847.
11. Barton JR: Views and treatment of an important injury of the wrist. Med Exam 1:365, 1838.
12. Thomas FB: Reduction of Smith's fracture. J Bone Joint Surg 39B:463, 1957.
13. Ellis J: Smith's and Barton's fractures. J Bone Joint Surg 47B:724, 1965.
14. Compère EL: Growth arrest in the long bones. JAMA 105:2140, 1935.
15. Aitken AP: End results of fracture dislocation of the radial epiphyses. J Bone Joint Surg 17:302, 1935.
16. Darrach W: Anterior dislocation of the head of the ulna. Ann Surg 56:802, 1912.
17. Dingman PVC: Resection of the distal end of the ulna in the Darrach operation. J Bone Joint Surg 34A:893, 1952.
18. Moore EM: Three cases illustrating luxation of the ulna in connection with Colles' fracture. Med Rec 17:305, 1880.
19. Tillmanns H: Lehrbuch der Algemeinen und Speziellen Chirurgie. Bund 2. S749, Leipzig, Veit, 1911.
20. van Lennep GA: Dislocation forward of the head of the ulna at the wrist joint and fracture of the styloid process of the ulna. Hahnemannian Monthly 32:350, 1897.
21. Baldwin WI: Surgery of the Hand and Wrist. In Jones R (ed): Orthopaedic Surgery of Injuries. London, 1921, pp 241–282.
22. Bunnell S: Surgery of the Hand, ed 3. Philadelphia, JB Lippincott, 1956.
23. Linscheid RL: Symposium on distal ulnar injuries. Contemp Orthop 7:81, 1983.
24. Madelung OW: Die spontane subluxation der hand nach vorne. Langenbecks Arch Klin Chir 23:395, 1879.
25. Dameron TB: Traumatic dislocation of the distal radio-ulnar joint. Clin Orthop 83:55, 1972.
26. Monteggia GB: Instituzioni Chirurgiche. Milan, Maspero, 5:130, 1814.
27. Galeazzi R: Uber ein besonderes syndrom bei verletsungen im bereich der unterarm knocken. Arch Orthop Unfallchir 35:557, 1935.
28. Essex-Lopresti B: Fractures of the head of the radius with distal ulnar dislocation. J Bone Joint Surg 33B:244, 1951.
29. Jones R, Lovat RW: Orthopaedic Surgery. Baltimore, William Wood, 1929.
30. Paget J: Lectures on Surgical Pathology. 50, ed 3. Philadelphia, Lindsay & Blakiston, 1865.
31. Marie et Foix P: Atrophie isolée de l'éminence thénar d'origine névritique: Rôle du ligament annulaire du carpe dans la pathologie de la lésion. Rev Neurol 26:647, 1913.
32. Woltman: Quoted by Phalen ES: Carpal tunnel syndrome. Clin Orthop 83:29, 1972.
33. Learmonth J: The principle of decompression in the treatment of certain diseases of peripheral nerves. Surg Clin North Am 13:905, 1933.
34. Brain WR, Wright AD, Wilkinson M: Spontaneous compression of both median nerves in the carpal tunnel: Six cases treated surgically. Lancet 1:277–282, 1947.
35. Phalen ES: The carpal tunnel syndrome: Seventeen years' experience in diagnosis and treatment of 654 hands. J Bone Joint Surg 48A:211, 1966.
36. Carroll RE, Green DP: The significance of the palmar cutaneous nerve at the wrist. Clin Orthop 83:24–28, 1972.
37. Ollier L: Traité des résections et des opérations conservatifs quand pratiqués sur le système osseux. Rev Chir 3, Paris, 1885.
38. Steindler A: Postgraduate Lectures on Orthopaedic Diagnosis and Indications, vol 3. Springfield, IL, Charles C Thomas, 1952.
39. Hodgson AR, Smith TK: Tuberculosis of the wrist. Clin Orthop 73:83, 1972.
40. Brittain HA: Architectural Principles in Arthrodesis, ed 2. Edinburgh, E & S Livingstone, 1952.
41. Kanavel AB: Infections of the Hand. Philadelphia, Lea & Febiger, 1912.
42. Preiser GKF: Zur frage der typischen traumatischen ernahrung storungen der kurzen hand und fuss wurzelknochen. Forschritte A. D. Gebiete der Rontgenstrahlen 17:360–362, 1911.
43. Crabbe WA: Excision of the proximal row of the carpus. J Bone Joint Surg 46B:708, 1964.
44. Dornan A: The results of treatment in Kienböck's disease. J Bone Joint Surg 42B:522, 1960.
45. Swanson AB: Flexible implant resection arthroplasty in the hand and extremities. St Louis, CV Mosby, 1973.
46. Gervis WH: Excision of the trapezium for osteoarthritis of the trapezio-metacarpal joint. J Bone Joint Surg 31B:537, 1949.
47. Murley AHG: Excision of the trapezium in osteoarthritis of the 1st carpo-metacarpal joint. J Bone Joint Surg 42B:502, 1960.
48. Tubby A: Surgical Treatment of Paralysis by Arthrodesis. London, 1901.
49. Colonna TC: Methods for fusion of the wrist. South Med J 37:195, 1944.
50. Steindler A: Traumatic deformities and disabilities of the upper extremity. Springfield, IL, Charles C Thomas, 1946.
51. Seddon HJ: Reconstruction surgery of the upper extremity in poliomyelitis. Papers and discussions presented at the 2nd International Poliomyelitis Conference. Philadelphia, JB Lippincott, 1952, p 226.
52. Smith-Petersen MN: A new approach to the wrist joint. J Bone Joint Surg 22:122, 1940.
53. Abbott LC, Saunders JB, Bost FC: Arthrodesis of the wrist. J Bone Joint Surg 24:883, 1942.
54. Steindler A: Operative treatment of paralytic conditions of the upper extremity. J Orthop Surg 1:608, 1919.
55. Durman DC: An operation for correction of deformities of the wrist following fracture. J Bone Joint Surg 17:1014, 1935.
56. Steindler A: Problems with reconstruction of the hand. Surg Gynaecol Obstet 27:317, 1918.
57. White JW, Stubbins SG: Flexion deformities of the wrist. J Bone Joint Surg 26:131, 1944.

58. O'Rahilly R: A survey of carpal and tarsal anomalies. J Bone Joint Surg 35A:626, 1953.

59. Schwartz S: Localised fusion at the wrist joint. J Bone Joint Surg 49A:1591, 1967.

60. Maguire WB: Carpal instability and its surgical management by scapho-lunate fusion. J Bone Joint Surg 62B:266, 1980.

61. Watson HK, Goodman ML, Johnson TR: Limited wrist arthrodesis. No 2. Intercarpal and radiocarpal combination. J Hand Surg 6:223, 1981.

62. Lichtman DM, Schneider JR, Swafford AR: Ulnar midcarpal instability: Clinical and laboratory analysis. J Hand Surg 6:515–523, 1981.

63. Callender GW: Fracture of the carpal end of the radius and of the scaphoid. Trans Pathol Soc 17:221, 1866.

64. Codman EA, Chase HM: The diagnosis and treatment of fractures of the carpal scaphoid with dislocation of the semilunar bone. Ann Surg 41:321, 1905.

65. Destot E: Fractures du scaphoïde. Lyon Chir 18:741, 1921.

66. Adams JD, Leonard RD: Fracture of the carpal scaphoid. N Engl J Med 198:401, 1928.

67. Berlin D: Position in the treatment of fractures of the carpal scaphoid. N Engl J Med 201:574, 1929.

68. London PS: The broken scaphoid bone: The case against pessimism. J Bone Joint Surg 43B:237, 1961.

69. Snodgrass LE: End results of carpal scaphoid fractures. Ann Surg 97:209, 1933.

70. Hosford JP: Prognosis in fractures of the carpal scaphoid. Proc R Soc Med 24:982, 1931.

71. Watson-Jones R: Carpal semilunar dislocations and other wrist dislocations with associated nerve lesions. Proc R Soc Med 22:1071, 1929.

72. Soto-Hall R, Haldeman KO: The conservative and operative treatment of fractures of the carpal scaphoid. J Bone Joint Surg 23:841, 1941.

73. Squire M: Carpal mechanics and trauma. J Bone Joint Surg 41B:210, 1959.

74. Watson-Jones R: Fractures and Joint Injuries, ed 4. Edinburgh, E & S Livingstone, 1955, p 610.

75. Murray G: Bone graft for non-union of the carpal scaphoid. Br J Surg 22:63, 1934.

76. Murray G: End results of bone grafting for non-union of the carpal navicular. J Bone Joint Surg 28:749, 1946.

77. Russe O: Fracture of the carpal navicular, diagnosis and operative treatment. J Bone Joint Surg 42A:759, 1960.

78. Risk GR: Wedge grafting of the ununited scaphoid. In Rob C, Smith R (eds): Operative Surgery (Orthopaedics, Part 2). London, Butterworths, 1979, p 540.

79. McLaughlin HL: Fracture of the carpal navicular (scaphoid). J Bone Joint Surg 36A:765, 1954.

80. Maudsley RH, Chen SC: Screw fixation in the management of fractured carpal scaphoid. J Bone Joint Surg 54B:432, 1972.

81. Herbert TJ, Fisher WE: Management of the fractured scaphoid using a new bone screw. J Bone Joint Surg 66B:114, 1984.

82. Lambrinudi C: Paper read at British Orthopaedic Association, 1943.

83. Guildford WW, Bolton RH, Lambrinudi C: Mechanism of the wrist joint with special reference to fractures of the scaphoid. Guy's Hospital Reports 92:52, 1943.

84. Landsmeer JMF: Studies in the anatomy of articulation. Acta Morphol Neerl Scand 3:304, 1961.

85. Fisk GR: Carpal instability and the fractured scaphoid (Hunterian Lecture 1968). Ann R Coll Surg London 46:63, 1970.

86. Linscheid RL, Dobyns JH, Beabout JW, Bryans RS: Traumatic instability of the wrist: Diagnosis, classification and pathomechanics. J Bone Joint Surg 54A:1612, 1972.

87. Armstrong GWD: Rotational subluxation of the scaphoid. Can J Surg 11:306, 1968.

88. Destot E: Le Poignet et les Accidents du Travail. London, Ernest Benn, 1925.

89. Conwell HE: Closed reduction of dislocation of the semilunar. Ann Surg 82:289, 1925.

90. Schnek F: Carpal dislocations. Ergeben D Chir u Orthop 23:1, 1930.

91. Watson-Jones R: Dislocation of the scaphoid. Proc R Soc Med 22.1084, 1928.

92. Johannson S: Dislocation of the os hamatum. Acta Radiol 7:9, 1926.

93. Watson-Jones R: Fractures and Other Bone and Joint Injuries, ed 2. Edinburgh, E & S Livingstone, 1941, p 424.

94. Russell TB: Intercarpal dislocations and fracture-dislocations: A review of 59 cases. J Bone Joint Surg 31B:524, 1949.

95. Bourgeois P: Contribution à l'Etude de l'Arthroplastie du Poignet. Algiers, Thèse, 1925.

96. Albee FH: Principles of arthroplasty. JAMA 96:245, 1931.

97. Swanson AB: Flexible implant resection arthroplasty in the hand and extremities. St Louis, CV Mosby, 1973.

98. Meuli HCh: Arthroplastie du poignet. Ann Chir 27:527, 1973.

99. Volz RG: Clinical experience with the new total wrist prosthesis. Arch Orthop Umfallchir 85:205, 1976.

100. Volz RG: Total wrist arthroplasty. Clin Orthop 128:180, 1978.

101. Alnot J-Y: Les arthroplasties du poignet. In Razemon J-P, Fisk GR (eds): Le Poignet. Paris, Expansion Scientifique Française, 1983, p 252.

102. Boyes JH: On the Shoulders of Giants: Notable Names in Hand Surgery. Philadelphia, JB Lippincott, 1976.

103. Rang M: Anthology of Orthopaedics. Edinburgh, E & S Livingstone, 1966.

104. Verdan C: L'histoire de la chirurgie de la main. Ann Chir 34:647, 1980.

105. Coleman HN: Injuries of the articular disc at the wrist. J Bone Joint Surg 42B:522, 1960.

106. Palmer AK, Werner FW: The triangular fibrocartilage complex of the wrist and function. J Hand Surg 6:153, 1981.

107. Vesalius A: De Humani Corporis Fabrica. Libre 7, Basle, Switzerland, 115, 1543.

108. Spigelius: Opera: Omnia Quae Extant. Amsterdam, 1645.

109. Bell C: The Hand, Its Mechanism and Vital Endowments as Evincing Design. London, William Pickering, 1833.

110. Bryce TH: On certain points in the anatomy and mechanism of the wrist joints. J Physiol 1896.

111. Destot E: Traumatismes du Poignet. Paris, Editions Masson, 1923.

112. Wood-Jones F: The Principles of Anatomy As Seen in the Hand. 195, London, Ballière, Tindal & Cox, 1919.

113. MacConaill MA: The mechanical anatomy of the carpus and its bearing on some surgical problems. J Anat 166:75, 1941.

114. Barnard L, Stubbins SG: Styloidectomy of the radius in the surgical treatment of non-union of the carpal navicular. J Bone Joint Surg 30A:98, 1947.

115. Lauenstein C von: Zur Behandlung der nach Karpalen Vorderarmfractur zurückbleibender Störung der Pro- und Supinations Bewegung. Zentralbl Chir 23:433, 1887.

116. Speed K: Traumatic Injuries of the Carpus. New York, D Appleton and Co, 1925.

117. Fisk GR: Traitement des pseudarthroses au scaphoïde carpien par greffe cunéiforme. In Razemon J-P, Fisk GR (eds): Le Poignet. Expansion Scientifique Française, 1983.

118. Matti H: Über die Behandlung der Naviculare-fraktur und der Refraktura Patellae durch Plombierung mit Spongiosa. Zentralbl Chir 64:23–53, 1937.

119. Cooper A: Treatise on Dislocations and on Fractures of the Joints. London, Longman, Hurst, Rees, Orme, and Brown, 1822.

120. Malgaigne JF: Considérations cliniques sur les fractures de la main et leur traitement par les griffes. J Connaissances Med Practiques 16:9, 1853–1854.

121. Parkhill C: Further observations regarding the use of bone clamps in ununited fractures, fractures with malunion and recent fracture with a tendency to displacement. Ann Surg 27:553, 1898.

122. Lambotte A: L'intervention Opératoire dans les Fractures. Lamartin, Brussels, 1907, p 3.

123. Anderson R: Treatment for fractures of tibia and fibula. Surg Gynecol Obstet 58:639–646, 1934.

124. Stader OH: A preliminary announcement of a new method of treating fractures. North Am Vet 18:37, 1937.

125. Hoffmann R: In Congrés Francais de Chirugie. 1938, p 601.

126. Anderson R, O'Neil G: Comminuted fractures of the distal end of the radius. Surg Gynecol Obstet 78:434–440, 1944.

127. Vidal J, Rabischong P, Bonnel F, Adrey J: Etude biomécanique due fixateur externe d'Hoffmann dans les fractures de jambe. Montpellier Clin 16:43, 1971.

128. Rigaud: Geciteerd door Feraud in de l'immobilization dans les fractures. Paris, 1870, p 630.

129. Böhler L: The Treatment of Fractures. New York, Grune & Stratton, 1929.

130. Böhler L: The Treatment of Fractures, ed 2. Vienna, Wilhelm Maudrich, 1930, pp 83–96.

131. Green DP: Pins and plaster treatment of comminuted fracture of the distal end of the radius. J Bone Joint Surg 57A:304–310, 1975.

132. Bacorn RW, Kurtzke JF: Colles' fracture: A study of two thousand cases from the New York State Workman's Compensation Board. J Bone Joint Surg 35A:643–658, 1953.

133. Gartland JJ, Werley CW: Evaluation of healed Colles' fractures. J Bone Joint Surg 22A:895–906, 1951.

134. DePalma AF: Comminuted fractures of the distal end of the radius treated by ulnar pinning. J Bone Joint Surg 34A:651–662, 1952.

135. Scheck M: Long-term follow-up of treatment of comminuted fracture of the distal end of the radius by transfixation with Kirschner wires and cast. J Bone Joint Surg 44A:337–351, 1962.

136. Cole JM, Obletz BE: Comminuted fractures of the distal end of the radius treated by skeletal transfixation in plaster cast. J Bone Joint Surg 48A:931–945, 1966.

137. Melone CP: Articular fractures of the distal radius. Orthop Clin North Am 15:217–236, 1984.

138. Cooney WP, Linscheid RL, Dobyns JH: External pin fixation for unstable Colles' fractures. J Bone Joint Surg 61A:840–845, 1979.

139. Nakata RY, Chand Y, Matiko JD, et al: External fixators for wrist fractures: A biomechanical and clinical study. J Hand Surg 10A:845–851, 1985.

140. Vaughan PA, Lui SM, Harrington IJ, Maistrelli G: Treatment of unstable fractures of the distal radius by external fixation. J Bone Joint Surg 67B:386–389, 1985.

141. Knirk JL, Jupiter JB: Intra-articular fractures of the distal end of the radius in young adults. J Bone Joint Surg 68A:647–659, 1986.

142. Bartosh RA, Saldana MJ: Intraarticular fractures of the distal radius: A cadaveric study to determine if ligamentotaxis restores radiopalmar tilt. J Hand Surg 15A:18–21, 1990.

143. Stevens CJ, Sun S, Beard CM, et al: Carpal tunnel syndrome in Rochester, Minnesota, 1960–1981. Neurology 38:134–138, 1988.

144. Carpal Tunnel Syndrome in Oregon, 1987–1991. Salem, OR, Oregon Department of Insurance and Finance, 1992.

145. Browne CD, Nolan BM, Faithfull DK: Occupational repetition strain injuries: Guidelines for diagnosis and management. Med J Aust 140:329–332, 1984.

146. Okutso I, Ninomiya S, Takatori Y, Ugawa Y: Endoscopic management of carpal tunnel syndrome. Arthroscopy 5:11–18, 1989.

147. Chow JCY: Endoscopic release of the carpal ligament: A new technique for carpal tunnel syndrome. Arthroscopy 5:19–24, 1989.

148. Chow JCY: Endoscopic release of the carpal ligament for carpal tunnel syndrome: 22-month clinical result. Arthroscopy 6:288–296, 1990.

149. Agee JM, McCarroll HR, Tortosa RD, et al: Endoscopic release of the carpal tunnel: A randomized prospective multicenter study. J Hand Surg 17A:987–995, 1992.

150. Brown RA, Gelberman RH, Seiler JG, et al: Carpal tunnel release: A prospective randomized assessment of open and endoscopic methods. J Bone Joint Surg 75A:1265–1275, 1993.

151. Agee JM, et al: Endoscopic carpal tunnel release: A prospective study of complications and surgical experience. J Hand Surg 20A:165–171, 1995.

152. Bromley GS: Minimal-incision open carpal tunnel decompression. J Hand Surg 19A:119–120, 1994.

153. Wilson KM: Double incision open technique for carpal tunnel release: An alternative to endoscopic release. J Hand Surg 19A:907–912, 1994.

154. Campbell CJ, Keokarn T: Total and subtotal arthrodesis of the wrist: Inlay technique. J Bone Joint Surg 46A:1520–1532, 1964.

155. Haddad RJ, Riordan DC: Arthrodesis of the wrist: A surgical technique. J Bone Joint Surg 49A:950–954, 1967.

156. Carroll RE, Dick HM: Arthrodesis at the wrist for rheumatoid arthritis. J Bone Joint Surg 53A:1365–1369, 1971.

157. Clayton ML: Surgical treatment of the wrist in rheumatoid arthritis: A review of thirty-seven patients. J Bone Joint Surg 47A:741–750, 1965.

158. Millender LH, Nalebuff EA: Arthrodesis of the rheumatoid wrist: An evaluation of sixty patients and a description of a different surgical technique. J Bone Joint Surg 55A:1026–1034, 1973.

159. Ryu J, Watson HK, Burgess RC: Rheumatoid wrist reconstruction utilizing a fibrous nonunion and radiocarpal arthrodesis. J Hand Surg 10A:830–836, 1985.

160. Larsson SE: Compression arthrodesis at the wrist: A consecutive series of 23 cases. Clin Orthop 99:146–153, 1974.

161. Richards RR, Patterson SD, Hearn TC: A special plate for arthrodesis of the wrist: Design considerations and biomechanical testing. J Hand Surg 18A:476–483, 1993.

162. Hastings H: Arthrodesis of the Osteoarthritic Wrist: Master Techniques in Orthopaedic Surgery, The Wrist. New York, Raven Press, 1994.

163. Fernandez DL: A technique for anterior wedge-shaped grafts for scaphoid nonunion with carpal instability. J Hand Surg 9A:733–737, 1984.

164. Mack GR, Bosse MJ, Gelberman RH, et al: The natural history of scaphoid non-union. J Bone Joint Surg 66A:504–509, 1984.

165. Ruby LK, Stinson J, Belsky MR: The natural history of scaphoid nonunion: A review of fifty-five cases. J Bone Joint Surg 67A:428–432, 1985.

166. Amadio PC, Berquist TH, Smith DK, et al: Scaphoid malunion. J Hand Surg 14A:679–687, 1989.

167. Nakamura R, Imaeda T, Miura T: Scaphoid malunion. J Bone Joint Surg 73B:134–137, 1991.

168. Green DP: The effect of avascular necrosis on Russe bone grafting for scaphoid nonunion. J Hand Surg 10A:597–605, 1985.

169. Stark HH, Richard TA, Zemel NP, Ashworth CR: Treatment of ununited fractures of the scaphoid. J Bone Joint Surg 70A:982–991, 1988.

170. Reinus WR, Conway WF, Totty WG, et al: Carpal avascular necrosis: MR imaging. Radiology 160:689–693, 1986.

171. Perlik PC, Guilford WB: Magnetic resonance imaging to assess vascularity of scaphoid nonunions. J Hand Surg 16A:479–484, 1991.

172. Braum RM: Pronator pedicle bone grafting in the forearm and proximal carpal row. Orthop Trans 7:25, 1983.

173. Kawai H, Yamamoto K: Pronator quadratus pedicled bone graft for old scaphoid fractures. J Bone Joint Surg 70B:829–831, 1988.

174. Hori Y, Tamai S, Okuda H, et al: Blood vessel transplantation to bone. J Hand Surg 4:23–33, 1979.

175. Pechlaner S, Hussl H, Künzel KH: Alternative operationsmethode bei kahnbeinpseudarthrosen: Prospektive studie. Handchirurgie 19:302–305, 1987.

176. Zaidemberg C, Seibert JW, Angrigiani C: A new vascularized bone graft for scaphoid non union. J Hand Surg 16A:474–478, 1991.

177. Sheetz KK, Bishop AT, Berger RA: The arterial blood supply of the distal radius and ulna and its potential use in vascularized pedicle bone grafts. J Hand Surg 20A:902–914, 1995.

178. Beckenbaugh RO: Noninvasive pulsed electromagnetic stimulators in the treatment of scaphoid nonunion. Orthop Trans 9:444, 1985.

179. Frykman GK, Taleisnik J, Peters GA, et al: Treatment of nonunited scaphoid fractures by pulsed electromagnetic field and cast. J Hand Surg 11A:344–349, 1986.

180. Adams BD, Frykman GK, Taleisnik J: Treatment of scaphoid nonunion with casting and pulsed electromagnetic fields: A study continuation. J Hand Surg 17A:910–914, 1992.

181. Palmer AK, Dobyns JM, Linscheid RL, et al: Management of

post-traumatic instability of the wrist secondary to ligament rupture. J Hand Surg 3:507–532, 1978.

182. Mayfield JK, Johnson RP, Kilcoyne RF: The ligaments of the human wrist and their functional significance. Anat Rec 186:417–418, 1976.

183. Mayfield JK, et al: Carpal dislocations: Pathomechanics and progressive perilunar instability. J Hand Surg 5:226–241, 1980.

184. Louis DS, et al: Central carpal instability, capitate lunate instability pattern: Diagnosis by dynamic displacement. Orthopaedics 7:1963–1969, 1984.

185. Johnson RP, Camera GF: Chronic capitolunate instability. J Bone Joint Surg 68A:1164–1176, 1986.

186. Dobyns JH, et al: Carpal instability, nondissociative. Presented to the Annual Meeting of The American Academy of Orthopaedic Surgeons, San Francisco, Jan 24, 1987.

187. Mikic ZD: Age changes in the triangular fibrocartilage of the wrist joint. J Anat 126:367–384, 1978.

188. af Ekenstam F, Hagert CG: Anatomical studies on the geometry and stability of the distal radio-ulna joint. Scand J Plast Reconstr Surg 19:17–25, 1985.

189. Palmer AK: Triangular fibrocartilage complex lesions: A classification. J Hand Surg 14A:594–606, 1989.

190. Darrow JC, Linscheid RL, Dobyns JH, et al: Distal ulnar recession for disorders of the distal radioulnar joint. J Hand Surg 10:482–491, 1985.

191. Watson HK, et al: Matched distal ulnar resection. J Hand Surg 11:812–817, 1986.

192. Bowers WH: Distal radioulnar joint arthroplasty: The hemiresection-interposition technique. J Hand Surg 10:169–178, 1985.

193. Feldon P, Terrono AL, Belsky MR: Wafer distal ulna resection for triangular fibrocartilage tears and/or ulna impaction syndrome. J Hand Surg 17:731–737, 1992.

194. Aptekar RG, Davie JM, Cattell HS: Foreign body reaction to silicone rubber: Complications of a finger joint implant. Clin Orthop 98:231–232, 1974.

195. Ferlic DC, Clayton ML, Holloway M: Complications of silicone implant surgery in the metacarpophalangeal joint. J Bone Joint Surg 57A:991–994, 1975.

196. Worsing RA, Engber WD, Lange TA: Reactive synovitis from particulate silastic. J Bone Joint Surg 64A:581–585, 1982.

197. Manes HR: Foreign body granuloma of bone secondary to silicone prosthesis: A case report. Clin Orthop 199:239–241, 1985.

198. Smith RJ, Atkinson RE, Jupiter JB: Silicone synovitis of the wrist. J Hand Surg 10A:47–60, 1985.

199. Peimer CA, Medige J, Eckert BS, et al: Reactive synovitis after silicone arthroplasty. J Hand Surg 11A:624–638, 1986.

200. Carter PR, Benton LJ, Dysert PA: Silicone rubber carpal implants: A study of the incidence of late osseous complications. J Hand Surg 11A:639–644, 1986.

201. Alexander AH, Turner MA, Alexander CE, Lichtman DM: Lunate silicone replacement arthroplasty in Kienböck's disease: A long term follow up. J Hand Surg 15A:401–407, 1990.

202. Chen YC: Arthroscopy of the wrist and finger joints. Orthop Clin 10:723–733, 1979.

203. Whipple TL, Marotta JJ, Powell JH: Technique of wrist arthroscopy. Arthroscopy 2:244–252, 1986.

204. Roth JH, Haddad RG: Radiocarpal arthroscopy and arthrography in the diagnosis of ulnar wrist pain. Arthroscopy 2:234–243, 1986.

205. Bora FW, Osterman AL, Maitin E, Bednor J: The role of arthroscopy in the treatment of disorders of the wrist. Contemp Orthop 12:28–36, 1986.

206. Koman LA, Poehling GC, Toby EB, Kammire G: Chronic wrist pain: Indications for wrist arthroscopy. Arthroscopy 6:116–119, 1990.

207. Osterman AL: Arthroscopic debridement of triangular fibrocartilage complex tears. Arthroscopy 6:120–124, 1990.

208. Wnorowski DC, Palmer AK, Werner FW, Fortino MD: Anatomic and biomechanical analysis of the arthroscopic wafer procedure. Arthroscopy 8:204–212, 1992.

209. Pederzini L, Luchetti R, Soragni D, et al: Evaluation of the triangular fibrocartilage complex tears by arthroscopy, arthrography, and magnetic resonance imaging. Arthroscopy 8:191–197, 1992.

210. Peste: Discussion. Paris Bull Soc Anat 18:169–170, 1843.

211. Kienböck R: Über traumatische malazie des mondbein und ihre fdgezustände: Entartungsformen und kompressionsfrakturen. Fortschr Geb Roentgen 16:77–103, 1910.

212. Baum EW: Über die traumatische affektion des os lunatum und naviculare carpi. Beit z Klin Chir 87:568, 1913.

213. Hultén O: Über anataomische variationen der hand-gelenkknochen: Ein beitrag zur kenntnis der genese zwei verschiedener mondbeinveranderungen. Acta Radiol 9:155–168, 1928.

214. Persson M: Pathogense und behandlung der kienböckshen lunatummalazie: Die frakturtheorie im liehte der erfolgeoperativen radiusverkürzung (Hultén) und einer neuen operationsmethode-ulnaverlängerung. Acta Chir Scand 98:1–138, 1945.

215. Stahl F: On lunatomalacia (Kienböck's disease), a clinical and roentgenological study, especially on its pathogenesis and the late results of immobilization treatment. Acta Chir Scand [Suppl] 126:1–133, 1947.

216. Lee MLH: The intraosseus arterial pattern of the carpal lunate bone and its relation to avascular necrosis. Acta Orthop Scand 33:43–55, 1963.

217. Gelberman RH, Bauman TD, Menon J, Akeson WH: The vascularity of the lunate bone and Kienböck's disease. J Hand Surg 5:272–278, 1980.

218. Lichtman DM, Mack GR, MacDonald RI, et al: Kienböck's disease: The role of silicone replacement arthroplasty. J Bone Joint Surg 59A:899–908, 1977.

219. Hori Y, Tamari S, Okuda H, et al: Blood vessel transplantation to bone. J Hand Surg 4:23–33, 1979.

CHAPTER 2

Anatomy of the Wrist

George P. Bogumill, PhD, MD

The wrist is the anatomic region that connects the hand to the distal forearm. The description of its boundaries and the components included are somewhat imprecise and depend on the purposes of the description.

The wrist consists of the distal radius and ulna, the proximal ends of the five metacarpals, and the intercalated carpal bones. The osseous elements are connected by a complex array of ligaments that are difficult to define, show a fair amount of variability from wrist to wrist, and are given a variety of names by different authorities.[1-4] The mobility of the wrist is determined by the shapes of the bones involved, as well as by the attachments and lengths of the various ligaments.[5] This complex osteoligamentous array allows a wide range of motion limited at the extremes by a combination of bone shape and ligamentous attachment. The fibrous capsule, lined by synovium, divides the complex into a series of joints that are separate from one another in the normal wrist but may communicate as the individual ages (e.g., the distal radioulnar joint may communicate with the radiocarpal joint).[6]

THE OSSEOUS ELEMENTS OF THE WRIST

The bony elements that make up the wrist joints consist of the distal end of the radius and ulna with their connecting ligaments and the distal radioulnar joint. Beyond this, there are the eight carpal bones, which are classically described as being in two rows: the scaphoid, lunate, triquetrum, and pisiform in the proximal row, and the trapezium, trapezoid, capitate and hamate in the distal row. Still more distal are the bases of the five metacarpals.

Distal Radius and Ulna

The distal radius is expanded from the cylindrical shape of the diaphysis to the triangular shape of the articular surface. The palmar face is flat, smooth, and covered with the pronator quadratus. The dorsal face has Lister's tubercle and other less prominent ridges for attachment of the dorsal retinaculum and extensor compartments (Fig. 2–1). The radial surface ends in the prominent radial styloid. The ulnar face has a concavity, the sigmoid notch, which is covered with hyaline cartilage for articulation with the distal ulna. The distal surface of the distal radius, covered with hyaline articular cartilage, is concave in both coronal and sagittal projections and has two recognizable facets for articulation with the scaphoid and lunate. These facets are separated and well-defined by an anterior-posterior ridge.

The distal ulna ends in an expansion that is covered with hyaline cartilage on its dorsal, lateral, and palmar surfaces as well as on its distal end.[7] The ulnar styloid projects from the posterior aspect of the distal ulna: There is a groove at the base of the styloid, known as the fovea, for attachment of the apex of the triangular fibrocartilage where it joins the head of the ulna. In this groove is a small synovium-containing recess. This synovium, when inflamed and hypertrophied, is the source of the erosions seen so commonly here in rheumatoid arthritis.

The Carpal Bones

The carpal bones are eight small, irregularly shaped ossicles conventionally described as being in two rows, proximal and distal (Fig. 2–2). With the exception of the pisiform, they have some common characteristics. Each is described in terms of its six surfaces: proximal, distal, anterior (palmar), posterior (dorsal), medial, and lateral.[8] For most of the carpal bones, the proximal and distal surfaces are articular. The medial and lateral surfaces may also be covered with articular cartilage to a variable extent. The anterior and posterior surfaces are usually roughened and irregular, reflecting attachments of the capsule and ligaments with openings for passage of nutrient vessels. Study of the dried bones with soft tissues removed provides a useful static picture of each bone, but one should keep in mind that the smooth surfaces are covered with hyaline articular cartilage in the intact wrist. The more articular cartilage–covered surface present on the bone, the less access for blood supply to enter the bone, with resultant disruption seen in fractures of the scaphoid (proximal pole) and in Kienböck's disease.

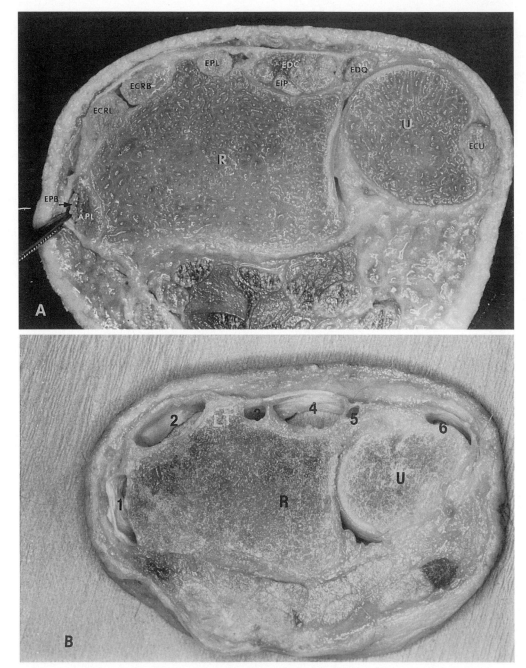

Figure 2–1. Cross-sections through the distal radioulnar joint. Note the incongruity of the ulnar head with the ulnar notch and also the loose capsule of the joint itself. *A,* With the forearm pronated, the extensor carpi ulnaris *(ECU)* lies on the ulnar aspect of the wrist and functions as an adductor, not extensor, of the wrist. *B,* Extensor tendons are removed from the retinacular compartments. With the forearm supinated, compartment 6 with the ECU is positioned dorsally and acts as an extensor. *APL* = abductor pollicis longus; *ECRB* = extensor carpi radialis brevis; *ECRL* = extensor carpi radialis longus; *EDC* = extensor digitorum communis; *EDQ* = extensor digiti quinti; *EIP* = extensor indicis proprius; *EPB* = extensor pollicis brevis; *EPL* = extensor pollicis longus; *LT* = Lister's tubercle; *R* = radius; *U* = ulna; 1,2,3,4,5,6 = extensor compartments at the wrist.

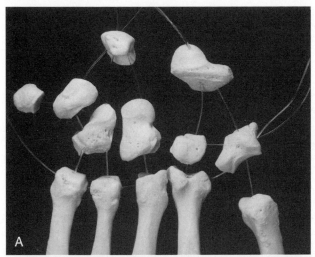

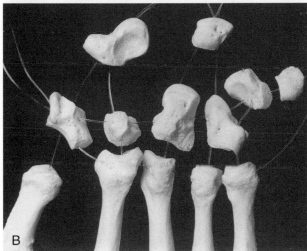

Figure 2–2. *A,* Dorsal view of carpal and metacarpal bones. *B,* Palmar view of carpal and metacarpal bones. The smooth areas seen in the dried bones are generally covered with hyaline cartilage in vivo, and the rough areas have ligament and capsular attachments in the intact wrist. Despite the irregularities of size, shape, and contour, each of the carpal bones can be assigned six surfaces for purposes of description.

SCAPHOID

The scaphoid is the most radially situated bone in the proximal row and is also the largest in that row. Its proximal surface is biconvex for articulation with the scaphoid facet on the distal radius. The distal surface is smooth and convex for articulation with the trapezium and trapezoid. The dorsal surface is rough and irregular and represents the site of attachment of the dorsal radiocarpal and radial collateral ligaments to the waist of the scaphoid. There are numerous perforations in this surface for small blood vessels to pass into the interior of the bone. The palmar surface has an irregular, roughened concavity that is filled with the radioscaphocapitate ligament, around which the scaphoid rotates.[7] There is also the rounded nonarticular projection of the scaphoid tubercle, to which the transversely oriented flexor

retinaculum is attached. The medial surface has a small, elongated semilunar surface for articulation with the lunate and a large concavity that occupies much of the medial surface of the bone for articulation with the head of the capitate.

The scaphoid articulates with five bones: the trapezium and trapezoid distally, the radius proximally, and the capitate and lunate medially.

LUNATE

The lunate is located between the scaphoid radially and the triquetrum medially. It is deeply concave on its distal surface for articulation with the head of the capitate; it is convex in two planes proximally for articulation with the lunate facet of the distal radius and the triangular fibrocartilage. Medially, there is a large, flattened facet for articulation with the triquetrum and usually a smaller facet for articulation with the hamate. Laterally, the lunate has a similar flattened facet for articulation with the proximal (medial) end of the scaphoid. The distal articular surface is narrower than the proximal; thus, the scaphoid and triquetral facets tilt toward each other, making the lunate wedge-shaped in two planes.[9] On coronal section, the planes converge distally, and on cross-section (axial section), the lunate is narrower dorsally. The palmar horn, almost triangular in outline, is broader than the dorsal horn, which allows for recognition of dorsal and palmar tilting, though not displacement, of the lunate on a posteroanterior (PA) film of the wrist.[8–11] Most of the bone is covered with articular cartilage, allowing only small areas on dorsal and palmar surfaces for ligamentous attachment. These small areas provide for a rather tenuous attachment of ligaments and an equally tenuous blood supply.

The lunate articulates with five bones: radius proximally, capitate and hamate distally, scaphoid laterally, and triquetrum medially.

TRIQUETRUM

The triquetrum, located on the ulnar side of the proximal row, is pyramid-shaped with its apex medial and distal and its base lateral. The convex proximal surface has a smooth portion that articulates with the triangular fibrocartilage of the wrist and a roughened surface for attachment of the ulnar collateral ligament. The distal surface of the bone is concave for articulation with the hamate and has a spiral configuration that exerts an important influence on relative motion between the two rows. The palmar surface has an oval facet for articulation with a similar facet on the pisiform. The remainder of the palmar surface as well as the entire dorsal surface is rough, permitting attachment of capsular ligaments. The smooth, flattened lateral surface is covered with hyaline cartilage, which allows for articulation with the lunate. The medial surface of the triquetrum, which is the apex of the pyramid, is roughened by the attachment of the ulnar collateral ligament.

The triquetrum articulates with three bones: the lunate laterally, the pisiform anteriorly, and the hamate distally. It also articulates with the triangular fibrocartilage proximally and occasionally with the distal radius, depending on the position of the wrist.

PISIFORM

The pisiform bone is small and rounded on most surfaces. It has a single articular facet by which it articulates with the anterior surface of the triquetrum. The remainder of the bone is rough, reflecting the attachment of the flexor carpi ulnaris tendon and its continuations, the pisohamate and pisometacarpal ligaments (see Fig. 2–14). The pisiform also provides attachment of origin for part of the abductor digiti minimi as well as medial attachment of the flexor retinaculum.

TRAPEZIUM (GREATER MULTANGULAR)

The trapezium is the most radially situated bone in the distal carpal row. On its palmar surface, there is a deep groove that is converted by a ligament into a tunnel for the flexor carpi radialis tendon. The proximal surface is smooth and somewhat flattened where it articulates with the distal end of the scaphoid. The distal surface is saddle-shaped for articulation with the base of the first metacarpal. The dorsal and palmar surfaces are rough and irregular, allowing for ligamentous and capsular attachments. The palmar surface, however, is somewhat smooth where it transmits the flexor carpi radialis tendon. On the lateral aspect of this deep palmar groove is a bony prominence, or tuberosity, that gives lateral attachment to the distal portion of the flexor retinaculum. The medial surface has two articular facets, the more proximal for articulation with the trapezoid, and the more distal for articulation with the base of the second metacarpal. This latter facet is very small but quite distinct.

TRAPEZOID

The trapezoid is the smallest bone in the distal row. It is wedge-shaped, with the apex on the palmar surface and the base located dorsally. The proximal surface is flattened and smooth where it articulates with the scaphoid. The distal surface is also smooth but has a longitudinal ridge that divides it into two facets. Both articulate with the proximal end of the second metacarpal. The dorsal and palmar surfaces are roughened by attachment of capsular ligaments; the lateral surface is smooth for articulation with the trapezium; and the medial surface is convex and smooth for articulation with the capitate. There is usually a fairly strong interosseous ligament between the capitate and the trapezoid in the center of this medial surface.

The trapezoid articulates with four bones: the scaphoid proximally, second metacarpal distally, trapezium laterally, and capitate medially.

CAPITATE

The capitate is the largest of the carpal bones. It is situated in the center of the wrist and is the center of wrist motion in all planes. Proximally, the surface is convex, smooth, and separated from the remainder of the bone by a relatively constricted area or neck. This proximal head articulates with the scaphoid and lunate bones. The distal surface is divided by two ridges into three facets for articulation with the second, third, and fourth metacarpals. The dorsal surface is broad and rough, permitting attachment of ligaments and capsules and penetration of blood vessels. The palmar surface of the capitate is likewise rough, allowing for attachment of the very thick, strong anterior ligaments and a portion of the origin of the adductor pollicis muscle. The lateral surface articulates with the trapezoid distally and the scaphoid proximally. There is a rough area in between that allows for attachment of ligaments. The medial surface articulates with the hamate by an elongated smooth facet that is somewhat irregular in shape but generally flattened (Fig. 2–3).

The capitate, therefore, articulates with seven bones: the scaphoid and lunate proximally; the second, third, and fourth metacarpals distally; the trapezoid radially; and the hamate on the ulnar side.

HAMATE

The hamate, the most medial bone in the distal row, is easily identified by the pronounced hook (hamulus) projecting from its palmar surface. The proximal surface is narrow, convex, and smooth for articulation with the lunate. The distal surface articulates with the fourth and fifth metacarpals by two facets that are separated by an anteroposterior ridge. The dorsal

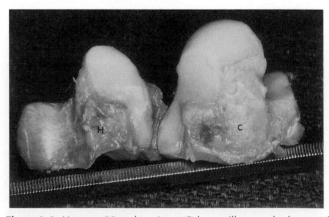

Figure 2–3. Hamate *(H)* and capitate *(C)* bones illustrate the long oval sliding joint they share, and the heavy capsular ligaments on their anterior surfaces. Note the large hook on the hamate, which is almost as extensive as the hamate itself.

surface is triangular, and roughened to provide for ligamentous attachment. The palmar surface has the pronounced hook that projects anteriorly and gives medial attachment at its apex to the distal portion of the flexor retinaculum as well as to the origin of the flexor digiti minimi and opponens digiti minimi. The palmar surface also provides insertion to the flexor carpi ulnaris through the pisohamate ligament. The lateral surface of the hamate has a deep concavity formed by the body and the hamulus. This concavity provides a pulley mechanism for the flexor tendons passing from the forearm to the fingers (see Figs. 2–8C, 2–13D, and 2–14). The ulnar surface articulates with the triquetrum by means of an oval, elongated, and flattened facet (Figs. 2–3 and 2–4). The spiral orientation of the triquetrohamate joint exerts an important influence on the relative motion between the two carpal rows.

The hook of the hamate makes up one of the four prominences on the palmar aspect of the carpus for attachment of the flexor retinaculum. The other three prominences are the pisiform, the tuberosity of the scaphoid, and the oblique ridge of the trapezium. The hamate articulates with five bones: the lunate proximally, the fourth and fifth metacarpals distally, the triquetrum medially, and the capitate laterally.

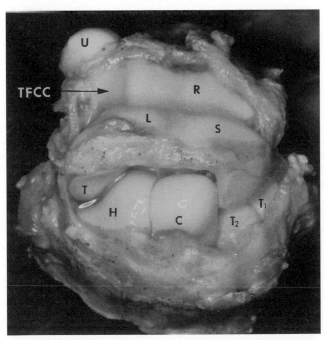

Figure 2–4. Dorsal view of opened radiocarpal and midcarpal joints illustrates their separation. Well illustrated is the smooth contour provided by the interosseous ligaments between lunate and scaphoid as well as between the radial articular surface and the triangular fibrocartilage. The distal radioulnar joint is separated from the radiocarpal joint by the triangular fibrocartilage. In the same way, the radiocarpal joint is separated from the midcarpal joint by the dorsal and volar capsule connecting the bones of the proximal carpal row, and by the interosseous ligaments between scaphoid and lunate, and lunate and triquetrum. *C* = capitate; *H* = hamate; *L* = lunate; *R* = radius; *S* = scaphoid; *T* = triquetrum; *T₁* = trapezium; *T₂* = trapezoid; *TFCC* = triangular fibrocartilage complex; *U* = ulna.

Metacarpals

The metacarpals participate in the wrist at their proximal ends. They are, in general, elongated bones that are flared both proximally and distally.

The *first metacarpal* has a concavoconvex proximal articular surface for articulation with the similar concavoconvex surface (saddle joint) of the trapezium. It is described in more detail elsewhere in this volume (see Chapter 25).

The *second metacarpal* is the longest of these bones. Its base is elongated medially by a projection that brings it into contact with the capitate. It has four articular surfaces; one on its medial surface for articulation with the third metacarpal and three on its proximal surface. The most medial of these is at the apex of the ridgelike projection of bone at the base of the metacarpal; this articulates with the base of the capitate. A concave surface of the center of the proximal end articulates with the trapezoid, and there is a small radial facet for articulation with the trapezium. The extensor carpi radialis longus inserts into the dorsal surface, and there may be a bony projection in this area at the tendinous attachment (metacarpal boss).

The *third metacarpal* is almost as large as the second. A dorsal projection on its base extends proximally to the distal surface of the capitate. It is just proximal to the insertion of the extensor carpi radialis brevis, and this metacarpal boss may be enlarged enough to cause concern about its being a tumor or to be confused with a ganglion. The proximal end of the third metacarpal articulates with the capitate through a flattened articular surface, and on the medial and lateral sides of the base there are articulations with the fourth and second metacarpals, respectively. The configuration of the second and third metacarpal bones together and the strong ligamentous attachment binding them to each other and to the trapezoid and capitate renders this region the so-called fixed point of the hand, with movements of the remainder of the hand described around these two bones as the axis.

The *fourth metacarpal* is smaller than the third but larger than the fifth; however, it usually has the narrowest medullary cavity of any of the metacarpal bones. The base is small and almost square. The medial and lateral surfaces are flattened and smooth, allowing for articulation with the fifth and third metacarpals, respectively. The proximal surface is smooth for articulation with the lateral portion of the base of the hamate, and the dorsal and palmar surfaces are rough, permitting attachment of ligaments.

The *fifth metacarpal* has an articular facet at its proximal end for the hamate and a flattened surface on its lateral side for articulation with the fourth metacarpal. The remainder of the base of the fifth metacarpal is rough, allowing for attachment of ligaments as well as for insertion of the flexor and extensor carpi ulnaris tendons.

WRIST JOINTS

Distal Radioulnar Joint

The distal radioulnar joint is a pivot joint formed between the head of the ulna and the ulnar (sigmoid) notch of the distal radius (see Fig. 2–1). The capsule of this joint is quite loose, in order to allow rotation of the radius about the ulna. Although anterior and posterior transverse fibers reinforce the capsule, they do not add stability to the joint. The bones are held together primarily by the interosseous membrane, which is present to the level of the joint, by the pronator quadratus, and by the triangular fibrocartilage complex (TFCC) or articular disk (Figs. 2–4 to 2–7). This latter structure is the chief uniting element of the joint.[6]

A synovial cavity extends between the distal radius and ulna and then across the distal ulna; it is, therefore, L-shaped in coronal section (Fig. 2–7). The synovial membrane of the radioulnar joint is usually completely separated from that of the radiocarpal joint. Occasionally, the center of the articular fibrocartilage is perforated. This usually occurs in older individuals and is so common that it may be due to normal wear and tear.[6]

Radiocarpal Joint

The radiocarpal joint is formed by the distal surface of the expanded end of the radius and the triangular

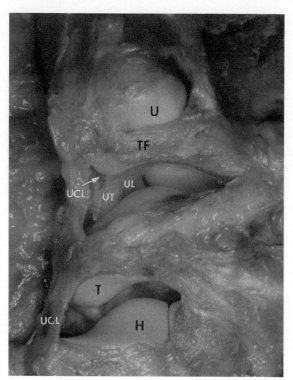

Figure 2–6. Dorsal view of ligaments and joint spaces on the ulnar aspect of the wrist. The ulnar collateral ligament is clearly shown as a separate, distinct entity from the triangular fibrocartilage complex. It extends from the outer aspect of the ulnar styloid to the triquetrum and continues to the hamate and the fifth metacarpal. The ulnolunate and ulnotriquetral ligaments originate from the anterior aspect of the triangular fibrocartilage and extend distally to attach to the lunate and triquetrum, respectively, on their anterior surfaces. The *arrow* points to the prestyloid recess. H = hamate; T = triquetrum; TF = triangular fibrocartilage; U = ulna; UCL = ulnar collateral ligament; UL = ulnolunate ligament; UT = ulnotriquetral ligaments.

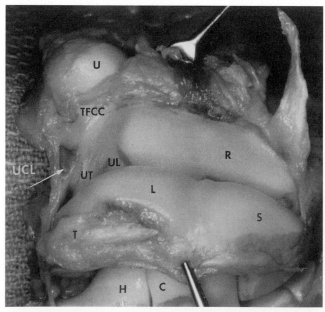

Figure 2–5. Dorsal view of the opened radiocarpal joint illustrating the triangular fibrocartilage complex and the anterior ligaments arising from it. The *arrow* indicates the prestyloid recess. C = capitate; H = hamate; L = lunate; R = radius; S = scaphoid; T = triquetrum; TFCC = triangular fibrocartilage complex; U = ulna; UCL = ulnar collateral ligament; UL = ulnolunate ligament; UT = ulnotriquetral ligament.

fibrocartilage proximally, and the scaphoid, lunate, and triquetrum distally (see Figs. 2–4 and 2–5). The bones of the proximal row are joined at their proximal edges by the interosseous ligaments (see Figs. 2–4, 2–5, and 2–7), forming a smooth biconvex surface that fits into the biconcave articular surface of the radius and articular disk. The loosely congruent surfaces allow free movement in flexion/extension, abduction/adduction, and circumduction. True rotation is not present. The articular capsule encloses the joint and is strengthened by dorsal and palmar radiocarpal ligaments and ulnocarpal ligaments. The radiocarpal ligaments are composed of fibers that run downward and toward the ulna from both the dorsal and palmar surfaces of the radius to the three carpal bones of the proximal row. This arrangement determines that the hand will follow the radius passively in movements of both pronation and supination of the radius.

The lax synovial membrane lines the deep surface of the capsule and presents numerous folds that may extend into the pisiform-triquetral joint, as shown by arthrography in approximately one third of normal wrists. The dorsal and palmar surfaces of the proxi-

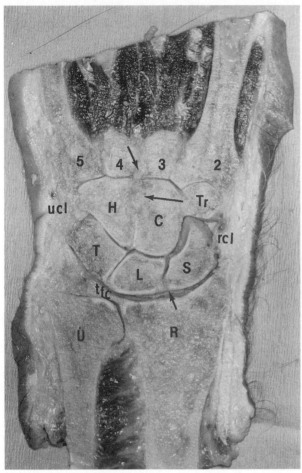

Figure 2–7. Coronal section through the carpus illustrating the separation of the distal radioulnar joint from the radiocarpal joint and of the radiocarpal joints from the midcarpal joint, as well as the continuity of the midcarpal joint with the carpometacarpal joints. *Arrows* indicate interosseous ligaments between the various carpal and metacarpal bones. *C* = capitate; *H* = hamate; *L* = lunate; *R* = radius; *rcl* = radial collateral ligament; *S* = scaphoid; *T* = triquetrum; *tfc* = triangular fibrocartilage complex; *Tr₂* = trapezoid; *U* = ulna; *ucl* = ulnar collateral ligament; *2,3,4,5* = second, third, fourth, and fifth metacarpals.

mal carpal row are sites of attachment of the dorsal and palmar capsule, respectively, thus sealing the radiocarpal joint into a single unit that does not communicate with other joints (see Figs. 2–4 through 2–6 and 2–8).

Midcarpal Joint

The midcarpal joint is formed by the scaphoid, lunate, and triquetrum in the proximal row, and the trapezium, trapezoid, capitate, and hamate in the distal row (Figs. 2–4, 2–7, and 2–8). The distal pole of the scaphoid articulates with the two trapezial bones as a gliding type of joint (Fig. 2–8A). The proximal end of the scaphoid combines with the lunate and triquetrum to form a deep concavity that articulates with the convexity of the combined capitate and ha-

mate in a form of diarthrodial, almost condyloid joint. (The importance of the triquetrohamate and the scaphotrapezial articulations in guiding intercarpal motion in both physiologic and pathologic conditions is discussed in Chapter 12.)

The cavity of the midcarpal joint is very extensive and irregular (see Figs. 2–7 and 2–8A). The major portion of the joint cavity is located between the distal surfaces of scaphoid, lunate, and triquetrum and the proximal surfaces of the four bones of the distal row. Proximal prolongations of the cavity occur between the scaphoid and lunate and between the lunate and triquetrum (see Figs. 2–7 and 2–8B). These extensions reach almost to the proximal surface of the bones in the proximal row and are separated from the cavity of the radiocarpal joint by the thin interosseous ligaments (see Fig. 2–7). There are three distal prolongations of the midcarpal joint cavity between the four bones of the distal row (Fig. 2–8C). The joint space between trapezium and trapezoid, or that between trapezoid and capitate, may communicate with the cavities of the carpometacarpal joints, most commonly the second and third. The cavity between the first metacarpal and carpus is always separate from the midcarpal joint; the joint cavity between the hamate and fourth and fifth metacarpals is a separate cavity more often than not, but it may communicate normally with the midcarpal joint.

Carpometacarpal Joints

The first carpometacarpal joint is quite complex and is described in Chapter 25. The second and third joints are also complex and extend between the bases of the metacarpals (see Chapter 26). The second and third carpometacarpal joints commonly communicate with the midcarpal joint or with the hamate-metacarpal joint.

Pisotriquetral Joint

The pisiform articulates with the palmar surface of the triquetrum in a flat, planar type of joint. It may occasionally communicate with the radiocarpal joint, as is shown in approximately one third of normal wrist arthrograms.

LIGAMENTOUS APPARATUS OF THE WRIST

The carpal bones are not interlocked solely by their shapes; rather, they are held together by interosseous ligaments and by volar, dorsal, radial, and ulnar ligaments.[5] The ligaments holding the carpal bones to each other, to the distal radius and ulna, and to the proximal ends of the metacarpals can be described as extrinsic, or capsular, and intrinsic, or interosseous

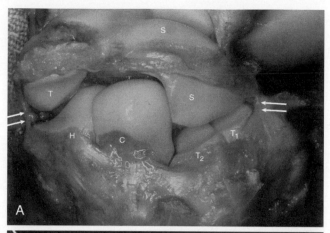

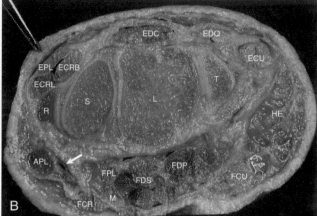

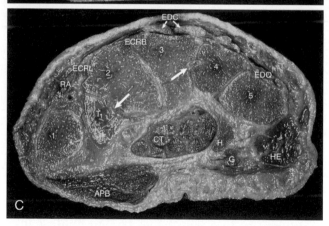

Figure 2–8. *A,* Dorsal view of the midcarpal joint, illustrating the condyloid nature of the articulation between the hamate and capitate bones, and the gliding articulation between the distal scaphoid and the trapezium-trapezoid combination. *Arrows* point to radial and ulnar collateral ligaments. *B,* Cross-section through the proximal carpal row, demonstrating the extensions of the midcarpal joint between the bones forming the proximal row. It also illustrates clearly the locations of the various tendons as they cross the wrist. The *arrow* indicates the position of the radial artery. *C,* Cross-section through the bases of the metacarpals to illustrate the extensions of the midcarpal and carpometacarpal joints between the metacarpal bases. The *large arrows* point out interosseous ligaments. The *small arrows* indicate divisions of the extensor digitorum communis tendon. *1,2,3,4,* and *5* indicate the respective metacarpal bones. Note that the wedge shape of the metacarpal bases provides for the dorsal carpal arch. *APB* = abductor pollicis brevis; *APL* = abductor pollicis longus; *C* = capitate; *CT* = carpal tunnel; *ECRB* = extensor carpi radialis brevis; *ECRL* = extensor carpi radialis longus; *ECU* = extensor carpi ulnaris; *EDC* = extensor digitorum communis; *EDQ* = extensor digiti quinti; *EPL* = extensor pollicis longus; *FCR* = flexor carpi radialis; *FCU* = flexor carpi ulnaris; *FDP* = flexor digitorum profundus; *FDS* = flexor digitorum superficialis; *FPL* = flexor pollicis longus; *G* = Guyon's canal; *H* = hamate; *HE* = hypothenar eminence; *L* = lunate; *M* = median nerve; *R* = radial styloid; *RA* = radial artery; *S* = scaphoid; *T* = triquetrum; *T₁* = trapezium; *T₂* = trapezoid.

(intercarpal).[1, 5] The function of the ligamentous system is guiding and constraining certain patterns of motion. Some portion of the ligaments are under tension in every position of the hand in relation to the forearm.

Interosseous Ligaments

The interosseous ligaments are those contained inside the joint capsule, extending directly from carpal bone to carpal bone and bathed in synovial fluid. The bones of the proximal carpal row are joined to each other by interosseous ligaments attached to the proximal articular surfaces of the scaphoid, lunate, and triquetrum (see Figs. 2–4, 2–5, and 2–7).

SCAPHOLUNATE INTEROSSEOUS LIGAMENT

The scapholunate interosseous ligament connects the proximal edges of the scaphoid and lunate from their palmar to dorsal surfaces and is regarded by some authorities as the major determinant controlling scapholunate relationships and motion.[12–15] The fibers are shorter, thicker, and thus stronger in their dorsal portion. They are longer with the fiber bundles separated by loose vascular connective tissue as they approach the palmar capsule.[14] On cross-section, the ligament is C-shaped, open distally, and attached to the proximal adjacent edges of the scaphoid and lunate. They are actually covered by a thin layer of hyaline cartilage that conceals, on gross inspection, the line between the contiguous bones (see Fig. 2–5).[5, 8]

Some authorities do not regard the scapholunate ligament as a major determinant of scapholunate stability[3, 16, 17]; rather they believe that the volar radioscapholunate ligament must be divided before scapholunate dissociation can occur. Others disagree[13, 18–20] and conclude that the very existence of a volar radioscapholunate ligament is questionable.

Studies of fetal wrists of different ages lead to the conclusion that the radioscapholunate ligament starts as a mesenchymal septum between the radioscaphoid and radiolunate joints and recedes toward the palm during development, finally giving the appearance of a ligament.[20] Landsmeer's studies of the radioscapholunate ligament indicate that it is merely a conduit for nerves and blood vessels surrounded by synovial tissues going to supply the scapholunate interosseous ligament. The vessels and nerves are intra-articular extensions of the anterior interosseous nerve and artery with contributions from the radial artery.[19] None of these vessels appears to penetrate into the bones, nor do vessels pass from the bones into the scapholunate interosseous ligament.[15] There are collagen fibers and an abundant blood vessel network, but no elastic fibers, in this structure on special stains.[15, 19]

LUNOTRIQUETRAL INTEROSSEOUS LIGAMENT

Fundamentally the same as the scapholunate interosseous ligament, the lunotriquetral interosseous ligament has been less thoroughly studied.

The dorsal and palmar ends of the ligaments of the proximal carpal row blend with the dorsal and volar capsular fibers that separate the radiocarpal and midcarpal joints from each other, as well as with the extrinsic ligaments, which provide added stability to intercarpal relationships.[21]

The distal carpal row has interosseous ligaments that unite the trapezium with the trapezoid, the trapezoid with the capitate, and the capitate with the hamate (see Figs. 2–7 and 2–8C), as well as strong ligaments between the bases of the metacarpals that unite them with each other and with the distal carpal row. These interosseous ligaments do not extend from the palmar to dorsal edges of the contiguous bones; consequently, the midcarpal joint spaces can communicate with the carpometacarpal joint spaces. The interosseous ligament between the capitate and hamate is the strongest in the distal row and is situated near the anterior distal portion of the two bones (see Figs. 2–3, 2–7, and 2–8C).

Extrinsic (Capsular) Ligaments

A great deal of study of the ligamentous system has been conducted during the past three decades.[1, 10, 14, 17, 19] Difficulties in description are encountered because the system consists of interwoven fiber bundles that differ in length, direction, and texture, making separation and definition problematic. The variability among individuals as well as the contrast between dissections of fresh and embalmed specimens also causes difficulty in coming to a consensus description.[21]

Some authorities regard the radial and ulnar collateral ligaments as being poorly developed and not deserving of the name radial or ulnar collateral[7, 8]; others believe that the radial collateral ligament is clearly defined but question the existence of an ulnar collateral.[21]

RADIAL COLLATERAL LIGAMENT

The radial collateral ligament of the wrist joint extends from the tip of the styloid process of the radius to attach to the waist of the scaphoid on its radial aspect. Some of the remaining fibers extend to the trapezium, where they blend with the transverse carpal ligament attachment to the scaphoid tuberosity. Other fibers blend with the radioscaphocapitate ligament and continue medial and distal to insert into the volar aspect of the capitate; in their course, these fibers provide support for the proximal pole of the scaphoid.[20] The more dorsal fibers are thin and clearly defined. The radial and volar borders are less well-defined but contain thick fascicles of fibrous connective tissue when seen from inside the joint (see Figs. 2–7, 2–8A, 2–10, and 2–11). Fibers blend with the sheath of the flexor carpi radialis and transverse carpal retinaculum.[22] The radial collateral ligament is crossed by the radial artery in its course around the lateral aspect of the wrist from palmar to dorsal. The ligament is fairly lax in the neutral position of the wrist joint and becomes tight only at the extreme of ulnar deviation.

ULNAR COLLATERAL LIGAMENT

Some investigators have questioned the very existence of a true ulnar collateral ligament, considering it to be poorly developed or merely a confluence of the dorsal retinaculum, floor of the extensor carpi ulnaris (ECU) compartment, and wrist joint capsule.[22] A readily identifiable group of collagen fibers attach to the base and body of the styloid process of the ulna and then pass distally to attach to the triquetrum, hamate, and fifth metacarpal. Usually, the tip of the styloid process is free of ligamentous attachments and projects into the prestyloid recess (see Figs. 2–5 through 2–8A, 2–9, and 2–11), a space between the ulnar collateral ligament and triangular fibrocartilage complex (TFCC). The proximal attachment of the ligament also extends into the anterior and posterior borders of the triangular fibrocartilage. As the fibers progress distally, they diminish in bulk and attach to the pisiform and transverse carpal ligament as well as to the triquetrum. The fibers then continue distally and insert into the ulnar border of the hamate and base of the fifth metacarpal (see Fig. 2–9). The ligament is lax and adds little support in most positions of the wrist except radial deviation of the hand.[1]

DORSAL RADIOCARPAL LIGAMENT

An obliquely placed thickening in the dorsal capsule, the dorsal radiocarpal ligament extends toward the ulna, as well as distally, from the dorsal lip of the articular surface of the radius toward the dorsal surface of the lunate and triquetrum (Fig. 2–9).[22] It blends with the ulnar collateral ligament medially. When the forearm pronates, the dorsal radiocarpal ligament draws the attached carpus and hand passively into pronation. This ligament also prevents the proximal row from excessive passive flexion as well as ulnar translation.

PALMAR RADIOCARPAL LIGAMENTS

The palmar radiocarpal ligaments are described in standard anatomy texts as a broad triangular band of fibers extending from the palmar edge and the styloid process of the distal radius to the palmar surfaces of the scaphoid, lunate, and triquetrum in the proximal row and in prolongation from there to the capitate

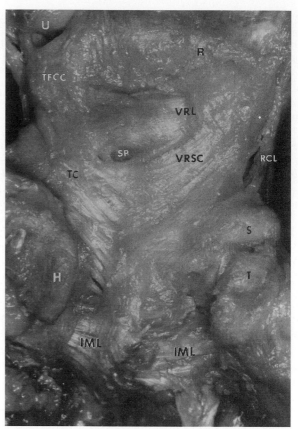

Figure 2–10. Volar aspect of wrist joint, illustrating the heavy interlacing fibers of the volar ligaments. The carpal tunnel is open, and its contents have been removed. The synovial lining covering the palmar aspect of the ligaments has also been removed. H = hamate; IML = intermetacarpal ligament; R = radius; RCL = radial collateral ligament; S = tuberosity of the scaphoid; SP = space of Poirier; T = oblique ridge of trapezium; TC = triquetral capitate ligament; TFCC = triangular fibrocartilage complex; U = ulna; VRL = volar radiolunate ligament; VRSC = volar radioscaphocapitate ligament.

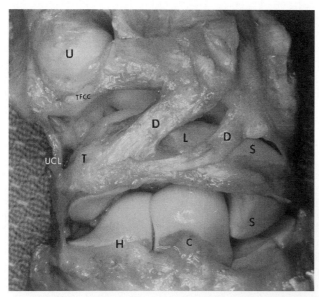

Figure 2–9. Dorsal view of the wrist showing clearly the dorsal radiocarpal ligament extending from the dorsal lip of the radius near Lister's tubercle to the dorsal aspect of the triquetrum. The dorsal capsule has been removed, leaving the reinforced fibers intact. C = capitate; D = dorsal radiocarpal ligament; H = hamate; L = lunate; S = scaphoid; T = triquetrum; TFCC = triangular fibrocartilage complex; U = ulna; UCL = ulnar collateral ligament.

and hamate of the distal row (Fig. 2–10). These ligaments have been assigned subdivisions after careful dissection of fresh specimens. These subdivisions have been shown to have functional value in terms of kinematics of the wrist and in appropriate treatment of injuries, and they are best visualized from inside the joint (Fig. 2–11).

The *palmar radiocapite ligament* is a strong intracapsular ligament that arises from the volar and radial aspects of the radial styloid process and extends distally and ulnarward. It fills a concavity in the waist of the scaphoid anteriorly and has an attachment there in most individuals.[7, 8] This ligament then continues to insert into the center of the volar aspect of the capitate; thus, it may be termed a radioscaphocapitate ligament.

The *radiolunate (radiolunatotriquetral) ligament* is medial to the palmar radiocapite. It is also an intracapsular ligament arising from the volar lip and styloid process of the radius. This ligament is directed toward the ulna across the volar aspect of the lunate, to which it has a variable attachment, and it ends in

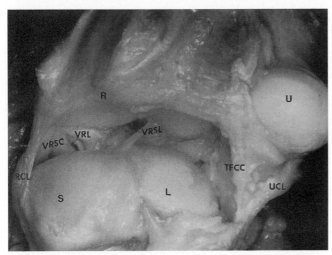

Figure 2–11. Open view of the radiocarpal joint illustrates the intracapsular portions of the volar radiocarpal ligaments. *L* = lunate; *R* = radius; *RCL* = radial collateral ligament; *S* = scaphoid; *TFCC* = triangular fibrocartilage complex; *U* = ulna; *UCL* = ulnar collateral ligament; *VRL* = volar radiolunate ligament; *VRSC* = volar radioscaphoid ligament; *VRSL* = volar radioscapholunate ligament.

the palmar surface of the triquetrum (see Figs. 2–10, and 2–11). The radiolunate ligament acts as a volar sling for the lunate. There may be a space between the radiolunate ligament and the preceding one, the space of Poirier (see Fig. 2–10), through which dislocations of the lunate occur.

The *volar radioscapholunate ligament* is the third component and the most controversial. Some believe it is the major stabilizer of the scapholunate joint,[2, 3, 4, 16] but others doubt its existence as a true ligament.[13, 19, 20] This ligament is more medial and slightly deeper than the radiolunatotriquetral ligament, originating from the volar lip of the radius at the ridge between lunate and scaphoid fossas of the radius. It inserts into the proximal volar surface of the scapholunate joint (see Fig. 2–11).

Special stains for elastic fibers fail to demonstrate any, even in the numerous blood vessels being carried in the volar radioscapholunate ligament to supply the interosseous scapholunate ligament.[15, 20] The palmar radioscapholunate ligament, however, is a variably sized structure that is consistently present and may require rupture or division before complete scapholunate dissociation can occur.

TRIANGULAR FIBROCARTILAGE COMPLEX

Studies have demonstrated that the TFCC is more complex than has previously been acknowledged or recognized.[6] The TFCC is thicker peripherally than centrally but is usually not perforated in younger individuals. The complex is attached by its base to the medial margin of the distal radius and by its apex to the lateral side of the base of the styloid process of the ulna (fovea). It is biconcave and articulates with

the distal ulna proximally and with the proximal carpal row, primarily the triquetrum, on its distal surface. The triangular fibrocartilage is reinforced anteriorly and posteriorly by fibrous bands that extend into the anterior and posterior capsule of the distal radioulnar joint. This capsule is only minimally reinforced and provides only minor support to the joint. It does not limit joint movement except at the extremes of forearm rotation. The triangular fibrocartilage is at maximum tension in approximately midposition between pronation and supination. At these positions, the interosseous membrane is under tension.

The *palmar ulnocarpal ligament* is formed by fibers that extend distally and radially from the anterior edge of the triangular fibrocartilage and the base of the ulnar styloid process and insert into the carpal bones (see Figs. 2–5, 2–6, and 2–10). The triangular fibrocartilage and adjacent ulnocarpal meniscus share a common origin from the attachment to the dorsal ulnar corner of the ulnar notch of the radius. The meniscus swings around the ulnar border of the wrist, attaching peripherally to the capsule and inserting into the triquetrum. There is a small triangular prestyloid recess filled with synovium surrounding the tip of the ulnar styloid and found between the meniscus and the triangular fibrocartilage (see Figs. 2–5 and 2–6).

Extending from the anterior border of the triangular fibrocartilage is the *ulnolunate ligament*, which inserts into the lunate. Medial to this is another diagonal band that attaches to the triquetrum and then extends onto the palmar aspect of the capitate and hamate (see Figs. 2–5, 2–6, and 2–10). This extension may represent the proximal ulnar arm of the arcuate ligament from the capitate to the triquetrum, described in Chapter 17. It adds stability to the ulnar aspect of the midcarpal joint. Because the triangular fibrocartilage is strongly attached to the radius, the ligaments arising from it attach the palmar aspect of the ulnar carpus to the radius as well as to the ulna.[1] Thus, the radiocarpal ligaments, the ulnocarpal ligaments, and the TFCC work together to provide stable pronation and supination of the hand and wrist.

FLEXOR RETINACULUM

The flexor retinaculum is a strong, broad ligament attached to the pisiform and hook of the hamate medially and to the tuberosities of the scaphoid and trapezium laterally (Fig. 2–12). Its primary function is to hold the flexor tendons of the digits in place during wrist flexion to prevent the loss of power that would occur with bow-stringing. The amount of support the flexor retinaculum provides the carpus is unknown, but it is under constant tension and is probably a factor in the maintenance of the contour of the carpal arch.

CARPOMETACARPAL LIGAMENTS

The joints between the distal carpal row and the second, third, fourth, and fifth metacarpals are rela-

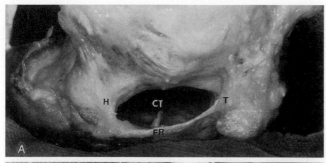
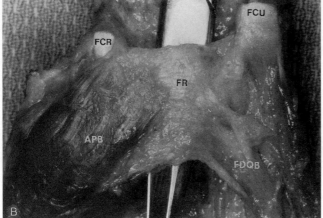
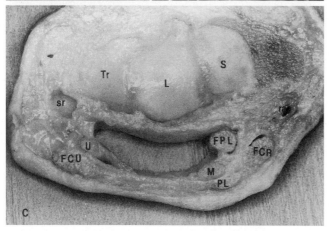

Figure 2–12. *A,* End-on view of carpal tunnel. *B,* Anterior view of flexor retinaculum, illustrating its attachment to the carpal bones and showing its extent. *C,* Cross-section through the radiocarpal joint to illustrate the carpal tunnel relationships. The finger flexor tendons have been removed for clarity. *APB* = abductor pollicis brevis; *CT* = carpal tunnel; *FCR* = flexor carpi radialis; *FCU* = flexor carpi ulnaris; *FDQB* = flexor digiti quinti brevis; *FPL* = flexor pollicis longus; *FR* = flexor retinaculum; *H* = hook of hamate; *L* = lunate; *M* = median nerve; *PL* = palmaris longus; *ra* = radial artery; *S* = scaphoid; *sr* = prestyloid recess; *T* = trapezium; *Tr* = triquetrum; *U* = ulnar nerve and artery.

tively complex when taken in their entirety. They are bound together by dorsal, palmar, and interosseous ligaments. The dorsal ligaments are the strongest and most distinct. Each of the central three metacarpals receives bands from two of the adjoining carpal bones. The fifth metacarpal receives one from the hamate. The palmar ligaments have a similar arrange-

ment, but they are less well-defined, although strong. The interosseous ligaments consist of short, thick fibers connecting contiguous distal margins of the capitate and hamate with the adjacent surfaces of the third and fourth metacarpals. Four short, strong interosseous ligaments are located between the bases of the five metacarpals. The ligament between the second and third metacarpal is the strongest. The somewhat block shape of the metacarpal bases, combined with the strong ligaments, provides for marked stability of the carpometacarpal joints, particularly the second and third.

PRIME MOVERS OF THE WRIST JOINTS

With the exception of the pisiform, which acts as a sesamoid bone in the tendon of the flexor carpi ulnaris, there are no carpal bones from which muscles or tendons arise or insert. Thus, any movement of the wrist is passive and dependent on muscle-tendon units that originate proximal, and insert distal, to the carpus. The shape of the bones, joint surfaces, and ligamentous attachments determines the effect of muscle pull on the wrist (see Chapters 4, 5, and 12).

For practical purposes and simplification, movements can be described as flexion/extension and abduction/adduction. The axes of these movements are considered to pass through the head of the capitate. Any muscle tendon unit crossing the wrist joint has an effect on these movements; thus, the long finger and thumb flexors and extensors can produce movements of the wrist as well as of the digits for which they are prime movers, unless countered by active contraction of antagonist wrist flexor and extensor muscles.

Active rotation of the hand-wrist unit occurs at the distal radioulnar joint. Active rotation of the carpus itself is negligible at best. The pronator teres and pronator quadratus muscles are the primary pronators of the forearm, pulling the attached hand and wrist into the palm-down position through the dorsal radiocarpal ligaments. The biceps brachii and supinator muscles are the primary supinators of the forearm, with the palmar radiocarpal ligaments passively pulling the wrist and hand into the palm-up position. The other forearm muscles play a minor role in rotation for the most part, unless the motion is vigorously resisted, at which point they may act to reinforce the primary movers.

Wrist flexion is done primarily by the flexor carpi radialis, palmaris longus, and flexor carpi ulnaris muscles, and secondarily by the long finger and thumb flexors. The abductor pollicis longus and extensor pollicis brevis muscles also cross volar to the axis of wrist flexion (see Figs. 2–1 and 2–13*C*) and often function as wrist flexors in cases of paralysis of the primary wrist flexors. The primary wrist flexor muscles have extensive origin from the medial humeral epicondyle, the deep forearm fascia, the intermuscular septa, and, in the case of the flexor carpi ulnaris, the shaft of the ulna throughout most of its length.

The tendon of the flexor carpi radialis muscle passes through a synovium-lined tunnel of its own in the carpal canal, where it lies in a groove or tunnel in the trapezium, and inserts into the bases of the second and third metacarpals opposite the insertions of the radial wrist extensors (Fig. 2–13). The flexor carpi ulnaris muscle inserts into the pisiform and is prolonged by the pisohamate and pisometacarpal ligaments to insert into the hamate and the base of the fifth metacarpal, respectively (Fig. 2–14). In addition to wrist flexion, the flexor carpi ulnaris muscle

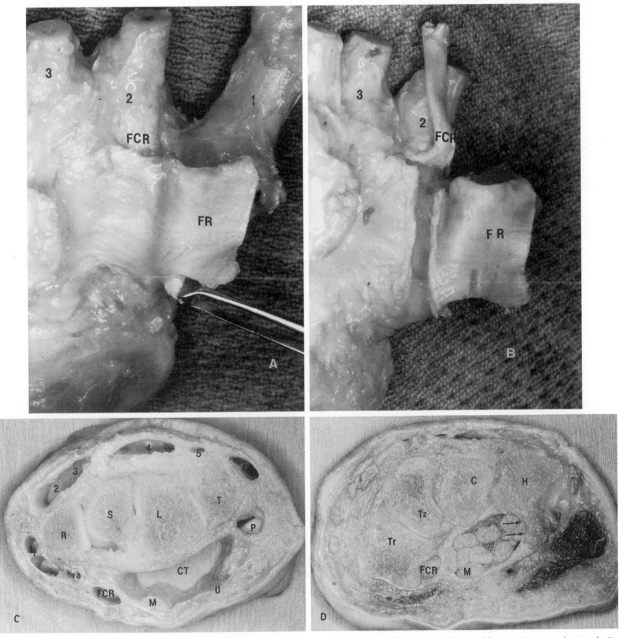

Figure 2–13. *A,* Flexor carpi radialis *(FCR)* with sheath intact and carpal tunnel opened. FCR is in carpal canal but not in carpal tunnel. *B,* Flexor carpi radialis sheath opened and tendon reflected distally. *C,* Cross-section of the wrist through the proximal carpal row with flexor and extensor tendons removed from their compartments. The FCR has its own compartment outside the carpal tunnel. *D,* Cross-section through the distal carpal row illustrating the groove in the trapezium for the FCR, converted into a tunnel by a covering ligament. *C* = capitate; *CT* = carpal tunnel; *FCR* = flexor carpi radialis; *FR* = flexor retinaculum (*1,2,* and *3* in views *A* and *B* indicate metacarpals); *H* = hamate (*arrows* indicate hamulus); *L* = lunate; *M* = median nerve; *P* = pisiform and pisotriquetral joint; *R* = radial styloid; *ra* = radial artery; *S* = scaphoid; *T* = triquetrum; *Tr* = trapezium; *Tz* = trapezoid; *U* = ulnar nerve dividing. (*1,2,3,4,5,* and *6* indicate extensor tendon compartments in view *C.* Note septation and volar position of first dorsal compartment; second and third compartments have merged into one distal to Lister's tubercle.)

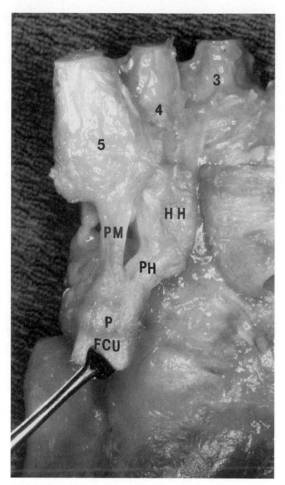

Figure 2–14. Flexor carpi ulnaris insertion. *FCU* = flexor carpi ulnaris tendon (in forceps); *HH* = hook of hamate; *P* = pisiform; *PH* = pisohamate ligament; *PM* = pisometacarpal ligament; 3, 4, and 5 = third, fourth, and fifth metacarpals.

muscle is located more ulnar than dorsal relative to the carpus and thus functions primarily as an adductor of the hand.

SUMMARY

The wrist is a pliable, osteoligamentous complex situated between the forearm and the palm of the hand. Its movements are permitted and restrained by the complex shape and ligamentous attachments of the various bones. Large portions of the surface of the involved bones are covered with articular cartilage. The ligamentous attachments are the sites for vascular access for the nourishment of the individual carpal bones. When these ligaments are disrupted, the vessels are commonly disrupted as well, with variable effects on the individual bones.

The *mobility* of the wrist results from its complex structure. The *stability* of the wrist is also a result of the complex shapes of the bones and the array of ligaments.

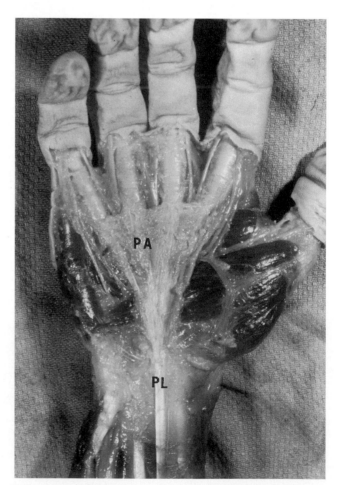

Figure 2–15. Palmaris longus insertion. *PA* = palmar aponeurosis; *PL* = palmaris longus tendon.

participates strongly in wrist adduction, and the flexor carpi radialis muscle is a strong wrist abductor. The palmaris longus muscle crosses the wrist superficial to the flexor retinaculum to insert into the palmar aponeurosis and palmar skin (Fig. 2–15).

Wrist extension is performed by the extensor carpi radialis longus, extensor carpi radialis brevis, and extensor carpi ulnaris muscles as well as the long finger and thumb extensors. All three wrist extensors proper originate from the distal humeral metaphysis and lateral epicondyle as well as from the deep forearm fascia covering their muscle bellies and from the fibrous septa between the muscle bellies. The muscles end in midforearm in tendons that insert into the bases of the second, third, and fifth metacarpals (Fig. 2–16). The extensor carpi ulnaris muscle participates with the flexor carpi ulnaris muscle to provide strong wrist adduction. The radial wrist flexors and extensors also combine to produce wrist abduction. With the forearm pronated, the extensor carpi ulnaris

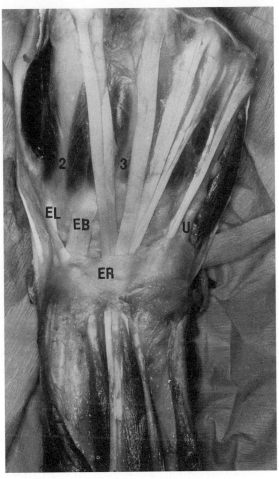

Figure 2–16. Wrist extensor insertions. *EB* = extensor carpi radialis brevis; *EL* = extensor carpi radialis longus; *ER* = extensor retinaculum; *U* = extensor carpi ulnaris; *2* and *3* = second and third metacarpals.

References

1. Taleisnik J: The ligaments of the wrist. J Hand Surg 1:110–118, 1976.
2. Mayfield JK, Johnson RP, Kilcoyne RF: The ligaments of the human wrist and their functional significance. Anat Rec 186:417–428, 1976.
3. Mayfield JK, Johnson RP, Kilcoyne RF: Carpal dislocations: Pathomechanics and progressive perilunar instability. J Hand Surg 5:226–241, 1980.
4. Mayfield JK: Wrist ligamentous anatomy and pathogenesis of carpal instability. Orthop Clin North Am 15:209–216, 1984.
5. Fisk G: Biomechanics of the Wrist Joint. In Tubiana R (ed): The Hand, volume I. Philadelphia, WB Saunders, 1981, pp 138–139.
6. Palmer AK, Werner FW: The triangular fibrocartilage complex of the wrist—anatomy and function. J Hand Surg 6:153–162, 1981.
7. Lewis OJ, Hamshere RJ, Bucknill TM: The anatomy of the wrist joint. J Anat 106:539–552, 1970.
8. Warwick R, Williams PL: Gray's Anatomy, 35th British ed. Philadelphia, WB Saunders, 1973, pp 336–341, 440.
9. Cantor RM, Braunstein EM: Diagnosis of dorsal and palmar rotation of the lunate on a frontal radiograph. J Hand Surg 13A:187–193, 1988.
10. Green DP: Carpal dislocations and instabilities. In Green DP (ed): Operative Hand Surgery, ed 3. London, Churchill-Livingstone, 1993.
11. Gillula LA: Carpal injuries: Analytic approach and case exercises. Am J Radiol 133:503–517, 1979.
12. Linscheid RL, Dobyns JN, Beabout JW, Bryan RS: Traumatic instability of the wrist: Diagnosis, classification and pathomechanics. J Bone Joint Surg 54A:1612–1632, 1972.
13. Ruby LK, An KN, Linscheid RL, et al: The effect of scapholunate ligament section on scapholunate motion. J Hand Surg 12A:767–771, 1987.
14. Kauer JMG: Functional anatomy of the wrist. Clin Orthop 149:9–20, 1980.
15. Hixson ML, Stewart C: Microvascular anatomy of the radioscapholunate ligament of the wrist. J Hand Surg 15A:279–282, 1990.
16. Taleisnik J: Wrist: anatomy, function and injury. AAOS Instr Course Lect 27:61–87, 1978.
17. Berger RA, Blair WF, Crowninshield RD, Flatt AE: The scapholunate ligament. J Hand Surg 7:87–91, 1982.
18. Blevens AD, Light TR, Jablonsky WS, et al: Radiocarpal articular contact characteristics with scaphoid instability. J Hand Surg 14A:781–790, 1989.
19. Berger RA, Kauer JMG, Landsmeer JMF: Radioscapholunate ligament: A gross anatomic and histologic study of fetal and adult wrists. J Hand Surg 16A:350–355, 1991.
20. Berger RA, Landsmeer JMF: The palmar radiocarpal ligaments: A study of adult and fetal human wrist joints. J Hand Surg 15A:847–854, 1990.
21. Kauer JMG, de Lange A: The carpal joint: Anatomy and function. Hand Clin 3:23–29, 1987.
22. Mizuseki T, Ikuta Y: The dorsal carpal ligaments: Their anatomy and function. J Hand Surg 14B:91–98, 1989.
23. Kaplan EB, Taleisnik J: The wrist. In Spinner M (ed): Kaplan's Functional and Surgical Anatomy of the Hand, ed 3. Philadelphia, JB Lippincott, 1984.

CHAPTER 3

Vascularity of the Carpus

Richard H. Gelberman, MD,
and Michael J. Botte, MD

Relatively few studies investigating the vascular patterns of the carpus have been performed. Technical difficulties in identifying small vessels in three dimensions and in determining their location within thick capsules and ligaments about the wrist have led to conflicting anatomic reports.[1, 5, 8, 19] Cadaver studies utilizing improved techniques with arterial injection, chemical débridement, and decalcification have allowed the arterial anatomy of the carpus to be more accurately delineated.[4–7, 16] This chapter discusses these arterial patterns, with attention to both the extraosseous and intraosseous vascularity.

EXTRAOSSEOUS VASCULAR PATTERNS

The extraosseous vascularity of the carpus consists of a series of dorsal and palmar transverse arches connected by anastomoses formed by the radial, ulnar, and anterior interosseous arteries.[6]

Dorsal Carpal Vascularity

The vascularity to the dorsum of the carpus consists of three dorsal transverse arches: the radiocarpal,[6, 8] the intercarpal,[2, 3, 6, 8, 13, 20] and the basal metacarpal[6] transverse arches (Figs. 3–1 and 3–2). These arches are approximately 1 mm in diameter; their branches are less than 1 mm. The presence of each arch is variable.

The dorsal radiocarpal arch, present in 80 percent of cadaver specimens studied,[6] is the most proximal. Located at the level of the radiocarpal joint, it lies deep to the extensor tendons. The radiocarpal arch provides the main nutrient vessels to the lunate and the triquetrum. It is usually supplied by branches of the radial and ulnar arteries and the dorsal branch of the anterior interosseous artery. Occasionally, the dorsal radiocarpal arch is supplied by the radial and ulnar arteries alone or by the radial and anterior interosseous arteries.[6]

The dorsal intercarpal arch is the largest of the dorsal transverse arches and is consistently present.[6] It runs transversely across the dorsal carpus between the proximal and the distal carpal rows, supplying

the distal carpal row and anastomosing with the radiocarpal arch to supply the lunate and the triquetrum. Like the radiocarpal arch, it receives variable contributions. It is supplied by the radial, ulnar, and anterior interosseous arteries in 53 percent of cadavers studied, by the radial and ulnar arteries alone in 20 percent, by the radial and anterior interosseous arteries in 20 percent, and by the ulnar and anterior interosseous arteries in 7 percent.[6]

The basal metacarpal arch is the most distal of the dorsal transverse arches and is located at the base of the metacarpals just distal to the carpometacarpal joints. It is the smallest of the dorsal arches and is actually a series of vascular retia; its presence is the most variable among these arches. It is complete in 27 percent of specimens, absent in 27 percent, and present in its radial aspect alone in 46 percent.[6] The

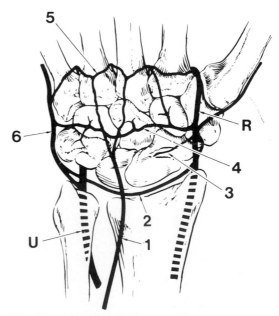

Figure 3–1. Schematic drawing of the arterial supply of the dorsum of the wrist. R = radial artery, U = ulnar artery; 1 = dorsal branch, anterior interosseous artery; 2 = dorsal radiocarpal arch; 3 = branch to the dorsal ridge of the scaphoid; 4 = dorsal intercarpal arch; 5 = basal metacarpal arch; 6 = medial branch of the ulnar artery. (From Gelberman RH, Panagis JS, Taleisnik J, et al: The arterial anatomy of the human carpus. Part I: The extraosseous vascularity. J Hand Surg 8:367–375, 1983.)

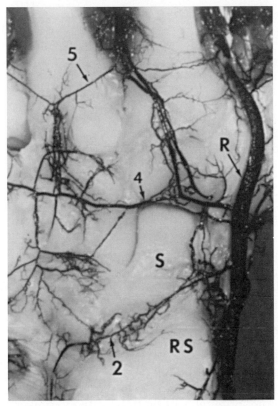

Figure 3–2. View of the three dorsal transverse arches. *RS* = radial styloid; *S* = scaphoid; *R* = radial artery; *2* = dorsal radiocarpal arch; *4* = dorsal intercarpal arch; *5* = basal metacarpal arch. (From Gelberman RH, Panagis JS, Taleisnik J, et al: The arterial anatomy of the human carpus. Part I: The extraosseous vascularity. J Hand Surg 8:367–375, 1983.)

arch supplies the palmar surface of the lunate and the triquetrum.

The intercarpal arch, located between the proximal and distal carpal rows, is the most variable in occurrence. Present in 53 percent of specimens, it is formed by branches of the radial, ulnar, and anterior interosseous arteries in 75 percent and by the radial and ulnar arteries alone in 25 percent. This arch is small and is not a major contributor of nutrient vessels to the carpus.

The deep palmar arch, the most distal of the palmar transverse arches, is located at the level of the metacarpal bases, 5 to 10 mm distal to the palmar carpometacarpal joints. It is consistently present and contributes to the radial and ulnar recurrent arteries and sends perforating branches to the dorsal basal metacarpal arch and to the palmar metacarpal arteries.

The three palmar arches are connected longitudinally by the radial, ulnar, anterior interosseous, and deep palmar recurrent arteries.

Specific Vessels

The five major arteries that supply the carpus are the radial artery, ulnar artery, anterior interosseous artery,

basal metacarpal arch is supplied by perforating arteries from the second, third, and fourth intraosseous spaces.[6] It contributes to the vascularity of the distal carpal row through anastomoses with the intercarpal arch.

The dorsal arches are connected longitudinally at their medial and lateral aspects by the ulnar and radial arteries. They are connected centrally by the dorsal branch of the anterior interosseous artery.

Palmar Carpal Vascularity

Similar to the dorsal vascularity, the palmar vascularity is composed of three transverse arches: the palmar radiocarpal, the palmar intercarpal, and the deep palmar arch (Fig. 3–3).

The palmar radiocarpal arch is the most proximal, extending transversely 5 to 8 mm proximal to the radiocarpal joint at the level of the distal metaphysis of the radius and the ulna. It lies within the wrist capsule. It is consistently present and is formed by branches of the radial, anterior interosseous, and ulnar arteries in 87 percent of specimens, and by the radial and ulnar arteries alone in 13 percent. This

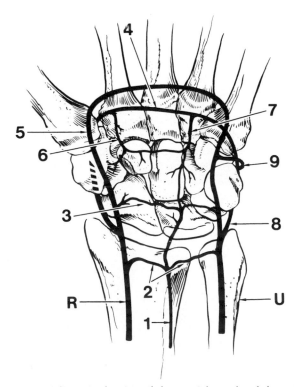

Figure 3–3. Schematic drawing of the arterial supply of the palmar aspect of the wrist. *R* = radial artery; *U* = ulnar artery; *1* = palmar branch, anterior interosseous artery; *2* = palmar radiocarpal arch; *3* = palmar intercarpal arch; *4* = deep palmar arch; *5* = superficial palmar arch; *6* = radial recurrent artery; *7* = ulnar recurrent artery; *8* = medial branch, ulnar artery; *9* = branch off ulnar artery contributing to the dorsal intercarpal arch. (From Gelberman RH, Panagis JS, Taleisnik J, et al: The arterial anatomy of the human carpus. Part I: The extraosseous vascularity. J Hand Surg 8:367–375, 1983.)

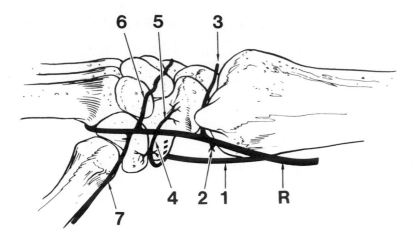

Figure 3–4. Schematic drawing of the arterial supply of the lateral aspect of the wrist. *R* = radial artery; *1* = superficial palmar artery; *2* = palmar radiocarpal arch; *3* = dorsal radiocarpal arch; *4* = branch to the scaphoid tubercle and trapezium; *5* = artery to the dorsal ridge of the scaphoid; *6* = dorsal intercarpal arch; *7* = branch to the lateral trapezium and thumb metacarpal. (From Gelberman RH, Panagis JS, Taleisnik J, et al: The arterial anatomy of the human carpus. Part I: The extraosseous vascularity. J Hand Surg 8:367–375, 1983.)

deep palmar arch, and accessory ulnar recurrent arteries.

RADIAL ARTERY

Of the major arteries supplying the carpus, the radial artery is the most consistent. It has seven major carpal branches: three dorsal, three palmar, and a final branch that continues distally (Figs. 3–4 and 3–5). The most proximal branch of the radial artery is the superficial palmar artery. It leaves the radial artery 5 to 8 mm proximal to the tip of the radial styloid, passes between the flexor carpi radialis and brachioradialis, and continues distally to contribute to the superficial palmar arch (see Fig. 3–4). The second branch contributes to the palmar radiocarpal arch. This branch leaves the radial artery approximately 5 mm distal to the superficial palmar artery and runs toward the ulna. A third branch originates at the level of the radiocarpal joint and runs dorsally and ulnarly, penetrating the radiocarpal ligament deep to the extensor tendons. This branch supplies the dorsal radiocarpal arch. The fourth branch arises palmarly at the level of the scaphotrapezial joint. It supplies the tubercle of the scaphoid and the radiopalmar surface of the trapezium. It then anastomoses with the superficial palmar artery. This vessel is absent in 25 percent of specimens; in 25 percent, it anastomoses with a branch of the superficial palmar artery prior to entering the scaphoid tubercle.[6] The fifth branch of the radial artery, the artery to the dorsal ridge of the scaphoid, originates directly from the radial artery in 75 percent of specimens and from the radiocarpal or intercarpal arch in 25 percent (see Fig. 3–4). It takes an ulnar retrograde course to supply the scaphoid. The sixth branch leaves the radial artery 5 mm distal to the branch to the scaphoid and contributes to the dorsal intercarpal arch. This arch courses ulnarly across the trapezoid and the distal half of the capitate prior to branching and anastomosing with both the dorsal branch of the anterior interosseous artery and the dorsal branches of the ulnar artery. The last branch of the radial artery originates at the level of the trapezium and courses radially and distally to

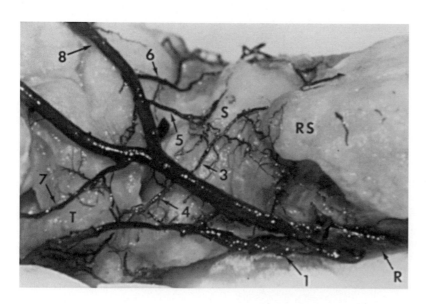

Figure 3–5. Vascularity of the lateral aspect of the wrist. *RS* = radial styloid; *S* = scaphoid; *T* = trapezium; *R* = radial artery; *1* = superficial palmar branch of the radial artery; *3* = dorsal radiocarpal arch; *4* = branch to the tubercle of the scaphoid and trapezium; *5* = artery to dorsal ridge of scaphoid; *6* = dorsal intercarpal arch; *7* = branch to the lateral trapezium and thumb metacarpal; *8* = medial branch of radial artery (seen in 22 percent of the specimens) penetrating the base of the index–long finger web space. (*Note:* In this view, *2*, the palmar radiocarpal arch, cannot be seen.) (From Gelberman RH, Panagis JS, Taleisnik J, et al: The arterial anatomy of the human carpus. Part I: The extraosseous vascularity. J Hand Surg 8:367–375, 1983.)

supply the trapezium and the lateral aspect of the thumb metacarpal.[6]

ULNAR ARTERY

At the level of the carpus, the ulnar artery gives off a latticework of fine vessels that span the dorsal and palmar aspects of the medial carpus (see Figs. 3–1 and 3–3). Proximal to the end of the ulna, there are three branches: a branch to the dorsal radiocarpal arch, one to the palmar radiocarpal arch, and one to the proximal pole of the pisiform and to the palmar aspect of the triquetrium. Several small branches supply the lateral aspect of the pisiform, and a single branch joins the palmar intercarpal arch. Distally, a branch supplies the distal pisiform and the medial hamate and continues dorsally between the pisohamate and the pisometacarpal ligaments to contribute to the dorsal intercarpal arch. At the midcarpal joint level, the medial branch of the ulnar artery contributes to the intercarpal arch (see Fig. 3–1). Distally, at the level of the metacarpal bases, the basal metacarpal arch receives its contribution from the medial branch of the ulnar artery. The medial branch of the ulnar artery then continues distally toward the base of the metacarpal of the little finger. A distal branch of the ulnar artery arises proximal to the origin of the superficial palmar arch and continues dorsally to supply the basal metacarpal arch. A deep palmar branch is given off distally that contributes to the deep palmar arch. The ulnar artery continues distally and radially to contribute to the superficial palmar arch.

ANTERIOR INTEROSSEOUS ARTERY

At the proximal border of the pronator quadratus muscle, the anterior interosseous artery bifurcates into dorsal and palmar branches. The dorsal branch continues distally on the interosseous membrane to the carpus, where it supplies the dorsal radiocarpal arch (89 percent of specimens).[6] Small branches extend radially to supply the lunate and to anastomose with several small radial artery branches supplying the dorsal ridge of the scaphoid. The dorsal branch of the anterior interosseous artery bifurcates at the intercarpal level, each branch contributing to the intercarpal arch (83 percent of specimens).[6] The dorsal branch of the anterior interosseous artery terminates by anastomosing with recurrent vessels from the basal metacarpal arch at the third and fourth interosseous spaces (70 percent of specimens) (see Fig. 3–1).[6]

The palmar branch of the anterior interosseous artery continues deep to the pronator quadratus and bifurcates 5 to 8 mm proximal to the radiocarpal arch. It usually contributes at least one branch to the palmar radiocarpal arch to supply the ulnar lunate and triquetrum and then terminates by anastomosing with recurrent vessels from the deep palmar arch.

DEEP PALMAR ARCH

The deep palmar arch provides the primary arterial supply to the distal carpal row by way of two branches—the radial and ulnar recurrent arteries (see Fig. 3–3). These branches run in a distal-to-proximal direction and are consistently present.[6] The radial recurrent artery is slightly smaller, originates from the arch just lateral to the base of the index metacarpal, and runs proximally to bifurcate on the palmar aspect of the trapezoid. It anastomoses with the ulnar recurrent artery in 45 percent of specimens.

The ulnar recurrent artery originates from the deep arch between the bases of the long and ring metacarpals. It courses proximally within the ligamentous groove between the capitate and the hamate, supplying both bones. It anastomoses with the terminal portion of the anterior interosseous artery in 80 percent of specimens.

ACCESSORY ULNAR RECURRENT ARTERY

In 27 percent of specimens, an accessory ulnar recurrent artery is present. It originates from the deep arch 5 to 10 mm medial to the ulnar recurrent artery and supplies the medial aspect of the hook of the hamate. When this vessel is not present, the medial aspect of the hamate is supplied by direct branches from the ulnar artery.[6]

POSTERIOR INTEROSSEOUS ARTERY

The posterior interosseous artery does not reach the carpus and does not directly contribute to its dorsal vascularity.[6, 20]

The contributions of the major arteries and arches to the carpus are summarized in Figures 3–6 and 3–7.

VASCULAR ANATOMY OF SPECIFIC CARPAL BONES

The specific vascular supply, including the intraosseous vascularity of each bone, is described here.[16] Nutrient arteries usually enter the bone through the noncartilaginous areas of ligamentous attachment and then branch to form an intraosseous vascular network within each bone.[4, 7, 8, 16, 20]

Scaphoid

The scaphoid receives its blood supply primarily from the radial artery (Fig. 3–8). Vessels enter palmarly and dorsally through nonarticular areas of ligamentous attachment.[1, 5, 8, 19]

The palmar vascular supply accounts for 20 to 30 percent of the internal vascularity, all in the region of the distal pole.[5] At the level of the radioscaphoid

Dorsal

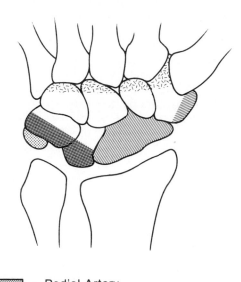

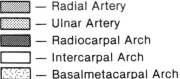

- Radial Artery
- Ulnar Artery
- Radiocarpal Arch
- Intercarpal Arch
- Basalmetacarpal Arch

Figure 3–6. Schematic drawing of the dorsum of the wrist, showing the major artery and arch contributions to the carpal bones. (From Gelberman RH, Panagis JS, Taleisnik J, et al: The arterial anatomy of the human carpus. Part I: The extraosseous vascularity. J Hand Surg 8:367–375, 1983.)

joint, the radial artery gives off the superficial palmar branch. Just distal to the origin of the superficial palmar branch, several smaller branches course obliquely and distally over the palmar aspect of the bone to enter the scaphoid through the region of the tubercle.[5, 8] These branches, the palmar scaphoid branches, divide into several smaller branches just prior to penetrating the bone. In 75 percent of specimens, these arteries arise directly from the radial artery.[5] In the remainder, they arise from the superficial palmar branch of the radial artery. Consistent anastomoses exist between the palmar division of the anterior interosseous artery and the palmar scaphoid branch of the radial artery, when the latter arises from the superficial palmar branch of the radial artery. There are no apparent communicating branches between the ulnar artery and the palmar branches of the radial artery that supply the scaphoid. Vessels in the palmar scapholunate ligament do not penetrate the scaphoid. The palmar vessels enter the tubercle and divide into several smaller branches to supply the distal 20 to 30 percent of the scaphoid. There are no apparent anastomoses between the palmar and dorsal vessels (Fig. 3–9).[5]

The dorsal vascular supply to the scaphoid accounts for 70 to 80 percent of the internal vascularity of the bone, all in the proximal region (Fig. 3–10).[5]

On the dorsum of the scaphoid, an oblique ridge lies between the articular surfaces of the radius and of the trapezium and trapezoid. The major dorsal vessels to the scaphoid enter the bone through small foramina located on this dorsal ridge (see Fig. 3–9).[1, 5] At the level of the intercarpal joint, the radial artery gives off the intercarpal artery, which immediately divides into two branches: a transverse branch to the dorsum of the wrist and a branch that runs vertically and distally over the index metacarpal. Approximately 0.5 cm proximal to the origin of the intercarpal vessel at the level of the styloid process of the radius, another vessel is given off that runs over the radiocarpal ligament to enter the scaphoid through its waist along the dorsal ridge. In 70 percent of specimens, the dorsal vessel arises directly from the radial artery. In 23 percent, the dorsal branch has its origin from the common stem of the intercarpal artery. In 7 percent, the scaphoid receives its dorsal blood supply directly from the branches of both the intercarpal artery and the radial artery. There are consistent major anastomoses between the dorsal scaphoid branch of the radial artery and the dorsal branch of the anterior interosseous artery in each specimen (see Fig. 3–8). No vessels enter the proximal dorsal region of the

Volar

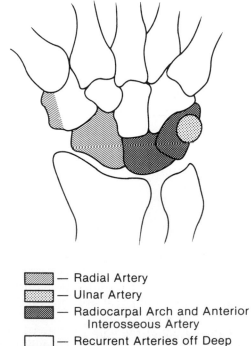

- Radial Artery
- Ulnar Artery
- Radiocarpal Arch and Anterior Interosseous Artery
- Recurrent Arteries off Deep Palmar Arch

Figure 3–7. Schematic drawing of the palmar aspect of the wrist, showing the major artery and arch contributions to carpal bones. (From Gelberman RH, Panagis JS, Taleisnik J, et al: The arterial anatomy of the human carpus. Part I: The extraosseous vascularity. J Hand Surg 8:367–375, 1983.)

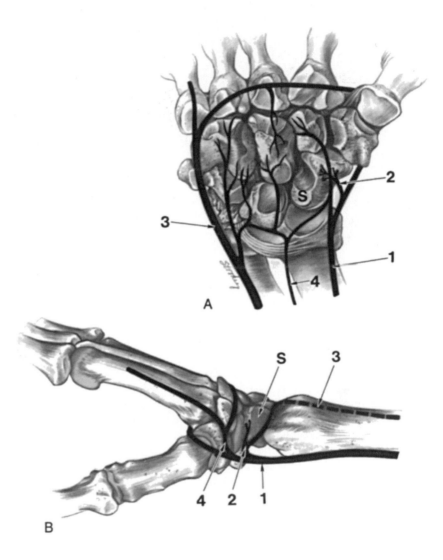

Figure 3–8. *A,* Schematic drawing of the volar external blood supply of the scaphoid. *S* = scaphoid; *1* = radial artery; *2* – volar scaphoid branches; *3* = ulnar artery; *4* = anterior division of the anterior interosseous artery. *B,* Schematic drawing of the dorsal blood supply of the scaphoid. *S* = scaphoid; *1* = radial artery; *2* = dorsal scaphoid branch; *3* = dorsal division of the anterior interosseous artery; *4* = intercarpal artery. (From Gelberman RH, Menon J: The vascularity of the scaphoid bone. J Hand Surg 5:508–513, 1980.)

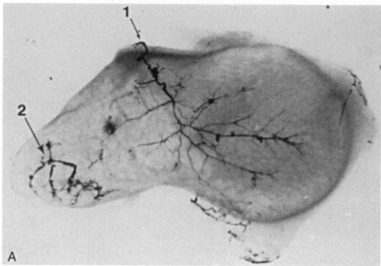
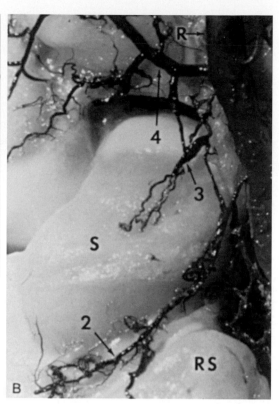

Figure 3–9. *A,* Photograph of a cleared specimen showing the internal vascularity of the scaphoid. (The vessels in the dorsal and volar scapholunate ligaments do not penetrate the bone.) *1* = dorsal scaphoid branch of the radial artery; *2* = volar scaphoid branch. *B,* Close-up view of the dorsoradial aspect of the wrist, demonstrating nutrient vessels entering the dorsal ridge of the scaphoid. *RS* = radial styloid; *S* = scaphoid; *R* = radial artery; *2* = dorsal radiocarpal arch; *3* = branch to the dorsal ridge of the scaphoid; *4* = dorsal intercarpal arch. *A,* From Gelberman RH, Menon JD: The vascularity of the scaphoid bone. J Hand Surg 5:508–513, 1980. *B,* From Gelberman RH, Panagis JS, Taleisnik J, et al: The arterial anatomy of the human carpus. Part I: The extraosseous vascularity. J Hand Surg 8:367–375, 1983.)

bone through the dorsal scapholunate ligament, and no vessels enter through dorsal cartilaginous areas.

The dorsal vessels usually enter the scaphoid through foramina located on the dorsal ridge at the level of the scaphoid waist; however, in a few of the specimens studied, they entered just proximal or distal to the waist. The dorsal vessels usually divide into two or three branches soon after entering the scaphoid. These branches run palmarly and proximally, dividing into smaller branches to supply the proximal pole as far as the subchondral region (see Fig. 3–9).

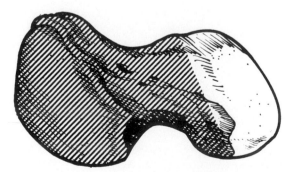

Figure 3–10. The proximal 70 to 80 percent of the bone is supplied by dorsal vessels *(shaded area).* The distal 20 to 30 percent is supplied by volar branches of the radial artery *(white area).* (From Gelberman RH, Menon J: The vascularity of the scaphoid bone. J Hand Surg 5:508–513, 1980.)

Trapezium

The trapezium receives vessels from distal branches of the radial artery (see Figs. 3–1, 3–3, and 3–4).

Nutrient vessels enter the trapezium through its three nonarticular surfaces (Fig. 3–11). These surfaces are the dorsal and lateral aspects, which are rough and serve as sites for ligamentous attachment, and the prominent palmar tubercle from which the thenar muscles arise. Dorsally, one to three vessels enter and divide in the subchondral bone to supply the entire dorsal aspect of the bone. Palmarly, one to three vessels enter the midportion and divide and anastomose with the vessels entering through the dorsal surface. Laterally, three to six very fine vessels penetrate the lateral surface and anastomose freely with the dorsal and palmar vessels. The dorsal vascular supply predominates. There are frequent anastomoses among all three systems.[16]

Trapezoid

The trapezoid is supplied by branches from the dorsal, the intercarpal, and the basal metacarpal arches and the radial recurrent artery (see Figs. 3–1 to 3–3).

The nutrient vessels enter the trapezoid through its two nonarticular surfaces (Fig. 3–12). These surfaces are the dorsal surface, which is broad and round, and the palmar surface, which is narrow and flat. Both surfaces are rough and serve as sites for ligament

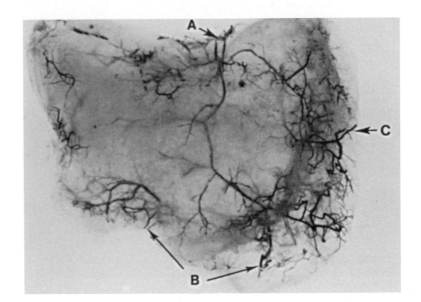

Figure 3–11. Trapezium: Distal view from articular surface at thumb trapeziometacarpal joint, showing dorsal *(A)*, palmar *(B)*, and lateral *(C)* nutrient vessels, with anastomoses of the three. (From Panagis JS, Gelberman RH, Taleisnik J, et al: The arterial anatomy of the human carpus. Part II: The intraosseous vascularity. J Hand Surg 8:375–382, 1983.)

attachment. Dorsally, three or four small vessels enter the central aspect of the rough, nonarticular surface. After penetrating the subchondral bone, the vessels branch to supply the dorsal 70 percent of the bone. Primarily, the dorsal vessels provide the vascularity of the trapezoid.[16]

Palmarly, one or two small vessels penetrate the central palmar area and branch several times to supply the palmar 30 percent of the bone. The palmar vessels do not anastomose with the dorsal vessels.[16]

Capitate

The capitate receives vessels from the dorsal intercarpal and the dorsal basal metacarpal arches and also from anastomoses between the ulnar recurrent and the palmar intercarpal arches.

The vessels enter through the two nonarticular surfaces on the dorsal and palmar aspects of the capitate. The dorsal surface is broad, deeply concave, and rough, serving for ligamentous attachment. Two to four vessels enter the distal two thirds of the concavity concavity (Fig. 3–13). Smaller vessels occasionally enter more proximally, near the neck. The dorsal vessels course palmarly, proximally, and ulnarly in a retrograde fashion to supply the body and head of the capitate. This dorsal supply predominates on the convex, rough palmar surface (Fig. 3–14).[16]

On the palmar surface, one to three vessels enter the distal half of the capitate and course proximally in a retrograde fashion. In 33 percent of the specimens, vascularity to the capitate head originates entirely from the palmar surface. There are significant anastomoses between the dorsal and the palmar blood supplies in 30 percent of specimens.[16]

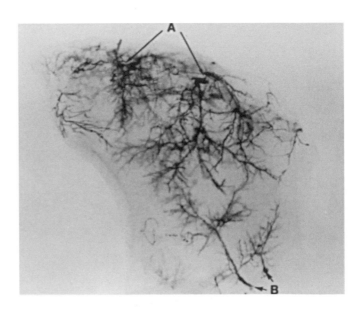

Figure 3–12. Trapezoid: Lateral view, showing dorsal nutrient vessels *(A)* supplying dorsal 70 percent of the bone and palmar vessels *(B)* supplying palmar 30 percent. There were no intraosseous anastomoses. (From Panagis JS, Gelberman RH, Taleisnik J, et al: The arterial anatomy of the human carpus. Part II: The intraosseous vascularity. J Hand Surg 8:375–382, 1983.)

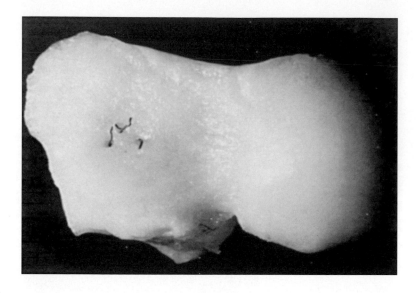

Figure 3–13. Capitate: Dorsal view prior to clearance with the Spalteholz technique, showing three arteries entering nutrient foramina in the distal one third of the bone. (From Panagis JS, Gelberman RH, Taleisnik J, et al: The arterial anatomy of the human carpus. Part II: The intraosseous vascularity. J Hand Surg 8:375–382, 1983.)

Hamate

The hamate receives vessels from the dorsal intercarpal arch, the ulnar recurrent artery, and the ulnar artery (see Figs. 3–1 and 3–3).

Vessels enter through the three nonarticular surfaces of the hamate: the dorsal surface, the palmar surface, and the medial surface, through the hamate hook (Fig. 3–15). The dorsal surface is triangular and receives three to five vessels. These branch in multiple directions to supply the dorsal 30 to 40 percent of the bone.[16]

The palmar surface is triangular and receives one large vessel that enters through the radial base of the hook. It then branches and anastomoses with the dorsal vessels in 50 percent of specimens studied.[16]

The hook of the hamate receives one or two small vessels that enter through the medial base and tip of the hook. These vessels anastomose with each other but usually not with the vessels to the body of the hamate.

Triquetrum

The triquetrum is supplied by branches from the ulnar artery, the dorsal intercarpal arch, and the palmar intercarpal arch. Nutrient vessels enter through its two nonarticular surfaces, the dorsal and the palmar.

The dorsal surface is rough and contains a ridge that runs from the medial to the lateral aspect. Two to four vessels enter this dorsal ridge and radiate in multiple directions to supply the dorsal 60 percent of the bone (Fig. 3–16). This network is the predominant blood supply to the triquetrum in 60 percent of specimens.[16]

The palmar surface contains an oval facet that articulates with the pisiform. One or two vessels enter proximal and distal to the facet. The vessels have multiple anastomoses with each other and supply the palmar 40 percent of the bone. This palmar vascular network is predominant in 20 percent of specimens studied (Fig. 3–17).[16]

The dorsal and the palmar vascular networks have

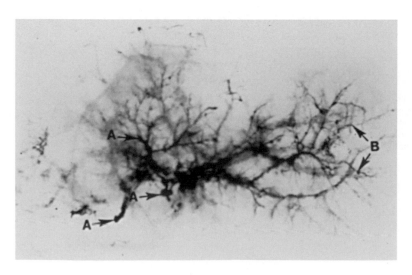

Figure 3–14. Capitate: Dorsal view, following clearing by Spalteholz technique. Nutrient vessels (A) enter distal third with retrograde course toward the proximal articular surface. Terminal vessels (B) in the head of the capitate. (From Panagis JS, Gelberman RH, Taleisnik J, et al: The arterial anatomy of the human carpus. Part II: The intraosseous vascularity. J Hand Surg 8:375–382, 1983.)

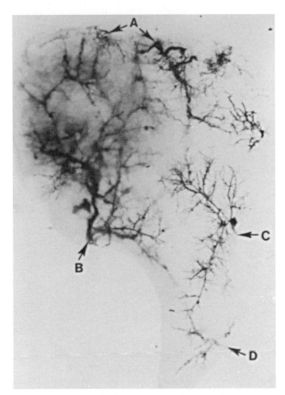

Figure 3–15. Hamate: End view from the distal surface, demonstrating dorsal *(A)* and palmar *(B)* supplies. Vessels to the hook enter at the medial base *(C)* and at the tip of the hook *(D).* (From Panagis JS, Gelberman RH, Taleisnik J, et al: The arterial anatomy of the human carpus. Part II: The intraosseous vascularity. J Hand Surg 8:375–382, 1983.)

significant anastomoses in 86 percent of specimens studied.[16]

Pisiform

The pisiform is a sesamoid bone within the tendon of the flexor carpi ulnaris. Dorsally, it articulates with the triquetrum. The remainder of the bone is rough and serves for ligament and muscle attachment. It receives its blood supply through the proximal and distal poles from branches of the ulnar artery. Proximally, one to three vessels enter inferior to the triquetral facet and divide into multiple branches. Two superior branches run parallel beneath the articular surface of the facet. One or two inferior branches run along the palmar cortex and anastomose with the superior branches.[16]

Distally, one to three vessels enter inferior to the facets, divide into superior and inferior branches, run parallel to the palmar cortex, and anastomose with the proximal vessels. The superior vessels run beneath the facet and anastomose with the proximal superior vessels, forming an arterial ring beneath the facet. There are multiple anastomoses between the proximal and the distal vascular networks (Fig. 3–18).[16]

Lunate

The lunate receives its nutrient vessels from both palmar and dorsal surfaces in 80 percent of specimens, and palmarly alone in 20 percent.[16] The remainder of the surface of the lunate is covered by articular cartilage. Dorsally, these nutrient vessels receive their supply from the dorsal radiocarpal arch, from the dorsal intercarpal arch, and occasionally from smaller branches of the dorsal branch of the anterior interosseous artery.[4, 6, 16] Palmarly, the lunate nutrient vessels are supplied by the palmar intercarpal arch, the palmar radiocarpal arch, and anastomosing vessels from the anterior interosseous artery and the ulnar recurrent artery (see Fig. 3–3).

The nutrient vessels that enter dorsally are slightly smaller than the palmar vessels. Major vessels branch proximally and distally after entering the bone and terminate in the subchondral bone. The dorsal and palmar vessels anastomose intraosseously just distal to the midportion of the lunate. The proximal pole is relatively avascular. There are three major intraosseous patterns forming Y, I, or X patterns (Figs. 3–19 to 3–21).[4] The Y pattern is the most common (59 percent), the stem of the Y occurring dorsally or palmarly with equal frequency. The I pattern, occurring in approximately 30 percent of specimens, consists of a single dorsal and a single palmar vessel that anastomose in a straight line. The X pattern, occurring in 10 percent, consists of two dorsal and two palmar vessels that anastomose in the center of the lunate.[4, 16]

In 20 percent of specimens studied, a single palmar supply was shown to be present. This consists of a single large vessel that enters on the palmar surface and branches within the bone to provide the sole blood supply (Fig. 3–22).

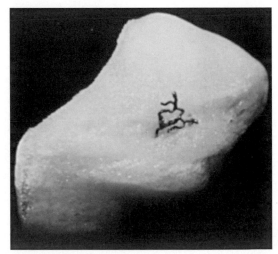

Figure 3–16. Triquetrum: Dorsal view prior to clearance with Spalteholz technique, showing a branching nutrient vessel entering the center of the obliquely running dorsal ridge. (From Panagis JS, Gelberman RH, Taleisnik J, et al: The arterial anatomy of the human carpus. Part II: The intraosseous vascularity. J Hand Surg 8:375–382, 1983.)

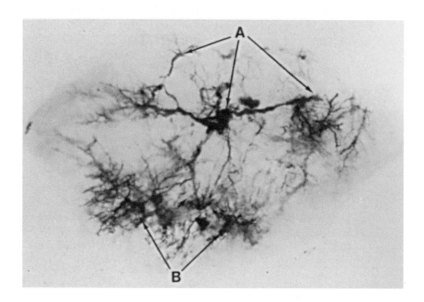

Figure 3–17. Triquetrum: Lateral view, showing three dorsal *(A)* and two palmar *(B)* nutrient vessels with intraosseous anastomoses in the middle one third of the bone. This pattern is seen in 80 percent of the specimens. (From Panagis JS, Gelberman RH, Taleisnik J, et al: The arterial anatomy of the human carpus. Part II: The intraosseous vascularity. J Hand Surg 8:375–382, 1983.)

Figure 3–18. Pisiform: Dorsal view looking onto the facet for the triquetrum, with the proximal superior *(A)* and distal superior *(B)* vessels forming an arterial ring beneath the facet. (From Panagis JS, Gelberman RH, Taleisnik J, et al: The arterial anatomy of the human carpus. Part II: The intraosseous vascularity. J Hand Surg 8:375–382, 1983.)

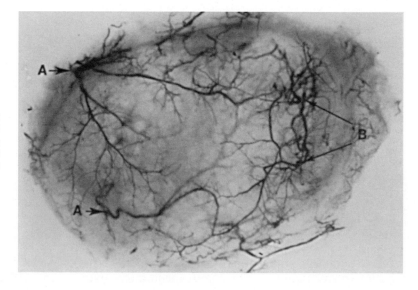

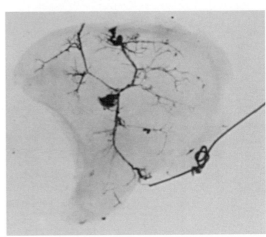

Figure 3–19. Lunate: The most common intraosseous vascular pattern—the Y pattern. (From Gelberman RH, Bauman RD, Menon J: The vascularity of the lunate bone and Kienböck's disease. J Hand Surg 5:272–278, 1980.)

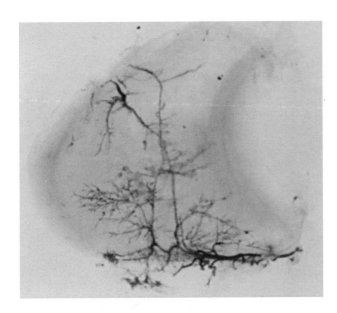

Figure 3–20. The X intraosseous vascular pattern formed by two dorsal and two volar vessels anastomosing in the midportion of the lunate. (From Gelberman RH, Bauman RD, Menon J: The vascularity of the lunate bone and Kienböck's disease. J Hand Surg 5:272–278, 1980.)

Figure 3–21. Schematic representation of I, X, and Y intraosseous vascular patterns. (From Gelberman RH, Bauman RD, Menon J: The vascularity of the lunate bone and Kienböck's disease. J Hand Surg 5:272–278, 1980.)

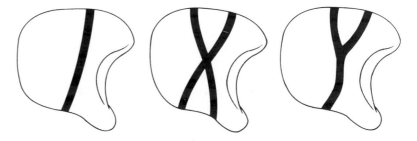

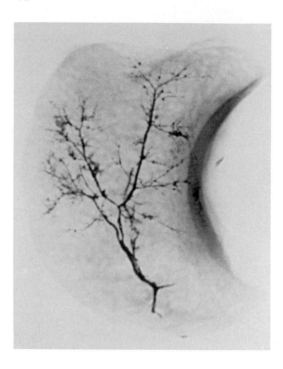

Figure 3–22. Lunate: Lateral view, showing single large vessel entering palmar surface and branching within the bone to provide the sole blood supply. This pattern is seen in 20 percent of the specimens. (From Panagis JS, Gelberman RH, Taleisnik J, et al: The arterial anatomy of the human carpus. Part II: The intraosseous vascularity. J Hand Surg 8:375–382, 1983.)

SUMMARY

The extraosseous arterial pattern is formed by an anastomotic network of three dorsal and three palmar arches connected longitudinally at their medial and lateral borders by the ulnar and radial arteries. Additional longitudinal anastomoses are provided by the dorsal and palmar branches of the anterior interosseous artery. The most distal of the palmar arches is the deep palmar arch, formed by the anastomosis of the radial artery and the deep palmar branch of the ulnar artery. Two consistent recurrent arteries, one radial and one ulnar, arise from the concavity of this arch and traverse proximally to frequently anastomose with the terminal branches of the anterior division of the anterior interosseous artery. This anastomosis provides the major collateral circulation about the wrist.

The bones of the carpus can be placed into three general groups on the basis of the size and location of nutrient vessels, the presence or absence of intraosseous anastomoses, and the dependence of large areas of bone on a single intraosseous vessel.[16] Group I consists of the scaphoid, the capitate, and, in approximately 20 percent of specimens, the lunate. Each has large areas of bone dependent on a single intraosseous vessel and is considered at greater risk to develop avascular necrosis following fracture. Group II contains the trapezoid and the hamate, both of which have two areas of vessel entry but lack intraosseous anastomoses. Group III are the trapezium, the triquetrum, the pisiform, and, in approximately 80 percent of specimens, the lunate; these bones receive nutrient arteries through two nonarticular surfaces, have consistent intraosseous anastomoses, and have no large area of bone dependent upon a single vessel. The clinical incidence of avascular necrosis in groups II and III is low.

The arterial anatomy of the carpus presents a technically demanding area of study. With improved techniques of investigation, the anatomy of this area can be more clearly defined. The results of a number of these recent studies have been summarized in this report.

References

1. Barber H: The intraosseous arterial anatomy of the adult human carpus. Orthopedics 5:1–19, 1972.
2. Coleman SS, Anson BJ: Arterial patterns in the hand. Surg Gynecol Obstet 113:409–429, 1961.
3. Edwards EA: Organization of the small arteries of the hand and digits. Am J Surg 99:837–846, 1960.
4. Gelberman RH, Bauman RD, Menon J: The vascularity of the lunate bone and Kienböck's disease. J Hand Surg 5:272–278, 1980.
5. Gelberman RH, Menon J: The vascularity of the scaphoid bone. J Hand Surg 5:508–513, 1980.
6. Gelberman RH, Panagis JS, Taleisnik J, et al: The arterial anatomy of the human carpus. Part I: The extraosseous vascularity. J Hand Surg 8:367–373, 1983.
7. Gelberman RH, Gross MS: The vascularity of the wrist—identifying arterial patterns at risk. Clin Orthop 202:40–49, 1986.
8. Grettve S: Arterial anatomy of the carpal bones. Acta Anat 25:331–345, 1955.
9. Hollingshead WH: Anatomy for Surgeons, vol 3. New York, Harper & Row, 1969.
10. Lawrence HW, Bachuber AE: The collateral circulation after ligature of both radial and ulnar arteries at the wrist [thesis]. University of Wisconsin, Department of Anatomy, 1923.
11. Lawrence HW: The collateral circulation in the hand. Indust Med 6:410–411, 1937.

12. Lee MCH: The intraosseous arterial pattern of the carpal lunate. Acta Orthop Scand 33:43–55, 1963.
13. Mestdagh H, Bailleu JP, Chambou JP, et al: The dorsal arterial network of the wrist with reference to the blood supply of the carpal bones. Acta Morphol Neerl Scand 17:73–80, 1979.
14. Meyers MH, Wells R, Harvey JP: Naviculocapitate fracture syndrome. J Bone Joint Surg 53:1383–1386, 1971.
15. Minne J, Depreux R, Mestdagh H, et al: Les pédicules artériels du massif carpien. Lille Méd 18:1174–1185, 1973.
16. Panagis JS, Gelberman RH, Taleisnik J, et al: The arterial anatomy of the human carpus. Part II: The intraosseous vascularity. J Hand Surg 8:375–382, 1983.
17. Quiring AP: Collateral Circulation. Philadelphia, Lea & Febiger, 1949.
18. Rockwood CA, Green DP: Fractures, vol 1. Philadelphia, JB Lippincott, 1975, pp 421–428.
19. Taleisnik J, Kelly PJ: Extraosseous and intraosseous blood supply of the scaphoid bone. J Bone Joint Surg 48:1125–1137, 1977.
20. Travaglini E: Arterial circulation of the carpal bones. Bull Hosp J Dis Orthop Inst 20:19–36, 1959.
21. Vance RM, Gelberman RH, Evans EF: Scaphocapitate fracture. J Bone Joint Surg 62:271–276, 1980.
22. Failla JM: Hook of hamate vascularity: vulnerability to osteonecrosis and nonunion. J Hand Surg 18A:1075–1079, 1993.
23. Handley RC, Pooley J: The venous anatomy of the scaphoid. J Anat 178:115–118, 1991.
24. Kuhlmann JN, Guerin-Surville H, Boabighi A: Vascularisation of the carpus, a systematic study. Surg Radiol Anat 10:21–28, 1988.
25. Oberlin C, Salon A, Pigeau I, et al: Three-dimensional reconstruction of the carpus and its vasculature: An anatomic study. J Hand Surg 17A:767–772, 1992.
26. Williams CS, Gelberman RH: Vascularity of the lunate. Anatomic studies and implications for the development of osteonecrosis. Hand Clin 9:391–398, 1993.

CHAPTER 4

Physiologic Bases for Wrist Function

Edward R. Weber, MD

The wrist functions as the final adjuster of the hand in a kinematic linkage with the rest of the body. To accomplish this task, the wrist possesses a large range of motion while maintaining enough stability to support the entire body mass. How the wrist accomplishes these goals has been the subject of inquiries for the past century.[1-10] This chapter combines the thinking of anatomists and bioengineers to form a theory on how the wrist functions.

WRIST ANATOMY

The wrist is defined by the articulation of the carpus with the forearm proximally and by the articulations with the metacarpals distally. It contains two transversely oriented rows of bones. The proximal row consists of the triquetrum, lunate, and scaphoid. The distal row contains the hamate and capitate. A third group of bones, the trapezoid, trapezium, and scaphoid, acts to support the thumb.

The proximal carpal row is devoid of any muscular attachment. Its motion and stability depend upon the geometry of the articular surfaces and its ligamentous constraints. The articulation of the scaphoid and lunate with the radius is accomplished through sulci in the distal radial articular surface. These depressions are separated by a ridge (the intersulcal or sagittal ridge). The sulcus for the scaphoid is teardrop-shaped, and its curvature is slightly greater than that of the sulcus for the lunate. The lunate sulcus is rectangular in shape and less curved than the scaphoid sulcus. Each sulcus represents about 50 percent of the distal radial articular surface. The ulnar third of the lunate and the triquetrum articulate with a fibrocartilaginous disk, which fills the space between the distal ulnar articular surface and the proximal carpal row. The distal articular surface of the proximal carpal row and the proximal articular surfaces of the capitate and hamate form the midcarpal joint. These articular surfaces are more complex than those of the radiocarpal joint. Of particular interest is the articulation between the triquetrum and hamate. The hamate's articular surface is helical in configuration. The most ulnar portion lies palmar to the radial portion. The surface is also twisted so that the ulnar facet faces in a palmar direction and the radial facet faces dorsally. The hamate surface presents an inclined plane for the triquetrum as it translates radial

dorsal to ulnar palmar. The capitate's proximal articular surface is dome-shaped, fitting into an acetabulum formed by the lunate and proximal pole of the scaphoid. Its radial surface is vertical, allowing flexion and extension motions of the scaphoid. The articulation between the capitate and hamate is also vertically oriented, but little motion is allowed at this joint.

The ligaments that control the proximal carpal row are divided into extrinsic (those with insertions on the proximal carpal row and on structures external to the proximal carpal row) and intrinsic (those with insertions exclusively within the proximal or distal carpal row). These ligaments are static structures that limit the motion of the bones of the proximal row through their range of motion. The ligaments directly controlling the proximal carpal row are primarily on the palmar surface. They have been classified by Taleisnik[11] as the deep extrinsic ligaments. They are the long radiolunate, radioscapholunate and the radioscaphocapitate ligaments. The long radiolunate ligament is an extremely stout structure arising from a sulcus just ulnar to the radial styloid on the volar lip of the radius. It courses obliquely to insert on the volar pole of the lunate. The radioscapholunate ligament arises from a small tubercle on the anterior margin of the radius and inserts primarily into the lunate and secondarily into the scaphoid. This ligament is weak and considered by many to be a vascular leash to the proximal carpal row. Berger[18] described a deep ligament separate from the radiolunate ligament that he called the short radiolunate ligament. It arises from the volar lip of the radius, ulnar to the radioscapholunate ligament, and inserts into the palmar pole of the lunate. This is a short, stout, broad ligament that tethers the palmar pole of the lunate to the radius (Fig. 4–1).

The ulnar ligamentous structures are complex. They consist of a strong fibrocartilaginous band of tissue that is attached to the dorsal ulnar corner of the radius. This ligament swings around the ulnar border of the wrist to insert into the palmar surface of the triquetrum. This ligament is called the meniscus homologue in recognition of the articulation of the ulnar styloid process with the triquetrum seen in the lower primates (Fig. 4–2). Sharing a common origin from the dorsal ulnar corner of the radius with the meniscus homologue is the triangular fibrocartilage. This structure passes volarly from the meniscus homologue to attach to the ulna near the base of the

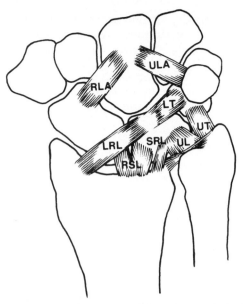

Figure 4–1. Ligaments: Palmar aspect of the wrist—extrinsic. *LRL* = long radiolunate ligament; *LT* = lunatriquetral ligament; *RLA* = radial arm of the arcuate ligament; *SRL* — short radiolunate ligament; *UL* = ulnolunate ligament; *ULA* = ulnar arm of the arcuate ligament; *UT* = ulnotriquetral ligament; *RSL* = radioscapholunate ligament.

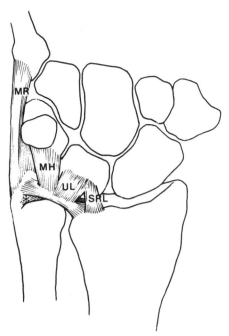

Figure 4–3. Palmar view: Ligaments of the ulnar side of the carpus. *MH* = meniscus homologue; *MR* = meniscus reflection; *SRL* = short radiolunate ligament; *UL* = ulnolunate ligament.

ulnar styloid. The triangular fibrocartilage and the ligament connecting it to the triquetrum are called the triangular fibrocartilage complex (TFCC) or the ulnar carpal complex. Arising from the palmar surface of the triangular fibrocartilage is another ligament that inserts into the lunate's palmar surface. This is called the ulnolunate ligament (Fig. 4–3). This

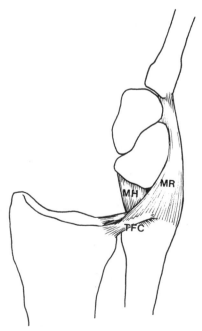

Figure 4–2. Dorsal view: Ligaments of the ulnar side of the carpus. *MH* = meniscus homologue; *MR* = meniscus reflection; *TFC* = triangular fibrocartilage.

ligament is considered by Berger[18] to be part of the short radiolunate ligament. Investing the TFCC on the dorsal and ulnar aspect is a thin ligamentous layer that attaches proximally to the TFCC and ulna and distally to the base of the fifth metacarpal. This structure is called the meniscal refraction.

The distal carpal row is firmly bound together by a group of short intrinsic ligaments. The volar intracarpal ligament, an intrinsic ligament, arises from the neck of the capitate and extends proximally to attach to the triquetrum ulnarly and to the scaphoid radially. This ligament is also called the arcuate, deltoid, or v ligament (see Fig. 4–1). The dorsal intrinsic ligament runs diagonally across the proximal carpal row, binding the dorsal surfaces of the scaphoid, lunate, and triquetrum together. This ligament is distinct from the dorsal radiocarpal ligament, which is an extrinsic ligament arising from the radius, in the region of Lister's tubercle, and coursing ulnarly to attach to the dorsal surface of the lunate and triquetrum (Fig. 4–4).

The radial collateral ligament arises from the radial styloid and attaches to the tuberosity of the scaphoid. The ulnar collateral ligament arises from the base of the ulnar styloid and attaches to the triquetrum. The collateral ligaments are poorly defined and do not function as true collateral ligaments because of the complexity of wrist motion. In modern terminology, the radial collateral ligament is included in the radial portion of the radioscaphocapitate ligament, and the ulnar collateral ligament is a portion of the meniscal reflection.

The last of the significant ligaments of the wrist are the radioscaphocapitate ligament, an extrinsic liga-

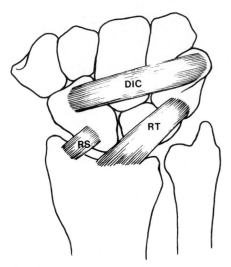

Figure 4–4. Dorsal wrist ligaments. *DIC*=dorsal intercarpal ligament; *RS*=radioscaphoid ligament; *RT*=radiotriquetral ligament (dorsal radiocarpal ligament).

ment, and the interosseous ligaments between the scaphoid and lunate and triquetrum. The radioscaphocapitate ligament is unique, in that it crosses two carpal articulations. It attaches proximally to a ridge on the volar surface of the radius and courses ulnarly and distally, over the scaphoid waist where it has a tenuous attachment, to insert into the capitate (Fig. 4–5). The more radial fibers inserting into the distal pole of the scaphoid were formerly called the radial collateral ligament.

The interosseous ligament between the lunate and triquetrum is thickened on its dorsal and palmar aspects, where it blends with the dorsal intrinsic carpal ligament and the palmar radiolunate ligament. The scapholunate ligament is a complex structure that is

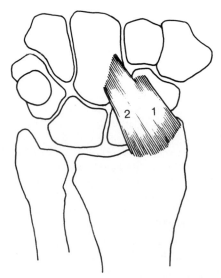

Figure 4–5. Palmar view: Components of the radioscaphocapitate ligament. *1*=radioscaphoid component; *2*=radiocapitate component.

thickened dorsally. Its fibers course from lunate to scaphoid and are thinner and more loosely bound toward the palmar surface. There is an attachment palmarly with the radiolunate ligament in some dissections. This ligament is distinct from the radioscapholunate ligament. In spite of its lack of bulk, this is one of the strongest of the wrist ligaments.

WRIST KINEMATICS

How the ligaments, articular surfaces, and motor units interact to produce the motions of the wrist is called wrist kinematics. One fact must be kept in mind when considering the function of ligaments: they are static structures and can only act to limit motion. The proximal carpal row flexes and extends in both dorsopalmar flexion and in radioulnar deviation motions of the wrist. Supination and pronation are primarily forearm motions. Because the proximal carpal row has no muscular or tendinous attachments, the flexion extension arc is governed by the contact surfaces and guided by the ligamentous constraints. During the motion of ulnar deviation, the proximal carpal row extends relative to the forearm bones and the distal carpal row (Fig. 4–6). The extension of the proximal carpal row is the result of a change in the alignment of the capitate and its complementary joint surfaces in the proximal row. The lunate and scaphoid form an acetabular joint conforming to the head of the capitate. As the capitate's axis is displaced dorsal to the axis of the lunate and proximal scaphoid pole, the compressive forces transmitted through the capitate drive the proximal row into extension. The change in axial alignment is produced by the descent of the triquetrum on the slope of the hamate as the triquetrum comes to rest in contact with the palmar ulnar facet of the hamate. Seventy-five percent of the force transmitted by the wrist comes through the head of the capitate, to the acetabulum formed by the scaphoid and lunate, then to the radius.[12] The placement of the mechanism governing the attitude of the proximal row outside the force-bearing axis and combining it with a simple lever, the inclined plane (the hamate slope), allows smaller forces to accomplish this task. The extension of the scaphoid is accommodated by the scaphotrapezotrapezoidal (STT) joint. Excision of the trapezium and trapezoid does not affect the extension of the proximal row in ulnar deviation. The radiocapitate ligament traverses the scaphoid waist and tightens in ulnar deviation, possibly aiding in the extension of the scaphoid. Sectioning of this ligament, however, increases the extension of the proximal row in ulnar deviation as the capitate is allowed to migrate even farther dorsally. It appears that one function of the radiocapitate ligament is to limit the dorsal migration of the capitate.

As the wrist is moved from ulnar deviation to radial deviation, the triquetrum moves up the slope of the hamate and partially onto the head of the capitate.

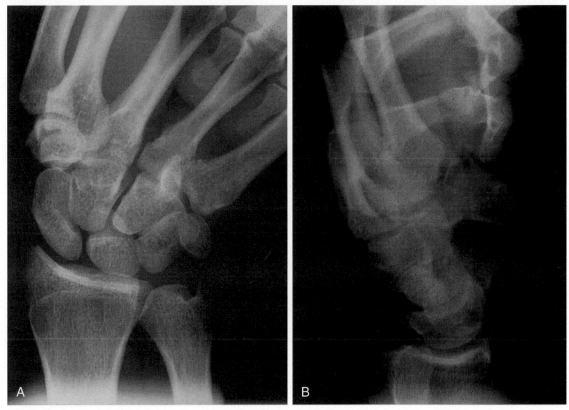

Figure 4–6. Radiographs of the wrist in ulnar deviation. *A,* Posteroanterior view. Note the elongated shape of the scaphoid, indicating the extension of this bone to fill the space between the radius and the thumb base. Note also the triangular shape of the lunate, indicating that it too has extended. *B,* Lateral view. Note the extension of the scaphoid and the dorsal facing stance of the lunate, indicating the extension of the entire proximal carpal row.

This action causes the head of the capitate to align with the lunate, thus producing relative flexion of the lunate[13] (Fig. 4–7). The radius of curvature of the scaphoid is greater than that of the lunate; therefore, more flexion is produced in the scaphoid by this change in axial alignment.[14] The scapholunate ligament is hinged dorsally, allowing the palmar portion of the scaphoid to separate from the lunate to accommodate this increase in flexion. Excision of the STT joint results in greater scaphoid flexion; this joint thus provides a constraint to scaphoid flexion rather than an initiation of this action.

Flexion and extension of the proximal carpal row during radial and ulnar deviation permits a marked increase in the range of motion of the wrist. As the wrist moves to radial deviation, the thumb base approaches the radius. As we have seen, this motion is accompanied by flexion of the scaphoid. Similarly, as ulnar deviation is achieved, the thumb base moves away from the radius. This increased distance is filled by extension of the scaphoid. Without flexion and extension of the proximal row, radial and ulnar deviation would be severely limited.

In flexion/extension motions of the wrist, the proximal row also flexes and extends, adding the motion of the proximal carpal joint to that of the midcarpal joint. The individual bones of the proximal row contribute unequally to the overall flexion/extension arch, depending on their various radii of curvature. The scaphoid, because of its greater curvature, must rotate more than the lunate to achieve the same arc of motion. The proximal row articulation provides more flexion, whereas the midcarpal articulation gives more extension, to the total arc of motion. In palmar flexion, the palmar extrinsic ligaments loosen, allowing greater mobility of the individual carpal bones. The dorsal radiocarpal ligament tightens during palmar flexion, guiding the triquetrum up the slope of the hamate, which maintains the alignment of the capitate and lunate. During dorsiflexion, the palmar ligaments tighten and the dorsal ligaments loosen. The taut palmar ligaments draw the bones of the proximal row together. This close-packed configuration of the carpus and the palmar-facing slope of the radius provides an extremely strong configuration for force transmission in this position.

FORCE TRANSMISSION

Gilford and colleagues,[5] Navarro,[15] Taleisnik,[16] and others have analyzed the wrist from the perspective of its injury patterns. They have viewed the wrist as a series of longitudinal columns with the capitate/

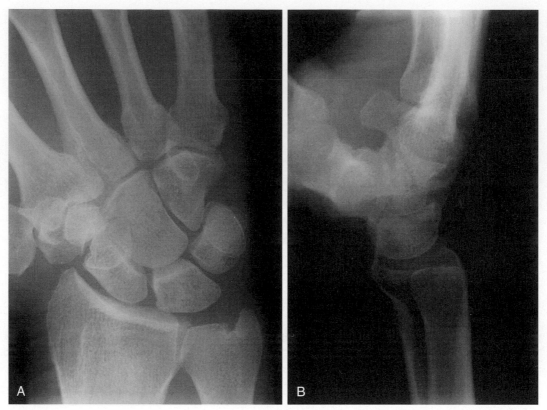

Figure 4–7. Radiographs of the wrist in radial deviation. *A*, Posteroanterior view. Note the foreshortened silhouette of the scaphoid and the quadrangular shape of the lunate, indicating flexion of the proximal row in radial deviation. *B*, Lateral view. Note the vertical stance of the scaphoid and coaxial alignment of the lunate with the radial sulcus. These findings indicate flexion of the proximal row when compared with the position of these bones in ulnar deviation.

lunate axis forming the central flexion/extension axis, the triquetrum providing rotation, and the scaphoid acting as a link between the proximal and distal rows. If the connection between the scaphoid and lunate is violated, the capitate forces its way between the scaphoid and lunate. The lunate rotates with the triquetrum into a dorsal-facing position, and the scaphoid flexes to accommodate the shortened distance between the thumb base and radius. In Chapter 12, the ring theory of Lichtman is described. He views the wrist as a series of transverse rows with the STT joint and the triquetrolunate joint as the links transmitting forces and guiding motion between the rows. A "break" in the proximal row permits uncoupling of these forces with predictable rotation of the respective components.[17]

It is helpful to view the wrist as longitudinal columns when considering force transmission. The majority of the forces passing through the carpus are transmitted to the radius. The principal force-transmitting chain consists of the capitate, lunate, and proximal pole of the scaphoid. The amount of force transmitted by the ulnar side of the wrist is limited by the mobility of the ring and small carpometacarpal joints, the slope of the hamate's proximal articular surface, and the compliance of the triangular fibrocartilage. Palmer and Werner[12] have shown that about 75 percent of the force is transmitted through the radius, and 25 percent through the ulna.

Much discussion has arisen between proponents of the vertical columnar view of the wrist and those who view the wrist as transverse rows. The wrist does move as two independent rows. However, the force is unevenly distributed between the radius and ulnar articulation. The previous section on wrist kinematics presents a unifying theory by which these facts are reconciled.

Those who propose that the proximal carpal row moves as a ring,[17] that is, tethered on the radial side at the STT joint and on the ulnar side at the triquetrohamate joint, are correct in a broad conceptual sense. When the proximal carpal row is viewed as a unit, it moves together. The amounts of rotation and twisting of the individual bones, however, are different. The amount of motion the individual bones undergo is the direct result of the geometry of their contact surfaces. Because all three bones of the proximal carpal row are uniquely shaped, their motions are also unique. Thus, the wrist moves as two rows of bones, the proximal and distal rows. Force transmission takes place in columns, however, with the central column sharing the greatest amount of load.

Proponents of the view that the wrist fails as if it were composed of columns are also correct. Force

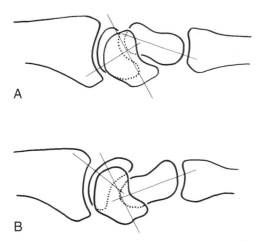

Figure 4–8. *A*, DISI deformity. Pattern of collapse with disruption of the scapholunate ligament. Note the vertical stance of the scaphoid, indicating shortening of the wrist. The lunate has assumed the stance normally seen in ulnar deviation, where extension of the proximal row is seen. The flexion of the scaphoid and extension of the lunate indicate the loss of connection between these bones. *B*, VISI deformity. Both the scaphoid and lunate have achieved a marked flexion stance. Because both bones have moved in unison, they have remained connected. The ligament damage leading to this deformity lies on the ulnar side of the wrist or at the midcarpal joint.

transmitted through the acetabulum, containing the capitate head, can become sufficient to break the connection between the scaphoid and lunate. The lack of connection within the proximal row allows for the individual units to act independently. In this case, the scaphoid undergoes abnormal flexion as force is transferred from the capitate head to the STT joint. The flexion of the scaphoid results in loss of carpal height. The shortening of the carpal unit causes the lunate and triquetrum, which remain connected, to displace ulnarward. Ulnar displacement of the triquetrum on the hamate also causes the descent of the triquetrum down the hamate slope; then the axis of the lunate falls volar to the axis of the capitate. Compressive forces from the capitate thus drive the lunate into extension. Thus, the hallmarks of the dorsal intercalated segment collapse described by Dobyns and colleagues[9] are established: (1) flexion of the scaphoid, (2) extension of the lunate, and (3) a gap between the scaphoid and lunate (Fig. 4–8*A*).

Disruption of the proximal carpal row between the medial column (triquetrum) and the central column (lunate) again leads to instability of the proximal row. In this instance, the triquetrum's descent on the hamate slope no longer influences the lunate. The axis of the capitate has lost its possibility of moving dorsal to that of the lunate. This imbalance eventuates in the permanent displacement of the capitate

axis volar to the lunate axis, producing flexion of both the lunate and scaphoid as carpal height is lost. Thus, the hallmarks of the volar intercalated segment collapse are produced: (1) reduction of the scapholunate angle to less than 40°, and (2) an increase in the lunocapitate angle to more than 10° (Fig. 4–8*B*).

The key to wrist function is that the force transmitted through the capitate head produces the movement of the proximal carpal row by positioning the axis of the capitate in relation primarily to the lunate and secondarily to the proximal pole of the scaphoid. The axial alignment of the two rows is controlled by the position of the triquetrum on the slope of the hamate. This theory attempts to resolve the differences between those who view the wrist as columns and those who view the wrist as rows.

References

1. Fick R: Handbuch der Anatomie und Mechanik der Gelenke. Jena, Fischer, 1911, part 3, p 357.
2. Cyriax EF: On the rotary movements of the wrist. J Anat 60:199–201, 1926.
3. Von Bonin G: A note on the kinematics of the wrist-joint. J Anat 63:259–262, 1929.
4. Destot E: Injuries of the Wrist: A Radiological Study. Atkinson FRB, trans. London, Ernest Benn Limited, 1925.
5. Gilford WW, Bolton RH, Lambrinudi C: The mechanism of the wrist joint with special reference to fractures of the scaphoid. Guy's Hosp Rep 92:52–59, 1943.
6. Landsmeer JMF: Studies in the anatomy of articulation. I: The equilibrium of the "intercalated" bone. Acta Morphol Neerl Scand 3:287–303, 1961.
7. Lindscheid RL: Scapholunate ligamentous instabilities (dissociations, subdislocations, dislocations). Ann Chir Main 3:323–330, 1984.
8. Dobyns JH, Perkins JC: Instability of the carpal navicular [abstract]. J Bone Joint Surg 49A:1014, 1967.
9. Dobyns JH, Linscheid RL, Chao EYS, et al: Tramatic instability of the wrist. In AAOS Instructional Course Lectures, vol 24. St Louis, 1975, pp 182–199.
10. Linscheid RL, Dobyns JH: The unified concept of carpal injuries. Ann Chir Main 3:35–42, 1984.
11. Taleisnik J: The ligaments of the wrist. J Hand Surg 1:110–118, 1976.
12. Palmer AK, Werner FW: Biomechanics of the distal radioulnar joint. Clin Orthop 187:26–34, 1984.
13. Ruby LK, Cooney WP III, An KN, et al: Relative motion of selected carpal bones: A kinematic analysis of the normal wrist. J Hand Surg 13A:1–10, 1988.
14. Kauer JMG, de Lange A: The carpal joint: Anatomy and function. Hand Clin 3:23–29, 1987.
15. Navarro A: Luxaciones del carpo. An Fac Med Montevideo, 6:113, 1921.
16. Taleisnik J: Classification of carpal instability. Bull Hosp Joint Dis 44:511–531, 1984.
17. Lichtman DM: Introduction to carpal instabilities. The wrist and Its Disorders. Philadelphia, WB Saunders, 1988, p 244.
18. Berger RA: Ulnocarpal translation. Presented at the Tenth International Wrist Investigator's Workshop. Rochester, Minnesota, May 22, 1994.

CHAPTER 5

Pathogenesis and Pathokinetics of Wrist Ligament Instability

Jack K. Mayfield, MD

Carpal instability represents persistent carpal bone malalignment, primarily as a result of ligamentous injury. A spectrum of ligamentous damage is now recognized, and various patterns of carpal instability have been elucidated. This chapter describes the pathogenesis and pathokinetics of the perilunate or dissociative carpal injuries. Midcarpal and nondissociative patterns are described elsewhere in the text (see Chapters 13 and 17).

In 1943, Gilford and associates[24] were the first to recognize carpal instability. They described the carpus as a link mechanism, with the scaphoid serving as the link between the proximal and the distal carpal rows. A disturbance of this connecting rod (the scaphoid) led to longitudinal carpal collapse. They noted that this phenomenon occurred primarily as a result of scaphoid fractures. Fisk[21] later described this same phenomenon of intercarpal instability as a "concertina deformity." He also recognized this instability pattern in other conditions, such as Kienböck's disease. This longitudinal collapse of the carpus is well-recognized on a lateral radiograph, and the associated scaphoid instability has been well-described by various authorities, using terms such as scaphoid subluxation and rotational subluxation.[3, 13, 14, 17, 19, 27, 32, 34, 42, 50, 66]

Kauer[35] thoroughly described the mechanism of the carpal joint. The intricate and complex movement of the carpal bones is governed by the longitudinal and transverse linkage, by the bone contours and joint contacts, and by ligamentous interconnections.

Linscheid and associates[44] later described a frequently observed post-traumatic intercarpal instability collapse deformity. Their classification was based primarily on the capitolunate angle seen on lateral radiographs. They described two basic patterns: dorsal intercalary segment instability, or DISI deformity (Fig. 5–1); and volar intercalary segment instability, or VISI deformity (Fig. 5–2). In their observations and analyses, they found that these collapse deformities of the carpus were due directly to the loss of various ligamentous restraints.

The concept of progressive ligamentous damage with progressive loading was described by Mayfield and associates.[46] Greater degrees of perilunar instability were noted with more extensive ligamentous damage. The degrees of associated perilunar instability were classified as stages I to IV. Taleisnik,[67] in addition, described the direct relationship between various patterns of carpal instability and overt tears or of attenuation or relaxation of wrist ligaments.

Attention in the literature has been focused principally on describing patterns of radiocarpal instability (perilunar and scapholunate instabilities). Alexander and Lichtman[2, 42, 43] described the phenomenon of midcarpal instability and the implications of ulnar carpal instability patterns. Now, much attention has been focused on injuries of specific ligaments and associated instability patterns. Furthermore, as a result of arthroscopy, we have gained a better understanding of the subtleties of these ligament injuries.

The mechanism of carpal injuries has been a subject of considerable controversy. Although some researchers have suggested that hyperflexion is an important mechanism,[21, 24] many authorities consider hyperextension to be the major mechanical factor leading to these injuries.[21, 29, 44, 59, 66, 69–71, 73] Many have been impressed with the wide spectrum of injuries that seem to occur about the carpus (perilunate and lunate dislocations; scaphoid fractures, trans-scaph-

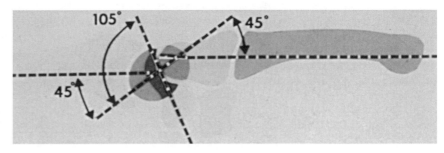

Figure 5–1. Dorsiflexion instability. Diagram of lateral radiograph of the wrist showing dorsiflexion of the lunate relative to the radius, a scapholunate angle of 105°, and palmar flexion of the capitate, relative to the lunate, of 45°. (From Linscheid RL, Dobyns JH, Beabout JW, et al: Traumatic instability of the wrist: Diagnosis, classification, and pathomechanics. J Bone Joint Surg 54A:1612–1632, 1972.)

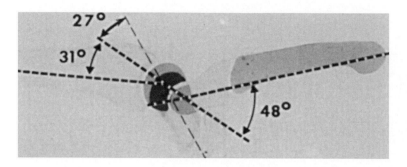

Figure 5–2. Palmar flexion instability. Diagram of lateral radiograph showing palmar flexion of the lunate, relative to the radius, of 31°, a scapholunate angle of 27° (somewhat less than normal), and dorsiflexion of the capitate, relative to the lunate, of 48°. (From Linscheid RL, Dobyns JH, Beabout JW, et al: Traumatic instability of the wrist: Diagnosis, classification, and pathomechanics. J Bone Joint Surg 54A:1612–1632, 1972.)

oid perilunate fracture-dislocations, radial styloid, triquetral, and, occasionally, capitate fractures). In addition, scapholunate diastasis and carpal instability are seen in distal radius fractures.[53, 65] Logically, it would seem unlikely that a single mechanism such as hyperextension could account for such a variety of fractures and dislocations. For this reason, investigators have looked for additional mechanisms.

Tanz[66] suggested that a rotational component might be important in perilunar dislocations. He considered lunate dislocations a result of compression, dorsiflexion, ulnar deviation, and pronation. He thought that perilunate dislocations were a result of the same mechanics, with the exception that supination, rather than pronation, of the hand was involved.

Explanations of the mechanism of scaphoid fractures have also been controversial. Fisk[21] suggested that extension and ulnar deviation were the principal mechanical components. Squire[64] was convinced that forced radial deviation would fracture the scaphoid over the tip of the radial styloid. Verdan and Narakas[70] showed that pronation and supination cause shearing forces at the scaphoid waist, implying that a rotational load would create shear stress in the scaphoid, leading to fracture, as suggested by Gilford and associates.[24] Experimental investigations have shown that the scaphoid can be fractured in cadaver specimens by hyperextension and ulnar deviation (Johnson RP, Mayfield JK, Kilcoyne RF: Scaphoid fractures and fracture-dislocations—pathomechanics and perilunar instability. Unpublished study, 1974).[34, 73] Knowledge of the mechanism of trans-scaphoid perilunate fracture-dislocations has been only speculative, although Fisk[21] was convinced that supination caused dorsal dislocation of the capitate. In 1974, Johnson and associates were able to create these complex injuries in fresh cadaver specimens with extension, ulnar deviation, and a rotational component, i.e., supination (Johnson RP, Mayfield JK, Kilcoyne RF: Scaphoid fractures and fracture-dislocations—pathomechanics and perilunar instability. Unpublished study, 1974).[34]

Perilunate fracture-dislocations are more common than perilunate dislocations at a ratio of two to one.[28] In addition to scaphoid fractures and perilunate dislocations, other associated injuries are common. Many authorities have noted the association of radial and ulnar styloid fractures with carpal injuries.[11, 13,] [17, 28, 72] The association of triquetral fractures with scaphoid fractures has been reported by Bartone and Grieco[5] and Borgeskov and colleagues.[12]

Because it has been difficult to identify a single planar mechanism as the cause of the many types of carpal injuries, investigations have focused on a three-dimensional mechanical concept to explain the pathogenesis of these enigmatic injuries.[21, 29, 30]

As our knowledge of carpal instability increases, we recognize that the role of the wrist ligaments in the development of this condition is extremely important. In order to understand the multitude of instability patterns that can develop with various combinations and degrees of ligamentous damage, a fundamental knowledge of wrist anatomy and wrist ligament biomechanics is essential.

WRIST LIGAMENT ANATOMY

Descriptive Anatomy

The intimate relationship between the carpal bones and the distal radius and ulna is maintained in all planes of motion by a complex arrangement of ligaments. Three types of ligaments are present across the wrist joint: intercarpal, capsular, and intracapsular.[47, 68]

The dorsal radiocarpal ligament is a thickening of the dorsal wrist capsule.[24–26, 63] It originates from the dorsal lip of the radial styloid process, passes obliquely across the dorsal surface of the lunate, to which it is also attached, and terminates in the dorsal aspect of the triquetrum. It also has connections to the hamate, but the major portion of the dorsal radiocarpal ligament is directed into the dorsal triquetrum (Fig. 5–3).

The proximal and distal rows of carpal bones are united by dorsal and volar intercarpal ligaments and by interosseous intercarpal ligaments.[26, 63]

The main functional ligaments of the wrist joint are volar and intracapsular.[35, 40, 46, 47, 49–51, 68, 69] In a functional sense, the complex intercarpal motion in radial and ulnar deviation and in dorsiflexion and volar flexion depends upon the specific arrangement and integrity of these volar intracapsular ligaments.

The volar or palmar radiocarpal ligament (ligamentum radiocarpeum palmare) is a large, thick intracapsular ligament seen only after the capsule is meticulously dissected from the volar aspect of the wrist or after the wrist joint is opened dorsally and the wrist is volarflexed (Figs. 5–4 and 5–5).[35, 47] This ligament is divided into three discrete ligaments, the first connecting the radius with the capitate (distal carpal row), the second connecting the radius with the triquetrum (proximal carpal row), and the third connecting the distal radius to the proximal scaphoid. The radiocapitate ligament (pars radiocapitate), the smaller and weaker of the first two, originates from the volar aspect of the radial styloid process, traverses a groove in the waist of the scaphoid, and terminates in the center of the volar aspect of the capitate body (see Fig. 5–4). The second ligamentous band is thick and tendinous in appearance and is the strongest of the volar intracapsular ligaments. This volar radiotriquetral ligament (pars radiotriquetral) originates from the volar aspect of the radial styloid process next to the radiocapitate ligament and, acting as a sling, passes under the lunate (to which it is also attached) and terminates in the volar surface of the triquetrum (see Figs. 5–4 and 5–5).

The separation of the radiocapitate ligament from the volar radiotriquetral ligament (known as the space of Poirier) over the volar aspect of the capitolunate joint is evident in most specimens (Fig. 5–6).[47, 57] The significance of this interligamentous space is evident when carpal motion is evaluated and after experimentally injured wrists are studied. A volar intracapsular ligament that is directed into the proximal pole of the scaphoid is consistently found. This ligament (the radioscaphoid ligament) actually

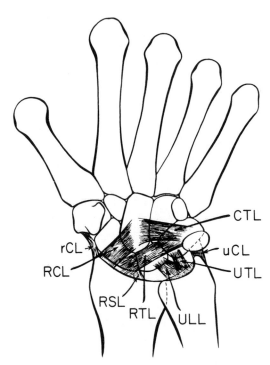

Figure 5–4. Volar view of the wrist joint, intracapsular and capsular collateral ligaments. Intracapsular ligaments: Lig. radiocarpeum palmare: *RCL* = pars radiocapitate; *RTL* = pars radiotriquetral; *RSL* = pars radioscaphoid. Lig. ulnocarpeum palmare: *ULL* = pars ulnolunate; *UTL* = pars ulnotriquetral. Lig. intercarpea palmaria; *CTL* = pars capitotriquetral. Capsular collateral ligaments: *rCL* = lig. collaterale carpi radiale; *uCL* = lig. collateral carpi ulnare. (From Mayfield JK, Johnson RP, Kilcoyne RK. Carpal dislocations: Pathomechanics and progressive perilunar instability. J Hand Surg 5:226–241, 1980.)

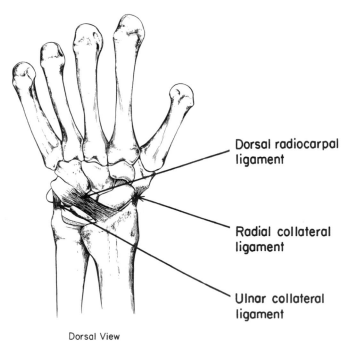

Figure 5–3. Dorsal view of the wrist joint. (From Mayfield JK, Johnson RP, Kilcoyne RK: The ligaments of the human wrist and their functional significance. Anat Rec 186:417–428, 1976.)

originates from the volar surface of the radial styloid process ulnar to the radiotriquetral ligament and is directed vertically to terminate in the proximal volar pole of the scaphoid (see Figs. 5–4 and 5–5). It also has some small attachments to the volar aspect of the lunate; hence, it is also known as the radioscapholunate ligament. It is classified as the third portion of the palmar radiocarpal ligament. The major portion (pars radioscaphoid) is separate from the interosseous intercarpal ligament connecting the scaphoid to the lunate.

In the unloaded wrist, sectioning of the scapholunate interosseous ligament (SLIL) does not allow the scaphoid to separate or rotate away from the lunate. Only after additional sectioning of the stabilizing radioscaphoid ligament from the scaphoid does it separate from the lunate on volar flexion and ulnar deviation.[47] In the loaded wrist, sectioning of the SLIL alone causes separation from the lunate plus proximal pole rotation of the scaphoid.[59] The size of the radioscaphoid ligament varies (it is frequently very large and massive), but it is consistently present.[6, 8, 47, 68]

A significant palmar intercarpal ligament, the capitrotriquetral ligament (pars capitotriquetral), is evident only after the overlying capsule is dissected away. It is directed from the volar surface of the

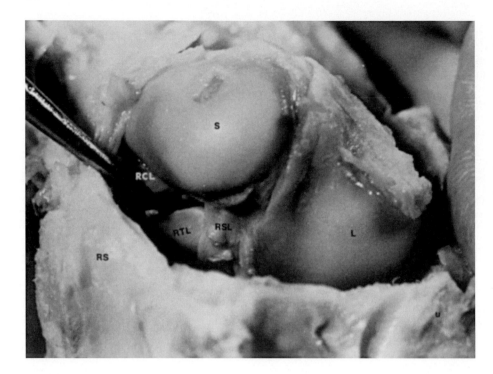

Figure 5–5. Intra-articular view of the radio-carpal joint. *S* = scaphoid; *L* = lunate; *RS* = radial styloid; *u* = ulna; *RCL* = radiocapitate ligament; *RTL* = radiotriquetral ligament; *RSL* = radioscaphoid ligament.

center of the capitate body across the volar surface of the hamate, to terminate in the volar surface of the triquetrum (see Fig. 5–4). This ligament is also known as the ulnar arm of the arcuate or deltoid ligament.

Ligamentous stabilization on the ulnar side of the wrist, in addition to the ulnar collateral ligament, is formed by the intracapsular ulnocarpal ligament. This is a thick, discrete ligament that originates from the volar aspect of the intra-articular triangular fibro-

cartilage complex (TFCC),[55] and continues in two separate directions, to the lunate (pars ulnolunate) and to the triquetrum (pars ulnotriquetral) (see Fig. 5–4).

This descriptive analysis of the wrist ligaments forms a model that is useful in the functional analysis of the wrist joint. These ligaments resemble parts of a puzzle, each of which has little significance alone, that when combined to form a unit, control complex carpal motion.

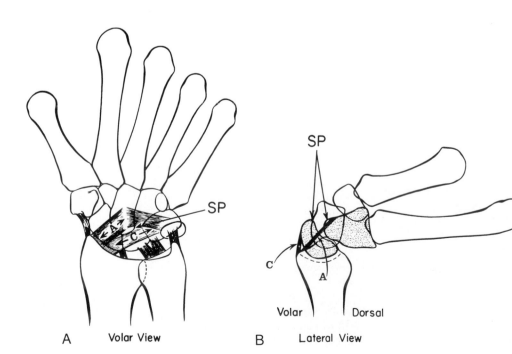

Figure 5–6. Space of Poirier volar *(A)* and lateral *(B)* views. *A* = radiocapitate ligament; *C* = radiotriquetral ligament; *SP* = space of Poirier. (From Mayfield JK, Johnson RP, Kilcoyne RK: The ligaments of the human wrist and their functional significance. Anat Rec 186: 417–428, 1976.)

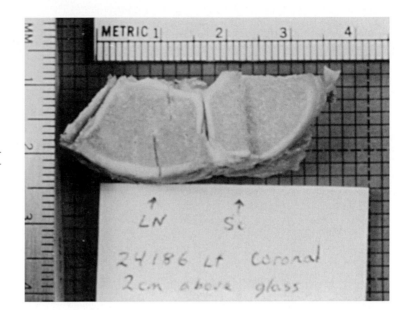

Figure 5–7. Cross-section of scapholunate joint. Note triangular shape and peripheral position of the scapholunate interosseous ligament. *LN* = lunate; *SC* = scaphoid.

The Ligamentous Anatomy of the Scapholunate Joint

Because fractures of the scaphoid are a common source of wrist instabilities, the scaphoid's ligamentous connections to the lunate and to the proximal carpal row have great significance.

In dissections of 34 cadaver wrists, Nash and Mayfield were able to differentiate the intricate ligamentous attachments of this joint (Nash D, Mayfield JK: The ligamentous anatomy of the scapholunate joint. Unpublished study, 1979). In their dissections, they found that the scapholunate interosseous ligament is triangular in cross-section, occupying nearly one third of the articular surface of this joint (Fig. 5–7), and peripherally attached at the joint (Fig. 5–8). A portion of the innermost aspect of the ligament is not attached to the bone but is free in the joint (see Fig. 5–8). The fibers of the scapholunate interosseous ligament run in several directions. The fibers at the dorsum of the joint run transversely or perpendicular to the joint and form a thick bundle that is tendinous in appearance (Nash D, Mayfield JK: The ligamentous anatomy of the scapholunate joint. Unpublished study, 1979).[36] The fibers of the peripheral portion of the ligament run peripherally and obliquely along the arc of the joint from the scaphoid downward to the lunate. The volar portion of the ligament runs obliquely between the volar aspects of the lunate and the scaphoid (Fig. 5–9). The orientation of these fibers

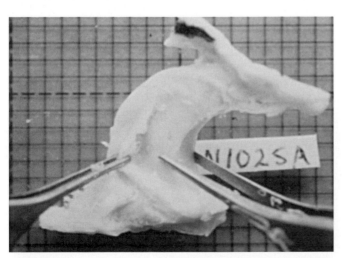

Figure 5–8. Intra-articular view of scapholunate joint, lunate side. Note peripheral aspect of interosseous ligament and dorsal thickening of the interosseous ligament. Tweezers are holding back the loose portion of the ligament.

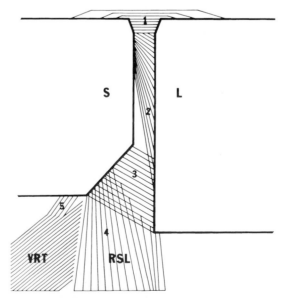

Figure 5–9. Drawing showing the direction of the fibers of the ligaments that stabilize the scapholunate joint. (Scapholunate interosseous ligament consists of portions *1*, *2*, and *3*.) *S* = scaphoid; *L* = lunate; *RSL* = radioscaphoid ligament; *VRT* = volar radiotriquetral ligament.

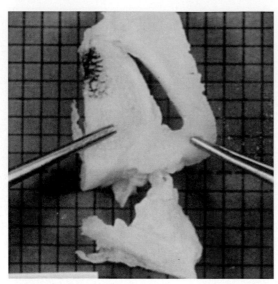

Figure 5–10. Transverse section through the base of the scapholunate joint. The blackened area marks the dorsum of the scaphoid. Note the mobility of the volar part of this joint.

is such that they allow mobility of the volar aspect of the joint about a fixed dorsal axis (Nash D, Mayfield JK: The ligamentous anatomy of the scapholunate joint. Unpublished study, 1979).[37, 59]

In addition to the three portions of the scapholunate interosseous ligament, the volar aspect of the proximal pole of the scaphoid and, to a lesser extent, the lunate, are stabilized to the distal radius by the radioscaphoid ligament, also called the radioscapholunate ligament (RSL) because of its attachment to both the scaphoid and lunate (see Figs. 5–5 and 5–9).[6, 47, 68] In some specimens, the volar radiotriquetral ligament (VRT) also has some fibrous attachments to the proximal inferior pole of the scaphoid (see Fig. 5–9).

The radioscaphoid ligament is consistently identified in adult and fetal wrist dissections (Nash D, Mayfield JK: The ligamentous anatomy of the scapholunate joint. Unpublished study, 1974).[6, 47, 68] However, there is some controversy whether this is an actual ligament. Lewis and associates[40] described it as a remnant of a mesenchymal septum that separated the radiocarpal and ulnocarpal joint cavities in fetal development. Berger and colleagues[6, 8] refer to this structure as a ligament that has a high vascularity, providing a vascular supply to the scapholunate interosseous ligament, and probably has little direct mechanical effect on the behavior of the carpus.

This unique arrangement of the directions of the fibers occurs in the three portions of the scapholunate interosseous ligament and, in conjunction with the radioscaphoid ligament, allows for certain movements at this joint. The joint is basically hinged at the dorsum by the transverse portion of the interosseous ligament, allowing volar opening of the joint (Figs. 5–10 and 5–11).[36, 37] In addition, the scaphoid can rotate on the lunate about a dorsal transverse axis. This fact has significance, because many carpal injuries are initiated by a hyperextension movement causing the scaphoid to rotate dorsally through a dorsal scapholunate axis. Because there is volar mobility at this joint, some of the load can be dissipated. If forced extension occurs, however, failure of the scapholunate interosseous ligaments begins in the volar region first.[48]

The Distal Ligamentous Complex of the Scaphoid

Drewniany and coworkers[18] studied the distal ligamentous complex of the scaphoid and trapezium anatomically and biomechanically. They describe four components of a scaphotrapezial trapezoidal ligament complex that stabilizes the distal pole of the scaphoid. Boabighi and associates[10] studied both the

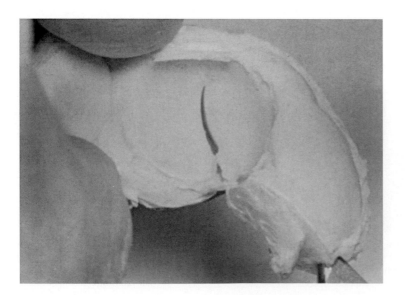

Figure 5–11. Distal view of the intact scapholunate complex with all ligaments attached. The triangle on the right at the bottom of the picture indicates the direction of force being applied to the distal scaphoid pole. Note the volar opening of the scapholunate joint.

distal scaphoid ligamentous complex and the scapho-lunate interosseous ligament. They found that the distal scaphoid ligamentous complex was twice as strong as the scapholunate interosseous ligament. They concluded from these biomechanical studies that the distal ligament complex had to fail first, before the scapholunate interosseous ligament (SCLN) failed in vivo. Unlike Landsmeer,[39] Mayfield and coworkers,[46–50] Kauer,[36, 37] and Ruby and associates,[59] Drewniany and coworkers[18] believed that the SCLN plays no important role in normal wrist movement.

WRIST LIGAMENT BIOMECHANICS

In order to understand the different patterns of injury that can occur in the different wrist ligaments, it is helpful to understand the biomechanics of the wrist ligaments themselves.

Investigations using 11 fresh or frozen human wrists have helped elucidate the biomechanical properties of these ligaments.[49] In this study, bone ligament–bone complexes for each ligament of the wrist were dissected free. The length of all ligaments was measured, and the cross-sectional area was determined using an area micrometer with a standardized blade pressure.[74] The ends were mounted in aluminum cups, fixed to an 810 MTS materials testing system, and tested in tension to failure with simultaneous graphic recordings. Cinematography provided correlative data during ligament elongation and failure. A strain rate of 1 cm/sec was utilized, because a strain rate of 50 to 100 percent of ligament length per second most closely approximates the strain rate of a physiologic injury. The strain rate used for the scapholunate interosseous ligament (SCLN) was 1 mm/sec because of its short length. Histologic analysis with light microscopy was performed on selected ligaments using both hematoxylin and eosin and elastin stains. The results of this study are particularly pertinent.

Failure Location and Mode

The radiocapitate ligament failed proximally between the radial styloid and the scaphoid waist in 80 percent of fresh specimens. There were no avulsions.

The radiotriquetral ligament failed distally more often than proximally, with 56 percent of specimens failing between the lunate and the triquetrum. Of the distal failures, four were ligament failures and one was a triquetral avulsion.

In testing of the radiotriquetral attachment to the lunate, it was found that less than half of specimens had strong ligamentous insertions, and most of the specimens (55 percent) experienced insertional failure (i.e., the ligament "pulled off" the lunate) with very low forces, averaging 64 newtons (N). This weak attachment to the lunate may explain the phenome-

non of dorsiflexion instability after hyperextension injuries.

The radioscaphoid ligament (RS) failed in its substance in all specimens, the failures being equally divided between proximal and distal ends.

The dorsal radiocarpal ligament (DRC) failed at its distal end in 90 percent of the specimens, eight in the ligament and one by triquetral avulsion.

The scapholunate interosseous ligament (SCLN) rarely failed in its substance, owing to its remarkable stiffness and strength. In 56 percent of specimens, ligament failure occurred at 359 N, and in 44 percent of specimens, bone avulsion or cement failure occurred at 410 N.

Tensile Properties

The radiocapitate and radiotriquetral ligaments were found to be approximately the same length (30 mm). The radioscaphoid was the shortest of all ligaments, except for the scapholunate interosseous ligament, which averaged 5.7 mm. The dorsal radiocarpal ligament, which is the dorsal proximal row stabilizer, was shorter than its volar mirror image, the radiotriquetral ligament. The ulnar collateral ligament was more than twice the length of the radial collateral ligament (Fig. 5–12).

No significant difference was found between the cross-sectional areas of the radiocapitate and radiotriquetral ligaments. The radioscaphoid was the smallest, the dorsal radiocarpal was smaller than the radiotriquetral, and the ulnar collateral was larger than the radial collateral ligament (Fig. 5–13).

Maximum Force. The maximum force required for failure of the volar radiotriquetral ligament was the greatest required for any of the volar intracapsular ligaments, significant at the 0.05 level. On the dorsal aspect of the wrist, the maximum force of 240 N for

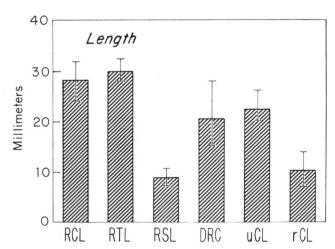

Figure 5–12. The length of the wrist ligaments. *DRC* = dorsal radiocarpal ligament; *RCL* = pars radiocapitate; *rCL* = lig. collaterale carpi radiale; *RSL* = pars radioscaphoid; *RTL* = pars radiotriquetral; *uCL* = lig. collaterale carpi ulnare.

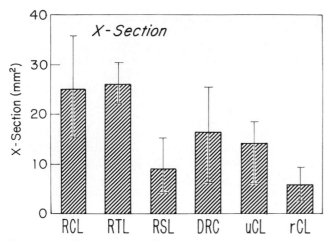

Figure 5–13. The cross-sectional area of the wrist ligaments. *DRC* = dorsal radiocarpal ligament; *RCL* = pars radiocapitate; *rCL* = lig. collaterale carpi radiale; *RSL* = pars radioscaphoid; *RTL* = pars radiotriquetral; *uCL* = lig. collaterale carpi ulnare.

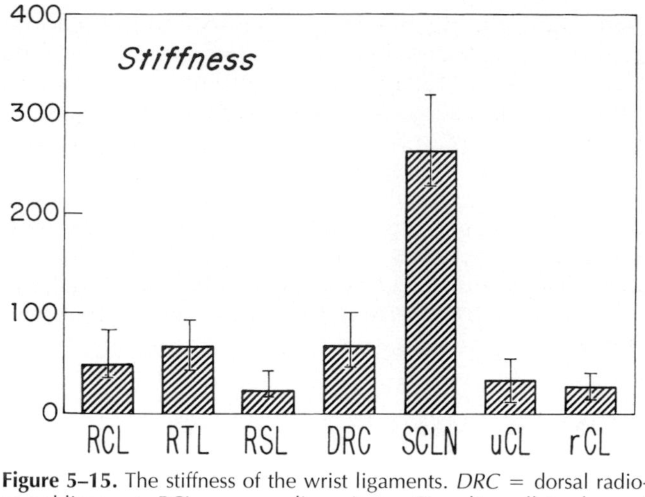

Figure 5–15. The stiffness of the wrist ligaments. *DRC* = dorsal radiocarpal ligament; *RCL* = pars radiocapitate; *rCL* = lig. collaterale carpi radiale; *RSL* = pars radioscaphoid; *RTL* = pars radiotriquetral; *SCLN* = scapholunate interosseous ligament; *uCL* = lig. collaterale carpi ulnare.

the dorsal radiocarpal ligament was not significantly different from that for the volar radiotriquetral ligament. The average radiocapitate ligament failed at 170 N, whereas the distal segment of this ligament required 190 N, supporting the clinical evidence that in carpal injuries, the scaphoid follows the capitate. The radioscaphoid ligament was the weakest of all volar ligaments, failing at 54 N. Of the two collateral ligaments, the radial collateral required the least force (70 N) to reach failure. The scapholunate interosseous ligament was the strongest of all ligaments tested in the wrist, with ligament failure occurring at a maximum force of 359 N (Fig. 5–14).

Stiffness. Of equal significance is the fact that the scapholunate interosseous ligament was found to be the stiffest of all wrist ligaments tested. The radiotri-quetral was significantly stiffer than the radiocapitate at the 0.01 significance level (Fig. 5–15).

Elastic Modulus. The elastic modulus of the radioscaphoid ligament was the lowest and that of the dorsal radiocarpal ligament was the highest, suggesting that the dorsal radiocarpal is the least elastic and the radioscaphoid is the most elastic of the carpal ligaments. The radial collateral ligament was more elastic than the ulnar collateral ligament (Fig. 5–16).

Maximum Stress. Maximum stress, or tensile strength, is the maximum force per unit cross-sectional area. Of interest, the dorsal radiocarpal ligament had the highest tensile strength, which may explain why lunate dislocations are less common than perilunate injuries when this ligament is ruptured (Fig. 5–17).

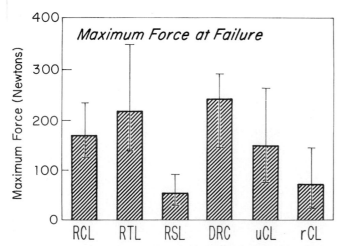

Figure 5–14. The maximum force at failure of the wrist ligament. *DRC* = dorsal radiocarpal ligament; *RCL* = pars radiocapitate; *rCL* = lig. collaterale carpi radiale; *RSL* = pars radioscaphoid; *RTL* = pars radiotriquetral; *uCL* = lig. collaterale carpi ulnare.

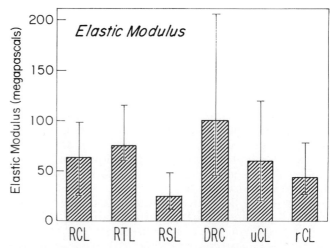

Figure 5–16. The elastic modulus of the wrist ligaments. *DRC* = dorsal radiocarpal ligament; *RCL* = pars radiocapitate; *rCL* = lig. collaterale carpi radiale; *RSL* = pars radioscaphoid; *RTL* = pars radiotriquetral; *uCL* = lig. collaterale carpi ulnare.

Maximum Strain. Maximum strain is the percent elongation at total failure. The two ligaments that elongated the most at failure were the radioscaphoid ligament and the scapholunate interosseous ligament. The scapholunate ligament doubled its length prior to total failure, with a maximum strain of 225 percent. The radioscaphoid ligament lost its continuity at 140 percent strain. The radiocapitate (RC) ligament, the distal carpal row stabilizer, had a maximum strain significantly greater than that of the radiotriquetral ligament at the 0.05 significance level (Fig. 5–18).

Partial Failure

Partial or sequential failure occurred in all ligaments to various extents. In every ligament filmed, there was evidence of partial failure (ligament elongation), even though the ligament appeared intact. The RC ligament, in particular, was grossly intact at 50 percent, 70 percent, and 80 percent strain, and only at approximately 100 percent strain was total failure evident. The gross continuity of a ligament, therefore, does not always reflect its biomechanical integrity.

Histology

Twenty-two ligaments from 10 fresh wrists were studied by light microscopy using hematoxylin and eosin and elastin stains (Nash D, Mayfield JK: The ligamentous anatomy of the scapholunate joint. Unpublished study, 1974). The wrist ligaments consist of collagen fibers and interstitial connective tissue that is rich in fat, vessels, and elastic fibers.[38] A relative abundance of elastic fibers was noted in the radioscaphoid liga-

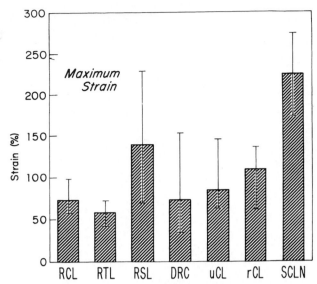

Figure 5–18. The maximum strain of the wrist ligaments. *DRC* = dorsal radiocarpal ligament; *RCL* = pars radiocapitate; *rCL* = lig. collaterale carpi radiale; *RSL* = pars radioscaphoid; *RTL* = pars radiotriquetral; *SCLN* = scapholunate interosseous ligament; *uCL* = lig. collaterale carpi ulnare. (From Mayfield JK. Wrist ligamentous anatomy and pathogenesis of carpal instability. Orthop Clin North Am 15:209–216, 1984.)

ment and less frequently in the scapholunate interosseous ligament.

The presence of elastic fibers in the radioscaphoid ligament has also been studied by Berger and associates.[6] Berger and Blair[8] described the presence of elastic fibers in the vascular structures of the ligament and not in the ligament itself. However, a later study of the microvascular anatomy of the radioscapholunate ligament by Hixson[30] revealed no uptake of elastin stain by the vessels in the ligament. Nevertheless, the presence of elastin in the scapholunate interosseous and radioscaphoid ligaments leads to speculation concerning the mechanics of the scapholunate articulation, because these two ligaments stabilize this joint, both have high strains at failure, and the radioscaphoid ligament is biomechanically elastic with very low elastic modulus (Fig. 5–19).

WRIST JOINT KINEMATICS AND CARPAL INJURY

Several investigators have studied the kinematics of the carpus.* The proximal carpus functions as an intercalated bone, and the specific shape of the intercalated bone creates a simultaneous movement in the radiocarpal and the midcarpal joints.[36]

In several studies using sonic digitalization and stereophotography, the apex of carpal rotation in the anteroposterior (AP) plane has been shown to be in the center of the capitate[20, 56] or at the junction of the radiocapitate and the capitotriquetral ligaments.[33, 47]

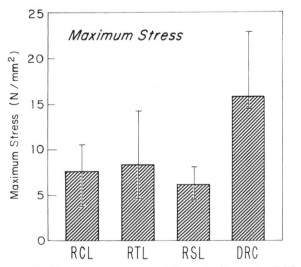

Figure 5–17. The maximum stress of the wrist ligaments. *DRC* = dorsal radiocarpal ligament; *RCL* = pars radiocapitate; *RSL* = pars radioscaphoid; *RTL* = pars radiotriquetral.

---

*References 9, 16, 20, 31, 33, 41, 46, 56, 58, 61, 62, 75, 77.

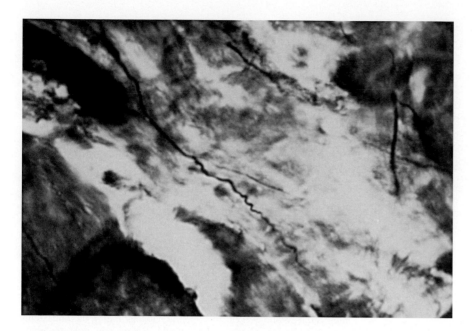

Figure 5–19. Histologic view of radioscaphoid ligament with elastin stain. Note numerous elastin fibers.

When the wrist moves from neutral position to maximum extension, the palmar ligaments become progressively more taut and achieve their maximum tautness in complete extension. Movement of the wrist in radial deviation relaxes the radiocapitate ligament. Movement of the wrist in ulnar deviation tightens the radiocapitate ligament (RCL) and relaxes the radiotriquetral ligament (RTL) (Fig. 5–20). When the wrist is progressively extended, an interligamentous space develops palmarly because of the separation of the radiocaptiate ligament and the radiotriquetral ligament. This space overlies the capitolunate joint primarily and is called the space of Poirier.[46, 47]

It is interesting to note that anatomic and kinematic studies have shown that the scapholunate joint has a dorsal axis of rotation (Fig. 5–21) (Nash D, Mayfield JK: The ligamentous anatomy of the scapholunate joint. Unpublished study, 1974).[58, 61] This is particularly pertinent, because most carpal injuries are initiated by hyperextension and intercarpal supination.[50] During impact loading over the thenar eminence, the scaphoid rotates dorsally on the lunate through a dorsal axis of the scapholunate joint. The anatomic arrangement of the fibers of the scapholunate interosseous and radioscaphoid ligaments in turn allows mobility of the volar inferior pole of the scaphoid

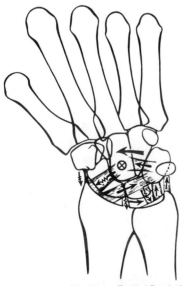

**Maximum Radial Deviation
Neutral Flexion**

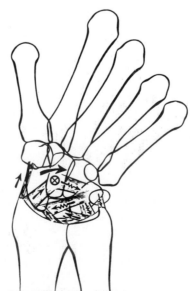

**Maximum Ulnar Deviation
Neutral Flexion**

Figure 5–20. Wrist kinematics. → = taut ligament, ⌇→ = loose ligament. (From Mayfield JK, Johnson RP, Kilcoyne RK: The ligaments of the human wrist and their functional significance. Anat Rec 186:417–428, 1976.)

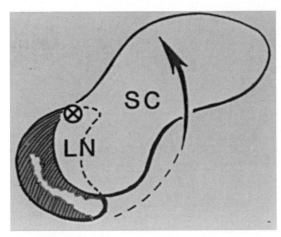

Figure 5–21. Dorsal axis of rotation of the scapholunate joint, side view. Note the volar, interosseous ligament tear. *LN* = lunate; *SC* = scaphoid; ⊗ = axis. (From Mayfield JK: Patterns of injury to carpal ligaments: A spectrum. Clin Orthop 187:36–42, 1984.)

(Nash D, Mayfield JK: The ligamentous anatomy of the scapholunate joint. Unpublished study, 1974),[36] allowing the inferior and proximal poles of the scaphoid to rotate about this dorsal axis. The ligamentous fiber orientation of this joint also allows separation of the scaphoid and the lunate at the inferior portion of this joint (see Figs. 5–9 to 5–11). Mechanically, the scapholunate joint has a specialized design that enhances stability but also allows load dampening when excessive loads are applied to the wrist in hyperextension and intercarpal supination.

The lunate and triquetrum seem to have a tight connection between them, as evidenced by close correlation of their axes of rotation with motion analysis.[62] The greatest motion between the lunate and triquetrum occurs from 45° to 35° of flexion, the greatest motion is seen between the scaphoid and lunate from 25° to 35° of extension.[61] The lunate is a pivot in the proximal carpal row intercalated between the distal carpal row and the forearm and also intercalated between the scaphoid and triquetrum.[61]

The following facts are useful in developing a mechanical concept of carpal injuries:

1. The weakest ligaments of the wrist are on the radial side
2. The radiocapitate ligament (RCL) is maximally taut in maximum extension and in ulnar deviation
3. The proximal carpal row is stabilized to the distal forearm by five ligaments, whereas the distal carpal row is stabilized to the forearm by only one, the radiocapitate ligament (RCL)
4. The weakest link between the distal carpal row and the distal forearm is the radiocapitate ligament.

MECHANISM OF CARPAL INSTABILITY

Carpal Dislocations

The actual mechanism of injury is difficult, if not impossible, to document in the clinical setting. Not infrequently, however, there is clinical evidence supporting a certain mechanism of injury, as shown in the following case studies.

Case 1

A 31-year-old male accountant suffered a hyperextension injury to his right wrist when he fell from a diving board. He sustained a dorsal perilunate dislocation and a radial styloid fracture. A large abrasion was noted over the thenar side of his palm in the area of the scaphoid tuberosity.

Case 2

A 25-year old man sustained a hyperextension injury to the left wrist and also a dorsal perilunate dislocation in a motorcycle accident. A large impact abrasion was noted over the thenar aspect of his palm.

These two cases and other similar ones would suggest that hyperextension was an important cause in these dislocations. Forced ulnar deviation and intercarpal supination could also be implicated, because the injuries were on the radial side of the palm. Experimental loading studies have helped to clarify these impressions.

EXPERIMENTAL LOADING

These studies have been described previously.[45]

Materials and Methods

Thirty-two fresh embalmed cadaver wrists were loaded to failure using two loading machines, one fast-loading and gravity-dependent, the other slow-loading and hydraulic. The average age of the specimens was 53 years (range 5 to 89 years). All specimens were stripped of soft tissue to within 2 cm of the wrist joint, leaving the interosseous membrane, radius, and ulna intact. They were then cemented in 2-inch steel pipes and secured in the loading machines with the wrist extended for various roentgenographic and loading studies. Specimens subjected to fast loading were loaded with an average of 19 kg from an average height of 68 cm. The force plate was placed across the metacarpal heads with the fingers free, and the angles of loading were varied with combinations of extension, ulnar deviation, and intercarpal supination (equivalent to pronation of the forearm on the carpus, as observed in actual clinical injuries). Specimens subjected to hydraulic slow loading were positioned in such a way that a 1-cm by 2-cm pressure plate engaged the scaphoid tuberosity in maximum extension. All loading studies included preloading radiographs, loading lateral cineradiographs at 60 and 120 frames/sec, and postloading radiographs. All specimens were dissected after loading to assess bony and ligamentous damage and carpal instability.

Results

Thirteen dorsal perilunate dislocations were produced. The mechanism of injury was extension, ulnar deviation, and intercarpal supination in 12 and extension alone in 1. Intercarpal supination was a major mechanical component, because all loading was on the radial side of the wrist. All specimens had rupture of the radioscaphoid and scapholunate interosseous ligaments. Scaphoid rotation was noted in 6 specimens. Two patterns of palmar ligamentous damage were noted.

One pattern was represented by radiocapitate and radial collateral ligament failure and scapholunate ligamentous failure (scapholunate interosseous and radioscaphoid ligaments) with capitate and scaphoid dislocation and opening of the space of Poirier (Fig. 5–22). The other pattern with more severe ligamentous damage had similar findings, except that radiotriquetral ligament failure between lunate and triquetrum was evident with triquetral dislocation (Fig. 5–23).

Two lunate dislocations were also produced, and the pathomechanics were the same as those of most of the perilunate dislocations (extension, ulnar deviation, and intercarpal supination). Scaphoid rotation and scapholunate diastasis were noted in both specimens (Fig. 5–24). The palmar ligamentous damage in the lunate dislocations was the same as that in the

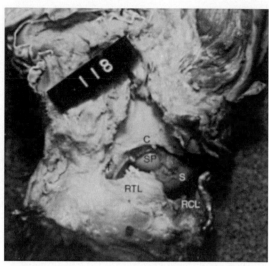

Figure 5–23. Volar view of stage III perilunate instability in an experimentally loaded wrist. Notice the scaphoid (S), capitate (C), and triquetral (T) dislocations. The space of Poirier (SP) is open wide. The torn ligaments are the radiocapitate (RCL) and the radiotriquetral (RTL) between the lunate and triquetrum. (From Mayfield JK: Mechanism of carpal injuries. Clin Orthop 143:45–54, 1980.)

severe perilunate dislocation, but in addition, dorsal radiocarpal ligament failure allowed palmar lunate rotation.

Scaphoid rotation was a direct result of progressive failure of the scapholunate ligamentous complex. Ligamentous failure began in the palmar aspect of the scapholunate joint and progressed dorsally, owing to the intercarpal supination component of the loading mechanics (Fig. 5–25).

Seven radial styloid fractures were produced by avulsion.

Triquetral fractures were associated with perilunate and lunate dislocations in five specimens; their mechanism was by avulsion of either the radiotrique-

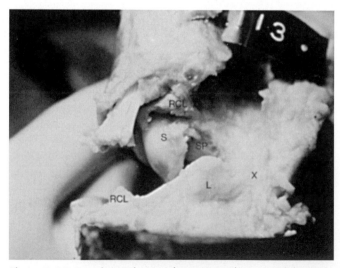

Figure 5–22. Carpal tunnel view of stage II perilunar instability in an experimentally loaded wrist. Notice the scaphoid and capitate dislocations, radiocapitate ligament (RCL) failure, and opening of the space of Poirier (SP). S = scaphoid; L = lunate; X = axis of intercarpal supination. (From Mayfield JK: Mechanism of carpal injuries. Clin Orthop 149:45–54, 1980.)

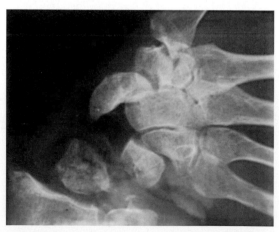

Figure 5–24. Experimentally loaded wrist with stage IV perilunate instability. The lunate has been reduced. Notice the scaphoid rotation and the triquetral avulsion fracture. (From Mayfield JK: Mechanism of carpal injuries. Clin Orthop 149:45–54, 1980.)

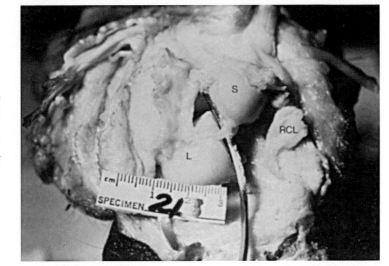

Figure 5–25. Experimentally loaded wrist showing the effects of intercarpal supination (dorsal view). Notice the dorsal rotational dislocation of the scaphoid. Probe is under the remaining portion of the scapholunate interosseous ligament. Notice also the failed radiocapitate ligament *(RCL)* avulsed from the capitate. *S* = scaphoid; *L* = lunate. (From Mayfield JK: Mechanism of carpal injuries. Clin Orthop 149:45–54, 1980.)

tral ligament (RTL) or the ulnotriquetral ligament (UTL) (see Fig. 5–24).

All dislocations had varying degrees of perilunar instability. As the loading forces of extension, intercarpal supination, and ulnar deviation progressed, the scaphoid, the capitate, and then the triquetrum were progressively dislocated from the lunate, creating progressive carpal instability. The degree of perilunar instability (PLI) has been divided into four stages, according to the degree of carpal dislocation and ligamentous damage that starts at the scapholunate joint and progresses around the lunate:

Stage I   PLI: Scaphoid dislocation or instability with scapholunate interosseous and radioscaphoid ligament injury
Stage II PLI: Capitate dislocation and opening of the space of Poirier
Stage III PLI: Triquetral dislocation and radiotriquetral ligament failure
Stage IV PLI: Radiocapitate, radiotriquetral, and dorsal radiocarpal ligament failure with lunate dislocation (Fig. 5–26).

Scaphoid Fracture and Fracture-Dislocation

It has long been recognized that in most carpal dislocations or fracture-dislocations, the scaphoid either fractures or dislocates from the lunate. Fracture of the waist of the scaphoid is the most common injury to the carpal bones. In reviewing carpal fractures, Borgeskov and coworkers[12] noted that of all carpal fractures, the scaphoid was the bone most commonly fractured (71.2 percent), but interestingly, the triquetrum was the next most frequently fractured bone (20.4 percent).[12] This association of scaphoid fractures with triquetral fractures has been a clinical curiosity, but the explanations for this association have been speculative. Seventy to 80 percent of scaphoid

fractures occur at the waist, with the remainder occurring equally often at the proximal pole and at the tubercle.[21, 45]

Displaced unstable fractures of the scaphoid associated with other carpal fractures and dislocations usually have a poor prognosis. This relationship between

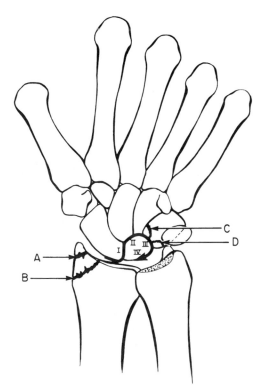

Figure 5–26. Progressive perilunar instability (PLI). Stage I—scapholunate failure; stage II—capitolunate failure; stage III—triquetrolunate failure; stage IV—dorsal radiocarpal ligament failure, allowing volar rotation of the lunate. *A* = radial styloid tip fracture, *B* = radial styloid body fracture; *C* = radiotriquetral ligament avulsion; *D* = ulnotriquetral ligament avulsion. (From Mayfield JK, Johnson RP, Kilcoyne RK: Carpal dislocations: Pathomechanics and progressive perilunar instability. J Hand Surg 5:226–241, 1980.)

scaphoid fractures and perilunar dislocations is well known clinically (Johnson RP, Mayfield JK, Kilcoyne RF: Scaphoid fractures and fracture-dislocations—pathomechanics and perilunar instability. Unpublished study, 1974).[21, 22, 29, 44, 52, 59, 72] The degree of instability of the scaphoid fracture seems to be directly related to the extent of ligamentous damage and associated perilunar instability, but this relationship has never been documented. Experimental work has aided our understanding of the pathomechanics of these fractures and fracture-dislocations (Johnson RP, Mayfield JK, Kilcoyne RF: Scaphoid fractures and fracture-dislocations—pathomechanics and perilunar instability. Unpublished study, 1974).[34, 75]

EXPERIMENTAL LOADING

The information described here has been described previously (Johnson RP, Mayfield JK, Kilcoyne RF: Scaphoid fractures and fracture-dislocations—perilunar instability. Unpublished study, 1974).

Materials and Methods

Twenty-nine fresh cadaver specimens, comprising hand, wrist, and forearm, were stripped of soft tissue within 2 cm of the distal articular surface of the radius and were cemented in steel pipes. Each prepared specimen was placed in a hydraulic machine and secured. A 1-cm by 2-cm pressure plate was positioned over the distal portion of the scaphoid with the wrist in maximum extension. Each wrist was subjected to progressive hydraulic loading. The loading sequence created extension, ulnar deviation, and intercarpal supination. All specimens were obtained fresh and were loaded within 72 hours postmortem. All specimens underwent preloading radiography (anteroposterior supination and lateral views, oblique and lateral views in flexion and extension). The loading sequence was recorded with the use of lateral cineradiography at 120 frames/sec. All wrists were loaded to either bone or ligament failure and then were dissected to assess the bony and ligamentous damage.

Results

Of the 29 wrists loaded, five scaphoid waist fractures, two proximal pole fractures, and six tuberosity fractures were produced. Five scaphoid fractures were associated with stage I perilunar instability (PLI), and three scaphoid fractures were associated with stage III PLI. In addition, seven fractures of the distal radius, three of the trapezium, and two of the triquetrum were produced as well as two scaphotrapezial dislocations.

Nonphysiologic hyperextension and ulnar deviation were the primary mechanisms of the scaphoid waist fractures, with the dorsal aspect of the scaphoid engaging the dorsal rim of the radius, thereby creating an anvil effect leading to fracture.

Scaphoid waist fractures were described according to their stability. Type I was stable, was not associated with significant ligamentous damage, and could not be displaced with extension, intercarpal supination, ulnar deviation, or distraction. Types II and III were unstable and were associated with moderate to severe degrees of ligamentous damage and perilunar instability (Fig. 5–27). They could be displaced with any of the preceding maneuvers and could be reduced by reversing the loading mechanism (i.e., radial deviation, flexion, or intercarpal pronation with compression).

The mechanism of fracture was hyperextension, with the scaphoid fracture beginning on the palmar side and progressing dorsally. In Type I fractures, the dorsal soft tissue hinge remained intact, and palmar flexion produced fracture stability. Type II and III scaphoid fractures had more severe ligamentous damage and associated carpal instability, and in these, the soft tissue hinge was lost.

Eight of the 12 scaphoid fractures were associated with varying degrees of perilunar instability as a result of associated ligamentous failure (trans-scaphoid perilunar fracture-dislocations) (see Fig. 5–27). Associated ligamentous damage and resultant perilunar instability were a direct result of the rotational component of intercarpal supination. This rotation of the scaphoid, distal carpal row, and triquetrum as a unit about the fixed lunate was also responsible for avulsion fracture of the triquetrum (avulsion of the radiotriquetral and ulnotriquetral ligaments) (see Fig. 5–27).

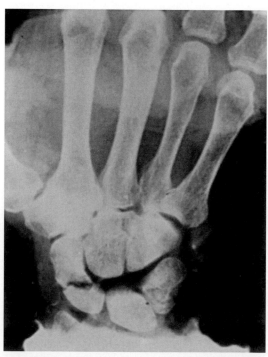

Figure 5–27. Displaced type III scaphoid waist fracture with stage III PLI (perilunar fracture-dislocation). Notice the triquetral fracture (avulsion of the ulnotriquetral ligament). (Courtesy of Roger P. Johnson, MD.)

Fractures of the proximal pole of the scaphoid were caused by subluxation of the scaphoid dorsally, before it was fractured over the dorsal rim of the radius. Scaphoid tuberosity fractures were caused by compression forces.

Cineradiography documented failure occurring first on the radial side of the wrist. This failure was either a scaphoid fracture or a scapholunate joint disruption (stage I PLI) or both. Any further degrees of perilunar instability (stage II–IV PLI) were a result of intercarpal supination. Virtually all of the scaphoid fractures had some scapholunate interosseous ligament failure. The spectrum stretched from a small tear palmarly to a complete disruption of the ligament.

A SPECTRUM OF WRIST LIGAMENT INJURY

Carpal injuries present a spectrum of bone and ligament damage. The name given to the various injuries (for example, lunate dislocation, perilunate dislocation, scaphoid fracture, and trans-scaphoid perilunate fracture-dislocation) only describe the resultant damage apparent on radiographs. Each injury is not a separate entity, but part of a continuum. The character of the final injury is determined by (1) the type of three-dimensional loading, (2) the magnitude and duration of the forces involved, (3) the position of the hand at the time of impact, and (4) the biomechanical properties of the bones and ligaments. Wrist arthroscopy can be invaluable in helping to delineate the exact ligamentous lesions.

Progressive Perilunar Instability

Impact on the thenar side of the wrist levers the wrist progressively into hyperextension, ulnar deviation, and intercarpal supination.[46, 50] The intercarpal injuries begin at the scapholunate joint and proceed around the lunate, progressively creating ligamentous injury as well as scapholunate, capitolunate, and triquetrolunate instability. In stage I perilunar instability (PLI), the primary instability is limited to the scapholunate joint. In stage II PLI, there is also ligamentous damage at the capitolunate articulation, and in Stage III PLI, ligamentous damage at the triquetrolunate joint is present in addition to the damage described for stages I and II (see Fig. 5–26).[46] Adolfsson[1] and Dautel and associates[15] have documented arthroscopically the common nature of scapholunate ligament lesions and associated carpal instability in patients with chronic post-traumatic wrist pain.

In stage IV PLI, dorsal disruption of the dorsal radiocarpal ligament (as a result of intercarpal supination) allows the lunate to rotate volarly on its volar radiotriquetral and ulnolunate ligamentous hinge. In stage I and II PLI, spontaneous reduction of the capitolunate and triquetrolunate joints frequently occurs as the wrist recoils from injury. In this situation,

persistent scapholunate diastasis may be the only manifestation of these more severe injuries. In stage IV PLI (lunate dislocation), the radiographic manifestations are more obvious. Experimental and clinical investigations have also shown that the spectrum of carpal instability previously described can also be expected and can be associated with scaphoid and capitate fractures as well as avulsion fractures of the radial and ulnar styloid processes and of the triquetrum.[46, 50]

Scapholunate Instability

Patients commonly complain of persistent pain over the radial aspect of the wrist joint after various hyperextension injuries of this joint. If scapholunate diastasis is present with or without stress radiographs, the diagnosis is clear. In many cases, however, no appreciable scapholunate diastasis can be clinically documented. This situation can be explained by two distinct types of incomplete ligamentous injury that occur at this joint.

In the first type, limited volar interosseous and radioscaphoid ligament failure occurs. Studies by Kauer[37] and Nash and Mayfield (Nash D, Mayfield JK: The ligamentous anatomy of the scapholunate joint. Unpublished study, 1974), have substantiated that the axis of motion of the scapholunate joint is in the dorsal part of the joint. Some wrist injuries can be associated with an intact dorsal interosseous ligament, along with volar interosseous ligament disruptions, because the scaphoid rotates on the lunate through the dorsal axis of this joint. This observation has been verified surgically in patients who had chronic wrist pain after a hyperextension injury.[48] Scapholunate diastasis was not present on stress roentgenograms (see Fig. 5–21 and Case 1).[48]

In the second type of limited scapholunate ligamentous injury, elongation of the scapholunate interosseous ligament and the radioscaphoid ligament occurs without complete ligament failure. Experimental studies have documented sequential elongation of these ligaments prior to failure (see Fig. 5–18).[49] This phenomenon has been substantiated in my clinical practice; such ligament elongation leads to varying degrees of persistent scapholunate instability (Fig. 5–28).

The syndrome of chronic wrist pain located about the scapholunate joint and associated with various degrees of scapholunate instability remains a common and vexing problem.

Anatomic studies by Kauer[37] and unpublished data of Nash have demonstrated the relative hypermobility of the volar aspect of the scapholunate joint. Biomechanical studies[49] have verified the relative weakness and elasticity of the radioscaphoid ligament. This information suggests that the weakest ligamentous attachments at this joint are volar. Because the axis of rotation of this joint is dorsal, wrist hyperex-

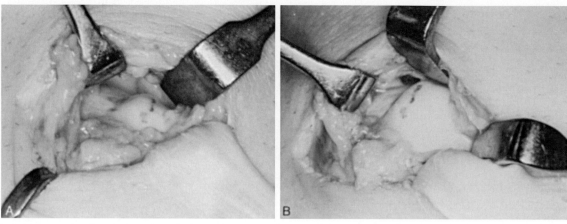

Figure 5–28. *A,* Intraoperative dorsal view of scapholunate joint. Note the step-off at this point. *B,* Surgeon is pushing longitudinally on the thumb, causing marked increase in the degree of step-off at the scapholunate joint. (From Mayfield JK: Wrist ligamentous anatomy and pathogenesis of carpal instability. Orthop Clin North Am 15:209–216, 1984.)

tension is accommodated to some degree by this volar scapholunate mobility. Conversely, in extremes of extension and intercarpal supination, this area is the first to tear. This subtle finding is illustrated in the following case.

Case 3

A 22-year-old male student was evaluated for chronic wrist pain after sustaining an extension injury a year earlier. Clinically, his pain was localized to the scapholunate joint area. Stress radiographs in ulnar deviation and extension under fluoroscopic control revealed only a minimal incongruity of the midcarpal scapholunate joint surfaces, suggesting mild instability. Surgical exploration verified a complete tear of the volar aspect of the scapholunate interosseous ligament. The dorsal aspect of the ligament was intact (see Fig. 5–21).[49]

The preceding case history suggests that a spectrum of ligament injury may be present at the scapholunate joint in stage I perilunar instability. The injury begins with a partial volar scapholunate interosseous ligament tear and proceeds to complete failure, or begins with ligament elongation and proceeds to complete failure.

It is my impression that many patients plagued by similar chronic wrist pain have partial interosseous ligament failure with volar tears or ligament elongation associated with minor degrees of scapholunate instability. These findings have been substantiated arthroscopically by Dautel and associates[15] and Adolfsson.[1] Not infrequently, these lesions can be associated with dorsal or volar ganglions. With careful dissection, the ganglions can be traced back to their origins in the torn interosseous ligaments.

Lunotriquetral Instability

Horii and colleagues[31] have demonstrated altered carpal kinematics after sectioning of the lunotriquetral ligaments, particularly the dorsal scaphotriquetral and radiotriquetral ligaments. A VISI pattern of carpal instability with volar lunate rotation was evident. It was their conclusion that injuries to this joint leading to lunotriquetral dissociation can produce synovitis, joint wear, abnormal ligament tension, and wrist pain associated with clicking on the ulnar side of the wrist. These findings have been substantiated arthroscopically.[59] Zachee and coworkers[77] arthroscopically described fraying of the ulnotriquetral and ulnolunate ligaments and signs of Palmer class 2D TFCC injury[54] as signs of long-standing triquetrolunate ligament rupture. Li and associates[41] studied the lunotriquetral joint by arthroscopically sectioning the lunotriquetral interosseous and volar radiolunotriquetral ligaments. The sectioning altered the motion of this joint. They concluded that the lunotriquetral interosseous ligament stabilized the joint in ulnar deviation and that the volar radiolunotriquetral ligament stabilized the joint in extension.

SUMMARY

Many advances have been made, since the first edition of this work, in our knowledge and understanding of the anatomy, biomechanics, kinematics, and mechanisms of injuries to the wrist joint and associated carpal instability patterns. Although the exact mechanics of injury are not completely known in all carpal injuries, it seems that the three-dimensional mechanics of extension, ulnar deviation, and intercarpal supination are fundamental. The resultant spatial vector, in conjunction with the magnitude and duration of loading, determines the combination of injuries produced. Carpal dislocations result from a force vector that emphasizes ulnar deviation and intercarpal supination. Scaphoid fractures are produced by a vector that emphasizes extension, and these bones are fractured over the dorsal rim of the radius.

A more thorough understanding of the anatomy of the ligaments of the wrist is now documented, and intense investigative effort has elucidated more completely our understanding of the anatomy, biomechanics, and function of the ligaments of the distal scaphoid as well as the scapholunate and lunotriquetral joints, all key components in carpal injuries.

The histology and biomechanical properties of the ligaments of the wrist joint have also been areas of laboratory investigation. New knowledge in these areas has helped us understand how their mechanical properties participate in the resultant injuries and residual carpal instability patterns.

The concept of progressive perilunar instability (PLI) (stages I through IV) with progressive ligamentous disruption around the lunate, starting at the scapholunate joint and progressing to the lunotriquetral joint, has been described. Arthroscopic documentation of residual ligamentous damage in wrist injuries at these joints has helped our understanding of the broad spectrum of ligament injuries and resultant carpal instabilities seen.

As our knowledge and understanding of this complex joint grow, more precise surgical procedures can be developed to solve the resultant carpal instability and abnormal kinematics. Nevertheless, much more laboratory and clinical research of the carpus is still needed to resolve present controversies. The next decade of work in this area should be even more impressive.

REFERENCES

1. Adolfsson L: Arthroscopic diagnosis of ligament lesions of the wrist. J Hand Surg 18B:65–69, 1993.
2. Alexander CE, Lichtman DM: Ulnar carpal instabilities. Orthop Clin North Am 15:307–320, 1984.
3. Andrews FT: A dislocation of the carpal bones—the scaphoid and the semilunar: Report of a case. Mich Med 31:269–271, 1932.
4. Armstrong BWD: Rotational subluxation of the scaphoid. Can J Surg 11:306–314, 1968.
5. Bartone NF, Grieco RV: Fractures of the triquetrum. J Bone Joint Surg 38A:353, 1956.
6. Berger RA, Kauer JMG, Landsmeer JMF: Radioscapholunate ligament: A gross anatomic and histologic study of fetal and adult wrists. J Hand Surg 16A:350–353, 1991.
7. Berger RA, Landsmeer JMF: The palmar radiocarpal ligaments: A study of adult and fetal wrist joints. J Hand Surg 15A:847–854, 1990.
8. Berger RA, Blair WF: The radioscapholunate ligament: A gross and histologic description. Anat Rec 210:393–405, 1984.
9. Berger RA, Crowinshield RD, Flatt AE: The three-dimensional rotational behaviors of the carpal bones. Clin Orthop 167:303–310, 1982.
10. Boabighi A, Kuhlmann JN, Kenesi C: The distal ligamentous complex of the scaphoid and the scapho-lunate ligament: An anatomic, histologic and biomechanical study. J Hand Surg 18B:65–69, 1993.
11. Bonnin JG, Greening WP: Fracture of the triquetrum. Br J Surg 31:278, 1943.
12. Borgeskov S, Christiansen B, Kjaer AM, et al: Fractures of the carpal bones. Acta Orthop Scand 37:276, 1966.
13. Campbell RD Jr, Lance EM, Yeoh CB: Lunate and perilunar dislocations. J Bone Joint Surg 46B:55–72, 1964.
14. Campbell RD Jr, Thompson RC, Lance EM, et al: Indications for open reduction of lunate and perilunate dislocations of the carpal bones. J Bone Joint Surg 47A:915–937, 1965.
15. Dautel G, Goudot B, Merle M: Arthroscopic diagnosis of scapho-lunate instability in the absence of x-ray abnormalities. J Hand Surg 18B:213–218, 1993.
16. DeLange A, Kauer JMG, Huiskes R: Kinematic behavior of the human wrist joint: A roentgenstereophotogrammetric analysis. J Orthop Res 3:56–64, 1985.
17. Destot E: Injuries of the Wrist: A Radiographic Study. New York, Paul B Koeker Co, 1926.
18. Drewniany JJ, Palmar AK, Flatt AE: The scaphotrapezial ligament complex: An anatomic and biomechanical study. J Hand Surg 10A(4):492, 1985.
19. England JPS: Subluxation of the carpal scaphoid. Proc R Soc Lond 63:581–582, 1970.
20. Erdman AG, Mayfield JK, Dorman F, et al: Kinematic and kinetic analysis of the human wrist by stereoscopic instrumentation. In 1978 Advances in Bioengineering. American Society of Mechanical Engineers, 1978, pp 79–82.
21. Fisk G: Carpal instability and the fractured scaphoid. Ann R Coll Surg Engl 46:63–76, 1970.
22. Friedenberg ZB: Anatomic considerations in the treatment of carpal navicular fractures. Am J Surg 78:379, 1949.
23. Gardner EE, Gray J, O'Rahilly R: Anatomy, ed 3. Philadelphia, WB Saunders, 1969, pp 160–163.
24. Gilford W, Bolton R, Lambrinudi C: The mechanism of the wrist joint. Guy's Hospital Report 92:52–59, 1943.
25. Grant JCB: An Atlas of Anatomy, ed 5. Baltimore, Williams & Wilkins, 1962, plates 90–94.
26. Goss CM: Gray's Anatomy of the Human Body, ed 29. Philadelphia, Lea & Febiger, 1973, pp 333–336.
27. Green DP, O'Brian ET: Classification and management of carpal dislocations. Clin Orthop 149:55–72, 1980.
28. Herzberg G, Comtet JJ, Linscheid RL, et al: Perilunate dislocations and fracture-dislocations: A multicenter study. J Hand Surg 18A:768–779, 1993.
29. Hill NA: Fractures and dislocations of the carpus. Orthop Clin North Am 1:275, 1970.
30. Hixson ML, Stewart M: Microvascular anatomy of the radioscapholunate ligament of the wrist. J Hand Surg 15A:279–282, 1990.
31. Horii E, Garcia-Elias M, An KN, et al: A kinematic study of the luno-triquetral dissociations. J Hand Surg 16A:355–362, 1991.
32. Howard FM, Fahey T, Wojcik E: Rotatory subluxation of the navicular. Clin Orthop 104:134, 1974.
33. Jackson WT, Hefky MS, Guo H: Determination of wrist kinematics using a magnetic tracking device. Med Eng Phys 16:123–133, 1994.
34. Johnson RP: The acutely injured wrist and its residuals. Clin Orthop 149:33–44, 1980.
35. Kauer JMG: The mechanism of the carpal joint. Clin Orthop 202:16–26, 1986.
36. Kauer JMG: Functional anatomy of the wrist. Clin Orthop 149:9–20, 1980.
37. Kauer JMG: The interdependence of carpal articulation chains. Acta Anat 88:481, 1974.
38. Kuhlman JN, Luboinski J, Laudet L, et al: Properties of the fibrous structures of the wrist. J Hand Surg 15B:335–341, 1990.
39. Landsmeer JMF: Les cohérences spatiales et l'équilibre spatial dans la région carpienne. Acta Anat 70(suppl 54):1–84, 1968.
40. Lewis OJ, Hamshere RJ, Bucknill TM: The anatomy of the wrist joint. J Anat 106:539–552, 1970.
41. Li G, Rowen B, Tokunaga D, et al: Carpal kinematics of lunotriquetral dissociations. Biomed Sci Instrum 27:273–281, 1991.
42. Lichtman DM, Noble WH, Alexander CE, et al: Dynamic triquetrolunate instability: Case report. J Hand Surg 9:186, 1984.
43. Lichtman DM, Schneider JR, Swofford AR, et al: Ulnar midcar-

pal instability—clinical and laboratory analysis. J Hand Surg 6:515–523, 1981.

44. Linscheid RL, Dobyns JH, Beabout JW, et al: Traumatic instability of the wrist: Diagnosis, classification, and pathomechanics. J Bone Joint Surg 54A:1612–1632, 1972.

45. London PS: The broken scaphoid bone. J Bone Joint Surg 43B:237, 1961.

46. Mayfield JK, Johnson RP, Kilcoyne RK: Carpal dislocations: Pathomechanics and progressive perilunar instability. J Hand Surg 5:226–241, 1980.

47. Mayfield JK, Johnson RP, Kilcoyne RK: The ligaments of the human wrist and their functional significance. Anat Rec 186:417–428, 1976.

48. Mayfield JK: Patterns of injury to carpal ligaments: A spectrum. Clin Orthop 187:36–42, 1984.

49. Mayfield JK, Williams WJ, Erdman AG, et al: Biomechanical properties of human carpal ligaments. Orthop Trans 3:143, 1979.

50. Mayfield JK: Mechanism of carpal injuries. Clin Orthop 149:45–54, 1980.

51. Mayfield JK: Wrist ligamentous anatomy and pathogenesis of carpal instability. Orthop Clin North Am 15:209–216, 1984.

52. Mazet R, Hoal M: Fractures of the carpal navicular. J Bone Joint Surg 45A:82, 1963.

53. Mudgal C, Hastings H: Scapho-lunate diastasis in fractures of the distal radius: Pathomechanics and treatment options. J Hand Surg [Br] 18:725–729, 1993.

54. Palmer AK: Triangular fibrocartilage complex lesions: A classification. J Hand Surg 14A:594–606, 1989.

55. Palmer AK, Werner FW: The triangular fibrocartilage complex of the wrist: Anatomy and function. J Hand Surg 6:153–162, 1981.

56. Peterson JW, Robbin ML, Erdman AG, et al: Screw axis measurement of the human wrist. In 1982 Advances in Bioengineering. American Society of Mechanical Engineers, 1982.

57. Poirier P, Charpy A: Traité de l'Anatomie Humaine, tome I. Paris, Masson et Cie, 1911, pp 226–231.

58. Robbin ML, Erdman AG, Mayfield JK, et al: Kinematic measurement of relative motion in the human wrist. In 1981 Advances in Bioengineering. American Society of Mechanical Engineers, 1981.

59. Ruby LK, An KN, Lindsheid RL, et al: The effect of scapholigament section on scapho-lunate motion. J Hand Surg 12A:767–770, 1987.

60. Russell TB: Intercarpal dislocations and fracture-dislocations. J Bone Joint Surg 31B:524, 1949.

61. Sennwald GR, Zdravkovic V, Jacob HAC, Kern HP: Kinematic analysis of relative motion within the proximal carpal row. J Hand Surg 18B:609–612, 1993.

62. Sennwald FR, Zdravkovic V, Kern HP, Jacob HAC: Kinematics of the wrist and its ligaments. J Hand Surg 18A:805–814, 1993.

63. Schaeffer JPL: Morris' Human Anatomy, ed 11. New York, McGraw-Hill, 1965, pp 339–347.

64. Squire M: Carpal mechanics and trauma. J Bone Joint Surg 41B:210, 1959.

65. Tang JB: Carpal instability associated with fracture in distal radius. Chinese J Surg 32:82–86, 1994.

66. Tanz SS: Rotational effect in lunar and perilunar dislocations. Clin Orthop 57:147–152, 1968.

67. Taleisnik J: Post-traumatic carpal instability. Clin Orthop 149:73–82, 1980.

68. Taleisnik J: The ligaments of the wrist. J Hand Surg 1:110–118, 1976.

69. Taleisnik J: Wrist anatomy, function and injury. In American Academy of Orthopaedic Surgeons, Instructional Course Lectures, vol XXVII. St Louis, CV Mosby, 1978, p 61.

70. Verdan C, Narakas A: Fractures and pseudarthrosis of the scaphoid. Surg Clin North Am 48:1083, 1968.

71. Wagner CJ: Perilunar dislocations. J Bone Joint Surg 38A:1198, 1956.

72. Wagner CJ: Fracture-dislocations of the wrist. Clin Orthop 15:181, 1959.

73. Weber ER, Chao EY: An experimental approach to the mechanism of scaphoid wrist fractures. J Hand Surg 3:142, 1978.

74. Williams WJ, Erdman AG, Mayfield JK: Design and analysis of a ligament cross-sectional area micrometer. In 1980 Advances in Bioengineering. American Society of Mechanical Engineers, 1980, pp 50–52.

75. Wright RD: A detailed study of movement of the wrist joint. J Anat 70:137, 1935.

76. Youm U, McMurtry RY, Flatt AE, Gillespie TE: Kinematics of the wrist: An experimental study of radial-ulnar deviation and flexion-extension. J Bone Joint Surg 60A:423, 1978.

77. Zachee L, Demet L, Fabry G: Frayed ulno-triquetral and ulno-lunate ligaments as an arthroscopic sign of longstanding triquetral-lunate ligament rupture. J Hand Surg 19B:570–571, 1994.

PART II

Evaluation and Special Procedures

CHAPTER 6

Physical Examination of the Wrist

Craig M. Torosian, MD, David E. Brown, MD,
Terri Skirven, OTR, CHT, and David M. Lichtman, MD

Successful examination of the wrist requires a thorough knowledge of topical anatomy and underlying structures. The ability to correlate the mechanism of injury with localized physical findings, such as tenderness, abnormal motion, and audible sounds, enables the examiner to formulate a differential diagnosis (Table 6–1) and to plan further investigative studies or treatments.

Many wrist disorders are readily identified during the first patient visit. Some, such as suspected carpal instability and ulnar-sided wrist pain, are conclusively diagnosed only after careful reexaminations supported by imaging studies.

CLINICAL HISTORY

If an acute injury has occurred, a careful history of the mechanism of injury is essential. Attention should be paid to the specific position of the wrist during the initial loading and to subsequent direction and amount of stress to which the wrist was subjected. Dorsiflexion and supination forces usually produce radially initiated perilunate injuries, whereas palmar flexion and pronation forces are more likely to produce ulnarly initiated perilunate injuries.[14]

The location, intensity, and duration of pain that occurred after the acute injury should be noted. Careful questioning of the patient often enables the examiner to more accurately localize the pain. Asking a patient whose "whole wrist hurts" to point to a single location of most intense and troublesome pain helps direct the physical examination. The period from the time of injury to the diagnosis and treatment can be divided into acute, subacute, and chronic phases to reflect various healing potentials. An acute or subacute injury would have a higher likelihood of healing with closed treatment than a chronic injury.[12]

Occasionally, the history can be almost pathognomonic. For example, an acute volar ulnar wrist pain in a golfer after hitting a large divot suggests a fracture of the hook of the hamate. Unfortunately, most histories are not as clear. Patients often require gentle probing by the examiner to obtain such histories.

When wrist pain is caused by a chronic or repetitive movement injury, the frequency with which it occurs and any particular movements or activities that aggravate or alleviate the discomfort must be determined. The extent to which occupational or avocational activities aggravate the symptoms should be ascertained and considered. Many repetitive-use injuries can be treated or eliminated by job modification, ergonomic changes, or temporary rest. If symptoms are brought on by an athletic activity, a sports professional's analysis of the patient's technique is occasionally necessary.

Information should be obtained about the presence of swelling, limitation of motion, burning, or tingling. The examiner should ascertain whether paresthesia, dysesthesia, or anesthesia is present. Does pain or discomfort follow a dermatomal distribution? Are the symptoms vague or precise? Do objective complaints correlate with objective findings?

The types and effects of previous immobilizations, medications, injections, or surgery should be defined. The efficacy of prior treatments is an important factor in choosing treatment alternatives.

The patient should be specifically questioned about the presence of abnormal sounds or sensation about the wrist with specific types of motion. These are often quite accurately described by patients as "grinding" (crepitus), "snaps," "clicks," or "clunks," each of which has a different qualitative sound and sensation.

A *click* usually represents a medium-pitched, medium-magnitude sensation such as that caused by two bones rubbing together, as in scapholunate or triquetrolunate instability. A *snap* represents a high-pitched sound with an intermediate intensity as caused by a subluxing tendon or plica. *Clunks* are low-pitched, highly perceivable sensations and often are presenting symptoms of midcarpal instability. *Grinding* is crepitus, a high-pitched, low-intensity sensation, usually representing synovitis (Table 6–2).

73

Table 6–1. DIFFERENTIAL DIAGNOSIS OF WRIST PAIN[3]*

I. Traumatic/degenerative
  A. Apparent fractures
  B. Occult fractures
     1. Distal radius
     2. Scaphoid
  C. Fracture nonunions
  D. Carpal instability
     1. Perilunate
        a. Scapholunate
        b. Lunotriquetral[19]
     2. Midcarpal
        a. Intrinsic[13]
        b. Extrinsic[21]
     3. Radiocarpal
        a. Ulnar translocation
        b. Dorsal subluxation
        c. Volar subluxation
        d. Distal radial ulnar joint disruption
           (1) Dislocation
           (2) Subluxation
           (3) Triangular fibrocartilage complex tears[18]
           (4) Ulnar abutment syndrome[17]
  E. Post-traumatic/postinstability arthrosis (SLAC)[25]
II. Congenital/developmental
  A. Madelung's deformity
  B. Radial or ulnar deficiency
  C. Simple bone cyst
  D. Kienböck's disease
  E. Osteoarthritis
III. Infectious
  A. Bacterial
  B. Granulomatous
IV. Neoplastic
  A. Enchondroma
  B. Osteoid osteoma
  C. Metastasis
V. Synovial inflammatory diseases
  A. Rheumatoid arthritis
  B. Systemic lupus erythematosus
  C. Gout
  D. Calcium pyrophosphate deposition disease (CPDD)
VI. Miscellaneous
  A. Peripheral nerve entrapment
     1. Carpal tunnel syndrome
     2. Ulnar tunnel (Guyon's canal) syndrome
     3. Superficial radial nerve entrapment at the wrist
        (Wartenberg's syndrome)
  B. Tendinitis
  C. Neuromata
  D. Ganglion
     1. Interosseous
     2. Extraosseous
  E. Subluxing extensor carpi ulnaris tendon[5]

*Superscript numbers in table refer to chapter references.

Table 6–2. SOUNDS EMANATING FROM THE WRIST

Sound	Pitch	Perceived Sensation Intensity	Example
Crepitus	Highest	Low	Wrist synovitis
Click	Medium	Moderate	Scapholunate instability
Snap	High	Moderate	Subluxing ECU tendon
Clunk	Low	High	Carpal instability

ECU = extensor carpi ulnaris.

After the history of the wrist problem is completed, a thorough medical history should be obtained from the patient, including information about other orthopedic or rheumatologic disorders. The presence of concurrent acute or chronic medical conditions such as diabetes or thyroid dysfunction should also be determined.

PHYSICAL EXAMINATION OF THE WRIST

It is important to obtain complete relaxation of the patient's forearm, wrist, and hand while performing an examination of the wrist. Following acute injury, the examination is performed with the involved extremity in a splint or lying flat on a soft examination table. For chronic wrist pain, it is important to examine the wrist with the forearm musculature relaxed. Relaxation is accomplished by having the patient rest the elbow on the thigh or a low table. The physician then gently holds the patient's distal forearm and hand to support the wrist (Fig. 6–1). This maneuver allows the examiner to carefully position the wrist as desired while permitting free and easy motion of the wrist and forearm.

A thorough and methodical examination is performed. It begins with inspection of the surface features and evaluation of range of motion of the extremity, followed by careful palpation of topographic anatomy. More specific provocative maneuvers can be performed as indicated by the history and physical examination.

It is our preference to avoid performing painful maneuvers early in the physical examination. Once a significant amount of pain has been elicited, by either motion, palpation, or a provocative maneuver, it is generally difficult to objectively test and rule out involvement of other areas. It is therefore a good idea to plan out the sequence of the examination in advance, testing all normal areas first and then focusing on the suspected pathologic area.

Accurate recording of the findings is critical for documentation and later reference. The recording can be facilitated by using a worksheet such as the one shown in Figure 6–2.

Inspection

Inspection should begin with a search for localized swelling, nodules or masses, erythema, abrasions, and lacerations. Bruising or incisions are identified, and their presence is recorded. Deformities of soft tissues or bony landmarks are noted.

Range of Motion

The wrist should be tested for active and passive motion in extension, flexion, radial deviation, and

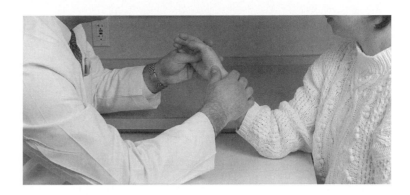

Figure 6–1. Patient positioning during wrist examination. The elbow, forearm, and hand must be supported to obtain relaxation of the forearm musculature. This can be achieved by having the patient rest the elbow on an examining table.

ulnar deviation (Fig. 6–3). Forearm pronation and supination as well as flexion and extension of the carpometacarpal joints are measured. Both active and passive motions should be recorded. It is especially important to note differences between passive and active motions when one is assessing a patient's response to therapy. Evaluating the range of motion of the hand, elbow, shoulder, and neck may be required. All values are compared with those of the opposite extremity. Particular attention is paid to any abnormal noises or pain that occurs during motion testing, because they help to localize the site of pathology.

Palpation and Topographic Anatomy

The osseous and soft tissue topographic anatomy should be systematically palpated to define areas of tenderness. Palpation should also be done to localize fine crepitance as well as any other previously described wrist noises or sensations.

A systematic approach to the topographic anatomic examination is achieved by dividing the wrist into five zones, three dorsal and two palmar. With an organized approach to osseous and soft tissue palpation, the physician can perform a comprehensive examination of the diffusely painful wrist or a precise regional examination when the symptoms are well localized.[3]

Prominent bony landmarks are utilized as reference points to begin the examination. The landmarks on the dorsal side are the radial styloid, Lister's tubercle, the ulnar styloid, and the base of the second and third metacarpals (Fig. 6–4). The landmarks on the palmar surface are the radial styloid, the pisiform, and the tubercle of trapezium (see Fig. 6–21); these prominences are easily palpable in most individuals.

RADIAL DORSAL ZONE

The bony features palpable in the radial dorsal zone are the radial styloid, the scaphoid, and the scaphotrapezial joint, the trapezium, the base of the first metacarpal, and the first carpometacarpal (CMC) joint. Soft tissue structures are the tendons of the first dorsal compartment (abductor pollicis longus and ex-

tensor pollicis brevis tendons) as well as the extensor carpi radialis longus (ECRL), extensor carpi radialis brevis (ECRB), and the extensor pollicis longus (Fig. 6–5). The scaphoid is present immediately distal to the radial styloid on both sides of the first dorsal compartment. The scaphoid tuberosity is just palmar and ulnar to the first compartment tendons and is more prominent in dorsiflexion and radial deviation. The anatomic snuffbox lies between the tendons of the first compartment and the extensor pollicis longus. The scaphoid waist is palpable deep in the snuffbox. Tenderness in the snuffbox may be caused by an occult scaphoid fracture or scaphoid non-union. In a patient with distal radius fractures and diffuse wrist pain and swelling, the eraser end of a pencil may be used to distinguish snuffbox tenderness (and a possible concomitant occult scaphoid fracture) (Fig. 6–6).

Distal to the scaphoid are the scaphotrapezial joint and the trapezium. Gentle rotation of the thumb allows the examiner to differentiate the trapezium from the first metacarpal.

The first CMC joint is easily identified. If the examiner's fingers slowly move in a proximal direction along the dorsal surface of the first metacarpal, a small depression can be felt, which represents the CMC joint. A similar depression exists palmarly, which can be easily palpated while distracting the thumb axially. Typically, the palmar surface of the joint is the most tender in arthritic conditions. Instability can be detected by axial distraction along with radial translation of the base of the metacarpal. The grind test is performed by applying axial compression on the thumb while palpating the first CMC joint (Fig. 6–7). Pain and crepitation reproduced by this test are commonly caused by CMC arthrosis.

An important part of the examination of the radial dorsal zone is palpation of the extensor pollicis brevis, abductor pollicis longus, and extensor pollicis longus tendons for tenderness, crepitation, or localized nodules. De Quervain's tenosynovitis (inflammation of the first dorsal compartment tendons) is a common cause of pain in this region. Pain, swelling, and tenderness over the first compartment tendons are aggravated by active thumb extension and abduction. Pain is best reproduced by asking the patient to passively grasp the thumb and ulnarly deviate the wrist (Finkelstein's test; Fig. 6–8).[6]

UPPER EXTREMITY ASSESSMENT WORKSHEET

NAME_____   AGE_____   DOMINANCE L/R   INDEX L/R

OCCUPATION_____   COMPANY_____   INJURED AT WORK Y/N

HISTORY_____

_____

_____

_____

PMH_____   PSH_____   MEDS_____

ALL: NKMA_____

RANGE OF MOTION

SHOULDER	RT.	LT.	WRIST	RT.	LT.	ELBOW	RT.	LT.	FOREARM	RT.	LT.
ELEVATION			DF			FLEXION			PRONATION		
ER AT SIDE			PF			EXTENSION			SUPINATION		
ER ELEVATED			RD								
IR			UD								

HAND		MP				PIP				DIP			
		RIGHT		LEFT		RIGHT		LEFT		RIGHT		LEFT	
		ACT.	PASS.	ACT.	PASS.	ACT.	PASS.	ACT.	PASS.	ACT.	PASS.	ACT.	PASS.
THUMB	FLEXION												
	EXTENSION												
INDEX	FLEXION												
	EXTENSION												
MIDDLE	FLEXION												
	EXTENSION												
RING	FLEXION												
	EXTENSION												
LITTLE	FLEXION												
	EXTENSION												

PINCH	RIGHT	LEFT	GRIP	RIGHT	LEFT
1			1		
2			2		
3			3		

Figure 6–2. An upper extremity worksheet such as this can facilitate documentation. (Courtesy Fox Valley Orthopaedic Institute, Geneva, Illinois.)

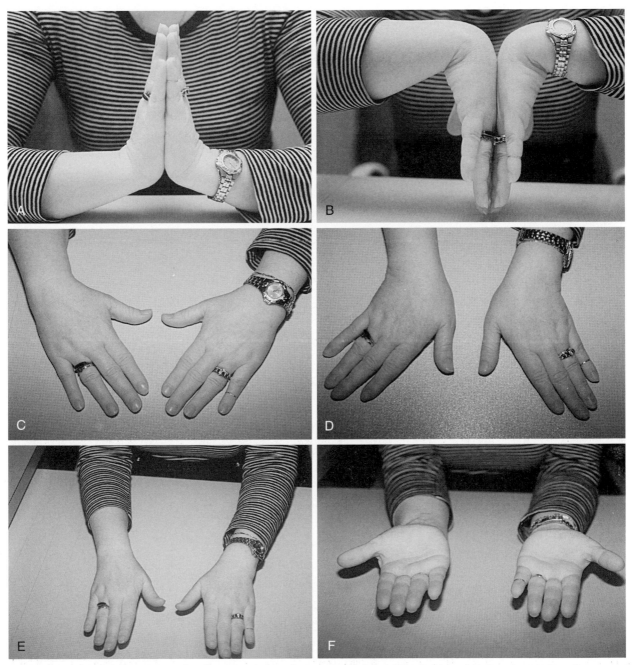

Figure 6–3. Wrist range of motion. *A,* dorsiflexion; *B,* palmar flexion; *C,* radial deviation; *D,* ulnar deviation; *E,* pronation; *F,* supination.

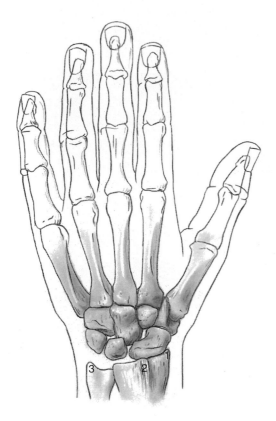

Figure 6–4. Landmarks of the dorsal side of the wrist. Identification of the radial styloid *(1)*, Lister's tubercle *(2)*, and ulnar styloid *(3)* provides an important starting point for the examination of the dorsal surface of the wrist.

Figure 6–5. Radial dorsal zone. On the radial side of the wrist lie the scaphoid, the trapezium, and the first metacarpal. The important tendons in the zone are the extensor pollicis longus, the extensor pollicis brevis, the abductor pollicis longus, and the extensor carpi radialis longus.

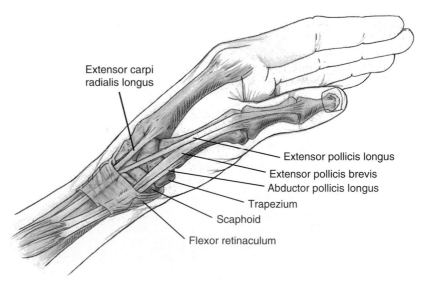

Extensor carpi radialis longus

Extensor pollicis longus

Extensor pollicis brevis

Abductor pollicis longus

Trapezium

Scaphoid

Flexor retinaculum

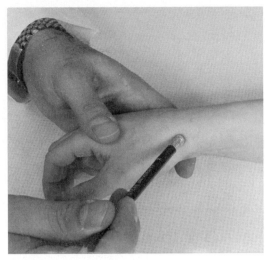

Figure 6–6. An eraser may be used to precisely pinpoint anatomic snuff-box tenderness in a patient with diffuse wrist pain and swelling.

Irritation of the superficial branch of the radial nerve (Wartenberg's syndrome) can occasionally occur from extrinsic compression (as from a tight wristband) or intrinsic pressure, usually due to the dorsal fascia of the brachioradialis muscle. Pain with ulnar deviation of the wrist occurs with stretch of this irritated nerve segment and may be confused with a positive Finkelstein's test. For this reason, tenderness and Tinel's sign over the superficial radial nerve must always be looked for in the examination of a patient with dorsoradial wrist pain.

Tenosynovitis of the second dorsal compartment tendons is also known as intersection syndrome. This syndrome manifests as pain and swelling 4 cm proximal to the wrist, with severe cases causing creptius and erythema as well. This syndrome is thought to represent inflammation in the area where the muscle

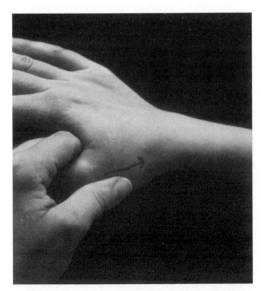

Figure 6–7. The grind test is performed by applying axial compression.

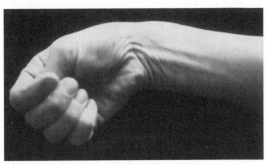

Figure 6–8. Finkelstein's test. The patient is asked to tuck the thumb under the fingers and ulnarly deviate the wrist.

belly of the abductor pollicis longus and extensor pollicis brevis cross the common wrist extensors of the second dorsal compartment.[9]

CENTRAL DORSAL ZONE

The central dorsal zone consists of Lister's tubercle, the scapholunate joint, the lunate, the capitate, the bases of the second and third metacarpals, and their CMC joints. The soft tissue structures in the zone are the distal aspects of the extensor carpi radialis longus and brevis, the extensor pollicis longus, and the extensor digitorum communis tendons (Fig. 6–9).

The lunate is present distal and ulnar to Lister's tubercle. It is more prominent with the wrist held in palmar flexion (Fig. 6–10). In the absence of trauma, lunate tenderness should raise a suspicion of Kienböck's disease (idiopathic osteonecrosis), especially when motion is limited secondary to pain. There is often associated local swelling or synovitis.

The scapholunate joint is detected as the depression between the lunate and the scaphoid. The examiner should begin palpating over the lunate and move radially until a depression is noted (Fig. 6–11). The wrist is moved in radial and ulnar deviation while an examining finger is placed over the scapholunate interval. The integrity of the joint is assessed. Tenderness, clicking, or an increase in the size of the scapholunate depression may indicate scapholunate disassociation. Tenderness may be due to an occult ganglion, a common cause of chronic wrist pain. These occult ganglia are often palpable as pea-sized, tender nodules dorsal to the scapholunate joint. Palmar flexion makes these ganglia more prominent (Fig. 6–12). The capitate is present just distal to the lunate and is located in a mild depression between the lunate and base of the third metacarpal.

Next, the examiner palpates the base of the second and third metacarpals, beginning over the dorsal surface of the metacarpal shafts and proceeding proximal. The metacarpal base is slightly more prominent than the shaft. The respective carpometacarpal joints are identified, and subluxation or carpal bossing is noted. The metacarpal stress test isolates pain to the CMC joint (Fig. 6–13). It is performed by distracting

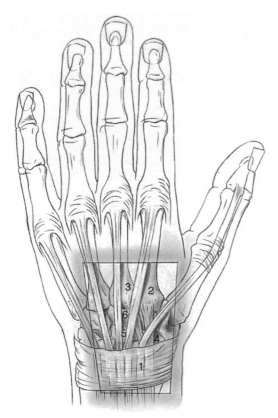

Figure 6–9. Central dorsal zone. In this zone are Lister's tubercle *(1)*, the proximal portions of the second and third metacarpal bases *(2* and *3)*, the proximal pole of the scaphoid *(4)*, the lunate *(5)*, and the capitate *(6)*.

the index and middle fingers with the metacarpophalangeal (MP) joints held in flexion. The fingers and metacarpals are then pronated and supinated.[7] Instability may occur after trauma. It may be detected by

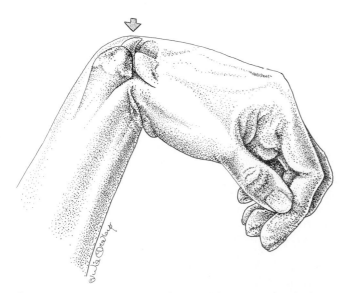

Figure 6–10. The lunate. Palmar flexion of the wrist makes the lunate *(arrow)* more prominent.

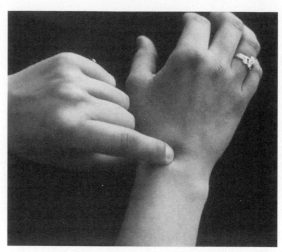

Figure 6–11. The scapholunate joint is palpated as a depression between the lunate and the scaphoid. Confirm by radially and ulnarly deviating the wrist.

axial compression and distraction, which may sublux and reduce the CMC joint.

The ECRL and ECRB tendons are located immediately radial and distal to Lister's tubercle. Just ulnar to Lister's tubercle is the extensor pollicis longus, which courses radially toward the thumb (Fig. 6–14). It becomes more prominent when the thumb metacarpophalangeal (MP) and interphalangeal (IP) joints are extended. Ulnar to the extensor pollicis longus is the extensor digitorum communis (Fig. 6–15). Tenderness over any of these tendons may be due to localized inflammation or to impingement beneath the extensor retinaculum.

The dorsal capsule can be tested by having the patient flex the wrist and extend the middle finger against resistance. Pain localized to the dorsum of the wrist indicates injury to the dorsal capsule, usually at the scapholunate interval.

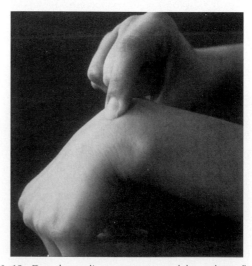

Figure 6–12. Dorsal ganglia are accentuated by palmar flexing the wrist.

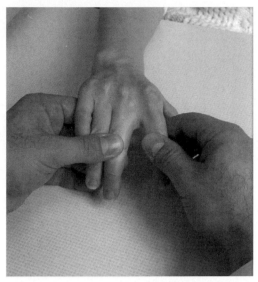

Figure 6–13. Metacarpal stress test. With the metacarpophalangeal joints held in flexion, the metacarpals are pronated and supinated. This maneuver isolates pain to the carpometacarpal joints.

Between the third and fourth dorsal compartments is the posterior interosseous nerve, which provides partial sensation to the radiocarpal, intercarpal, and carpometacarpal joints. Burning pain associated with a positive Tinel's sign here, as often occurs with recurrent dorsal ganglia, may represent a neuroma or a neuroma-in-continuity of the posterior interosseous nerve.

ULNAR DORSAL ZONE

The ulnar dorsal zone comprises the ulnar styloid, distal radioulnar joint, triquetrum, hamate, and bases of the fourth and fifth metacarpals. The principal soft tissue structures located in this zone are the triangular fibrocartilage complex and the extensor carpi ulnaris tendon (Fig. 6–16).

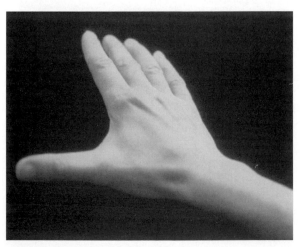

Figure 6–14. The extensor pollicis longus is more prominent with the thumb metacarpophalangeal and interphalangeal joints extended.

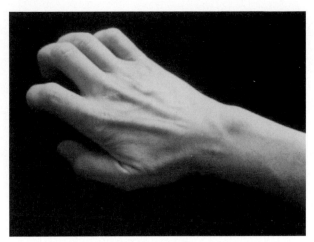

Figure 6–15. The extensor digitorum communis.

The distal radioulnar joint (DRUJ) is located just radial to the prominent ulnar head. The patient's forearm should be rotated to maximum pronation and supination, and any changes in the relationship between the distal ulna and the radius should be noted. The distal ulna is normally more prominent in full pronation. Pain that occurs with forearm rotation may indicate DRUJ disease. Squeezing the radius and the ulna together will cause pain in a patient

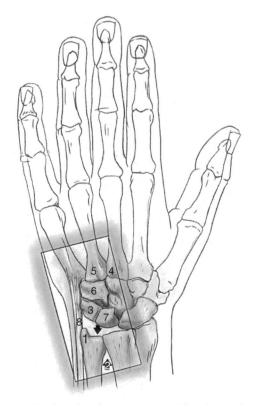

Figure 6–16. The ulnar dorsal zone consists of the ulnar styloid (1), the triquetrum (3), the hamate (6), the proximal fourth and fifth metacarpals (4 and 5), the extensor carpi ulnaris (8), the distal radioulnar joint (2), and the triangular fibrocartilage complex (arrow).

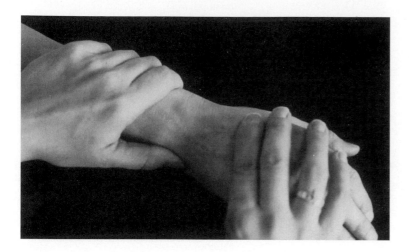

Figure 6–17. The triquetrum can be palpated in the sulcus between the ulnar styloid and the hamate.

with distal radioulnar joint disease. Dorsal or palmar instability can be tested by gently translating the distal ulna with thumb-tip pressure. DRUJ arthrosis can be elicited by these provocative maneuvers.

The examiner should check for symmetry between the patient's wrists. Subtle deformities in the length and rotation of the distal radius and carpus create apparent visual alterations in the prominence of the ulnar head and styloid.

Immediately distal to the ulnar head lies the triangular fibrocartilage complex (TFCC). Exquisite tenderness is noted with acute tears of the TFCC or when ulnar carpal abutment causes triquetral chondromalacia. Either of these disorders may be associated with clicking in the wrist. Tenderness over the dorsal TFCC generally represents TFCC avulsions off the ulnar styloid (Palmar type IB lesion) or tears near the radius (Palmar Type ID lesion).[18] Unlike in the DRUJ disorders, forearm rotation is generally pain free, unless the examiner rotates the arm passively by turning the hand and wrist.

The hamate is palpable proximal to the base of the fifth metacarpal. With the wrist in radial deviation, the triquetrum can be found in an apparent sulcus between the hamate and the ulnar styloid (Fig. 6–17). In the patient with midcarpal instability, localized pain, swelling, and tenderness are most noticeable in this area. In addition, the wrist seems to sag on the ulnar side. As the wrist is moved from neutral to ulnar deviation, a pronounced clunk signals the reduction of the midcarpal subluxation (the midcarpal shift test; see later).

The lunotriquetral joint should be identified and is tender in the presence of sprains or dislocations. There may be an associated wrist click. The lunotriquetral ballottement test[19] is positive in the unstable joint. To perform this test, the examiner stabilizes the lunate with the thumb and index finger of one examining hand while attempting to displace the triquetrum dorsally with the other (Fig. 6–18). A positive result consists of excessive laxity, pain, and crepitus.

The extensor carpi ulnaris (ECU) tendon is located ulnar to the ulnar styloid, becoming quite prominent dorsally in supination and in active ulnar deviation. A recurrent subluxation of the tendon can be detected by a sudden palpable snap when the forearm is actively supinated and the wrist is slightly flexed and ulnarly deviated (Fig. 6–19).

RADIAL VOLAR ZONE

In the radial volar zone, the examiner should locate the scaphoid tuberosity, the tubercle of the trapezium, the flexor carpi radialis, the palmaris longus (if present), the long finger flexors, and the median nerve (Fig. 6–20). The scaphoid tuberosity can be detected just distal to the radial styloid. It is most prominent when the wrist is radially deviated. Distal to the scaphoid is the trapezial ridge, which is palpable with the wrist in all positions and tender when fractured. A carpal tunnel radiographic view is usually

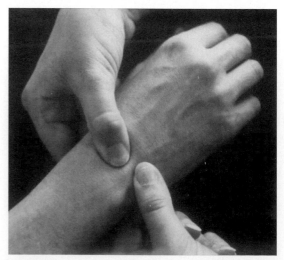

Figure 6–18. The lunotriquetral ballottement test. The lunate is fixed between the examiner's index finger and thumb, and the triquetrum is displaced dorsally and palmarly.

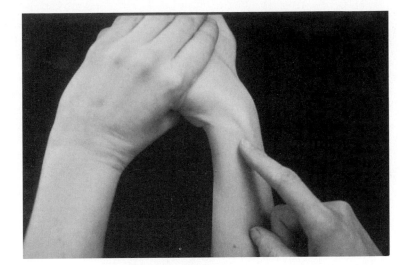

Figure 6–19. The extensor carpi ulnaris tendon. The examiner tests for subluxation by having the patient actively supinate and ulnarly deviate the wrist with the examiner's finger over the sheath.

necessary to demonstrate fracture of the trapezial ridge. The volar aspect of the first CMC joint lies next to the trapezial ridge. When CMC joint inflammation is present, this area is exquisitely sensitive.

Ulnar to the scaphoid tuberosity is the prominent flexor carpi radialis (FCR) tendon, which enters a fibro-osseous tunnel at the proximal border of the trapezium.[1] Tenderness along the FCR tendon at the proximal margin of the trapezial crest with resisted palmar flexion or radial deviation indicates FCR tendinitis.[8]

The palmaris longus tendon, which lies ulnar to the FCR, and is present in 87 percent of limbs.[20] If present, it can be identified best when active wrist flexion is accompanied by opposition of the thumb and small finger.

The median nerve is present immediately deep and radial to the palmaris longus tendon. Carpal tunnel syndrome can be tested for by performing a nerve percussion test. When light percussion is applied to the area over the median nerve from proximal to distal, the patient with carpal tunnel syndrome reports a tingling sensation. Phalen's test can be performed by having the patient flex both wrists for 60 seconds. Numbness in the median nerve distribution should occur within 60 seconds in the presence of carpal tunnel syndrome. Prolonged extension of the wrist can elicit similar symptoms. In the median nerve compression test, the examiner presses with the thumb directly over the median nerve at the wrist. If the patient's symptoms are exacerbated within 2 minutes, the test is considered positive.

ULNAR VOLAR ZONE

In this zone are located the pisiform, the hook of the hamate, the ulnar nerve and artery, and the tendon of the flexor carpi ulnaris (Fig. 6–21). The pisiform is the bony prominence located at the base of the hypothenar eminence. When the wrist is relaxed, the pisiform is mobile and can be palpated using ballottement against the triquetrum. This maneuver causes pain and possibly crepitation in cases of pisotriquetral arthrosis. If the examiner palpates at a slightly radial and distal direction, the hook of the hamate is easily located. It can fracture when the loaded wrist is suddenly dorsiflexed, such as when a golfer strikes a tree or firm ground with a golf club. A carpal tunnel radiograph, an oblique radiograph, or a computed tomography (CT) scan confirms the diagnosis. The

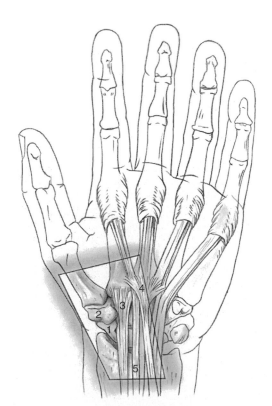

Figure 6–20. Structures identified in the radial volar zone zone are the scaphoid tuberosity (1), tubercle of the trapezium (2), flexor carpi radialis (3), palmaris longus (4), and the long finger flexors (5).

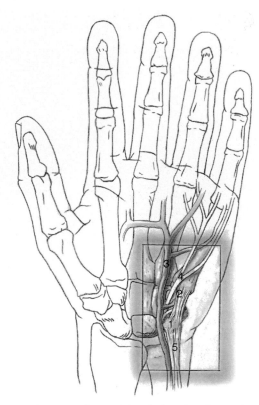

Figure 6–21. Structures that are identified in the ulnar volar zone are the pisiform (1), hook of the hamate (2), ulnar artery and nerve (3 and 4), and flexor carpi ulnaris tendon (5).

presence of isolated tenderness should prompt the astute clinician to order these special radiographs or a CT scan.

Between the pisiform and the hook of the hamate lie the ulnar nerve and artery within Guyon's canal. Usually the ulnar nerve can be detected under the palpating finger with a gentle rolling motion over this canal. In this area, small ganglia or pulsatile masses should be sought, especially when vascular or neurologic symptoms are present in a distal ulnar nerve distribution.

Peripheral TFCC tears off the ulna (Palmar Type IB lesions) result in tenderness over the ulnar styloid process. TFCC avulsions of the ulnolunate and ulnotriquetral ligaments (Palmar Type IC lesions) cause tenderness over the palmar aspect of the distal ulna (Fig. 6–22).[18]

The flexor carpi ulnaris (FCU) tendon is identified by having the patient flex and ulnarly deviate the clenched fist. FCU tendon inserts into the pisiform, the hook of the hamate (through the pisohamate ligament), and the fifth metacarpal (through the pisometacarpal ligament).

Provocative Maneuvers

Following palpation of each of the bony or soft tissue structures just described, attention should be focused on any area of pain that is produced by palpation or by gentle movement of the involved area. If possible, the patient should repeat the motions and positions that reproduce the wrist discomfort while the examiner palpates over the area of pain.

Several provocative maneuvers have been described to help identify wrist disease. These tests should be performed in patients with suspected radiocarpal or intercarpal wrist pathology.

SCAPHOID SHIFT TEST

As originally described by Watson and associates,[23, 25, 26] the scaphoid shift test (scaphoid test, Watson's test, radial stress test) is a provocative maneuver used to assess periscaphoid ligamentous support. The main stabilizers of the scaphoid are the radioscaphocapitate, scaphoid-trapezium-trapezoid (STT), and scapholunate interosseous ligaments.[2, 15]

The patient places the flexed elbow on the examining table "as if to arm-wrestle." If the right wrist is being examined, the examiner's right-hand fingers are wrapped dorsally on the distal radius, and the right thumb is placed on the distal pole of the scaphoid (Fig. 6–23A). The examiner's left hand is used to put the ulnarly deviated and slightly extended wrist into radial deviation and slight flexion.

With radial deviation, the scaphoid flexes to accommodate the decreased space between the trapezium, trapezoid, and distal radius. The examiner's thumb obstructs this scaphoid motion. In a patient with normal scaphoid restraints, the scaphoid continues to flex, and the examiner feels this flexion as pressure on the thumb (Fig. 6–23B). With lax periscaphoid ligaments, the proximal pole displaces dorsally out of the scaphoid fossa and over the dorsal rim. When the examiner releases the pressure, the scaphoid reduces back into the scaphoid fossa (Fig. 6–23C). In a positive test, a clunk is appreciated by

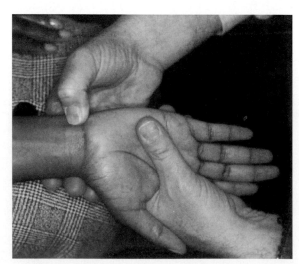

Figure 6–22. Triangular fibrocartilage complex lesions may cause tenderness over the palmar aspect of the distal ulna.

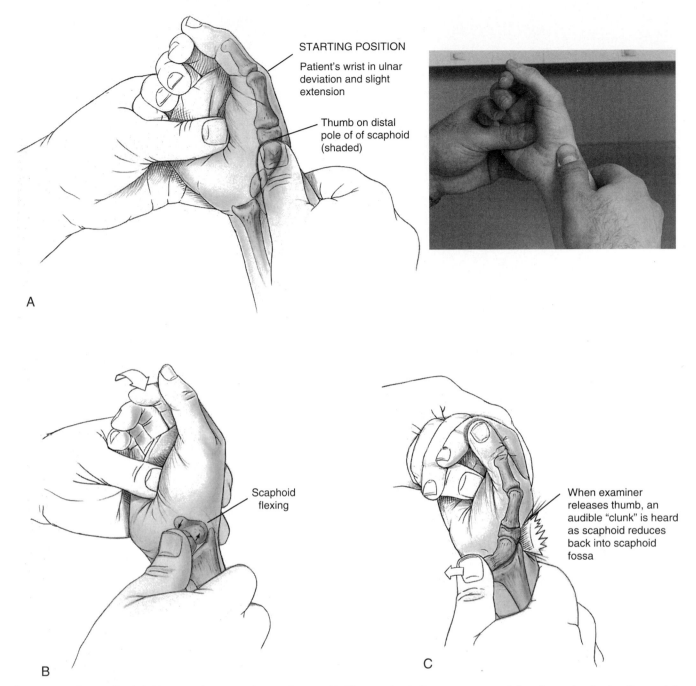

STARTING POSITION

Patient's wrist in ulnar deviation and slight extension

Thumb on distal pole of of scaphoid (shaded)

A

Scaphoid flexing

B

When examiner releases thumb, an audible "clunk" is heard as scaphoid reduces back into scaphoid fossa

C

Figure 6–23. The scaphoid shift test. *A* (drawing and inset photograph), The examiner's fingers are wrapped dorsally on the distal radius, and the examiner's thumb is placed on the distal pole of the scaphoid. *B*, With radial deviation, the scaphoid flexes to accommodate the decreased space between the trapezium, the trapezoid, and the distal radius. *C*, With lax periscaphoid ligaments, the proximal pole displaces dorsally out of the scaphoid fossa, over the dorsal rim. When the examiner releases the pressure, the scaphoid reduces back into the scaphoid fossa.

both the examiner and the patient. To be significant, it should (1) cause pain, (2) reproduce the patient's symptoms, and (3) be asymmetric.

Lane[11] described a variation of the scaphoid shift test in which the scaphoid is suddenly pressed dorsally by the examiner's thumb. This maneuver causes some amount of shifting of the scaphoid, which is noted and compared with the other side.

The significance of a positive scaphoid shift test

result in assessing periscaphoid ligamentous support is a subject of current debate. Watson and associates[25] noted 20 percent of the general population had a unilateral increase in that scaphoid mobility. Easterling and Wolfe[4] noted a positive result prevalence of one-third in an uninjured, asymptomatic population; they also correlated a positive scaphoid shift test with generalized ligamentous laxity. In a companion study, Wolfe and Crisco[27] demonstrated a significant differ-

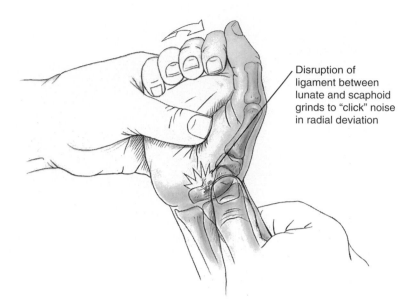

Disruption of ligament between lunate and scaphoid grinds to "click" noise in radial deviation

Figure 6–24. In patients with incompetence of the scapholunate interosseus ligament (i.e., carpal instability–dissociative, or CID), there is clicking between the scaphoid, which is fixed by the examiner's thumb, and the lunate, which is flexing as the wrist is radially deviated.

ence in scaphoid displacement, when measured in a load-displacement apparatus, between subjects with and without a positive scaphoid shift test. These researchers noted that ligament stiffness is "significantly decreased among subjects who demonstrate a positive scaphoid shift, indicating laxity, but not necessarily pathology of the carpal ligaments."[27]

Rotary subluxation of the scaphoid and a scaphoid shift test result are not "all-or-none" phenomena, but constitute a spectrum of instability that represents either ligamentous disruption and/or ligamentous laxity. We believe that there are two components to this examination. In patients with incompetence of the scapholunate interosseus ligament (i.e., with carpal instability–dissociative [CID]), there is clicking between the scaphoid, which is fixed by the examiner's thumb, and the lunate, which is flexing as the wrist is radially deviated (Fig. 6–24). The second component of the examination tests for carpal instability–nondissociative (CIND), in which the scapholunate ligament is intact and therefore the scaphoid and the lunate are moving synchronously. In the presence of periscaphoid ligamentous laxity, the scaphoid can be subluxed over the dorsal rim of the distal radius when pressure is exerted by the examiner's thumb. As this pressure is released, the scaphoid reduces back into the scaphoid fossa with a clunk.

The scaphoid shift test must be interpreted within the context of the presence or absence of acute injury, the test recreating the patient's symptoms, and asymmetry. The clinician must also test for general ligamentous laxity and must be aware that 20 to 32 percent of the general population have a "positive" scaphoid shift, and that two thirds of them are asymptomatic.[4, 25]

TESTS FOR LUNOTRIQUETRAL INSTABILITY

A common cause of ulnar-sided wrist pain is lunotriquetral ligament tears. These injuries can result from acute injury, degenerative changes, or ulnar abutment. Such ligamentous disruptions can range from partial tears of the lunotriquetral interosseous ligament alone to complete disruption of the lunotriquetral interosseous ligament as well as the dorsal and palmar lunotriquetral ligaments. The following tests may help elucidate these injuries.

Lunotriquetral Ballottement Test. The lunate is fixed between the examiner's thumb and index finger while the triquetrum and pisiform are displaced dorsally and palmarly with the examiner's other hand (see Fig. 6–18). A wrist with lunotriquetral instability demonstrates pain, crepitus, and asymmetric laxity compared with the patient's other side.

The Shuck Test. The lunate is stabilized in the same manner as in the lunotriquetral ballottement test, but the wrist is both actively and passively, radially and ulnarly deviated. In a positive test, such movements cause pain at the lunotriquetral joint.

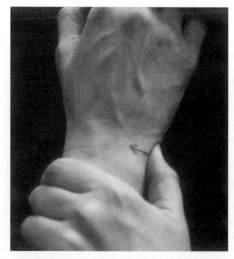

Figure 6–25. The lunotriquetral squeeze test.

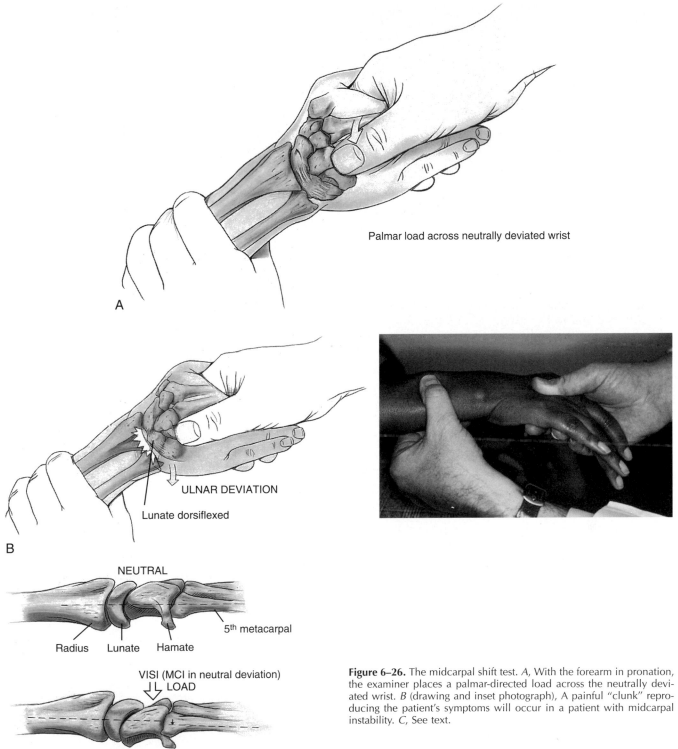

Palmar load across neutrally deviated wrist

A

ULNAR DEVIATION

Lunate dorsiflexed

B

NEUTRAL

Radius   Lunate   Hamate   5th metacarpal

VISI (MCI in neutral deviation)

LOAD

DISI (MCI in ulnar deviation)

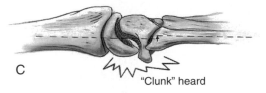

C

"Clunk" heard

Figure 6–26. The midcarpal shift test. *A,* With the forearm in pronation, the examiner places a palmar-directed load across the neutrally deviated wrist. *B* (drawing and inset photograph), A painful "clunk" reproducing the patient's symptoms will occur in a patient with midcarpal instability. *C,* See text.

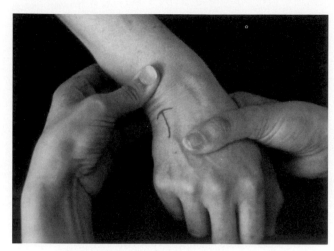

Figure 6–27. Triangular fibrocartilage load test.

The Squeeze Test. The triquetrum is palpated in the sulcus distal to the ulnar styloid and is displaced radially and distally (Fig. 6–25). In a patient with lunotriquetral instability, the test produces pain.

TESTS FOR MIDCARPAL INSTABILITY

Patients with lax ligaments spanning the midcarpal joint may present with a painful wrist clunk.[13] Progressive ligament disorders range from laxity or tears of the dorsal triquetrum-hamate ligament to laxity or tears of the heavier volar arcuate (triquetrum-hamate-capitate) ligaments.

The midcarpal shift test reproduces this painful clunk in patients with midcarpal instability. With the forearm in pronation, the examiner places a palmar-directed load across the neutrally deviated wrist (Fig. 6–26A). In the pathologic condition, when the ligamentous support to the midcarpal joint is stretched or disrupted, the lunate assumes a flexed posture (Fig. 6–26C). The wrist is then ulnarly deviated. A painful clunk reproducing the symptoms occurs in the patient with midcarpal instability (Fig. 6–26B). This catch-up clunk represents sudden flipping of the the flexed lunate into extension (see Fig. 6–26C). Many normal individuals with hyperlax ligaments may also have a positive midcarpal shift test. In these individuals, the clunk does not reproduce the patient's symptoms.

TRIANGULAR FIBROCARTILAGE (TFC) LOAD TEST

In the TFC test, the ulnar column of the wrist is stressed in order to detect tears in the TFC (Fig. 6–27). An axial load is applied across the patient's ulnarly deviated wrist. Patients with TFC tears have pain, although pain may also be caused by ulnar abutment or chondral defects of the proximal pole of the hamate. Supination and pronation of the hand on

Table 6–3. DIFFERENTIAL INJECTION

To Distinguish:	Recommended Site of Injection
de Quervain's tenosynovitis vs. occult scaphoid fracture	First dorsal compartment
FCR tendinitis vs. STT joint arthrosis	FCR tendon sheath
ECU tendinitis vs. TFCC tear	Ulnocarpal or distal radioulnar joint
FCU tendinitis vs. pisotriquetral arthrosis	Pisotriquetral joint

the fixed forearm also provokes pain in TFC disorders.

DRUJ PROVOCATIVE TESTS

Maneuvers provoking DRUJ disorders are discussed in the section on examination of the ulnar volar zone.

Differential Injections

Differential injections of specific structures with short-acting local anesthetic agents with or without corticosteroids can be performed to confirm the location and source of a patient's pain. Such measures are also useful in a patient with pain in several distinct anatomic areas of the wrist. In these patients, injection of a specific region often determines the proportion of the symptoms that arise from that location. The patient should then be asked to estimate what percentage, if any, of the pain was relieved by the injection. Following the injection, the patient should be carefully reexamined.

Differential injections can be especially useful in distinguishing inflammation of the tendon sheaths from arthrosis of adjacent joints. Examples of such approaches are given in Table 6–3.

SUMMARY

Advances in imaging modalities such as magnetic resonance (MR) imaging and wrist arthroscopy have

Table 6–4. COSTS OF DIAGNOSTIC TESTS IN CHICAGO AS OF JANUARY 1996

Test	Cost ($)*
Routine wrist radiographic series	67
Lidocaine injections	102
Bone scan of wrist	516
Trispiral tomography without contrast	629
CT scanning	740
Triphase wrist arthrogram	190
Cineradiograph	154
MR imaging	998
Evaluation and management new patient level 2 of 5	98

*Physician Fee Analyzer Plus, Medicode, Salt Lake City, Utah, 1995.

greatly expanded our knowledge of the wrist. The diagnosis of a "wrist sprain" no longer adequately describes the myriad wrist disorders that affect our patients today.

As third-party payors of medical expenses demand more cost-effective treatment, and employers as well as employees demand prognostic information, it is critical to arrive at the correct diagnosis and spare our patients unnecessary treatment while offering help to those who may benefit from it.

Table 6–4 lists the costs, as of January 1996, of diagnostic tests that can be used in cases of wrist pain. If all patients who presented with wrist pain underwent two or more of the diagnostic tests listed, health care funds would quickly be depleted. In most cases, appropriate diagnostic information can be obtained from a physical examination conducted according to the guidelines described in this chapter, the January 1996 cost of which is also shown in the table.

References

1. Bishop AT, Gabel G, Carmichael SW: Flexor carpi radialis tendinitis. Part I: Operative anatomy. J Bone Joint Surg 76A:1009–1014, 1994.
2. Blevens AD, Light TR, Jablonsky WS, et al: Radiocarpal articular contact characteristics with scaphoid instability. J Hand Surg 14A:781–790, 1989.
3. Brown DE, Lichtman DN: The evaluation of chronic wrist pain. Orthop Clin North Am 15:184, 1984.
4. Easterling KJ, Wolfe SW: Scaphoid shift in the uninjured wrist. J Hand Surg 19A:604–606, 1994.
5. Eckhardt WA, Palmer AK: Recurrent dislocation of the extensor carpi ulnaris tendon. J Hand Surg 6:629, 1981.
6. Finkelstein H: Stenosing tenovaginitis at the radial styloid process. J Bone Joint Surg 12:509–540, 1930.
7. Fusi S, Watson HK, Cuono CB: The carpal boss: A 20 year review of operative management. J Hand Surg 208:405–408, 1995.
8. Gabel G, Bishop AT, Wood MB: Flexor carpi radialis tendinitis. J Bone Joint Surg 76A:1015–1018, 1994.
9. Grundberg AB, Reagan DS: Pathologic anatomy of the forearm: Intersection syndrome. J Hand Surg 10A:299–302, 1985.
10. Hodge JC, Gilula LA, Larsen CF, Amadio PC: Analysis of carpal instability—clinical applications. J Hand Surg 20A:767–776, 1995.
11. Lane LB: Scaphoid shift test. J Hand Surg 18A:366–368, 1993.
12. Larsen CF, Amadio PC, Gilula LA, and Hodge JC: Analysis of carpal instability: description of the scheme. J Hand Surg 20A:757–764, 1995.
13. Lichtman DM, Schneider JR, Swafford AR, et al: Ulnar midcarpal instability—clinical and laboratory analysis. J Hand Surg 6:515, 1981.
14. Mayfield JK: Mechanisms of carpal injuries. Clin Orthop 149:45–54, 1980.
15. Mayfield JK, Johnson RP, Kilcoyne RF: Carpal dislocations: Pathomechanics and progressive pisilunar instability. J Hand Surg 5A:226–241, 1980.
16. Palmar AK: Triangular fibrocartilage disorders: Injury patterns and treatment. Arthroscopy 6:125–132, 1990.
17. Palmer AK, Glisson RR, Werner FW: Ulnar variance determination. J Hand Surg 7:376, 1982.
18. Palmer AK, Werner FW: The triangular fibrocartilage complex of the wrist—anatomy and function. J Hand Surg 6:153, 1981.
19. Reagin DS, Linscheid RL, Dobyns JH: Lunotriquetral sprains. J Hand Surg 9A:502–514, 1984.
20. Reimann RF, et al: The palmaris longus muscle and tendon: A study of 1600 extremities. Anat Rec 89:495, 1944.
21. Taleisnik J, Watson HK: Midcarpal instability caused by malunited distal radius fractures. J Hand Surg 9:350, 1984.
22. Viegas SF, Patterson RM, Mokanson JA, et al: Wrist anatomy: Incidence, distribution, and correlation of anatomic variations, tears, and arthrosis. J Hand Surg 18A:463–475, 1993.
23. Watson HK, Ashmead D IV, Makhlouf MV: Examination of the scaphoid. J Hand Surg 13A:657–660, 1988.
24. Watson HK, Ballet FL: The SLAC wrist: Scapholunate advanced collapse pattern of degenerative arthritis. J Hand Surg 9:358, 1984.
25. Watson H, Ottoni L, Pitts EC, Handal AG: Rotary subluxation of the scaphoid: A spectrum of instability. J Hand Surg 18B:62–64, 1993.
26. Watson HK, Ryu J, Akelman E: Limited triscaphoid intercarpal arthrodesis for rotatory subluxation of the scaphoid. J Bone Joint Surg 68A:345–349, 1986.
27. Wolfe SW, Crisco JJ: Mechanical evaluation of the scaphoid shift test. J Hand Surg 19A:762–768, 1994.

CHAPTER 7

Post-Traumatic Wrist Pain and Instability: A Radiographic Approach to Diagnosis

Frederick A. Mann, MD, and
Louis A. Gilula, MD

The wrist is an anatomically compact and biomechanically complex region that is commonly subject to injury.[31] There is substantial overlap of the signs and symptoms caused by the diverse etiologies of wrist debility, and effective treatment begins with accurate diagnosis.[2, 4, 9, 28, 35, 57]

This chapter describes an imaging approach to the efficient evaluation of the symptomatic traumatized wrist. Pertinent radiographic techniques and image assessment (including the analysis of soft tissue contours, bony alignment, and metrics) are presented.

The patient with a subacute or chronic wrist injury, but without an obvious clinical or radiographic abnormality to explain the pain, remains a great diagnostic challenge to both the hand clinician and the radiologist. In some cases, a normal variant, such as a negative ulnar variance, places a patient at greater risk for injury.[69] Additional radiologic studies, such as an instability series or magnetic resonance imaging (MR imaging, MRI), may demonstrate the associated symptomatic pathology (e.g., lunatomalacia).[65, 66] Further, the potential of secondary gain in many injuries that are work-related and compensatable under current labor laws demands exclusion or careful documentation of any abnormality.

Radiographic evaluation of the wrist should not proceed until a careful history describing the mechanism of injury is obtained and a complete physical examination has been performed.[1, 50] An important step in the physical examination is to relate the site of maximum tenderness to an underlying anatomic structure, such as a particular carpal bone or ligament. If a diagnosis is not made following the physical examination, we believe the preferred and most cost-effective imaging strategy begins with conventional radiographs. Subsequent studies must be selected and tailored to address unanswered clinical questions and usually can proceed according to an algorithm (Fig. 7–1). Asymmetric progression through the algorithm should result in a definitive roentgenographic diagnosis, if one is possible.

IMAGING TECHNIQUES

The imaging tools available are (1) the four-view wrist survey, (2) specific carpal bone views, (3) targeted tangential or fluoroscopically positioned spot radiographs, (4) an instability series, (5) bone scintigraphy, (6) conventional or computed tomography, (7) wrist arthrography, and (8) MR imaging.

Wrist Survey

The four standard views centered on the wrist, not the hand, are the neutral ("zero") posteroanterior (PA) view, neutral ("zero") lateral views, scaphoid view (ulnarly deviated PA with proximally angled beam or radiocarpal extension), and semipronated oblique view.[74]

NEUTRAL PA VIEW

The neutral PA view may be obtained in one of two ways: (1) with the shoulder *ab*ducted and the elbow flexed 90° with the palm and cassette flat on the radiography table at the level of the shoulder or (2) with the elbow *ad*ducted to the trunk and flexed 90° with the ulnar side of the hand and the edge of the cassette resting on the radiography table. In both projections, the palm is held in the plane of the forearm and flat on the film cassette. The long axes of the third metacarpal and distal radius are parallel. The central ray of the x-ray beam is centered on the cassette and directed through the back of the carpus at the midpoint of a line connecting the distal extents of the radial and ulnar styloid processes (the inter-styloid line). When the arm is *ad*ducted, the x-ray beam is horizontal (parallel to the top of the radiography table). When the arm is *ab*ducted, the x-ray beam is vertical (perpendicular to the top of the table). A well-positioned neutral PA view shows the carpometacarpal joints in profile and the ulnar styloid in a most

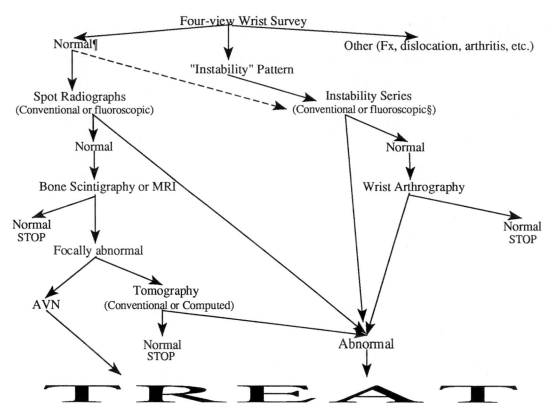

§ Abnormal motion or "popping" should be observed fluoroscopically.
¶ If "instability" suspected, get Instability Series

Figure 7–1. Roentgenographic approach to the painful wrist. *AVN* = avascular necrosis; *Fx* = fracture; *MRI* = magnetic resonance imaging.

medial (ulnar) position, and has less than 3 mm of osseous overlap at the distal radioulnar joint. Such standardization ensures reproducibility of positioning and makes metrics, such as evaluation of ulnar variance at the distal end of the ulna,[37, 48] more precise.

NEUTRAL LATERAL VIEW

We also obtain the neutral lateral view in one of two ways: (1) the arm is *ab*ducted in the coronal plane until the elbow is at the level of the shoulder and the elbow flexed 90° or (2) the elbow is *ad*ducted to the trunk and flexed 90°. In both positions, the ulnar margin of the wrist should be on the cassette, and the flat surface of the cassette should be perpendicular to the palm. The long axes of the third metacarpal and distal radius are parallel in the sagittal and coronal planes. The central ray of the x-ray beam is centered in the middle of the cassette and passes through the radial styloid. When the arm is *ad*ducted, the x-ray beam is vertical (perpendicular to the top of the radiography table). When the arm is *ab*ducted, the x-ray beam is horizontal (parallel to the top of the table).

Mere supination of the pronated hand from the PA to the lateral position does not provide a true lateral view of the ulna. A well-positioned lateral view of the wrist can be recognized by identifying the position of

radial- and ulnar-sided bones of the carpus. The distal pole or distal third of the scaphoid should be ventral to the palmar surface of the pisiform, and the palmar surface of the pisiform should project approximately halfway between the palmar surfaces of the capitate head and the distal scaphoid tubercle (Fig. 7–2).

If the pisiform is visible ventral to or overlaps the distal scaphoid pole, the wrist is off-lateral or semisupinated. The ulna may be more ventral in this position. Also, in this position, the lunate may falsely appear abnormally tilted. With semipronation, the pisiform is not readily, if at all, apparent, and more than the distal one third to one half of the scaphoid projects free of the other carpal bones, as in the standard semipronated oblique view. The ulna is more dorsal in this view. Although much emphasis has been placed on the position of the dorsal surface of the ulna lying over the dorsal surface of the radius to indicate a good lateral wrist view, variations in the shape and position of the distal ulna make the method of checking the relative position of various carpal bones just described more reliable for recognizing true laterality of the wrist on a radiograph.

SCAPHOID VIEWS

We obtain our scaphoid views in one of two positions. Most commonly, we initially position the wrist as for a neutral PA view and then maximally ulnar-deviate the carpus. The central ray of the x-ray beam is angled 15° to 20° toward the elbow and centered at the scaphoid waist. Alternatively, the cassette may be placed on a 20° angled sponge with the palm of the hand flat on the cassette, the carpus in maximal ulnar deviation, and the wrist extended at the radiocarpal joint. The central ray of the x-ray beam is perpendicular to the table top and centered at the scaphoid waist.

SEMIPRONATED OBLIQUE VIEW

The semipronated PA oblique view is obtained by elevating the radial side of the wrist 45° from the initial neutral PA position. The central ray of the x-ray beam is centered at the midpoint of the interstyloid line.

READING THE RADIOGRAPHS

Soft Tissue Evaluation

On each view, one should first survey the soft tissues to identify focal swelling indicative of an underlying abnormality.[13, 17] Such swelling, in the absence of an obvious abnormality, should guide a directed search of the region for "occult" bony or soft tissue injury. Although often difficult to appreciate on conventional films, soft tissue detail on computed radiographs, with their greater latitude, may be specifically enhanced.

Soft tissue swelling is most easily identifiable on the lateral view, especially along the dorsal surface of the wrist. Normally, the dorsal soft tissues of the wrist are concave, and any straightening or convexity in this region is abnormal, albeit nonspecific. The pronator quadratus fat stripe along the palmar aspect of the wrist should be straight or minimally palmar-convex and should appear to contact the palmar surface of the distal radius 2 to 4 mm proximal to its articular margin. In our experience, this fat stripe is present in more than 90 percent of neutral lateral views of normal wrists. Bulging, palmar displacement, or obliteration (partial or complete) of this stripe implies a local hematoma and suggests injury to the distal radius, ulna, or adjacent soft tissues.

The navicular fat stripe is best seen on neutral PA or scaphoid views as a thin, radiolucent line that parallels the lateral surface of the scaphoid.[62] In our experience, it is present in less than 70 percent of normal PA projections. Obliteration or bowing of this fat stripe in comparison with a previously normal appearance indicates localized hemorrhage or edema around the scaphoid, a finding that may occasionally be the only sign of an acute scaphoid fracture (Fig. 7–3). Although the absence of a scaphoid fat pad may not be diagnostic of a scaphoid or periscaphoid fracture, a normal scaphoid fat pad is strong evidence against a fracture of the scaphoid waist.

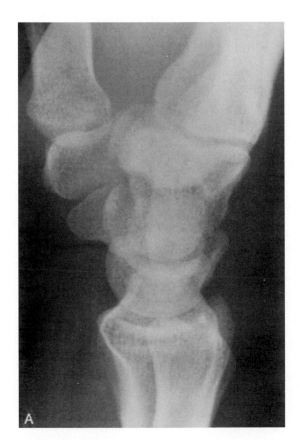

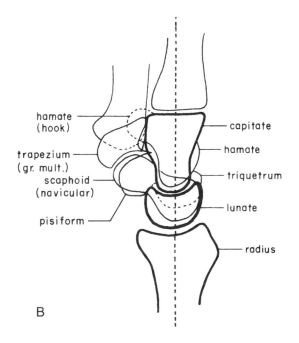

Figure 7–2. A and B, Normal lateral view with the carpal bones labeled. (B from Gilula LA: Carpal injuries: Analytic approach and case exercises. AJR 133:503–517, © 1979 by The Endocrine Society.)

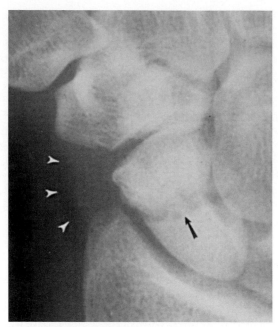

Figure 7–3. An acute, nondisplaced scaphoid waist fracture *(arrow)* causes bowing of the scaphoid fat stripe *(arrowheads)*.

Soft tissue contours along the radial and ulnar margins of the wrist are quite variable. Nonetheless, when focal convexity is seen in conjunction with obliteration of the subcutaneous fat stripe, local edema or hematoma may be suspected and subsequent search for underlying injury directed accordingly.

Bony Evaluation

Subsequent examination of the bones for fracture and malalignment should be systematic.

Neutral PA View. On the neutral PA view, a lambda-shaped zone of vulnerability (Fig. 7–4) contains those carpal structures that have been involved in more than 90 percent of all carpal fractures, fracture-dislocations, dislocations, sprains, and "instabilities" we have seen. Minimally displaced or nondisplaced carpal bone fractures are relatively common. To optimize diagnostic accuracy, one should verify the cortical integrity of the most commonly fractured carpals (e.g., scaphoid, triquetrum, trapezium, and hamate) on all views.[25] If no abnormalities are found during this primary survey, we switch to our "stealth mode" and evaluate the less commonly injured carpals, such as the pisiform, trapezoid, and distal capitate.

On the neutral PA view, findings for static malalignment may be direct (abnormal step-off or widening at a joint) or indirect (unexpected conformation of a carpal bone). The radiocarpal and midcarpal joints normally form three smooth arcs on the neutral PA view (Fig. 7–5). Disruption of these arcs or abnormal overlapping of adjacent bones (adjacent cortices profiled that should be parallel) on the neutral PA view

commonly indicates carpal malalignment, i.e., subluxation or dislocation (Fig. 7–6).[17] There are, however, two common normal variants that mimic step-offs within the carpal arcs: (1) a triquetrum shorter in its proximal-distal dimension than the adjacent lunate creates a lunotriquetral step-off of the first carpal arc and a normal second carpal arc and (2) a proximally prominent hamate with an apposing hamate facet on the lunate (type II lunate)[68] that produces a bilobate third carpal arc and a smooth second carpal arc *if* the radial portion ("capitate facet"), rather than the hamate facet, of the distal lunate articular surface is used to create the second carpal arc.[47] Also, there is a caveat: On other views, such as the semipronated or semisupinated oblique views, or on radially or ulnarly deviated PA views, the carpal arcs are not diagnostically reliable.[49]

The normal scapholunate joint (SLJ) space width is the same as the width between pairs of the other carpal bones. The dorsally convex transverse carpal arch results in scapholunate and lunotriquetral articulations that are slightly oblique and convergent palmarly to the sagittal plane. Therefore, the scapholunate and lunotriquetral joints are rarely both in profile on neutral PA views. To more reliably profile the scapholunate joint, one should position the hand as for a neutral PA view and elevate the ulnar aspect of the hand 10° to 15° or obtain a neutral anteroposterior (AP) view. When measured in its midportion, this space normally measures 2 mm or less and usually remains constant within the normal range of radial or ulnar deviation of the wrist.[55] In lunotriquetral coalition, however, a measurable change in the SLJ space between the extremes of ulnar and radial deviation is normal.[44] Abnormal widening to more than 3 to 4 mm suggests a scapholunate ligament tear or laxity (Fig. 7–7). Disruption of the intrinsic

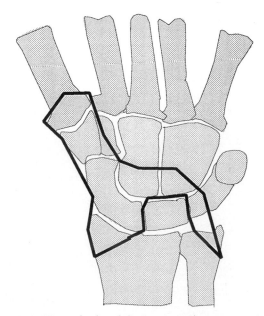

Figure 7–4. "Zone of vulnerability" on neutral posteroanterior view.

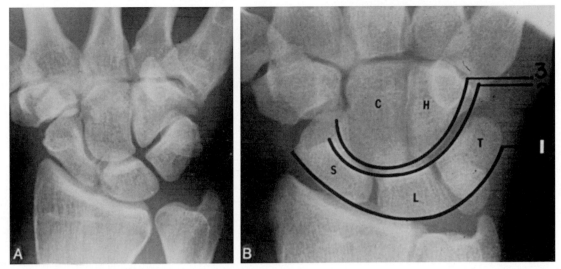

Figure 7–5. *A,* Posteroanterior view of a normal wrist. *B,* Same view with the three arcs drawn. Arc *1* connects the proximal articular surfaces of the scaphoid *(S),* lunate *(L),* and triquetrum *(T).* Arc *2* joins the distal concave surfaces of these same carpal bones. Arc *3* outlines the proximal convexities of the capitate *(C)* and hamate *(H).*

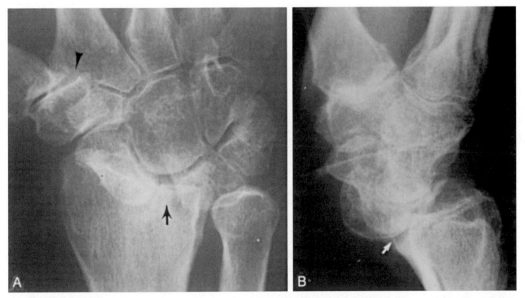

Figure 7–6. Chronic right wrist pain is present 3 years after injury. *A,* Posteroanterior view shows ulnar translocation of the entire carpus with respect to the distal radius. The scapholunate joint is abnormally wide *(arrow)* from disruption of the scapholunate ligament. Overlap of the scaphoid and lunate bones and the distal articular surface of the radius indicates dislocation at the radiocarpal joint. Degenerative spurring of the trapezial first metacarpal joint *(arrowhead)* is evident. *B,* The lateral projection shows ventral dislocation of the carpus with pseudojoints *(arrow)* suggested at the radiolunate and radioscaphoid junctions. (From Bellinghausen HW, Gilula LA, Young LV: Post-traumatic palmar carpal subluxation. J Bone Joint Surg 65A:998–1006, 1983.)

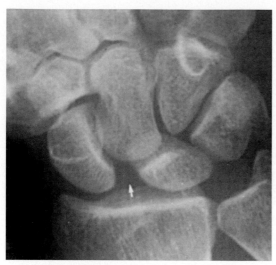

Figure 7–7. Abnormal widening of the scapholunate joint *(arrow)* and signet ring appearance (foreshortening) of the scaphoid bone indicate scapholunate ligament disruption with resultant rotary subluxation of the scaphoid.

scapholunate interosseous ligament may be confirmed with arthroscopy, arthrography, or MR imaging.

Abnormal conformation of either the scaphoid ("signet ring" sign) or the lunate (triangle shape) or both suggests pathologic flexion of a portion or all of the proximal carpal row (PCR) relative to the radius and distal carpal row (DCR). Similarly, pathologic extension of the lunate relative to the radius and DCR is suggested by a broad rhomboid shape.

Metrics on Neutral PA View. *Ulnar variance (UV)* quantifies the apparent difference in length between the radius and ulna. We generally use the "method of perpendiculars."[37] This method measures the shortest distance between two lines perpendicular to the long axis of the radius. These lines are tangential to the ulnarmost extent of the subchondral white line of the distal radius and the distalmost extent of the distal articular surface of the ulnar dome.

Carpal height (CH) is the distance between the base of the third metacarpal and the subchondral white line of the distal radius measured along the proximal extension of the long axis of the third metacarpal.[37] Measurement of carpal height allows comparative quantification of carpal collapse in an individual patient over time. A CH ratio allows comparison between individuals and can be calculated by dividing the CH by the length of the third metacarpal.[37] Similarly, a CH index may be obtained by dividing the CH ratio of the diseased wrist by that of the normal hand. Some investigators believe the CH index to be the most sensitive for detection of abnormal carpal height in a specific hand.[38]

Ulnar translocation (UT) of the carpus is pathologic ulnarward displacement of the carpus due to disruption or attenuation of radiocarpal and intercarpal ligaments.[20, 37] Three techniques have been de-

scribed to quantify UT: (1) radial-carpal distance,[14] (2) index of carpal translation,[21] and (3) carpal-ulnar distance ratio.[40] The radial-carpal distance is measured as the shortest distance between the long axis of the radius and the center of rotation in the head of the capitate (normal, 5.7 ± 1.4 mm). The index of carpal translation is calculated by dividing the shortest distance between the long axis of the capitate and the tip of the radial styloid by the length of the third metacarpal (normal, 0.28 ± 0.03). Finally, the carpal-ulnar distance ratio is obtained by dividing the shortest distance between the long axis of the ulna and the center of rotation in the head of the capitate by the length of the third metacarpal (normal, 0.30 ± 0.03).

Neutral Lateral View. In our experience, a "squashed H"–shaped zone of vulnerability seen on the neutral lateral view (Fig. 7–8) contains those carpal structures that are involved in more than 90 percent of all carpal fractures, fracture-dislocations, dislocations, sprains, and "instabilities." First, one should verify the cortical integrity of those carpals most commonly seen fractured on the lateral view: scaphoid tubercle and dorsal margins of the triquetrum or, less commonly, the hamate. When no osseous abnormality is detected during this primary survey, we go to our "stealth mode" and search for the less common and often palmar fractures, especially of the pisiform, tubercles of the trapezium and scaphoid, and hook of the hamate.

At times, the overlap of the carpal bones on the lateral view makes it difficult to identify all the carpal bones and their interrelationships. However, this

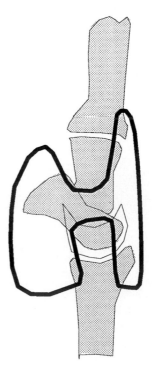

Figure 7–8. "Zone of vulnerability" on neutral lateral view.

view is essential to detect and classify many significant carpal injuries and ligament instabilities.[1] The neutral lateral view shows the amount of apparent displacement between the dorsal margins of the distal ulna and radius, the articulations between the radius, carpus, and metacarpals as well as alignment of the scaphoid, lunate, and capitate (see Fig. 7–2). Although it can be readily suspected from the PA view, final classification of lunate, perilunate, or radiocarpal dislocation is best made using the lateral projection (see Fig. 7–6).[1, 13, 17] When one is evaluating the position of the carpal rows on the lateral view, the lunate may be used to identify the proximal carpal row, whereas the capitate can represent the position and attitude of the distal carpal row. When an intercarpal dislocation occurs, usually either the lunate or the capitate remains centered over the radius. Therefore, with a lunate dislocation, the capitate head remains centered over the radius. Conversely, with a perilunate dislocation, the capitate is dorsal (rarely ventral) to the lunate and the distal radius, but the lunate normally remains aligned with the radius.[17, 36, 39] In both of these conditions, the triquetrum, hamate, trapezium, trapezoid, and distal portion of the scaphoid (if there is a scaphoid fracture present) typically move as a unit with the capitate, away from the lunate. The presence or absence of parallel articulating surfaces (seen best on the PA view) allows the physician to detect dissociation or probable normal articulation between adjacent carpal bones.[17]

On the lateral view, the scaphoid can be identified with its proximal convexity overlapping the midportion of the lunate and its distal pole (tubercle) projecting proximal to the trapezium.

Metrics on the Neutral Lateral View. *Carpal bone axes* are determined on the neutral lateral view. The long axis of the scaphoid can be drawn by passing a line tangent to the distal and proximal palmar convexities of the scaphoid.[20] This line serves as a reproducible axis of the scaphoid and is helpful in evaluating rotary subluxation of the scaphoid (see Fig. 7–7).[12, 20] The long axis of the lunate is drawn as a perpendicular to a line connecting the dorsal and palmar lips of the lunate at the lunocapitate joint.

The long axis of the capitate passes through the midportion of its base with the third metacarpal and bisects the head at the lunocapitate joint. Not infrequently, the distal anatomy of the capitate is difficult to appreciate; therefore, the long axis of the third metacarpal may be used as a substitute for the long axis of the capitate. We determine the long axis of the radius by connecting two points that bisect its distal shaft and metaphysis at 5 cm and 3 cm proximal to the subchondral white line of the distal radial articular surface.

Dorsal radio-ulnar overlap that exceeds 4 mm when the carpus is in a true lateral projection (i.e., the palmar surface of the pisiform is midway between the palmar surfaces of the capitate and scaphoid tubercle) is suggestive of distal radioulnar subluxation.

There are several *intercarpal angles*; however, we principally use the scapholunate, lunocapitate, and radiolunate angles. These are measured as the subtended angles at the intersections of their respective long axes.

Scaphoid View. Because the scaphoid bone is usually foreshortened on the PA view, scaphoid views better profile the scaphoid waist (Fig. 7–9).[12] Detection of truly nondisplaced fractures is greatly enhanced when the central ray of the x-ray beam is parallel to the fracture plane.[63] Thus, the detection of nondisplaced scaphoid fractures can be significantly improved through the use of multiple different and

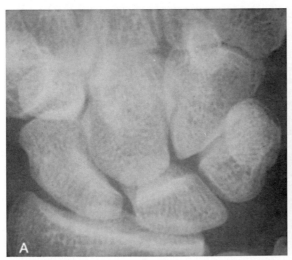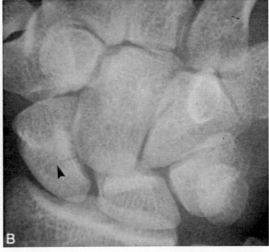

Figure 7–9. *A,* Posteroanterior view of the wrist appears normal in this young patient with pain over the snuffbox. On second inspection, after examination of the scaphoid view *(B),* one can see a subtle lucency evident at the junction of the proximal and middle thirds of the scaphoid. *B,* A scaphoid view of the hand in ulnar deviation profiles the scaphoid waist and reveals a subtle, nondisplaced fracture *(arrowhead):* The ulnar edges of the lunate and radius are in line, the distal end of the triquetrum is closer to the distal end of the hamate, and the proximal pole of the hamate has moved radially toward the central portion of the lunate.

reproducible views of the scaphoid.[63] In fact, subtle scaphoid fractures may be evident on only one of these views (see Fig. 7–9).

Semipronated Oblique View. The semipronated oblique view profiles the scaphotrapeziotrapezoidal and the trapeziotrapezoidal joints as well as the scaphoid tubercle along the radial aspect of the wrist. The dorsoulnar margins of the hamate, triquetrum, lunate, and radius are also put in profile. In addition, portions of the scaphocapitate and lunocapitate joints may be profiled in this view. Pronated oblique views generally show fractures of the scaphoid tubercle and the dorsal margin of the triquetrum when present. Osteoarthritis involving the base of the thumb and processes involving the trapeziotrapezoidal joints are commonly best visualized on this view.

Specific Carpal Bone Views

To evaluate cortical margins of carpal bones not routinely shown on the four-view wrist survey, targeted examinations, such as the carpal tunnel view (Fig. 7–10), the carpal boss view,[11] and semisupination (off-lateral) and reverse oblique views, may be obtained. For example, the carpal tunnel view is useful in detecting fractures of the hook of the hamate, pisiform, or tubercles of either the scaphoid or trapezium in patients with focal palmar pain and a normal four-view wrist series. In a similar clinical setting, the carpal boss or supinated off-lateral view better shows the dorsal margins of the index and long finger carpometacarpal joints (carpal boss region).

CARPAL TUNNEL VIEW

The carpal tunnel view is obtained with the wrist dorsiflexed and either the ventral aspect of the wrist or the palm placed on the film cassette.[74] The x-ray beam is angled to profile the carpal tunnel. The hamate hook, trapezium, pisiform, and palmar surface of the capitate or lunate are revealed.

OFF-LATERAL VIEW

A slightly semisupinated off-lateral view to show the dorsal carpal boss on a tangent enables distinction among (1) a separate os styloideum, (2) a bony prominence attached to the second or third metacarpal base or apposing surface of the trapezoid or capitate bones, and (3) degenerative osteophytes in this same area.[74] Palmarly, the semisupination oblique view demonstrates the pisotriquetral joint, pisiform, triquetrum, and hook of the hamate.

REVERSE OBLIQUE VIEW

With the PA "reversed" (hyper-pronated) oblique view (thenar eminence on the table and hypothenar eminence elevated off the table or film cassette), avulsion fractures of the dorsum of the scaphoid waist and ulnar aspect of the hamate and triquetrum can be detected.[74]

Tangential Conventional Radiographs and Fluoroscopic Spot Films

If focal tenderness is detected and the previous views are not revealing, multiple conventional or fluoroscopically positioned views at progressive 5° to 10° of obliquity can be obtained to radiographically characterize the point of tenderness or focal hot spot noted on a bone scan. Similarly, angulation of the x-ray beam with respect to the long axes of individual carpal bones may occasionally provide new information (i.e., it may profile a fracture line not shown on routine views).

When detailed carpal views fail to demonstrate an abnormality in a clinically suspicious area, the wrist may be studied with fluoroscopy, and special attention can be paid to particular areas of tenderness and to popping or grinding. Specifically, precisely profiled spot radiographs of cortical surfaces and joints can easily be accomplished with good fluoroscopic techniques. In patients with midcarpal pain in

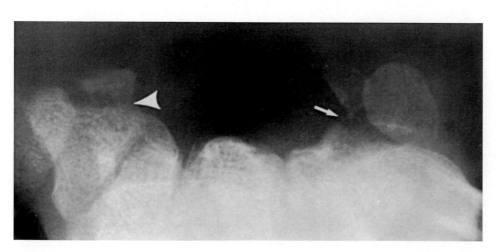

Figure 7–10. On a carpal tunnel view, fractures of the trapezium *(arrowhead)* and the hook of the hamate *(arrow)* are evident.

whom routine films are normal, manipulation under fluoroscopy (see next section) may reveal dynamic intercarpal instability.[71]

Conventional and Videofluoroscopic Ligament Instability Series

We believe that an instability series[18, 20, 54, 56] is indicated to detect abnormal carpal motion if one or more of the following criteria are present: (1) abnormal carpal alignment on the four-view wrist survey radiographs, (2) scapholunate joint or ligament pain on physical examination, (3) reproducible painful popping or clicking, and (4) capitolunate instability.[66]

Our conventional 17-view radiographic ligament instability series for each wrist consists of anteroposterior (AP) clenched fist and PA views in neutral, radial, and ulnar deviation; radial and ulnar translation views in PA position; a 30° semipronated oblique view; lateral views in neutral, full flexion, and full extension; lateral views with ulnar and radial deviation; dorsal and volar capitolunate instability pattern (CLIP) wrist stress views; and 30° semisupinated off-lateral oblique views.[54, 66, 67, 71] Comparison views of the unaffected wrist are helpful for detecting motion abnormalities and normal variations. Modification of this full instability series is performed as directed by one of the four indications just listed.[67]

Active and assisted carpal motions may also be studied using fluoroscopy with videotape record. Motions should include active and passive flexion/extension, radial-ulnar deviation, and idiosyncratic maneuvers that recreate an individual patient's symptoms. This method of examination is of particular use in detecting dynamic ligament instabilities and for the patient with a history of clicking or popping whose wrist appears normal on plain films. The movement that causes the sound should be reproduced as closely as possible.[18] Videotape facilitates full assessment of intercarpal motion because it enables repeated review of all motions, and slow-motion or step-motion review of the study.

Scintigraphy

Technetium Tc 99m (^{99m}Tc) bone scans are extremely sensitive physiologic studies that can be divided into at least three phases: vascular (angiographic), equilibrium (blood pool), and delayed (bone).[24] Although the anatomic resolution is limited, this modality's exquisite sensitivity to new bone production makes it especially valuable for excluding osteochondral or osseous abnormalities when the preceding radiographic work-up is normal. Close monitoring of the technical aspects, especially the type of collimator used, facilitates recognition of abnormal areas and the identification of individual abnormal carpal bones.

The bone scan must be detailed enough to examine both wrists in dorsal and ventral views with additional lateral or oblique views to enable localization of any hot spots to a specific carpal bone or to a particular site in the wrist (Fig. 7–11A). When correlated with the locus of the clinical complex, detection of such an abnormal area can direct more detailed spot films or tomography.

Radioisotope uptake occurs in specific sites of increased bone turnover secondary to an osseous or chondral fracture or to one of the various causes of local hyperemia, i.e., infection or synovitis. Broader areas of increased uptake are seen in synovitis as well as other inflammatory processes involving the soft tissues. It is uncertain whether purely ligamentous injuries without bone involvement can produce hot spots.

Conventional and Computed Tomography

Tomography is indicated to characterize and stage any questionable bone abnormality found on conventional radiographs or fluoroscopy, especially if there is clinical correlation with a focally abnormal bone scan.[75]

Although conventional tomography has been essentially supplanted by computed tomography (CT) in ease and ready availability, it remains a valuable adjunct in selected patients. Sections are taken at 2-mm or 3-mm intervals in two positions at 90° to each other. Occasionally, 1-mm sections may be necessary to show an abnormality such as a small osseous component of an osteochondral fracture. The best position for polytomography is determined by the specific bone in question, and the wrist should be placed in the position that optimally profiles this bone (Fig. 7–11B). Fluoroscopy can facilitate optimal wrist positioning prior to tomography.

Computed tomography is a substitution technology for conventional tomography. The technical factors of the examination must be tailored to the clinical question and to the anatomic focus of interest. Detection of nondisplaced carpal bone fractures and assessment of fracture union status may necessitate contiguous thin (1-mm to 2-mm) sections through the affected carpal bone(s) in two orthogonal planes (e.g., parallel with and perpendicular to the long axis of the scaphoid). The choice of scanning plane should minimize the number of slices necessary to "cover" the area of clinical concern and should be oriented perpendicular to the plane of fracture or other pathology, if possible. In our opinion, spiral (helical or slip-ring) CT currently does not have a routine role in imaging the wrist.

Fractures, including those of the hamate hook, can be easily demonstrated with CT.[15, 16, 29, 60, 75] However, CT is not often necessary to demonstrate such fractures, because directed conventional radiographic examinations detect fractures at much lower expense.

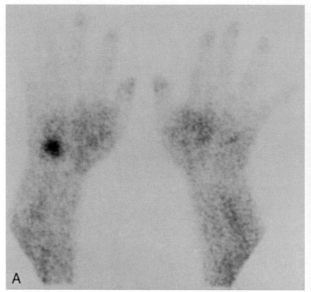

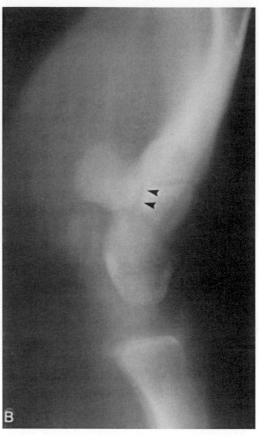

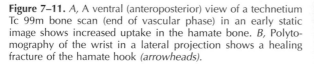

Figure 7–11. *A,* A ventral (anteroposterior) view of a technetium Tc 99m bone scan (end of vascular phase) in an early static image shows increased uptake in the hamate bone. *B,* Polytomography of the wrist in a lateral projection shows a healing fracture of the hamate hook *(arrowheads).*

Similarly, the extent of lunate fragmentation in Kienböck's disease is readily shown by CT scan. CT is also valuable when pain or cast immobilization prevents optimal positioning of the wrist for plain radiographs, and in situations in which, even with adequate radiographs, the diagnosis is still uncertain.[7, 10, 46, 60] Both wrists should be symmetrically positioned with the palms flat on the table top inside the CT scanner for transaxial plane sections. If direct acquisition of the desired orthogonal plane cannot be obtained, contiguous or overlapping thin sections are required to obtain diagnostic-quality reformations of the images.

Distal radioulnar joint instability may be difficult to diagnose both clinically and radiographically. Thin (2-mm to 3-mm) axial contiguous CT sections of both wrists obtained in the extremes of pronation and supination, or in some other position that produces pain of the presenting type, best demonstrate the alignment of the ulnar dome within the sigmoid notch and allow use of the unaffected wrist as control.

As a general rule, CT of the wrist, except when used for distal radioulnar, lunate, and hamate hook problems, can be performed in other positions to show the margins of the carpal bones for better osseous detail. The coronal plane is obtained with the wrist elevated off the CT table and dorsiflexed and the gantry tilted toward the patient's elbow, or with the patient prone with the forearm and hand, thumb up, above the head and nearly perpendicular to the CT table. The resultant CT sections display the carpus in the coronal plane, which provides sections looking like PA tomograms of the wrist. These sections allow much easier interpretation of subtle and gross wrist abnormalities.[5, 6, 60] The oblique sagittal plane, with the long axis of the scaphoid in the plane of the CT section, is valuable to show the sagittal long axis of the scaphoid.[60, 75] Need for other information may lead to direct sagittal plane images or oblique views of the scaphotrapeziotrapezoidal joint.[60]

Wrist Arthrography

When a patient's history, plain films, and ligament instability series suggest an intercarpal ligamentous problem, arthrography may be used to confirm the diagnosis. Arthrography may also demonstrate nonunion of carpal bone fractures as the flow of contrast medium through a fracture defect.

In young normal patients, there are four or five noncommunicating joints within the wrist: the distal radioulnar joint (DRUJ), the radiocarpal joint (RCJ), the midcarpal joint (MCJ), the first metacarpal trapezial joint, and the pisotriquetral joint. In our experience, the pisotriquetral joint communicates with the

RCJ in about 75% of normal wrists. In almost all patients, carpometacarpal (CMC) joints 2 through 5 commonly communicate with the MCJ. As a normal variant, the fourth and fifth CMC joints occasionally do not fill when the second and third CMC joints fill. Communications with the first metacarpotrapezial joint are statistically abnormal but of uncertain clinical significance.

Contrast medium may be injected into one or more of the three principal noncommunicating spaces in the carpus: DRUJ, RCJ, and MCJ. The decision to perform single versus three-compartment arthrography rests upon the specific clinical questions that need answering and the recognized limitations of wrist arthrography.

A small number (less than 5 percent) of interjoint communications appear to be robustly unidirectional, that is, they are shown only on injection of one but not both joints divided by an interosseous ligament or triangular fibrocartilage (TFC).[72] Most "one-way" communications seem to be related to technical factors, especially the volume of contrast injected into a joint, rather than to a peculiar morphology and related pathophysiology ("ball-valve" effect). Similarly, some capsular detachments of the foveal margin of the DRUJ may be shown only by DRUJ arthrography.[32] Moreover, normal or postinflammatory joint partitioning may necessitate a direct attempt at injection of the sequestered or unfilled joint. For example, if a patient is symptomatic at a pisotriquetral joint space not filled during RCJ arthrography, the joint may be injected directly. Finally, interjoint communications appear to be a normal accoutrement of aging,[45] frequently are bilaterally symmetric,[8, 23] and often are clinically silent.[8, 42, 43]

TECHNIQUE

Techniques for individual and multiple compartment wrist arthrography have been described in the literature.[19, 23, 32, 52, 64] We inject the radiocarpal joint to maximal distention at either the radioscaphoid or radiolunate joints away from the site of utmost tenderness, using a dilute, water-soluble contrast material such as Conray 43 (iothalamate meglumine) diluted 2:1 with anesthetic as lidocaine 1% (Fig. 7–12A). Filling of the distal radioulnar joint after injection of the radiocarpal joint indicates a perforation in the triangular fibrocartilage complex (TFCC). When contrast material injected into the radiocarpal joint enters the midcarpal joint, the site of communication indicates a perforation of that structure, i.e., the scapholunate ligament, the lunotriquetral ligament, or the radial or ulnar capsule (Fig. 7–12B).

Fluoroscopic spot films should be obtained during injection in order to determine which ligament is perforated, because on the complete filling phase, the anatomy may be obscured by overlying contrast material.[19] Alternatively, the injection may be recorded with videotape or digital fluoroscopy.[52] We commonly use digital acquisition of images (so that digital subtraction can be applied), because it more accurately depicts the routes of contrast passage between joints during injections; however, nonsubtraction images are necessary for reliable detection of postexercise communications.[76]

Because the scapholunate ligament is commonly abnormal and it is the wrist joint that is most commonly diastatic, the wrist is maintained in a position with the scapholunate joint profiled during the filling phase (Fig. 7–12C). If no perforations have been detected after injection of contrast material, stress views are obtained under fluoroscopic control to facilitate visualization of communicating defects that may not fill during routine injection. Radial- and ulnar-deviated views with the wrist in both PA and AP positions are diagnostically valuable maneuvers to create moderate stress in a wrist distended with contrast material. An abnormal scapholunate (SL) or lunotriquetral (LT) ligament can falsely appear normal when it has been bridged with scar tissue.[41] However, replacement of the normal undulating shouldered contour of the ligament at its origin or insertion as seen on RCJ arthrography by a sharp edge is very suggestive of ligamentous rupture, with or without posttraumatic scarring.[47] MCJ injection is excellent to show an abnormal SL or LT ligament that has a noncommunicating defect.[41]

If no abnormalities are detected to explain the patient's problem and the patient has ulnar-sided wrist pain, a distal radioulnar joint injection to maximal distention may be performed to diagnose partial proximal surface disruptions of the triangular fibrocartilage complex. This is best performed following a temporal delay sufficient to allow significant dilution and resorption of contrast in the RCJ.

We inject the MCJ to maximal distention either at the "four corners" junction of the lunotriquetral and capitohamate joints or along the distal scaphocapitate joint. The SL joint is usually maintained in profile during contrast instillation. The postinjection examination, including the radial and ulnar deviation "stress" views and postexercise filming, is identical to that for RCJ arthrography.

MCJ arthrography detects a few more interjoint communications, especially radial-sided capsular communications, than RCJ arthrography.[64, 72] Thus, when we are performing three-compartment wrist arthrography, we initially inject the MCJ and, if no RCJ communication is shown, the DRUJ. Following an appropriate temporal delay, we inject the RCJ. As mentioned previously, MCJ injections are preferable to RCJ injections to identify scarring or other abnormality of the SL ligament and noncommunicating avulsions of the SL or LT ligaments from their attachments to the scaphoid, lunate, or triquetrum.

Given the frequency of interjoint communications in normal wrists, it is not surprising that there is a poor correlation between individual interjoint communications and patient symptoms.[8, 42, 43] However, specific arthrographic findings do seem to correlate with patient symptoms. Periscaphoid transcapsular

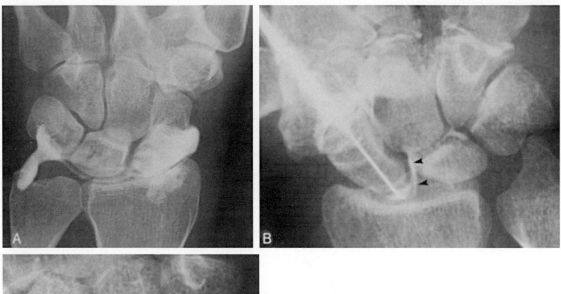

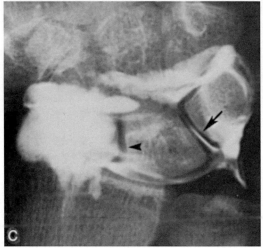

Figure 7–12. *A,* Posteroanterior view of the wrist following a normal radiocarpal joint arthrogram. Contrast remains confined to the radiocarpal space. *B,* Following a radiocarpal joint space injection, contrast tracks *(arrowheads)* through a disrupted scapholunate ligament to fill the midcarpal and carpometacarpal joint spaces. *C,* Following a radiocarpal joint space arthrogram, the scapholunate ligament is intact, because contrast has not yet filled the scapholunate space *(arrowhead)*; however, contrast tracks through the lunotriquetral joint space *(arrow)* as a result of lunotriquetral ligament disruption.

interjoint communications have not been described in normal wrists and seem to be associated with radial-sided pain.[38] Capsular detachments of the foveal margin of the DRUJ[33] and combined TFC-LT perforations (especially with ulnar-positive variance)[42, 43] correlate with ulnar-sided symptoms. It has been suggested that asymmetric communications (those present on the patient's affected wrist but not on his or her normal wrist) may have greater diagnostic significance.[8, 23] Finally, loss of the palmar interligamentous sulcus is associated with disruption of the radioscaphocapitate ligament and may be seen in some cases of rotary subluxation of the scaphoid and palmar intercalated segment instability.[47]

Additional information as to the origin of pain may be gained by mixing a small amount of anesthetic with the contrast agent and, after injection of one or more of these wrist compartments, noting whether the patient's presenting symptoms have been relieved (RL Linscheid, MD, personal communication, 1986). As mentioned previously, we perform this step routinely.

Magnetic Resonance Imaging

Unlike other imaging modalities, MR imaging does not rely on ionizing radiation.[65] Instead, using a magnetic field, it generates a proton map of the patient's anatomy. This mapping may have different appearances, depending on the manner in which the scan is performed. Scans may be performed to take advantage of different tissue characteristics, e.g., relative fat and water concentrations in the tissue examined.

Patients with wrist pain, for whom plain films are normal and a bone scan is abnormal are especially suited for MR imaging. In patients with unexplained wrist pain, MR imaging aids in the diagnosis of avascular necrosis with a high degree of specificity, and its use suggests a more specific diagnosis than does bone scan in a significant proportion of the cases.[51] MR imaging is particularly useful in patients suspected of having stage I Kienböck's disease[26, 30, 65] and in patients with scaphoid fracture for whom a diagnosis of proximal pole avascular necrosis or nonunion is considered (Fig. 7–13).[27, 65] Additionally, MR imaging can exclude occult scaphoid fractures in the acute setting when plain films are normal and clinical findings strongly suggestive.

Although MR imaging has been reported as an effective modality to evaluate the integrity of the TFC as well as the SL and LT interosseous ligaments,[22, 65] not all investigators have been able to reproduce the optimistic early reports. Extrinsic ligaments are commonly demonstrable,[59, 65] but specific ligaments are not reliably shown on each examination. Further, MR imaging has not been reported to show normal variations in ligament course that can be recognized anatomically. Therefore, we believe this modality should be applied only with caution in the diagnosis of intrinsic and extrinsic ligamentous abnormalities.

Nevertheless, MR imaging can clearly demonstrate synovial proliferation and distinguish "synovitis" from synovial fibrosis.[65] The adjunctive use of intravenous gadolinium-DTPA may allow accurate quantification of synovial inflammation in arthritis and thereby facilitate the early assessment of response to therapy.

Currently, we infrequently recommend MR imaging for post-traumatic wrist symptoms unless lunatomalacia, unrecognized fracture, or another process affecting the marrow (such as a bone bruise) is a leading diagnostic consideration.

CARPAL INSTABILITY

The joints of the wrist are superbly congruent, and pathologic subluxation may lead to "giving out" (instability) and to accelerated and potentially disabling osteoarthritis. Common end-stage conditions, such as scapholunate advanced collapse (SLAC), may occur from loss of integrity of a carpal bone (scaphoid nonunion) or ligament (scapholunate interosseous or radioscaphocapitate ligament). Although physiologic insufficiency may be evident as a resting deformity, resting deformity commonly does not reflect the severity and extent of underlying soft tissue injury. However, the range of transarticular displacement found under physiologic or "stress" loading that exceeds that seen in a normal joint directly reflects the magnitude of disruption to the supporting soft tissue skeleton.[34]

Carpal instabilities are conditions in which carpal bones have lost normal alignment and intercarpal

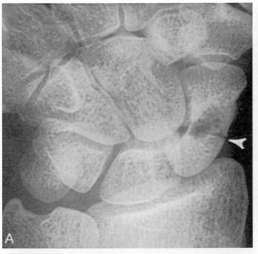
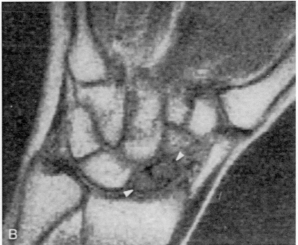
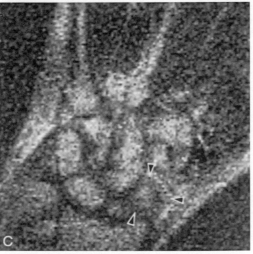

Figure 7–13. *A,* Ulnar deviation posteroanterior view of the left wrist shows a transverse scaphoid waist fracture *(arrowhead)* with an accompanying oval lucency. An adjacent band of sclerosis is present in the distal pole. *B,* T$_1$-weighted magnetic resonance image of the same wrist shows decreased signal (darker areas) about the fracture and the proximal two thirds of the scaphoid (between *arrowheads*), indicating replacement of marrow fat. *C,* T$_2$-weighted magnetic resonance image (compared with adjacent carpal bones) demonstrates decreased signal proximal *(arrowheads)* and normal signal distal to the fracture line. The combination of abnormal T$_1$- and T$_2$-weighted images, both with decreased signal in the proximal pole, appears to be specific for avascular necrosis.[52, 66] Even in retrospect, the plain film does not suggest the diagnosis of avascular necrosis.

Table 7–1. LIGAMENTOUS INSTABILITY OF THE WRIST

Ligamentous Instability	Scapholunate Angle	Capitolunate Angle	Comments
Normal (Fig. 7–14A and B)	30°–60°	0–30°	—
Dorsiflexion (DISI) (lateral view) Lunate tilts dorsally and scaphoid tilts palmarly (Fig. 7–14C and D)	60°–80° = ? abnormal >80° = abnormal	Normal or increased	Present when the scapholunate and/or the capitolunate angle is abnormal and abnormal intercarpal motion exists
Palmar flexion (VISI) (lateral view) Both lunate and scaphoid tilt palmarly (Fig. 7–14E and F)	<30°	<30° or normal	Present when abnormal intercarpal motion exists
Ulnar translocation (PA view) Carpal bones are ulnar in position (Fig. 7–2A)	Normal	Normal	Space increases between scaphoid and radial styloid; over 50 percent of lunate is medial to radius on neutral PA hand position
Dorsal subluxation (lateral view) Carpal bones are dorsal to midplane of the radius (Fig. 7–14G)	Normal	Normal	Usually this has an associated dorsally impacted distal radius fracture
Palmar subluxation (lateral view) Carpal bones are palmar to midplane of the radius (Figs. 7–14H and 7–2B)	Normal	Normal	In reported cases, there is associated ulnar translocation

Modified from Gilula LA, Destouet JM, Weeks PM, et al: Roentgenographic diagnosis of the painful wrist. Clin Orthop Relat Res 187:56, 1984.

motion because of osseous fracture, or interruption of some of the intrinsic or extrinsic ligaments or both, resulting in hand dysfunction.[3, 20, 56, 58] Recognition of these conditions is necessary for proper patient treatment. At times, patients can have instability patterns with minimal symptoms; however, in many cases, this instability progresses to further disruption between carpal bones.

Delayed recognition or unsuccessful conservative treatment of carpal ligament instabilities can lead to irreversible scar formation in and about the carpus, with atypical alignment and abnormal function of the carpal bones. Malaligned carpal bones may be associated with early degenerative arthritis and the formation of pseudojoints (see Fig. 7–6). In fact, carpal instability may be the single reason a patient receives major compensation for loss of hand and wrist function.

Carpal malalignment may be static (i.e., recognizable on neutral PA and lateral radiographs) or dynamic (i.e., abnormal alignment and motion between carpal bones recognizable only during either active or passive maneuvers, whether observed clinically or fluoroscopically).

The majority of static carpal malalignments can be classified into one of six radiographic patterns.[3, 20, 36] They are: (1) ulnar translocation, (2) palmar carpal subluxation, (3) dorsal carpal subluxation, (4) rotary subluxation of the scaphoid (RSS), (5) dorsiflexion or dorsal collapse (DISI—dorsal intercalated segmental instability), and (6) palmar flexion or palmar collapse (VISI—ventral intercalated segmental instability) (Table 7–1) (Fig. 7–14). A complete classification of carpal instabilities can be found in Chapter 12.

The key to recognizing each of these malalignment patterns is to identify the interrelationships between the scaphoid, lunate, capitate, and radius on neutral PA and lateral radiographs. The systematic search (see discussions of neutral PA and neutral lateral views) for malalignment using the analysis of carpal arcs, apparent joint width, lunate and scaphoid conformation, and intercarpal angles allows the assignment of a wrist as radiographically normal, abnormal, or indeterminant for a static malalignment.

Except for ulnar translocation, the neutral lateral wrist radiograph is more reliable in detecting malalignment patterns than is the PA or AP view. On the lateral view, the scapholunate angle ranges from 30°

Figure 7–14. A to H, Ligament instability patterns of the wrist (see Table 7–1); C = capitate axis; L = lunate axis; S = scaphoid axis. A, The scapholunate angle is normal between 30° and 60° and is sometimes normal up to 80°. Although here the scaphoid axis (S) is drawn through the center of the scaphoid, it is easier and is also adequate to draw a scaphoid axis line tangent to the proximal and distal ventral convexities of the scaphoid.[20] (See axis S in view E.) B, The capitolunate angle is normally less than 30°. C, Dorsiflexion instability (DISI) is suspected when there is dorsal tilting of the lunate and ventral tilting of the scaphoid with resultant increased scapholunate angle, with or without an increased capitolunate angle. D, Dorsiflexion instability. As the lunate tilts dorsally and the scaphoid tilts ventrally, the lunate tends to move ventrally and the capitate dorsally. E, Palmar flexion instability (VISI) is suspected with a scapholunate angle decreased to less than 30° and/or a capitolunate angle of 30° or more. F, In palmar flexion instability, the scaphoid and lunate both tilt ventrally. The lunate tends to move or slide dorsally; and although the distal pole of the capitate tends to tilt dorsally, the head (or proximal end) tends to move ventrally. G, With dorsal carpal subluxation, the center of the carpus is dorsal to the center of the midaxis of the radius. H, Palmar carpal subluxation is recognized when the central axis of the carpus and lunate is ventral to the midaxis of the radius. (From Gilula LA, Weeks PM: Post-traumatic ligamentous instabilities of the wrist. Radiology 129:641–651, 1978.)

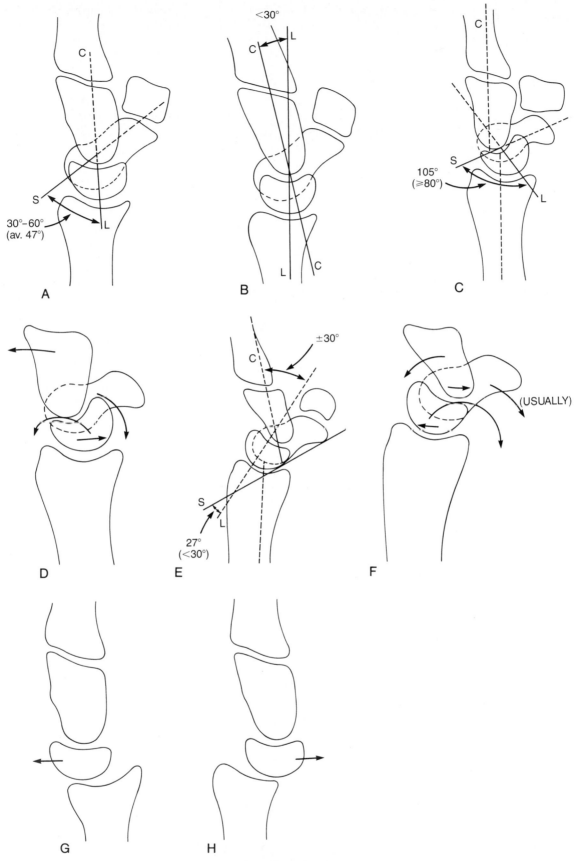

Figure 7–14 *See legend on opposite page*

to 60° and is borderline abnormal up to 80° (Fig. 7–14A), and the normal absolute capitolunate angle is less than 30° (Fig. 7–14B) (see Table 7–1).

Ulnar Translocation

In ulnar translocation (UT), the carpus has subluxed ulnarly, so that on the neutral PA view, more than half of the proximal articular surface of the lunate lies ulnar to the radius, and there may be more space (more than the width of other intercarpal spaces) either between the radial styloid process and scaphoid (type I; see Fig. 7–6A) or between the scaphoid and lunate (type II). In other words, in type I translocation, the entire carpus is subluxed ulnarly and in type II translocation, the scaphoid remains in the scaphoid fossa and the rest of the carpus is subluxed ulnarly.[20, 61] Concomitant palmar translocation is expected as the magnitude of UT increases. UT may also be reproducibly quantified by application of indices developed by McMurtry and colleagues[40] or Chamay.[21] Although uncommon following trauma, ulnar translocation is common in synovium-based processes, such as rheumatoid arthritis.

Subluxation

In dorsal carpal subluxation, the carpus displaces dorsally onto the distal articular surface of the radius (Fig. 7–14G; see Table 7–1). It is usually associated with a dorsally impacted malunion of the distal radius. Over time, a so-called adaptive carpus with a "pseudo-VISI" pattern may develop.[15]

In the uncommon palmar carpal subluxation,[3] the carpus often has an associated ulnar carpal subluxation (Fig. 7–14H). This condition is recognized on the lateral radiograph when the central axis of the lunate and carpus is ventral to the midaxis of the shaft of the radius.

Rotary subluxation of the scaphoid (RSS) is a pathologic displacement of the scaphoid following partial or complete disruption of its ligamentous attachments.[70] Most commonly, the proximal pole subluxes dorsally at the radioscaphoid joint in association with pathologic palmar rotation of the distal pole relative to the lunate (SL angle greater than 80°), capitate and radius (see Chapter 15). Unlike in DISI, this ventral tilting of the scaphoid in RSS is accompanied by normal alignment and motion of the lunate on an instability series.

Flexion Malalignments

Dorsiflexion malalignment (DISI) may be suspected when the PA view shows scaphoid foreshortening, a rhomboid-shaped lunate profile,[8] and an increased overlap of the proximal and distal carpal rows, partic-

ularly of the lunate over the capitate.[20] On the neutral lateral view, the DISI pattern is recognized as dorsal tilting of the lunate; that is, the lunate tilts so that its distal articular surface faces more dorsally than normal (Fig. 7–14C and D; see Table 7–1). A so-called dissociated carpal instability (CID) is present if there is an associated scapholunate dissociation (RSS, SL diastasis, SL angle greater than 80°) or an LT dissociation. Alternatively, a nondissociated carpal instability (CIND) with DISI is present if relations within the proximal carpal row are normal and there is abnormal capitolunate alignment.[73]

Palmar flexion malalignment is a condition also known as VISI (see Table 7–1). The diagnosis may be suspected from the PA view when (1) there is both foreshortening of the scaphoid and a triangular shape to the lunate and (2) adjacent dorsal articular surfaces of the scaphoid and lunate are parallel. The lateral view shows palmar flexion of both the lunate and the scaphoid, so that the scapholunate angle is decreased (usually less than 30°), the capitolunate angle is increased (absolute CL angle almost always greater than 30°), or both (Fig. 7–14E and F). The distal carpal row, as identified by the capitate, is usually displaced palmarly so that the lunate overlaps the capitate, and on the PA view, this overlap appears to be greater than that on the opposite, normal side. If there is an associated LT and/or SL dissociation, a VISI-CID is present (see Chapter 16); however, if the relationships within the proximal carpal row are normal, a VISI-CIND is diagnosed (see Chapter 17).

When either DISI or VISI is suspected, the scapholunate and capitolunate angles should be measured, and, at minimum, the three lateral views listed in the discussion of the ligament instability series (neutral, full flexion, and extension) should be performed. The lateral neutral view should be obtained with the dorsum of the metacarpals and the radius in a straight line. With flexion and extension, carpal motion should be normal. The lunate can be used to identify the proximal, and the capitate the distal, carpal rows.[20, 36] On flexion, the capitate axis should be flexed palmar to the lunate axis, and the lunate axis should be flexed with respect to the long axis of the radius. On extension, the capitate axis should be extended with respect to the lunate axis, and the lunate axis should be extended with respect to the radius axis. These extension and flexion views should be abnormal in a patient with DISI and normal in a patient with RSS. Similarly, the ulnar and radial deviation views of the wrist in lateral position should demonstrate normal lunate motion in a patient with RSS and abnormal motion in a patient with DISI. The normal lunate tilts palmarly with radial deviation and dorsally with ulnar deviation.[61] When evaluation of carpal motion is performed, comparison views of the opposite side are mandatory.

DISCUSSION

A thorough clinical history and physical examination form the most solid basis for reaching a definitive diagnosis of wrist pain. When a definite clinical diagnosis can be made, a radiographic examination may not be necessary. However, such diagnoses as ganglion, tenosynovitis, and de Quervain's disease may be associated with underlying, unsuspected disease.

A wrist survey is recommended in all patients in order to exclude anatomic variants,[18, 69] osteophytes, ischemic necrosis, degenerative joint disease, and even old, non-united fractures that are not clinically suspected. This survey may change the surgical approach to the patient's problem and may alter expectations for full recovery.

If after the initial clinical investigation no definitive diagnosis is made, plain films of the wrist should be obtained. When the plain films are normal, the work-up should proceed as described in the algorithm (see Fig. 7–1), depending on whether bony or soft tissue abnormality is suspected.

If a bony abnormality is suspected, detailed spot views or fluoroscopic spot films of a tender site may be helpful. If these do not reveal the cause of the patient's problem, MR imaging or bone scanning is the next step used to localize and verify subtle bone abnormalities, such as hairline fractures, avulsion injuries, and chondral-osteochondral abnormalities. Once the bone scan or MR image has detected an abnormal region, plain films, fluoroscopic detailed views, or tomography (plain or CT) may be useful for further definition of the abnormality.

If a ligamentous injury is suspected, an instability series may demonstrate static malalignments and abnormal intercarpal motion. Dynamic motion studies or stress views may detect dynamic ligamentous instabilities or may define the cause of popping or clicking. Wrist arthrography may then be used to further define the nature of the ligamentous or capsular abnormality, particularly when the patient has point tenderness localized over the dorsum of the wrist. As with bone abnormalities, if these radiographic measures fail to demonstrate an anatomic abnormality, a bone scan may reveal an area of abnormal uptake of radioisotope. In the patient with a persistent focal bone scan abnormality (especially if the bone scan is prominently or markedly abnormal) and clinically significant debility, a practical clinical and radiologic evaluation should be done to try to explain the abnormality, because such findings are rarely, if ever, meaningless. In this situation, MR imaging is strongly recommended to evaluate for bone marrow abnormality such as unrecognized fracture or bone marrow edema.

Acknowledgement

We are grateful to Drs. Judy M. Destouet and William R. Reinus for their original contributions to this work.

References

1. Ashmead D, Watson HK: Physical examination of the wrist and hand. II. Examination of the hand and wrist. In Gilula LA, Yin Y (eds): Imaging of the Wrist and Hand. Philadelphia, WB Saunders, 1996, pp 19–21.
2. Beckenbaugh RD: Accurate evaluation and management of the painful wrist following injury: An approach to carpal instability. Orthop Clin North Am 15:289–306, 1984.
3. Bellinghausen HW, Gilula LA, Young LV: Post-traumatic palmar carpal subluxation. J Bone Joint Surg 65A:998–1006, 1983.
4. Berger RA, Dobyns JH: Physical examination and provocative maneuvers of the wrist. In Gilula LA, Yin Y (eds): Imaging of the Wrist and Hand. Philadelphia, WB Saunders, 1996, pp 23–42.
5. Biondetti PR, Vannier MD, Gilula LA, Knapp R: Three-dimensional surface reconstruction of the carpal bones from CT scans: Transaxial versus coronal technique. Comput Med Imaging Graph 12:67–73, 1988.
6. Biondetti PR, Vannier MW, Gilula LA, Knapp R: Wrist: Coronal and transaxial CT scanning. Radiology 163:149–151, 1987.
7. Bowers WH: Problems of the distal radioulnar joint. Adv Orthop Surg 7:289–303, 1984.
8. Cantor RM, Stern PJ, Wyrick JD, Michaels SE: The relevance of ligament tears or perforations in the diagnosis of wrist pain: An arthrographic study. J Hand Surg [Am] 19A:945–953, 1994.
9. Chernin MM, Pitt MJ: Radiographic disease patterns at the carpus. Clin Orthop 187:72–80, 1984.
10. Cone RO, Szabo R, Resnick D, et al: Computed tomography of the normal radioulnar joints. Invest Radiol 18:541–545, 1983.
11. Conway WF, Destouet JM, Gilula LA, et al: The carpal boss: An overview of radiographic evaluation. Radiology 156:29–31, 1985.
12. Cope JR: Rotatory subluxation of the scaphoid. Clin Radiol 35:495–501, 1984.
13. Curtis DJ: Injuries of the wrist: An approach to diagnosis. Radiol Clin North Am 19:625–644, 1981.
14. DiBenedetto MR, Lubbers LM, Coleman CR: A standardized measurement of ulnar carpal translocation. J Hand Surg [Am] 15A:1009–1010, 1990.
15. Doig SG, Rao SG, Carvell JE: Late carpal instability with dorsal distal radial fracture. Injury 22:486–488, 1991.
16. Egawa M, Asai T: Fracture of the hook of the hamate: Report of six cases and the suitability of computerized tomography. J Hand Surg 8:393–398, 1983.
17. Gilula LA: Carpal injuries: Analytic approach and case exercises. AJR 133:503–517, 1979.
18. Gilula LA, Destouet JM, Weeks PM, et al: Roentgenographic diagnosis of the painful wrist. Clin Orthop Relat Res 187:52–64, 1984.
19. Gilula LA, Totty WG, Weeks PM: Wrist arthrography: The value of fluoroscopic spot viewing. Radiology 146:555–556, 1983.
20. Gilula LA, Weeks PM: Post-traumatic ligamentous instabilities of the wrist. Radiology 129:641–651, 1978.
21. Green DP: Carpal dislocations and instabilities. In Green DP (ed): Operative Hand Surgery, ed 3. New York, Churchill-Livingstone, 1992, pp 861–928.
22. Greenan T, Zlatkin MB: Magnetic resonance imaging of the wrist. Semin Ultrasound CT MR 11:267–287, 1990.
23. Herbert TJ, Faithfull RG, McCann DJ, Ireland J: Bilateral arthrography of the wrist. J Hand Surg [Br] 15B:233–235, 1990.
24. Holder LE: Bone scintigraphy. In Gilula LA, Yin Y (eds): Imaging of the Wrist and Hand. Philadelphia, WB Saunders, 1996, pp 319–350.
25. Hu CH, Kundel HL, Nodine CF, et al: Searching for bone fractures: A comparison with pulmonary nodule search. Acta Radiol 1:25–32, 1994.
26. Imaeda T, Nakamura R, Miura T, Makino N: Magnetic resonance imaging in Keinböck's disease. J Hand Surg [Br] 17B:12–19, 1992.
27. Imaeda T, Nakamura R, Miura T, Makino N: Magnetic reso-

nance imaging in scaphoid fractures. J Hand Surg [Br] 17B:20–27, 1992.

28. King GJW, McMurtry RY: Physical examination of the wrist and hand. I: Physical examination of the wrist. In Gilula LA, Yin Y (eds): Imaging of the Wrist and Hand. Philadelphia, WB Saunders, 1996, pp 5–18.

29. Kreitner V K-F: Die isolierte fraktur des hamulus ossis hamatieine leicht zu ubersehende handwurzelverletzung. Fortschr Roentgenstr 159:398–399, 1993.

30. Kuzma GR: Kienböck's disease. Adv Orthop Surg 8:250–263, 1985.

31. Larsen CF, Lauritsen J: Epidemiology of acute wrist trauma. Int J Epidemiol 22:911–916, 1993.

32. Levinsohn EM, Palmer AK: Arthrography of the traumatized wrist. Radiology 146:647–651, 1983.

33. Levinsohn EM, Palmer AK, Coren AB, Zinberg E: Wrist arthrography: The value of the three compartment injection technique. Skeletal Radiol 16:539–544, 1987.

34. Logan SE, Nowak MD: Intrinsic and extrinsic wrist ligaments: Biomechanical and functional differences. Biomed Sci Instrum 23:9–13, 1987.

35. Linscheid RL, Dobyns JH: Athletic injuries of the wrist. Clin Orthop 198:141–151, 1985.

36. Linscheid RL, Dobyns JH, Beabout JW, et al: Traumatic instability of the wrist. J Bone Joint Surg [Am] 54A:1612–1632, 1972.

37. Mann FA, Wilson AJ, Gilula LA: Radiographic evaluation of the wrist: What does the hand surgeon want to know? Radiology 184:15–24, 1992.

38. Mann FA, Wilson AJ, Gilula LA: Triple-injection wrist arthrography: A study of pathology or technique? J Hand Surg [Am] (accepted).

39. Mayfield JK: Patterns of injury to carpal ligaments: A spectrum. Clin Orthop 187:36–42, 1984.

40. McMurtry RY, Youm Y, Flatt AE, Gillespie TE: Kinematics of the wrist. II: Clinical applications. J Bone Joint Surg [Am] 60A:955–961, 1978.

41. Metz VM, Gilula LA: Is this scapholunate joint normal? J Hand Surg [Am] 18A:746–755, 1993.

42. Metz VM, Mann FA, Gilula LA: Three compartment wrist arthrography: Correlation of pain site with location of uni- and bidirectional communications. AJR 160:819–822, 1993.

43. Metz VM, Mann FA, Gilula LA: Lack of correlation of wrist pain and location of noncommunicating defects shown by three compartment wrist arthrography. AJR 160:1239–1243, 1993.

44. Metz VM, Schimmerl SM, Gilula LA, et al: Wide scapholunate joint space in lunotriquetral coalition: A normal variant? Radiology 188:557–559, 1993.

45. Mikic ZD: Age changes in the triangular fibrocartilage of the wrist joint. J Anat 126:367–384, 1978.

46. Mino DE, Palmer AK, Levinsohn EM: Radiography and computerized tomography in the diagnosis of incongruity of the distal radioulnar joint. J Bone Joint Surg [Am] 67A:247–252, 1985.

47. Obermann WR: Radiology of Carpal Instability. Amsterdam, Elsevier, 1994, pp 131–172.

48. Palmer A, Glisson RR, Werner FW: Ulnar variance determination. J Hand Surg [Am] 7A:376–379, 1982.

49. Peh W, Gilula LA: Normal disruption of carpal arcs. J Hand Surg [Am] 21:561–566, 1996.

50. Polley HF, Hunder GG: The wrist and carpal joints. In Rheumatologic Interviewing and Physical Examination of the Joints, ed 2. Philadelphia, WB Saunders, 1978, pp 90–111.

51. Reinus WR, Conway WF, Totty WG, et al: Carpal avascular necrosis: MR imaging. Radiology 160:689–693, 1986.

52. Resnick D, Andre M, Kerr R, et al: Digital arthrography of the wrist: A radiographic-pathologic investigation. AJR 142:1187–1190, 1984.

53. Ruby LK, Stinson J, Belsky MR: The natural history of scaphoid nonunion: A review of fifty-five cases. J Bone Joint Surg [Am] 67A:428–432, 1985.

54. Schernberg F: Radiography for wrist instabilities. In Gilula LA, Yin Y (eds): Imaging of the Wrist and Hand. Philadelphia, WB Saunders, 1996, pp 169–188.

55. Schimmerl SM, Metz VM, Totterman SMS, et al: Anatomic variation of the scapholunate joint: Where should the SL joint be measured? Presented at the annual oration of the Radiological Society of North America (RSNA), Chicago, IL, 1993.

56. Sebald JR, Dobyns JH, Linscheid RL: The natural history of collapse deformities of the wrist. Clin Orthop 104:140–148, 1974.

57. Sennwald G, Fischer W, Stahelin A: Malunion of the distal radius and its treatment. Int Orthop 16:45–51, 1992.

58. Sennwald G, Kern HP, Jacob HAC: Die arthrose dos handgelenks als folge der karpalen instabilitat: Therapeutische alternativen. Orthopade 22:65–71, 1993.

59. Smith DK: Dorsal carpal ligaments of the wrist: Normal appearance on multiplanar reconstructions of three-dimensional Fourier transform MR imaging. AJR 161:119–125, 1993.

60. Stewart NR, Gilula LA: Computed tomography of the wrist: A tailored approach. Radiology 183:13–20, 1992.

61. Taleisnik J: Proximal carpal instability. In The Wrist. New York, Churchill-Livingstone, 1995, pp 305–326.

62. Terry DW, Ramin JE: The navicular fat stripe: A useful roentgen feature for evaluating wrist trauma. AJR 124:25–28, 1975.

63. Tiel-van Buhl MMC, van Beek EJR, Dijkstra PF, et al: Radiography of the carpal scaphoid: Experimental evaluation of "the carpal box" and first clinical results. Invest Radiol 27:954–959, 1992.

64. Tirman RM, Weber ER, Snyder LL, et al: Midcarpal wrist arthrography for detection of tears of the scapholunate and lunotriquetral ligaments. AJR 144:107–108, 1985.

65. Totterman SMS, Miller RJ: MRI of the hand and wrist. In Gilula LA, Yin Y (eds): Imaging of the Wrist and Hand. Philadelphia, WB Saunders, 1996, pp 441–478.

66. Truong NP, Mann FA, Gilula LA: Indications for wrist instability series and its cost-effectiveness. In Gilula LA, Yin Y (eds): Imaging of the Wrist and Hand. Philadelphia, WB Saunders, 1996, pp 188–202.

67. Truong NP, Mann FA, Gilula LA, Kang S-W: Wrist instability series: Increased yield with clinical-radiologic screening criteria. Radiology 192:481–484, 1994.

68. Viegas SF, Wagner K, Patterson R, Peterson P: Medial (hamate) facet of the lunate. J Hand Surg [Am] 15A:564–571, 1990.

69. Voorhees DR, Daffner RH, Nunley JA, et al: Carpal ligamentous disruptions and negative ulnar variance. Skeletal Radiol 13:257–262, 1985.

70. Watson HK, Ryu J: Evolution of arthritis of the wrist. Clin Orthop 202:57–67, 1986.

71. White SJ, Louis DS, Braunstein EM, et al: Capitate-lunate instability: Recognition by manipulation under fluoroscopy. AJR 143:361–364, 1984.

72. Wilson AJ, Gilula LA, Mann FA: Unidirectional joint communication in wrist arthrography: An evaluation of 250 cases. AJR 157:105–109, 1991.

73. Wright TW, Dobyns JH, Linscheid RL, et al: Carpal instability non-dissociative. J Hand Surg [Br] 19:763–773, 1994.

74. Yin Y, Mann FA, Gilula LA: Positions and techniques. In Gilula LA, Yin Y (eds): Imaging of the Wrist and Hand. Philadelphia, WB Saunders, 1996, pp 93–158.

75. Yin Y, McEnery KW, Gilula LA: Computed tomography: Applications and tailored approach. In Gilula LA, Yin Y (eds): Imaging of the Wrist and Hand. Philadelphia, WB Saunders, 1996, pp 411–440.

76. Yin Y, Wilson AJ, Gilula LA: Three-compartment wrist arthrography: Direct comparison of digital subtraction with nonsubtraction images. Radiology 197:287–290, 1995.

CHAPTER 8

Soft Tissue Radiography of the Wrist

Edward F. Downey, Jr, DO, and David J. Curtis, MD

The soft tissue structures are intimately involved in trauma to the hand and wrist yet are often ignored in the evaluation of radiographs. Most descriptions of trauma deal strictly with bony abnormalities. When soft tissue abnormalities are described, the descriptions usually refer to the deep structures of the wrist.[2, 8, 11, 14]

A systematic approach to soft tissue abnormalities of the hand and wrist can be helpful in avoiding misdiagnosis.[3, 4, 6] This approach evaluates soft tissues as well as bone and joint abnormalities and correlates the findings. If discrepancies arise, additional imaging may be necessary for resolution. Good film quality is necessary so that all structures may be adequately visualized. The evaluation of the soft tissue is most useful when reviewing the posteroanterior (PA) and lateral radiographs of the wrist. The relevance of these soft tissue abnormalities can be confirmed by correlating other anatomic findings with the observed distribution of the swelling.[5, 9, 10]

RADIOGRAPHIC ANATOMY

The Deep Fat Planes

Two deep fat planes useful in the radiographic evaluation of wrist trauma are the pronator quadratus fat pad and the scaphoid fat pad. The pronator quadratus fat pad lies between the pronator quadratus muscle and the volar tendon sheaths. This fat plane is seen on the lateral radiograph of the wrist as a lucent crescent closely applied to the volar aspect of the normal distal radius (Fig. 8–1). It can be obliterated in trauma to the distal radius or ulna (Fig. 8–2A). The scaphoid fat plane lies between the radial collateral capsular ligament and the abductor pollicis brevis tendon. This fat plane is seen on the PA radiograph as a lucent stripe extending from the radial styloid to the trapezium and almost paralleling the radial aspect of the scaphoid (Fig. 8–2B).

The Superficial Fat Planes

Seven superficial fat planes, which include the continuous skin–subcutaneous fat zones, are useful in localizing the site of bony abnormality.[3, 4] Four of these fat planes are visualized on the PA view (Fig. 8–3A). These are the thenar fat plane, overlying the proximal aspect of the first metacarpal; the hypothenar fat plane, at the level of the proximal fifth metacarpal and the hamate; the paraulnar fat plane, superficial to the distal aspect of the ulna; and the pararadial fat plane, superficial to the distal aspect of the radius. The remaining three fat planes involve the dorsal aspect of the hand and wrist on the lateral radiograph (see Figs. 8–1 and 8–3B). The normal dorsal superficial skin-fat zones appear to be continuous; however, fresh cadaver dissections have demonstrated the existence of superficial compartmentalization of the soft tissues deep to the skin–subcutaneous fat zone.[5, 6, 10] Three distinct anatomic areas are created by fascial planes that connect the dorsal retinaculum to the skin; these are the dorsal hand, dorsal wrist, and dorsal forearm compartments. This anatomic configuration makes the localization of swelling useful in determining the site of bony injury.

ANALYSIS OF SOFT TISSUE CHANGES

Swelling that conforms to an observed fracture or dislocation is present within the acute period of injury. This relationship of soft tissue swelling that conforms to a specific bony abnormality lasts approximately 8 hours. After that time, the swelling may become more diffuse and nonspecific but is still present.[4, 6] Also, absence of swelling in the acutely injured wrist denotes absence of significant bony abnormality in the vast majority of cases. However, this is not a completely accepted concept, particularly in reference to the scaphoid fat plane.[2, 7, 13, 16]

A fracture or dislocation must be excluded with particular care in the presence of soft tissue swelling of two or more complementary fat planes (Fig. 8–4). Also, the presence of unequivocal soft tissue swelling in one location should be considered strongly suggestive of a fracture, even though evaluation of the associated bony structures may not show an obvious abnormality. Additional views should be taken in this situation, especially if the morbidity is high for the suspected injury. For example, missed scaphoid fractures may result in significantly higher cost and greater disability to the patient. Re-examination with

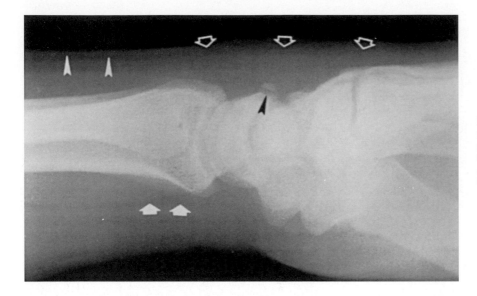

Figure 8–1. Triquetral fracture, lateral wrist. A normal dorsal forearm *(white arrowheads)*, dorsal hand, and pronator fat pad *(white arrows)* are seen. Dorsal wrist swelling only is seen *(open arrows)*. An avulsion of the triquetrum explains this swelling *(black arrowhead).*

radiographs after immobilization should be performed when swelling exists without a detectable fracture, particularly when the soft tissue swelling is in the scaphoid fat pad (Fig. 8–5).

A statistical analysis of soft tissue swelling in wrist trauma has revealed practical associations between the soft tissue changes and bone abnormalities (Table 8–1).[4] The criteria for swelling in these fat planes depend on the fat plane involved (Table 8–2).[6] Subtle obliteration of the skin–subcutaneous fat interface can be confirmed by following the interface where it is well seen into the area under question. A short subtle change in the skin–subcutaneous fat interface demands attention to the deeper tissues. If the anatomic region normally has a sharp margin because of underlying tendons (pararadial, paraulnar), indistinctness of this fat-tendon interface adds credence to the more superficial changes. These fat planes may become completely obliterated. The deep scaphoid and pronator fat planes will be convexly bowed away from the underlying bone prior to loss of fat plane distinctness.[6]

Evaluation of fat planes in the lateral view can narrow the search for abnormality to the area affected by the swelling (Fig. 8–6A). Careful inspection of the PA view directs attention to the radial side (thenar,

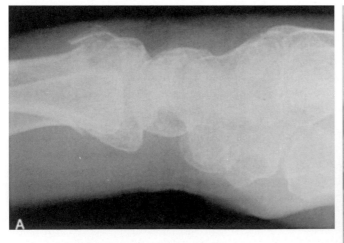

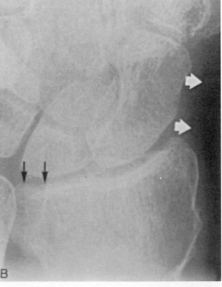

Figure 8–2. Lateral and posteroanterior (PA) views of wrist with intra-articular distal radius fracture. *A,* Lateral view of the wrist. The pronator fat pad is obliterated, and dorsal forearm swelling is seen. Dorsal and volar cortical radial fractures are noted, explaining these soft tissue abnormalities. *B,* PA view. A normal scaphoid fat plane is seen *(white arrows).* A comminuted fracture of the distal radius is seen with a depressed medial articulating surface *(black arrows).*

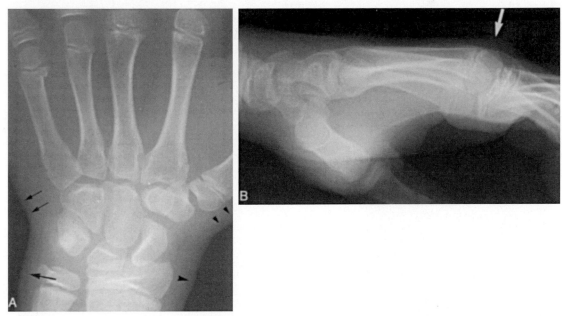

Figure 8–3. Posteroanterior (PA) and lateral views of hand and wrist with fifth metacarpal head fracture. *A,* PA view of the hand. Radial deviation makes the scaphoid fat plane difficult to interpret. Normal pararadial *(large arrowhead)* and paraulnar *(large arrow)* skin–subcutaneous fat interfaces are seen. The hypothenar region also appears normal *(small arrows)*. The thenar region is also normal *(small arrowheads)*. Salter-Harris II fracture of the fifth metacarpal is seen. *B,* Lateral view of the hand. Localized soft tissue swelling is seen over the head of the metacarpals *(arrow)*.

scaphoid, and pararadial fat planes) or ulnar aspect (hypothenar and paraulnar fat planes) if further swelling is detected (Fig. 8–6*B*). A routine oblique view helps evaluate the radial side of the wrist, as does the scaphoid view. The reverse oblique (ballcatcher's) view assists in the evaluation of the ulnar aspect injuries. Stress views assist in the evaluation of midcarpal wrist injuries (Fig. 8–7). Traction radiographs may demonstrate ligamentous injuries that can explain soft tissue swelling seen in the absence of a fracture.

SPECIFIC SWELLING ASSOCIATED WITH SPECIFIC INJURIES

Scaphoid Fat Pad

The most important and one of the most common post-traumatic soft tissue abnormalities of the wrist is swelling of the scaphoid fat pad. However, without good film technique it may be difficult to appreciate. In one third of all carpal fractures, there is associated

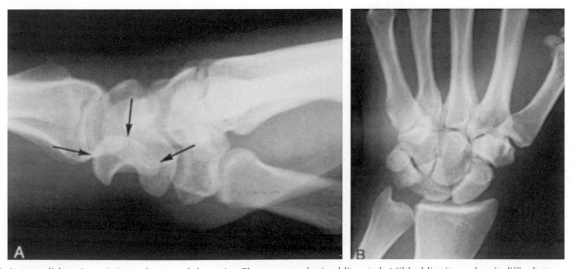

Figure 8–4. Lunate dislocation. *A,* Lateral view of the wrist. The pronator fat is obliterated. Mild obliquity makes it difficult to confirm dorsal forearm and dorsal wrist swelling. The lunate is dislocated volarly *(arrows)*. *B,* Posteroanterior view of the wrist. Minimal scaphoid swelling is noted. There is loss of normal scapholunate, radiolunate, and proximal carpal row joint spaces, and the lunate appears to have a triangular shape.

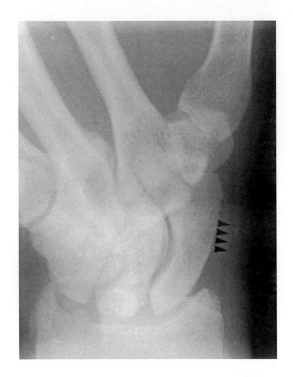

Figure 8–5. Wrist sprain. Scaphoid view shows partial loss of distinct scaphoid fat pad *(arrowheads)*. No fracture is noted. Mild scapholunate joint diastasis is seen (the space appears triangular rather than parallel). Immobilization and re-examination may be helpful in this type of case.

Table 8–1. POSSIBLE ASSOCIATIONS BETWEEN SOFT TISSUE SWELLING AND BONE FRACTURES AND DISLOCATIONS*

Bone Injury	Soft Tissue (Fat Plane) Swelling								
	Dorsal Hand	*Dorsal Wrist*	*Dorsal Forearm*	*M. Pronator Quadratus*	*Thenar*	*Hypothenar*	*Scaphoid*	*Pararadial*	*Paraulnar*
Fracture									
Thumb (first metacarpal)					U		RS		
Second to fifth metacarpal	U	DMB				O			
Scaphoid		U					U		
Greater multangular (trapezium)		O			O		O		
Lunate		U							
Capitate		O							
Triquetrum		U							O
Hamate		O				O			
Pisiform									O
Radius			U	U			RS	U	O
Ulna			O	O					U
Dislocation									
Radiocarpal		O	O	O			O	O	O
Second to fifth metacarpal	U	O			O	O			
Thumb					U				

*DMB = associated with dislocated metacarpal base only; O = occasionally; RS = radial styloid only; U = usually.
Adapted from Curtis DJ, Downey EF Jr, Brower AC, et al: Importance of soft tissue evaluation in hand and wrist trauma: Statistical evaluation. AJR 142:781–788, 1984.

Table 8–2. SWELLING CRITERIA FOR FAT PLANE

Type Fat Plane	Fat Planes	Criteria for Diagnosing Swelling		
		Mild	*Moderate*	*Severe*
Skin–subcutaneous interface	Dorsal hand Dorsal wrist Dorsal forearm Thenar Hypothenar* Pararadial Paraulnar	Subtle silhouette that requires close comparison with normal areas (usually less than 1 cm affected)	Cloudy, deeper fat Obvious loss of skin–subcutaneous fat interface	Solid white from skin to bone Thickening of tissues
Deep fat/tendon	Pararadial	Fluffy, indistinct Less than 1 cm affected	Fuzzy fat-tendon margin may be over 1 cm long Overlying fat cloudy Skin–subcutaneous fat interface may be subtly involved or normal	No tendon separable from white overlying soft tissues to skin Thickening of tissue
Deep fat/variable deep soft tissue	Dorsal wrist Thenar Hypothenar Paraulnar	Strandlike increases in soft tissue densities within fat	Fluffy, confluent area of increased density in fat	Uniformly dense soft tissue
Deep fat overlying fascial compartment	Dorsal hand Dorsal wrist Dorsal forearm†	Flat, mildly uniformly white, deep to fat	Convex, uniformly white, ill-defined soft tissue deep to fluffy fat	Convex bulging of very dense soft tissue poorly delineated from skin
Deep fat lying between tendons or ligaments	Pronator quadratus Scaphoid	Convex displacement of fat plane with indistinctness of a portion of the fat plane	Indistinctness of the entire fat plane	No fat plane discernible Uniformly white soft tissues with thickening of tissues

*Least distinct interface and the hardest to image because of excessive soft tissue of hypothenar eminence and oblique orientation of skin–subcutaneous fat (less than 0.5 cm of this interface is tangential with the x-ray beam).
†Forearm fascia is more tightly applied than other dorsal regions of the skin–subcutaneous fat interfaces.

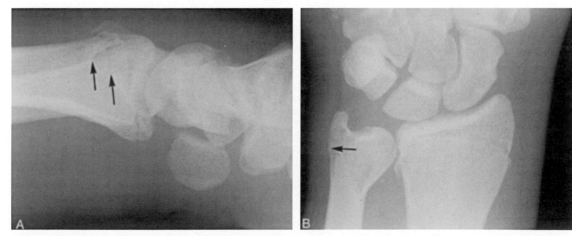

Figure 8–6. Minimally displaced extra-articular fractures of distal radius and ulna. *A,* Lateral view of the wrist. Normal dorsal hand soft tissue is seen. The dorsal wrist and forearm fat planes are obliterated. No pronator is seen. A dorsal cortical fracture of the radius is noted. Less distinctly seen is a volarly displaced ulnar fracture *(arrows)*. *B,* Posteroanterior view. Normal thenar and hypothenar fat planes are seen. Pararadial, paraulnar, and scaphoid fat planes are obliterated. Cortical fractures are noted medially and laterally on the radius. What appears to be a cortical fracture is also seen medially on the ulna *(arrow)*. Dorsal wrist and scaphoid swelling are not well explained by the radioulnar fracture.

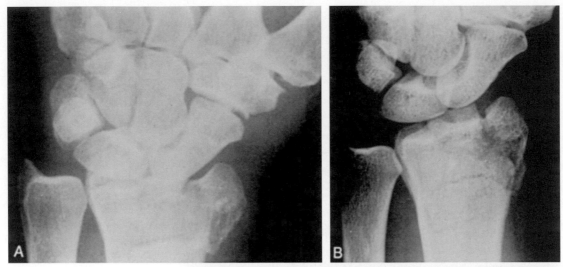

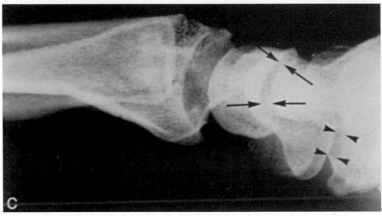

Figure 8–7. Comminuted radial styloid fracture with capitate fracture and carpal ligamentous injuries. *A*, Nondistracted posteroanterior (PA) view of the wrist shows radial styloid comminuted fracture with some scapholunate widening, a nonparallel midintercarpal row, and a triangular scapholunate joint space, which suggest disrupted intercarpal ligaments. The capitate appears irregular, and there is intercarpal joint widening. A distraction view should help illustrate the carpal injuries. *B*, PA view of the wrist with distraction. The severely comminuted radial styloid and radius articulating surface fragments are more anatomically aligned. There is widening of the radiocarpal joint, midintercarpal row, and ulnar scaphotrapezial joints. The scapholunate joint is not parallel (the proximal scaphoid surface is seen; no lunate articulating surface is seen). *C*, Lateral distraction view shows radiocarpal, volarly asymmetric capitolunate joint *(arrows)*, and symmetric scaphotrapezial joint widening *(arrowheads)*. These ligamentous disruptions better explain the distribution of subsequent posttraumatic osteoarthritis than do the fractures themselves.[9]

swelling of this fat pad. Most of these are scaphoid fractures (Fig. 8–8).

The best position for observing this swelling is the ulnarly deviated PA view. This position allows the contour of the scaphoid fat pad to be visualized in its entirety, from the radial styloid to the trapezium. The ulnarly deviated PA view also facilitates the diagnosis of subtle changes in the scaphoid fat pad caused by edema deep to the fat pad. Displacement of the fat pad without its obliteration may be seen in scaphoid fractures that otherwise might not be apparent. This is another reason that the ulnarly deviated PA view of the wrist should be part of the wrist trauma series.[6, 12]

Other fat planes may be swollen in association with scaphoid fractures, most often in the dorsal wrist region (Figs. 8–8*C* and 8–9). In one series, two thirds of isolated scaphoid fractures were associated with dorsal wrist swelling.[4] Another series suggested that if the dorsal soft tissues were normal, a scaphoid fracture could be excluded.[2] A third report noted that

65 percent of patients with scaphoid fractures had a normal dorsal wrist fat plane.[16] Therefore, in the evaluation of scaphoid fractures, abnormality of the scaphoid fat pad is the most important soft tissue finding, with the dorsal wrist fat plane having secondary significance.

Other carpal fractures may cause swelling of the scaphoid fat pad, often in association with swelling of other compartments. Trapezoid fractures are one example. Any intra-articular fracture of the distal radius may also cause this finding, as may acute injury to the scapholunate ligaments (Fig. 8–10*A*). The most important fact about scaphoid fat pad swelling following trauma is that a fracture, usually of the scaphoid, is almost always present, whether visible on plain radiographs or not. One study demonstrated a false predictive value for scaphoid fat pad swelling of only 3.4 percent.[16] Immobilization followed by subsequent re-examination in 10 to 14 days is then indicated.

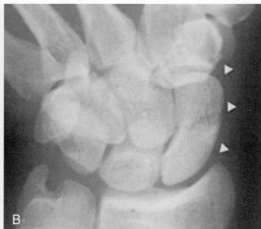

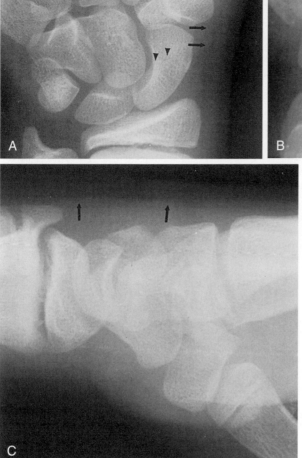

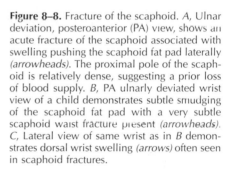

Figure 8–8. Fracture of the scaphoid. *A*, Ulnar deviation, posteroanterior (PA) view, shows an acute fracture of the scaphoid associated with swelling pushing the scaphoid fat pad laterally *(arrowheads)*. The proximal pole of the scaphoid is relatively dense, suggesting a prior loss of blood supply. *B*, PA ulnarly deviated wrist view of a child demonstrates subtle smudging of the scaphoid fat pad with a very subtle scaphoid waist fracture present *(arrowheads)*. *C*, Lateral view of same wrist as in *B* demonstrates dorsal wrist swelling *(arrows)* often seen in scaphoid fractures.

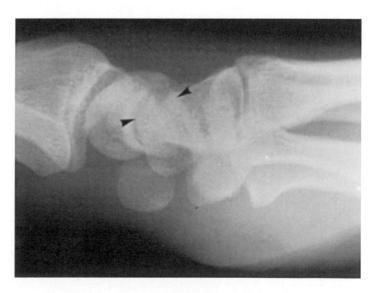

Figure 8–9. Fracture of the scaphoid. Mildly obliqued lateral view. Significant dorsal wrist swelling is seen. An angulated scaphoid waist fracture is shown *(arrowheads)*.

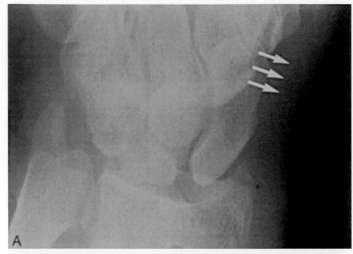

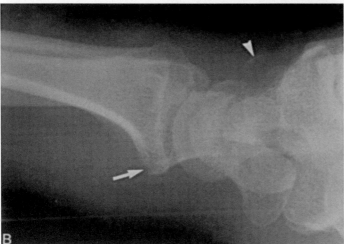

Figure 8–10. Radial styloid fracture, triquetral fracture, and scapholu-nate ligamentous injury. *A,* Angled scaphoid view shows radial styloid fracture and scapholunate diastasis. Pararadial swelling is prominent. The proximal scaphoid fat plane is obliterated. Only the distal portion of the scaphoid fat pad is normal *(arrows). B,* Lateral view. Wrist swelling is present. An avulsion of the dorsal triquetrum is seen *(arrowhead).* The pronator fat pad is bowed and almost obliterated. Dorsal forearm swelling is present. A volar radial cortical break is barely visible *(arrow).* Dorsal hand swelling is not seen.

Pronator Quadratus Fat Pad

Swelling of the other deep fat plane in the wrist, that of the pronator quadratus, is also a good indicator of bony abnormality.[4, 6, 8, 11] The fracture is usually of the radius or, less frequently, the ulna (see Figs. 8–2*A,* 8–4*A,* 8–6*A,* and 8–10*A*). Swelling of the pronator quadratus fat pad in the absence of an obvious frac-ture should be considered presumptive evidence of a fracture. This is especially true in children, because the fat pad disruption may be the only radiographic abnormality in Salter-Harris I or II fractures of the distal radius (Fig. 8–11). A poor lateral radiograph may create a false-positive impression owing to rota-tion, and a repeat true lateral radiograph may be indicated in questionable cases.

Palmar bulging is also suggestive of fracture (Fig. 8–12). This is a less useful indicator of fracture than radiographic obliteration of the fat pad, however. One study of the pronator quadratus fat pad determined pronator values in normal subjects.[16] The pronator value is the distance between the pronator quadratus fat pad and the volar surface of the radius. A wide variation existed, but in this study, only 7 of 384

females had a pronator value greater than 7 mm, and only 5 of 389 males had a pronator value of greater than 10 mm among the normal subjects. This varia-tion makes evaluation of palmar bowing less sensitive as an indicator of fracture. In addition, this study found pronator quadratus fat pad swelling, in general, to be less sensitive in forearm fractures than dorsal wrist swelling in radius and/or ulna fractures, and significantly less sensitive than scaphoid fat pad swelling as an indicator of fracture.[16]

Dorsal Hand Fat Plane

Swelling of the dorsal hand fat plane is strongly asso-ciated with a fracture of the second through fifth metacarpals (Fig. 8–13). If swelling is localized over the metacarpal heads, close attention to the distal metacarpal often reveals the fracture (see Fig. 8–3*B*). However, swelling of the dorsal hand fat plane or any of the other superficial fat planes can be present from direct soft tissue trauma without fracture.

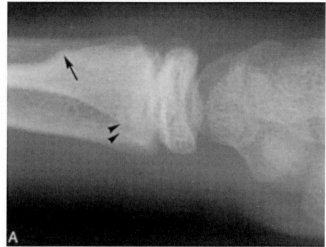

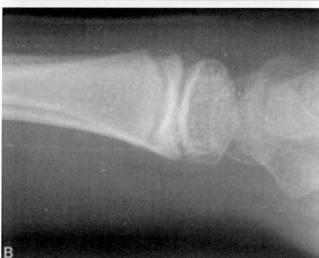

Figure 8–11. Comparison views of minimally displaced wrist fracture in a child. *A,* Lateral view of the wrist. No pronator fat pad is seen. There is dorsal forearm and dorsal wrist swelling as well. A minor dorsal radius cortical fracture is seen *(arrow).* A volar ulnar fracture is also present, suggesting a Salter-Harris II fracture component *(arrowheads). B,* Lateral view of the opposite wrist shows a normal pronator fat pad. Minimal wrist swelling is seen. No fracture or definite diastasis is seen.

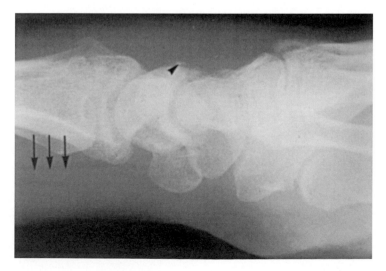

Figure 8–12. Cortical fracture of radius with triquetral avulsion. Lateral view of the wrist. Dorsal wrist and dorsal forearm swelling are seen. The pronator is minimally bowed volarly *(arrows).* A dorsal radius cortical fracture is evident, with loss of the normal articulating angle of the distal radius. An avulsion of the dorsum of the triquetrum is also visible *(arrowhead).*

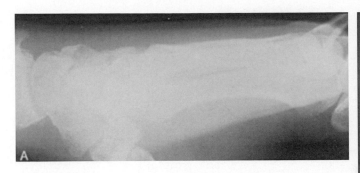

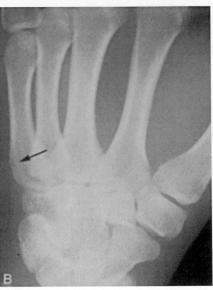

Figure 8–13. Fracture of the base of the fifth metacarpal. *A,* Lateral view of the hand and wrist shows swelling of the dorsum of the hand. *B,* Oblique view of the hand. A nondisplaced fifth metacarpal fracture is visible *(arrow).*

Dorsal Wrist Fat Plane

Swelling in the dorsal wrist region is strongly associated with carpal fractures or dislocations (see Figs. 8–1, 8–2A, 8–6A, 8–8C, 8–9, 8–10A, 8–11A, 8–12, and 8–14). As in all the subcutaneous fat planes, however, swelling may be observed without a fracture present. In two different studies, dorsal wrist swelling was the most commonly observed without a fracture.[4, 16] Several authorities discuss the importance of dorsal wrist and scaphoid fat plane swelling

in scaphoid fractures,[2, 4, 15] whereas another found this combination less often.[16]

When both dorsal hand and dorsal wrist swelling are present, the cause is (1) a carpometacarpal dislocation, (2) an intra-articular fracture of the base of one or more of the second through fifth metacarpals, or (3) both metacarpal and carpal fractures. Longitudinally oriented radial fractures that involve the radiocarpal articular surface accounted for all dorsal wrist swelling seen in isolated forearm fractures (Figs. 8–2 and 8–15A). If a nonarticular fracture of the

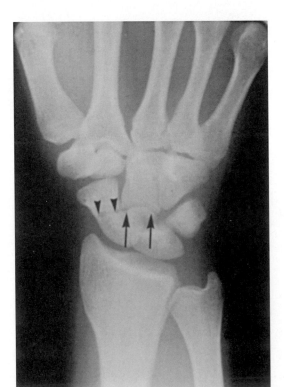

Figure 8–14. Transscaphoid, transcapitate fracture. Distraction posteroanterior view shows radiocarpal and midcarpal distraction. The scaphoid waist fracture *(arrowheads)* was not seen prior to distraction. An associated capitate fracture with inversion of the fragment is present *(arrows).*

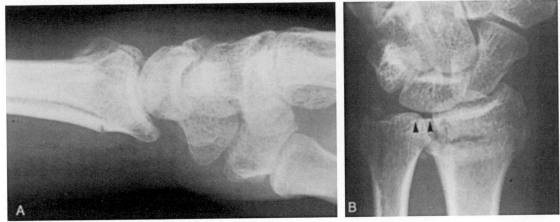

Figure 8–15. Intra-articular distal radius and ulna fracture. *A*, Lateral view of the wrist shows bowing and near-obliteration of the pronator fat pad. Dorsal forearm and dorsal wrist swelling are seen. There is a reversal of the normal distal radius angle because of an impacted fracture. *B*, Posteroanterior view of the wrist. Pararadial and paraulnar swelling is noted. A comminuted radial fracture is seen with a depressed medial fragment *(arrowheads).* An ulnar styloid fracture is shown.

radius is seen and dorsal wrist swelling is present, a carpal fracture or dislocation should also be sought.

Dorsal Forearm Fat Plane

Swelling in this area is common, with two thirds[4] to 80 percent[16] of distal radius and ulnar shaft fractures associated with this swelling. Radial or ulnar fractures accounted for all cases reported in two series with dorsal forearm swelling when only one bone was fractured.[4] When both dorsal wrist and dorsal forearm swelling are present, the cause is (1) a radial fracture involving the radiocarpal articular surface, (2) a dislocation (Figs. 8–4 and 8–16), or (3) a carpal fracture associated with a forearm fracture (see Figs. 8–9 and 8–12). Dorsal forearm swelling may be the only radiographic finding in nondisplaced Salter-Har-

ris I or II fractures, as has been seen with swelling of the pronator quadratus fat pad.

Thenar Fat Plane

Swelling of the thenar fat plane usually indicates a first metacarpal base fracture or first metacarpal-carpal subluxation (Fig. 8–17). Occasionally, this fat plane may be disrupted by a more distal injury to the first metacarpophalangeal joint or proximal first phalanx (Fig. 8–18). Rarely, it is associated with a trapezius fracture.

Hypothenar Fat Plane

Swelling of the hypothenar fat plane is mainly due to second through fifth metacarpal fractures (Fig. 8–19*A*). However, it may be subtle or unidentified in

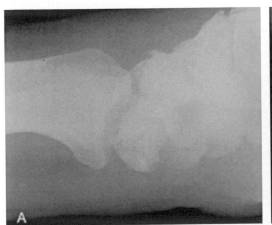

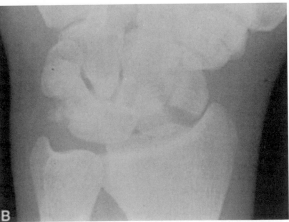

Figure 8–16. Transscaphoid perilunate dislocation. *A*, Lateral view of the wrist. There is dorsal wrist, dorsal forearm, and pronator fat pad swelling. A perilunate dislocation is seen. *B*, Posteroanterior view of a "clenched fist" wrist. There is mild widening of the capitohamate and hamatotriquetral joints. Radiolunate widening is seen. Scaphoid, pararadial, and paraulnar fat plane swelling is prominent. A nonaligned midscaphoid fracture is present. No joint is visible between the lunate and capitate. Bone fragments in the ulnar aspect of the wrist were avulsed from the triquetrum.

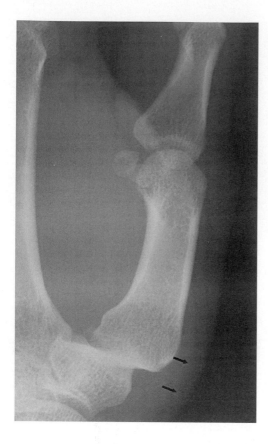

Figure 8–17. Posteroanterior view of the first metacarpal joint, demonstrating an avulsion fracture from the base of the first metacarpal as well as subluxation of the first metacarpal joint. Note the thenar fat plane swelling *(arrows)*.

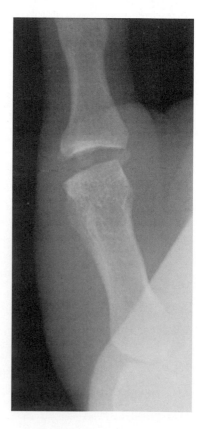

Figure 8–18. Radial collateral ligament tear. Posteroanterior view of thumb shows loss of skin–subcutaneous fat interface. A widened first metacarpal phalangeal joint is evident with medial deviation of the phalanx.

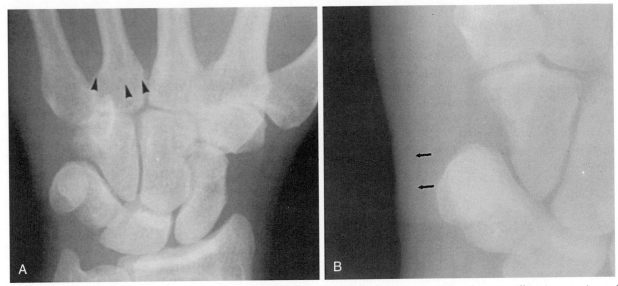

Figure 8–19. *A,* Fracture of the fourth metacarpal base on posteroanterior (PA) view of the wrist. Hypothenar swelling is seen. A careful look shows the metacarpal fracture *(arrowheads).* A reverse (ballcatcher's) oblique view would further elucidate this and help to determine whether the fifth metacarpal base is subluxed or fractured. *B,* PA view of wrist demonstrating subtle hypothenar fat plane swelling *(arrows)* in a patient with nondisplaced triquetral fracture.

such fractures. Swelling in the hypothenar region may indicate a hamate or triquetral fracture, especially when dorsal wrist swelling is present and dorsal hand swelling is absent (Fig. 8–19B). Hamate fractures are often difficult to diagnose, and the presence of hypothenar fat pad swelling can help direct attention to the hamate, with additional evaluation performed if needed.

Pararadial Fat Plane

Swelling of the pararadial fat plane is strongly indicative of a radial fracture (Figs. 8–6, 8–10A, 8–15B, and 8–20). However, carpal dislocations may show swelling adjacent to the radial styloid without fracture of the radius (see Fig. 8–16B). In children, pararadial swelling is presumptive evidence of a Salter-Harris I or II fracture in the appropriate clinical setting, even in the absence of definite bone abnormality.[4] Lack of soft tissue swelling in children does not exclude a fracture, however, because in one study, 36 percent of greenstick fractures of the radius or ulna were associated with normal soft tissues.[16] In adults, in the presence of pararadial swelling and a radial fracture, an ulnar fracture should also be sought, because radial fractures are isolated less than 20 percent of the time.[4]

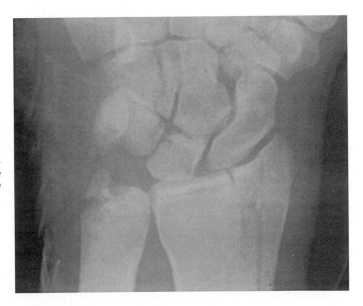

Figure 8–20. Severely comminuted intraarticular radius fracture with lunate and capitate waist fracture on posteroanterior view of the wrist. There is pararadial, paraulnar, and scaphoid swelling. A comminuted, longitudinally oriented radius fracture is noted disrupting the articulating surface of the radius. The ulnar styloid has been fractured. The distal articulating surface of the lunate is fragmented. The waist of the capitate shows a nondisplaced fracture.

Paraulnar Fat Plane

Swelling of the paraulnar fat plane is strongly indicative of a forearm fracture (see Figs. 8–6, 8–15*B*, 8–16*B*, and 8–20). It is rarely present without swelling in some other soft tissue compartment. When no other soft tissue swelling is seen, paraulnar fat pad swelling suggests a pisiform fracture (the result of a direct blow to the volar surface of the wrist). When an ulnar styloid fracture is present, another fracture should be sought, because only 6 percent of ulnar styloid fractures occur alone.[4]

CONCLUSION

The importance of soft tissue evaluation in wrist trauma cannot be overstated. High-quality radiographs are needed as well as a systematic evaluation of the soft tissues. Fractures are rare in the absence of soft tissue swelling, and the location and combinations of fat plane abnormalities help to localize the bony abnormality. This is especially true in subtle or occult fractures, particularly of the scaphoid, because missing a fracture can lead to significant disability.

References

1. Andersen JL, Gron P, Langhoff O: The scaphoid fat stripe in the diagnosis of carpal trauma. Acta Radiol 29:664–668, 1988.
2. Carver RA, Barrington NA: Soft tissue changes accompanying scaphoid injuries. Clin Radiol 36:423–425, 1985.
3. Curtis DJ: Injuries of the wrist: An approach to diagnosis. Radiol Clin North Am 19:625–644, 1981.
4. Curtis DJ, Downey EF Jr, Brower AC, et al: Importance of soft tissue evaluation in hand and wrist trauma: Statistical evaluation. AJR 142:781–788, 1984.
5. Curtis DJ, Downey EF Jr, Brahman SL: Compartmentalized swelling in hand and wrist trauma [letter to the editor]. AJR 145:195, 1985.
6. Curtis DJ, Downey EF Jr: Soft tissue evaluation in trauma. In Gilula LA (ed): The Traumatized Hand and Wrist: Radiographic and Anatomic Correlation. Philadelphia, WB Saunders, 1992, pp 45–63.
7. Diaz JJ, Finlay DB, Brenkell J, et al: Radiographic assessment of soft tissue signs in clinically suspected scaphoid fractures: The incidence of false negative and false positive results. J Orthop Trauma 1:205–208, 1987.
8. Harris JH Jr: The significance of soft tissue injury in the roentgen diagnosis of trauma. CRC Crit Rev Diagn Imaging 6:295–298, 1975.
9. Kursunoglu-Brahme S, Gundry CR, Resnick D: Advanced imaging of the wrist. Radiol Clin North Am 28:307–320, 1990.
10. Lewis OJ, Hanshere RJ, Bucknil TM: The anatomy of the wrist joint. Anatomy 106:539–541, 1970.
11. MacEwan DW: Changes due to trauma in the fat plane overlying the quadratus muscle: A radiographic sign. Radiology 82:879–886, 1964.
12. Rockwell WB, Destouet JM, Gilula LA, et al: Radiographic approach to the painful wrist. Orthop Rev 14:270–279, 1985.
13. Schunk K, Weber W, Strunk H, et al: Traumatology and diagnosis of scaphoid fracture. Radiologe 29:61–67, 1989.
14. Terry DW Jr, Ramin JE: The navicular fat stripe: A useful roentgen feature for evaluating wrist trauma. AJR 124:25–28, 1975.
15. Yousefzadeh DK: The value of traction during roentgenography of the wrist and metacarpophalangeal joints. Skelet Radiol 4:29–33, 1979.
16. Zammit-Maempel I, Bisset RAL, Morris J, Forbes WS: The value of soft tissue signs in wrist trauma. Clin Radiol 39:664–668, 1988.

CHAPTER 9

Advanced Imaging of the Carpus

Gordon A. Brody, MD, and David W. Stoller, MD

Magnetic resonance (MR) imaging of the wrist and hand, to identify both normal anatomy and pathology, has received increasing attention at hand and radiologic society meetings. For the first time, MR imaging makes it possible for the radiologist to accomplish accurate, noninvasive imaging of specific ligamentous injuries, rendering the vague diagnosis "wrist sprain" obsolete. As new data on the biomechanics of the carpus are collected, applications are developed for kinematic imaging. As techniques for dynamic MR imaging of the carpus advance, these methods may well become the standard for evaluating instability from a physiologic viewpoint. This *instability* can be best defined as the inability of two bones or groups of bones to maintain a normal physiologic relationship.

STATUS OF IMAGING TECHNIQUES

Standard Radiography

Standard radiographic evaluation of the wrist and hand is restricted primarily to demonstrating the osseous structures. With the localization of certain pathologic processes, select views, such as the scaphoid and carpal tunnel views, may provide additional information. The scaphoid fat stripe, which can be identified radial to the scaphoid, and the pronator quadratus line, which is commonly obscured by fracture, are shown in posteroanterior and lateral radiographic views, respectively. The usefulness of the scaphoid fat stripe in diagnosing acute scaphoid fractures has been challenged. The static bony relationships of the radius, lunate, and capitate can be measured in longitudinal axes in a lateral radiograph.

Arthrography

Wrist arthrography has been used to evaluate the integrity of the triangular fibrocartilage (TFC) and the scapholunate (SL) and lunotriquetral (LT) interosseous ligaments.[1–4] The three-compartment (i.e., triple-injection) arthrogram, in which contrast agent is in-

troduced into the radiocarpal, distal radioulnar, and midcarpal joints, is considered the standard technique.[5, 6] Although arthrographic findings correlate quite well with ulnar-sided wrist pain, the technique is far less effective for radial-sided problems. Manaster and colleagues[7] found that, although 88 percent of patients with ulnar pain had LT ligament perforations, only 26 percent of patients with SL dissociation had SL ligament perforations. Thus, arthrography does not appear to be useful in assessing the physiologic integrity of the interosseous ligaments on the radial side of the wrist. Another limitation is that, because of the nature of the technique, it is impossible to differentiate pinhole perforations from perforations that are large and biomechanically significant.[8, 9] Anatomic studies of aging wrists have shown that degenerative perforations in both the interosseous ligaments and the triangular fibrocartilage complex (TFCC) are quite common in people older than 35 years of age.[10, 11] Therefore, arthrography is less diagnostically useful for these patients.

Computed Tomography

Computed tomography (CT) has limited but well-defined application in the wrist. Primarily, it is used to evaluate the carpal tunnel and the non-osseous structures about the wrist and hand. Although subtle differences in closely related soft tissue attenuation values cannot be optimally resolved with CT, it is an excellent modality for defining the location and extent of carpal bone fractures and complex intra-articular fractures of the distal radius.[12, 13] Reformatted coronal and sagittal scans, direct coronal scans, and three-dimensional (3D) CT renderings are useful for evaluating fractures and for displaying fracture morphology displacement, non-union, and alignment through specific anatomic areas (e.g., the hook of the hamate).[14, 15] Small chip fractures and loose bodies may be identified in thin-section (i.e., 1.5-mm) CT scans. Axial CT scans of the distal radioulnar joint can be diagnostic for distal radioulnar joint subluxation or dislocation.

Ultrasound and Miscellaneous Techniques

Ultrasonography has been used to study the gross motion of the tendons in the carpal tunnel during

Portions of this chapter, including the illustrations, have been adapted from Stoller DW: *Magnetic Resonance Imaging in Orthopaedics and Sports Medicine.* Philadelphia, JB Lippincott, 1993; written with Gordon Brody, MD.

flexion.[16] Videofluoroscopy and cinematographic CT studies of wrist motion may provide indirect evidence of pathology in tendons, ligaments, and cartilage without direct imaging or arthroscopy of these structures. Videofluoroscopy enables diagnosis of midcarpal instability and can be helpful in evaluating the pathogenesis of other carpal instabilities.

Magnetic Resonance Imaging

Magnetic resonance imaging of the wrist provides the high spatial and contrast resolution of soft tissue and osseous components needed for evaluation of the small and complex anatomy of the wrist and hand.[12, 17–27] Supporting muscles, ligaments, tendons, tendon sheaths, vessels, nerves, and marrow are demonstrated on MR images with excellent spatial resolution using small fields of view (FOVs) and uniform signal-intensity penetration.[28–32] Magnetic resonance has the potential to replace conventional wrist arthrography in diagnosing tears involving the intercarpal ligaments and the TFCC. Multiplanar images permit direct anatomic and pathologic discrimination in axial, coronal, sagittal, and oblique planes without the delayed reconstructions or reformatting required for CT. Sagittal MR images display bone and ligamentous anatomy in a selective "tomographic-like" section, without the overlapping of carpal bones seen in lateral radiographs. This facilitates a more accurate assessment of carpal instabilities. Three-dimensional volume imaging allows for image acquisition with retrospective reformatting of additional orthogonal or nonorthogonal oblique images.[33] Kinematic imaging in coronal and sagittal orientations provides information regarding carpal bone motion and synchrony with supporting ligamentous structures. MR imaging used in conjunction with intra-articular contrast can improve soft tissue contrast visualization of the TFC and intrinsic carpal ligaments.

Magnetic resonance imaging is currently used in the evaluation of trauma (i.e., fracture), avascular necrosis (AVN), and Kienböck's disease, as well as the TFC and carpal tunnel. In addition, the status of articular cartilage and the cortical and subchondral bone response in arthritis can be assessed and categorized.

MAGNETIC RESONANCE IMAGING TECHNIQUES

The wrist and hand are imaged using a dedicated circumferential design coil to optimize the signal-to-noise ratio (SNR) and obtain high-resolution images (Fig. 9–1). With this coil design, the patient's arm may be positioned at the side. Proper positioning requires alignment of the long axis of the distal radius and central metacarpal axis with the wrist in neutral position. Radial or ulnar deviation and dorsal or volar angulation should be avoided to maintain consistent alignment of the carpus. The wrist is studied in pronation, with the fingers held in extension. The posi-

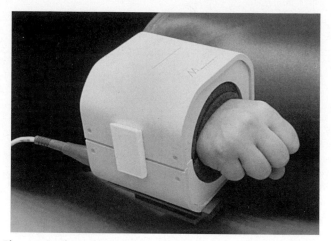

Figure 9–1. The coil is correctly positioned at a patient's side; normally, however, the wrist is studied with the fingers relaxed and held in extension.

tion of the wrist may change relative to the design of the surface coil used.

T_1-weighted images are obtained with a short T_R (recovery time) and short T_E (echo time) spin-echo pulse sequence. Tissues characteristically bright on a T_1-weighted sequence include fat and paramagnetic substances (e.g., gadolinium-DTPA, subacute hemorrhage). Tissues with characteristic low signal intensity on T_1-weighted images include those with a lack of mobile protons (e.g., calcium, fibrous tissue) and liquid (e.g., cerebrospinal fluid, joint fluid, cysts). Tissues with intermediate signal intensity include muscle, solid organs, and hematopoietic bone marrow.

T_2-weighted images are obtained with a long T_R and long T_E. The major advantage of T_2-weighted images is that areas containing liquid or excess free water are bright in signal intensity. Other types of T_2-like techniques are gradient-echo (T_2*) and fast spin-echo (FSE; commonly used in association with fat suppression). Short T_1 inversion recovery (STIR) sequences are very sensitive to fluid (which is bright) and suppress signal from normal subcutaneous or medullary fat. These sequences are very sensitive to edema and hemorrhage in fractures and to neoplasms and show ligaments as dark structures in contrast to adjacent bright fluid.

In the axial plane T_1-weighted images are used as the initial localizer (Fig. 9–2). A small FOV is routinely used to facilitate the resolution required to visualize the TFC and intrinsic ligaments. Either T_2*-weighted or STIR axial images may be substituted for T_1-weighted images when tenosynovitis, ganglia, carpal tunnel syndrome, or neoplasm is suspected. Gradient-echo axial images through the phalanges optimally differentiate between the flexor digitorum superficialis and the profundus tendons. Coronal T_1-weighted 3-mm images are acquired with a small FOV. Coronal T_2 or T_2* images display the anatomy of the TFC and SL and LT ligaments (Fig. 9–3A). Alignment of the carpus, including capitolunate and

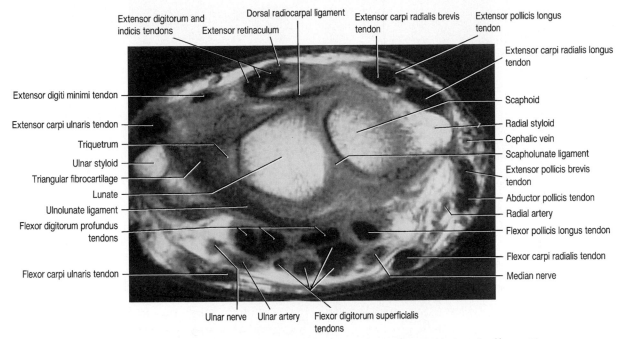

Figure 9–2. T_1-weighted axial image at the level of the proximal carpal row and triangular fibrocartilage.

scapholunate angle measurements, is best evaluated on sagittal images (Fig. 9–3B).

T_{2^*}-weighted and T_2 fast spin-echo coronal images produce superior contrast between the intercarpal ligaments and the TFCC. Three-dimensional volume acquisitions, which use gradient-echo protocols, are not limited by slice thickness and can be used to reformat anatomy in other planes of section. FSE T_2 fat suppression images provide the highest contrast between ligaments and fluid (Fig. 9–4). Coupled 3-inch circular surface coils positioned in a kinematic wrist device have been used to track distal and carpal row motion with radial and ulnar deviation of the wrist. This information is displayed in a cine-loop format and can be recorded on video or photographed.

Dorsiflexion and palmar flexion motions are best studied in the sagittal plane and require either greater degrees of freedom from the surface coil or pivoting of the coil to accommodate the increased range of motion. Image quality considerations need to be balanced in designing a surface coil with greater diameter or anatomic coverage. Separate axial imaging sequences in positions of pronation and supination may be useful in the evaluation of subluxation patterns in the distal radioulnar joint (DRUJ). Developments in hyperscan technology may facilitate true dynamic joint imaging, which would be able to more accurately describe carpal translations and impingement in various instability patterns.

MR IMAGING VISUALIZATION OF CARPAL INSTABILITIES
Stable and Unstable Equilibrium in the Wrist

With radial deviation, the radial border must shorten; this is accomplished by rotation of the scaphoid into a flexed position (Fig. 9–5). The ulnar border is lengthened as the triquetrum slides out from beneath the hamate. On plain radiographs or coronal MR images of the wrist in this position, the scaphoid is foreshortened and the joint space is evident between the hamate and triquetrum; no superimposition of these bones occurs. The lunate is linked or associated with the scaphoid and triquetrum through the interosseous ligaments, which are displayed as homogeneous low-signal-intensity structures on coronal MR images. The SL ligament has a triangular morphology, whereas the LT ligament is more linear. Lunate motion is thus a reflection of this proximal carpal row linkage as well as the compressive forces placed on it by the capitate. At extreme radial deviation, the summation of these forces produces slight volar flexion of the lunate. Because a condition of stable equilibrium exists, the bones of the proximal row return to their neutral position when the radial deviating force is removed.

With ulnar deviation, the radial side of the flexible spacer must lengthen, and the ulnar side must shorten. Therefore, the scaphoid becomes more horizontal or extended to lengthen the radial side, and the triquetrum slides beneath the hamate to shorten the ulnar side. Posteroanterior radiographs show an elongated scaphoid and superimposition of the hamate on the triquetrum. Coronal MR images demonstrate the triquetral movement in an ulnar direction on the slope of the hamate (Fig. 9–6). Palmar movement of the triquetrum in relationship to the hamate results in palmar position of the lunate axis relative to the capitate. Compressive forces transmitted by the capitate produce dorsal rotation or dorsiflexion of the lunate. Associated volar shift of the lunate maintains colinear alignment of the capitate and radius. During

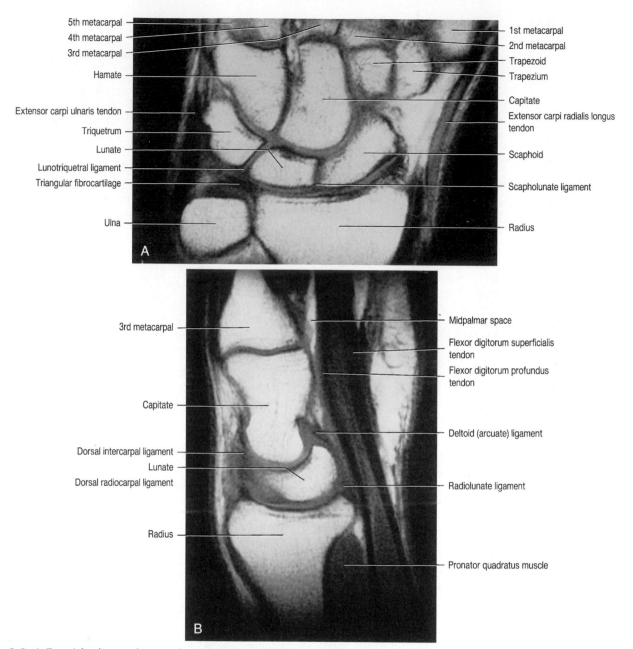

5th metacarpal

4th metacarpal

3rd metacarpal

Hamate

Extensor carpi ulnaris tendon

Triquetrum

Lunate

Lunotriquetral ligament

Triangular fibrocartilage

Ulna

1st metacarpal

2nd metacarpal

Trapezoid

Trapezium

Capitate

Extensor carpi radialis longus tendon

Scaphoid

Scapholunate ligament

Radius

3rd metacarpal

Capitate

Dorsal intercarpal ligament

Lunate

Dorsal radiocarpal ligament

Radius

Midpalmar space

Flexor digitorum superficialis tendon

Flexor digitorum profundus tendon

Deltoid (arcuate) ligament

Radiolunate ligament

Pronator quadratus muscle

Figure 9–3. *A*, T$_1$-weighted coronal image showing the intrinsic ligaments and triangular fibrocartilage. *B*, T$_1$-weighted sagittal image in the plane of the capitate and lunate.

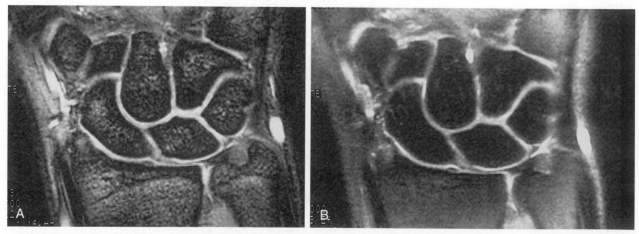

Figure 9–4. *A*, T$_2$*-weighted gradient echo coronal image. *B*, Fast spin-echo T$_2$-weighted coronal image showing improved ligament-fluid contrast.

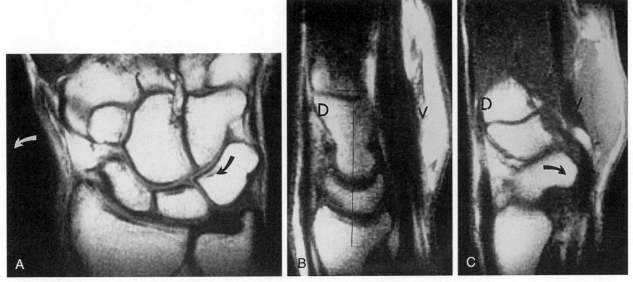

Figure 9–5. *A,* Radial deviation of the wrist *(white arrow)* produces radial and dorsal translation of the triquetrum relative to the slope of the hamate *(black arrow). B,* Colinear alignment of the capitate and lunate *(straight line).* There may be mild palmar flexion of the lunate in extreme radial deviation. *C,* Palmar flexion of the scaphoid *(black arrow).* D = dorsal; V = volar.

lunate dorsiflexion, there is elevation of the distal pole of the scaphoid (i.e., scaphoid extension).

Interosseous Ligament Pathology

If an injury to these constraints occurs, such as a tear of the SL ligament, the linkage between the scaphoid and lunate is removed, and these bones are dissociated. An SL ligament tear, however, may exist without a static instability (Fig. 9–7). The lunate is no longer under the influence of the scaphoid and instead follows the triquetrum, and the loading force of the capitate is not opposed by torque transmitted through the SL ligament from the flexed scaphoid. Similarly, the lunate no longer exerts force on the scaphoid, and there is less opposing force to its flexion.

In this situation, radial deviation produces an exaggeration of the normal motions of the bones of the

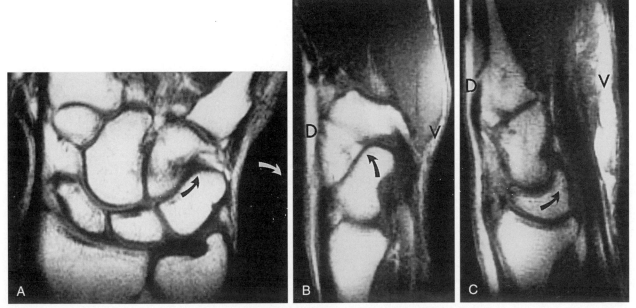

Figure 9–6. *A,* Ulnar deviation of the wrist *(white arrow)* produces ulnar translation of the triquetrum relative to the slope of the hamate *(black arrow). B,* Dorsiflexion of the lunate (i.e., dorsal tilt) with associated volar shift *(arrow)* allows the capitate to remain colinear with the radius. *C,* Elevation (i.e., extension) of the distal pole of the scaphoid *(arrow).* D = dorsal; V = volar.

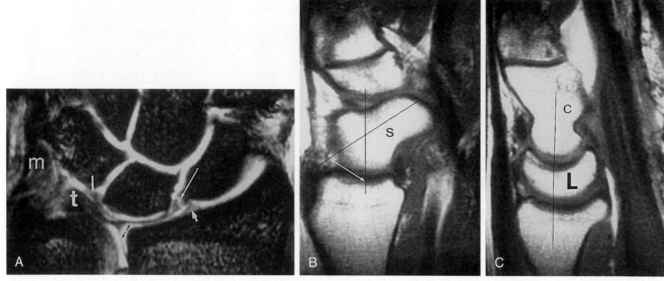

Figure 9–7. *A,* A T_2^*-weighted coronal image demonstrates a vertical, high-signal-intensity tear of the scapholunate ligament *(long white arrow)* without static carpal instability. A proximal portion of the radial scapholunate *(short white arrow),* the lunotriquetral ligament (l), the meniscus homologue (m), and the triangular fibrocartilage (t) with its radial attachments *(black arrows)* are shown. There is positive ulnar variance with an intact triangular fibrocartilage. *B,* The normal scapholunate angle *(double-headed arrow)* is shown. S = scaphoid. *C,* Colinear (i.e., coaxial) alignment of the capitate (C), lunate (L), and radius, with normal capitolunate angle. There is no instability pattern.

proximal row. With SL interosseous ligament disruption, the scaphoid becomes more flexed in relation to the lunate, and the SL angle, which is normally less than 30° to 60°, increases to more than 70° (Fig. 9–8). The SL angle is determined from two sagittal images to demonstrate the separate lunate and scaphoid axes, which are not shown together in the same sagittal image. The lunate, free of the influence of the scaphoid, tips into a dorsiflexed position in relation to the axis of the capitate. As the scaphoid flexes, a gap appears between the scaphoid and the lunate, and in time, the capitate will fall into this gap, contributing to a reduction in carpal height.

Rotatory subluxation of the scaphoid, which begins as an SL dissociation, has been described. In its final stages, as the lunate is dorsiflexed, a dorsal intercalary segment instability (DISI) pattern is established. On lateral radiographs, there is 10° or more of lunate dorsiflexion relative to the radius. On sagittal MR images, dorsal tilting of the lunate is associated with proximal migration of the capitate and loss of colinear alignment of the capitate, lunate, and radius. The capitolunate angle, normally 0° to 30°, can be directly measured on sagittal images and may be increased in dorsiflexion ligamentous instability.

Disruption of the SL ligament is shown on the FSE T_2- or T_2^*-weighted images as complete ligamentous disruption or as a discrete area of linear bright signal intensity in a partial or complete tear. In complete tears, synovial fluid communication between the radiocarpal and midcarpal compartments may be identified. Associated stretching (i.e., redundancy) or tearing of the radiolunate ligament and the radioscaphocapitate (RSC) ligament is shown in sagittal

images. A loss of linkage (i.e., dissociation) between the triquetrum and the lunate—due to a tear of the LT ligament—allows the lunate to follow the scaphoid. Under this influence, volar flexion of the lunate occurs and gives rise to a volar intercalatry segment instability (VISI) pattern (Fig. 9–9). *Volar intercalatry segment instability* may be defined as a carpal instability characterized by dorsal migration and flexion of the lunate. Sagittal MR images characterize the palmar tilting of the lunate and scaphoid. The SL angle is decreased to less than 30°. Disruption of the LT ligament is commonly identified by its loss of signal on T_2^*-weighted coronal images.

DIAGNOSIS BY MR IMAGING

In evaluating SL interosseous ligament pathology, MR imaging was shown to have a sensitivity rate of 93 percent, specificity of 83 percent, and accuracy of 90 percent compared with arthrography.[23] In the diagnosis of ligamentous tears, with arthroscopy as the gold standard, MR imaging was 86 percent sensitive, 100 percent specific, and 95 percent accurate. In the diagnosis of LT interosseous ligament tears, MR imaging was 56 percent sensitive, 100 percent specific, and 90 percent accurate compared with arthrography,[23] and 50 percent sensitive, 100 percent specific, and 80 percent accurate compared with arthroscopy. The LT ligament is less substantial than the SL ligament; therefore, three-dimensional coronal images may be needed to improve the sensitivity of diagnosis. Osseous widening of the LT articulation is uncommon in comparison with SL ligament dissociations, which may make the detection of LT ligament pathology

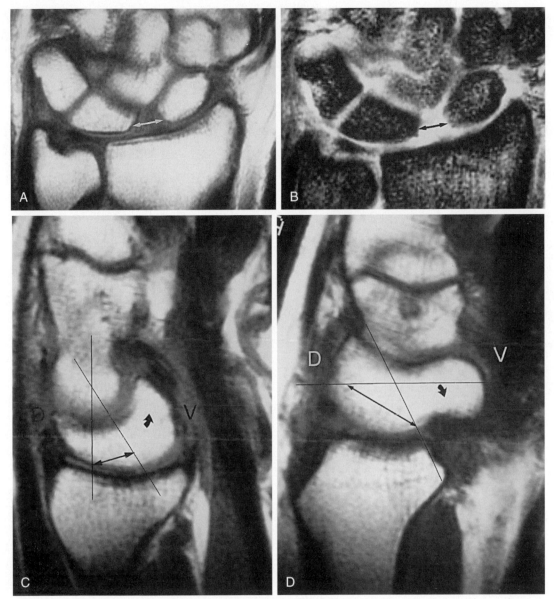

Figure 9–8. Coronal T₁-weighted *(A)* and T₂*-weighted *(B)* images show scapholunate dissociation *(double-headed arrows)* with complete disruption of the scapholunate interosseous ligament in dorsal intercalated segmental instability. *C,* Dorsal tilting of the lunate *(curved arrow)* without volar shift is present. Note the dorsal displacement of the capitate relative to the radius. The capitolunate angle *(double-headed arrow)* measures 32 °. *D,* Palmar tilting of the scaphoid *(curved arrow)* causes an abnormally increased scapholunate angle *(double-headed arrow)* of 124 °. D = dorsal; V = volar.

more difficult, especially in the presence of an effusion or synovitis. Thin-section axial images may further improve the identification of both SL and LT ligament pathology.

Midcarpal Instabilities

Midcarpal instabilities are recognized more commonly, and there is greater experience with MR imaging of the these wrist injuries. In palmar midcarpal subluxation, first studied by Lichtman and associates,[34] patients present with palmar subluxation at the midcarpal joint and a painful clunk with ulnar deviation of the wrist. These researchers found that this instability is due mainly to laxity of the ulnar arm of the volar arcuate ligament.[34] There is also evidence of increased ligamentous laxity in these patients, and sagittal MR images show palmar flexion of the lunate, as in the VISI pattern.

DISTAL RADIOULNAR JOINT

Ulnar Variance

The concept of ulnar variance is critical in the management of distal radial fractures, in the pathogenesis of Kienböck's disease, and in triangular fibrocartilage

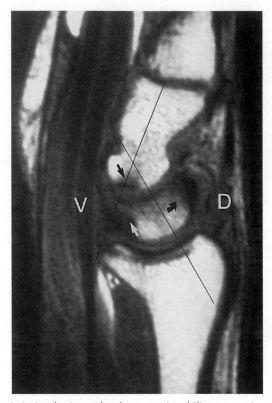

Figure 9–9. A volar intercalated segment instability pattern is apparent in clinical midcarpal instability. A sagittal T_1-weighted image shows the volar tilt of the lunate *(curved black arrow)*, increased capitolunate angle, and subchondral sclerosis of the opposing surfaces of the capitate *(straight black arrow)* and lunate *(white arrow)*. The ulnar arm of the arcuate ligament was not visible in this midcarpal instability. MR imaging was the first modality able to document degeneration of the proximal pole of the capitate in subluxation of the capitate on the lunate. D = dorsal; V = volar.

(TFC) pathology. *Ulnar variance* refers to the relative lengths of the radius and ulna and can be defined as the level of the distal end of the ulna relative to that of the radius. If the ulna is short, ulnar variance is considered negative (Fig. 9–10). If the ulna is long, the variance is referred to as positive (Fig. 9–11). Neutral ulnar variance occurs when the lengths of the radius and ulna are relatively equal. Radiographically, the relative lengths of the radius and ulna are measured from the centers of their distal articular surfaces. There are three commonly used methods for measuring ulnar variance; all are similarly accurate and reliable.[35] It should be noted that wrist position is an important determinant of ulnar variance. Supination causes relative ulnar shortening, and pronation causes lengthening.[36] For this reason, it is critical that ulnar variance be determined with the forearm and wrist in zero pronation and supination.

Ulnolunate Impingement Syndrome

The syndrome of ulnolunate impingement occurs when positive ulnar variance is excessive (see Fig.

9–11).[37] In this condition, there is a painful compression of the distal ulna on the medial surface of the lunate. It is not unusual to see full-thickness defects of the cartilage of the lunate as well as tears of the TFC. In extreme cases of excessive ulnar length—common in patients with rheumatoid arthritis—dorsal subluxation of the ulna occurs, and supination is blocked. Severe dorsal subluxation with supination of the carpus is common. Attritional ruptures of the extensor tendons of the fourth and fifth compartments often occur from erosion caused by this prominent ulna.

FINDINGS ON MR IMAGING

With the exception of positive ulnar variants or a prominent ulnar styloid, plain radiographs in patients with early ulnolunate (i.e, ulnocarpal) impingement are unremarkable. Later, subchondral sclerosis and cystic degeneration can be seen along the proximal, adjacent borders of the triquetrum and lunate. Bone scintigraphy may show nonspecific uptake in the ulnolunate region. Magnetic resonance imaging shows central perforations of the TFC in association with neutral or positive ulnar variance; these tears occur between contact surfaces of the lunate and ulna. With MR imaging, it is also possible to detect the earliest changes of subchondral sclerosis on the ulnar aspect of the lunate. Sclerotic changes demonstrate low signal intensity on T_1-, T_2-, or T_2*-weighted

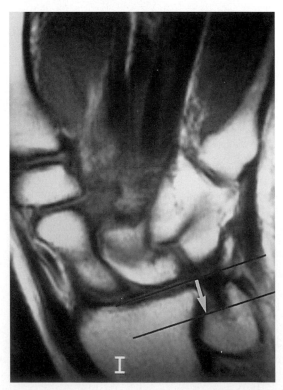

Figure 9–10. Negative ulnar variance with the articular surface of the ulna projecting proximal to the articular surface of the radius *(arrow)*. Note the secondary deformity of the triangular fibrocartilage.

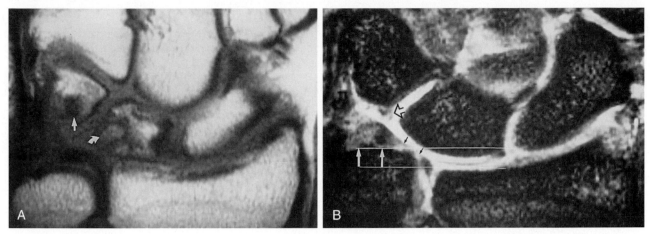

Figure 9–11. Ulnolunate impingement syndrome. *A,* A T₁-weighted coronal image shows low-signal-intensity subchondral degenerative sclerosis involving the ulnar aspect of the lunate *(straight arrow)* and triquetrum *(curved arrow). B,* Positive ulnar variance *(white arrows),* triangular fibrocartilage perforations *(black arrows),* and a torn lunotriquetral ligament *(open arrow)* are features of ulnolunate (i.e., ulnocarpal) impingement syndrome.

images. The cysts demonstrate low or low-to-intermediate signal intensity on T_{2^*}-weighted images. Coronal images reveal the initial degenerative changes in the articular cartilage surfaces of the distal ulna, proximal lunate, or proximal triquetrum. These degenerative changes are indicated either by attenuation of articular cartilage or by irregularity or denuding of the articular cartilage surface. Another feature of the ulnolunate impingement syndrome that can be documented on coronal and sagittal MR images is lunotriquetral ligament disruption and resultant instability. Treatment with TFCC débridement and ulnar shortening may be necessary to relieve pain and halt progression of impingement.

Instability of the Distal Radioulnar Joint

Both CT scanning and MR imaging of both wrists in full pronation and full supination have been shown to be useful in the diagnosis of distal radioulnar subluxation.[38, 39] A new technique to evaluate instability at this joint uses a frame that places a calibrated degree of stress on the distal ulna and radius in conjunction with CT scanning.[40] The controlled load placed on the joint is supposed to simulate the physiology of dynamic subluxation, a condition that is difficult to diagnose. Useful quantitation of the degree of subluxation may also be possible with this technique.

The advantage of axial MR imaging in maximum pronation and supination is the identification of the relative positions of the distal radius and ulna with soft tissue contrast information (Fig. 9–12). Axial images display the condition of the dorsal and volar radioulnar ligaments, and volar radioulnar ligament tears may be associated with dorsal instability of the DRUJ. The normal volar distal radioulnar ligament is maximally taut when the wrist is studied in pronation. Ulnar styloid avulsions, TFCC tears, or distal

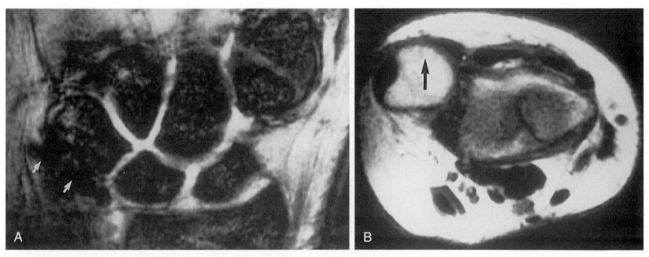

Figure 9–12. Postoperative repair of the triangular fibrocartilage. *A,* A T_{2^*}-weighted coronal image shows low-signal-intensity artifact over the triangular fibrocartilage complex *(arrow). B,* A T₁-weighted axial image shows associated dorsal displacement of the ulna *(arrow).*

radial fractures may lead to DRUJ instability with subluxation, and these structures can be assessed during the same examination with MR imaging in the coronal plane. Compared with CT scanning, MR imaging is more accurate in the characterization of associated effusions of the DRUJ, which are secondary signs of TFC pathology. Axial and sagittal images are useful in demonstrating displacement of the distal ulna in relationship to the TFCC.

MR IMAGING EVALUATION OF THE TRIANGULAR FIBROCARTILAGE COMPLEX

Anatomy

Both the distal and proximal surfaces of the TFC are depicted with MR imaging; this information is not available through wrist arthroscopy or single-compartment radiocarpal arthrography. On T_1-, T_2-, or T_2^*-weighted images taken in the coronal plane, the TFC is depicted as a biconcave disk of homogeneous low signal intensity. The tendon of the extensor carpi ulnaris is seen on the radial aspect of the ulnar styloid process. Coronal plane images of the TFC disk demonstrate the lateral attachment to the ulnar aspect of the distal radius with separate superior and inferior radial attachments. The inferior radial attachment is not seen in arthroscopic evaluation restricted to the radiocarpal surface of the TFC.

The contours of the TFC (i.e., proximal and distal surfaces) and ulnar variance are best assessed in coronal images. The distribution of force across the radial plate is increased by negative ulnar variance and is reduced by positive ulnar variance. The TFC is thus an important contributor in the stabilization of the medial aspect of the radiocarpal joint. Disruption of the TFC is associated with various extents of DRUJ instability. Small tears can lead to pain, clicking, and a subjective feeling of instability. Massive tears can produce subluxation or dislocation in either direction. Volar instability occurs with the wrist in supination, and dorsal instability with the wrist in hyperpronation.

On axial images, the TFC is shaped like an equilateral triangle. The apex of the TFCC converges on the ulnar styloid, with the base of the triangle attached on the superior margin of the distal radial sigmoid notch. Sagittal images show the TFC in sections through the triquetrum. In this plane, the TFC has discoid morphology as seen from anterior to posterior. The TFC is located immediately distal to the dome of the ulna and is thinned centrally with broader volar and distal margins (i.e., peripheral thickening). This peripheral thickening is composed of lamellar collagen and gives rise to the dorsal and volar radioulnar ligaments. The ulnocarpal ligament arises from the volar distal surface of the TFC and passes distally to the bones of the ulnar carpus.

Pathology

Magnetic resonance imaging of the TFCC reveals many tears that previously went undetected.[41] These include intrasubstance (i.e., horizontal) tears and peripheral lesions of the insertions of the TFCC that do not show contrast leakage.

Central perforations of the TFC are unusual in the first two decades of life. By the fifth decade of life, however, symptomatic perforations can be identified in 40 percent of TFC studies, and by the sixth decade, perforations are found in 50 percent of patients studied.[10, 42] This finding may explain the poor correlation between clinical findings of wrist pain and the communication of contrast across the TFC seen in radiocarpal arthrograms. The fact that radiocarpal compartment communication with the inferior radioulnar compartment is found more frequently in anatomic dissections than with arthrographic injection can be explained by the existence of partial tears and unidirectional flap tears (Fig. 9–13).

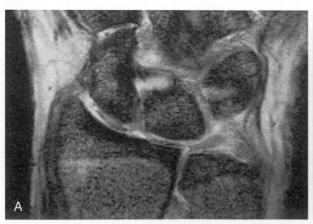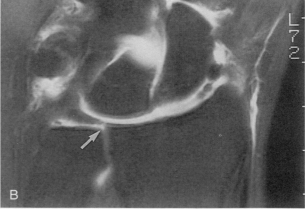

Figure 9–13. T_2^*-weighted coronal image of the wrist without intraarticular contrast (A). Compare this image with B, the same wrist with an intra-articular MR contrast agent. Fluid across a perforated triangular fibrocartilage is visible (arrow).

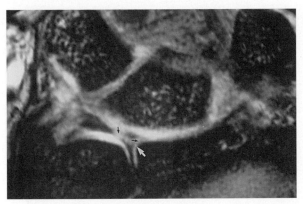

Figure 9–14. A T$_2$*-weighted coronal image shows a high-signal-intensity linear triangular fibrocartilage tear with distal surface and radial extension *(black arrows)*. Note the normal, high-signal-intensity hyaline articular cartilage at the ulnar aspect of the distal radius *(white arrow)*.

The thin layer of hyaline articular cartilage proximal to the radial attachment of the TFC along the ulnar aspect of the distal radius is seen on MR images as bright signal intensity on T$_2$*-weighted images and should not be mistaken for fluid communication with the inferior radioulnar joint or detachment of the radial aspect of the TFC (Fig. 9–14). Intrasubstance degeneration of the TFC is best depicted on T$_2$*-weighted images and appears as regions of increased signal intensity without extension to the superior or inferior margins of the TFC. The meniscal homologue demonstrates greater signal intensity than does the TFC on T$_2$*-weighted images. Partial tears in this area may be more difficult to identify owing to the increased signal intensity and inhomogeneity of the meniscal homologue. Tears of the TFC may occur either as an isolated injury or in association with subluxations of the DRUJ or perilunate dislocations. Patients with TFC pathology often present with pain, clicking, or both on the ulnar aspect of the wrist. An unstable flap of tissue from a torn TFC causes catching on the ulnar aspect of the wrist, especially when loaded in extension or ulnar deviation. TFC tears, demonstrated as discontinuity or fragmentation, are most commonly located near or adjacent to the radial attachment.[43] Contour irregularities, especially with associated regions of increased signal intensity, can be identified on T$_1$-, T$_2$-, or T$_2$*-weighted images. Tears on the radial aspect of the TFC frequently have a dorsal-to-volar orientation extending to both its proximal and distal surfaces.

Associated synovitis presents as a localized fluid collection or radiocarpal joint effusion on T$_2$- or T$_2$*-weighted images and may be associated with chondromalacia of the lunate, triquetrum, or ulna. In younger patients, there is a higher incidence of tears on the ulnar aspect of the TFC. Peripheral tears are usually secondary to traumatic avulsion, whereas central perforations may be associated with findings of TFC degeneration.[44] These degenerative changes of the TFC include increased signal intensity on T$_1$- and

T$_2$*-weighted images and thinning or attenuation of the articular disk. Whereas deformity of the TFC is common in patients with negative ulnar variance, TFC tears are associated with positive ulnar variance.

Magnetic resonance imaging can be used in assessing postoperative TFC repairs and associated distal joint instability. Accuracy of this modality for detecting TFC tears is reported to be 95 percent compared with arthrography and 89 percent compared with arthroscopy and arthrotomy.[23, 41]

FRACTURES OF THE DISTAL RADIUS AND CARPUS

Conventional radiography is limited in the detection of nondisplaced or partially displaced fractures of the carpus and distal radius. Trispiral tomography depends on correct planar positioning, without which carpal fractures may be underdiagnosed. Early bone scintigraphy, performed within 72 hours of an acute fracture, may be negative or equivocal. Computed tomography using thin (1.5-mm) sections in either direct coronal or axial planes with reformatting and 3D rendering is the most accurate modality for identifying fractures and for characterizing morphology and associated comminution or displacement. Chip fractures have been detected by CT in patients with negative MR imaging studies. Fracture extent and adjacent marrow hyperemia are well seen in MR images. In subacute and chronic fractures, sclerosis demonstrates low signal intensity on T$_1$-weighted images. The temporal stage of a fracture (e.g., acute, subacute, chronic) and its location determine the optimal diagnostic imaging plane (e.g., coronal, axial, sagittal). Magnetic resonance shows associated ligamentous injury in isolated or multiple carpal bone trauma. If initial imaging is inadequate, delayed diagnosis and treatment may lead to poor anatomic reduction and function.

Colles' Fractures

Colles' fractures occur secondary to a fall on the outstretched hand, with a pronated forearm in dorsiflexion. The fracture commonly occurs in adult females more than 50 years of age. The fracture line occurs within 2 to 3 cm of the articular surface of the distal radius. The distal fracture segment may demonstrate dorsal displacement, angulation, or both. Medial or lateral displacement may also be present. The transmission of force across the transverse carpal ligament may result in an associated ulnar styloid fracture.

With MR imaging, it is possible to assess the articular surface of the distal radius and to document precise angulation deformities in sagittal, axial, and coronal planes. The median and ulnar nerves, which may be involved at the time of injury, are best seen on axial MR images.

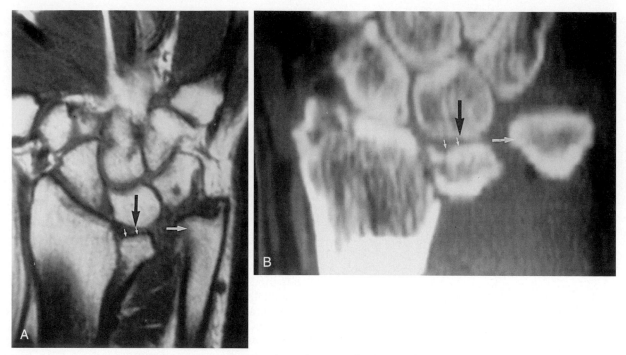

Figure 9–15. Die-punch fracture. T_1-weighted MR image (*A*) and two-dimensional reformatted CT image (*B*) show splitting and depression of the lunate fossa *(small white arrows)* of the distal radius, with proximal migration of the lunate *(black arrows)*. Associated diastasis *(large white arrows)* of the distal radioulnar joint is present, with complete disruption of the triangular fibrocartilage complex.

Die-Punch Fractures

In a die-punch fracture, the lunate impacts the distal radius, splitting its fossa in both the coronal and sagittal planes and depressing the articular surface, much like a tibial plateau fracture (Fig. 9–15).[45, 46] It is critical to restore the articular surface to anatomic continuity following this injury to prevent the development of late traumatic arthritis.

Clinical studies have shown that more than 90 percent of young adult patients with incongruity (defined as more than 2 mm of displacement) develop arthritis.[47] Because the die-punch lesion is a common cause of incongruity, surgeons have increased their efforts to reestablish normal articular anatomy following these injuries. Newer surgical techniques that show some promise include arthroscopic percutaneous pinning and reduction. Once the depressed articular fragments are reduced, they can be augmented with buttressing bone grafts placed via an extra-articular approach. Thin-section (1.5-mm) CT scans or multiplanar MR images can be used to assess the intra-articular extent of fracture as well as fracture morphology. Coronal and sagittal images are especially helpful in measuring cortical depression or offset.

Carpal Fractures

SCAPHOID FRACTURES

On MR imaging studies of scaphoid fractures, the low-signal-intensity fracture line is clearly displayed and may persist, contrasting with the surrounding bright signal intensity of marrow during healing (Fig. 9–16). The identification of extension to cortical bone is necessary to accurately differentiate acute from chronic fractures, and it allows MR imaging to be more sensitive than CT scanning or conventional radiography in evaluating the progress of subacute or chronic fractures.

Sagittal images demonstrate the abnormal morphology of the scaphoid, secondary to fracture fragmentation or suboptimal healing (i.e., humpback deformity). This foreshortening of the scaphoid is associated with DISI instability (Fig. 9–17). Herbert screws are imaged with minimal artifact. The articular cartilage surface of the scaphoid and the congruity of adjacent coronal surfaces should be assessed. T_{2*}-weighted images are not as sensitive to the range of contrast as conventional T_1-weighted images and may not identify a nonacute, nondisplaced fracture. Gradient-echo images are, however, useful in demonstrating the integrity of the adjacent SL ligament. The volar capsule (the RSC ligament and radiolunotriquetral ligament) is shown on sagittal images, and adjacent synovitis or edema of ligamentous structures may be identified on T_1- or T_{2*}-weighted images at the level of the scaphoid. STIR imaging is more sensitive to hyperemia in the proximal pole or in bone adjacent to the fracture site, which may be misdiagnosed as sclerosis, necrosis, or both on conventional T_1-, T_2-, or T_{2*}-weighted images.

TRIQUETRUM FRACTURES

Fractures of the triquetrum represent the second most common fracture of the carpus.[48] Correct positioning

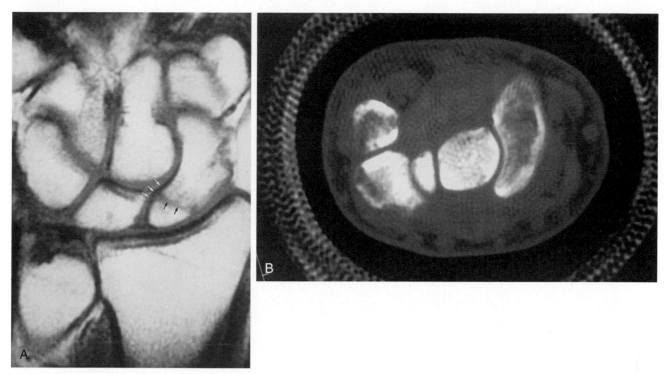

Figure 9–16. *A,* T_1-weighted coronal image shows a low-signal-intensity healing fracture line located across the proximal pole of the scaphoid *(black arrows),* with intact cortical margins *(white arrows).* Normal fat marrow is present in the proximal pole. *B,* The corresponding axial image does not show cortical or trabecular fracture. This is consistent with the continuity of the cortex seen on corresponding MR images, which are more sensitive in the initial and healing stages of scaphoid fractures. Small chip fractures of other carpal bones, however, are still best evaluated with thin-section CT.

in lateral and pronated oblique projections is usually required to identify fractures of the triquetrum on standard radiography. Computed tomography examination of the triquetrum is not limited by overlapping of proximal and distal carpal rows, which may obscure identification of a fracture line. Triquetral fractures include chip fractures that involve the dorsal surface and occur secondary to an avulsion injury at the insertional site of the ulnotriquetral ligament, or to trauma to the wrist positioned in hyperextension and ulnar deviation (Fig. 9–18). Fracture through the body of the triquetrum is less common. Triquetral body fractures may be associated with perilunate dislocations or ulnar carpal dissociation.

Multiple fracture lines and acute fracture through the triquetrum may obscure fracture morphology secondary to reactive hyperemia of subchondral bone. T_1-weighted images in the axial, coronal, and sagittal imaging planes identify low signal intensity in the area of the fracture. In our experience, CT scanning has been more useful in displaying cortical detail and fracture morphology.

LUNATE FRACTURES

Fracture of the lunate is an uncommon injury that usually occurs secondary to a fall with the wrist in dorsiflexion.[48] Acute fractures of the lunate associated with Kienböck's disease may be related to single or multiple episodes of compression forces. However, fracture of the lunate is more commonly seen during the advanced stages of this disease, as a pathologic fracture through areas of necrotic bone. Associated perilunate dislocation with ligamentous trauma should be evaluated.

PISIFORM FRACTURES

The pisiform is a sesamoid bone within the flexor carpi ulnaris tendon.[48] Pisiform fracture is caused by direct or blunt trauma, such as occurs when the heel of the hand is used as a hammer. It appears as a comminuted or simple fracture. Pisotriquetral arthritis may develop secondary to pisiform fracture. Sagittal and axial T_1-weighted images display a larger surface area of the pisiform bone, minimizing the partial-volume effect that may complicate coronal images.

HAMATE FRACTURES

Fractures of the hamate, which account for approximately 2 percent of carpal fractures,[48] may involve either the body or the hook (i.e., the hamulus).[49] Fracture of the hook of the hamate may involve an avulsion injury of the transverse carpal ligament. Direct trauma to the volar aspect of the wrist, the most common mechanism of injury, usually occurs in activities that require a grasping movement, such as holding a

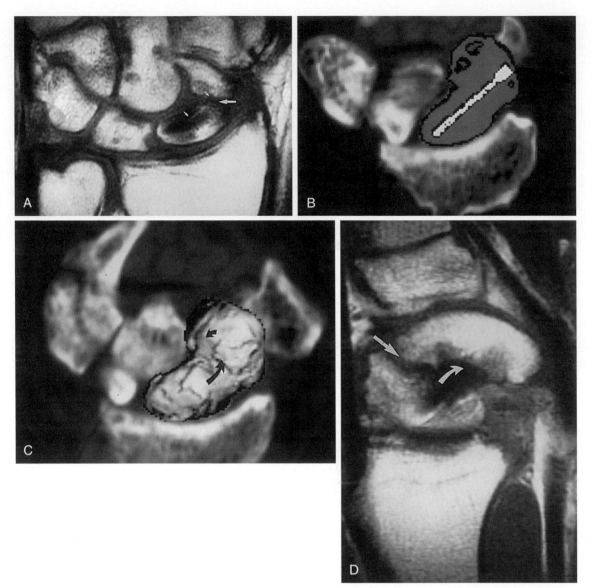

Figure 9–17. Scaphoid fracture with dorsal intercalated segment instability (DISI). *A,* A T_1-weighted coronal image shows minimal artifact adjacent to the screw *(small arrows).* A low-signal-intensity fracture line *(large arrow)* is seen in the middle one-third of the scaphoid, without development of avascular necrosis of the proximal pole. *B,* Two-dimensional reformatted CT image showing titanium screw. *C,* Three-dimensional representation of scaphoid with flexion of the distal pole *(arrow).* *D,* T_1-weighted sagittal image demonstrating humpback deformity of flexed scaphoid *(curved arrow)* at fracture site *(straight arrow).*

bat, club, or racquet. Conventional radiographic imaging is often negative for hamate fracture; diagnosis may require the use of a carpal tunnel or supinated oblique projection. For MR imaging studies, T_1-weighted axial and sagittal images are best suited for display of the anatomy of the hook of the hamate (Fig. 9–19). Thin (1.5-mm) CT scans, however, more accurately identify the extent and location of fractures of the hamate, especially the hook of the hamate. The proximity of the ulnar nerve to the hamate may contribute to the presentation of ulnar finger and hand pain in patients sustaining hamate trauma.

CAPITATE FRACTURES

Fractures of the capitate, which account for 1 to 3 percent of carpal bone fractures,[48] are similar to scaphoid fractures in that the blood supply of the capitate extends from distal to proximal through the waist of the capitate, making the proximal pole susceptible to AVN. Capitate fractures are caused by either direct trauma or forced dorsiflexion and may be associated with perilunate dislocation. The most common site of fractures involves the waist or neck of the capitate. Sagittal MR images are helpful in assessing rotation at the fracture site.

TRAPEZIUS AND TRAPEZOID FRACTURES

Fractures of the trapezius involve either the body or the volar margin.[48] The trapezoid is the least commonly fractured bone of the carpus.

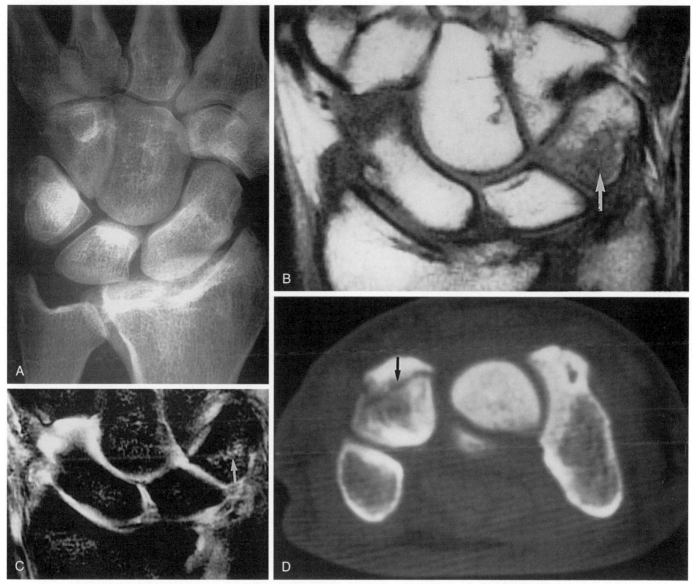

Figure 9–18. *A,* Standard anteroposterior projection radiograph negative for triquetral fracture. *B,* T$_1$-weighted coronal image with low-signal-intensity marrow hyperemia in triquetrum *(arrow). C,* T$_2$*-weighted coronal image with hyperintense marrow edema and hemorrhage *(arrow). D,* Axial CT scan identifies dorsal fracture morphology directly *(arrow).*

AVASCULAR NECROSIS OF THE SCAPHOID

Avascular necrosis of the scaphoid is primarily a post-traumatic event that occurs secondary to the proximal pole or waist fractures that endanger the dominant blood supply of the scaphoid. There often is sclerosis of the proximal pole related to osteopenia and hyperemia of adjacent nonnecrotic bone. By the time resorption and collapse are evident on plain radiographs, however, the disease is in an advanced state. Avascular necrosis of the scaphoid may also occur in the absence of fracture and is then referred to as Preiser's disease.

The application of MR imaging to the detection and evaluation of AVN is facilitated by the bright-signal-intensity contrast generated from the normal fatty marrow content of the carpal bones. MR imaging has been reported to be as sensitive as bone scintigraphy in the detection of AVN and to possess even greater specificity in diagnosis.[17, 18, 50–53] On T$_1$-weighted (i.e., short T$_R$/T$_E$ sequences), MR imaging's sensitivity rate for the detection of decreased marrow signal associated with AVN is 87.5 percent. With the addition of T$_2$-weighted sequences, specificity is reported to be 100 percent.

The most common MR imaging appearance of AVN of the scaphoid is low signal intensity in the proximal pole on both and T$_1$- and T$_2$-weighted images (Fig. 9–20). In diffuse marrow necrosis, low-signal-intensity marrow may not be restricted to the proximal pole. T$_2$-weighted images may demonstrate localized

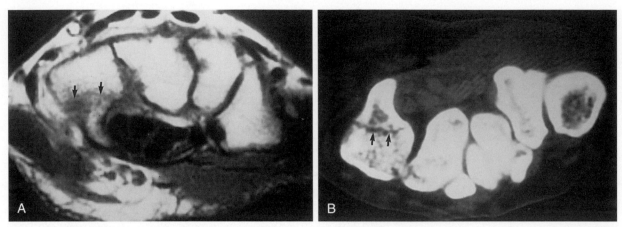

Figure 9–19. Hamate fracture. *A*, A T₁-weighted axial image shows a low-signal-intensity transition *(arrows)* between a fractured hook of the hamate and normal fat marrow signal intensity. Guyon's canal is also seen. *B*, Corresponding axial image of the carpal tunnel shows a transverse undisplaced fracture *(arrows)* with greater cortical edge detail. MR imaging, however, allows visualization of Guyon's canal and assessment of the ulnar neurovascular structures, which may be secondarily compromised. Fractures of the hook of the hamate are more common than body fractures and may be overlooked on clinical examination or standard radiographs, because a carpal tunnel view is required for their identification.

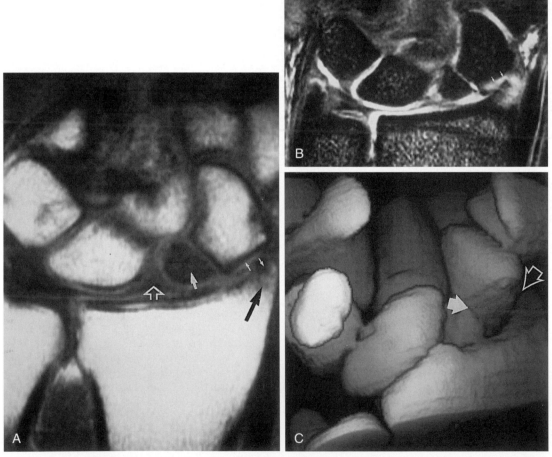

Figure 9–20. Avascular necrosis (AVN) of the scaphoid, with early scapholunate advanced collapse (SLAC) wrist. *A*, A low-signal-intensity "corner sign" of radial styloid subchondral sclerosis *(black arrow)* is seen in the presence of scaphoid non-union and AVN of the proximal pole *(large white arrow)* on a T₁-weighted coronal image. There is mild narrowing of the radioscaphoid articulation with respect to the distal pole *(small white arrows)*. The scapholunate interosseous ligament is intact *(open arrow)*. *B*, Attenuated articular cartilage is seen in the proximal aspect of the distal pole of the scaphoid in early SLAC degeneration *(arrows)* on a T₂*-weighted coronal image. The radiolunate joint is characteristically unaffected. *C*, A three-dimensional CT image shows the fracture site *(solid arrow)* and narrowing of the radioscaphoid articulation at the level of the distal pole of the scaphoid *(open arrow)*.

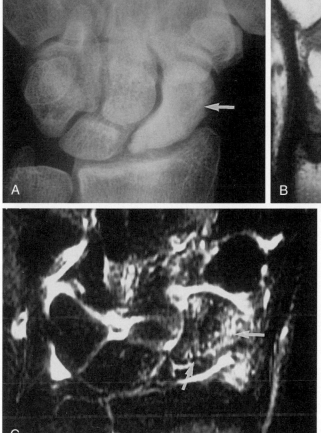
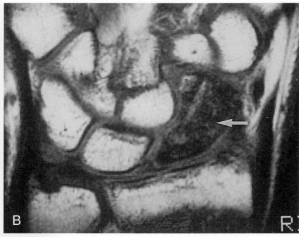

Figure 9–21. Scaphoid avascular necrosis. *A,* An anteroposterior radiograph shows diffuse sclerosis of the scaphoid. The deformity of the proximal aspect of the proximal pole is known as the "nipple sign" and is sometimes seen in association with scaphoid fractures. There is relatively little sclerosis of the distal pole *(arrow)* compared with that present in the proximal pole. *B,* A T_1-weighted coronal image shows diffuse low-signal-intensity sclerosis *(arrow). C,* A short TI inversion recovery (STIR) coronal image most accurately depicts hyperintense hyperemic marrow in the waist and distal pole of the scaphoid *(arrows);* these hyperintensities are not seen on the T_1-weighted image. A scaphoid fracture is not identified.

fluid accumulation and limited marrow edema of the proximal pole. Reactive marrow hyperemia of the distal pole may be confused with diffuse changes of necrosis (Fig. 9–21). *Short TI inversion recovery* (STIR) images can be used to document increased hyperemia of the distal pole marrow, which may not be appreciated on conventional T_1-, T_2-, or T_{2^*}-weighted images. Accurate assessment of vascularity may be limited to gradient-echo sequences. Vascularized pedicle graft is a treatment option prescribed for scaphoid non-union with a nonviable proximal fragment.

Kienböck's Disease

Although the MR imaging of Kienböck's disease was discussed in detail earlier, a few comments are in order here concerning the early presentation of the disease. In stage I, plain films are normal; before MR imaging became readily available, the standard test at this stage was the three-phase-technetium Tc 99m-methylene disphosphonate (^{99m}Tc-MDP) study.[54] When there is abnormal uptake of ^{99m}Tc, especially in the third or delayed phase, a CT scan should be performed to assess trabecular bone morphology and to identify fractures. The three-phase ^{99m}Tc-MDP study is extremely sensitive but does not provide detail about physiologic changes in the marrow, which can be seen on MR images. Magnetic resonance imaging is potentially the best first imaging examination to be done after routine radiographs. It not only allows assessment of the lunate, but also facilitates ruling out or adding other possibilities in the differential diagnosis. MR imaging studies may reveal occult ganglion cysts as well as inflammatory arthritides with synovitis.

FINDINGS ON MR IMAGING

MR imaging findings in Kienböck's disease can also be grouped according to the stage of disease.[53]

Stage I

As mentioned, conventional radiographs are usually normal in stage I Kienböck's disease, although an associated fracture line or compression fracture may be present. At this early stage, bone scintigraphy is both sensitive and nonspecific for the diagnosis of this disorder. However, bone scintigraphy is poor in differentiating fractures, osteochondral lesions, ero-

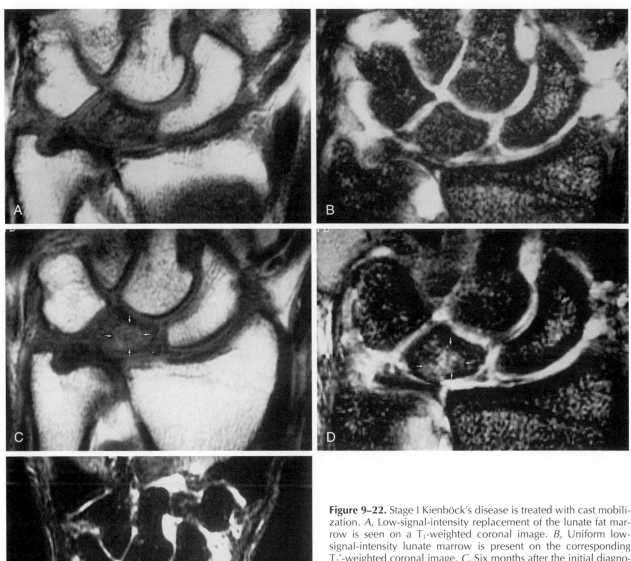

Figure 9–22. Stage I Kienböck's disease is treated with cast mobilization. *A,* Low-signal-intensity replacement of the lunate fat marrow is seen on a T_1-weighted coronal image. *B,* Uniform low-signal-intensity lunate marrow is present on the corresponding T_2^*-weighted coronal image. *C,* Six months after the initial diagnosis, central fat marrow signal intensity *(arrows)* is seen on a T_1-weighted coronal image. The corresponding T_2^*-weighted image and (*D*) short TI inversion recovery (STIR) image (*E*) show lunate hyperintensity *(arrows).* The STIR image is more sensitive to marrow hyperemia.

sions, and the spectrum of degenerative changes that manifest as subchondral sclerosis. Magnetic resonance imaging offers comparable or greater sensitivity and better specificity compared with scintigraphy or radiographs (Fig. 9–22).

With MR imaging, it is possible to characterize the extent of necrosis and the morphology of marrow involvement as well as the overall morphology of the lunate cortical surfaces, including articular cartilage. Focal or diffuse low signal intensity is seen on T_1-weighted images in affected areas of marrow involvement. Coronal plane images best display the largest anteroposterior surface area of involvement. The addition of sagittal or axial images provides more accurate assessment of the volume of marrow involvement. On T_{2^*}-weighted images, the lunate demonstrates uniform low signal intensity. Normal lunate marrow or recovering marrow vascularity usually displays a central region of mildly increased signal intensity or inhomogeneity in gradient-echo images. STIR sequences are more sensitive to hyperemia or vascular dilation and demonstrate increased signal intensity restricted to the lunate. In contrast, T_{2^*}-weighted images are likely to demonstrate faint vascular signal intensity from all carpal bones, especially the scaphoid and lunate in the noninjured carpus.

In early Kienböck's disease, T$_1$-weighted images show unaffected marrow with the high signal intensity of fat, isointense with the other carpal bones of the wrist. The distribution of low-signal-intensity necrosis may be restricted to a portion of the volar or dorsal coronal plane or may demonstrate an eccentric or central region of involvement. Radiocarpal joint effusion or more localized synovitis demonstrates bright signal intensity on T$_2$-weighted, T$_{2*}$-weighted, and STIR sequences.

Interval MR imaging can be used to show the progression of Kienböck's disease or to document healing with the return of normal marrow signal intensity in stage I disease (Figs. 9–22 and 9–23). The relative osteopenia of the remaining carpus is not seen using MR imaging techniques.

Stage II

In stage II Kienböck's disease, plain film radiographs show sclerosis of the lunate, which demonstrates low signal intensity on T$_1$-weighted MR images. STIR images demonstrate areas of increased signal intensity in patients who have sclerosis on corresponding radiographs. Generally, although morphology and size are preserved, decreased height of the radial aspect of the lunate may be seen in late stage II disease (Fig. 9–24).

Stage III

The lunate undergoes distal-to-proximal collapse in the coronal plane and elongation in the sagittal plane in stage III Kienböck's disease (Fig. 9–25). There is reciprocal proximal migration of the capitate. The absence or presence of SL dissociation with rotatory subluxation of the scaphoid divides patients into stage IIIA and stage IIIB, respectively. Rotation of the scaphoid may be accompanied by ulnar deviation of the triquetrum. With scaphoid rotation, the inability to see the entire long axis of the scaphoid in a single coronal image is the MR imaging equivalent of the radiographic "ring" sign in conventional anteroposterior radiographic projections.

Stage IV

Stage IV Kienböck's disease is characterized by degenerative arthrosis of the lunate and carpus. There are no regions of increased signal intensity on T$_{2*}$-weighted or STIR images in this advanced stage of disease. Lunate collapse can be defined in all three orthogonal planes with MR imaging. With splaying of the volar and dorsal poles of the lunate, there are extrinsic effacement and convex bowing of the flexor tendons in the sagittal plane. This may contribute to symptoms of carpal tunnel syndrome, especially if there is associated proximal migration of the flexor retinaculum with wrist shortening. Fragmented portions of the lunate are usually identified with low signal intensity on T$_1$- and T$_{2*}$-weighted images. Thin-section (1.5-mm) CT scans provide more accurate assessment of cortical fragmentation. Kienböck's disease has also been associated with Madelung's de-

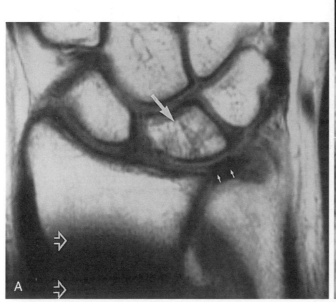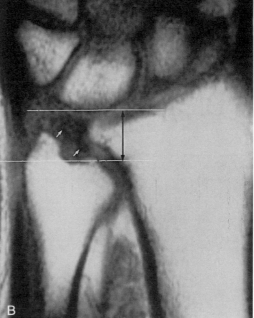

Figure 9–23. *A,* Recovering fat marrow signal intensity *(large arrow)* is present after treatment of stage I Kienböck's disease of the wrist. The triangular fibrocartilage *(small arrows)* is normal. A low-signal-intensity postoperative artifact secondary to radial shortening is present *(open arrows). B,* The untreated left wrist shows severe negative ulnar variance *(black double-headed arrow)* and deformed but intact triangular fibrocartilage *(white arrows).* The lunate marrow is unaffected.

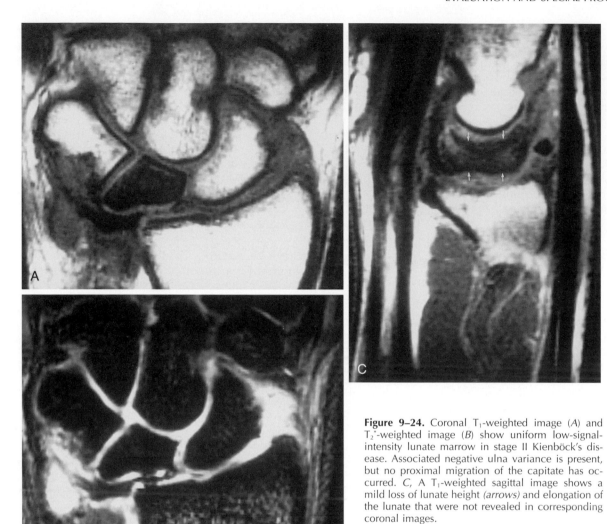

Figure 9–24. Coronal T_1-weighted image (*A*) and T_2^*-weighted image (*B*) show uniform low-signal-intensity lunate marrow in stage II Kienböck's disease. Associated negative ulna variance is present, but no proximal migration of the capitate has occurred. *C*, A T_1-weighted sagittal image shows a mild loss of lunate height *(arrows)* and elongation of the lunate that were not revealed in corresponding coronal images.

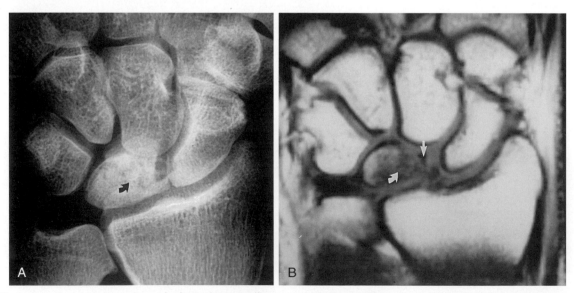

Figure 9–25. *A*, An anteroposterior radiograph shows lunate collapse *(curved arrow)* and proximal migration of the capitate in early stage III Kienböck's disease. *B*, A T_1-weighted coronal image better depicts necrotic marrow *(curved arrow)* and lunate collapse in the radial border *(straight arrow)*.

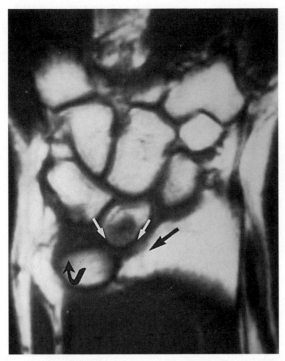

Figure 9–26. Madelung's deformity. A T_1-weighted coronal image shows medial angulation of the distal radial articular surface *(straight black arrow)*, dorsal subluxation of the ulna *(curved black arrow)*, and triangular configuration of the carpus with the lunate at the apex *(white arrows)*, all of which constitute Madelung's deformity. Associated Kienböck's disease is shown as central low-signal-intensity marrow.

formity, a developmental anomaly involving the distal radius and carpus (Fig. 9–26).

MR IMAGING FINDINGS IN CARPAL TUNNEL SYNDROME

The ability to display the cross-sectional anatomy of the median nerve and adjacent structures on axial images and to trace the flexor tendons on coronal plane images makes MR imaging valuable in characterizing normal anatomy and pathology in the carpal tunnel.[55–59] Early detection of the cause of carpal tunnel syndrome requires soft tissue discrimination not possible with standard radiographs or CT scanning. Axial and coronal MR imaging of the wrist has shown potential for evaluating patients with a clinical presentation of median nerve deficits.

Axial MR images demonstrate bowing of the flexor retinaculum in patients with flexor tenosynovitis, and inflamed synovium and tendon sheaths demonstrate low signal intensity on T_1-weighted images and increased signal intensity on T_2-weighted, T_{2^*}-weighted, and STIR sequences (Fig. 9–27).

Changes in the median nerve are present regardless of the etiology of carpal tunnel syndrome.[57] These findings include the following:

1. Diffuse swelling or segmental enlargement of the median nerve, best evaluated at the level of the pisiform.
2. Flattening of the median nerve, best demonstrated at the level of the hamate.
3. Palmar bowing of the flexor retinaculum, assessed at the level of the hamate.[58]
4. Increased signal intensity within the median nerve on T_2-weighted images.

Comparison with the contralateral wrist may be misleading, because involvement is bilateral in one half to two thirds of patients with carpal tunnel syndrome.

Alterations in median nerve signal intensity are nonspecific and may represent edema or demyelination without neural fibers. Signal intensity may be decreased when fibrosis is the primary median nerve pathology. Compression and flattening of the median nerve may be demonstrated at the level of the hamate along with bowing of the flexor retinaculum. Ratios of swelling can be calculated by dividing the cross-sectional area of the median nerve at the level of the pisiform and the hamate by the cross-sectional area of the median nerve at the level of the distal radius.[56, 57] Significant differences, with doubling of ratios of swelling, have been shown in patients with carpal tunnel syndrome, despite the subjective flattening of the median nerve at the lateral and distal carpus. Ratios of flattening have been used to document statistically significant flattening of the median nerve at the level of the hamate.[57, 58] The median nerve may display enlargement or dilation at the level of the pisiform, and compression with flattening at the level of the hook of the hamate.

Increased signal intensity of the median nerve, best demonstrated on gradient-echo axial or STIR images, may be accompanied by an increase in its cross-sectional diameter. Degenerative arthritis and instabilities in advanced arthrosis may cause a decrease in cross-sectional area of the carpal tunnel and produce symptoms of carpal tunnel disease. These attempts to correlate median nerve diameter with clinical pathology, however, require further study. Magnetic resonance imaging is most useful in characterizing space-occupying lesions, whether tenosynovitis, ganglia, lipomas, or granulomatous infections (Fig. 9–28).

Enlargement or swelling of the median nerve proximal to the carpal tunnel, referred to as a *pseudoneuroma*, has also been documented with MR imaging. This condition may actually be associated with constriction of the median nerve within the carpal tunnel, distal to the point of swelling.

Chronic induration after transverse carpal ligament release is seen on MR images as an area of neural constriction. Residual hyperintensity of the median nerve within the carpal tunnel may occur with incomplete release of the flexor retinaculum. Release of the transverse carpal ligament from the hook of the hamate may cause the flexor tendons or contents of the carpal tunnel to demonstrate a greater volar convexity because of the loss of the normal roof support of the flexor retinaculum. Widening of the fat stripe

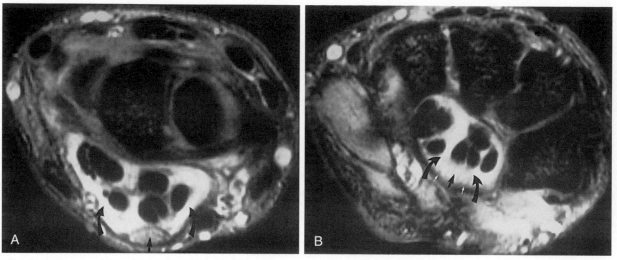

Figure 9–27. In carpal tunnel syndrome, T_2^*-weighted axial images show (A) severe, high-signal-intensity flexor tenosynovitis *(curved arrows)*, swelling of the median nerve proximal to the carpal tunnel *(black arrow)*, and (B) hyperintense synovitis *(curved black arrows)* and median nerve *(straight black arrow)*. The flexor retinaculum is bowed *(white arrows)*.

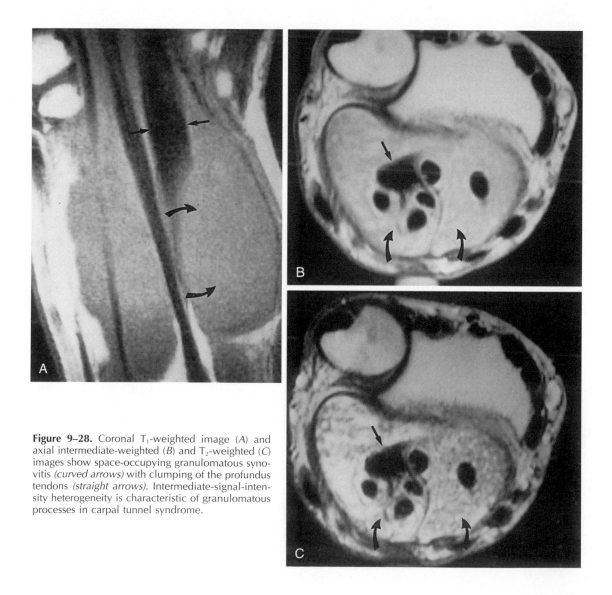

Figure 9–28. Coronal T_1-weighted image (A) and axial intermediate-weighted (B) and T_2-weighted (C) images show space-occupying granulomatous synovitis *(curved arrows)* with clumping of the profundus tendons *(straight arrows)*. Intermediate-signal-intensity heterogeneity is characteristic of granulomatous processes in carpal tunnel syndrome.

is normally seen posterior to the flexor digitorum profundus tendons postoperatively.

ARTHRITIS

Conventional radiography has been the cornerstone of evaluation and follow-up of arthritides involving the wrist. The superior soft tissue discrimination achieved by MR imaging, however, has proved useful in evaluating patients in both the initial and advanced stages of arthritis. Magnetic resonance imaging achieves noninvasive, accurate delineation of hyaline articular cartilage, ligaments, tendons, and synovium as distinct from cortical bone.[18, 60, 61] Alterations in joint morphology or structure can be identified with MR imaging studies before changes can be seen in standard radiographs. Although MR imaging should never replace radiography nor be used in every patient receiving rheumatologic evaluation, it can, in selected cases, offer specific information that may modify the patient's diagnosis or treatment.

Degenerative Arthritis

Joint space narrowing, loss of articular cartilage, subchondral sclerosis, and cyst formation characterize degeneration patterns of the carpus. Scapholunate advanced collapse (SLAC) develops from incongruent loading and degeneration across the radioscaphoid articulation, related to malalignment of the scaphoid.[62] The SLAC wrist represents the most common form of degenerative arthritis and is associated with the gradual collapse and loss of ligamentous support. Scapholunate advanced collapse degeneration may occur with carpal collapse, including that caused by scaphoid non-union, scapholunate instability, calcium pyrophosphate deposition disease (CPDD), and Kienböck's disease. The earliest changes seen in the SLAC wrist involve spiking at the junction of the articular and nonarticular surfaces on the radial side of the scaphoid, sharpening at the radial styloid tip, and loss of cartilage. Early cartilage loss can be seen clearly on MR images, and the low-signal-intensity initial changes in subchondral sclerosis of the radial styloid appear on MR images prior to any visible changes on conventional radiographs. Later in the disease, there is narrowing of the radioscaphoid joint, and the capitolunate joint begins to degenerate. Once the articular space between the capitate and lunate is lost, the hamate impinges against the lunate, and degeneration also occurs at this site (Fig. 9–29).

Triscaphe arthritis, the second most common form of degenerative arthritis, involves the scaphoid, trapezius, and trapezoid articulation.[62] Isolated scaphotrapezial involvement is more common than isolated scaphotrapezoidal involvement. An SLAC wrist may occur in combination with triscaphe degenerative arthritis. Other locations of degenerative arthritis include between the distal ulna and the lunate, and the LT joints.[62]

Rheumatoid Arthritis

Small joint involvement of the wrist in rheumatoid arthritis characteristically involves the carpus and the metacorpophalangeal (MP) and proximal interphalangeal (PIP) joints.[63] Soft tissue swelling includes joint effusion, edema, and tenosynovitis. Swan-neck and boutonnière deformities are common, and in advanced disease, there are subluxations, dislocations, ulnar deviation in the MP joints, and radial deviation in the radiocarpal articulation. Destructive changes include "main en lorgnette" (i.e., telescoping of the fingers), ulnar erosions, SL dissociation, and DRUJ incongruity.

Gadolinium contrast has been used in MR imaging to selectively enhance pannus tissue in synovitis involving the DRUJ; the ulnar styloid process; the radiocarpal, intercarpal, and MP joints; and the flexor and extensor tendons. Synovial involvement of ligamentous structures commonly affects the ulnolunate and ulnotriquetral ligaments, TFCC, DRUJ, ulnocarpal meniscal homologue, as well as the ulnar collateral, radioscaphocapitate (RSC), radioscapholunate (RSL), long radiolunate (LRL), and short radiolunate (SRL) ligaments.[64] The differential diagnosis of rupture of the extensor tendons at the wrist includes MP synovitis, posterior interosseous nerve palsy from rheumatoid disease of the elbow, and extensor tendon subluxation overlying the metacarpal heads.[65] With MR imaging, it is possible to identify rupture of the extensor pollicis longus tendon, which may be difficult to assess clinically.[64] Triangular fibrocartilage tears, dorsal displacement of the ulna, carpal tunnel pathology, and SL dissociation are also assessed on routine coronal, axial, and sagittal studies (Fig. 9–30).

In patients with chronic rheumatoid disease, both plain film radiography and MR imaging studies document the subluxations and erosions affecting the phalanges, carpals, metacarpals, and ulnar styloid. The changes are more pronounced on MR images. Both T_1 and T_2 tissue relaxation times are prolonged in acute inflammation with edema and in joint effusion; therefore, both conditions demonstrate low signal intensity on T_1-weighted images and high signal intensity on T_2-weighted images. Inflammatory edema may also extend into the subcutaneous tissues. In contrast, chronically inflamed tissue remains low in signal intensity on both T_1- and T_2-weighted images. In more advanced rheumatoid disease, pannus formation can be identified and demonstrates low to intermediate signal intensity on both T_1- and T_2-weighted images. Adjacent areas of fluid collection demonstrate increased signal intensity on T_2-weighted acquisitions. Although the signal intensity of localized edematous or inflammatory tissue may be similar to that of synovial fluid, noninflammatory effusions in the wrist do not, when imaged on T_2-weighted sequences, display an irregular pattern or focal distribution at multiple sites.

Cystic carpal erosions are better delineated on MR images than on corresponding anteroposterior radio-

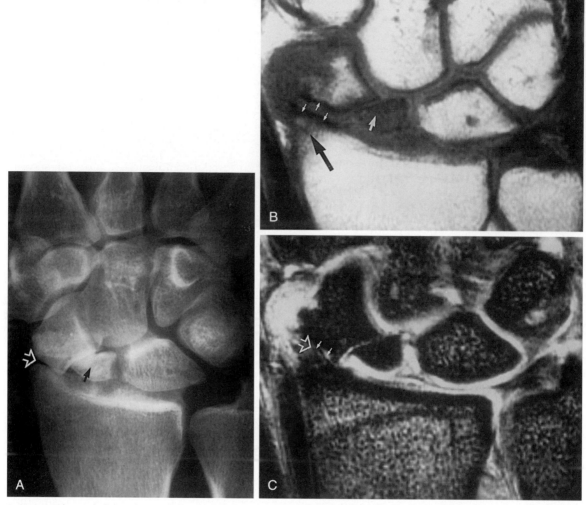

Figure 9–29. Wrist with scapholunate advanced collapse (SLAC). *A,* An anteroposterior radiograph shows non-union of a scaphoid fracture with degenerative joint space narrowing between the distal pole of the scaphoid and radius *(open arrow).* Sclerosis is present in avascular necrosis (AVN) of the proximal pole *(solid arrow).* Coronal T_1-weighted (*B*) and T_2^*-weighted (*C*) images of SLAC wrist reveal degeneration at the radioscaphoid joint *(open arrow)* and subchondral low-signal-intensity sclerosis in the radiostyloscaphoid area. Denuded articular cartilage *(small white arrows)* extends proximally only to the level of the non-union. The proximal pole of the scaphoid functions as a second lunate with preserved articular cartilage. In (*B*), note the low-signal-intensity "corner sign" of the radial styloid, which is characteristic of early SLAC degeneration *(large black arrow).* AVN of the proximal pole is indicated *(large white arrow).* Increased loading of the capitolunate joint is associated with loss of radioscaphoid cartilage.

graphs. Destruction of the cartilage and joint arthrosis can be distinctly seen on T_1-weighted images. Marrow changes (e.g., subchondral sclerosis), present on both sides of the joint or carpal articulation, helped to differentiate arthrosis from intramedullary edema.

In patients with juvenile rheumatoid arthritis with wrist involvement, early fluid collections along tendon sheaths, subarticular erosions, and cysts, as well as attenuated intercarpal articular cartilage, were detected on MR images but were not revealed on conventional radiographs. Subluxations and areas of bone destruction were equally evident on MR images and plain film radiographs.

Magnetic resonance imaging has the potential to become an important adjunct in diagnosing and monitoring patients with rheumatoid disease. Further

studies with larger patient populations and comparisons with conventional radiographic studies are required before standard indications can be implemented in rheumatoid arthritis. Magnetic resonance imaging may also prove to be valuable in monitoring response to drug therapy, including remittative agents such as methotrexate and gold in juvenile and adult rheumatoid disease.

Miscellaneous Arthritides

In evaluating non-rheumatoid arthritic disease, we have had the opportunity to study patients with psoriatic arthritis, Lyme disease, intraosseous sarcoid,

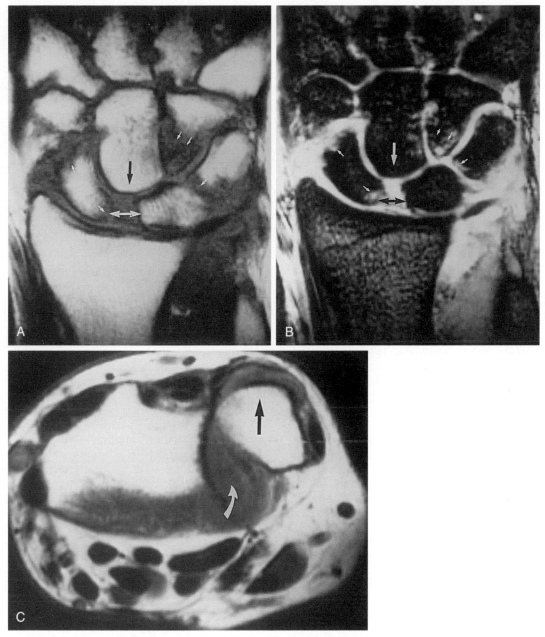

Figure 9–30. Rheumatoid arthritis T$_1$-weighted coronal (*A*) and T$_2^*$-weighted (*B*) images show rheumatoid changes of scapholunate dissociation *(double-headed arrows)*, proximal migration of the capitate *(large single arrow)*, and multiple erosions involving the scaphoid, triquetrum, and hamate *(small white arrows)*. Erosions of the intermetacarpal joints are also present. Note that the carpus has begun to migrate toward the ulna, and the distance between the radial styloid and the scaphoid is increased. *C,* An axial T$_1$-weighted image shows dorsal subluxation of the ulna *(straight arrow)* and distal radioulnar joint effusion and pannus *(curved arrow)*.

hemophilia, calcium pyrophosphate deposition disease, and the more commonly found osteoarthritis.

Magnetic resonance imaging studies in psoriatic arthritis demonstrate destruction of the TFC with pancompartmental joint space narrowing, erosions, SL ligament disruption, and subchondral low-signal-intensity sclerosis of the carpus. Synovitis of the flexor carpi radialis tendon and the inferior radioulnar compartment, intermediate-signal-intensity inflammatory tissue, and dorsal subluxation of the distal ulna can be identified on T$_1$- and T$_2$-weighted axial images. In diffuse soft tissue swelling of a single digit secondary to psoriatic arthritis, MR imaging may be successful in excluding osteomyelitis (Fig. 9–31).

Magnetic resonance imaging studies of Lyme arthritis of the wrist reveal information not available on conventional radiographs. Pockets of fluid collection, characterized by high signal intensity on T$_2$-weighted images, can be detected, and a scalloped contour of fluid interface can be demonstrated adjacent to inflamed synovium. Joint deformities or cartilaginous erosions are not usually detected.

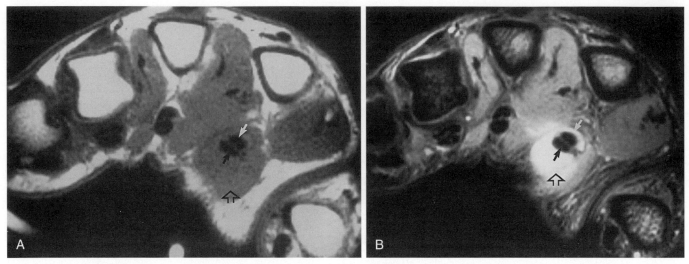

Figure 9–31. Psoriatic arthritis. T_1-weighted (A) and T_{2^*}-weighted (B) images show tenosynovitis *(open arrows)* of the flexor digitorum superficialis *(black arrows)* and profundus *(white arrows)* tendons involving the entire second digit (i.e., sausage digit).

The hand is a predominant site of involvement in patients who have the relatively rare disorder skeletal sarcoidosis. In one of our cases, conventional radiographs demonstrated lytic changes characteristic of sarcoid in both the middle and distal phalanges. Although MR images did not provide any additional diagnostic information, the extent of soft tissue granulomatous proliferation in the cystic defects and areas of cortical destruction were more accurately demonstrated on coronal and axial MR images. The noncaseating, granulomatous tissue typical of sarcoidosis demonstrates low to intermediate signal intensity on T_1-weighted sequences and high signal intensity on T_2-weighted images.

In hemophilia, acute hemorrhage into the soft tissues may be seen with a fluid-fluid level. Higher-signal-intensity serum layers above hemorrhagic sediment. More subacute or chronic hemorrhage demonstrates hemosiderin (i.e., dark) signal intensity on T_1-, T_2-, or T_{2^*}-weighted images.

We have studied one patient with CPDD. On T_1-weighted images, areas of intra-articular calcification were not satisfactorily demonstrated compared with high-quality magnification radiographs. T_2 and T_{2^*} weighting and photography at high contrast settings may prove useful in identifying areas of calcified crystalline depositions. Subchondral carpal sclerosis, erosions, and intraosseous cysts are better characterized on MR images than conventional radiographs. Thin (1.5-mm) section CT scans show greater detail of the peripheral outline of the cystic bony involvement. Cystic deposition to ligaments can lead to their rupture. Thus, degenerative changes and SLAC wrist deformity can be seen in CPDD.

OTHER ABNORMALITIES OF THE SYNOVIUM

In addition to changes seen in arthritis, other abnormalities of the synovium, such as synovial cysts, ganglia, tenosynovitis, and capsular synovitis, have been characterized on MR images of the wrist.

Ganglions

Cystic swellings overlying a joint or tendon sheath are referred to as *ganglions*, and are thought to be secondary to protrusions of encapsulated synovial tissue.[66-68] On MR images, ganglions generate uniform low signal intensity on T_1-weighted images and high signal intensity on T_2-weighted images. Fibrous septations may cause loculation of the ganglion. Even with infiltration or edema of adjacent tissues, these lesions are well demarcated on MR imaging. Intercar-

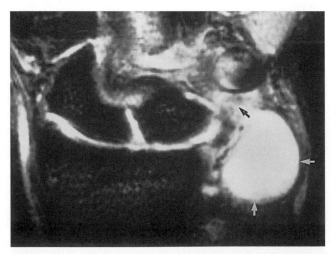

Figure 9–32. T_2-weighted image shows a large cystic ganglion *(white arrows)* projecting from the ulnar aspect of a torn triangular fibrocartilage *(black arrow)*.

pal communication of the ganglion is more common than communication with the radiocarpal joint.

Magnetic resonance imaging is used to identify the joint or tendon of origin and to exclude other soft tissue masses, such as neoplasm, when an accurate preoperative clinical assessment is difficult and wrist arthrography is not satisfactory (Fig. 9–32). Wrist ganglions may also be associated with the first carpometacarpal joint, the STT joint, the volar wrist capsule, or the flexor carpi radialis tendon. The stalk of the ganglion commonly can be discerned on MR images.

Pigment villonodular synovitis of the tendon (i.e., giant cell tumor of the tendon sheath) manifests as an extra-articular soft tissue swelling that may be mistaken for a ganglion. Low to intermediate signal intensity on T_1- and T_2-weighted images is characteristic.

Tenosynovitis and Capsular Effusion

Tenosynovitis and capsular synovitis may occur together as part of the spectrum of rheumatoid disease, or they may exist as isolated conditions with a traumatic or infectious etiology. Thickening, swelling, or fluid associated with an irritated synovial tendon sheath may be demonstrated on MR images. An edematous sheath appears as a rim of increased signal intensity on T_2-weighted images. Both flexor and extensor tenosynovitis may occur without a history of infection. Carpal distention may be evident in the small interphalangeal or metacarpal joints when small amounts of synovial fluid accumulate.

References

1. Manaster BJ: Digital wrist arthrography: Precision in determining the site of radiocarpal-midcarpal communication. AJR 147:563, 1986.
2. Braunstein EM, et al: Fluoroscopic and arthroscopic evaluation of carpal instability. AJR 144:1259, 1985.
3. Tirman RM, et al: Midcarpal wrist arthrography for detection of tears of the scapholunate and lunotriquetral ligaments. AJR 144:107, 1985.
4. Hall FM: Wrist arthrography. Radiology, 175:585, 1990.
5. Palmer A: Arthrography of the wrist. J Hand Surg [Am] 8:15–23, 1983.
6. Zinberg E, et al: The triple injection wrist arthrogram. J Hand Surg [Am] 13A:803–809, 1988.
7. Manaster B, Mann R, Rubenstein S: Wrist pain: Correlation of clinical and plain film findings with arthrographic results. J Hand Surg [Am] 14:466–473, 1989.
8. Manaster BJ: The clinical efficacy of triple-injection wrist arthrography. Radiology 178:267–268, 1991.
9. Metz VM, Mann FA, Gilula LA: Lack of correlation between site of wrist pain and location of noncommunicating defects shown by three-compartment wrist arthrography. AJR 160:1239–1243, 1993.
10. Mikic Z: Age changes in triangular fibrocartilage of the wrist joint. J Anat 126:367–384, 1978.
11. Mikic Z: Arthrography of the wrist joint. An experimental study. J Bone Joint Surg 66A:371–378, 1984.
12. Quinn SF, et al: Advanced imaging of the wrist. Radiographics 9:229, 1989.
13. Hindman BW, et al: Occult fractures of the carpals and metacarpals demonstrated by CT. AJR 153:529, 1989.
14. Pennes DR, et al: Direct coronal CT of the scaphoid bone. Radiology 171:870, 1989.
15. Biondetti PR, et al: Three-dimensional surface reconstruction of the carpal bones from CT scans: Transaxial versus coronal technique. Comput Med Imag Graph 12:67, 1988.
16. DeFlaviis L, et al: High resolution ultrasonography of wrist ganglia. J Clin Ultrasound 15:17, 1987.
17. Weiss KL, et al: High field strength surface coil imaging of the hand and wrist. Part I: Normal anatomy. Radiology 160:143, 1986.
18. Baker LL, et al: High resolution magnetic resonance imaging of the wrist: Normal Anatomy. Skeletal Radiol 16:128, 1987.
19. Middleton WD, et al: High resolution surface coil imaging of the joints: Anatomic correlation. Radiographics 7:645, 1987.
20. Koenig H, et al: Wrist: Preliminary report of high resolution MR imaging. Radiology 160:463, 1986.
21. Mark S, et al: High resolution MR imaging of peripheral joints using a quadrature coil at 0.35T. ROFO 146:397, 1987.
22. Fisher MR, et al: MR imaging using specialized coils. Radiology 157:443, 1985.
23. Zlatkin MB, et al: Chronic wrist pain: Evaluation with high resolution MR imaging. Radiology 173:723, 1989.
24. Greenan T, et al: Magnetic resonance imaging of the wrist. Semin Ultrasound CT MR 11:267, 1990.
25. Gundry CR, et al: Is MR better than arthrography for evaluating the ligaments of the wrist? In vitro study. AJR 154:337–341, 1990.
26. Binkovitz LA, et al: Magnetic resonance imaging of the wrist: Normal cross sectional imaging and selected abnormal cases. Radiographics 8:1171, 1988.
27. Heuck A, et al: Possibilities of MR tomography of diseases of the hand and wrist. Radiologue 29:53–60, 1989.
28. Rominger MB, Bernreuter WB, Kenney PJ, Lee DH: MR imaging of anatomy and tears of wrist ligaments. Radiographics, 13:1233–1246, 1003.
29. Totterman SM, Miller R, Wasserman B, et al: Intrinsic and extrinsic carpal ligaments: Evaluation by three-dimensional Fourier transform MR imaging. AJR 160:117–123, 1993.
30. Smith DK: Volar carpal ligaments of the wrist: Normal appearance on multiplanar reconstructions of three-dimensional Fourier transform MR imaging. AJR 161:353–357, 1993.
31. Smith DK: Dorsal carpal ligaments of the wrist: Normal appearance on multiplanar reconstructions of three-dimensional Fourier transform MR imaging. AJR 161:119–125, 1993.
32. Zeiss J, Jakab E, Khimji T, Imbriglia J: The ulnar tunnel at the wrist (Guyon's canal): Normal MR anatomy and variants. AJR 158:1081–1085, 1992.
33. Foo TK, Shellock FH, et al: High resolution MR imaging of the wrist and eye with short TR, short TE, and partial-echo acquisition. Radiology 183:277–281, 1992.
34. Lichtman D, et al: Ulnar midcarpal instability: Clinical and laboratory analysis. J Hand Surg [Am] 9:350–357, 1981.
35. Steyers C, Blair W: Measuring ulnar variance: A comparison of techniques. J Hand Surg [Am] 14:607–612, 1989.
36. Epner R, et al: Ulnar variance: The effect of wrist positioning and roentgen filming technique. J Hand Surg [Am] 7:298–305, 1982.
37. Palmer AC: The distal radioulnar joint. In Lichtman D (ed): The Wrist and Its Disorders. Philadelphia, WB Saunders, 1988, pp 220–243.
38. Olerud C, et al: The congruence of the distal radioulnar joint: A magnetic resonance imaging study. Acta Orthop Scand 59:183–185, 1988.
39. Wechsler R, et al: Computed tomography diagnosis of distal radioulnar subluxation. Skeletal Radiol 16:1–5, 1987.
40. Pirela-Cruz M, et al: Stress computed tomography analysis of the distal radioulnar joint: A diagnostic tool for determining translational motion. J Hand Surg [Am] 16:75–82, 1991.
41. Golimbu CN, et al: Tears of the triangular fibrocartilage of the wrist: MR imaging. Radiology 173:731, 1989.
42. Lewis OJ, et al: The anatomy of the wrist joint. J Anat 106:539–552, 1970.

43. Weber ER: Wrist mechanics and its association with ligamentous instability. In Lichtman D (ed): The Wrist and Its Disorders. Philadelphia, WB Saunders, 1988, pp 41–52.

44. Greenan T, et al: Magnetic resonance imaging of the wrist. Semin Ultrasound CT MR 11:267, 1990.

45. Scheck M: Long term follow up of treatment for comminuted fractures of the distal end of the radius by transfixation with Kirschner wires and cast. J Bone Joint Surg 44A:337, 1962.

46. Stevens J: Compression fractures of the lower end of the radius. Ann Surg 71:594, 1962.

47. Knirk J, Jupiter J: Intraarticular fractures of the distal end of the radius in young adults. J Bone Joint Surg 68(A):647–659, 1986.

48. O'Brien ET: Acute fractures and dislocations of the carpus. In Lichtman D (ed): The Wrist and Its Disorders. Philadelphia, WB Saunders, 1988, p 129.

49. Gillespy T III, et al: Dorsal fractures of the hamate: Radiographic appearance. AJR 151:351, 1988.

50. Ruby LK, et al: Natural history of scaphoid nonunion. Radiology 156:856, 1985.

51. Reinus WR, et al: Carpal avascular necrosis: MR imaging. Radiology 160:689, 1986.

52. Cristiani G, et al: Evaluation of ischaemic necrosis of carpal bones by magnetic resonance imaging. J Hand Surg [Br] 15: 249–255, 1990.

53. Desser TS, et al: Scaphoid fractures and Kienböck's disease of the lunate: MR imaging with histopathologic correlation. Magn Reson Imag 8:357, 1990.

54. Duong R, et al: Kienböck's disease: Scintigraphic demonstration in correlation with clinical, radiographic and pathologic findings. Clin Nucl Med 7:418–420, 1982.

55. Middleton WD, et al: MR imaging of the carpal tunnel: Normal anatomy and preliminary findings in the carpal tunnel syndrome. AJR 148:307, 1987.

56. Mesgarzadah M, et al: Carpal tunnel: MR imaging. Part I: Normal anatomy. Radiology 171:743–748, 1989.

57. Mesgarzadah M, et al: Carpal tunnel: MR imaging. Part II: Carpal tunnel syndrome. Radiology 171:749–754, 1989.

58. Healy C, et al: Magnetic resonance imaging of the carpal tunnel. J Hand Surg [Br] 15:243–248, 1990.

59. Zeiss J, et al: Anatomic relations between the median nerve and flexor tendons in the carpal tunnel: MR evaluation in normal volunteers. AJR 153:533–536, 1989.

60. Yulish BS, et al: Juvenile rheumatoid arthritis: Assessment with MR imaging. Radiology 165:149, 1987.

61. Meske S, et al: Rheumatoid arthritis lesions of the wrist examined by rapid gradient echo magnetic resonance imaging. Scand J Rheumatol 19:235–238, 1990.

62. Watson KH: Degenerative disorders of the carpus. In Lichtman D (ed): The Wrist and Its Disorders. Philadelphia, WB Saunders, 1988, pp 286–292.

63. Renner WR, et al: Early changes of rheumatoid arthritis in the hand and wrist. Radiol Clin North Am 26:1185, 1988.

64. Ellstein JL, et al: Rheumatoid disorders of the hand and wrist. In Dee R (ed): Principles of Orthopaedic Practice, vol 1. New York, McGraw-Hill, 1989, pp 646–665.

65. Rubens DJ, et al: Rheumatoid arthritis: Evaluation of wrist extensor tendons with clinical examination versus MR imaging—a preliminary report. Radiology 187:831–838, 1993.

66. Hollister AM, et al: The use of MRI in the diagnosis of an occult wrist ganglion cyst. Orthop Rev 18:1210–1212, 1989.

67. Feldman F, et al: Magnetic resonance imaging of para-articular and ectopic ganglia. Skeletal Radiol 18:353–358, 1989.

68. Louis DS, et al: Magnetic resonance imaging of the collateral ligaments of the thumb. J Hand Surg [Am] 14:739–741, 1989.

CHAPTER 10

Wrist Arthroscopy

Gregory I. Bain, MBBS, Robert S. Richards, MD, and
James H. Roth, MD

HISTORY

Arthroscopy was first reported by Professor Kenji Takagi[1] in 1920, but it was not until 1979 that small
joint instrumentation was perfected and Yung-Cheng
Chen[2] described the procedure in the wrist. Wrist
arthroscopy has developed into an accepted diagnostic and therapeutic tool that is well into its second
decade. The therapeutic indications have been extended as the principles of open surgical procedures
have been adapted to the arthroscope.

PRINCIPLES AND GOALS

The goals of arthroscopy are to provide an accurate
anatomic diagnosis of wrist pathology and to treat
those patients with an anatomic lesion. The superior
visualization provided by arthroscopy enables the
anatomy to be seen in a magnified form and allows
instruments to be placed with precision. New techniques and instrumentation have extended the therapeutic possibilities of wrist arthroscopy. The introduction of suction punches and smaller motorized
resectors and burs has facilitated arthroscopic removal, or "-ectomy," of bone and soft tissue.[3, 4]
Arthroscopy is a minimally invasive technique that
enables the patient to rehabilitate quickly with less
morbidity and fewer complications. Using the anatomic principles that have been developed for open
surgical procedures, arthroscopic techniques are producing good long-term results.

INDICATIONS FOR WRIST ARTHROSCOPY

The indications for wrist arthroscopy are both diagnostic and therapeutic. Wrist arthroscopy has become
the gold standard for diagnosis of intra-articular pathology. The probe can be used as the "palpating
index finger" so that greater detail of the contour,
stability, and texture of the soft tissues and bone can
be obtained. This gives the surgeon a more accurate
understanding of the pathology. Wrist arthroscopy
is indicated to confirm findings suggested by other
diagnostic modalities or for the diagnosis of wrist
pain of unknown etiology. Wrist arthroscopy can be
used to assess the severity of degenerative changes
prior to other surgical procedures; this would include
assessing the midcarpal joint before proceeding to a
proximal row carpectomy or the status of an interosseous ligament prior to reconstruction. A list of
indications for wrist arthroscopy is presented in
Table 10–1.

Many of the indications for wrist arthroscopy are
relative, so the surgeon must weigh the benefits of
surgery against the possible risks.

DIAGNOSTIC VALUE OF ARTHROSCOPY

Wrist arthrography has historically been the gold
standard for the diagnosis of soft tissue wrist pathology. The introduction of arthroscopy and later of magnetic resonance (MR) imaging has significantly
changed this situation.

Table 10–1. INDICATIONS FOR WRIST ARTHROSCOPY*

Diagnostic arthroscopy	Assessment of ligamentous injuries of the wrist
	Scapholunate ligament disruption
	Lunotriquetral ligament disruption
	TFCC disorders
	Assessment of chondral defects
	Assessment of chronic wrist pain of unknown etiology
Therapeutic arthroscopy	ARIF of scapholunate and lunotriquetral ligament tears
	ARIF of distal radial fractures
	Débridement and repair of TFCC tears
	ARIF of scaphoid fractures
	Lavage of septic arthritis
	Synovectomy
	Removal of loose bodies
	Débridement of chondral defects
	Débridement of degenerative arthritis
	Excision of ganglion
	Resection arthroplasty
	Distal ulnar resection

*ARIF = Arthroscopically assisted reduction and internal fixation; TFCC =
triangular fibrocartilage complex.

Arthroscopy versus Arthrography

Arthrography has a number of limitations. There is a high incidence of false-negative studies, for several reasons: Perforations may be obstructed by synovitis or fibrosis. A tear may act as a flap valve and prevent communication of contrast agent between compartments. Arthrography does not quantify the size or type of the perforation, so an extensive tear and a small perforation may have the same arthrographic appearance. Arthrography does not provide adequate information about adjacent structures, such as the articular cartilage and synovium. A further concern

is that patients with a positive arthrogram have up to a 74 percent chance of having a positive arthrogram on the other, asymptomatic wrist.[5]

Comparison of three-compartment arthrography with arthrotomy revealed a false-positive rate from 10 to 20 percent.[6] Assessments of radiocarpal arthrography versus arthroscopy have shown similar weakness in the diagnostic accuracy and anatomic information provided.[7]

In contrast, arthroscopy provides detailed anatomic information. Palpation with the arthroscopic probe allows assessment of the stability and texture of intra-articular structures and measurement of defects. The

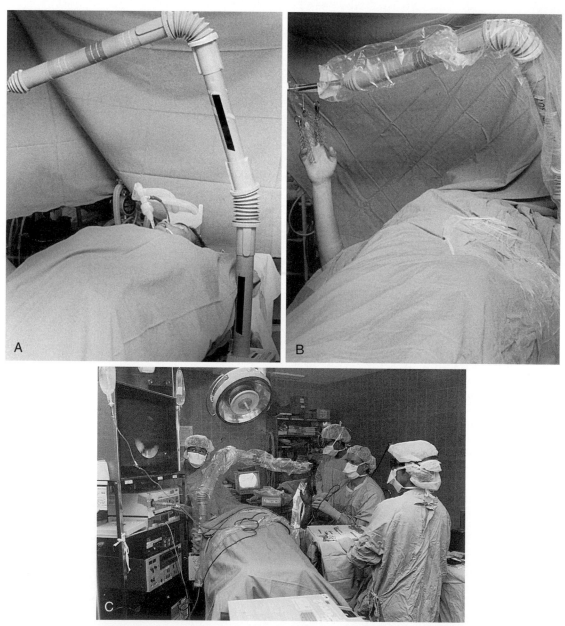

Figure 10–1. *A* and *B*, Setup for wrist arthroscopy: The patient's arm is suspended with finger traps from an articulated arm. The arm is abducted from the patient's side. A tourniquet is applied, and a sling with traction weights is attached to the upper arm. The surgeon sits in a chair with armrests to prevent fatigue. For ease of viewing, the video monitor is placed on the side of the bed opposite to the operative side. A fluoroscopy unit is valuable for the management of distal radial fractures and carpal instability.

stability of ligaments can be assessed under direct vision while the joint is stressed with a probe or by external manipulation. The adjacent structures such as the synovium and articular cartilage can be clearly seen, allowing a more thorough assessment of the wrist. The surgeon can then treat the abnormalities that are seen.

Arthroscopy versus Magnetic Resonance Imaging

MR imaging is a noninvasive diagnostic modality that can quickly visualize the wrist. Kang and associates[8] have shown that MR imaging can distinguish triangular fibrocartilage complex (TFCC) degeneration from perforation. Sensitivity rates for diagnosis of TFCC tears range from 72 to 93 percent,[9, 10] which are similar to the sensitivity rate reported for conventional radiocarpal arthrography but less than that for three-compartment arthrography.[9] MR imaging produces false-negative images, but generally there are only a few false-positives. False-positive images are due to irregularities of the central portion of the TFCC.[10]

A weakness of MR imaging is the inability to detect the cartilage erosions often associated with TFCC tears.[8, 11] Cerofolini and colleagues[11] reported that in none of their 10 cases was MR imaging able to visualize cartilaginous lesions later seen at arthroscopy.

Despite theoretic advantages and promising early results, MR imaging has not established itself as the investigation of choice for all circumstances. Currently, the most accepted use of MR imaging in the wrist is to assess the vascularity of the lunate and the proximal pole of the scaphoid.

SURGICAL TECHNIQUE OF ARTHROSCOPY

Anesthesia

We prefer general or regional anesthesia for wrist arthroscopy. Regional anesthesia can be axillary or intravenous regional (Bier) block. Unlike for knee arthroscopy, local anesthesia is insufficient for wrist arthroscopy. Merely distending the joint with fluid does not give sufficient exposure to perform satisfactory wrist arthroscopy. The greater relaxation and distraction allowed by regional or general anesthesia are essential for optimal visualization.

Setup and Traction

With the use of a general or regional anesthetic, the patient is positioned supine on the operating table. The shoulder is placed along the edge of the table to allow the arm to hang free when the shoulder is abducted. A tourniquet is placed above the elbow

and inflated to 250 mm Hg. A sling is placed over the tourniquet. Distraction of the wrist is obtained by hanging 7 to 10 lb of weight from the sling. Distraction rather than distention of the wrist is needed for visualization. The small volume and tight wrist capsule make distention impractical. The hand and forearm are prepared with alcohol-based tincture of iodine to prevent the fingers slipping in the finger traps.

Generally, two or three fingers are placed in the finger traps. In patients with fragile skin, the risk of skin damage can be decreased by placing more fingers in the traps. For most cases of diagnostic arthroscopy, distraction is obtained by placing the index and long fingers in the finger traps. For therapeutic arthroscopy, the finger traps are attached to the ulnar or radial three digits to distract the side with the suspected pathology. The finger traps may be suspended from intravenous poles, overhead hooks, static arms attached to the table, or a distraction tower on a hand table. Our preference is for an articulated arm system attached to the operating room table, which allows easy positioning of the patient's arm during the procedure (Fig. 10–1A). The articulated arm system is pneumatic, and the multiple joints allow easy positioning of the arm. The finger traps are suspended from the articulated arm (Fig. 10–1B and 1C). Use of an articulated arm system allows pronation and supination of the wrist by an assistant, which make visualization easier. Tower distraction devices placed on the hand table are also easy to use but make it more difficult to pronate and supinate the patient's arm. We use a chair with arm rests to support the elbows and prevent fatigue.

Instrumentation

For wrist arthroscopy, a 2.5- to 3.0-mm scope is used (Fig. 10–2). The 1.7-mm arthroscope does not provide an adequate field of view. The 4.0-mm arthroscope is

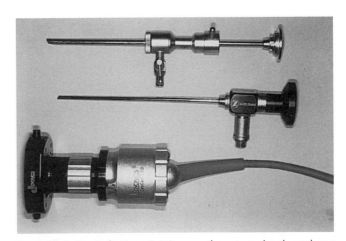

Figure 10–2. Top to bottom: A 2.5-mm arthroscope, sheath, and camera.

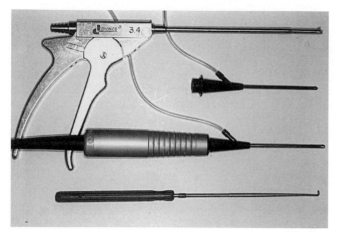

Figure 10–3. Instruments required for intra-articular wrist surgery. Suction punch, motorized full-radius resector, motorized bur, arthroscopic hook probe.

difficult to introduce and increases the risk of articular damage. Shorter arthroscopes with a lever arm of 100 mm are much easier to control in the wrist joint. An oblique viewing angle of 30° allows good visualization.

The instruments used to perform arthroscopic "-ectomy" surgery are many and varied (Figs. 10–3 and 10–4). Palpation with the angled probe enables the surgeon to manipulate the tissues so that a better appreciation of the texture, contour, and stability can be obtained. It also allows measurement of chondral defects and ligament tears. An 18-gauge needle may be used to spear or manipulate loose bodies. Basket forceps and suction punches are cutting instruments that are valuable for resecting tears of the TFCC and chondral defects. The suction punch has largely replaced the basket forceps, because the suction helps deliver the tissues into the jaws of the forceps and removes the debris from the joint. Rongeurs are useful for removal of loose bodies and excision of carpal

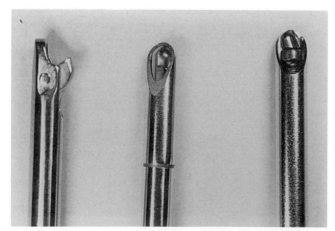

Figure 10–4. Close-up view *(from left to right)* of a suction punch, full-radius resector, and bur.

bones. Curettes and knives are now rarely used because of the development of motorized instruments.

Motorized resectors permit a more rapid removal of soft tissue than a manual cutting instrument. The full-radius resectors are best for small-joint arthroscopy, because they provide a large aperture. Motorized resectors work most efficiently at low speeds, such as 400 rpm. At higher speeds, there is insufficient time for the soft tissue to enter the cutting mechanism, effectively closing the aperture.[4] The 3.5-mm, full-radius resector is used in the radiocarpal joint, and the 2-mm resector in the midcarpal joint. Motorized burs are effective for removing bone. It is best to use the suction intermittently to clear debris, because with continuous suction, the bone swirls in the turbulence and restricts visibility. Burs perform best in bone at high speeds, such as 1200 rpm.[4] New instrumentation has allowed the surgeon to extend the indications of wrist arthroscopy to include therapeutic procedures.[12, 13]

Portals

All arthroscopic examinations of the wrist should include both the midcarpal and radiocarpal joints. Midcarpal arthroscopy provides valuable information about the stability and alignment of bones in the proximal carpal row. A systematic approach allows complete examination of both radiocarpal and midcarpal joints in a very short time.

Multiple dorsal portals are described (Fig. 10–5). The radiocarpal portals are numbered according to their relation to the extensor tendons. For example, the 1-2 portal is situated between the first and second extensor compartments.

RADIOCARPAL PORTALS

1-2 Portal

The 1-2 portal is located in the extreme dorsum of the anatomic snuffbox, just radial to the extensor pollicis longus tendon, to avoid the radial artery.[14] It is recommended for access to the radial styloid, scaphoid, and articular surface of the distal radius. Its uses include reduction and Kirschner (K) wire fixation of radial styloid fractures as well as insertion of K wires for pinning of the scapholunate ligament.

3-4 Portal

The 3-4 portal is used most commonly for radiocarpal arthroscopy. This portal is established by palpating first Lister's tubercle and then the extensor pollicis longus and extensor digitorum communis tendons. The portal is 1 cm distal to Lister's tubercle, between the tendons of the third and fourth compartments.

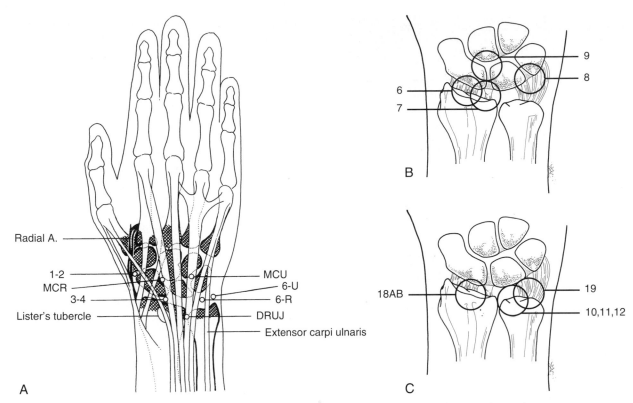

Figure 10–5. *A,* Portals for wrist arthroscopy. Numbering of the radiocarpal portals is based on their relationship to the extensor compartments of the wrist. Midcarpal portals are identified by their position in relationship to the capitate. *A.* = artery; DRUJ = distal radioulnar joint; MCR = midcarpal radial; MCU = midcarpal ulnar. *B,* Diagram of the wrist showing precise locations of the actual arthroscopic views illustrated in Figures 10–6, 10–7, 10–8, 10–9, and 10–15. *C,* Diagram of the wrist showing precise locations of the actual arthroscopic views illustrated in Figures 10–10, 10–11, 10–12, 10 18, and 10–19.

4-5 Portal

Use of either the 4-5 or the 6-R portal allows access to the ulnar side of the wrist. Use of one or the other is a personal preference. There is no need to establish both during radiocarpal arthroscopy. The 4-5 portal is just ulnar to the fourth compartment and 1 cm distal to Lister's tubercle.

6-R Portal

The 6-R portal is located distal to the ulnar head and radial to the extensor carpi ulnaris (ECU) tendon. The portal is made just proximal to the triquetrum to avoid damaging the TFCC. The 4-5 or 6-R portal is established under direct vision after the arthroscope is advanced to transilluminate the ulnar side of the wrist. Transillumination allows the superficial veins to be avoided.

6-U Portal

The 6-U portal is also established under direct vision, much like the 6-R portal. The needle is inserted distal to the ulnar styloid on the ulnar side of the ECU tendon. The 6-U portal can be used as an inflow or outflow portal but generally is not required.

Midcarpal Radial (MCR) Portal

The MCR portal is established 1 cm distal to the 3-4 portal, along a line bordering the radial edge of the third metacarpal. A soft depression between the proximal and distal carpal rows can be palpated.

Midcarpal Ulnar (MCU) Portal

The MCU portal is best located under direct vision after the MCR portal is established. A gap between the proximal and distal carpal rows can be palpated along the midline of the fourth metacarpal.

Distal Radioulnar Joint (DRUJ) Portal

The DRUJ portal is located by palpating the radial edge of the ulnar head. The wrist is supinated to relax the dorsal capsule and to facilitate entry. The arthroscope can be introduced into the angle between the ulna and radius or just beneath the TFCC. It is easier to insert the scope in the most proximal portal.

Technique of Wrist Arthroscopy

RADIOCARPAL JOINT EXAMINATION

After traction is applied, examine the external wrist and palpate the landmarks. It is helpful to mark the

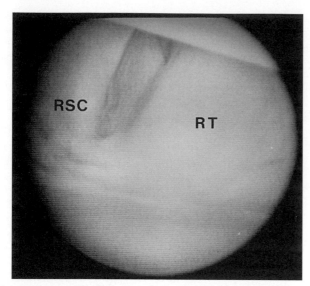

Figure 10–6. Starting from the radial side of the wrist, the radiocapho-capitate (RSC) and the radiolunotriquetral (RT) volar ligaments are clearly seen with the arthroscope in the 3-4 portal. (Precise localization of this view is shown in the diagram in Figure 10–5*B*.)

position of Lister's tubercle, the tendons of the third and fourth compartments, and the ECU tendon. Establish the 3-4 portal first. Insert an 18- to 21-gauge needle 1 cm distal to Lister's tubercle as previously discussed. Angle the needle 10° volarly to conform to the slope of the radiocarpal joint and to decrease the risk of articular damage. Following distal radius fracture, adjust the inclination of the needle appropriately. Distend the joint with 5 to 7 mL of lactated Ringer's solution. To maintain orientation, avoid moving your thumb from Lister's tubercle. Use a No. 15 blade to make a longitudinal stab incision at the 3-4 portal site. A longitudinal incision minimizes the risk to soft tissue structures. Through the use of blunt dissection with a mosquito forceps, identify the joint capsule. Then use the blunt trocar to penetrate the capsule to avoid injury to the articular cartilage.

Lactated Ringer's solution or normal saline should be used for distention and irrigation. We prefer lactated Ringer's solution, as it is more physiologic and is rapidly absorbed. Inflow is gravity fed through the arthroscope sheath. This arrangement provides more effective cleansing of the joint than a separate inflow. Unlike for other joints, infusion pumps have not been necessary, because wrist distraction avoids the need for high-pressure distention.[17] A small finger-squeeze pump attached to the inflow tubing can clear bubbles and small debris from in front of the arthroscope.

After introduction of the arthroscope into the 3-4 portal, establish the 6-R portal. Use the arthroscope to transilluminate the ulnar side of the wrist so that the extent of the joint can be seen and the veins avoided.

Establish the 6-R portal just proximal to the triquetrum and radial to the ECU tendon. Palpate the triquetrum, and insert an 18-gauge needle at its proximal edge. Visualize the needle via the arthroscope,

and make a stab incision at the needle entry site. Dissect the soft tissue. Then enter the capsule with the tips of a mosquito clamp. The return of irrigation fluid confirms entry into the joint. An adequate capsular incision provides sufficient outflow without the use of accessory portals. Insert a hook probe into the 6-R portal, and orient the camera.

The examination should start radially with the arthroscope in the 3-4 portal. Visualize the radial styloid, then the radioscaphocapite, radiolunatotriquetral, and radioscapholunate (RSL) ligaments (Fig. 10–6). An important anatomic landmark is the synovial fold associated with the radioscapholunate ligament (Fig. 10–7). Previously, this structure has been referred to as a fat pad, but in reality, it is a synovial fold or tuft. Examine the articular surfaces of the scaphoid, lunate, and radius. The scapholunate ligament initially may not be clearly seen, but its soft pliable texture and slight concavity (when normal) make it easily identified with a probe.

After completing the examination of the radial side of the joint, insert the arthroscope into the 6-R portal and the hook probe into the 3-4 portal. The lunate, triquetrum, and lunotriquetral ligament are seen (Fig. 10–8). The ulnocarpal ligament can be seen radiating from the volar TFCC to the triquetrum and lunate. Ulnar to the ulnotriquetral ligament is the pisotriquetral recess, which in 30 percent of cases allows visualization of the pisiform.[15, 16] A tear of the ulnotriquetral ligament is demonstrated by localized synovitis, visualization of the pisiform and pisotriquetral joint, and ballooning of the ulnar capsule with separation of the most ulnar aspect of the TFCC. This separation is different from the normal pisotriquetral recess location on the palmar-ulnar aspect of the TFCC.

An intact TFCC has a firm surface much like that of a trampoline. In contrast, a torn TFCC loses the

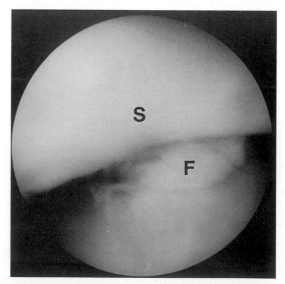

Figure 10–7. The synovial fold *(F)* is easily seen from the 3-4 portal and is a landmark for the scapholunate ligament *(S)* seen above it. (Precise localization of this view is shown on the diagram in Figure 10–5*B*.)

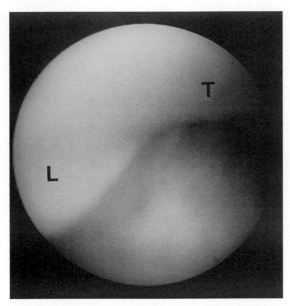

Figure 10–8. A normal lunate *(L)*, triquetrum *(T)*, and lunotriquetral ligament seen through the 6-R portal. (Precise localization of this view is shown on the diagram in Figure 10–5*B*.)

normal tension. Diagnosis of incomplete tears of the interosseous ligaments and TFCC can be made easily with the hook probe. The radiocarpal joint can be arthroscopically examined while it is manipulated to assess the stability of the distal radioulnar joint, TFCC, and intercarpal ligaments.[16]

MIDCARPAL JOINT EXAMINATION

A diagnostic arthroscopy should also examine the midcarpal joints. Establish the MCR portal 1 cm distal to the 3-4 portal. The MCR portal is located along the radial border of the third metacarpal and is palpable as a small depression or "soft spot" between the proximal and distal carpal rows, just radial to the index extensor tendons. This portal overlies the distal scaphocapite joint. Again, slight volar angulation of both the needle and the arthroscope aids in entering the joint space. The MCU portal is located in a depression between the proximal and distal carpal rows along the midline of the fourth metacarpal. Establish the MCU portal using the same transillumination technique as described for the radiocarpal joint. The scaphotrapeziotrapezoid (STT) joint can be visualized from the MCR portal, with the trapezoid being dorsal to the trapezium. The scapholunate interval, capitate, and lunate can also be visualized (Fig. 10–9). Carefully examine the lunate facets and the articulation with the proximal pole of the hamate for arthrosis, as suggested by Viegas.[18] A type II lunate with a medial lunate facet is present in 60 percent of patients and may show arthrosis of the proximal pole of the hamate. Fractures of the scaphoid, as well as separation at the scapholunate joint and triquetrolunate joints, are better seen and reduced via the mid-

carpal joint than the radiocarpal joint. When seen through the midcarpal joint, the scapholunate and lunotriquetral intervals are not covered by interosseous ligaments. These three bones form a smooth acetabulum. Normally, it is not possible to introduce a probe into the scapholunate or triquetrolunate joint. However, instability produces laxity and a stepoff between these joints. A probe or sometimes the arthroscope can then be inserted at the site of instability.

THERAPEUTIC ARTHROSCOPY

Tears of the TFCC

The fibrocartilage disk of the TFCC is a unique structure that has similarities to the menisci of the knee (Fig. 10–10). It attaches to the sigmoid notch of the distal radius and spans the ulnar head to attach to the base of the ulnar styloid.[19] The ulnocarpal ligaments extend from the disk to the lunate and triquetrum, to give stability to the carpus. The dorsal and volar radioulnar ligaments border the disk and become taut during rotation. These ligaments must be preserved to maintain stability of the DRUJ (Fig. 10–11). Biomechanical studies have demonstrated that approximately 20 percent of the load across the wrist is borne by the distal ulna.[19] (See Chapter 20 for details of TFCC anatomy and biomechanics.)

Only the peripheral 25 percent of the triangular fibrocartilage on the dorsal, volar, and ulnar margins is vascularized.[20] The central and radial portions remain avascular and so do not have the potential to heal readily. Therefore, lesions of the avascular cen-

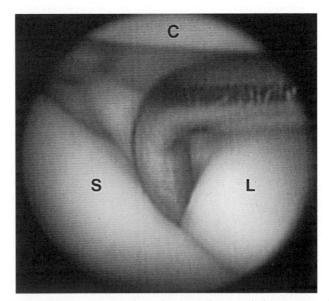

Figure 10–9. A normal midcarpal joint with a scapholunate interval that will not admit a probe. *C* = capitate; *L* = lunate; *S* = scaphoid. (Precise localization of this view is shown on the diagram in Figure 10–5*B*.)

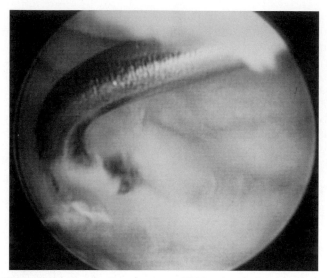

Figure 10–10. Examination of an acute TFCC tear with the arthroscopic hook probe. (Precise localization of this view is shown on the diagram in Figure 10–5C.)

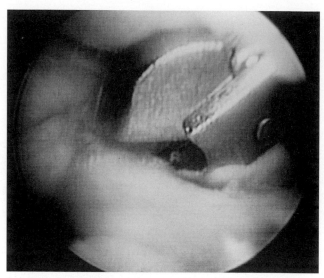

Figure 10–12. Débridement of the TFCC tear with the suction punch. (Precise localization of this view is shown on the diagram in Figure 10–5C.)

tral and radial portions of the TFCC are usually managed with débridement. Lesions of the vascular peripheral 25 percent of the disk do have the potential to heal. It is only these tears for which suture repair has been routinely advocated.

Acute tears of the TFCC are often seen in association with fractures of the radius and have been reported to occur in up to 45 percent of distal radial fractures.[21] Most acute tears are from the avascular radial attachment, so we manage them with débridement of the radial and central portions of the TFCC. However, it is possible to treat them with open means, by suturing the TFCC to a trough created in the ulnar aspect of the distal radius, which may allow introduction of blood supply.[22] Cooney and associates[22] report good early results of radial TFCC repair, but theirs is the first large series to address this problem. Patients with chronic tears often have a history of previous trauma and/or have a positive ulnar vari-

ance. Our goal is to débride the radial and central portions of the TFCC without causing instability.

We perform arthroscopic débridement of TFCC tears with the arthroscope in the 6-R portal and the instruments in the 3-4 portal. We use the suction punch in débriding the central and radial portions of the torn TFCC (Figs. 10–11 and 10–12). The 3.5-mm, full-radius resector is used for resecting the degenerative fibrocartilage and the adjacent synovitis. If there is positive ulnar variance, we sometimes remove the distal 2 mm of the ulnar head (wafer procedure), through the enlarged perforation in the TFCC (Fig. 10–13).[23] The forearm is pronated and supinated to enable visualization and resection of the full circum-

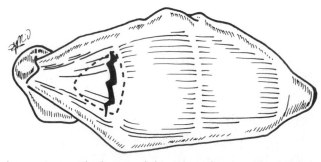

Figure 10–11. Débridement of the TFCC. The avascular radial and central portions are débrided. The vascularized volar, dorsal, and ulnar portions are important stabilizers of the DRUJ and should not be violated. (Precise localization of this view is shown on the diagram in Figure 10–5C.)

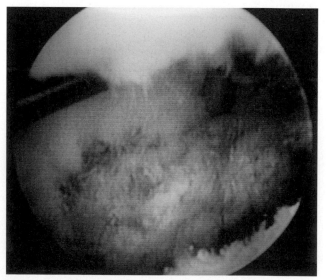

Figure 10–13. The head of the ulna following an arthroscopic "wafer procedure." The edge of the débrided TFCC can be seen.

ference of the ulnar head. Fluoroscopic examination in supination and pronation is required to ensure that adequate resection has been performed. For advanced arthritis or when triquetrolunate, midcarpal, or DRUJ instability is associated with positive ulnar variance, we prefer open methods of ulnar shortening (see later discussion of ulnar impaction syndrome).

Osterman[24] reported a prospective study of 52 consecutive patients with isolated tears of the TFCC that were diagnosed with arthrography and treated by arthroscopic débridement. The locations of the TFCC tears were: central, 46 percent; radial, 34 percent; and ulnar, 20 percent. Ulnar synovitis was present in 90 percent of patients, and a lunotriquetral tear (not identified by arthrography) in 15 percent. Chondromalacia and positive ulnar variance were treated by limited arthroscopic resection of the ulnar head in 25 percent of patients. A powered bur was used to remove between 1 and 2 mm of ulnar head, once the TFCC had been débrided. Pain was completely relieved in 73 percent of patients and improved in another 12 percent. Range of motion improved in all but 1 patient, and Jamar grip strength improved in the majority of patients. There was no clinical or radiographic instability of the distal radioulnar joint or carpus. These results are similar to the 78 percent good results reported for ulnar shortening,[25] but do not require an open surgical procedure or immobilization or involve the risk of a non-union.

REPAIR OF TEARS OF THE ULNAR ASPECT OF THE TFCC

When a tear of the ulnar aspect of the TFCC is visualized arthroscopically, localized synovitis is often present and must be resected to allow adequate visualization of the ulnar side of the wrist. The tear opens with pronation and supination. We repair the ulnar tear arthroscopically as follows: Introduce a 20-gauge Tuohy (epidural) needle through the 1-2 or 3-4 portal while the arthroscope is in the 6-R portal. Pass the needle through the ulnar edge of the TFCC, capsule, and skin. Withdraw the obturator and advance a suture through the needle and hold it. Withdraw the needle into the wrist and again advance it through the TFCC and skin. This places a loop of suture on either side of the tear with the two free ends protruding through the skin. Tie the ends of the suture over the capsule or a button. Insert one to three sutures.

The technique of repair is shown in Figure 10–14. The dorsal cutaneous branch of the ulnar nerve needs to be protected.[26] This can be done by incising the skin first, isolating the nerve, and tying the sutures at an exit point near the base of the ulnar styloid.

Ulnar Impaction Syndrome

Ulnar impaction syndrome is a degenerative condition characterized by ulnar wrist pain, swelling, crepitus, and limited wrist motion caused by excessive load-bearing across the ulnar aspect of the wrist.[24, 27, 28] Patients with positive ulnar variance are predisposed to develop ulnar impaction syndrome. Positive ulnar variance is often idiopathic but can be caused by malunion of a distal radial fracture, premature physeal arrest of the distal radius, or an Essex-Lopresti injury.[28]

Radiographs may demonstrate positive ulnar variance, subchondral sclerosis, or cyst formation in the ulnar head, lunate, or triquetrum. At arthroscopy, degenerative tears of the TFCC are usually seen as oval or circular with an irregular frayed edge, and are located in the central avascular portion.[24] The distal ulna can be seen if the perforation is large. There may be chondromalacia or degenerative arthritis of the ulnar head or carpus, and the lunotriquetral ligament may be perforated.[27]

Ulnar impaction syndrome has been successfully treated by unloading the distal ulna. Treatment options have included débridement of the TFCC,[28] wafer procedure,[29] hemiresection of the distal ulna,[30] and ulnar shortening osteotomy.[31] All except the ulnar shortening osteotomy can be performed via the arthroscope.

Feldon and associates[23] stated that the wafer procedure is contraindicated if there is carpal instability or degenerative arthritis of the distal radioulnar joint. Palmer and coworkers[32] believe that this procedure is contraindicated if there is an associated lunotriquetral tear, because it unloads the ulnocarpal joint and increases the carpal instability. If instability is present, we prefer an open ulnar shortening osteotomy to prevent the ulnar impaction and tighten the ulnar carpal ligaments. A lunotriquetral fusion may be required in some patients.

Wnorowski and colleagues[33] reported a biomechanical study of the arthroscopic wafer procedure in nine cadaveric forearms with positive ulnar variance. There was a statistically significant unloading of the ulnar side of the wrist following excision of the TFCC, and resection of the ulnar head, to the depth of the subchondral bone. Those wrists with advanced TFCC pathology required more resection to unload the distal ulnar.[33] The technique of arthroscopic ulnar head resection was discussed previously.

Carpal Instability

There are two main classes of carpal instability: carpal instability–dissociative (Mayo), or perilunar instability (Lichtman), and carpal instability–nondissociative (Mayo), or midcarpal and/or proximal carpal instability (Lichtman) (see Chapter 12). In cases of perilunate or dissociative instability, the interosseous ligaments of the proximal row are torn. Arthroscopy provides the best means to evaluate the ligaments and joint surfaces and allows the surgeon to visualize these joints while they are stressed by external manipulation or with an arthroscopic probe.[17] In midcarpal,

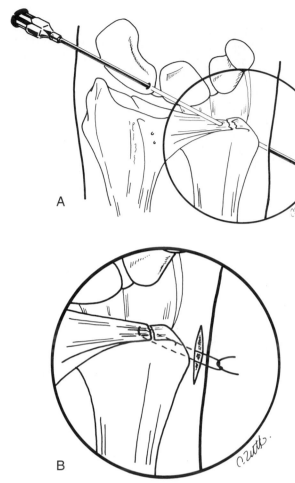

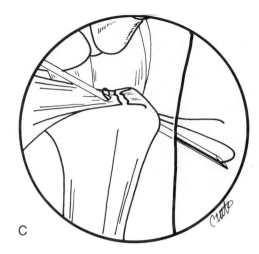

Figure 10–14. *A,* A 20-gauge Tuohy needle is inserted into the 3-4 portal and through the ulnar edge of the TFCC, capsule, and skin. The suture is advanced through the needle, and the free end is held. *B,* The needle tip is withdrawn into the wrist and again advanced through the TFCC. The suture remains in the lumen of the needle and is passed through the TFCC a second time to complete the loop. The free end is then withdrawn from the needle to allow the ends to be tied. *C,* The two ends of the suture are tied over the capsule or a button. One to three sutures can be inserted.

proximal carpal, or nondissociative instability, the ligaments are usually normal or lax but not grossly disrupted.

SCAPHOLUNATE TEARS

Scapholunate tears may be as common as scaphoid fractures.[34] Treatment, during the first 6 weeks when the soft tissues are healing, provides the best opportunity for ligamentous healing to prevent instability and the subsequent degeneration to scapholunate advanced collapse (SLAC wrist).[35] Unfortunately, early diagnosis can be difficult. Clinically, scapholunate ligament tears manifest, like scaphoid fractures, with pain, swelling, and tenderness over the dorsum of the wrist and anatomic snuffbox. Watson and associates[36] have described a provocative test for scapholunate ligament disruption, but it should not be performed until a scaphoid fracture is excluded. Widening of the scapholunate gap may not appear until the secondary ligamentous restraints become lax.[37] Arthrography of soft tissue structures has multiple problems, as outlined previously. MR imaging has been reported to have a sensitivity of only 25 percent, with an accuracy of 64 percent in assessing the scapholunate ligament tears.[38] Neither arthrography nor MR imaging is

a satisfactory method of identifying scapholunate tears.

The simple immobilization of acute scapholunate tears in a cast does not reduce the scapholunate interval.[39] It is only with anatomic reduction and fixation that the normal articulation can be recreated and the natural history of this injury changed.

A tear of the scapholunate or lunotriquetral ligament can be seen as irregular frayed tissue on radiocarpal arthroscopy. A tear is confirmed with midcarpal arthroscopy. A better appreciation of the carpal alignment is obtained from the midcarpal joint. If a tear is present, there is loss of the normal alignment of the scaphoid and lunate that is not obscured by ligaments. Normally, a probe is not admitted into the scapholunate interval (Fig. 10–15). Open interosseous ligament repair has been advocated, but it is difficult to perform because of the small size of the ligament.

Technique of Arthroscopy-Assisted Scapholunate Reduction and Fixation

If scapholunate instability is confirmed, we recommend percutaneous fixation of the joint, as follows: After the traction is released, introduce two or three smooth 0.062-inch K wires into the scaphoid just distal to the radial styloid and advance them under fluoroscopic control. Place K wires into the dorsum of the scaphoid and lunate to act as "joysticks." With the arthroscope in the midcarpal joint, use the "joysticks" to reduce the scapholunate interval. Then, advance the K wires into the lunate, and assess the final position with fluoroscopy. Neither the radiocarpal nor the midcarpal joint is crossed, to maintain movement between each carpal row and the radius. The K wires are normally removed at 12 weeks.

In our series of 14 patients with acute traumatic wrist pain, 9 had scapholunate tears (unpublished data). These 9 patients were treated with arthroscopic reduction and percutaneous K-wire fixation. Seven were pain free and returned to their previous occupation. Only 1 patient developed subsequent widening of the scapholunate interval. Percutaneous fixation in subacute or chronic scapholunate instability is less likely to be successful.

Whipple and associates[40] report 80 percent good results at 4 years for arthroscopic reduction and percutaneous fixation of scapholunate and lunotriquetral tears. Results were superior for those patients who underwent repair less than 3 months after injury and in whom no static scapholunate diastasis developed on plain radiographs.[40] Before this technique can be routinely recommended, however, it must undergo controlled studies comparing these results with those of simple immobilization of acute, nonradiographically evident tears.

LUNOTRIQUETRAL TEARS

A lunotriquetral injury may occur following forced ulnar deviation or pronation of the wrist[34] or as part of a healed perilunate injury.[39] Clinical assessment may identify localized tenderness, pain, and instability with triquetrolunate ballottement (see Chapter 18).[41] Plain radiographs are often normal, although classically there may be proximal migration of the triquetrum on the ulnar-deviation anteroposterior radiograph. Clinical diagnosis can be difficult, and the differential diagnosis includes other causes of ulnar-sided wrist pain. Assessment of lunotriquetral ligament tears with MR imaging is more difficult than that of scapholunate ligament injuries because of the small size and the oblique orientation of the lunotriquetral ligament. The reported sensitivity of MR imaging ranges from 23 to 50 percent.[38] Arthroscopic diagnosis and reduction of lunotriquetral tears are performed using the same techniques as described for a scapholunate tear (Fig. 10–16). The disruption is best visualized through the 6-R portal.

Lunotriquetral ligament dissociation with instability must be distinguished from stable minor tears secondary to impaction syndrome. Limited débridement is all that is required for symptomatic degenerative tears due to impaction syndrome or excessive wear.

Fractures of the Distal Radius

Arthroscopy is gaining popularity for the treatment of distal radial fractures, for the following reasons:

1. It enables a thorough assessment of the articular surface of the distal radius.
2. It provides a unique opportunity to assess associated injuries of the carpus, intercarpal ligaments and TFCC.
3. It aids in obtaining an anatomic reduction of the distal radius and carpus.
4. It can be used with percutaneous K-wire fixation to minimize the soft tissue injury.

Knirk and Jupiter[42] established the causal relationship between intra-articular displacement and subsequent degenerative arthritis. The surgeon should aim for an anatomic reduction, because a 2-mm stepoff leads to subsequent degenerative arthritis.[42] Open reduction of comminuted unstable fractures is often difficult, requiring extensive soft tissue stripping, which leads to slow rehabilitation. Arthroscopy is a minimally invasive technique that enables a superior examination and a more accurate reduction of the joint. To perform arthroscopy-assisted reduction of distal radial fractures, the surgeon should be experienced in wrist arthroscopy. A larger arthroscope (3.0-mm), with the inflow through its sheath, provides a greater volume of fluid for washing blood away from the surgical field. Inflow is gravity fed through the arthroscope sheath. Infusion pumps will produce extravasation of fluid into the soft tissues with the risk of compartment syndrome.[43] Wrapping the forearm with an elastic wrapping such as an Ace bandage or Coban wrap helps to minimize extravasation. A

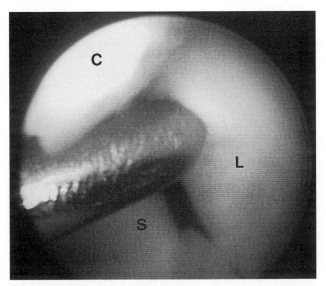

Figure 10–15. Disruption of the scapholunate interval seen through the midcarpal radial portal. Normally, the proximal carpal row forms a smooth acetabulum that will not admit a probe. *C* = capitate; *L* = lunate; *S* = scaphoid. (Precise localization of this view is shown on the diagram in Figure 10–5*B*.)

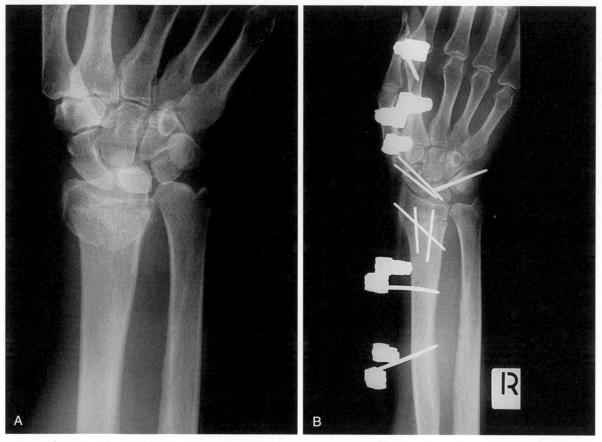

Figure 10–16. *A,* This patient has a McMurtry three-part distal radial fracture. The scapholunate interval appears normal but the lunotriquetral interval appears wide. *B,* The fracture has been treated with intrafocal pin fixation and an external fixator. Wrist arthroscopy revealed a TFCC tear, which was débrided, and scapholunate and lunotriquetral tears, which were reduced with arthroscopic assistance and fixed with percutaneous K wires.

motorized resector is useful to clear the hemarthrosis. Fluoroscopy is essential for arthroscopy-assisted reduction and fixation.

Traction applied to the arm reduces many fractures by ligamentotaxis but will not reduce most depressed intra-articular fragments. Applying excessive distraction in an attempt to reduce fractures leads to problems of extensor tendon tightness and secondary stiffness. Arthroscopy-guided external manipulation with percutaneous K-wire "joysticks" aids in reduction and avoids the need for excessive distraction. The arthroscopic probe can be used to manipulate intra-articular fragments and to test the stability of fragments following fixation. A greater understanding of the fracture pattern can be obtained by viewing the fracture from two portals. Small osteochondral fragments that may block reduction can be removed.

Radial Styloid Fractures: McMurtry Two-Part Fractures[44]

The radial styloid fracture pattern is ideally suited to arthroscopic reduction and fixation. The trans-radial styloid pins have been advocated by Mah and Atkin-

son.[45] First, we place a K wire in the radial styloid for manipulation of the styloid fragment under arthroscopic visualization. The K wires are advanced once the fracture is reduced. With this fracture pattern, it is common for there to be an associated scapholunate ligament tear, which may be part of a perilunate instability (see Fig. 10–16).

McMurtry Three- and Four-Part Fractures

The same principles are used for these fractures as those used for two-part fractures. It is the involvement of the lunate fossa that makes these fractures difficult to manage. Transulnar pin fixation techniques have been developed to try to control the lunate fossa fragments. Such transulnar pins included an extra-articular pin described by DePalma[46] and the multiple pins described by Rayhack and colleagues.[47] The Rayhack technique uses wires that cross from the ulna to the distal radius and are left in situ for 6 weeks. Some wires cross the distal radioulnar joint. Rayhack and colleagues[46] state that pronation and supination are not compromised after use of this technique.

We have modified the Rayhack pin technique to fix lunate fossa fractures as follows: Introduce two wires into the ulna head under fluoroscopic control so that when advanced they will enter the subchondral bone of the distal radius (Fig. 10–17A). Reduce the articular surface under arthroscopic vision with the "joysticks" and the arthroscopic probe (Fig. 10–17B). Then, advance the transulnar K wires into the subchondral bone of the distal radius. Withdraw the

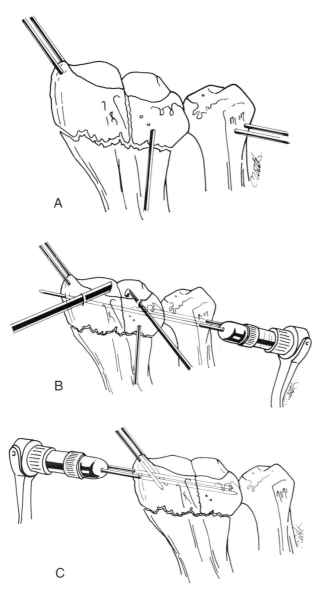

Figure 10–17. Modified Rayhack technique for fixation of distal radial fractures. *A,* "Joysticks" are placed in the radial styloid and lunate fossa fragments. Kirschner wires are placed in the distal ulna so that, when advanced, they will pass through the subchondral bone of the distal radius. *B,* The articular surface is reduced, under arthroscopic vision, with the "joysticks" and the arthroscopic probe. *C,* The transulnar pins are advanced into the subchondral bone of the distal radius. They are withdrawn from the radial side so that they do not impinge upon the DRUJ.

wires from the radial side, under fluoroscopic control, until they do not impinge upon the DRUJ (Fig. 10–17C). Placement of the pins from the ulnar side of the wrist avoids distraction of the fracture and helps to close any gap between the scaphoid fossa and the lunate fossa.

Another technique that we have found useful for lunate fossa fractures is to introduce a K wire into the joint just above the free fragment. This wire acts as a guide to the position and direction of the definitive wire, which is introduced just proximal to the first wire.

With these new techniques, intra-articular stepoffs can be reduced to less than 1 mm in all but the most comminuted fractures (Fig. 10–18). Instability of osteochondral fragments following attempted percutaneous pin fixation is an indication for limited open reduction and bone grafting.

Following reduction and fixation of the distal radial fracture, the carpus and TFCC should be assessed. The association between extra-articular radius fractures and wrist ligamentous injury has been recognized for some time. Arthrography has shown the incidence of TFCC disruption in extra-articular distal radius fractures to range up to 45 percent,[21] and clinical symptoms have been reported in 5 to 15 percent of fractures.[48, 49] Jupiter and Masem[50] reported that preservation of distal radioulnar joint function is preferable to secondary arthroplasty. In our series of 105 acute distal radial fractures, the TFCC was acutely torn in 54 percent of extra-articular fractures and 33 percent of intra-articular fractures (unpublished data). Of these tears, 77 percent were central, 15 percent volar, and 8 percent dorsal in location. A **d**orsal **u**lnar **r**adial **f**racture (DURF), avulsed from the lunate fossa of the radius, was present in 62 percent of the intra-articular fractures. This fragment was attached to the TFCC. We found that patients with this fracture pattern were less likely to have a tear of the TFCC due to force dissipation through the lunate fossa. The majority of TFCC tears occur in the avascular radial or central portion and are thus, in our opinion, best treated by débridement, because open repair in the acute fracture setting is difficult.

We have found interosseous ligament tears to be common with intra-articular distal radial fractures. The details of their management were discussed along with carpal instability. Certain distal radial fractures are better managed with open techniques. These include fractures with a large volar fragment that impinges upon the carpal tunnel, volar or dorsal Barton's fracture-dislocations, some open fractures, and pathologic fractures. Fractures that cannot be reduced or held with percutaneous techniques should be managed with open reduction. Arthroscopy-assisted reduction and fixation can be combined with small dorsal incisions and application of cancellous bone grafts for comminuted metaphyseal fractures.

With comminuted fractures, there is a risk of compartment syndrome from extravasation of irrigation

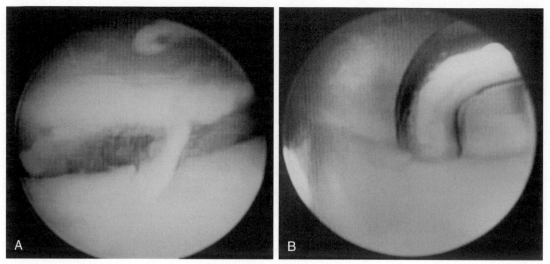

Figure 10–18. *A,* An intra-articular fracture of the distal radius seen through the 3-4 portal. *B,* Following arthroscopic reduction and fixation of the articular surface, the arthroscopic probe is used to assess the reduction and to test the stability of the fracture fragments. (Precise localization of these views is shown on the diagram in Figure 10–5C.)

fluid. This has not been a problem in our experience, but the surgeon should be aware of the possibility.

Scaphoid Fractures

Open reduction with internal fixation has become the gold standard for management of acute displaced fractures of the scaphoid. However, the volar approach breaches the important volar ligament, and the dorsal approach may compromise the blood supply to the scaphoid. Arthroscopy-assisted reduction and fixation of scaphoid fractures avoid these problems.[51, 52]

We perform arthroscopy-assisted reduction via the (MCR) portal using joysticks in the proximal and distal poles and the arthroscopic probe as follows: Identify the tuberosity of the scaphoid though a volar approach, and excise the volar lip of the trapezium with a rongeur in preparation for insertion of the internal fixation. Insert the hook of the Herbert-Whipple alignment guide through the 1-2 portal into the dorsal articular surface of the proximal scaphoid. Next, place the barrel of the alignment guide on the distal pole of the scaphoid and use it to compress the fracture and guide the screw.

Septic Arthritis

Septic arthritis is a condition that has been managed successfully with arthroscopy in the knee. Arthroscopy of the wrist facilitates a thorough lavage of the joint and enables a biopsy of the synovium to be obtained. The surgeon can visualize the articular surface and the reactive synovitis. Because of the less invasive nature of arthroscopy, patients are rehabilitated more quickly.[53]

SYNOVECTOMY

Synovectomy has historically been the first-line surgical treatment of joints affected by rheumatoid arthritis for which medical management has failed. Synovectomy for rheumatoid arthritis appears to slow down and, in some cases, halt progression of the disease.[54, 55] Experience with other joints has shown that synovectomy should be performed during the early stages of the disease, before severe joint destruction develops. The concerns with open synovectomy are the prolonged rehabilitation and the possibility of loss of motion.

Arthroscopy provides us with a magnified view of the pathologic synovium (Fig. 10–19), which typically accumulates on the volar ligaments of the radiocarpal joint.[56, 57] Usually, we perform complete synovectomy by alternating the resector between the 3-4 and 6-R portals. Occasionally, the 1-2 or 6-U portal is required if there is extensive synovitis. When indicated, we also perform midcarpal synovectomy, although this joint is commonly spared in rheumatoid arthritis.[56]

Adolfsson and Nylander[56] reported the results of arthroscopic synovectomy in 16 patients (18 wrists) with rheumatoid arthritis. All patients experienced a reduction in pain at rest, during activity, and at night. The average arc of extension and flexion improved from 69° to 90°, and no patient experienced a decrease in the range of motion. The average grip strength improved 87 percent after 6 months. There were no complications in this series.[56]

Arthroscopic synovectomy of the wrist is now an established procedure that offers superior visualization, easy access, and effective removal of the pathologic synovium in an outpatient setting.[12, 56, 58] However, patients with dorsal tenosynovitis require an open procedure.

Loose Bodies

Arthroscopy is a valuable technique to remove loose bodies. Loose bodies usually occur following chondral defects or degenerative osteoarthritis and cause symptoms such as pain and locking. Other causes are intra-articular fractures, cartilage nutrition disorders, and infection.[59] Small loose bodies can be difficult to visualize with plain radiographs but are clearly demonstrated with computed tomographic (CT) arthrography.

We routinely obtain repeat radiographs on the day of surgery. We prefer to use an arthroscopic portal close to the loose body and a separate inflow so that the flow is toward the arthroscope. We find that the addition of suction to the arthroscope is often helpful. A hypodermic needle is useful to maneuver or skewer the loose body. Loose bodies that cannot be retrieved are morcellated with a mechanical bur or resector.[59]

Ganglion

Dorsal ganglia of the wrist often originate from the dorsal aspect of the scapholunate ligament. The ganglion and the adjacent synovitis can be visualized on the scapholunate ligament and the adjacent dorsal capsule.[12, 60] We place the arthroscope in the 6-R or 1-2 portal and the mechanical resector in the 3-4 portal in order to excise the ganglion.[51] The ganglion and adjacent dorsal capsule are resected until the extensor tendons are visualized.

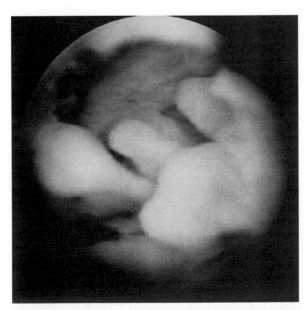

Figure 10–19. Extensive synovitis on the ulnar side of the radiocarpal joint, which can be excised with a motorized resector. (Precise localization of this view is shown on the diagram in Figure 10–5C.)

Chondral Defects

Chondral defects are far more common than might be expected, and are a frequent source of occult wrist pain.[59, 61] Clinical diagnosis of chondral defects is difficult, because the patient often has only diffuse tenderness. Chondral defects are poorly diagnosed by standard imaging modalities, including MR imaging.[11] If wrist pain persists despite conservative measures, wrist arthroscopy offers diagnosis and treatment. Arthroscopy is also valuable for assessment of the joint surfaces to determine whether more definitive procedures, such as proximal row carpectomy or limited carpal fusion, are indicated.

Partial-thickness cartilage lesions have some potential to heal, but full-thickness cartilage defects have no such potential.[61] The fate of articular cartilage adjacent to a defect depends on the strength of its edges and the mechanical stability of the joint.[61] If the subchondral bone is disrupted, granulation tissue is formed, which is transformed into fibrocartilage.[62] The clinical application of this phenomenon is abrasion and drill chondroplasty. Unfortunately, the fibrocartilage produced becomes soft and is poorly resistant to wear.[62]

At arthroscopy, we establish the size and stability of the chondral defects. Chondral lesions are smoothed to reduce mechanical symptoms and to minimize the production of intra-articular debris that would facilitate the degenerative process. Thick chondral flaps are débrided with a suction punch or basket forceps; thin lesions are débrided with a motorized resector. Whipple[59] advises that patients often have symptomatic relief following abrasion arthroplasty for lesions in the wrist less than 5 mm in diameter.[59] Abrasive arthroplasty is unlikely to be successful if extensive changes are present; however, the lavage of debris and lysomal enzymes from the joint will provide temporary relief of symptoms in some patients.[61] In patients with full-thickness lesions less than 5 mm, we perform abrasion chondroplasty to bleeding bone. In those patients with defects greater than 5 mm, abrasion chondroplasty is less likely to result in symptomatic relief, and we only excise the loose chondral flap.

Poehling and Roth[61] reported a multicenter study of chondral defects in the wrist diagnosed with arthroscopy. Cartilage lesions were classified as primary if the source of symptoms was judged to be the articular cartilage and secondary if it was from another cause (e.g., ligament instability or fracture). Eighty-three percent of patients with primary lesions improved, but only 55 percent with secondary lesions improved.[61]

Degenerative Arthritis

Arthroscopic débridement of degenerative arthritis of the knee has been reported to produce good results in two thirds of patients.[63–65] Similar results could be expected in the non–weight-bearing wrist joint. Arthroscopic débridement is most likely to be successful in patients with mechanical symptoms and minimal radiographic changes. Lavage and débridement of chondral flaps, osteophytes, and synovitis can be rewarding.[63–65]

The scaphotrapeziotrapezoid (STT) joint is a common site of degenerative osteoarthritis. We perform arthroscopic débridement with a 2-mm, full-radius resector using the STT or the radial MCR portal.

Resection Arthroplasty

Many procedures that were previously performed through an arthrotomy can now be performed arthroscopically, with the advantages of decreased postoperative pain and less stiffness.

Proximal row carpectomy has been performed arthroscopically.[13] Arthroscopy also allows accurate assessment of the articular surfaces of the capitate and the lunate fossa prior to the proximal row carpectomy. We resect the lunate first, followed by the triquetrum and proximal pole of the scaphoid. Resection is carried out using a rongeur. We readily utilize intraoperative radiographs to confirm the desired bony resection.

Hemiresection of the distal ulna has also been performed.[13] We pronate and supinate the forearm to ensure an adequate ulnar head resection. Intraoperative radiographs are important to ensure that an adequate amount of bone has been resected.[13]

Other arthroscopic procedures that have been reported are radial styloidectomy and excision of the proximal pole of the scaphoid for a scaphoid nonunion.[66] Resection of the lunate for Kienböck's disease could also be performed arthroscopically. Arthroscopic arthrodesis of the ankle has been reported.[67] Similar techniques could be developed for full or limited wrist fusion. Many of these techniques should be regarded as investigational at this stage, as there are no reported series for their evaluation.

Chronic Wrist Pain

Chronic wrist pain can be considered mechanical or dystrophic.[25] Patients with mechanical symptoms, such as catching, clicking, locking, and pain that increases with activity and decreases with rest, are more likely to have a good result following wrist arthroscopy. In contrast, patients with dystrophic symptoms, such as burning pain that is often worse at night, exacerbated by minimal activity, or associated with cold insensitivity, dysesthesia, paresthesia, or vasomotor changes, are less likely to obtain symptomatic relief following arthroscopy.[25]

Ligamentous and cartilage injuries are seen with arthroscopy in 70 to 96 percent of patients.[68, 70] Conventional studies, including MR imaging, often fail to delineate the problem.[71] Arthroscopy resulted in a change in the diagnosis in up to 40 percent of patients.[72] However, correlation of the arthroscopic findings with the clinical symptoms is important. The final caution is that extra-articular causes of chronic wrist pain, such as neuromas and tendinitis, need to be excluded prior to the arthroscopy.

Depending on the arthroscopic findings, débridement of loose osteochondral flaps, or of partial ligamentous injuries, or abrasion chondroplasty can be performed.

POSTOPERATIVE CARE

All arthroscopies are performed on an outpatient basis. The tourniquet is released and 10 mL of 0.5% bupivacaine (Marcaine) is injected into the joint, portal sites, and the region of the posterior interosseous nerve in the base of the fourth extensor tendon compartment. The portals are not sutured, to allow drainage of fluid into the dressing. The arm is placed in a below-elbow bulky dressing for 7 days, and the patient is instructed to mobilize the fingers, elbow, and shoulder. After the dressing is removed, the patient is advised to commence mobilizing the wrist and begin performing activities of daily living. Patients with ligament injuries are immobilized for 6 to 8 weeks in a below-elbow cast.

COMPLICATIONS

Complications of arthroscopy are rare, and wrist arthroscopy is no exception. Major national surveys in France and the United States have revealed an overall complication rate of 0.56 percent.[73, 74] In the wrist, the major potential complications are infections, neuromas, tendon injuries, reflex sympathetic dystrophy (RSD), dorsal skin slough, tourniquet neurapraxia, compartment syndromes, and finger joint injury or skin slough from the finger traps. With the exception of the occasional patient with RSD, none of these complications have occurred in our patients. Adequate precautions taken during arthroscopy prevent most of the listed complications.

During arthroscopy of distal radial fractures, the risk of compartment syndrome is a concern. However, few cases of compartment syndrome following arthroscopy have actually been reported.[75, 76] All reported cases occurred following knee arthroscopy. Safety measures to minimize fluid extravasation include the use of gravity-fed systems, wrapping the forearm with an elastic bandage, and using large portals to allow free egress of fluid.[76] Irrigation pumps are likely to increase fluid extravasation. If surgery is delayed for 48 hours following a distal radial fracture, the fracture hematoma will have clotted, minimizing intra-articular bleeding and fluid extravasation. Simple elevation of the arm and cessation of arthroscopy will relieve the problem of fluid extravasation.[25]

The radial artery is at risk during the establishment of the 1-2 portal. To prevent injury to the radial artery, the portal should be just volar to the extensor pollicis longus tendon. The dorsal cutaneous branch of the ulnar nerve and the superficial radial nerve are at risk when the portals are established. The 6-R portal places the dorsal cutaneous branch of the ulna at risk.[77] Appropriate precautions, as previously described, should minimize the occurrence of complications.

UNRESOLVED ISSUES

The major unresolved issue of wrist arthroscopy is, What are its limits?

In the last 10 years, wrist arthroscopy has progressed from diagnostic modality to therapeutic tool. Wrist arthroscopy is becoming increasingly valuable in the evaluation and treatment of distal radial fractures and acute carpal injuries. In the near future, the exact role of wrist arthroscopy in this patient population will be better defined. The indications for arthroscopy in chronic wrist problems will continue to be defined.

CONCLUSION

Arthroscopy provides the surgeon with a magnified view of all intra-articular structures, including those areas difficult to access via an arthrotomy. Advances in arthroscopic techniques and instrumentation have enabled the surgeon to extend the therapeutic possibilities of wrist arthroscopy. Suction punches and smaller, lighter motorized resectors and burs have enabled intra-articular surgery to be performed more efficiently. The wrist arthroscopist can now effectively manage scaphoid and distal radius fractures, TFCC tears, interosseous ligament tears, septic arthritis, chondral defects, and degenerative arthritis. The surgeon can use the anatomic principles that have been developed for open procedures and adapt them for the arthroscope. Arthroscopic surgery is minimally invasive; hence, patients rehabilitate quickly with fewer complications. Arthroscopic surgery requires a high level of skill from the surgeon but, when mastered, provides considerable benefit to the patient. The indications and limitations of therapeutic wrist arthroscopy are being established. The role of wrist arthroscopy in distal radius fractures, scaphoid fractures, ligament injuries, chondral defects, and degenerative arthritis is still evolving.

References

1. Takagi K: The classic arthroscope. Clin Orthop 167:6–8, 1982.
2. Yung-Cheng C: Arthroscopy of the wrist and finger joints. Orthop Clin North Am 10:723–733, 1979.
3. Roth JH: Hand instrumentation for small joint arthroscopy. Arthroscopy 4:126–128, 1988.
4. Whipple TL: Powered instruments for wrist arthroscopy. Arthroscopy 4:290–294, 1988.
5. Herbert TJ, Faithfull RG, McCann DJ, et al: Bilateral arthrography of the wrist. J Hand Surg [Br] 15:233–235, 1990.
6. Levinsohn EM, Rosen DI, Palmer AK: Wrist arthrography: value of the three-compartment injection method. Radiology 179:231–239, 1991.
7. Roth JH, Haddad RG: Radiocarpal arthroscopy and arthrography in the diagnosis of ulnar wrist pain. Arthroscopy 2:234–243, 1986.
8. Kang HS, Kindynis P, Brahme SK, et al: Triangular fibrocartilage and intercarpal ligaments of the wrist: MR imaging: Cadaveric study with gross pathologic and histologic correlation. Radiology 181:401–404, 1991.
9. Gundry CR, Kursunoglu-Brahme S, Schwaighofer B, et al: Is MRI better than arthrography for evaluating the ligaments of the wrist? In vitro study. AJR 154:337–341, 1990.
10. Golimbu CN, Firooznia H, Melone C, et al: Tears of the triangular fibrocartilage of the wrist: MR imaging. Radiology 173:731–733, 1989.
11. Cerofolini E, Luchetti R, Pederzini L, et al: MRI evaluation of triangular fibrocartilage complex tears in the wrist: Comparison with arthrography and arthroscopy. J Comput Assist Tomogr 14:963–967, 1990.
12. Whipple TL: Arthroscopic Surgery of the Wrist. Philadelphia, JB Lippincott, 1992.
13. Roth JH, Poehling GG: Arthroscopic "-ectomy" surgery of the wrist. Arthroscopy 6:141–147, 1990.
14. Whipple TL, Marotta JJ, Powell JH: Techniques of wrist arthroscopy. Arthroscopy 2:244–252, 1986.
15. North RE, Thomas S: An anatomic guide for arthroscopic visualization of the wrist capsular ligaments. J Hand Surg [Am] 13:815–822, 1988.
16. Cooney WP, Dobyns JH, Linscheid RL: Arthroscopy of the wrist: Anatomy and classification of carpal instability. Arthroscopy 6:133–140, 1990.
17. Oretorp N, Elmersson S: Arthroscopy and irrigation control. Arthroscopy 2:46–50, 1986.
18. Viegas SF: The lunatohamate articulation of the midcarpal joint. Arthroscopy 6:5–10, 1990.
19. Palmer AK: Triangular fibrocartilage disorders: Injury patterns and treatment. Arthroscopy 6:125–132, 1990.
20. Mikic Z: The blood supply of the human distal radioulnar joint and the microvasculature of its articular disk. Clin Orthop 187:26–35, 1984.
21. Mohanti RC, Kar N: Study of triangular fibrocartilage of the wrist joint in Colles' fracture. Injury 11:321–324, 1980.
22. Cooney WP, Linscheid RL, Dobyns JH: Triangular fibrocartilage tears. J Hand Surg [Am] 19:143–154, 1994.
23. Feldon P, Terrono AL, Belsky MR: Wafer distal ulna resection for triangular fibrocartilage tears and/or ulna impaction syndrome. J Hand Surg [Am] 17:731–737, 1992.
24. Osterman AL: Arthroscopic debridement of the triangular fibrocartilage complex tears. Arthroscopy 6:120–124, 1990.
25. Darrow JC, Linscheid RL, Dobyns JH, et al: Distal ulnar recession for disorders of the distal radioulnar joint. J Hand Surg [Am] 10:482–491, 1985.
26. Poehling GP, Chabon SJ, Siegel DB: Diagnostic and operative arthroscopy. In Gelberman RH (ed): The Wrist: Master Techniques in Orthopedic Surgery. New York, Raven Press, 1994, pp 21–48.
27. Friedman SL, Palmer AK: Ulnar impaction syndrome. Hand Clin 7:295–310, 1991.
28. Menon J, Wood VE, Schoene HR, et al: Isolated tears of the triangular fibrocartilage of the wrist: Results of partial excision. J Hand Surg [Am] 9:527–530, 1984.
29. Feldon P, Terrono AL, Belsky MR: The "wafer" procedure; partial distal ulnar resection. Clin Orthop 275:124–129, 1992.
30. Bowers WH: Distal radioulnar joint arthroplasty: The hemiresection-interposition technique. J Hand Surg [Am] 10:169–178, 1985.
31. Milch H: Cuff resection of the ulna for malunited Colles' fracture. J Bone Joint Surg 23:311–313, 1941.

32. Palmer AK, Werner FW, Glisson RR, et al: Partial excision of the triangular fibrocartilage complex. J Hand Surg [Am] 13:391–394, 1988.

33. Wnorowski DC, Palmer AK, Werner FW, et al: Anatomic and biomechanical analysis of the arthroscopic wafer procedure. Arthroscopy 8:204–212, 1992.

34. Jones WA: Beware the sprained wrist: The incidence and diagnosis of scapholunate instability. J Bone Joint Surg 70B:293–297, 1988.

35. Watson HK, Ballet FL: The SLAC wrist: Scapholunate advanced collapse pattern of degenerative arthritis. J Hand Surg [Am] 9:358–365, 1984.

36. Watson K, Ashmead D IV, Makhlouf MV: Examination of the scaphoid. J Hand Surg [Am] 13:657–660, 1988.

37. Meade TD, Schneider LH, Cherry K: Radiographic analysis of selective sectioning at the carpal scaphoid: A cadaveric study. J Hand Surg [Am] 15:855–862, 1990.

38. Schweitzer ME, Brahme SK, Hodler J, et al: Chronic wrist pain: Spin-echo and short tau inversion recovery MR imaging and conventional and MR arthrography. Radiology 182:205–211, 1992.

39. Mayfield JK, Johnson RP, Kilcoyne RK: Carpal dislocations: pathomechanics and progressive perilunar instability. J Hand Surg 5:226–241, 1980.

40. Whipple TL, Schengel D, Caffrey D, Ellis F: Treatment of scapholunate dissociation by arthroscopic reduction and internal fixation. Presented at Int Wrist Investigators Workshop, Long Beach, CA, May 1990.

41. Reagan DS, Linscheid RL, Dobyns DH: Lunotriquetral sprains. J Hand Surg 9:502–513, 1984.

42. Knirk JL, Jupiter JB: Intra-articular fractures of the distal end of the radius in young adults. J Bone Joint Surg 63A:647–659, 1986.

43. Fruensgard S, Holm A: Compartment syndrome complicating arthroscopic surgery: Brief report. J Bone Joint Surg 70B:146–147, 1988.

44. McMurtry RY, Jupiter JB: Fractures of the distal radius. In Browner BD, Jupiter JB, Levine AM, Trafton PG (eds): Skeletal Trauma: Fractures, Dislocations, Ligamentous Injuries. Philadelphia, WB Saunders, 1992, pp 1063–1093.

45. Mah E, Atkinson R: Percutaneous Kirschner wire stabilization following closed reduction of Colles' fractures. J Hand Surg [Br] 17:55, 1992.

46. DePalma A: Comminuted fractures of the distal end of the radius treated by ulnar pinning. J Bone Joint Surg 34A:651–662, 1952.

47. Rayhack J, Langworthy J, Belsole R: Transulnar percutaneous pinning of displaced distal radial fractures: A preliminary report. J Orthop Trauma 3:107, 1989.

48. Lidstrom A: Fractures of the distal end of the radius: A clinical and statistical study of end results. Acta Orthop Scand Suppl 41:7–118, 1959.

49. Cooney WP, Dobyns JH, Linscheid RL: Complications of Colles' fractures. J Bone Joint Surg 62A:613–619, 1980.

50. Jupiter JB, Masem M: Reconstruction of post-traumatic deformity of the distal radius and ulna. Hand Clin North Am 4:377–390, 1988.

51. Whipple TL: The role of arthroscopy in the treatment of wrist injuries in the athlete. Clinics Sports Med 11:227–238, 1992.

52. Zimmer product information. Herbert/Whipple bone screw system. Surgical techniques for the scaphoid and other small bone fractures. Zimmer Inc., Warsaw, IN.

53. Thiery JA: Arthroscopic drainage in septic arthritides of the knee: A multicentre study. Arthroscopy 5:65–69, 1989.

54. Smiley P, Wasilewski SA: Arthroscopic synovectomy. Arthroscopy 6:18–23, 1990.

55. Taylor AR: Synovectomy of the knee in rheumatoid arthritis patients. J Bone Joint Surg 61B:121, 1979.

56. Adolfsson L, Nylander G: Arthroscopic synovectomy of the rheumatoid wrist. J Hand Surg [Br] 18:92–96, 1993.

57. Richards RS, Roth JH: Wrist arthroscopy: Advances in diagnosis and treatment. Advances in Operative Orthopaedics, 203–225, 1993.

58. Roth JH: Radiocarpal arthroscopy: Techniques and selected cases. In Lichtman DM (ed): The Wrist and Its Disorders. Philadelphia, WB Saunders, 1988, pp 108–117.

59. Whipple TL: Articular surface defects and loose bodies. In Arthroscopic Surgery of the Wrist. Philadelphia, JB Lippincott, 1992, pp 93–102.

60. Viegas SF: Intraarticular ganglion of the dorsal interosseous scapholunate ligament: A case for arthroscopy. Arthroscopy 2:93–95, 1986.

61. Poehling GG, Roth JH: Articular cartilage lesions of the wrist. In McGinty JB (ed): Operative Arthroscopy. New York, Raven Press, 1991, pp 635–639.

62. Johnson LL: Arthroscopic abrasion arthroplasty historical and pathological perspective: Present status. Arthroscopy 2:54–69, 1986.

63. Bert JM, Maschka K: The arthroscopic treatment of unicompartmental gonarthrosis: A five year follow-up study of abrasion arthroplasty plus arthroscopic debridement and arthroscopic debridement alone. Arthroscopy 5:25–32, 1989.

64. Dandy DJ: Arthroscopic debridement of the knee [editorial]. J Bone Joint Surg 73B:877–878, 1991.

65. McLaren AC, Blokker CP, Fowler PJ, et al: Arthroscopic debridement of the knee for osteoarthritis. Can J Surg 34:595–598, 1991.

66. Whipple TL: Clinical applications of wrist arthroscopy. In Lichtman DM (ed): The Wrist and Its Disorders. Philadelphia, WB Saunders, 1988, pp 118–128.

67. Ogilvie-Harris DJ, Lieberman I, Fitsialos D: Arthroscopically assisted arthrodesis for osteoarthritic ankles. J Bone Joint Surg 75A:1167–1174, 1993.

68. Koman LA, Poehling GG, Toby EB, et al: Chronic wrist pain: Indications for wrist arthroscopy. Arthroscopy 6:116–119, 1990.

69. Adolfsson L: Arthroscopy in the diagnosis of post traumatic wrist pain. J Hand Surg [Br] 17:46–50, 1992.

70. North ER, Meyer S: Wrist injuries: Correlation of clinical and arthroscopic findings. J Hand Surg [Am] 15:915–920, 1990.

71. Levy HJ, Gardner RD, Lemak LJ: Bilateral osteochondral flaps of the wrists. Arthroscopy 7:118–119, 1991.

72. Kelly EP, Stanley JK: Arthroscopy of the wrist. J Hand Surg [Br] 15:236–242, 1990.

73. Kieser CH: A review of complications of knee arthroscopy. Arthroscopy 8:79–83, 1992.

74. Small NC: Complications in arthroscopy: The knee and other joints. Arthroscopy 2:253–258, 1986.

75. Nillium A, Rosser B: Akut compartment syndrom vid knaartroskopi. Lakartidningen 80:590, 1983.

76. Peek RD, Haynes DW. Compartment syndrome as a complication of arthroscopy: A case report and a study of interstitial pressures. Am J Sports Med 12:464–468, 1984.

77. Pianka G: Wrist arthroscopy. Hand Clin 8:621–630, 1992.

CHAPTER 11

Clinical Applications of Wrist Arthroscopy

Terry L. Whipple, MD

Although wrist arthroscopy is a modality of relatively recent development, it is rapidly gaining widespread application. The wrist is a complex joint composed of 15 bones and 27 articular surfaces. It is crossed by 24 tendons, two major arteries, and five primary nerves and branches. This anatomic complexity provides numerous opportunities for the development of joint symptoms that are often difficult to attribute to a specific anatomic structure. The diagnostic aids conventionally used to evaluate wrist pain are radiography, arthrography, cineradiography, and computed tomography (CT). Magnetic resonance (MR) imaging has been employed as a potential modality for wrist evaluation.[1] The design of smaller MR imaging coils and refinement of image clarity have increased the value of this diagnostic modality, but the scarce availability of the better coils and relatively limited expertise in the interpretation of wrist MR images limit its suitability. With the exception of MR imaging, the ancillary techniques listed primarily display the skeletal tissues of the wrist and are of limited use in the evaluation of soft tissue disorders. The numerous subtle instability patterns and intra-articular soft tissue disorders involving the ligaments, the triangular fibrocartilage complex (TFCC), the articular cartilage, and the synovium are impossible to diagnose or confirm without the advantage of direct tissue inspection.

Arthroscopy of the wrist provides this advantage.[2, 3] As a minimally invasive technique, wrist arthroscopy affords a means of direct visualization of intra-articular tissues with magnification and remarkable clarity. These structures may be explored by palpation and manipulation using various accessory instruments (Fig. 11–1).[4] The procedure can be performed using regional anesthesia and causes virtually no morbidity.

Disruptions of intercarpal ligaments can be demonstrated by wrist arthrography when dye passes from one isolated compartment of the wrist to another. However, it is not possible by use of arthrography to identify the pattern or size of a tear in a specific ligament or in the TFCC, nor is arthrography helpful in discerning the mechanical significance of a ligament tear in relation to wrist function or symptoms.[5]

These latter considerations have important implications in the formulation of prognoses and appropriate treatment regimens. Central perforations of the triangular fibrocartilage occurring from attrition may be of little long-term significance and require no surgical intervention. An unstable flap tear of the triangular fibrocartilage, however, may cause symptoms of impingement or limitation of motion if the flap is displaced, or may even contribute to subtle instabilities of the distal radioulnar joint.[6] Although the arthrographic appearances of these two lesions are similar, arthroscopic examination of the TFCC can disclose the size, shape, and precise location of the tear as well as its functional significance in relation to position and stress (Fig. 11–2).

The volar radiocarpal and ulnocarpal ligaments represent specific bulky condensations of fibers in the volar wrist capsule.[7, 8] These concentrated bundles protrude into the joint, standing in relief from the volar capsule, and can be seen clearly on arthroscopic examination. When these ligaments are torn, palpation of the volar side of the wrist displaces the fiber bundles farther into the joint, confirming the specific location and severity of the injury (Fig. 11–3). Chondromalacia and other lesions of articular cartilage without underlying bone sclerosis or osteopenia are best revealed by direct visual inspection of the articular surfaces but do not necessarily require arthrotomy (Fig. 11–4).[9–12]

Precise indications for wrist arthroscopy are still evolving. Experience in the past decade has defined certain specific circumstances in which the procedure is extremely useful.[13] Certain surgical procedures may also be performed under arthroscopic control, with the advantage of reduced operative morbidity compared with similar procedures performed through arthrotomy. In the evaluation of wrist symptoms, there can be no substitute for a thorough physical examination based on discovery of the mechanism of injury, localization of symptoms, and complete familiarity with wrist anatomy.[3] Conventional diagnostic imaging techniques should then be employed to the greatest possible advantage. When these techniques are insufficient to provide the necessary information for a definitive treatment plan, however, arthroscopy can provide critical anatomic data.

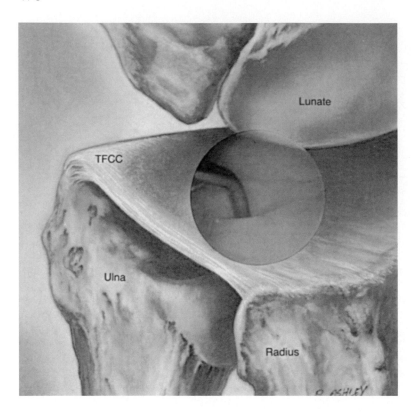

Figure 11–1. Exploration of the soft triangular fibrocartilage complex (TFCC) with a hook probe. Viewed through a 1.9-mm arthroscope from a dorsal approach between the third and fourth extensor compartments.

SPECIFIC INDICATIONS

Through extensive clinical experience with wrist arthroscopy, certain specific indications for the procedure have become apparent. The first group of indications pertains to lesions of soft tissue.

Soft Tissue Lesions

If a patient suspected of having an injury to one of the intercarpal ligaments or to the TFCC has a positive arthrogram that demonstrates communication between normally isolated intra-articular spaces, arthroscopy is indicated to assess the size of the defect and to determine whether or not an open procedure is necessary for definitive repair. If, on clinical examination, cineradiography, or stress radiography, intercarpal instability is proved to be severe enough to warrant surgical stabilization or ligament reconstruction, arthroscopy is indicated for evaluation of articular surfaces. The condition of these surfaces may influence the selection of preferred stabilization procedures. Carpal instability invariably produces abnormal stress on articular surfaces; therefore, certain stabilization procedures that may result in additional stress to already worn articulations would be contraindicated. It is useful, as well, to know of any associated pathologic conditions of soft tissue that may be present in the wrist when an open procedure is contemplated.

Many patients have a history of allergic reactions to iodine-based radiographic contrast material or to shellfish or other foods with significant iodine content. In these individuals, contrast arthrography is contraindicated. However, if intercarpal ligament tears or injury to the TFCC is suspected in such a patient, arthroscopic examination can demonstrate the presence of these disorders.[9, 14, 15]

Finally, in undiagnosed cases of monarticular synovitis, or when a wrist is the largest joint involved with synovial hypertrophy, arthroscopy provides a convenient and straightforward means of synovial biopsy or limited therapeutic synovectomy.[16–18]

A few case examples help illustrate these points.

Case 1

A 32-year-old male fell on his pronated outstretched left hand, causing severe dorsoradial pain and swelling in the wrist. His radiographs demonstrated a minimally displaced fracture of the radial styloid process and widening of the scapholunate interval that was not obviously acute (Fig. 11–5). An arthrogram showed dye passing through the scapholunate interval. Arthroscopy confirmed that the scapholunate ligament was completely ruptured from its dorsal to its volar aspect and that the injury was indeed acute.

Under arthroscopic control, the scapholunate joint was reduced and pinned with Kirschner (K) wires, and the radial styloid fracture was managed in a short-arm cast (see next section).

The patient's radial styloid fracture was managed adequately in the short-arm thumb spica cast. Four years postoperatively, the scapholunate joint remained stable and asymptomatic.

Figure 11–2. *A,* Central perforation of the TFCC viewed from the ulnar side of the wrist. The ulnar head is seen through the perforation. The lesion is smooth and stable, however, and no surgical treatment is indicated. *B,* Unstable flap tear of the TFCC adjacent to its insertion on the ulnar notch of the radius. Turned-up flap of cartilage catches beneath the lunate, causing impingement and pain aggravated by pronation and ulnar deviation. Viewed arthroscopically from dorsal radial approach between first and second extensor compartments.

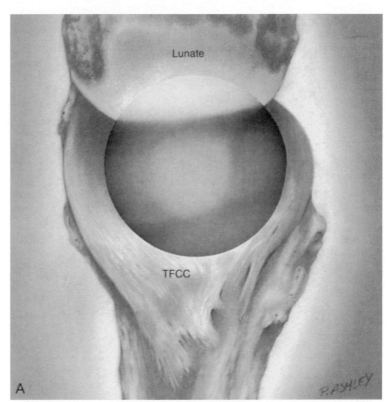

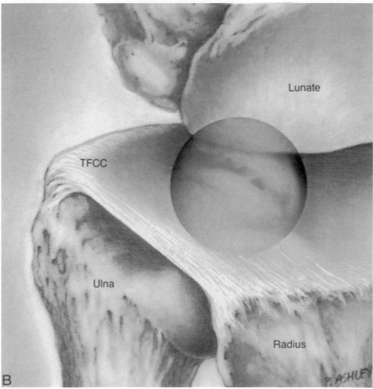

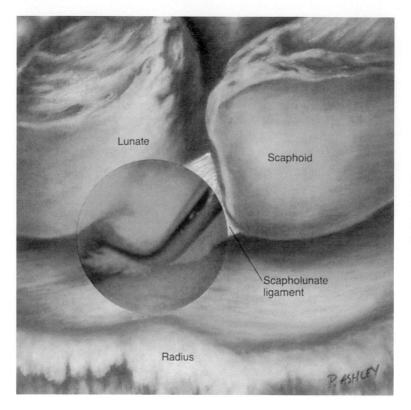

Figure 11–3. A tear of the volar radiolunate triquetral ligament is viewed from a dorsal approach between the third and fourth extensor compartments with a hook probe introduced between the fourth and fifth extensor compartments. Palpation of the volar side of the wrist displaces this ligament into the radiocarpal space.

Figure 11–4. Articular cartilage changes on the distal pole of the scaphoid and the proximal articular surface of trapezoid are explored and palpated with a 23-gauge needle. The triscaphe joint is examined through a 1.9-mm arthroscope introduced in the midcarpal space between the scaphoid and capitate.

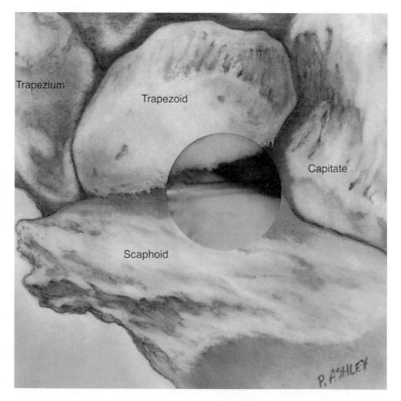

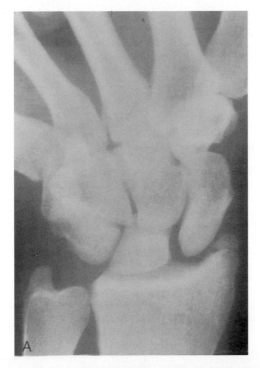

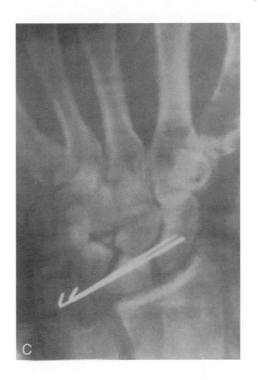

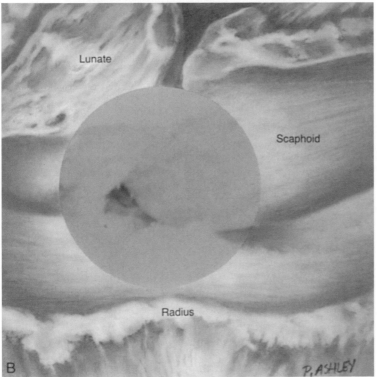

Figure 11–5. *A,* Radiograph shows separation between the scaphoid and lunate association, with transverse fracture of the radial styloid. *B,* Arthroscopic view of proximal edge of the scapholunate interval. Freshly torn tissue confirms acute nature of injury. The defect is viewed arthroscopically through a dorsal approach between the third and fourth extensor compartments. *C,* Radiograph of two K wires used to reduce and stabilize, under arthroscopic control, the scapholunate interval.

SURGICAL TECHNIQUE FOR ARTHROSCOPIC REDUCTION AND INTERNAL FIXATION OF SCAPHOLUNATE DISSOCIATION[15, 19]

The wrist is distracted by means of flexible nylon finger traps applied to the index and long fingers, then attached to a wrist Traction Tower (Linvatec, Inc, Largo, FL) with a distraction force of 8 to 12 lb, depending on the size and flexibility of the extremity. An inflow cannula is placed in the 6-U portal just ulnar to the extensor carpi ulnaris tendon, and the joint is distended with lactated Ringer's solution. A 2.7-mm arthroscope is introduced in the 3-4 portal. This provides visualization of the scapholunate ligament distally and the articular surface of the radius proximally. With the radial joint capsule adjacent to the proximal pole of the scaphoid in view, two 0.045-inch K wires are introduced through the dorsal aspect of the anatomic snuffbox through 14-gauge hypodermic needles. The hypodermic needles serve as inexpensive cannulae that will prevent the K wires from injuring cutaneous branches of the radial nerve. The K wires are drilled into the proximal pole of the scaphoid, aiming toward the lunate.

The arthroscope is then transferred to the midcarpal ulnar (MCU) portal, and the inflow is attached to the arthroscope sheath to provide ample distention in the midcarpal space. Accurate reduction of the scapholunate interval is best seen from the midcarpal joint, because there is no interosseous ligament to obscure visualization of this articulation on its distal surface. The Traction Tower is adjusted to place the wrist in slight extension and ulnar deviation. The two K wires can then be used to manipulate the scaphoid into anatomic relationship with the lunate. If the lunate is in extreme dorsal intercalary segment instability (DISI) posture, an additional K wire can be inserted percutaneously into the dorsal aspect of the lunate to facilitate the reduction. Once the scapholunate interval is completely closed, and with the field of view in the midcarpal space, the two K wires are advanced through the proximal pole of the scaphoid into the lunate. The reductions, the position of the K wires, and their depth of penetration are then confirmed by intraoperative fluoroscopy. Two additional K wires are inserted roughly parallel to the first two, giving additional security to the fixation.

Great care is taken to ensure that the K wires do not violate any articular surface other than the scapholunate interval. The K wires are bent 90° adjacent to the skin and are cut short. It is not necessary to débride the scapholunate ligament unless there is a large flap of ligament that might fold on itself and become pinched between the radius and the proximal carpal row. Neither is it necessary to débride the articular cartilage between the scaphoid and the lunate; the passage of four or five K wires provides ample excoriation of these surfaces to produce a fibrous ankylosis that will maintain reduction in most acute cases.

The pins are covered with an antiseptic gauze, and the wrist is immobilized in slight extension in a short-arm thumb spica cast for 7 to 8 weeks, after which time the pins can be removed without anesthesia. It is prudent to inspect the pins every two weeks to cleanse them and reapply antiseptic gauze.

Case 2

A 45-year-old female had scapholunate dissociation that caused pain on flexion and radial deviation. Symptoms were chronic and progressive. A triscaphe or scaphocapitate arthrodesis[20] was considered, but arthroscopy showed moderately advanced chondromalacic changes on the proximal pole of the scaphoid and early degenerative changes on the radial

styloid articular surface. A dorsal reconstruction of the radioscapholunate ligament was performed using a free tendon graft. Although this procedure is not as durable as intercarpal arthrodesis, it does not transfer excessive axial load to the radioscaphoid articulation.

Case 3

A 27-year-old professional football player injured his dominant wrist early in the playing season, and an arthrogram showed leakage of dye across the triangular fibrocartilage complex into the distal radioulnar joint. His wrist had slight positive ulnar variance, pain with pronation against resistance, and tenderness over the triangular fibrocartilage complex. The presence of positive ulnar variance raised a question about the significance and acuteness of the TFCC defect demonstrated on the arthrogram. However, if arthrotomy had been performed to explore and possibly resect the fibrocartilage, it would have eliminated the patient from playing for the remainder of the football season and would have caused him significant loss of income. Arthroscopy was performed instead, revealing a flap tear of the TFCC near its attachment to the radius. The unstable portion of the TFCC was resected under arthroscopic control (see next section), and the patient returned to play within 4 weeks (see Fig. 11–2B).

SURGICAL TECHNIQUE FOR CENTRAL EXCISION OF THE TRIANGULAR FIBROCARTILAGE COMPLEX[6, 14, 21]

The wrist is distracted through nylon finger traps applied to the index and long fingers. Alternatively, in extremely stiff wrists, the finger traps may be applied to the ring and little fingers. The finger traps are then secured to a Traction Tower, and 10 to 12 lb of distraction force is applied. An inflow cannula is placed in the 1-2 portal in the dorsal aspect of the anatomic snuffbox near the intersection of the extensor pollicis longus and the extensor carpi radialis longus tendons.

A 2.7-mm arthroscope is introduced through the 3-4 portal. Looking proximally and ulnarward, the surgeon identifies the triangular fibrocartilage. Squeezing the distal radioulnar joint causes tears in the central disk of the TFCC to billow open. It may be necessary to introduce a hook probe through the 6-R portal to palpate the triangular fibrocartilage disk and appreciate fully the size and mechanical significance of a tear.

A small powered shaver can be introduced through the 6-R portal to débride thin filmy cartilage tissue from the TFCC tear margins. For thicker flaps of tissue, a miniaturized suction punch (Smith and Nephew Dyonics, Inc, Norwood, MA) is introduced through the 6-R portal, and the unstable margins of the central TFCC disk can be excised adjacent to the radius and parallel to the thickened volar radioulnar ligament.

The arthroscope is then transferred to the 6-R portal, and the suction punch to the 3-4 portal, for resection of the ulnar and dorsal aspects of the central disk. Care is always taken to preserve the integrity of the thickened dorsal and volar ligamentous portions of the triangular fibrocartilage disk, because these portions of the disk confer some of the stability to the distal radioulnar joint.

Postoperatively, the wrist is bandaged in a soft compressive dressing, and early range of motion is encouraged. Return to function can be permitted as comfort allows. In the presence of significant positive ulnar variance, formal ulnar shortening procedures should be considered as well, although performing them will significantly compound the recuperation process. It is possible to resect slightly prominent portions of the seat of the ulna under arthroscopic control using a powered bur, if one is very meticulous about leaving no bone fragments or prominent cortical ridges of the ulna behind.

Case 4

A 34-year-old sheet metal worker injured the ulnar aspect of his right wrist when a power drill bound in a metal block, forcefully pronating his wrist. He demonstrated tenderness to palpation over the triangular fibrocartilage complex dorsally and had pain in that location with passive wrist pronation, but radiographs were normal and an arthrogram of the radiocarpal space and distal radioulnar joint showed no leakage of dye across the TFCC. The patient wore a splint for 6 weeks, but 4 months later, he still had pain with rotational motion or hyperflexion of the wrist.

An arthroscopic examination revealed the dorsal aspect of the TFCC to be detached from the dorsal wrist capsule, although there was no communication between the radiocarpal space and the distal radioulnar joint. Under arthroscopic control, the central articular disk of the TFCC was reattached to the dorsal capsule (see next section).

The patient's power grip returned, as well as full range of wrist motion. He has remained at work at the same job for the 4 years since his injury.[19]

SURGICAL TECHNIQUE FOR ARTHROSCOPICALLY ASSISTED REPAIR OF THE TFCC

The wrist is placed in the Traction Tower and 10 lb of axial traction is applied through nylon finger traps attached to the index and long fingers. An inflow cannula is inserted through the 1-2 portal in the dorsal aspect of the anatomic snuffbox. A 2.7-mm arthroscope is inserted in the 3-4 portal. Through the 6-R portal, a probe is used to test the tension on the central articular disk. If the disk is not taut, it can be presumed to be detached at the periphery. Close inspection of the dorsal margin of the disk often discloses a peripheral detachment extending from the prestyloid recess dorsally and radially. Hypertrophic

synovium at the dorsal rim of the central disk can be débrided with a powered shaver through the 6-R portal. A small suction punch is used to débride the dorsal edge of the TFC in the pathologic defect.

A longitudinal incision is made extending 15 mm proximally from the 6-R portal. The extensor retinaculum is incised, and the extensor carpi ulnaris (ECU) tendon is retracted to one side.

The Inteq (Linvatec, Inc, Largo, FL) offers the easiest means of reattaching the TFC disk to the dorsal capsule. The cannulated needle of the Inteq device is passed through the floor of the ECU tendon sheath at the level of the distal radioulnar joint and is directed distally to perforate the dorsal edge of the TFC disk under arthroscopic visualization. The wire loop of the Inteq device is inserted through the dorsal capsule at the radiocarpal level and placed over the cannulated needle. A length of 2-0 PDS suture is threaded through the needle and is then withdrawn by the suture retriever through the dorsal capsule.

A series of such sutures are placed about 2 to 3 mm apart and are then tied snugly over the floor of the ECU tendon sheath. The retinaculum is closed, the skin edges are approximated with a subcuticular suture, and the wrist is immobilized in slight extension in a long-arm cast for 3 weeks and then in a short-arm cast for 3 weeks longer.

Other Indications for Wrist Arthroscopy

Certain cases of intra-articular fractures, such as displaced die-punch fractures and comminuted intra-articular fractures of the radius, are also indications for arthroscopy. Arthroscopy provides a means of thoroughly evacuating hemarthrosis and fibrin precipitate. It also permits reduction of individual fracture fragments to restore a more normal contour to the articular surfaces. In addition, small osteochondral loose bodies can be removed with minimal surgical morbidity through the use of arthroscopic techniques. Case examples help illustrate the advantages of arthroscopy in such circumstances.

Case 5

A 34-year-old male sustained a nondisplaced distal radius fracture 16 years previously. He complained of pain in the midcarpal space on wrist extension and on radial deviation, aggravated particularly by lifting or power grip. He had full range of motion, but his wrist was tender to palpation in the midcarpal space. Radiographs showed a small osseous loose body between the distal pole of the scaphoid and the radial side of the capitate (Fig. 11–6A). Under arthroscopic control, the loose body was identified (Fig. 11–6B) and then extracted from the midcarpal space. The results were complete relief of the patient's discomfort and full restoration of pain-free function. The wrist required only a protective splint for 5 days postoperatively.

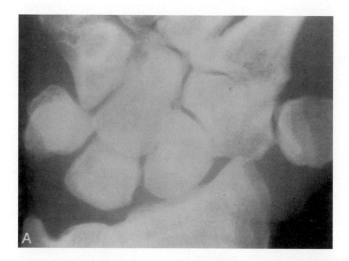

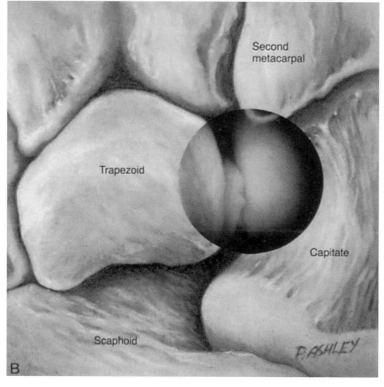

Figure 11–6. A, Radial deviation radiograph shows small osseous loose body in the interval between capitate, scaphoid, and trapezoid. B, Arthroscopic view of loose body between capitate and trapezoid, seen through a 1.9-mm arthroscope introduced dorsally between capitate and scaphoid.

Case 6

A 21-year-old male roofer fell from a ladder, injuring both wrists. He had a displaced Colles' fracture on the nondominant side and a three-part intra-articular fracture of the distal radius on the dominant side with a transverse fracture of the ulnar styloid. With conventional management, these fractures would have required bilateral long-arm casts, and the likelihood of achieving nonoperative reduction of the radial articular surface on the dominant side would have been small. At arthroscopy, the dominant wrist was cleansed of hemarthrosis and small cartilaginous loose bodies. An occult fracture of the waist of the scaphoid was identified. With transcutaneous K wires, the articular fragments of the radius were reduced anatomically to restore a near-perfect relationship of the articular surfaces, and the unstable fragments were pinned with a transcutaneous

K wire. A short-arm thumb spica cast on the dominant side permitted bending at the elbow postoperatively, enabling the patient to manage independent feeding and personal hygiene, and the scaphoid fracture healed uneventfully (Fig. 11–7).

SURGICAL TECHNIQUE FOR ARTHROSCOPIC REDUCTION AND INTERNAL FIXATION OF DISTAL RADIUS FRACTURES

The ideal time for arthroscopic examination of a wrist with an acute intra-articular fracture is 48 to 72 hours after injury. Earlier intervention usually encounters too much bleeding from the fracture site to maintain a clear visual surgical field; after longer delays, fibrin precipitate from the hemarthrosis becomes tenacious and more difficult to clear from the joint.

An initial attempt at closed reduction is made using anesthesia. If articular fragments are not anatomically reduced, flexible nylon finger traps are applied to the index, long, and ring fingers, and 15 lb of axial traction is applied through the wrist Traction Tower. The tower is angulated to flex or extend the wrist in the direction opposite the mechanism of injury. An inflow cannula is placed in the 6-U portal, and a 2.7-mm arthroscope is introduced in the 3-4 portal. A few seconds are spent lavaging the joint to clear the hemarthrosis. A Coban wrap on the forearm will help to prevent proximal extravasation of fluid.

The articular surface of the radius is then explored to identify all fracture planes. (A preoperative CT scan is often helpful.) A small powered shaver is introduced through the 6-R or 4-5 portal to remove fibrin clot and particulate fracture debris from the joint. Then, a thorough examination is conducted to identify any concomitant soft tissue injury, such as tears in the TFCC or injuries to the intrinsic or extrinsic ligaments. It is advisable also to transfer the arthroscope to the 1-2 portal to ensure that all fracture planes have been identified. Dorsal rim fractures are easy to miss when viewed from the 3-4 portal.

An arthroscopic dissecting probe can be inserted through any standard portal to pry impacted fracture fragments apart. Hypodermic needles are then inserted percutaneously and perpendicular to the fracture lines and are used as guides to direct percutaneous K-wire insertions. Then, 0.045-inch K wires are drilled into each major fracture fragment but not across the fracture planes. Beginning with the largest fragments, the pieces of articular surface are then reassembled. When the fracture fragments are reduced, the K wires are advanced across the fracture planes to stabilize them. The surgeon should always begin with the larger fragments and proceed sequentially to the smaller ones. External finger pressure helps to close the fracture gaps. Numerous K wires may be necessary. Intraoperative radiographs or fluoroscopy should confirm reduction of the articular surface. If necessary then, a dorsal or volar plate can be applied to stabilize the metaphysis of the radius. I have found the use of external fixators rarely necessary.

Postoperatively, a short-arm cast or splint is applied. It can be removed at 2 weeks in most cases for controlled gentle passive range-of-motion exercises. The fracture fragments should remain stable for these early exercises. Pins are typically removed 3 to 4 weeks postoperatively.[22, 23]

Case 7

Shortly before the state championship game, a 17-year-old high school football lineman fractured his dominant scaphoid. Under arthroscopic control, a Herbert-Whipple screw was placed across the fracture, compressing the fragments (see next section). The patient was comfortable enough with a 0.25-inch skin incision and stabilization of the fracture to play in the championship game wearing a latex thumb spica cast (Fig. 11–8).

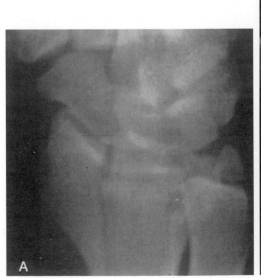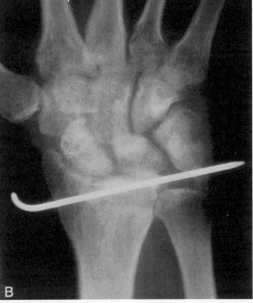

Figure 11–7. *A,* Radiograph of comminuted intra-articular distal radius fracture and ulnar styloid fracture. Dorsal fragment of lunate facet is displaced proximally, and ulnar fragment of distal radius is displaced medially. Scaphoid appears normal but has an occult transverse fracture confirmed on arthroscopic examination. *B,* Radiograph following arthroscopic reduction and K-wire fixation. Articular surface of distal radius has been restored by transcutaneous manipulation of individual fragments.

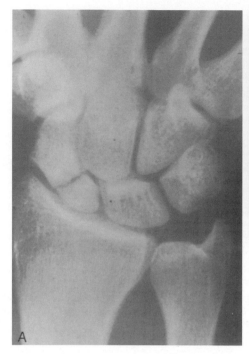

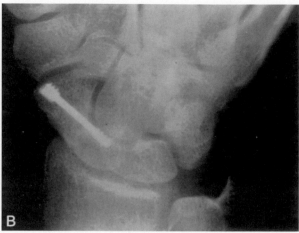

Figure 11–8. *A*, Nondisplaced fracture of right scaphoid. *B*, Appearance of scaphoid compression and internal fixation following arthroscopic placement of a Herbert screw. The procedure was performed with 1.9-mm arthroscope introduced dorsally between the third and fourth extensor compartments, the Herbert screw guide introduced radially between the first and second extensor compartments, and the screw inserted through a small incision over the scaphoid tubercle.

SURGICAL TECHNIQUE FOR ARTHROSCOPICALLY ASSISTED INTERNAL FIXATION OF SCAPHOID FRACTURES

A radially curved 15-mm incision is centered over the scaphotrapezial joint with the proximal end of the incision paralleling the radial border of the flexor carpi radialis tendon. The scaphotrapezial joint is exposed by deeper dissection, and the joint capsule is reflected from the trapezium attachment. The volar tubercle of the trapezium is excised with a 5-mm osteotome. Enough trapezium must be removed to expose the margin of the articular cartilage on the distal pole of the scaphoid. A point on the articular margin is marked at 30 to 40 percent of the distance ulnar to the most radial aspect of the scaphoid using a skin marker.

A self-retaining retractor is left in the incision, and the wrist is placed in the Traction Tower by means of flexible nylon finger traps on the index and long fingers to apply 10 to 12 lbs of axial traction.

A 2.7-mm or 1.9-mm arthroscope is inserted into the midcarpal radial (MCR) portal, and the fracture of the scaphoid is examined along the concave surface of the scaphoid. The proximal or distal pole of the scaphoid is manipulated with a transcutaneous K wire, if necessary, to accomplish reduction of the fracture.

The arthroscope is then transferred to the 4-5 portal. Looking in a radial direction, the surgeon inserts target hook of the Herbert-Whipple fracture reduction jig into the radiocarpal space through the 1-2 portal. The target hook is advanced ulnarward between the scaphoid and the radius to a point 1 mm radial to the scapholunate ligament on the most proximal horizon of the scaphoid. Here, the target hook is implanted into the articular cartilage by palmar rotation of the handle of the target hook. The guide barrel of the fracture reduction jig is assembled to the target hook handle, and the guide barrel is centered on the point previously marked along the articular cartilage margin of the distal pole of the scaphoid through the volar incision. The fracture is compressed. Two guide wires are placed through the jig, and their position is confirmed by intraoperative fluoroscopy. The central guide wire is then overdrilled with a cannulated step drill, and the Herbert-Whipple screw is inserted over the guide wire, compressing the fracture fragments. The purpose of the secondary guide wire is to control rotation of the fracture fragments during the drilling process and insertion of the Herbert-Whipple screw.[23]

Postoperative immobilization requires only a volar plaster splint or short-arm cast for 2 to 3 weeks, after which early gentle range of motion can be initiated.

Case 8

A 58-year-old amateur golfer with a chronic non-union of an old scaphoid fracture had developed increased wrist pain. Now he had an opportunity to play in a "Pro-Am" tournament as a representative of his prestigious corporation. Although he had already developed end-stage arthritic changes typical of "scapholunate advanced collapse," or SLAC wrist, he was not willing to undergo definitive intercarpal fusion (Fig. 11–9). After considerable counseling, the patient agreed to an arthroscopic resection of the small proximal pole fragment of the scaphoid and an arthroscopic radial styloidectomy (see next section). He was able to play in the "Pro-Am" golf tournament 3 weeks later with much greater comfort, and has required no additional surgical treatment in the ensuing 4 years.

SURGICAL TECHNIQUE FOR ARTHROSCOPIC RADIAL STYLOIDECTOMY

The wrist is suspended in the Traction Tower by finger trap traction applied through the index and long fingers. An inflow cannula is placed in the 6-U portal, and a 2.7-mm arthroscope is introduced through the 3-4 portal. A 1-2 portal is created, and a powered bur is used to mark a sagittal line on the articular surface of the radius half the distance between the sagittal ridge and the tip of the radial styloid. The bur is then used to remove all of the bone radial to the sagittal line until the resected surface is perfectly horizontal, or perpendicular to the long axis of the radius. Postoperatively, a sterile compressive bandage is applied for 3 to 5 days. Then, range of motion and use are permitted as comfort allows.

DISCUSSION

Although these illustrative case histories may seem to involve extenuating circumstances, they are not atypical of cases encountered in a busy hand surgery

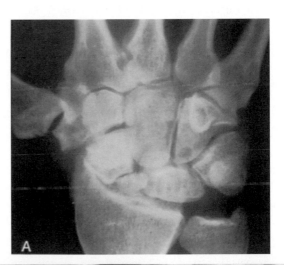

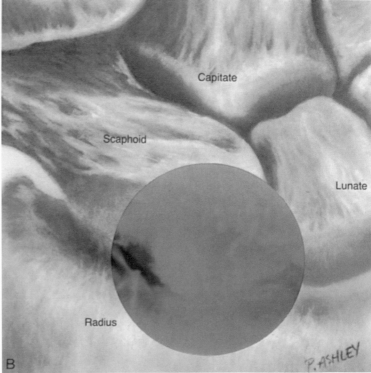

Figure 11–9. *A,* Radiographic appearance of arthritic radiocarpal interval resulting from chronic non-union of scaphoid fracture. The radial styloid is enlarged and impinges upon the distal scaphoid fragment. *B,* Arthroscopic appearance of the loose proximal scaphoid fragment. Articular surface of radius is eburnated and devoid of cartilage. Viewed arthroscopically through a dorsal approach between the third and fourth extensor compartments.

practice. Arthroscopic examination of the wrist has proved to be useful in symptomatic individuals who have an unconfirmed diagnosis despite thorough conventional work-up. Patients with persistent symptoms but no reliable objective evidence for diagnosis should undergo arthroscopy for direct visual examination of intra-articular tissues. Patients in whom conventional work-up results are equivocal, i.e., in whom objective findings are inconsistent with the stated symptoms and history, are candidates for arthroscopy. Patients who have been diagnosed by use of conventional techniques may become candidates for wrist arthroscopy when the definitive treatment has a high morbidity or complication rate and the necessity or urgency of surgical intervention is in question.[24] Such cases typically involve a need to evaluate the status of the articular cartilage or the size and mechanical significance of lesions of the TFCC, as previously noted.

In such circumstances, arthroscopy of the wrist provides a safe, simple, and convenient means of direct inspection of the joint as an adjunctive diagnostic technique with virtually no surgical morbidity. If it is practiced beforehand in a surgical skills laboratory and performed with appropriate instrumentation, this minimally invasive technique will continue to open new vistas in the surgical treatment of many wrist disorders.

References

1. Koman LA: Magnetic resonance imaging of the wrist. Presented at Orthopaedic Research of Virginia: The Carpal Connection—Diagnostic and Therapeutic Approaches to the Painful Wrist, Orlando, FL, May 22, 1986.
2. Whipple TL, Marotta JJ, Powell JH III: Techniques of wrist arthroscopy. Arthroscopy 2:244–252, 1986.
3. Whipple TL: Preoperative evaluation and imaging. In Arthroscopic Surgery: The Wrist. Philadelphia, JB Lippincott, 1992 pp. 11–36.
4. Whipple TL: Instrumentation. In Arthroscopic Surgery: The Wrist. Philadelphia, JB Lippincott, 1992, pp. 37–48.
5. Roth JH, Haddad RG: Radiocarpal arthroscopy and arthrography in the diagnosis of ulnar wrist pain. Arthroscopy 2:234–243, 1986.
6. Whipple TL: Triangular fibrocartilage complex. In Arthroscopic Surgery: The Wrist. Philadelphia, JB Lippincott, 1992, pp. 103–118.
7. Bowers WH: The distal radioulnar joint. In Green DP (ed): Operative Hand Surgery, ed 2, vol 1. New York, Churchill Livingstone, 1988, pp. 939–990.
8. Whipple TL: Extrinsic ligaments. In Arthroscopic Surgery: The Wrist. Philadelphia, JB Lippincott, 1992, pp. 131–142.
9. Moskowitz RW: Which comes first: Inflammation or osteoarthritis? J Rheumatol Suppl 9:57–58, 1983.
10. Poehling GG, White M: Partial thickness defects of articular cartilage. Orthop/Arthrosc 2:1–5, 1983.
11. Brandt KD: Management of osteoarthritis. In Kelley WN, Harris ED Jr, Ruddy S, Sledge CB (eds): Textbook of Rheumatology, ed 2, vol 2. Philadelphia, WB Saunders, 1985, pp. 1448–1458.
12. Whipple TL: Articular surface defects and loose bodies. In Arthroscopic Surgery: The Wrist. Philadelphia, JB Lippincott, 1992, pp. 93–102.
13. Whipple TL: Diagnostic arthroscopic examination. In Arthroscopic Surgery: The Wrist. Philadelphia, JB Lippincott, 1992, pp. 73–90.
14. Osterman AL: Arthroscopic debridement of triangular fibrocartilage tears. Arthroscopy 2:120–124, 1990.
15. Whipple TL: Intrinsic ligaments and carpal instability. In Arthroscopic Surgery: The Wrist. Philadelphia, JB Lippincott, 1992, pp. 119–130.
16. Chin Y-C: Arthroscopy of the wrist and finger joints. Orthop Clin North Am 10:723–733, 1979.
17. Ferlic DC: Inflammatory and rheumatoid arthritis. In Lichtman DM (ed): The Wrist and Its Disorders. Philadelphia, WB Saunders, 1988.
18. Ferlic DC, Cooney WP: Inflammatory arthritis of the wrist. In McGinty JB (ed): Operative Arthroscopy. New York, Raven Press, 1991, pp. 641–645.
19. Whipple TL, Corso SJ, Savoie FH: Arthroscopic repair of peripheral tears of the triangular fibrocartilage complex. Presented at the American Academy of Orthopaedic Surgeons Annual Meeting, New Orleans, February 1994.
20. Watson KH, Ryu J: Degenerative disorders of the carpus. Orthop Clin North Am 15:337–344, 1984.
21. Bednar JM, Osterman AL: The role of arthroscopy in the treatment of traumatic triangular fibrocartilage injuries. Hand Clin 10:605–614, 1994.
22. Whipple TL, Cooney WP, Poehling GG: Intraarticular fractures. In McGinty JB (ed): Operative Arthroscopy. New York, Raven Press, 1991, pp. 651–654.
23. Whipple TL: Intraarticular fractures of the distal radius and carpals. In Arthroscopic Surgery: The Wrist. Philadelphia, JB Lippincott, 1992, pp. 143–156.
24. Whipple TL: Arthroscopy of the distal radioulnar joint: Indications, portals, and anatomy. Hand Clinics 10:589–592, 1994.

PART III

Carpal Bones

CHAPTER 12

Introduction to the Carpal Instabilities

David M. Lichtman, MD

The subject of carpal instability has been undergoing constant reevaluation ever since Navarro[4] attempted to describe carpal mechanics in 1919 with the columnar theory. Since that time, many authorities have contributed to the understanding and visualization of carpal kinematics and pathomechanics. This chapter explores and analyzes these theories and presents a new concept for carpal kinematics—the "ring" model. We have outlined a new classification system of carpal instabilities based on this model.

THE WRIST AS A LINK MECHANISM

In 1943, Gilford and colleagues[1] popularized Lambrinudi's concept of the wrist as a "link" mechanism in which the radius, the proximal carpal row, and the distal carpal row constitute the individual links. The link mechanism is stable in tension but collapses with axial compression (Fig. 12–1). In order to explain the deformity noted in certain cases of scaphoid non-union, Gilford and colleagues[1] likened the scaphoid to a control rod linking the proximal and distal rows.

The Scaphoid as a Slider-Crank

Later, Linscheid and associates[2] introduced the "slider-crank" analogy to explain the scaphoid's role in preventing intercarpal collapse and controlling intercarpal motion (Fig. 12–2). A slider-crank is a machine that transforms reciprocal motion into rotatory motion or rotatory motion into reciprocal motion. Examples of this action are the piston and drive shaft of an internal combustion engine and the piston and crankshaft of a compressor. According to Linscheid's theory, the scaphoid acts as a bridge between the two rows, stabilizing them and transforming radial and ulnar deviation of the distal row into flexion and extension of the proximal row.

DISI and VISI

In 1970, Fisk[3] expanded on Gilford's link theory while stressing the importance of the volar ligamentous structures. Fisk[3] described the intercarpal collapse that occurred after trauma or as a result of Kienbock's disease as a "concertina deformity." Linscheid and associates[2] noted two distinct patterns of intercalary collapse and named them *dorsal intercalary segment instability* (DISI) and *volar intercalary segment instability* (VISI). Their classification was based upon the capitolunate angle seen on the lateral radiograph. In the DISI pattern, the lunate is displaced anteriorly and extended in relation to the capitate, whereas in the VISI pattern, the lunate is displaced dorsally and flexed (Fig. 12–3). This classification is still a good way to subdivide perilunate or dissociative instabilities.

THE COLUMNAR WRIST CONCEPT

In 1919, Navarro[4] introduced a model for wrist kinematics based on the concept of a columnar carpus

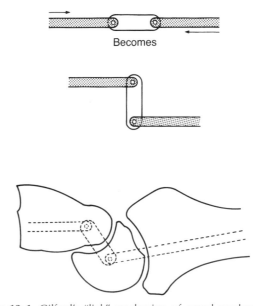

Figure 12–1. Gilford's "link" mechanism of carpal mechanics shows that the carpus is stable in tension but collapses in compression. (From Gilford W, Boltar R, Lambrinudi C: The mechanism of the wrist joint. Guy's Hospital Report 92:52–59, 1943.)

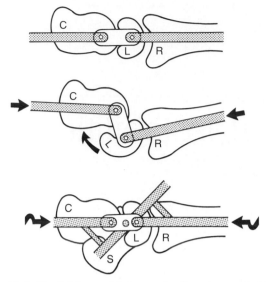

Figure 12–2. The "slider-crank" theory visualizes the scaphoid acting as a bridge between the proximal and distal carpal rows, controlling intercarpal motion much as the piston and crankshaft do in a compressor. (From Linscheid RL, Dobyns JH, Bebout JW: Traumatic instability of the wrist: Diagnosis, classification, and pathomechanics. J Bone Joint Surg 54A:1612–1632, 1972.)

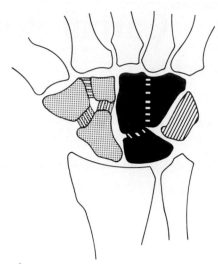

Figure 12–4. The columnar carpus of Navarro, showing three vertical columns: central or flexion-extension column, formed by the lunate, capitate, and hamate; lateral or mobile column, with the scaphoid, trapezium, and trapezoid; medial or rotation column, consisting of the triquetrum and pisiform (see reference 4). Dotted area = lateral (mobile) column; solid area = central (flexion-extension) column; striped area = medial (rotation) column.

(Fig. 12–4). The model was amplified in detail by Scaramuzza[5] in 1969. In 1976, Taleisnik[6] modified Navarro's model in order to accommodate clinically recognized patterns of carpal instability. In Taleisnik's model, the central flexion/extension column consists of the entire distal row and the lunate (Fig. 12–5). The scaphoid is the mobile lateral column, and the triquetrum is the rotatory medial column. This concept has led to the belief that many carpal instabilities occur in columnar or longitudinal patterns, e.g., "radial column instability" and "ulnar column instability." Consequently, scapholunate dissociation has been classified as a radial instability and triquetrolunate dissociation as an ulnar instability. In many ways this is a useful concept, but it fails to account for the transverse (perilunar) patterns of instability produced in vitro by Mayfield and coworkers[7, 8] as well as for the well-established clinical patterns of transverse midcarpal and transverse proximal carpal instabilities.[9–12]

DISI—Dorsiflexion Intercalary Segment Instability

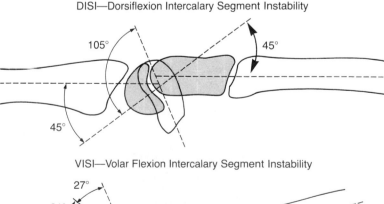

VISI—Volar Flexion Intercalary Segment Instability

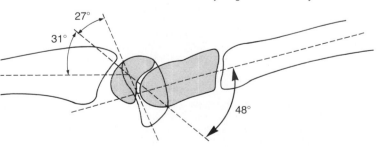

Figure 12–3. Dorsiflexion intercalary segmental instability *(top)* shows the lunate displaced anteriorly and dorsiflexed 45°. Volar flexion intercalary segmental instability *(bottom)* shows the lunate dorsal to the capitate and palmar flexed. (From Linscheid RL, Dobyns JH, Bebout JW: Traumatic instability of the wrist: Diagnosis, classification, and pathomechanics. J Bone Joint Surg 54A:1612–1632, 1972.)

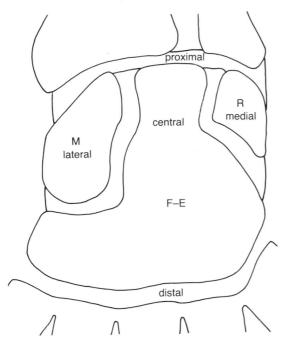

Figure 12–5. Taleisnik's modification of Navarro's columnar model. The entire distal carpal row, along with the lunate, becomes the central flexion-extension column. The scaphoid forms the lateral mobile column and the triquetrum the medial rotatory column (see ref. 5). *R* = rotatory column; *M* = mobile column; *F-E* = flexion-extension column.

PATHOMECHANICS OF CARPAL INSTABILITIES

Perilunate Pattern of Injury

The work of Mayfield and coworkers[7, 8] established the perilunate pattern of injury to the stabilizing ligaments of the wrist in an experimentally produced in vitro simulation of a fall on the outstretched hand (Fig. 12–6). As the wrist was forced into progressive dorsiflexion, ulnar deviation, and intercarpal supination, a reproducible pattern of ligament failure occurred, starting with the radial collateral ligament and progressing to the radiocapitate and the radioscapholunate ligaments, and then to the scapholunate interosseous ligament. These initial ligament failures were manifested dynamically by scapholunate instability (stage I). With continued force, the capitolunate ligaments failed (stage II). Next, the volar radiotriquetral ligament failed, resulting in triquetrolunate instability (stage III). Finally, the dorsal radiocarpal ligaments gave way, permitting volar lunate dislocation or dorsal perilunate dislocation (stage IV) (Fig. 12–7). Interestingly, it was observed that if the force vector took a wider arc around the lunate, it would create a variety of perilunate fracture dislocations. One example is the trans-scaphoid transcapitate perilunate dislocation (naviculocapitate syndrome). It has been suggested that a "greater arc" injury is more likely to occur if the hand is radially deviated when the forced

transmission is initiated.[13] Thus, depending on the relative position of the hand with respect to radial and ulnar deviation at the time of impact, a lesser arc (ligamentous) or greater arc (bone) perilunate instability can be created (Fig. 12–8). Several combinations of the greater and lesser arc instabilities are also possible (e.g., trans-scaphoid perilunate dislocation).

The previously described perilunate pattern occurs most typically in the ulnar-neutral or ulnar-negative wrist. In the ulnar-positive wrist, where a greater proportion of transmitted stress is absorbed by the ulnar carpus, a fall on the outstretched hand can produce a primary triquetrolunate or triangular fibrocartilage complex (TFCC) tear. This is one possible explanation for the relatively rare, isolated lunotriquetral dissociation.

Newly Recognized Instability Patterns

MIDCARPAL INSTABILITIES

In 1980, a series of patients were studied who had palmar subluxation at the midcarpal joint and a painful clunk with ulnar deviation of the wrist.[14] Experimental and clinical studies suggested that the midcar-

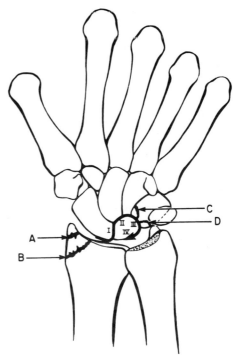

Figure 12–6. The perilunate pattern of injury to the volar ligaments of the wrist is divided into four stages. Stage I is a partial disruption of the scapholunate joint. Stage II is a complete disruption of the scapholunate joint. Stage III is a disruption of the scapholunate, capitolunate, and triquetrolunate joints. Stage IV is a disruption of all the preceding stages and the dorsal radiocarpal ligaments, allowing volar lunate dislocation or dorsal perilunate dislocation. Occasionally, radial styloid (*A, B*) or triquetrum (*C, D*) fractures accompany perilunate ligament injuries. Other fracture patterns also occur (see Fig. 12–8). (From Mayfield JK, Johnson RP, Kilcoyne RF: Carpal dislocations: Pathomechanics and progressive perilunar instability. J Hand Surg 5:226–241, 1980.)

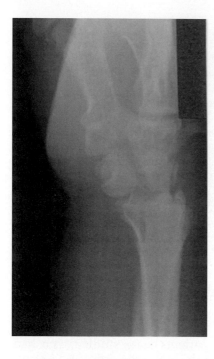

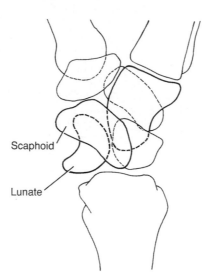

Figure 12–7. A volar lunate dislocation (Stage IV perilunate dissociation) caused by disruption of the radiocarpal ligaments. *A,* radiograph; *B,* line drawing.

Scaphoid

Lunate

pal subluxation was due to laxity of the ulnar arm of the volar arcuate ligament.[15, 16] Subsequent information has implicated laxity of the dorsal radiotriquetral ligament as well.[17] Originally, midcarpal instability (MCI) was classified as an ulnar instability, but this led to some confusion, because the ulnar longitudinal column, as described by Taleisnik,[6] is not affected in this type of instability. Instead, it is truly a transverse laxity, the pathokinetics occurring transversely across the entire proximal row.[18, 19]

In addition to the *volar midcarpal pattern,* a few patients have now been identified with the reverse pattern, or *dorsal midcarpal instability* (J Taleisnik, MD, personal communication, 1985). Other patterns of dorsal instability are described in Chapter 17. MCI has also been seen following dorsally displaced fractures of the distal radius.[10] In 1984, Taleisnik and Watson[10] described this pattern, which I call *extrinsic midcarpal instability* to differentiate it from the intrinsic variety described previously. In extrinsic MCI, the dorsally displaced distal radial fracture induces a Z deformity in the carpus, which eventually results in laxity of the midcarpal ligaments. Correction of the extrinsic instability is achieved by osteotomy of the distal radius.

PROXIMAL CARPAL INSTABILITIES

Another group of carpal instabilities occurs at the radiocarpal and ulnocarpal joints. Ulnar translocation of the carpus is the most widely recognized entity in this group. It can be due to rheumatoid arthritis or can result from surgical resection of the distal ulna.[20, 21] A series of post-traumatic cases has also been described.[22] It is generally believed that the volar radiolunate ligament must be torn to create a traumatic ulnar translocation, but in all likelihood,

most of the other radiocarpal ligaments, including the dorsal radial triquetral, must be disrupted in order for this to happen.[23]

Other entities in the proximal group are dorsal and palmar carpal dislocations secondary to malunited intra-articular rim fractures of the distal radius (so-called Barton's variants) (Fig. 12–9). Collectively, this group is called the *proximal carpal instabilities.*

MISCELLANEOUS INSTABILITIES

Several miscellaneous patterns of carpal instability have been described. Among them are axial instabili-

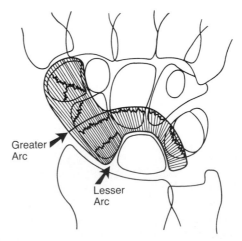

Greater Arc

Lesser Arc

Figure 12–8. The greater arc and lesser arc paths of carpal injury. The greater arc injuries tend to occur with the hand radially deviated, transmitting the force through the scaphoid and creating primarily a bony (perilunate) instability. The lesser arc injuries occur with the hand less radially deviated, creating primarily a ligamentous perilunate instability. (From Weber ER, Chao EV: An experimental approach to the mechanism of scaphoid wrist fractures. J Hand Surg 3:142–148, 1978.)

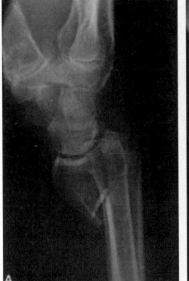
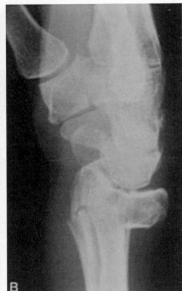

Figure 12–9. *A*, A volar Barton's fracture, showing the carpus in a volar subluxed position. *B*, A dorsal Barton's fracture, showing the carpus in a dorsal subluxated position.

tics, in which the carpal bones are separated longitudinally along an ulnar or radial axis with continuation of the diastasis between adjacent metacarpal bones. These instabilities are most likely due to crush injuries in which a strong longitudinal (axial) force also occurs. Trans-scaphoid instabilities have also been described,[24] possibly due to a force entering at the radioscaphoid joint and exiting distally through the scaphotrapeziotrapezoid (STT) joint. Other miscellaneous instabilities are triquetral dislocation, triquetrum *and* lunate dislocation, and trapezoid dislocation. No consistent mechanism has been accepted for these unusual patterns.

THE RING CONCEPT

In light of the experimental findings about the pathogenesis of perilunate carpal instabilities as well as the clinical recognition of transverse midcarpal and proximal instability patterns, I find it difficult to adhere to the columnar wrist concept and the longitudinal classification system of carpal instabilities that derives from it. It is also difficult to continue to visualize the scaphoid as a slider-crank, linking and controlling motion between the proximal and distal rows. In reality, the entire proximal row—*including the scaphoid*—moves passively as a unit in response to the resultant compressive and tensile forces acting on its articular surfaces. This motion is guided and restrained by the unique arrangement of bone contacts and ligament supports of the wrist. It is well known that radial deviation of the hand and distal carpus causes palmar flexion of the entire proximal row and that ulnar deviation of the hand and distal row causes proximal row extension (Fig. 12–10). Key components in this reciprocal motion between the carpal rows are the two physiologic "links": the mo-

bile STT joint and the rotary triquetrohamate joint (Fig. 12–11). Without these two mobile links, the two transverse rows of the ring could not move relative to each other. Radial deviation compresses the STT link, forcing the scaphoid into flexion (Fig. 12–12). With intact interosseous ligaments, the entire proximal row follows the scaphoid into flexion. Ulnar deviation forces the triquetrum to glide into its extended position against the hamate (Fig. 12–13). With intact ligaments, the entire proximal row now follows the triquetrum into extension. In neutral deviation, these opposing forces are dissipated if the wrist is relaxed, and they are neutralized by intact bone and ligamentous supports if the wrist is stressed, as by a clenched fist.

Utilizing this transverse "ring" model of carpal ki-

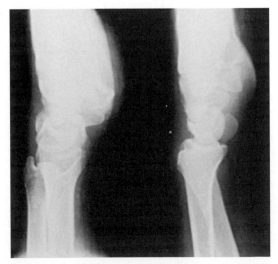

Figure 12–10. In radial deviation *(left)* and ulnar deviation *(right)*, the normal wrist displays a "physiologic" VISI and DISI pattern.

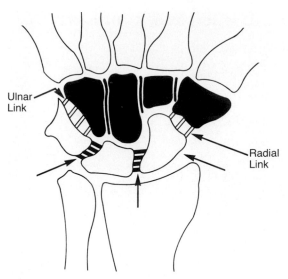

Figure 12–11. The "ring" model of carpal kinematics. The distal arc proximal carpal rows are joined by two physiologic "links," thus allowing reciprocal motion. These links are the mobile scaphotrapezial joint *(radial link)* and the rotatory triquetrohamate joint *(ulnar link).*

ULNAR DEVIATION

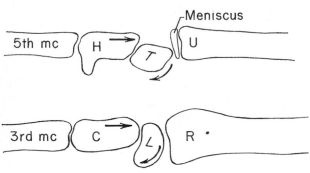

Figure 12–13. The ulnar link (triquetrohamate joint). With ulnar deviation, the hamate glides radially on the triquetrum at the midcarpal joint. Because of the helicoid shape of the triquetrohamate articulation, the triquetrum rotates into extension. The mechanism of triquetrum rotation is similar to a toboggin moving up and down a sinuous track. As the triquetrum extends, the lunate follows via intact triquetrolunate ligaments. Secondary forces act at the capitolunate joint to assist in proximal row extension. *C* = capitate; *L* = lunate; *MC* = metacarpal; *R* = radius; *T* = triquetrum; *U* = ulna.

netics enables a clearer visualization of the pathomechanics of perilunate and midcarpal instabilities (see Fig. 12–11). A break (dissociation) anywhere in the proximal row unbalances the neutralized forces across the proximal row and sets in motion a predictable kinematic pattern. With a "break" in the ring through the triquetrolunate joint, the bones on the radial side of the break (i.e., the scaphoid and the lunate) palmar-flex in response to the flexion moment

RADIAL DEVIATION

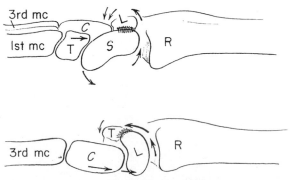

Figure 12–12. The radial link (STT joint). With radial deviation, the distal pole of the scaphoid is forced into flexion by proximal movement of the trapezium and trapezoid. The proximal pole of the scaphoid rotates dorsally and carries with it the lunate via intact scapholunate ligaments. The lunate thus assumes a flexed (VISI) posture. Secondary forces act at the palmar capitolunate articulation to assist in flexing the lunate and triquetrum. *C* = capitate; *L* = lunate; *MC* = metacarpal; *R* = radius; *S* = scaphoid; *T* (upper) = trapezium; *T* (lower) = triquetrum.

at the STT joint. The triquetrum extends as it is pushed ulnarward along the helicoid slope of the hamate by the descending head of the capitate. A static VISI deformity (flexion of the lunate) is seen on routine lateral radiographs.

With a break in the ring through the scapholunate joint, a similar sequence occurs. However, the lunate is now on the ulnar side of the "break" and follows the triquetrum as it rotates into its low, extended position. Even though the scaphoid flexes in response to forces on the radial side, routine lateral radiographs show a DISI deformity (extension of the lunate). With an unstable trans-scaphoid fracture, a DISI pattern again results, except that the proximal pole of the scaphoid also extends because it, too, is on the ulnar side of the break and is carried along with the lunate and triquetrum.

In midcarpal instability, laxity of the ulnar arm of the arcuate ligament and the dorsal capsule decreases the influence of the geometric configuration of the triquetrohamate joint on the proximal carpal row. This allows the proximal carpal row to assume a gravity-induced palmar-flexed position (VISI), which persists until the last few degrees of ulnar deviation, at which point the proximal row suddenly snaps into its reduced, extended position.

Thus, unstable scaphoid fractures or scapholunate ligament disruptions result in a DISI pattern, whereas triquetrolunate injury and midcarpal laxity create a VISI deformity. If the tear is small or incomplete, the instability does not manifest clinically unless significant stress is applied to the wrist. When a DISI or VISI pattern can be seen only with stress views, the pattern has been termed *dynamic instability*, whereas when the pattern is present without additional stress, it is called *static instability*.[25] Static deformities are usually due to unstable complete ligament or bone injuries, whereas dynamic instabilities are most likely due to partial ligament tears. The term predynamic instability has been introduced to subclassify dynamic instabilities, but I do not find it a useful concept.

CID AND CIND

Carpal instabilities have also been classified into those caused by torn ligaments with dissociation of adjacent bones (carpal instability–dissociative, or CID) and those caused by lax or overstretched ligaments with intermittent carpal subluxation (carpal instability–nondissociative, or CIND). Scapholunate and triquetrolunate dissociations have been placed in the CID category, and midcarpal and radiocarpal instabilities have been placed in the CIND category. However, in some "dynamic" scapholunate or triquetrolunate instabilities, the ligaments may be stretched but not actually torn. Also, in traumatic midcarpal instability, there may be a true dissociation or tear of the volar midcarpal or dorsal radiocarpal ligaments rather than a laxity or stretch. Thus, the terms CIND and CID lack anatomic and etiologic precision. Nevertheless, these terms have become a popular way to categorize the carpal instabilities described.

CLASSIFICATION OF CARPAL INSTABILITIES

In order to integrate what we have now learned about carpal kinematics, clinical instability patterns, and the pathogenesis of carpal ligament disruptions, a new classification system of carpal instabilities is presented (Table 12–1). This system is based on the transverse pattern of carpal instabilities, as visualized by the carpal ring concept, rather than on the more traditional longitudinal or columnar carpus concept. It also assumes that the reader accepts the scaphoid as a full-fledged member of the proximal row rather than as a mechanical linkage between the two.

In the miscellaneous group are trapezioscaphoid and capitolunate instabilities, which are probably subdivisions of midcarpal instability. Sooner or later, every articulation of the wrist will have its own reported instability, of either traumatic or congenital origin. However, until these entities can be studied carefully to establish their possible relationship to existing instability patterns, I think that they should remain in the miscellaneous category.

In the next few chapters, established carpal instability patterns are reviewed in greater depth. The reader is reminded that the classification scheme presented here has evolved from a synthesis of experimental studies, case reports, and personal experience. It does not necessarily represent the thought processes of each of our contributors. Brian Tobias and Gerald Blatt's chapter on scapholunate injuries

Table 12–1. CLASSIFICATION OF CARPAL INSTABILITIES*

I. Perilunate instabilities (CID)
   A. Lesser arc pattern
      1. Scapholunate instability
         a. Dynamic—partial
         b. Static—complete (DISI)
         c. Rheumatoid/inflammatory
      2. Triquetrolunate instability
         a. Dynamic—partial
         b. Static—complete (VISI)
         c. Rheumatoid/inflammatory
      3. Complete perilunate dislocation
         a. Dorsal perilunate dislocation
         b. Palmar lunate dislocation
   B. Greater arc pattern
      1. Scaphoid fracture
         a. Stable
         b. Unstable (DISI)
      2. Naviculocapitate syndrome
      3. Trans-scaphoid transtriquetral perilunate dislocations
      4. Variations and combinations of 1 through 3
II. Midcarpal instabilities (midcarpal CIND)
   A. Intrinsic (ligamentous laxity)
      1. Palmar midcarpal instability (VISI)
      2. Dorsal midcarpal instability (DISI)
      3. Combined
   B. Extrinsic (dorsally displaced radial fracture)
III. Proximal carpal instabilities (proximal carpal CIND?)
   A. Ulnar translocation of the carpus
      1. Rheumatoid
      2. Posttraumatic
      3. Iatrogenic (after excision of the ulnar head)
   B. Dorsal instability (after dorsal rim distal radial fracture—dorsal Barton's fracture)
   C. Palmar instability (after volar rim distal radial fracture—volar Barton's fracture)
IV. Miscellaneous
   A. Axial
   B. Periscaphoid

*CID = carpal instability–dissociative; CIND = carpal instability–nondissociative; DISI = distal intercalary segment instability; VISI = volar intercalary segment instability.

(Chapter 15) and Charlotte Alexander's chapter on triquetrolunate injuries (Chapter 16) cover the perilunate instabilities. Eric Gaenslen, Garry Pollock, and I review the midcarpal and proximal carpal instabilities (Chapter 17). The proximal instabilities also are discussed individually in several other areas of the book, including Chapter 33 on rheumatoid arthritis, by Donald Ferlic, and Chapter 19 on intra-articular carpal fractures, by Charles Melone.

References

1. Gilford W, Boltan R, Lambrinudi C: The mechanism of the wrist joint. Guy's Hosp Rep 92:52–59, 1943.
2. Linscheid RL, Dobyns JH, Bebout JW: Traumatic instability of the wrist: Diagnosis, classification, and pathomechanics. J Bone Joint Surg 54A:1612–1632, 1972.
3. Fisk G: Carpal instability and the fractured scaphoid. Ann R Coll Surg Engl 46:63–76, 1970.
4. Navarro A: Luxaciones del carpo. An Fac Med (Montevideo) 6:113, 1921.
5. Scaramuzza RFJ: El movimiento de rotation en el carpo y su

relacion con la fisiopathologia de sus lesiones traumaticas. Bolentines y trabjos de la Sociedad Argentina de parthopedia y Traumatologia 34:337, 1969.

6. Taleisnik J: The ligaments of the wrist. J Hand Surg 1:110–118, 1976.

7. Mayfield JK, Johnson RP, Kilcoyne RF: The ligaments of the human wrist and their functional significance. Anat Rec 186:417–428, 1976.

8. Mayfield JK, Johnson RP, Kilcoyne RF: Carpal dislocations: Pathomechanics and progressive perilunar instability. J Hand Surg 5:226–241, 1980.

9. Jackson WT, Protas JM: Snapping scapholunate subluxation. J Hand Surg 6:590–594, 1981.

10. Taleisnik J, Watson K: Midcarpal instabilities caused by malunited fractures of the distal radius. J Hand Surg 9A:350–357, 1984.

11. Lichtman DM, Noble WH, Alexander CE: Dynamic triquetrolunate instability: Case report. J Hand Surg 9A:185–187, 1984.

12. Weeks PM, Young VL, Gilula LA: A case of painful clicking wrist: A case report. J Hand Surg 4:522–525, 1979.

13. Weber ER, Chao EV: An experimental approach to the mechanism of scaphoid wrist fractures. J Hand Surg 3:142–148, 1978.

14. Lichtman DM, Swafford AR, Schneider JR: Midcarpal instability. Presented at the thirty-fifth annual meeting of the American Society for Surgery of the Hand, Atlanta, Feb 4–6, 1980.

15. Lichtman DM, Schneider JR, Swafford AR, et al: Ulnar midcarpal instability—clinical and laboratory analysis. J Hand Surg 9A:350–357, 1981.

16. Trumble T, Bour CJ, Smith RJ, Glisson RR: Kinematics of the ulnar carpus related to the volar intercalated segment instability pattern. J Hand Surg 15A:384–392, 1990.

17. Viegas SE, Patterson RM, Peterson PD, et al: Ulnar sided perilunate instability: An anatomic and biomechanic study. J Hand Surg 15A:268–278, 1990.

18. Alexander CE, Lichtman DM: Ulnar carpal instabilities. Orthop Clin North Am 15:307–320, 1984.

19. Lichtman DM, Bruckner JD, Culp RW, Alexander CE: Palmar midcarpal instability: Results of surgical reconstruction. J Hand Surg 18A:307–315, 1993.

20. Gainor BJ, Schaberg J: The rheumatoid wrist after resection of the distal ulna. J Hand Surg 10A:837–844, 1985.

21. Linscheid RL, Dobyns JH: Radiolunate arthrodesis. J Hand Surg 10A:821–829, 1985.

22. Rayhack JM, Linscheid RL, Dobyns JH: Post-traumatic ulnar translocation of the carpus. J Hand Surg 12A:180–189, 1987.

23. Viegas SF, Patterson RM, Eng M, Ward K: Extrinsic wrist ligament in the pathomechanics of ulnar translation instability. J Hand Surg 20A:312–318, 1995.

24. Szabo RM, Newland CC, Johnson PG, et al: Spectrum of injury and treatment options for isolated dislocation of the scaphoid. J Bone Joint Surg 77A:608–615, 1995.

25. Lichtman DM, Taleisnik J, Watson K: Symposium on wrist injuries. Contemp Orthop 4:1, 107–144, 1982.

CHAPTER 13

Carpal Fractures and Dislocations

Andrew D. Markiewitz, MD, Leonard K. Ruby, MD,
and Eugene T. O'Brien, MD

Carpal fractures and dislocations represent a spectrum of injury ranging from isolated fractures or dislocations to complex combinations. At the mild end of the spectrum, the patient presents with a history of a wrist injury that continues to be painful despite normal radiographs and conservative treatment. At the severe end of the spectrum, the patient sustains a high-energy injury, as in a fall from a height or a motor vehicle accident, and the wrist fracture or dislocation is only one component of the patient's injuries. Both types of injury demand prompt attention. Regardless of accurate diagnosis and appropriate intervention, some patients may be left with wrist pain that can be chronic and disabling. Treatment options become more limited and less satisfactory, however, the longer the patient remains untreated and undiagnosed.

In this chapter, we discuss the more common fractures, dislocations, and combinations thereof with the understanding that, depending on the mechanism of injury, any combination may be possible. More subtle forms of wrist injury are discussed in other chapters.

INITIAL EVALUATION

When a patient presents with an injury, the initial evaluation should consist of a thorough history and physical examination and appropriate imaging studies, which have been discussed earlier in this book. If the diagnosis is not evident, one needs to immobilize the patient's wrist, to reevaluate frequently, and to utilize any special radiographic views necessary to visualize fractures or dislocations. Special radiographic tests include distraction views, stress views, nonlinear tomography, computed tomography (CT), bone scans, and even magnetic resonance (MR) imaging. Owing to poor visualization of fracture lines in carpal bone injuries, a multitude of projections and preferences fill the literature. Fracture planes may affect the visualization of the fracture. The burden of proof lies in the examiner's ability to visualize the fracture. Therefore, it is helpful for orthopedists and hand surgeons to develop a close rapport with their radiology colleagues in order to better diagnose carpal fractures and dislocations.

CARPAL FRACTURES

The Scaphoid

MECHANISM OF FRACTURE

The unique position of the scaphoid in relation to the radius, distal row, and volar carpal ligaments makes it more susceptible to injury than any other carpal bone. Scaphoid fractures can represent up to 78.8 percent of carpal fractures, according to a literature review.[7]

Elucidation of the mechanism of fracture has provided a rational basis for determining the position of immobilization most conducive to union. Weber and Chao[251] produced experimental scaphoid waist fractures by loading the radial aspect of the palm of fresh cadaver specimens, with the wrist in 95° to 100° of extension (Fig. 13–1). Mathematical analysis of the forces about the scaphoid showed that the scaphoid waist fracture resulted from bending forces applied to the distal pole of the scaphoid as the proximal pole was strongly stabilized against the radius by the radiocapitate and radioscaphoid ligaments. Because of the physiologic flexion moment created by compression at the scaphoid-trapezoid-trapezium articulation, the distal pole of the scaphoid flexes when freed from the stabilized proximal pole. Weber and Chao[251] recommended immobilizing waist fractures in slight radial deviation and slight palmar flexion to prevent malalignment.

Experimental scaphoid fractures were also produced by Mayfield.[140] He loaded fresh cadaver wrists in nonphysiologic hyperextension and ulnar deviation, and noted that the dorsal aspect of the scaphoid engaged the dorsal rim of the radius, thus creating an anvil effect leading to fracture. Fractures of the proximal pole resulted when the scaphoid first subluxed dorsally before being fractured over the dorsal rim of the radius. Mayfield[140] concluded that the position of immobilization for these injuries should be the reverse of their mechanism of production, that is, flexion, radial deviation, and intercarpal pronation.

VASCULARITY

Three extraosseous vascular systems were noted by Taleisnik and Kelly[222] in their injection studies. There

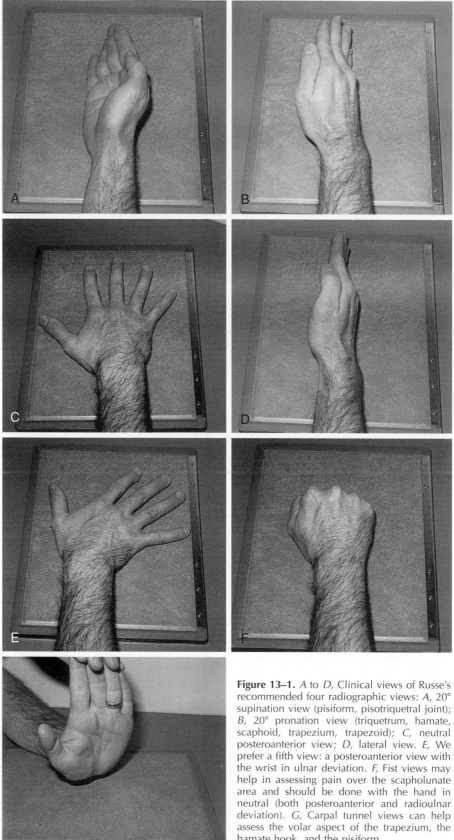

Figure 13–1. *A* to *D,* Clinical views of Russe's recommended four radiographic views: *A,* 20° supination view (pisiform, pisotriquetral joint); *B,* 20° pronation view (triquetrum, hamate, scaphoid, trapezium, trapezoid); *C,* neutral posteroanterior view; *D,* lateral view. *E,* We prefer a fifth view: a posteroanterior view with the wrist in ulnar deviation. *F,* Fist views may help in assessing pain over the scapholunate area and should be done with the hand in neutral (both posteroanterior and radioulnar deviation). *G,* Carpal tunnel views can help assess the volar aspect of the trapezium, the hamate hook, and the pisiform.

was a predominant laterovolar group of vessels entering the scaphoid volar and lateral to its radial articular surface; a dorsal group penetrating the narrow grooved dorsal surface of the scaphoid; and a distal group supplying a circumscribed area in the tuberosity (see Chapter 3). Gelberman and Menon,[86] also using injection studies, noted two major arterial systems: dorsal ridge vessels, which entered dorsally between the articular surfaces of the scaphoid and of the trapezium and trapezoid to supply the proximal 70 to 80 percent of the scaphoid, and scaphoid tubercle branches, which supply the remaining 20 to 30 percent of the internal vascularity of the bone in the region of the distal pole (Fig. 13–2). Gelberman and Menon[86] believed that their dorsal ridge vessels were analogous to Taleisnik and Kelly's[222] laterovolar vessels. Neither study found a proximal pole blood supply, the absence of which explains the high incidence of delayed healing and avascular necrosis of proximal pole scaphoid fractures.

DIAGNOSIS

Despite a high level of awareness, acute scaphoid fractures are frequently missed, especially because the initial radiographs may be unremarkable. Clinically, patients present with radial wrist and anatomic snuffbox pain. There may also be pain on first ray compression. Swelling rarely obliterates the normal concavity of the snuffbox. If the examination is suggestive, the patient should be immobilized in a thumb spica cast and reexamined within 2 to 3 weeks. Repeat radiographs including scaphoid views should be done. Although isolated fractures do occur commonly, one should verify the absence of associated carpal instabilities.

On plain radiographs, Terry and Ramin[227] noted a normal triangular or linear fat collection located between the radial collateral ligament and the tendon sheaths of the abductor pollicis longus and the extensor pollicis brevis. They coined the term *navicular fat stripe* (NFS) for this finding and noted its absence or displacement in 29 of 33 acute scaphoid fractures. They believed the NFS to be a useful radiographic sign alerting one to the presence of an underlying scaphoid fracture.[41] (For a full discussion, see Chapter 8).

Russe[191] recommended four radiographic views: 20° supination, 20° pronation, and neutral posteroanterior and lateral views (see Fig. 13–1). Many authorities have recommended taking posteroanterior and oblique radiographs with the patient making a fist in some degree of ulnar deviation, so that the scaphoid profile is maximal and the beam is more apt to parallel the fracture line. Daffner and colleagues[56] recommend a proximal tilt view in which the beam is 30° off the vertical toward the elbow, which elongates the scaphoid and capitate, allowing visualization of certain fracture patterns. Additionally, one can perform a distal tilt view, which would be 30° off the vertical toward the fingers and would elongate the capitate.[56] These views enable visualization of transverse fracture patterns. However, horizontal fracture patterns may be hidden, as the x-ray beams would not pass through this plane. Daffner and colleagues[56] suggest that one can also try ulnar deviation of the wrist in a posteroanterior view in combination with either of these views.

Trispiral tomography or CT with axial and paraaxial views is very helpful in delineating hard-to-visualize fractures and is quite valuable in assessing the presence or absence of healing. We recommend the use of bone scans or CT if repeat radiographs at follow-up are negative (Fig. 13–3) but one remains suspicious of a fracture (see Fig. 13–2).

In our opinion, CT is very useful not only to identify scaphoid fractures but also to diagnose displacement, angulation, and intercarpal instability. It is helpful for the physician to develop a good rapport with the radiologist, who can provide axial views of the scaphoid when the physician's objectives are understood.

Positive bone scans are nonspecific, because soft tissue injury or other adjacent bony injury may cause increased activity. A negative bone scan 72 hours after injury, however, effectively rules out an occult fracture of the scaphoid.[79, 167, 209, 215]

Fractures of the scaphoid in children are uncommon and differ significantly from those in adults.[79, 98, 99, 162, 232] Scaphoid fractures in children more commonly involve the distal pole. Small avulsion fractures of the dorsoradial aspect of the bone are common. Overall, less than 10 percent are displaced, and up to 25 percent involve only one cortex. Larson and associates[125] reported on a proximal pole fragment that appeared to have undergone ischemic necrosis and non-union. A full discussion of pediatric carpal fractures can be found in Chapter 30.

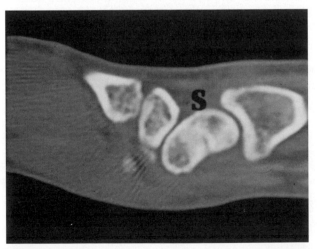

Figure 13–2. CT scans provide excellent visualization of bony bridging for assessing the healing or detailing the status of scaphoid fractures. With its similar cost and availability, CT scans have replaced bone scans to investigate vague scaphoid pain.

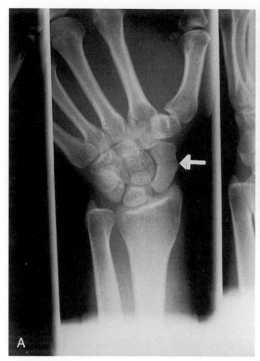

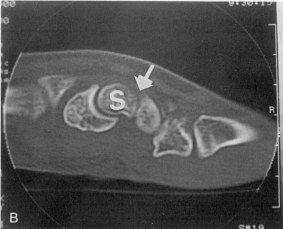

Figure 13–3. *A,* Plain radiographs may remain questionable despite continued snuffbox pain. *B,* A CT scan reveals a persistent fracture line *(arrow).* (S = scaphoid.)

CLASSIFICATION

Russe[191] proposed classification of scaphoid fractures by location—tuberosity, distal pole, waist, and proximal pole—and by direction of the fracture line—horizontal oblique, vertical oblique, or transverse. Several others have classified scaphoid fractures according to stability.[49, 114, 140, 250] Displacement implies instability, and these fractures most often result from incomplete or spontaneously reduced perilunate dislocation, as evidenced by the frequently associated dorsiflexion

instability of the lunate. Cooney and associates[49] define a displaced unstable fracture as one having more than 1 mm of step-off or more than 15° of lunocapitate angulation (Fig. 13–4). Weber[250] added the concept of an angulated scaphoid fracture hinged open dorsally on the intact (volar) radioscaphocapitate ligament in association with dorsiflexion instability of the lunate.

Uncorrected displacement (instability) is associated with a marked increase in the rate of pseudarthrosis. Eddeland and associates[62] noted the failure of union in 23 of 25 scaphoid fractures (92 percent) in which the displacement exceeded 1 mm. In their study, delay in treatment of more than 4 weeks and location of the fracture in the proximal pole were the other two factors adversely affecting healing.

Uncomplicated scaphoid fractures have a union rate approaching 95 percent when diagnosed early and properly immobilized (Table 13–1).

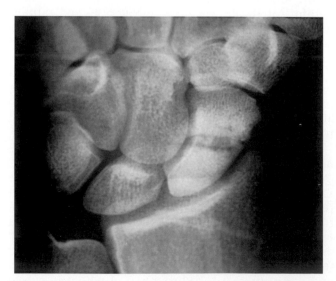

Figure 13–4. Unstable fractures may show a 1-mm stepoff or more than 15° of lunocapitate angulation.

Table 13–1. HEALING IN FRESH FRACTURES OF THE SCAPHOID

Study	Number of Cases	Percentage Healed
Shands (1944)[197]	198	98.5
Stewart (1954)[213] (1968)[214]	323	85
Bohler et al (1954)[22]	734	96.6
Russe (1960)[191]	220	99.5
Eddeland et al (1975)[62]	92	95
Cooney et al (1980)[49]	32	94
Morgan and Walters (1984)[158]	100	97.6

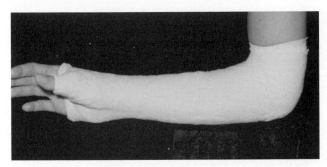

Figure 13–5. Our preferred cast treatment is 6 weeks of immobilization in a long-arm thumb spica cast followed by 6 weeks of immobilization in a short-arm thumb spica cast.

TREATMENT

Cast Application

Every conceivable position of the wrist has at one time or another been recommended as the best position for immobilization to achieve union of a scaphoid fracture.[14, 32, 57, 75, 121, 204] Cadaver studies demonstrate that passive pronation and supination of the forearm result in motion of the two fragments of an artificially created scaphoid fracture.[228, 238, 239] Theoretically, an above-elbow cast should improve the rate of union of scaphoid fractures, particularly those fractures that are unstable. Several studies have been performed to compare healing times with a long-arm cast and with a short-arm cast in comparable types of scaphoid fractures.[5, 33, 91]

Although the type of cast used remains controversial, we prefer to use a long-arm thumb spica cast for the first 6 weeks in treating a patient with a nondisplaced fracture or a fracture that has been reduced by manipulation.[49, 52, 158] After 6 weeks, we use a short-arm thumb spica cast (Fig. 13–5). Frequent cast changes, every 2 to 3 weeks, are necessary to prevent loosening of the cast and loss of fixation. We do not stop immobilization until CT scans demonstrate at least 50 percent bridging or healing[128] or until the patient has undergone 4 to 6 months of treatment.

A short-arm cast with the wrist in slight palmar flexion (10° or so) and radial deviation (the metacarpal of the middle finger aligned with the radial shaft) may close any palmar fracture gap (Fig. 13–6). The thumb is placed in full palmar abduction, and the interphalangeal joint is left free. Casts must be snugly applied and well molded between the thenar and the hypothenar eminences to maintain the normal arches of the hand.

If serial radiographs or CT scans show that progress toward union is lacking or has ceased, consideration may be given to bone grafting at 4 to 6 months after injury. Despite some reports to the contrary, electrical stimulation, both in the literature and in our practice, has not been shown to be of value.[26, 27, 77, 200] Fisk[71] coined the term "peanut fractures" for those asymptomatic, radiologically non-united fractures that have united centrally by fibrous tissue and are surrounded by a shell of healed articular cartilage. Although patients who have a persistent fracture line despite adequate immobilization may tolerate a clinical trial with the arm out of the cast, it is our belief that a high percentage of these patients will have a subsequent injury that will "fracture" the fibrous union (see Fig. 13–3). In any event, nearly all scaphoid non-unions (Fig. 13–7) eventually develop arthritis,[133, 190, 237] and the patient should be advised accordingly. Avascular necrosis of the proximal pole certainly delays the union of the fracture but is not an indication for bone grafting as long as there is evidence of progress toward union.[191]

With the potential of being missed initially, scaphoid fractures may manifest late. An affected patient may benefit from immobilization if the fracture re-

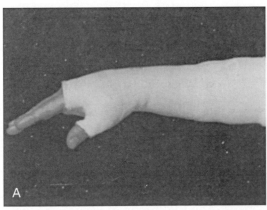
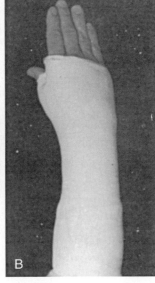

Figure 13–6. Position of immobilization with slight flexion and radial deviation. (From O'Brien ET: Acute fractures and dislocations of the carpus. Orthop Clin North Am 15:237–258, 1984.)

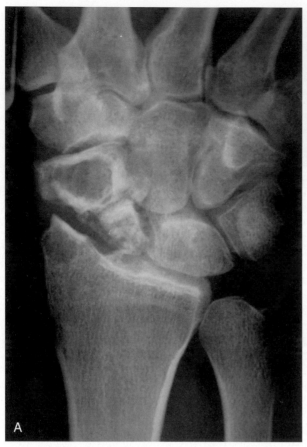

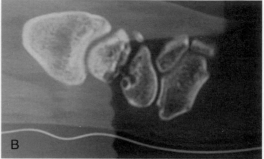

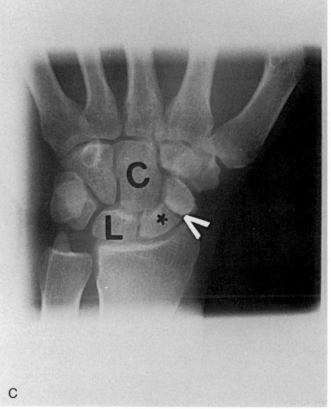

Figure 13–7. Although the progression to arthritis remains controversial, scaphoid non-unions eventually become symptomatic. *A,* Further arthritis may develop if the non-union is left untreated. *B,* Joint space narrowing, squaring of articular surfaces, and cysts may be evidence of this progression. *C,* Early non-unions show sclerotic, rounded borders. (C = capitate; L = lunate; * = proximal pole; and arrow = non-union.)

mains nondisplaced; however, the chances of healing are diminished. After 6 months without evidence of healing, the patient can be described as having a non-union, and a more aggressive approach is indicated. Non-union and malunion can occur uncommonly in the acute nondisplaced scaphoid fracture. Thus, some authorities have advocated internal fixation even in nondisplaced fractures.[103, 104] We believe, however, that a trial of cast immobilization is warranted in most of these cases.

Although reports indicate that healing of the acute nondisplaced fracture is the rule in pediatric fractures, non-union or malunion can occur.[177, 202] Open reduction with internal fixation has been suggested by Mintzer and Waters[152] for displaced fractures and by Suzuki and Herbert[217] if malunion exists in the presence of limited remaining growth.

In summary, we use cast treatment for acute, non-displaced scaphoid tuberosity, waist, or proximal pole fractures without carpal instability.

Internal Fixation

Displaced scaphoid fractures require accurate reduction by either a closed or open method. Closed reduction, achieved by employing traction on the thumb while molding the anatomic snuffbox, was advised by Soto-Hall.[200] Cooney and associates[49] attempted closed reduction of a displaced scaphoid fracture by longitudinal traction combined with manual pressure on the proximal carpal row, with the wrist in flexion to reduce the proximal scaphoid fragment and the maltrotated lunate. A long-arm cast with the wrist in flexion and radial deviation was used to maintain the reduction. Four of the seven displaced fractures in their series that healed had been reduced and then immobilized in a long-arm cast. Two other fractures that were initially nondisplaced became displaced during treatment. Cooney and associates[49] recommended obtaining radioulnar deviation stress views and traction oblique views if there was doubt initially about the stability of the fracture. King and colleagues[121] compared the trapezium and distal radius to a carpenter's C clamp holding the scaphoid. Positioning the wrist in mid-dorsiflexion, full ulnar deviation, and full supination enables the "clamp" to tighten and reduce the scaphoid fragments. These researchers achieved union within 4 to 6 weeks in 22 of 23 scaphoid fractures they treated using this method.[121]

Weber[250] attempted closed reduction of a dorsally angulated fracture of the scaphoid by maximal radial deviation of the wrist in neutral flexion. This maneuver was chosen to help abolish the accompanying

dorsiflexion instability to the lunate by causing the lunate to flex, avoiding scaphoid malunion. Extreme wrist positions for extended periods are counterproductive, especially if the reduction may be lost.

We believe that operative intervention is necessary for acute, displaced fractures. Additionally, patients who would suffer economically or who have medical contraindications to prolonged immobilization may be considered for surgery. Accurate reduction and internal fixation may decrease the non-union rate. Some surgeons use a Herbert screw; however, we recommend smooth Kirschner (K) wire fixation (Fig. 13–8). If bone grafting is not required, one or two wires can be placed through a volar approach percutaneously, passing distal to proximal. We bury our wires to have the option of keeping them in place for more than 6 weeks. A short arm thumb spica cast is used in conjunction with all of our operative ap-

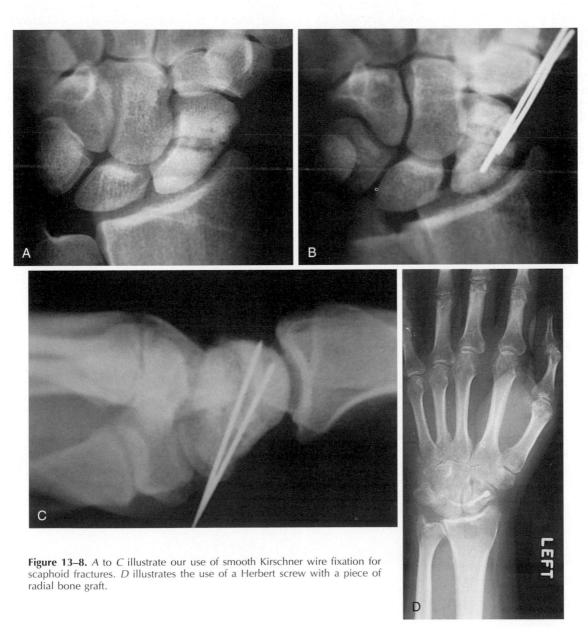

Figure 13–8. *A* to *C* illustrate our use of smooth Kirschner wire fixation for scaphoid fractures. *D* illustrates the use of a Herbert screw with a piece of radial bone graft.

proaches until healing is 90 percent complete by CT scanning. Our technique is as follows.

After adequate axillary block or general anesthesia, we prepare and drape the arm as for any hand procedure. The surgeon attempts reduction by palmar translation of the distal carpal row (and metacarpals) on the proximal carpal row with one hand as the forearm is stabilized by the surgeon's other hand (Fig. 13–9); this is the midcarpal shift maneuver. Then, we radially deviate the wrist (metacarpals) to compress the fracture site while simultaneously maintaining the palmar shift position. The assistant then drives one or two, 0.054-inch or 0.062-inch, smooth Kirschner wires from distal to proximal across the fracture site, trying to engage the subchondral bone of the proximal fragment. Accurate reduction and K-wire placement are checked with a sterile draped C-arm mini-fluoroscan or plain x-ray machine. A short-arm cast is then applied, and casts are changed every 2 weeks until the fracture is healed on CT scan.

In proximal pole fractures representing a quarter or less of the scaphoid, we prefer an open dorsal approach and use a Herbert screw as described by De-Maagd and Engber.[57A] We obtain reduction by the same manipulation as in closed reduction and place a provisional K wire first, followed by a screw of appropriate length (Fig. 13–10).

If open reduction is required, scaphoid fractures can be approached dorsally, palmarly, or radially, depending on one's preference for fixation and bone grafting and the location of the fracture. Baldy Dos Reis and coworkers[10] and DeMaagd and Engber[57A] describe a dorsal approach to scaphoid fractures. The dorsal approach achieved a 100 percent healing rate in acute fractures and an 87 percent healing rate in delayed union and non-union, with a time of 8.3 weeks to union.[10] Postoperative cast immobilization averaged 18 days.[10]

Bone Grafting. Bone grafting techniques are usu-ally the first line of treatment and remain the gold standard of care for treatment of non-unions and comminuted fractures. Grafting may be done with or without fixation, with an 80 to 90 percent success rate. Graft techniques include the Matti technique, which uses cancellous graft from a dorsal approach,[189] and the Russe approach, which uses cancellous and cortical cancellous struts from a volar approach.[140, 189] Typically, the wrist assumes a dorsal intercalated segment instability (DISI) pattern when the scaphoid has angulated. A dorsal approach can be helpful when one needs to reduce the lunate onto the capitate, and for proximal pole fractures. We rarely use the dorsal approach for waist or distal pole fractures, however, because the use of a small spreader or "joysticks" through a volar approach can wedge open the scaphoid in acutely angulated or old fractures to reduce the DISI pattern. The volar approach facilitates placement of a corticocancellous wedge graft. A complete discussion of bone grafting techniques for scaphoid non-union is presented in Chapter 14.

Screws. Herbert and Fisher[104] describe the use of the Herbert headless screw, which provides interfragmentary compression when used with a jig. Use of the Herbert screw in acute nondisplaced and acute displaced scaphoid fractures demonstrates a 92 percent success rate.[35A] The Herbert screw itself has a differential pitch between its heads and is buried in the scaphoid. Herbert and Fisher[104] found a 100 percent union rate in all acute fractures.

Improper placement of the jig can alter screw placement and represents a common problem with the application of the Herbert screw.[1A] Additionally, as noted by Bunker et al,[35A] the scaphotrapezium joint must be entered to allow barrel placement. Jig manipulation may alter reduction and may cause fracture malalignment in cases with comminution. Cannulated AO screws allow placement of guide wires,

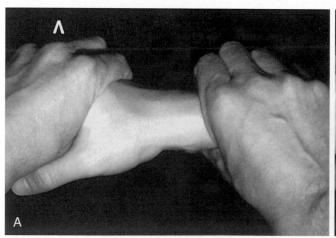
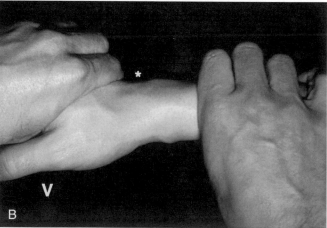

Figure 13–9. The midcarpal shift allows palmar translation of the distal carpal row on the proximal carpal row for reduction or assessment of laxity. The examiner's proximal hand stabilizes the forearm while the distal hand shifts the carpus dorsally *(A)* and volarly *(B)*. *Arrowheads* indicate direction of the shift. Comparison with the uninvolved wrist allows evaluation for laxity. This maneuver can also be used for intraoperative carpal reduction. Asterisk highlights area of interest.

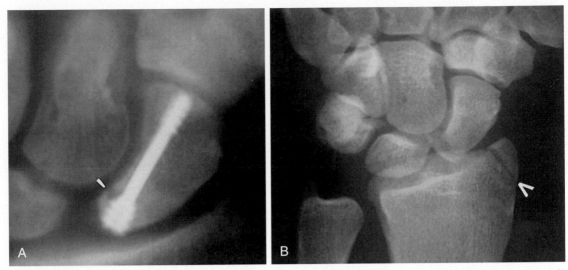

Figure 13–10. *A,* Proximal pole scaphoid fracture fixed with a Herbert screw *(arrow). B,* A concurrent radial styloid fracture *(arrowhead)* may also be present.

which minimizes dissection and manipulation. If fixation is satisfactory, early motion (approximately 6 weeks) may be allowed in a protective splint. Adams and colleagues[1A] report a lower success rate for the Herbert screw, of 67 percent, if non-unions and acute fractures are combined. Screws cannot be used with very small distal or proximal fragments. We have used 3.5-mm AO cannulated screws or Kirschner wires with great success.

Our preference is to use Kirschner wires whenever feasible. If the proximal fracture is angulated or displaced, we prefer to use the Herbert screw through a dorsal approach. An anterior approach with the 3.5-mm AO cancellous screw or a 2.7-mm AO compression screw is preferred if the fracture is angulated, displaced, or comminuted and cannot be reduced and fixed by closed means. In addition, the scaphoid must be large enough and relatively straight to accommodate a screw.[57B] It is technically easier to use K wires in the small or highly curved (C-shaped) scaphoid. One disadvantage of the K-wire fixation is that it must be removed after healing, whereas a screw rarely requires removal. Another is that K wires prevent aggressive early motion.

COMPLICATIONS

Complications of scaphoid fractures are numerous, including malunion, non-union, delayed union, avascular necrosis, and arthritis. Proximal third fractures have an avascular necrosis rate of 14 to 39 percent by radiographic assessment.[50] Middle third fractures, if displaced, have high rates of slow and delayed healing[6] as well as of non-union (20 percent).[50] Nonunions or malunions may result in and be caused by carpal instability. Arthritis results from non-union and malunion.[133, 190, 237]

Although the initial injury causing scaphoid fracture may often go unnoticed, patients with scaphoid non-unions present in a variety of ways. Pain and stiffness often force patients to seek medical advice. Following minor injuries, patients may present with radiographs showing sclerosis, avascular necrosis, malalignment, and arthritis. These findings are typically inconsistent with an acute injury but indicate that the patient suffered an injury in the past. Treatment of old scaphoid non-unions varies, but the goal is to achieve a pain-free, functional wrist.

The literature is replete with treatments of scaphoid non-union. Bone grafting with or without internal fixation remains the standard of care if there is no arthritis. Watson and associates[248] describe a dorsal approach with bone grafting and K-wire fixation that produces an 89 percent rate of healing. This approach preserves the volar ligaments, and these surgeons are able to correct the carpal malalignment and the scaphoid malalignment. Updates of procedures initially described by Matti and Russe for bone grafting through either a volar or dorsal approach without supplementary fixation have been published.[189, 206]

No discussion of scaphoid non-union and delayed union would be complete without mention of the use of pulsed electromagnetic fields (PEMF). Adams and coworkers[1] report that healing rates with PEMF are worse than previously reported, yielding a 69 percent overall success rate. This indicates to us that use of a bone grafting technique would be preferable over prolonged immobilization with the addition of a PEMF. Adams and coworkers[1] recommend using pulsed electromagnetic fields as a secondary option to bone grafting techniques in patients with nondisplaced fractures without angulation or pseudarthrosis. Healing rates, according to these researchers, decrease to 50 percent when the proximal pole is involved.[1] We do not use this technique in our practice.

Jiranek and associates[113] did not find scaphoid malunions to have statistically significant subjective results, despite lower objective scores. This finding, after an average follow-up of 11 years, suggests that bony union is more important than alignment in preventing symptomatic wrist degeneration. Amadio and colleagues[6] found that as the angulation of the scaphoid increased, the clinical success rate decreased and the risk of post-traumatic arthritis increased. Although malunion does result in altered wrist dynamics and a worse objective result, we do not routinely recommend corrective osteotomy for scaphoid malunion in asymptomatic patients (Fig. 13–11).

Children appear able to remodel scaphoid malunions if they have significant growth potential remaining. If limited or no growth potential remains, Suzuki and Herbert[217] recommend reduction. We prefer to treat teenagers as adults. Avascular necrosis appears to be rare in children.

Salvage procedures are indicated in patients in whom operative or nonoperative treatment has failed and arthritis is too severe to correct with scaphoid reconstructive techniques (Fig. 13–12). Multiple procedures for wrist salvage have been proposed, including proximal row carpectomy, intercarpal wrist fusion, total wrist fusion, radial styloidectomy, Bentzon's procedure (pseudarthrosis procedure), and proximal and distal scaphoid excision with or without tendon interposition.[189] Use of silicone scaphoid replacement has not been successful and has been abandoned. Proximal row carpectomy preserves functional motion[54]; however, some pain typically remains. Total wrist fusion is more dependable in relieving pain and can be done through a dorsal approach as described by Weil and Ruby.[252] Radial styloidectomy typically requires additional procedures at a later date, and we do not recommend it as a definitive treatment, although it may be useful as an adjunctive procedure.

Limited fusions such as scaphocapitate and lunate-capitate-hamate-triquetrum with scaphoid excision are advocated by some, but early reports have not shown uniform success,[7, 189] and the long-term results are unknown.

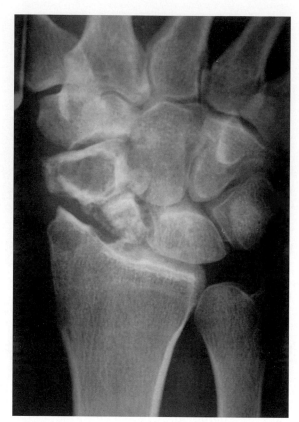

Figure 13–12. Wrists with scaphoid non-unions reveal an advanced collapse pattern.

SCAPHOID TUBEROSITY FRACTURES

Crush injuries of the hand can lead to avulsion fractures of the scaphoid tuberosity. Treatment for nondisplaced avulsion fractures remains nonoperative, cast application being continued until healing is seen radiographically. Displaced fractures require fixation to avoid non-union or malunion, which may be symptomatic as described by Moody and colleagues.[153] Late diagnosed fractures may require a volarly placed bone graft or excision.

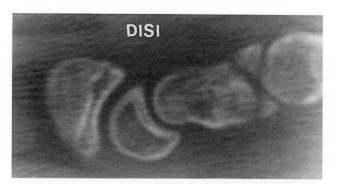

Figure 13–11. We have not routinely recommended osteotomy for malunion, although dorsal intercalary segment instability (DISI) patterns may occur.

SUMMARY

For nondisplaced acute fractures of the scaphoid, we prefer a long-arm cast for 6 weeks followed by a short-arm cast until healing is complete as shown by CT scan. For acute displaced or angulated fractures, we prefer open or closed reduction and internal fixation with or without bone graft. We use bone grafting only for acute comminuted fracture in which collapse and angulation are probable. For non-union or delayed union, we recommend open reduction, internal fixation with K wires or screws, and bone grafting. For asymptomatic malunion of the scaphoid we recommend observation.

The Triquetrum

MECHANISM OF INJURY AND DIAGNOSIS

Small fractures of the dorsal aspect of the triquetrum are commonly seen after hyperextension injury of the wrist. Triquetrum fracture is the second most common carpal fracture, representing 13.8 percent of carpal fractures.[7] Triquetrum fractures are typically secondary to ulnar styloid impingement on the dorsal proximal aspect of the bone. These represent a shear or chisel type pattern of fracture.[80A, 126A] Forced dorsiflexion and ulnar deviation of the wrist drive the triquetrum against the ulnar styloid and can result in fracture. Levy and associates[126A] believe that a prominent ulnar styloid is associated with these fractures. Small fractures of the dorsal triquetrum are best seen in lateral or oblique radiographs as a fleck of bone raised off dorsally.

Most fractures of the main body of the triquetrum, especially if displaced, are associated with perilunate dislocations, crush injuries,[81] or other associated carpal injuries. Because of the attachments of strong palmar and dorsal radiocarpal ligaments (palmar lunotriquetral and dorsal radiotriquetral ligaments, respectively), carpal instability may occur following triquetral fractures. In particular, a volar intercalated segment instability (VISI) pattern can occur if the dorsal ligaments are avulsed with a fragment of triquetrum (Fig. 13–13).[242]

TREATMENT

Four to 6 weeks of immobilization in a short-arm cast usually relieves the patient's pain, and even though non-union of the small fragment is common,[25] it is rarely of clinical significance.[11] If symptomatic, the bone chip may be excised.

Main body fractures require accurate reduction and internal fixation. Avascular necrosis (AVN) of the triquetrum has not been reported. Nondisplaced body fractures may be treated in a cast. Any VISI deformity must be looked for and corrected by appropriate fracture reduction and/or ligament repair.

The Trapezium

MECHANISM OF INJURY AND DIAGNOSIS

In 1960, Cordrey and Ferrier-Torells[53] reviewed 75 trapezial fractures in the literature, added five new cases, and noted the incidence to be about 5% of all carpal bone fractures. Amadio and Taleisnik[7] noted the incidence to be closer to 2.3%. Later literature has focused on two main fracture types: a split fracture of the trapezium with lateral subluxation of the first metacarpal, which remains attached to the lateral trapezial fragment, and a fracture of the trapezial ridge (base or tip).

An isolated trapezial fracture results from a direct blow to the abducted thumb or from a fall on the hyperextended hand in radial deviation, which compresses the trapezium between the first metacarpal and the radial styloid.[35] Body fractures are commonly intra-articular and are associated with ligament injuries,[66, 81] especially of the thumb. A fall on the outstretched hand results in a fracture of the trapezial ridge either by direct trauma or through tension applied through the attached transverse carpal ligament as the thenar and hypothenar eminences diverge.[173] Jensen and Christiansen[112] believe that traction force through the transverse carpal ligament can lead to ridge fractures.

Trapezial fractures can best be visualized in an oblique radiograph obtained with the ulnar border of the hand on the cassette and with the forearm pronated 20° from vertical.[53] Trapezial ridge fractures, like fractures of the hook of the hamate, are more apt to be missed, because they can be seen only on the carpal tunnel view, not a pronated lateral view (Fig. 13–14).[144] CT scans can be very useful (Fig. 13–15). Chip fractures may be larger than radiographs indicate.[72A]

Clinically, ridge fractures are characterized by localized tenderness at the base of the thenar eminence and pain elicited on resisted wrist flexion; associated carpal tunnel and ulnar tunnel syndromes can occur.

TREATMENT

Displaced vertical fractures of the trapezium with lateral subluxation of the first metacarpal require accurate reduction and internal fixation, similar to Bennett's fracture-dislocation (Fig. 13–16). Cordrey and Ferrer-Torells[53] achieved excellent results in five such injuries treated by open reduction and smooth Kirschner wire fixation. The first Kirschner wire was introduced into the lateral fragment and used to manipulate it, and then was used to hold the reduction while a second wire was drilled through both fragments. Normal function was noted by Freeland and

Figure 13–13. Volar intercalary segment instability (VISI) pattern. Chip fractures off the triquetrum can represent destabilizing ligament avulsion and should be investigated.

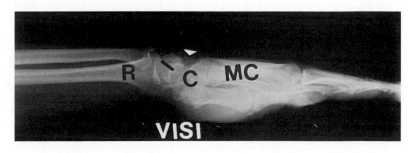

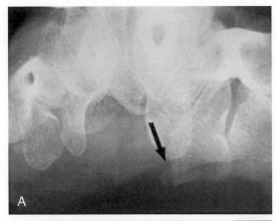

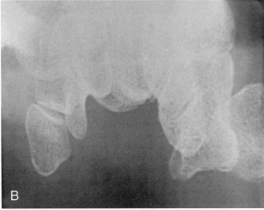

Figure 13–14. *A,* Radiograph taken 2 months after a 61-year old professor sustained a trapezial ridge fracture in a fall onto her outstretched hand. The arrow points to the trapezial ridge fracture. She had volar wrist pain, but no symptoms or signs of carpal tunnel syndrome. *B,* Follow-up radiograph taken 6 months after the injury showed apparent healing despite the lack of any immobilization.

Finley[74] after open reduction with cancellous bone grafting and lag screw fixation in one patient who had a vertical trapezial fracture with lateral subluxation of the first metacarpal. If the fracture is unreduced, thumb metacarpal subluxation, arthritis, and impaired pinch may occur.[66, 72A] If nerve compression is evident, tunnel release should be performed as an emergency procedure. Observation is key in fractures related to crush injuries.

As with fractures of the hamate hook, non-union of a trapezial ridge fracture is not uncommon. Palmer[173] recorded one case of fracture through the wider base of the trapezial ridge that healed after thumb spica immobilization with the first ray in abduction. If painful non-union occurs, excision of the non-united fragment usually relieves the patient's symptoms after a prolonged recovery.[144]

The Hamate

MECHANISM OF INJURY AND DIAGNOSIS

Hamate fractures, although unusual (1.5% of carpal fractures), can involve either the body or the hook

(see Fig. 13–15). More common than body fractures, hook fractures can occur following many injury patterns, such as falls, direct trauma, and striking a ball with a tennis racquet or soft club. All radiographs must be viewed carefully, as many hamate fractures are not diagnosed early.[255] Bishop and Beckenbaugh[17] report that standard radiographs, including 20° supination oblique and carpal tunnel views, are unreliable and recommend CT scans or tomograms (Figs. 13–15 and 13–17).[19, 39, 63, 178] The clinician should be suspicious when a patient presents with pain distal to the pisiform, a painful grip, and pain with palpation over the hook. This pressure can be applied either volarly or dorsally. Failla and Amadio[66] note that resisted distal interphalangeal flexion of the ring and little fingers with an ulnarly deviated wrist causes pain in a hamate hook fracture. In this position, the hook acts as a pulley for the flexor tendons of the ulnar digits.

TREATMENT

Although several surgeons have recommended excision of the fractured hamate hook, acute fractures that are nondisplaced may be treated nonoperatively with short-arm cast immobilization for 6 to 8 weeks. Stark and associates[207] recommend early subperiosteal removal of all hook fractures. Non-unions of the hook can have complications, including flexor tendon synovitis or rupture (profundus-ring, little), ulnar nerve irritation, and chronic pain.* Removal of a displaced comminuted fracture or non-union usually relieves these symptoms. Even with early open reduction and internal fixation, hook healing is not guaranteed.[19] Because of the potential for late healing,[194] we

---

*References 9, 35, 43, 55, 107, 170, 207, 219.

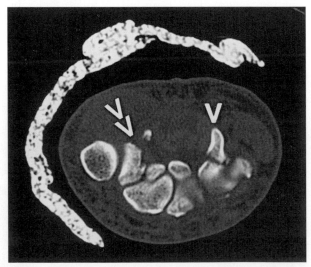

Figure 13–15. Use of CT scans improves one's ability to define hamate *(arrowhead)* or trapezium *(double arrowheads)* fractures, as seen here, in a patient who suffered a heavy compressive blow to the back of the wrist.

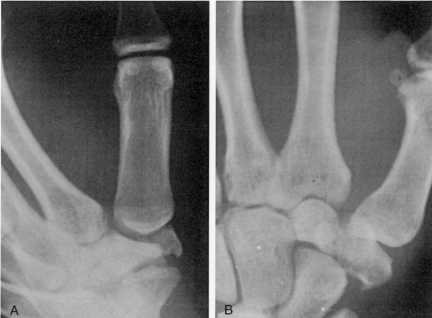

Figure 13–16. *A* and *B,* This 20-year old man sustained a displaced fracture of the trapezium in a motorcycle accident. *C,* An open reduction and internal fixation carried out 3 days after injury restored the articular surface of the trapezium, and healing was noted 10 weeks later.

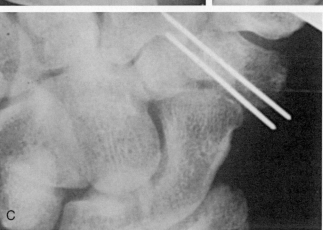

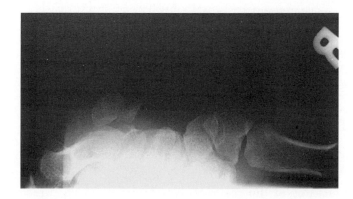

Figure 13–17. Carpal tunnel view illustrating trapezium and hamate fractures. Such radiographs are technically difficult to obtain in patients whose wrists are swollen and tender.

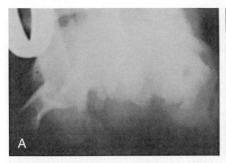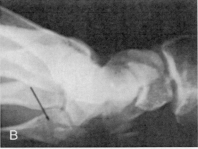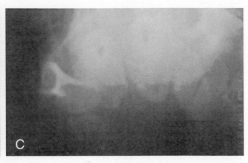

Figure 13–18. Radiographs had been made on several occasions of this 31-year-old man, who had hypothenar pain for 2 years after injuring his wrist playing racquetball, but they were interpreted as normal. *A,* A non-united fracture of the hook of the hamate can be seen on the carpal tunnel and oblique views. *B* and *C,* Excision of the non-united fragment relieved the patient's pain. (*A* and *C* from O'Brien ET: Fractures and dislocations of the carpal bones. In Kane WJ (ed): Current Orthopaedic Management. New York, Churchill-Livingstone, 1981, by permission. *B* from O'Brien ET: Acute fractures and dislocations of the carpus. Orthop Clin North Am 15:237–258, 1984.)

prefer to treat patients with a short-arm cast if seen within 3 weeks of the injury. Failing this course of therapy, we excise the fragment (Fig. 13–18).

Body fractures of the hamate are usually in the coronal plane and angled 20° dorsally.[135, 229] They may be associated with dorsal dislocations of the metacarpals,[135, 229] crush injuries,[81] or perilunate dislocations[64] (Fig. 13–19). Milch[149] classifies body fractures according to whether they are medial (ulnar) or lateral (radial) to the hook. CT scans may be necessary to define the fracture plane. Body fractures need to be reduced and fixed if unstable. Cast immobilization for 6 weeks is sufficient for a stable fracture. The dislocations, if present, must be reduced and fixed at the same time.

Failla[65] notes, from a cadaver investigation, that the blood supply predominantly enters the radial base of the hamate hook, with a smaller and more variable supply entering the ulnar tip of the hook. This distribution of blood supply is postulated to be the reason that hook fractures are at risk for non-union.

Internal fixation of hamate body fractures may be done with Kirschner wires or a small T plate applied dorsally as described by Marck and Klasen.[135] Old unrecognized fracture-dislocations of the fourth and fifth carpometacarpal joints may require reduction and fusion (see Fig. 13–19).

The Lunate

MECHANISM OF INJURY AND DIAGNOSIS

Isolated acute lunate fractures are rarely discussed because lunate fractures are usually associated with Kienböck's disease. Thus, an incidence for lunate fractures of 1.4 percent of carpal fractures may be too high. In reviewing the literature, Teisen and Hjarbaek[225] found that acute lunate fractures account for between 1.1 and 6.5 percent of all carpal bone fractures. Although these researchers attempted to classify 17 fractures into five groups, the limited number of acute cases prevents validation of this scheme.

One should note that volar pole fractures appear to be most common. In contrast to the report by Armistead and colleagues,[8] Teisen and Hjarbaek[225] did not find a progression to Kienböck's disease in their follow-up of treated lunate fractures; they argue that untreated lunate fractures may progress to Kienböck's disease. (Kienböck's disease is discussed in Chapter 18.) Diagnosis requires close attention to the area of a patient's pain and radiographs. CT scanning or tomography is often necessary because the fracture plane frequently is coronal.

TREATMENT

Treatment of acute nondisplaced lunate fractures should be cast immobilization. Displaced fractures, especially palmar pole fractures, should undergo open reduction and internal fixation. The vascular work of Gelberman and colleagues indicates a rich network of surface vessels producing both volar and dorsal nutrient vessels in a variety of patterns. Thus, a dorsal or volar approach is possible for surgical repair.

Despite early appropriate treatment, complications may occur. Gelberman and Gross[85] hold that compression fractures of the lunate that are dependent on a single nutrient artery (Y version) are at greatest risk of avascular necrosis with horizontal fractures. Unfortunately, this information is not available clinically at this time, as these fractures are seldom seen. MR imaging remains one of the best ways to evaluate AVN.[231A] We do not have any experience with isolated lunate fractures.

The Pisiform

MECHANISM OF INJURY AND DIAGNOSIS

Fractures of the pisiform usually result from direct trauma to the volar ulnar aspect of the wrist. Pisiform fractures, although uncommon (1% of carpal fractures[7]), can occur in conjunction with dorsal radius,

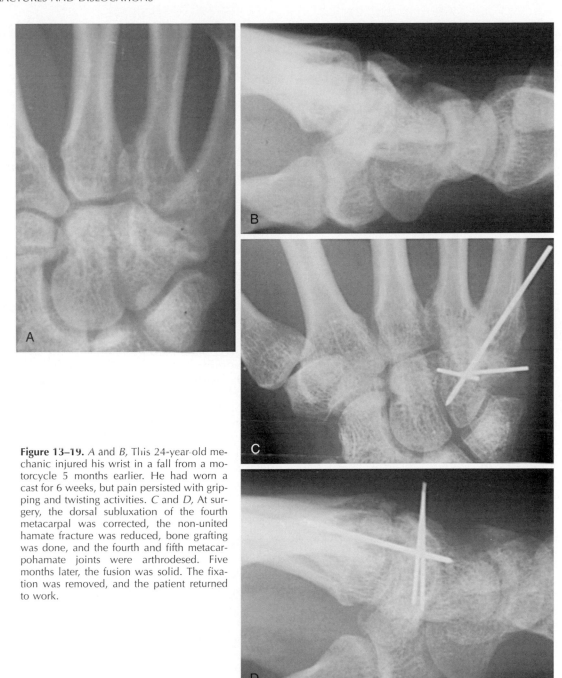

Figure 13–19. *A* and *B,* This 24-year-old mechanic injured his wrist in a fall from a motorcycle 5 months earlier. He had worn a cast for 6 weeks, but pain persisted with gripping and twisting activities. *C* and *D,* At surgery, the dorsal subluxation of the fourth metacarpal was corrected, the non-united hamate fracture was reduced, bone grafting was done, and the fourth and fifth metacarpohamate joints were arthrodesed. Five months later, the fusion was solid. The fixation was removed, and the patient returned to work.

hamate, and triquetrum fractures or dislocations. The pisiform maintains a close relationship with the triquetrum throughout its range of motion.[35] Therefore, the force required to damage or dislocate the pisiform is significant. The fracture line may be transverse (usually a chip fracture of the distal end of the bone) or longitudinal; occasionally the bone is comminuted. The fracture is best visualized in the 30° supination palm-up view or the carpal tunnel view (see Fig. 13–1). Most fractures are revealed by standard radiographs, although CT scans or bone scans may be of use.[69] Patients may have pain, swelling, and tenderness localized to the proximal hypothenar eminence.[69] Because the pisiform makes up the medial (ulnar) wall of Guyon's canal, ulnar neuritis may occur.

TREATMENT

Displacement of the fragments in a pisiform fracture is rare, and Vasilas and associates[236] noted healing after 3 to 6 weeks of immobilization in all but 1 of their 13 patients with pisiform fractures. Most patients are asymptomatic after 3 to 6 weeks of cast immobilization. Non-union or malunion with post-traumatic arthritis is an indication for excision, as is an acute fracture involving the articular surface in which there is significant displacement.[100] The hand should be casted in 30° of flexion with slight ulnar deviation. Repair of this small intratendinous bone is not necessary. We prefer subperiosteal excision if nonoperative treatment fails.

The Capitate

MECHANISM OF INJURY AND DIAGNOSIS

The incidence of capitate fracture varies from 1.3 percent[183] to 14 percent[18] of carpal fractures. Amadio and Taleisnik[7] put the incidence at closer to 1 percent. Capitate fractures have been classified by Rand and associates[183] into isolated fractures, fractures associated with perilunate dislocation (scaphocapitate syndrome), and fractures associated with other carpal injury. The mechanism of injury may be direct trauma to the dorsal wrist, dorsiflexion in neutral or ulnar deviation, dorsiflexion in radial deviation (scaphocapitate syndrome), or trauma to the heads of the second and third metacarpals with the wrist palmar-flexed.[3] Richards and Bell[187] have postulated that when the patient falls on a dorsiflexed wrist, the radius impacts on the dorsum of the capitate and fractures it (Fig. 13–20).

A fracture of the capitate is similar in several ways to a fracture of the scaphoid. Because the blood sup-ply enters mainly through the palmar waist, avascular necrosis and non-union of the proximal pole in proximal capitate fractures occur rather frequently.[85, 235] Dorsal waist arterial contributions are less significant. Nondisplaced fractures may also be missed initially, so follow-up radiographs and perhaps even lateral tomography[3] may be necessary to make the diagnosis. One should look at the three arcs formed on postero-anterior (PA) radiographs of the wrist as described by Bellinghausen and coworkers.[12A] The smaller distal arc is centered on the capitate (see Fig. 13–20).

TREATMENT

Nondisplaced capitate fractures without associated injuries can be treated with cast immobilization for 6 weeks or until healed as shown on CT. Displaced capitate fractures require open reduction and internal fixation.

Fixation methods include use of Herbert screws and Kirschner wires. Fixation is best accomplished through a dorsal incision (Fig. 13–21), which allows excellent visualization. Transient avascular changes are common in proximal pole fractures, but collapse and resorption after fracture seem to be quite unusual.[183] Most reported cases of avascular necrosis of the capitate have involved the proximal pole and were not associated with a definite fracture.[161] The report by Vander Grend and associates[235] is an exception: They found non-union and proximal avascular necrosis in four patients, only two of whom could recall a specific injury. Curettage with cancellous bone grafting was successful in achieving union in

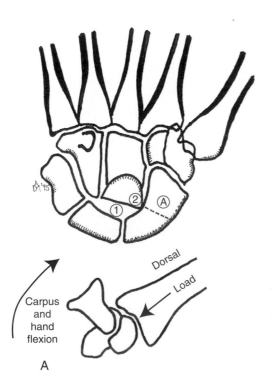

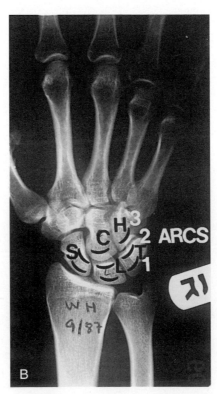

Figure 13–20. *A*, Capitate impacts on the radius, creating fracture fragment, which then flips 180°. If the PA radiograph is not properly centered, the arcs may blur, and the new irregular capitate margin may go unnoticed unless the arcs are drawn. (1 = irregular gap; 2 = fracture fragment; A = scaphoid.) *B*, As described by Gilula, three arcs may be superimposed on the normal wrist. The greater one can be noted along the proximal row between carpus and radius. The other two arcs line the proximal and distal edges of the midcarpal row. Disruption of these arcs indicates displacement of carpal bones from their normal alignment. (1 = proximal arc of proximal row; 2 = distal arc of proximal row; S = scaphoid; L = lunate; T = triquetrum; C = capitate; H = hamate.) (Modified from Bellinghausen HW, Gilula LA, Young LV, Weeks PW: Post-traumatic palmar carpal subluxation: Report of two cases. J Bone Joint Surg 65A:998–1006, 1983.)

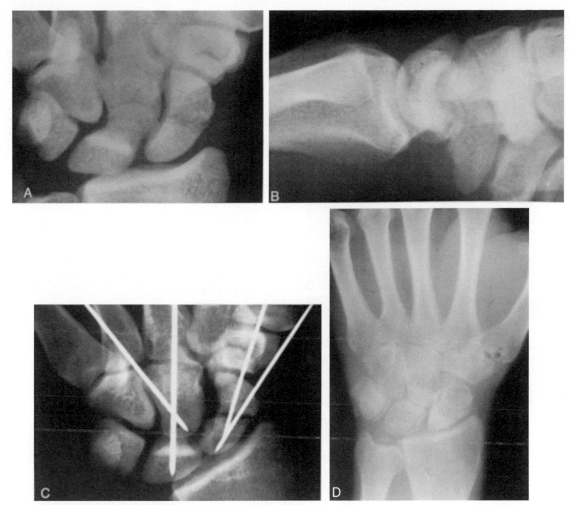

Figure 13–21. *A* and *B,* This 22-year-old student fell while playing basketball and was seen on the day of injury in an emergency room, where a cast was applied for a fracture of the scaphoid. *C,* Two weeks later, orthopaedic consultation was obtained, and the displaced capitate fracture and the fracture of the scaphoid were opened and fixed with Kirschner wires. *D,* Transient avascular changes were noted in both proximal fragments; however, healing occurred, and the results were excellent 4 years later.

three patients with non-union. Rand and associates[183] achieved union in two patients with non-union of the capitate and emphasized the need for an intercalary bone graft to restore the length of the shortened bone. They noted a significantly high incidence of arthrosis in the late follow-up of isolated capitate fractures as well as capitate fractures associated with trans-scaphoid perilunate dislocation.

Capitate fractures that rotate 180° or those associated with scaphoid fractures need to be reduced. We prefer a dorsal approach with internal fixation. Malalignment of the fracture may lead to early arthritis and midcarpal collapse. Patients with collapse and pericapitate arthritis may benefit from midcarpal fusion.

The Trapezoid

The trapezoid is infrequently injured (0.2 percent of carpal fractures) because of its protected position in

the wrist. Strong ligaments fasten it in place. Bryan and Dobyns[35] report that avascular necrosis occurs only with dislocation. As we have no experience with trapezoid fractures, we concur with Bryan and Dobyns'[35] recommendation to use cast immobilization for up to 6 weeks and to consider fusion for late arthritis.

INTERCARPAL DISLOCATIONS AND FRACTURE-DISLOCATIONS

Carpal dislocations usually require considerable force, such as in a fall from a height or a motor vehicle accident. These injuries can be associated with fractures of carpal bones as well as forearm or metacarpal fractures. Additionally, there are often life-threatening injuries that distract one's attention. Injuries to the head, neck, abdomen, pelvis, and lower extremity obviously require immediate attention and intervention before the patient can be reas-

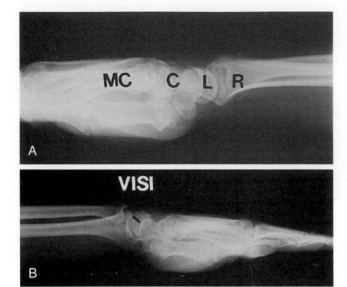

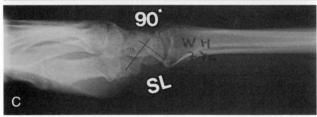

Figure 13–22. The lunate's position on lateral radiographs should alert one to wrist pathology regardless of the scapholunate angle. *A,* Normal/colinear nature of radius (R), lunate (L), capitate (C), and third metacarpal (MC). SL 30° to 60°, SL angles between 60° and 80° are in a gray zone. *B,* VISI deformity. SL < 30°. *C,* DISI deformity. SL > 80°.

sessed for less lethal injuries. This portion of the chapter discusses carpal fracture-dislocations and intercarpal dislocations. Carpometacarpal fractures and dislocations also occur and are discussed elsewhere (see Chapters 25 and 26).

The contributions of Mayfield and associates,[139–142] Taleisnik,[221] and Taleisnik and Kelly[222] have helped to clarify the mechanism and sequence of injury in intercarpal dislocations. Tanz[224] first pointed out the importance of intercarpal rotation in determining the direction of displacement of the distal carpal row. Mayfield[142] defined four stages of increasing dorsal perilunar instability observed when they loaded cadaver wrists experimentally in extension, ulnar deviation, and intercarpal supination. These stages were scapholunate instability (stage I) progressing through scapholunate dislocation (stage II) to triquetrolunate diastasis (stage III) before terminating in volar dislocation of the lunate (dorsal perilunate dislocation) (stage IV). These injuries can be associated with fractures of the scaphoid or triquetrum.

The exact mechanism of loading that results in volar perilunate dislocations and/or dorsal dislocation of the lunate has not been defined. Forced hyperflexion from a fall on the back of the hand has been proposed as the mechanism of injury by Aitken and Nalebuff.[4] O'Brien[168] has reported volar perilunate

dislocation from a fall onto a dorsiflexed wrist with supination of the forearm and proximal carpal row on the distal carpal row and hand. These reports underscore the fact that dislocations and fracture-dislocations of the wrist can occur from many different mechanisms.

Chapter 12 provides a full discussion of the classification of carpal injuries and instabilities. The clinician must be alert to almost any combination of injury requiring treatment plan modification.

Scapholunate Dissociation

DIAGNOSIS

Patients with scapholunate dissociation present with a history of a fall or motor vehicle accident along with pain, swelling, and decreased motion. Early diagnosis is important for successful treatment. Ruby[189] has highlighted the need to treat these dissociations early. Physical examination should include the elbow, forearm, and hand as well as the wrist, because associated injuries are not uncommon. The examiner should attempt to pinpoint the most painful area, which typically is the dorsal scapholunate area. Pain

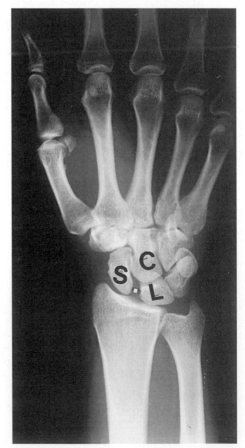

Figure 13–23. A scapholunate gap of greater than 3 or 4 mm indicates interosseous ligament injury. (S = scaphoid; C = capitate; and L = lunate.)

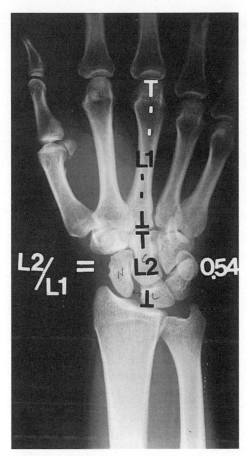

Figure 13–24. Use of the carpal height ratio allows one to evaluate carpal height *(L2)* compared with the third metacarpal length *(L1)*. Normal ratio (L2/L1) is 0.54 ± 0.03. Abnormal ratios indicate shortening of the carpus, found in dislocations and fractures. (Modified from Youn Y, Flatt A: Kinematics of the wrist. Clin Orthop 149:21–32, 1980.)

over third metacarpal length;[259A] Fig. 13–24), a wider appearance of the triquetrum as it acquires a dorsiflexed position, a foreshortened appearance of the scaphoid, and a double-density projection of the cortical waist of the scaphoid (the "ring" sign) indicate scapholunate dissociation[168] (Fig. 13–25). Abnormal carpal alignment and scapholunate gapping can be recreated by placing the wrist in radial or ulnar deviation or by loading the wrist as with a fist view (on an anteroposterior view) (Fig. 13–26). Moneim[155] has found that a tangential PA view with the ulnar border of the hand elevated 20° off the cassette is particularly helpful in demonstrating the scapholunate gap in subtle cases (Fig. 13–27).

Attention to the lateral view is also important. Chip fractures may be seen, especially on the lateral views (Fig. 13–28). A dorsal chip may indicate a ligament avulsion; therefore, special attention should be paid to the bony stability in the area of the chip. The alignment of the radius, lunate, and capitate should be colinear on the lateral view. In scapholunate dissociation, the scaphoid assumes a more vertical orientation with respect to the radius, and the proximal pole

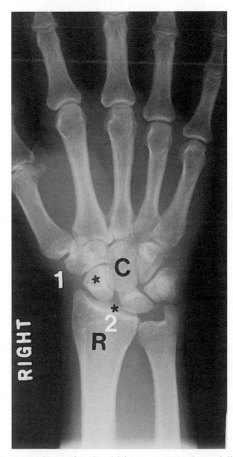

Figure 13–25. Radiographs should be investigated carefully for clues to carpal injuries, such as a foreshortened scaphoid appearance (*1*, flexed) and a ring sign (*) representing a double density projection of the scaphoid cortices. Scapholunate gaps may be visible (*2**) without stress or wrist deviation. (C = capitate; R = radius.)

is accentuated by dorsiflexion. Swelling is minimal. Pressure over the scaphoid tuberosity may be painful. Radiographs are especially helpful.

Dobyns and coworkers[58] describe six wrist views for evaluating the "sprained wrist," as follows: posteroanterior and lateral views in neutral, lateral views in maximal dorsiflexion and in palmar flexion, and posteroanterior views in maximal radial deviation and in ulnar deviation. We recommend PA radiographs in neutral, radial deviation, and ulnar deviation combined with a lateral radiograph. The lateral radiograph should be taken with the hand in neutral and the third metacarpal aligned with the radius. Deviation from this position alters the scapholunate angle. Comparison views can help erase any doubts about the involved side (Fig. 13–22). Three concentric arcs should be seen on the PA radiograph at the proximal and distal edges of the proximal carpal row and the distal proximal edge of the midcarpal row (see Fig. 13–20).[12A]

A scapholunate gap of more than 4 mm[73] may indicate disruption of the scapholunate interosseous ligament (Fig. 13–23). Additionally, a decreased carpal height ratio (< 0.54 ± 0.02, ratio of carpal height

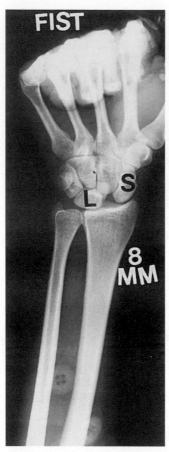

Figure 13–26. If suspected scapholunate injuries are not apparent on standard radiographs, stress views such as this one can produce a load across the carpus, highlighting a scaphoid-lunate gap. Abnormal gap is greater than 3 mm; here it is 8 mm. (S = scaphoid; L = lunate.)

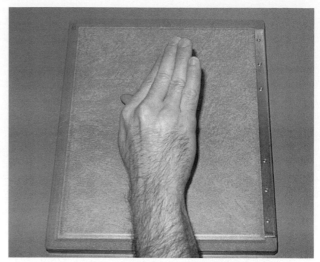

Figure 13–27. Example of a tangential view taken with the wrist in pronation with the ulnar border of the wrist elevated 20° off the film cassette and the radial border resting on the cassette.

is dorsal to the lunate and radius. Taleisnik[221] has described a "V" sign. In the lateral view, the normal, wide C-shaped line along the volar margins of the scaphoid and the radius becomes a sharper, V-shaped pattern when the scaphoid is subluxed. Abnormal lunate angulation is a key finding (see Fig. 13–22).

Gilula and associates[89A] discuss radiographic values for scapholunate angulation as follows. 30° to 60° is normal; more than 80° indicates DISI (scaphoid tilts volarly; lunate tilts dorsally); and less than 30° indicates VISI (scaphoid and lunate tilt volarly). In borderline cases (scapholunate angles 60° to 80°), comparison views can be very helpful. Further views may be necessary, including dynamic studies. No one set of radiographs is fully conclusive in all injury patterns. Therefore, one should continue to investigate wrist pain when radiographs are questionable.

Clinical stress tests may be used to define the amount of carpal instability. Watson and colleagues[245A] describe a test in which the examiner stabilizes the distal pole of the scaphoid and deviates the wrist. If instability exists, the proximal pole of the scaphoid can be forced out of its radial facet over the dorsal lip of the radius. The "clunk" appreciated

represents reduction of the scaphoid into its facet as the wrist is brought into ulnar deviation. The midcarpal shift test evaluates laxity of the distal row on the proximal row. In order for a valid test result to be obtained, the patient must be able to rest the elbows on the examination table and relax the forearm musculature. Normally, the examiner should be able to shift the carpus volarly, but not dorsally (see Fig. 13–9).

Wrist arthrography, cineradiography, trispiral tomography, and CT scans are sometimes useful adjuvant diagnostic techniques in the more chronic carpal instabilities. Magnetic resonance imaging's role remains to be defined because bony alignments are better seen on radiography. MR images may show ligament damage but are more reliable in diagnosing avascular necrosis. Arthroscopy is showing promise in diagnosis, allowing full examination of the ligamentous architecture of the wrist. It can also be used

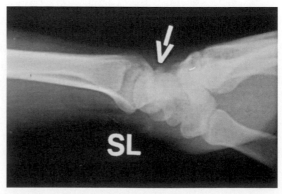

Figure 13–28. This lateral radiograph reveals a small dorsal chip (arrow), which correlates with the lunate and indicates a scapholunate ligament avulsion.

to help débride, reduce, and pin a scapholunate or triquetrolunate dissociation.

TREATMENT

If there is tenderness over the scapholunate joint but no radiographic evidence of separation or carpal malalignment, we treat the injury as a ligament sprain, with a short-arm cast for 6 weeks.

Complete scapholunate dissociation results when the entire scapholunate interosseous ligament, including its volar portion, is torn.[189] Prompt diagnosis, along with reduction and internal fixation to allow ligamentous healing, results in a high rate of success.[126] Unfortunately, the diagnosis is often missed, and the golden opportunity for restoring alignment is lost. Reduction, however, is feasible with some hope of ligamentous healing even as late as 3 months after injury.[29, 52, 126]

If the injury is very fresh (within the first few days), it is sometimes possible to close the scapholunate gap and to restore the colinear alignment of the lunate and capitate by dorsiflexing and radially deviating the wrist. We prefer to reduce the capitolunate joint by volar translocation and radial deviation of the hand and distal carpal row while stabilizing the forearm (Fig. 13–29). A 0.054-inch or 0.062-inch smooth Kirschner wire is driven across the capitolunate joint or radiolunate. The scaphoid can then be reduced to the lunate by 15° to 20° of radial deviation and volarly directed pressure to the proximal pole of the scaphoid. Two smooth Kirschner wires (0.054 or 0.062 inch) are driven through the scaphoid, one into the capitate and one into the lunate, under radiographic guidance. Advanced through the skin by pressure, the wires should not be drilled until they rest on bone, to avoid wrapping up neurovascular structures. Before multiple passes are made, a cutdown may be preferable, because of the presence of vital structures

in this area, as described by Steinberg and colleagues.[210A] A short-arm splint is applied postoperatively for 1 week, followed by a short-arm cast.

We prefer to cut our wires subcutaneously so that we can minimize the risk of pin tract infections. We leave the pins in for 8 weeks (see Fig. 13–29). A short-arm cast is worn full time for the first 8 weeks; then the pins are removed, and a removable splint is worn for 4 weeks. If there is any question about the adequacy of reduction, or if the injury has been present for more than 2 to 3 weeks, an open reduction is performed.

If the patient is a good surgical candidate, we open the wrist using our standard dorsal approach through the third dorsal compartment, taking care to avoid undermining the skin and injuring the superficial radial nerve (Fig. 13–30).

The extensor pollicis longus tendon is exposed in the third dorsal compartment and retracted radially. Lister's tubercle is then osteotomized, and the second compartment is reflected subperiosteally and radially. The fourth compartment is elevated subperiosteally and retracted ulnarly. Care is taken not to expose the fourth compartment tendon, which would increase postoperative morbidity. The longitudinal incision through the floor of the third compartment is continued distally to open the capsule and expose the scaphoid, lunate, and capitate.

If the injury is fresh, no sutures are necessary in the scapholunate ligament. Blood clot is removed from the scapholunate space. If the injury is subacute, we place drill holes in the edge of the scaphoid using a .063-inch Kirschner wire as a drill bit before reduction. We then pass 1-0 nonabsorbable sutures through these holes using a straight needle in retrograde fashion. The suture is then passed through the ligament and left untied.

The dorsiflexion instability of the lunocapitate joint is corrected by either the palmar shift maneuver

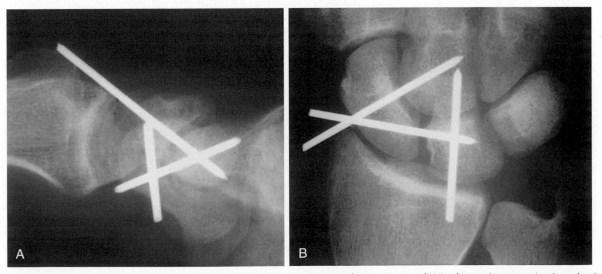

Figure 13–29. *A* and *B,* If fracture can be reduced closed and pinned, we prefer to use smooth Kirschner wires to maintain reduction.

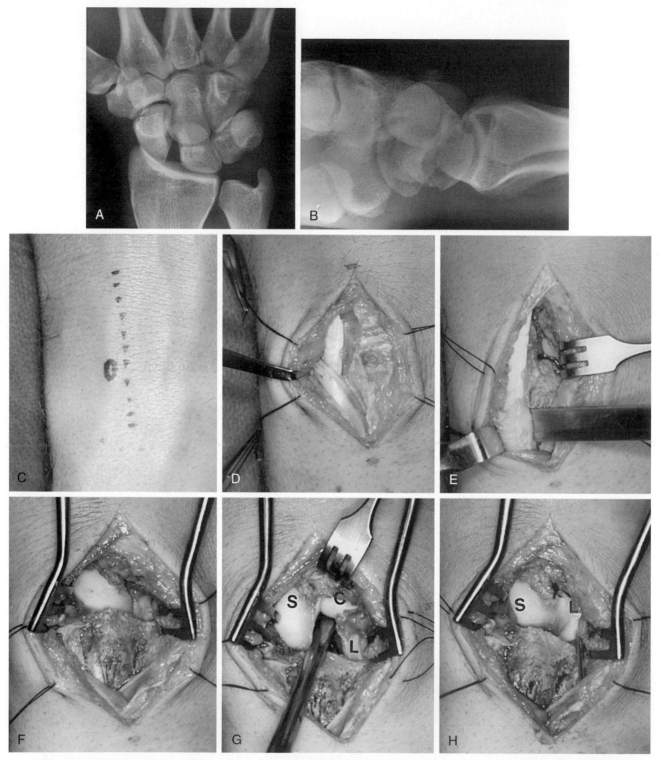

Figure 13–30. *A* and *B,* Our preferred technique for scapholunate ligament repair. *C,* Incision along the ulnar border of Lister's tubercle. The extensor pollicis longus tendon is identified and retracted *(D)* to allow osteotomy of the tubercle *(E).* F, Dissection and retraction of the fourth compartment allow wrist exposure. *G,* A joker is used to reduce the carpus after the articular surfaces are checked for injury. Reduction is peformed using joysticks as needed and is held with Kirschner wires before ligament repair (if possible) or after scaphoid-lunate sutures are placed but before they are tied. *H,* Repair of the scapholunate (SL) ligament is done; otherwise, sutures are passed with straight needles.

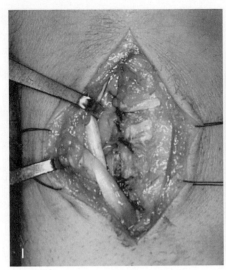
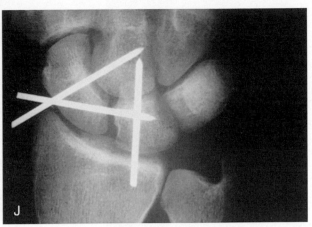

Figure 13–30 *Continued I,* A dorsal capsulorrhaphy is performed to complete the closure. *J,* The completed repair is verified radiographically. (S = scaphoid; L = lunate; C = capitate.)

or the joystick method. The joystick method uses 0.045-inch Kirschner wires placed in the waist of the scaphoid and the lunate to function as levers to reduce the scapholunate and lunocapitate joints. While the surgeon holds the reduction, an assistant drills the Kirschner wires across the lunocapitate, scapholunate, and scaphocapitate joints. The sutures are then tied in a horizontal mattress fashion over the ligament after reduction and pinning. This maneuver positions the knots off the articular surfaces. A dorsal capsulodesis is performed, which may include tightening of the radiotriquetral ligament. Suture anchors may be used for capsulodesis.[231B]

The postoperative course is the same as that for closed reduction and pinning. We position the wrist in neutral for casting. The treatment of chronic or irreducible scapholunate dissociations is covered in Chapter 15.

Dorsal Perilunate and Volar Lunate Dislocations

DIAGNOSIS

If the hyperextension force on the wrist continues, the radioscaphocapitate ligament tears (or an avulsion fracture of the radial styloid occurs), and the capitate dislocates dorsally from the lunate (stage II perilunate instability).[139–142] Further hyperextension and intercarpal supination tear the dorsal and volar radiotriquetral ligaments (stage III), and volar dislocation of the lunate results when the distal carpus spontaneously reduces, pushing the lunate volarly (stage IV perilunate instability).[139–142]

The patient with a dorsal perilunate dislocation has considerable swelling, and a mini-silver fork deformity is often present.[168] If the swelling is not too great, it may be possible to palpate the edge of the capitate dorsally. Dislocation of the lunate causes volar swelling, and two-point discrimination is commonly diminished in the median nerve distribution secondary to acute carpal tunnel syndrome. The patient holds the fingers in semiflexion, and active and passive extension of the fingers are incomplete and painful. Both perilunate and trans-scaphoid perilunate dislocations have been reported to occur in children.[88, 174]

In a dorsal perilunate dislocation, the lateral radiograph shows the longitudinal axis of the capitate dorsal to the longitudinal axis of the radius, and the scaphoid is flexed (Fig. 13–31). In the anteroposterior projection, the carpus is foreshortened, with overlapping of the proximal capitate and distal lunate margins, and there is an abnormal gap between the scaphoid and the lunate.

In a lunate dislocation, the longitudinal axis of the capitate is colinear with that of the radius, and the lunate is displaced volarly, with its distal articular surface tilted anteriorly (the "spilled teacup" sign). In the AP view, the lunate assumes a triangular shape instead of its normal quadrilateral shape (the "piece of cheese" sign[181]) (see Fig. 13–31). Occasionally, the entire lunate may be displaced volarly and proximally under the anterior margin of the distal radius.

In both perilunate and trans-scaphoid perilunate dislocations, there is also an intermediate stage of injury, in which the carpal displacements are halfway between a perilunate and a lunate dislocation. The capitate is slightly dorsal to the longitudinal axis of the radius, and the lunate is angulated volarly but has not fully dislocated. Distraction views made during finger-trap traction are often helpful in determining the extent of ligamentous damage and the presence of associated fractures in patients with perilunate or lunate dislocations.

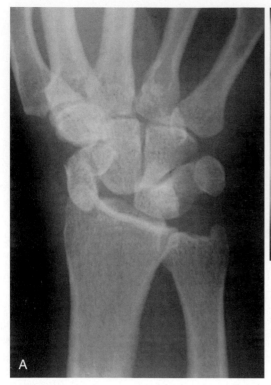

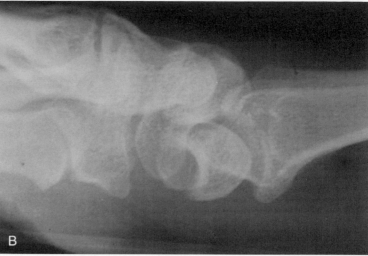

Figure 13–31. The triangular shape of the lunate when dislocated is shown as is a dorsal perilunate dislocation or volar lunate dislocation. Alignments are altered with abnormal gaps, bony overlap (capitate or lunate), scaphoid flexion, and the capitate lying dorsal to the radius. The lunate is dislocated volarly.

TREATMENT

Acute perilunate and lunate dislocations are usually relatively easy to reduce if the patient is seen early. After a thorough neurovascular evaluation of the extremity, closed reduction of the dislocation is attempted. Once adequate anesthesia (axillary block or general) has been achieved, vertical finger-trap traction is applied, with 10 to 15 lbs of counterweight across the upper arm, and is left undisturbed for about 5 minutes. Anteroposterior and lateral distraction radiographs are obtained during this time.

Manipulation, consisting of dorsiflexion followed by gradual palmar flexion and pronation to reduce the capitate back into the lunate, is then performed. If the lunate is dislocated volarly, the operator's thumb stabilizes the lunate as the capitate is brought into palmar flexion. Often, the initial stages of reduction of the lunate reproduce the dorsal perilunate stage prior to final reduction.

With traction maintained, the reduction is checked with anteroposterior and lateral radiographs. Sometimes, the dislocation is completely reduced, and there is no residual scapholunate dissociation. If this is the case, the hand and wrist are prepared for surgery, and the scapholunate and scaphocapitate joints are fixed in the reduced position with smooth percutaneously inserted 0.062-inch Kirschner wires, with use of the image intensifier, as in fixation for scapholunate dissociation. Two percutaneous pins are placed—one from scaphoid to capitate and one from scaphoid to lunate (see Fig. 13–31). Under no circum-

stances should one rely on a cast alone to maintain the reduction.

The postoperative course is the same as that described previously for closed or open pinning of scapholunate dissociation. The torn volar ligaments are approximated by reduction of the dislocation. Mild carpal tunnel symptoms usually resolve promptly after the reduction, and formal carpal tunnel release is not usually necessary.

If anatomic reduction cannot be achieved, open reduction with pin fixation through a dorsal approach, as described previously, is necessary (Fig. 13–32). The dorsiflexion instability of the lunate is often greater than in an isolated scapholunate dissociation. Two 0.045-inch smooth Kirschner wires, one in the dorsal nonarticular surface of the lunate and one in the dorsal nonarticular surface of the scaphoid, help manipulate the carpus. With use of these "joysticks," the reduction can be obtained and then held while smooth Kirschner wires are drilled sequentially from the lunate into the capitate, the scaphoid to the lunate, and the scaphoid to the capitate. The lunocapitate wire is the key wire to place first, to maintain alignment. If extra force is necessary, traction combined with placement of a blunt Freer elevator between the capitate and lunate will rotate the lunate back into alignment. We have found the short radiolunate ligament usually to be intact in these injuries.

Through the dorsal exposure, the lunocapitate relationship is restored and maintained with a 0.062-inch smooth Kirschner wire inserted from the lunate into the capitate. The dorsally subluxed scaphoid is reduced and is held while one Kirschner wire is drilled through the scaphoid into the lunate, and a second wire into the capitate; this is the same technique as already described.

The postoperative management is the same as that described for other carpal dislocations. We typically place a fourth 0.062-inch smooth Kirschner wire from the triquetrum into the lunate to fix the joint between them. This wire is more important when a lunotriquetral step-off or triquetral avulsion fracture is visualized. Posteroanterior radiographs of the wrist in radial and ulnar deviation may highlight the step-off.

After closed reduction of a volar lunate dislocation or an intermediate dislocation, residual scapholunate

dissociation as well as considerable dorsal instability of the lunate may be present. Treatment is the same as previously discussed to maintain reduction.

Occasionally, because the injury involves more ligamentous damage and tends to be quite unstable, a second, volar incision is needed to achieve reduction of the lunate and restoration of a colinear lunocapitate joint. We find that a volar incision is necessary only if the patient has worsening or unimproving complaints of neurologic impairment (median nerve distribution) or if reduction is impossible through the dorsal approach. The volar approach, an extended standard carpal tunnel incision, reveals a transverse tear in the volar capsule through the space of Poirer with the lunate volarly subluxed or dislocated

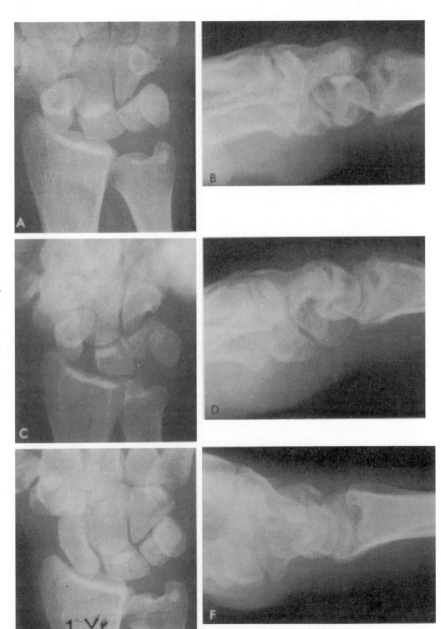

Figure 13–32. *A* and *B*, A 28-year old man sustained this dorsal perilunate dislocation in a car accident. *C* and *D*, Closed manipulation reduced the perilunate dislocation, but an obvious scapholunate dissociation is present. Open reduction and Kirschner wire fixation were performed through a dorsal approach, and the pins were left in for 8 weeks. *E* and *F*, Function was excellent at 1 year, and the radiographs were normal. (From O'Brien ET: Acute fractures and dislocations of the carpus. Orthop Clin North Am 15:237–258, 1984.)

through the defect into the carpal canal. Radiocarpal instability can occur after this injury. It is possible that a volar approach in suspected cases may prevent this complication. A radiocarpal pin may be an alternative solution. Unsuspected small osteochondral fractures, usually of the capitate and the lunate, are often found and require removal. If they are large, reduction and fixation are recommended. This can be done from the dorsal approach. When both incisions are utilized, the lunate is reduced and the volar capsular rent is repaired with 2-0 nonabsorbable sutures. These rents in the capsule do not usually involve the long radiolunate or short radiolunate ligament.

Dorsal Trans-Scaphoid Perilunate Dislocation

In dorsal trans-scaphoid perilunate dislocation, the intercarpal dislocation is accompanied by a fracture through the waist of the scaphoid. The distal scaphoid fragment is displaced dorsally with the rest of the distal row and the triquetrum, leaving the proximal fragment attached to the lunate. There is often considerable radial displacement of the scaphoid fracture and the distal carpus on the anteroposterior radiograph. The proximal scaphoid fragment and the lunate often tend to translate ulnarly. Concomitant avulsion fractures involving the radial styloid process and the triquetrum are often present.

The initial clinical evaluation and closed reduction techniques are identical to those described previously for a perilunate dislocation without fracture. Reduction of the intercarpal dislocation is usually easily accomplished, but residual scaphoid malalignment is the rule rather than the exception. The oblique radiograph shows the displacement best. Even if perfect alignment of the fractured scaphoid is achieved by closed reduction, it is very difficult to maintain with plaster immobilization in these inherently unstable injuries. Adkinson and Chapman[2] noted that 13 of 19 trans-scaphoid perilunate dislocations that were initially reduced anatomically by closed methods subsequently lost position and required late open reduction. Satisfactory closed pinning of the scaphoid fracture is difficult, and distraction may result. For these reasons, we prefer to reduce and fix the scaphoid by open reduction.[2, 73, 106, 156, 157, 175, 258] Prompt accurate reduction and internal fixation also seem to speed healing, and revascularization of the commonly associated increased density of the proximal scaphoid fragment is more rapid. True avascular necrosis is probably uncommon.[95–97]

The open reduction of the scaphoid fracture can be performed either through a dorsal or a volar incision. If the perilunate dislocation is well reduced, as it often is, the fracture can be approached volarly using the Russe incision paralleling the flexor carpi radialis tendon. Fixation can be accomplished with Kirschner wires or with a Herbert screw. The latter achieves excellent fixation with some compression of the frag-

ments (Fig. 13–33). Union was achieved with the screw in all 15 acute fracture-dislocations treated by Herbert and Fisher.[104] It is a demanding technique to master and requires a significant exposure of the normal scapho-trapezial joint; also, as Herbert and Fisher[104] noted themselves, unstable fractures associated with intercarpal dislocations are technically the most difficult ones to fix. Herbert screw fixation does allow earlier discontinuation of cast immobilization (at 6 weeks when ligamentous healing is satisfactory) than Kirschner wire fixation.

If difficulty is experienced in inserting the screw, one should not hesitate to abandon it in favor of Kirschner wire fixation. Two 0.045-inch smooth Kirschner wires are drilled in a parallel manner through the distal fragment, so that their position can be checked prior to reduction. The fracture is then reduced and held with a towel clip or reduction clamp, while the wires are advanced into the proximal fragment as far as the subchondral bone. We cut off our Kirschner wires subcutaneously and leave them in place for a minimum of 8 weeks.

If serial radiographs fail to show progress toward union by about 4 months, consideration should be given to bone grafting. Supplemental bone grafting is indicated during the initial procedure if there is comminution of the fracture that compromises stability.[95, 104] Our preference is the standard dorsal approach, because it makes the reduction of the scaphoid and the carpus easier. A Herbert screw can be placed in retrograde fashion freehand across the scaphoid. Smooth Kirschner wires are then used to fix the triquetrolunate joint.

If an avulsion fracture of the radial styloid exists and needs repair, a smooth Kirschner wire or screw can be used for fixation. If the fragment is small and displaced, excision is an option. If, however, the origins of the radioscaphocapitate and long radiolunate ligaments are involved, either the fragment must be anatomically fixed or the ligaments must be reattached to bone. Such fracture-dislocations are termed transradial trans-scaphoid perilunate fracture-dislocations. The observation of ulnar and radial styloid fragments should alert the examiner to the presence of a more severe carpal injury.

Volar Perilunate and Volar Trans-Scaphoid Perilunate Dislocation

Only a few isolated cases of volar perilunate and volar trans-scaphoid perilunate dislocation, rare injuries, have been reported in the literature.[4, 68, 180, 193, 257] Volar perilunate dislocation, like its more common dorsal counterpart, is always accompanied by either a scaphoid fracture or scapholunate dissociation. The lunate is palmar flexed, and the capitate is displaced volarly. Because of the rarity of this injury, the proper diagnosis is liable to be missed. Although

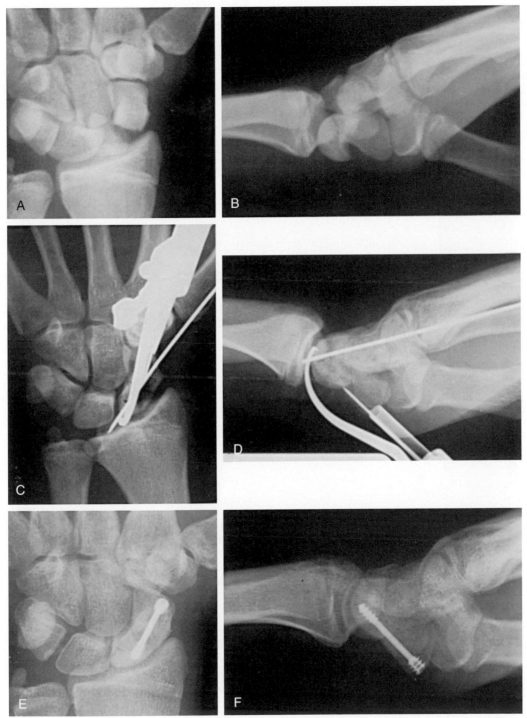

Figure 13–33. *A* and *B,* This 17-year-old student sustained a dorsal trans-scaphoid perilunate dislocation when he fell while playing baseball. Closed reduction was successful in reducing the perilunate dislocation. *C* and *D,* Through a volar Russe approach, the scaphoid was reduced and temporarily fixed with a Kirschner wire, and a Herbert screw was inserted. Plaster immobilization was continued for only 6 weeks. *E* and *F,* Three and a half months after injury, the patient had regained most of his wrist motion, and union was almost complete.

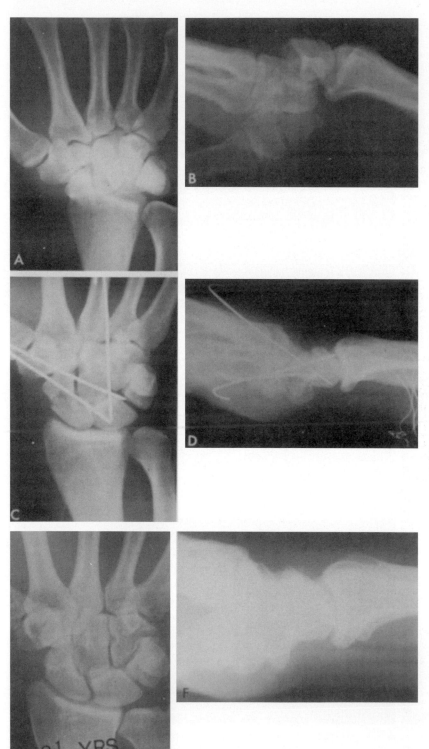

Figure 13–34. *A* and *B,* A 25-year-old man sustained a volar trans-scaphoid perilunate dislocation when he tripped over a fallen teammate while playing basketball. *C* and *D,* Closed reduction with finger-trap traction reduced the perilunate displacement; however, residual displacement of the scaphoid fracture necessitated open reduction and Kirschner wire fixation through a volar Russe approach. The pins were left in place for 8 weeks, and plaster immobilization was continued for 13 weeks. *E* and *F,* Two and a half years after injury, the patient had 90% of normal wrist motion and only a 20-lb diminution of grip strength. (From O'Brien ET: Fractures and dislocations of the carpal bones. In Kane WJ (ed): Current Orthopaedic Management. New York, Churchill-Livingstone, 1981, by permission.)

the PA radiograph shows overlapping carpal rows, the lunate dislocation is best seen on the lateral radiograph (Fig. 13–34).

Closed reduction of a volar perilunate dislocation utilizing finger-trap traction, with supination of the hand and distal carpal row, is sometimes successful. Reduction and fixation of the residual scapholunate dislocation can be performed through a dorsal approach if they cannot be achieved in a closed manner. Kirschner wire fixation must be maintained for 8 weeks.

A volar trans-scaphoid perilunate dislocation is apt to be widely displaced and may be more unstable than the more common dorsal variety.[193] Open reduction and internal fixation of the scaphoid fracture can be accomplished either through a volar Russe incision or through a dorsal approach, once the perilunate dislocation is reduced (Fig. 13–34). We prefer to use a dorsal approach for its versatility and better exposure. We also add triquetrolunate pinning.

Dorsal Dislocation of the Lunate

Dorsal dislocation of the lunate is even more uncommon than volar perilunate dislocation (Fig. 13–35). Fisk[72] postulated that the injury resulted from forced palmar flexion of the wrist, but the mechanism is unknown.

Seidenstein[195] reported that a patient with a dorsal dislocation of the lunate was treated by delayed excision of the bone at 2 weeks and had a satisfactory result 1 year after surgery. We would prefer open reduction and internal fixation. Bilos and Hui[16] reported on two patients with dorsal dislocation of the lunate, both of whom were treated by open reduction and pin fixation. Each achieved a satisfactory clinical result, although increased density of the lunate without collapse was noted in one of the patients at 1 year. Dorsal dislocation of the lunate may be associated with rupture of the long and short radiolunate ligaments. Repair of these ligaments as well as decompression of the median nerve can be done through a volar approach.[97] Small suture anchors may

be useful. We recommend a volar approach for open reduction and internal fixation, followed by immobilization for 8 weeks. Loss of the radiolunate ligaments may allow ulnar translation of the carpus.

Variants of Trans-Scaphoid Perilunate Dislocation

SCAPHOCAPITATE SYNDROME

In scaphocapitate syndrome, a relatively uncommon variation of trans-scaphoid perilunate dislocation, the head of the capitate is fractured and rotated 180°. The squared-off contour of the proximal end of the capitate, best seen in a PA distraction view, is the key to making the proper diagnosis.[254] Fenton[67] coined the term "naviculocapitate syndrome" in 1956, postulating that the fracture resulted from a force transmitted from the radial styloid through the waist of the scaphoid. Stein and Seigel[210] presented what appears to be the most logical mechanism of injury, that is, direct compression of the capitate on the lip of the proximal radius with the wrist in acute hyperextension. The proximal capitate fragment is rotated 90° secondary to its dorsiflexion, and return of the hand to the neutral position completes the 180° rotation (Fig. 13–36).

At least half of the reported cases have been associated with a dorsal trans-scaphoid perilunate dislocation, and two cases of volar trans-scaphoid perilunate dislocation with fracture of the proximal capitate have been reported.[147, 154] When a scaphocapitate syndrome is seen without a perilunate dislocation, diagnosis of the capitate fracture is often missed. Presumably, perilunate dislocation occurred at the time of injury and spontaneously reduced.[86, 115] We have not found capitate head fractures displaced into the carpal tunnel.

Fenton[67] advocated excision of the proximal pole as primary treatment, because he believed that avascular necrosis and non-union were inevitable. Although Jones[115] and Adler and Shaftan[3] have reported cases in which the fragment healed in its malrotated posi-

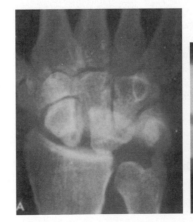
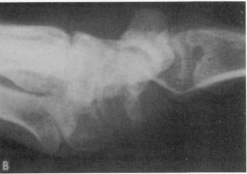

Figure 13–35. *A* and *B,* This dorsal dislocation of the lunate resulted from a fall from a wheelchair. The patient, who suffered from a paralytic neuromuscular disorder, eventually had the lunate excised because of a long delay in diagnosis. (Case courtesy of Richard Eaton, MD.)

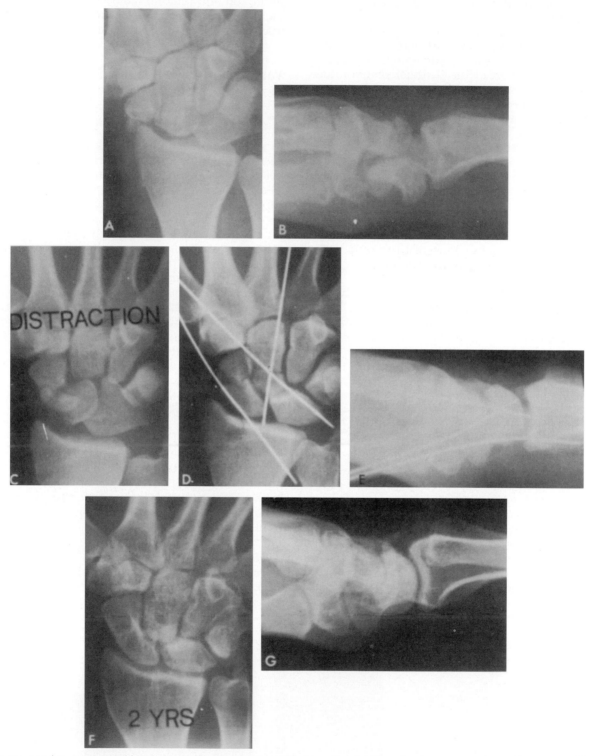

Figure 13–36. *A* and *B,* A 21-year-old man sustained a dorsal trans-scaphoid perilunate dislocation in a motorcycle accident. *C,* In addition, there is a displaced fracture of the proximal end of the capitate, seen best on a distraction view. *D* and *E,* Open reduction and internal fixation of the capitate and scaphoid fractures were performed through a dorsal approach on the day of injury. Pin fixation was continued for 8 weeks, and plaster immobilization was discontinued at 20 weeks. *F* and *G,* Two years later, radiographs showed good healing of the scaphoid and capitate fractures, and function was good. (From O'Brien ET: Fractures and dislocations of the carpal bones. In Kane WJ (ed): Current Orthopaedic Management. New York, Churchill Livingstone, Inc, 1981, by permission.)

tion, Marsh and Lampros[136] subsequently demonstrated that the fragment may undergo necrosis if left unreduced. Healing of the capitate fracture with good restoration of function has been achieved by open reduction and internal fixation.[64, 147, 185, 233, 254] Transient avascular changes are usually seen, but collapse and non-union are unusual (Fig. 13–36).[183] Even late reduction and fixation of a capitate fracture that was initially missed may be achieved if the articular cartilage looks healthy, though this is unlikely. We agree that open reduction with internal fixation through a dorsal approach is the treatment of choice. A volar approach is used if a dorsal approach is unsuccessful for reduction or neurologic symptoms are present.

TRANSTRIQUETRAL TRANS-SCAPHOID PERILUNATE DISLOCATION

Small avulsion fractures from the dorsal aspect of the triquetrum are seen fairly commonly in association with perilunate dislocations (Fig. 13–37). A transverse or oblique fracture through the bone is occasionally seen in conjunction with a trans-scaphoid perilunate dislocation or a scaphocapitate syndrome.[254] The line of cleavage in this case extends through the triquetrum, leaving its proximal half

attached to the lunate and allowing the distal fragment to be displaced with the capitate. The fracture fragments may reduce as the perilunate dislocation is reduced. If open reduction and fixation are required for persistent displacement, the standard dorsal incision is extended so that the triquetrum can be exposed. Additionally, the subperiosteal dissection of the fourth compartment is extended more ulnarly, with care taken not to detach the dorsal radioulnar ligament nor enter the distal radioulnar joint. If further exposure is required, the dissection proceeds in a plane superficial to this ligament. Rarely is this dissection necessary.

VOLAR DISLOCATION OF THE PROXIMAL SCAPHOID FRAGMENT (WITH OR WITHOUT DISLOCATION OF THE LUNATE)

Weiss and associates[253] reported treating a patient with a dorsal trans-scaphoid perilunate dislocation that could not be reduced because the proximal fragment was dislocated anteriorly and rotated 180°. The displaced proximal scaphoid fracture had a rounded appearance on the posteroanterior view. Open reduc-

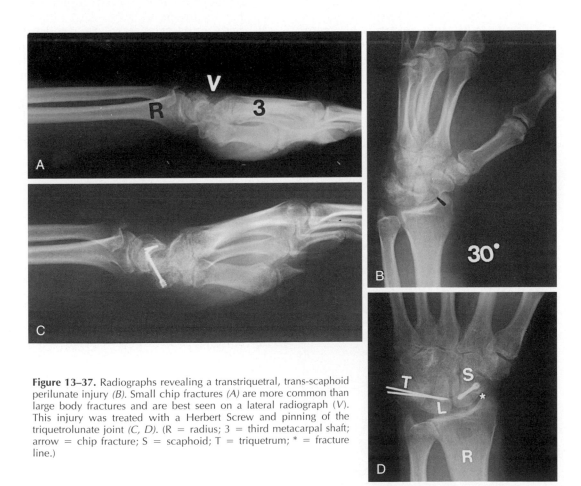

Figure 13–37. Radiographs revealing a transtriquetral, trans-scaphoid perilunate injury (B). Small chip fractures (A) are more common than large body fractures and are best seen on a lateral radiograph (V). This injury was treated with a Herbert Screw and pinning of the triquetrolunate joint (C, D). (R = radius; 3 = third metacarpal shaft; arrow = chip fracture; S = scaphoid; T = triquetrum; * = fracture line.)

tion through a volar Russe approach was followed by union without evidence of avascular necrosis.

This injury most likely results when a scapholunate dissociation and a waist fracture of the scaphoid occur together. The displaced bone should be approached volarly to avoid injuring any remaining soft tissue attachment (Fig. 13–38). O'Carroll and Gallagher[169] reported a patient with an irreducible dorsal trans-scaphoid perilunate dislocation in which the proximal scaphoid was displaced dorsally and rotated 180°. Open reduction performed through a dorsal incision 5 days after injury was followed by healing.

A fractured scaphoid is rarely encountered in association with a volar dislocation of the lunate. When these injuries coexist, the proximal scaphoid fragment is apt to be displaced volarly with the lunate as a single unit. The injury is more likely to be open than is the usual trans-scaphoid perilunate or lunate dislocation.[96] As Russell[192] noted in the six cases he reported, reduction is more difficult than in the routine case, and in two of his cases, the displaced lunate and scaphoid fragments were excised when reduction failed. Unsatisfactory results (non-union and avascular necrosis of the proximal scaphoid) followed open reduction and fixation in both patients with this injury, as cited in the report by Green and O'Brien.[95] Stern,[211] however, achieved satisfactory results in two patients with this injury who were treated with immediate open reduction and internal fixation. Although complications may occur, the results still depend on early recognition and accurate reduction; therefore, we recommend open reduction and internal fixation.

Individual Carpal Bone Dislocations

DISLOCATION OF THE SCAPHOID (WITH OR WITHOUT DISLOCATION OF THE LUNATE)

Dislocation of the scaphoid can occur alone[36, 70, 124, 134, 160, 230, 245] or in association with a volar dislocation of the lunate.[34, 37, 44, 123] If both bones are dislocated, they may have become so as a unit or separately. The mechanism of injury is unknown, but loading in dorsiflexion and ulnar deviation seems most likely. The high force required to dislocate a scaphoid should alert the examiner to look for associated injuries.

In isolated dislocations of the scaphoid, the bone dislocates radially, and often there is an accompanying fracture of the radial styloid (Fig. 13–39). The scaphoid may dislocate without any intercarpal displacement, but commonly there is also a radial displacement of the distal carpal row, with the head of the capitate displaced between the dislocated scaphoid and the lunate. Closed reduction using longitudinal traction and radial deviation often successfully reduces the scaphoid, but a residual scapholunate dissociation is often present. Avascular necrosis following replacement of the scaphoid is usually transient, if it occurs at all.[245]

Taleisnik and associates[223] reported treating a patient with simultaneous volar dislocation of the scaphoid and lunate as a unit. Closed reduction was successful, but lunotriquetral dissociation and palmar flexion instability of the lunate were noted 6 weeks after injury. These researchers collected five

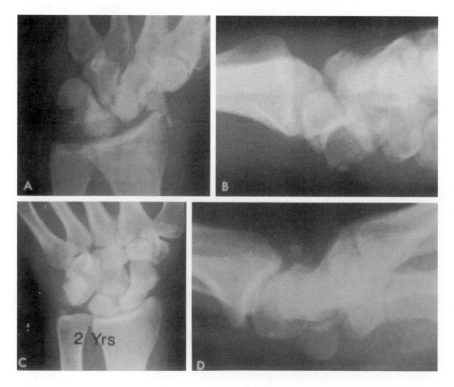

Figure 13–38. A 23-year-old man sustained a dorsal trans-scaphoid perilunate dislocation in a motorcycle accident. *A*, In the posteroanterior view, the proximal scaphoid fragment is displaced and overlapped by the capitate. *B*, In the lateral view, the proximal scaphoid fragment is volarly displaced and rotated forward. Closed reduction failed. Open reduction was therefore performed through a volar incision. Casting was continued for 6 months. *C, D,* At 2 years, the scaphoid fracture was well healed, and function was excellent. (From Kane WJ [ed]: Current Orthopaedic Management. New York, Churchill Livingstone, Inc, 1981.)

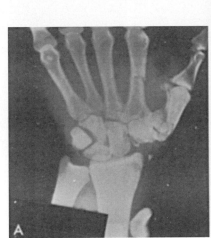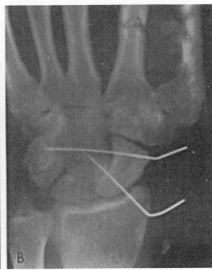

Figure 13–39. *A,* A 19-year-old man sustained this open, markedly displaced dislocation of the scaphoid and fractures of the first and second metacarpals in a motorcycle accident. The capitate is displaced proximal and radial to the lunate. The scaphoid was replaced and fixed with Kirschner wires. *B,* Two months later, there is slightly increased density of the scaphoid. The pins were removed at this time, and unfortunately, the patient was lost to follow-up. (From O'Brien ET: Acute fractures and dislocations of the carpus. Orthop Clin North Am 15:237–258, 1984.)

similar cases from the literature, but only one had an adequate follow-up. The patient in this case, as reported by Dunn,[60] had a good result 2 years after open reduction and Kirschner wire fixation. In the patient reported by Kupfer,[123] a dorsal intercalated segment instability followed an open reduction and internal fixation performed 90 days after volar dislocation of the scaphoid and the lunate as a unit. Cleak[44] and Kupfer[123] both emphasized the need for early reduction and internal fixation of this injury.

Gordon[94] described a patient who had simultaneous volar dislocation of the scaphoid and the lunate in which the bones were dissociated from each other. Open reduction and cast immobilization for 4 weeks were followed by chronic scapholunate dissociation of the scaphoid a year after injury (Fig. 13–40). Although the rarity of this dislocation prevents a large series from addressing treatment options, we agree with the recommendation by McNamara and Corley[146] for open reduction and internal fixation using Kirschner wires.

DISLOCATION OF THE TRAPEZOID

Twenty cases of trapezoid dislocation (16 dorsal and 4 volar) have been recorded.[122] Volar dislocations are commonly associated with metacarpal injuries. Open reduction of the volarly dislocated trapezoid is usually necessary because of its wedge shape, the area of palmar surface being more than 50 percent larger than that of the dorsal surface.[208] Open reduction may require only a dorsal incision, but late volar dislocation of the trapezoid requires both dorsal and volar incisions. Acute dorsal dislocations of the trapezoid can usually be reduced by closed manipulation.[13, 148] Avascular necrosis may follow open reduction of either type of dislocation.[186, 208] Anticipating this problem, Goodman and Shankman[92, 93] performed a primary limited arthrodesis after relocation of a volarly dislocated trapezoid and reduction of an associated index and middle carpometacarpal dislocation.

DISLOCATION OF THE TRAPEZIUM

Complete dislocation of the trapezium is a rare injury that is usually produced by direct trauma. Volar dislocations[30, 90, 196, 198] predominate over dorsal dislocations,[21, 60] and open injury is common. Several methods of treatment have been reported, including acceptance of the dislocation,[192] closed reduction,[60] and primary excision.[90, 176] Open reduction and internal fixation of the displaced trapezium may be followed by complete loss of thumb carpometacarpal motion.[196, 198] Good results, however, have been achieved by open reduction,[21, 30] which is the method of choice when closed reduction is unsuccessful.

DISLOCATION OF THE PISIFORM

Dislocation of the pisiform is an uncommon injury, usually resulting from sudden violent contraction of the flexor carpi ulnaris muscle and only occasionally from direct injury. Proximal,[137] distal,[150] ulnar,[78] and volar[45] dislocations have been reported. Closed reduction may be successful but is likely to be followed by persistent or recurrent dislocation after removal of the cast.[109, 137] Re-displacement has resulted even after open reduction and pin fixation with immobilization for 8 weeks.[150] Excision of this bone is the best treatment for an acute or recurrent pisiform dislocation.[168] Although the pisiform itself is expendable, proper reapproximation of its many attachments is essential to maintain the balance of structures on the ulnar border of the hand and wrist.

DISLOCATION OF THE HAMATE

Dislocation of the hamate is an exceedingly rare injury. In the nine published cases in which the di-

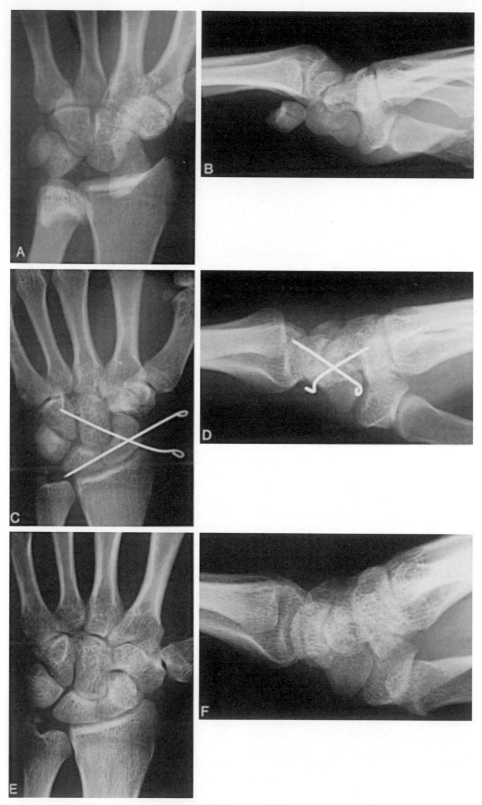

Figure 13–40. *A* and *B,* This 25-year-old man sustained a volar dislocation of the lunate and scaphoid in a fall from a motorcycle. Decreased sensation was noted in the median distribution. *C* and *D,* Closed reduction was unsuccessful, so open reduction and internal fixation were carried out through dorsal and volar incisions. *E* and *F,* Four months later, bone density was unchanged, but early narrowing of the lunocapitate and scapholunate joints was present. The patient regained full sensibility, had no pain, and returned to work.

rection of dislocation is known, five dislocations were volar and four dorsal. Duke[59] achieved a stable closed reduction of a volarly dislocated hamate by pronating the forearm without anesthesia. If closed reduction fails, open reduction and temporary Kirschner wire fixation should achieve a satisfactory result.[78, 84, 101]

DISLOCATION OF THE TRIQUETRUM

Only three cases of isolated triquetral dislocation have been reported, two volar[76, 201] and one dorsal.[15] Both volar dislocations were missed initially—one was discovered 7 weeks and one 4 months after injury—and required late excision. The chronic median nerve compression was relieved, and essentially full motion was restored 19 months and 34 months, respectively, after excision. Open reduction of a dorsal triquetral dislocation 7 days after injury was followed by full return of motion and grip strength 8 months later in the patient reported by Bieber and Weiland.[15]

DISLOCATION OF THE CAPITATE

Russell[192] reported a patient who had an open dorsal dislocation of the capitate with the third and fourth metacarpals, and a dorsal dislocation of the trapezoid with the second metacarpal. Open reduction and plaster immobilization for 10 weeks were followed 6 months later by a return of one third of normal wrist motion and a powerful grip. Two total volar dislocations of the capitate have been reported, both associated with other carpal injuries. Open reduction was carried out in both patients, and carpometacarpal degenerative changes were noted 10 months[131] and 20 months[60] later.

Other Intercarpal Dislocations

SCAPHOTRAPEZIOTRAPEZOID DISLOCATIONS

Gibson[89] reported a patient with a dorsal dislocation of the scaphotrapeziotrapezoid joint in which full motion was restored by open reduction with Kirschner wire fixation for 6 weeks. He made a reference to a patient reported by Tachakara[218]—a 13-year-old boy with a diastasis of the scaphotrapezial joint that closed spontaneously after 4 weeks of plaster immobilization. Two patients who had chronic (6 months and 8 months) dorsal dislocation of the trapezium and trapezoid with their attached first and second metacarpals on the scaphoid ("radial hand dislocation") were reported by Watson and Hempton.[246] Satisfactory function was restored in both cases by trapezial-trapezoid-scaphoid arthrodesis.

TRIQUETROLUNATE DISSOCIATION

Diagnosis

Triquetrolunate dissociation represents a carpal instability with abnormal alignment between the lunate and triquetrum. It occurs secondary to a tear of the triquetrolunate interosseous ligament, dorsal radiotriquetral ligament, and/or volar lunotriquetral ligament following a dorsiflexion or hyperpronation injury to the wrist.[168, 184] Patients typically present with dorsal ulnar-sided wrist pain. Stressing of the triquetrolunate dissociation reveals pain and point tenderness as well as increased motion, reproducing the patient's symptoms. Reagan and colleagues[184] described the physical finding triquetral balottement, wherein the lunate is stabilized with the examiner's one hand while the triquetrum is shifted both dorsally and palmarly with the other. Radiographs reveal a step-off between the two bones on the PA view. Deviation views may increase the step-off. The carpal bones assume a VISI pattern on the lateral view in complete cases. Arthroscopy reveals a tear or increased laxity of the triquetrolunate ligament, a step-off between the triquetrum and lunate on midcarpal arthroscopy, or abnormal motion between these two carpal bones.

On the basis of cadaver studies, Viegas and colleagues[242] classified triquetrolunate dissociations as a progression of ligament disruptions producing no abnormal carpal pattern (lunotriquetral interosseous ligament only), a dynamic VISI pattern (interosseous and volar lunotriquetral ligament), or a static VISI pattern (interosseous, volar lunotriquetral, and dorsal radiocarpal ligaments).

Treatment

Nonoperative treatment may be tried first. Splinting, nonsteroidal anti-inflammatory medication, and occupational therapy for range of motion and strengthening can be used.

For acute injuries without a resulting VISI pattern, we agree with use of an arthroscopically or radiographically guided closed pinning of the triquetrolunate joint. If a VISI pattern is present, however, indicating considerable ligamentous injury, we prefer a volar and dorsal approach with reduction, internal fixation of the triquetrum to the lunate, and ligamentous repair (both volar and dorsal). If this repair fails, we prefer a midcarpal arthrodesis including the scaphoid, capitate, lunate, hamate, and triquetrum (Fig. 13–41). One approach to failure of conservative treatment is to perform ulnar shortening, which results in tightening of the ulnar carpal ligaments and may help stabilize the triquetrolunate joint. We use this treatment in chronic cases only if no VISI is present.

Several reviews of lunotriquetral fusions have found the fusion to predictably relieve pain and allow patients to return to work.[121A, 164A, 177A, 177B] Nelson and associates[164A] recommend wire and Herbert screw fixation over Kirschner wire fixation alone.

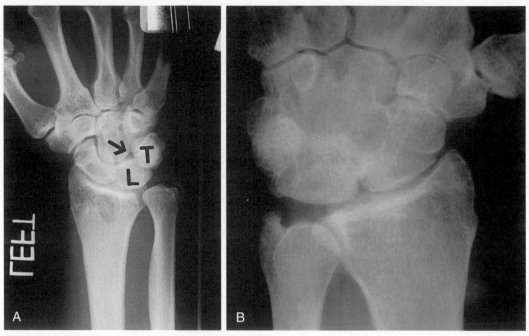

Figure 13–41. A, The *arrow* indicates the triquetrolunate stepoff following TL ligament injuries. Closed reduction and pinning is recommended, if possible. B, Late arthritis can be salvaged with a midcarpal arthrodesis. (T = triquetrum; L = lunate.)

Taking a minimum of 8 weeks, fusion should be verified with CT scan or tomogram before therapy is started.[164A] Approximately 80 percent of range of motion may be preserved as compared with the other arm.[121A, 177B] Recovery of grip strength is quite variable (60 and 90 percent).[121A, 177B] Our experience with triquetrolunate fusions does not confirm these results. Therefore, we do not routinely perform fusion.

TRANSTRIQUETRAL PERILUNATE FRACTURE-DISLOCATION

The natural continuation of a perilunate injury propagates around the lunate and toward the triquetrum. It may occasionally propagate through the triquetrum itself. With this type of injury, the proximal portion of the triquetrum stays with the lunate as the triquetrolunate interosseous ligament is undisturbed. The distal fragment displaces dorsally with the capitate and distal row. This fracture should be reduced anatomically, and we recommend internal fixation using K wires or a screw for fixation. We have not found non-union to be a problem in this injury.

Axial Carpal Dislocations

CRUSH INJURY OF THE CARPUS

Mechanism of Injury and Diagnosis

Garcia-Elias and associates[81] coined the term "crush injury of the carpus" to describe an injury characterized by disruption of the carpal arch through the capitohamate joint distally and the pisotriquetral

joint proximally. These researchers reviewed nine similar cases from the literature[3, 181] and added the details and outcomes of four new cases.

Disruption of the capitohamate joint distally with ulnar and volar dislocation of the hamate and its

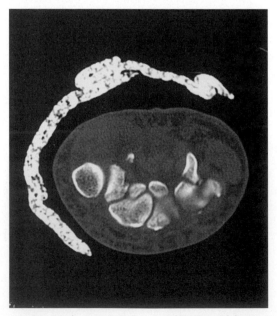

Figure 13–42. Crush injuries are a combination of bone and soft tissue injuries with poorer prognoses than isolated injuries. The injury illustrated here occurred when a dumpster fell on this man's hand, leading to hamate hook and trapezium fractures, with the development of an acute carpal tunnel syndrome due to hematoma that necessitated emergency decompression.

attached fourth and fifth metacarpals, with disruption of the pisotriquetral joints proximally, results from a severe crush with flattening of the carpal arch. The capitate and hamate bones are normally tightly associated, requiring considerable force to be displaced. Clinically, the ring and little finger are ulnarly deviated and malrotated, and there is often an associated bursting-type laceration of the thenar eminence. Three different variations of medial capitohamate dislocation were described by Garcia-Elias and associates[81]: fracture of the hamate with pisotriquetral dislocation, dislocation of the capitohamate and pisotriquetral joints without fracture, and dislocation with a displaced fracture of the triquetrum. The injury is best seen using PA and partially supinated oblique views of the wrist.

Additionally, crush injuries produce diffuse swelling and soft tissue trauma (Fig. 13–42). Immobiliza-

tion for fracture healing further increases the severity of adhesions, complicating rehabilitation. Additionally, nerve compromise may occur acutely from swelling, hematoma, or inflammation. Serial neurologic assessments are necessary, and patient education allows for monitoring if early discharge is considered.

Treatment

Closed reduction may be successful if done early; however, the initial diagnosis is apt to be missed, necessitating open reduction and internal fixation (Fig. 13–43).[181] The goal of reduction is to recreate the transverse arch and prevent rotational malalignment.

Late Treatment of Missed Dislocations

Intercarpal dislocations continue to be missed even though patients usually present for treatment shortly

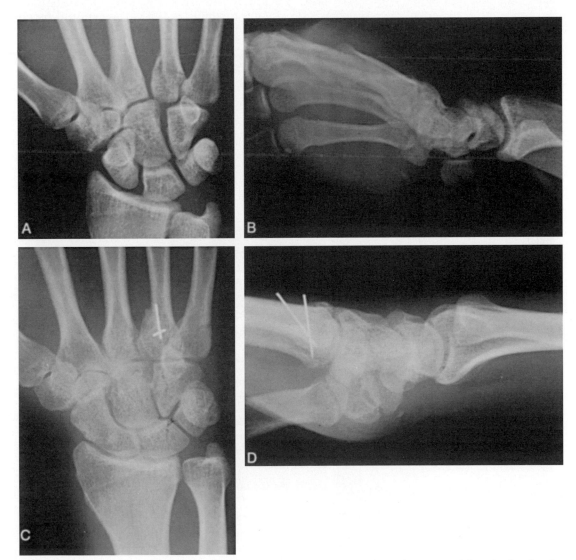

Figure 13–43. *A* and *B,* This 19-year old laborer sustained a crush injury of the carpus when a heavy pipe fell on his hand. A large wound was present over the proximal palm. Open reduction and internal fixation of the disrupted capitohamate joint and fourth metacarpal fracture were performed 6 days after injury. *C* and *D,* Four months later, the fracture had healed, and intercarpal relationships were normal. (Case courtesy of William E. Sanders, MD.)

after injury and wrist radiographs are ordered. The radiographs are usually difficult to interpret, however, having overlying shadows. Life-threatening injuries associated with the severe dislocations and fracture-dislocations prevent accurate initial examination and divert attention from the wrist injury. Scapholunate dislocation is the most commonly missed acute intercarpal injury, and its late management is discussed in Chapter 15.

Volar dislocation of the lunate is the next most commonly missed carpal dislocation. Fortunately, the dislocated bone can usually be replaced with a fair chance of success up to 6 months[37] and possibly even up to a year[23] after injury. Campbell and associates[38] reported satisfactory results in three late open reductions of the lunate performed 6 weeks, 3.5 months, and 6 months after injury. They emphasized the rarity of avascular necrosis following this injury and believed strongly that reduction gives a more satisfactory result than excision. We agree with their findings.

In open reduction, the median nerve is released, and the lunate is inspected through a long carpal tunnel incision. If the bone is not damaged and its cartilage surfaces appear healthy, the lunate is carefully mobilized using a Freer elevator, with care taken not to disrupt the consistently intact, short radiolunate ligament. A dorsal incision is usually required to clean the fibrous tissue from the space between the radius and capitate formerly occupied by the lunate. The lunate is then replaced by means of longitudinal traction and direct manipulation, utilizing the two incisions. Kirschner wire fixation of the scapholunate and the scaphocapitate and triquetrolunate joints is maintained for 8 weeks (Fig. 13–44). If the lunate cartilaginous surfaces are not healthy and too much time has elapsed since the dislocation occurred, excision of the bone without the insertion of a Silastic implant may yield an acceptable clinical result.[214] A collagen spacer ("anchovy") may be used. If fixed scaphoid rotation (flexion) is present, a midcarpal fusion to stabilize the carpus should be considered.

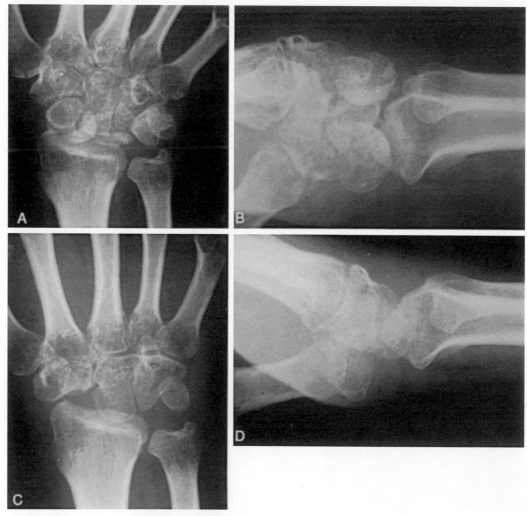

Figure 13–44. *A* and *B*, A 21-year-old man injured his wrist in a fall from a motorcycle. The volar lunate dislocation remained undiagnosed for 4 months. Open reduction was performed through dorsal and volar incisions. *C* and *D*, At 1 year, motion had almost returned to normal, and grip strength was equal to that of the uninjured side. (From O'Brien ET: Fractures and dislocations of the carpal bones. In Kane WJ (ed): Current Orthopaedic Management. New York, Churchill Livingstone, 1981, by permission.)

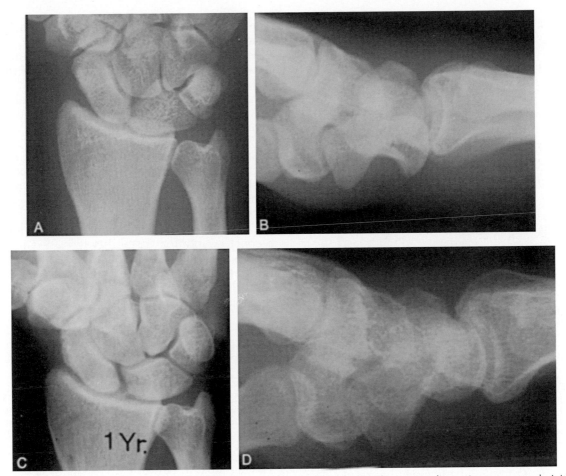

Figure 13–45. *A* and *B,* A 21-year-old man injured his wrist in a motor vehicle accident. The correct diagnosis was not made initially, and he presented 4 months later with unreduced dorsal perilunate dislocation. A proximal row carpectomy was performed. *C* and *D,* At 1 year, dorsiflexion was 40°, palmar flexion was 50°, and grip strength was two-thirds normal. Symptoms were minimal. (From O'Brien ET: Fractures and dislocations of the carpal bones. In Kane WJ (ed): Current Orthopaedic Management. New York, Churchill Livingstone, 1981, by permission.)

Late open reduction of a neglected dorsal perilunate dislocation can be attempted up to 6 or 8 weeks after injury, if the cartilage covering the displaced bones is healthy. Through a dorsal incision, a Freer elevator is used to carefully dissect around the capitate, lunate, and proximal pole of the scaphoid. Temporary Kirschner wire handles in the scaphoid and lunate are useful in securing and maintaining the reduction while smooth K wires for fixation are inserted. With a delay of 4 to 6 weeks after injury, consideration can be given to triscaphoid fusion at the same time that the reduction is performed. We prefer a midcarpal fusion (scaphoid-lunate-capitate-hamate-triquetrum). Pin fixation is continued for 8 weeks.

If the reduction is delayed more than 6 to 8 weeks, or if the condition of the bones precludes reduction, then proximal row carpectomy is a possible salvage procedure.[37, 54, 110, 117, 165] Pain relief is good, and instability has not been a problem. Motion and grip strength are surprisingly good, and the results do not seem to deteriorate with time (Fig. 13–45). If arthritis has occurred in both the radiocarpal and intercarpal joints, a complete wrist arthrodesis should be performed, correcting the deformity at the same time.

The same principles apply to the neglected trans-scaphoid perilunate dislocation; however, success in reducing and obtaining union of the displaced scaphoid fracture is less likely than for neglected lunate and perilunate dislocations. If delayed open reduction is performed, bone grafting of the scaphoid should be done at the same time. The indications for proximal row carpectomy and radiocarpal arthrodesis are the same as in perilunate dislocations. Both fragments of the scaphoid should be excised if proximal row excision is performed.

Complications of Intercarpal Dislocations and Fracture-Dislocations

Scaphoid non-union, delayed union, and avascular necrosis of the proximal fragment of the scaphoid are more commonly encountered with trans-scaphoid

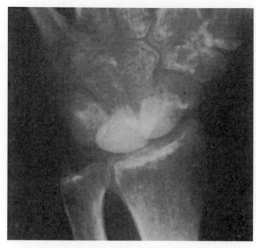

Figure 13–46. This radiograph, taken 12 weeks after closed reduction of a dorsal trans-scaphoid perilunate dislocation, shows increased density of the lunate proximal pole of the scaphoid. Healing occurred without collapse or fragmentation of either bone, and function was good. (From O'Brien ET: Acute fractures and dislocations of the carpus. Orthop Clin North Am 15:237–258, 1984.)

seem to be progressive, and revascularization occurred (Fig. 13–46).

Median neuritis accompanying perilunate and lunate dislocations has a good prognosis if the dislocation is reduced early. Delayed treatment may result in persistent symptoms, even if a carpal tunnel release is performed. Sympathetic dystrophy is a rare complication of intercarpal dislocations.[143]

Owing to the extensive damage of the ligamentous architecture of the wrist following fracture-dislocations, it is not surprising that stiffness is a common postoperative problem. Many surgical procedures intentionally sacrifice motion to achieve stability.[37, 38] Losses of range of motion (up to 50 percent) and grip strength have been reported following ligament reconstruction for instability.[37, 38, 105] Clinical retrospective reviews note increased stiffness with delayed treatment.[105] Patients need to be aware that some loss of mobility must be accepted to achieve the objectives of surgery.

perilunate dislocations than with simple scaphoid fractures. Scaphoid malunion usually results in subsequent painful arthritis and should be avoided by maintenance of accurate reduction until healing is complete. Osteotomy can occasionally salvage a malunited scaphoid fracture.[68] Because malunion does not necessarily produce a bad subjective result, however, we do not routinely recommend it.

Recurrence of scapholunate dissociation following closed or open reduction and fixation is sometimes noted after the fixation is removed and mobility of the wrist is regained. Although the scapholunate gap may recur, we find that the patient may still have a good result if the carpal alignment is preserved. Patients with recurrent dorsal trans-scaphoid perilunate dislocation were reported by Lowdon and associates.[130] One of these patients, a 20-year-old man, underwent closed reduction of a dorsal trans-scaphoid perilunate dislocation, and his wrist was immobilized for 3 months. Non-union was noted 8 months after injury, and 5 years later, after he sustained another dorsiflexion injury, recurrent closed trans-scaphoid perilunate dislocation occurred through the non-union. Open reduction and scaphoid bone grafting corrected the deformity, but union was not achieved.

Avascular necrosis of the lunate is rarely encountered following closed or open reduction of dislocations of this bone. Wagner[244] and Cave[40] each reported a single case of avascular necrosis of the lunate following closed reduction, but neither case showed the collapse and fragmentation typical of Kienböck's disease. Avascular necrosis involving the lunate and the proximal pole of the scaphoid has been seen in several cases of trans-scaphoid perilunate dislocation reported in the literature.[256] The changes did not

References

1. Adams BD, Frykman GK, Taleisnik J: Treatment of scaphoid nonunion with casting and pulse electromagnetic fields: A study continuation. J Hand Surg 17A:910–914, 1992.
1A. Adams BD, Blair WF, Reagan DS, Grundberg AB: Technical factors related to Herbert screw fixation. J Hand Surg 13A:893–899, 1988.
2. Adkinson JW, Chapman MW: Treatment of acute lunate and perilunate dislocations. Clin Orthop 164:199–207, 1982.
3. Adler JB, Shaftan GW: Fractures of the capitate. J Bone Joint Surg 44A:1537–1547, 1962.
4. Aitken AP, Nalebuff EA: Volar transnavicular perilunar dislocations of the carpus. J Bone Joint Surg 42A:1051–1057, 1960.
5. Alho A, Kanhaanjaa U: Management of fractured scaphoid bones: A prospective study of 100 fractures. Acta Orthop Scand 46:737–743, 1975.
6. Amadio PC, Berquist TH, Smith DK, et al: Scaphoid malunion. J Hand Surg 14A:679–687, 1989.
7. Amadio PC, Taleisnik J: Fractures of the carpal bones. In Green DP (ed): Operative Hand Surgery, vol 1. New York, Churchill-Livingstone, 1993, pp 799–860.
8. Armistead RB, Linscheid RL, Dobyns JH, Beckenbaugh RD: Ulnar lengthening in the treatment of Kienböck's disease. J Bone Joint Surg 64A:170–178, 1982.
9. Baird DB, Friedenberg ZB: Delayed ulnar nerve palsy following fracture of the hamate. J Bone Joint Surg 50:570–572, 1968.
10. Baldy Dos Reis F, Koeberle G, Leite NM, Katchburian MV: Internal fixation of scaphoid injuries using the Herbert screw through a dorsal approach. J Hand Surg 18A:792–797, 1993.
11. Bartone NF, Grieco RV: Fracture of the triquetrum. J Bone Joint Surg 38A:353–356, 1956.
12. Beckenbaugh RD: Accurate evaluation and management of the painful wrist following injury: An approach to carpal instability. Orthop Clin North Am 15:289–306, 1984.
12A. Bellinghausen HW, Gilula LA, Young LV, Weeks PM: Post-traumatic palmar carpal subluxation: Report of two cases. J Bone Joint Surg 65A:998–1006, 1983.
13. Bendre DV, Baxi VK: Dislocation of trapezoid. J Trauma 21:899–900, 1981.
14. Berlin D: Position in the treatment of fracture of the carpal scaphoid. N Engl J Med 201:574, 1929.
15. Bieber EJ, Weiland AJ: Traumatic dorsal dislocation of the triquetrum: A case report. J Hand Surg 9A:840–842, 1984.

16. Bilos J, Hui PW: Dorsal dislocation of the lunate with carpal collapse. J Bone Joint Surg 63A:1484–1486, 1981.

17. Bishop AT, Beckenbaugh RD: Fracture of the hook of the hamate. J Hand Surg 13A:135–139, 1988.

18. Bizairo AH: Traumatology of the carpus. Surg Gynecol Obstet 34:574–588, 1922.

19. Blair WF, Kilpatrick WC, Over GE: Open fracture of the hook of the hamate: A case report. Clin Orthop 163:180–184, 1982.

20. Blatt G: Capsulodesis in reconstructive hand surgery: Dorsal capsulodesis for the unstable scaphoid and volar capsulodesis following excision of the distal ulna. Hand Clin North Am 3A:81–102, 1987.

21. Boe S: Dislocation of the trapezium (multangulum majus). Acta Orthop Scand 50:85–86, 1979.

22. Bohler L, Trojan E, Jahna H: Die Behandlungsergebnisse von 734 frischen Bruchen des Kahnbeinkörpers der Hand. Widerherst, Traumatology 2:86–111, 1954.

23. Bohler L: The Treatment of Fractures. New York, Grune & Stratton, 1956.

24. Bolton-Maggs BG, Held BH, Ravell PA: Bilateral avascular necrosis of the capitate: A case report and a review of the literature. J Bone Joint Surg 66B:557–559, 1984.

25. Bonnin JG, Greening WP: Fractures of the triquetrum. Br J Surg 31:278–283, 1943.

26. Bora FW, Osterman AL, Brighton CT: The electrical treatment of scaphoid nonunion. Clin Orthop 161:33–38, 1981.

27. Bora FW Jr, Osterman AL, Woodbury Dr, et al: Treatment of nonunion of the scaphoid by direct current. Orthop Clin North Am 15:107–112, 1984.

28. Bowen TL: Injuries of the hamate bone. Hand 5:235–238, 1973.

29. Boyes JG: Subluxation of the carpal navicular bone. South Med J 69:141–144, 1976.

30. Brewood AFM: Complete dislocation of the trapezium: A case report. Injury 16:303–304, 1985.

31. Brighton CT: Semi-invasive method of treating non-union with direct current. Orthop Clin North Am 15:33–45, 1984.

32. Brittain HA: Fracture of the carpal scaphoid. Br Med J 2:671–673, 1938.

33. Broome A, Oedell CA, Coleen S: High plaster immobilization for fracture of the carpal scaphoid bone. Acta Chir Scand 128:42–44, 1964.

34. Brown RHL, Muddu BN: Scaphoid and lunate dislocation: A report on a case. Hand 13:303–307, 1981.

35. Bryan RS, Dobyns JH: Fractures of the carpal bones other than lunate and navicular. Clin Orthop 149:107–111, 1980.

35A. Bunker TD, McNamee PB, Scott TD: The Herbert screw for scaphoid fractures. J Bone Joint Surg 69B:631–634, 1987.

36. Buzby BF: Isolated radial dislocation of carpal scaphoid. Ann Surg 100:553–555, 1934.

37. Campbell RD Jr, Lance EM, Yeoh CB: Lunate and perilunar dislocations. J Bone Joint Surg 46B:55–72, 1964.

38. Campbell RD Jr, Thompson TC, Lance EM, et al: Indications for open reduction of lunate and perilunate dislocations of the carpal bones. J Bone Joint Surg 47A:915–937, 1965.

39. Carter PR, Eaton RG, Littler JW: Ununited fracture of the hook of the hamate. J Bone Joint Surg 59A:583–588, 1977.

40. Cave EF: Fractures and Other Injuries. Chicago, Year Book Medical Publishers, 1958, p 388.

41. Cetti R, Christensen SE: The diagnostic value of displacement of the fat stripe in fracture of the scaphoid bone. Hand 14:75–79, 1982.

42. Clay NR, Dias JJ, Costigan PS, et al: Need the thumb be immobilized in scaphoid fractures? A randomized prospective trial. J Bone Joint Surg 73B:828–832, 1991.

43. Clayton ML: Rupture of the flexor tendon in carpal tunnel (non-rheumatoid) with specific reference to fracture of the hook of the hamate. J Bone Joint Surg 51A:798–799, 1969.

44. Cleak DK: Dislocation of the scaphoid and lunate bones without fracture: A case report. Injury 14:278–281, 1982.

45. Cohen I: Dislocation of the pisiform. Ann Surg 75:238–239, 1922.

46. Connell MC, Dyson RP: Dislocation of carpal scaphoid: Report of a case. J Bone Joint Surg 37B:252–253, 1955.

47. Conway WF, Gilula LA, Manske PR, et al: Translunate, palmar perilunate fracture-subluxation of the wrist. J Hand Surg 14A:635–639, 1989.

48. Cooney WP, Bussey R, Dobyns JH, Linscheid RL: Difficult wrist fractures: Perilunate fracture-dislocations of the wrist. Clin Orthop 214:136–147, 1987.

49. Cooney WP, Dobyns JH, Linscheid RL: Fractures of the scaphoid: A rational approach to management. Clin Orthop 149:90–97, 1980.

50. Cooney WP, Dobyns JH, Linscheid RL: Nonunion of the scaphoid: Analysis of the results from grafting. J Hand Surg 5A:343–353, 1980.

51. Cooney WP, Linscheid RL, Dobyns JH: Scaphoid fractures: Problems associated with nonunion and avascular necrosis. Orthop Clin North Am 15:381–391, 1984.

52. Cope JR: Rotatory subluxation of the scaphoid. Clin Radiol 35:495–501, 1984.

53. Codrey LJ, Ferrer-Torells M: Management of fracture of the greater multangular. J Bone Joint Surg 42A:111–118, 1980.

54. Crabbe WA: Excision of the proximal row of the carpus. J Bone Joint Surg 46B:706–711, 1964.

55. Crosby EB, Linscheid RL: Rupture of the flexor profundus tendon of the ring finger secondary to ancient fracture of the hook of the hamate: Review of the literature and report of two cases. J Bone Joint Surg 56A:1076–1078, 1974.

56. Daffner RM, Emmerling EW, Buterbaugh GA: Proximal and distal oblique radiography of the wrist: Value in occult injuries. J Hand Surg 17A:499–503, 1992.

57. Dehno E, Deffer PA, Feighney RE: Pathomechanics of the fracture of the carpal navicular. J Trauma 4:96–114, 1964.

57A. DeMaagd RL, Engber WD: Retrograde Herbert screw fixation for treatment of proximal pole scaphoid nonunions. J Hand Surg 14A:996–1003, 1989.

57B. Diao G, Hatano I, Ishimoto T, Peimer CA: Anatomic scaphoid classification: An algorithm for management of scaphoid fractures. Presented at the American Society for Surgery of the Hand, Phoenix, AZ, November 11–14, 1992.

58. Dobyns JH, Linscheid RL, Chao EYS, et al: Traumatic instability of the wrist. American Academy of Orthopaedic Surgeons Instructional Course Lectures 24:182–199, 1975.

59. Duke R: Dislocations of the hamate bone: Report of a case. J Bone Joint Surg 45B:744, 1963.

60. Dunn AW: Fractures and dislocations of the carpus. Surg Clin North Am 52:1513–1538, 1972.

61. Duppe H, Johnell O, Lundborg G, et al: Long term results of fracture of the scaphoid. J Bone Joint Surg 76A:249–252, 1994.

62. Eddeland A, Eiken O, Hellgren E, et al: Fractures of the scaphoid. Scand J Plast Reconstr Surg 9:234–239, 1975.

63. Egawa M, Asai T: Fractures of the hook of the hamate: Report of six cases and the suitability of computerized tomography. J Hand Surg 8:393–398, 1983.

64. ElKhoury G, Usta HY, Blair WF: Naviculocapitate fracture-dislocation. AJR 139:385–386, 1982.

65. Failla JM: Hook of the hamate vascularities: Vulnerability to osteonecrosis and nonunion. J Hand Surg 18A:1075–1079, 1993.

66. Failla JM, Amadio PC: Recognition and treatment of uncommon carpal fractures. Hand Clin 4:469–476, 1988.

67. Fenton RL: The naviculo-capitate fracture syndrome. J Bone Joint Surg 38A:681–684, 1956.

68. Fernandes HJA Jr, Koberle G, Ferreira GHS, et al: Volar transscaphoid perilunar dislocation. Hand 15:276–280, 1983.

69. Fleege MA, Jebson PJ, Renfre DL: Pisiform fractures. Skeletal Radiol 20:169–172, 1991.

70. Fishman MC, Dalinka MK, Osterman L: Case report 309. Skeletal Radiol 13:245–247, 1985.

71. Fisk GR: An overview of injuries of the wrist. Clin Orthop 149:137–144, 1980.

72. Fisk GR: The wrist. J Bone Joint Surg 66B:396–407, 1984.

72A. Foster RJ, Hastings H 2d: Treatment of Bennett, Rolando, and vertical intra-articular trapezial fractures. Clin Orthop 214:121–129, 1987.

73. Frankel VH: The Terry-Thomas sign. Clin Orthop 129:321–322, 1977.

74. Freeland AE, Finley JS: Displaced vertical fracture of the trapezium treated with a small cancellous lag screw. J Hand Surg 9A:843–845, 1984.

75. Friedenberg ZB: Anatomic considerations in the treatment of carpal navicular fractures. Am J Surg 78:379–381, 1949.

76. Frykman E: Dislocation of the triquetrum. Scand Plast Reconstr Surg 14:205–207, 1980.

77. Frykman G: Pulsing electromagnetic field treatment of nonunion of the scaphoid: A preliminary report. Orthop Trans 6:160, 1982.

78. Gainor BJ: Simultaneous dislocation of the hamate and pisiform: A case report. J Hand Surg 10A:88–90, 1985.

79. Gamble JF, Simmons SC III: Bilateral scaphoid fractures in a child. Clin Orthop 162:125–128, 1982.

80. Ganel A, Engel J, Oster Z, et al: Bone scanning in assessment of fractures of the scaphoid. J Hand Surg 4:540–543, 1979.

80A. Garcia-Elias M: Dorsal fractures of the triquetrum—avulsion or compulsion fractures? J Hand Surg 12A:266–268, 1987.

81. Garcia-Elias M, Abanco J, Salvador E, et al: Crush injury of the carpus. J Bone Joint Surg 67B:286–289, 1985.

82. Garcia-Elias M, Bishop AT, Dobyns JH, et al: Transcarpal carpometacarpal dislocations, excluding the thumb. J Hand Surg 15A:531–540, 1990.

83. Garcia-Elias M, Dobyns JH, Cooney WP, Linscheid RL: Traumatic axial dislocations of the carpus. J Hand Surg 14A:446–457, 1989.

84. Geist DG: Dislocation of the hamate bone. J Bone Joint Surg 21:215–217, 1939.

84A. Gelberman RH, Bauman TD, Menon J, Akeson WH: The vascularity of the lunate bone and Kienböck's disease. J Hand Surg 5:272–278, 1980.

85. Gelberman RH, Gross MS: The vascularity of the wrist: Identification of arterial patterns at risk. Clin Orthop 202:40–49, 1986.

86. Gelberman RH, Menon J: The vascularity of the scaphoid bone. J Hand Surg 5:508–513, 1980.

87. Gelberman RH, Wolock BS, Siegel DB: Fractures and nonunions of the carpal scaphoid. J Bone Joint Surg 71A:1560–1565, 1989.

88. Gerard FM: Post-traumatic carpal instability in a young child: A case report. J Bone Joint Surg 62A:131–133, 1980.

89. Gibson PH: Scaphoid-trapezium-trapezoid dislocation. Hand 3:267–269, 1983.

89A. Gilula LA, Destouet JM, Weeks PM, et al: Roentgenographic diagnosis of the painful wrist. Clin Orthop 187:52–64, 1984.

90. Goldberg I, Amit S, Bahar A, et al: Complete dislocation of the trapezium (multangulum majus). Hand Surg 6:193–195, 1981.

91. Goldman S, Lipscomb PR, Taylor WF: Immobilization for acute carpal scaphoid fractures. Surg Gynecol Obstet 129:281–284, 1969.

92. Goodman ML, Shankman GB: Palmar dislocation of the trapezoid: A case report. J Hand Surg 8:606–609, 1983.

93. Goodman ML, Shankman GB: Update: Palmar dislocation of the trapezoid: A case report. J Hand Surg 9A:127–131, 1984.

94. Gordon SL: Scaphoid and lunate dislocation: Report of a case in a patient with peripheral neuropathy. J Bone Joint Surg 54A:1769–1772, 1972.

95. Green DP, O'Brien ET: Open reduction of carpal dislocations: Indications and operative techniques. J Hand Surg 3:250–265, 1978.

96. Green DP, O'Brien ET: Classification and management of carpal dislocations. Clin Orthop 149:55–72, 1980.

97. Green DP: Carpal dislocations and instabilities. In Green DP (ed): Operative Hand Surgery, vol 1. New York, Churchill-Livingstone 1993, pp 861–928.

98. Green MH, Hadied AM, LaMont RL: Scaphoid fractures in children. J Hand Surg 9A:536–541, 1984.

99. Greenspan A, Posner MA, Tucker M: The value of carpal tunnel trispiral tomography in the diagnosis of fracture of the hook of the hamate. Bull Hosp Joint Dis Orthop Inst 45:74–79, 1985.

100. Grundy M: Fractures of the carpal scaphoid in children. Br J Surg 56:523–524, 1969.

101. Gunn RS: Dislocation of the hamate bone. J Hand Surg 10B:107–108, 1985.

102. Heim U, Pfeiffer KM, in collaboration with Meuli HC: Small Fragment Set Manual. Technique Recommended by the ASIF Group (Swiss Association for Study of Internal Fixation). New York, Springer-Verlag, 1974.

103. Herbert TJ: Internal fixation of the carpus with the Herbert bone screw system. J Hand Surg 14A:397–400, 1989.

104. Herbert TJ, Fisher WE: Management of the fractured scaphoid using a new bone screw. J Bone Joint Surg 66B:114–123, 1984.

105. Herzberg G, Comtet JJ, Linscheid RL, et al: Perilunate dislocations and fracture-dislocations: A multicenter study. J Hand Surg 18A:768–779, 1993.

106. Hill NA: Fractures and dislocations of the carpus. Orthop Clin North Am 1:275–284, 1970.

107. Howard FM: Ulnar nerve palsy in wrist fractures. J Bone Joint Surg 43A:1197–1201, 1961.

108. Imbraglia JE, Broudy AS, Hagberg WC, McKernan D: Proximal row carpectomy: Clinical evaluation. J Hand Surg 15A:426–430, 1990.

109. Immermann EW: Dislocations of the pisiform. J Bone Joint Surg 30A:489–492, 1948.

110. Inglis AE, Jones EC: Proximal row carpectomy for diseases of the proximal row. J Bone Joint Surg 59A:460–463, 1977.

111. James ETR, Burke FD: Vibration disease of the capitate. J Hand Surg 9B:169–170, 1984.

112. Jensen BV, Christiansen C: An unusual combination of simultaneous fracture of the tuberosity of the trapezium and hook of the hamate. J Hand Surg 15A:285–287, 1990.

113. Jiranek WA, Ruby LK, Millender B, et al: Long term results after Russe bone grafting: The effect of malunion of the scaphoid. J Bone Joint Surg 74A:1216–1229, 1992.

114. Johnson RP: The acutely injured wrist and its residuals. Clin Orthop 149:33–44, 1980.

115. Jones GB: An unusual fracture-dislocation of the carpus. J Bone Joint Surg 37B:146–147, 1955.

116. Jones JA, Pellegrini VS Jr: Transverse fracture-dislocation of the trapezium. J Hand Surg 14A:481–485, 1989.

117. Jorgensen EC: Proximal row carpectomy: An end result study of twenty-two cases. J Bone Joint Surg 51A:1104–1111, 1969.

118. Jupiter JB: Scaphoid fractures: In Manske PR (ed): Hand Surgery Update. Englewood, NJ, American Society for Surgery of the Hand, 1994, pp 8.1–8.10.

119. Kerluke L, McCabe SJ: Nonunion of the scaphoid: A critical analysis of recent natural history studies. J Hand Surg 18A:1–3, 1993.

120. Kimmel RB, O'Brien ET: Surgical treatment of avascular necrosis of proximal pole of capitate: A case report. J Hand Surg 7:284–286, 1982.

121. King RJ, Machenney RP, Elnur S: Suggested method for closed treatment of fractures of the carpal scaphoid: Hypothesis supported by dissection and clinical practice. J R Soc Med 75:860–867, 1982.

121A. Kirschenbaum D, Coyle MP, Leddy JP: Chronic lunotriquetral instability: Diagnosis and treatment. J Hand Surg 18:1107–1112, 1993.

122. Kopp JR: Isolated palmar dislocation of the trapezoid. J Hand Surg 10A:91–93, 1985.

123. Kupfer K: Palmar dislocation of scaphoid and lunate as a unit: Case report with special reference to carpal instability and treatment. J Hand Surg 11A:130–134, 1986.

124. Kuth JR: Isolated dislocation of the carpal navicular. J Bone Joint Surg 21:479–483, 1939.

125. Larson B, Light TR, Ogden JA: Fracture and ischemic necrosis of the immature scaphoid. J Hand Surg 12A:122–127, 1987.

126. Lavernia CJ, Cohen MS, Taleisnik J: Treatment of scapholunate dissociation by ligamentous repair and capsulodesis. J Hand Surg 17A:354–359, 1992.

126A. Levy M, Fischel RE, Stern GM, Goldberg I: Chip fractures of the os triquetrum: The mechanism of injury. J Bone Joint Surg 61B:355–357, 1979.

127. Light TR: Injury to the immature carpus. Hand Clin 4:415–424, 1988.

128. Linscheid RL, Dobyns JH, Younge DK: Trispiral tomography in the evaluation of wrist injury. Bull Hosp J Dis 44:297–308, 1984.

129. London PS: The broken scaphoid bone: The case against pessimism. J Bone Joint Surg 43B:237–244, 1961.

130. Lowdon IMR, Simpson AHRW, Burge P: Recurrent dorsal trans-scaphoid perilunate dislocation. J Hand Surg 9B:307–310, 1984.

131. Lowrey DG, Moss SH, Wolff TW: Volar dislocation of the capitate. J Bone Joint Surg 66A:611–613, 1984.

132. Lowry WE, Cord SA: Traumatic avascular necrosis of the capitate bone: A case report. J Hand Surg 6:245–248, 1981.

133. Mack GR, Bosse MJ, Gelberman RH, Yu E: The natural history of scaphoid nonunion. J Bone Joint Surg 66A:504–509, 1984.

134. Maki NJ, Chuinard RG, D'Ambrosia R: Isolated, complete radial dislocation of the scaphoid. J Bone Joint Surg 64A:615–616, 1982.

135. Marck KW, Klasen HJ: Fracture-dislocation of the hamato-metacarpal joint: A case report. J Hand Surg 11A:128–130, 1986.

136. Marsh AP, Lampros PJ: The naviculo-capitate fracture syndrome. AJR 82:255–256, 1959.

137. Mather JH: Dislocation of the pisiform bone. Br J Radiol 29:17–18, 1924.

138. Maudsley RH, Chen SC: Screw fixation in the management of the fractured scaphoid. J Bone Joint Surg 54B:432–441, 1972.

139. Mayfield JK, Johnson RP, Kilcoyne RK: Carpal dislocations: Pathomechanics and progressive perilunar instability. J Hand Surg 5:226–241, 1980.

140. Mayfield JK: Mechanism of carpal injuries. Clin Orthop 149:45–54, 1980.

141. Mayfield JK, Johnson RP, Kilcoyne RF: The ligaments of the human wrist and their functional significance. Anat Rec 186:417–428, 1976.

142. Mayfield JK: Patterns of injury to carpal ligaments. Clin Orthop 187:36–42, 1984.

143. McBride ED: An operation for late reduction of the semilunar bone. South Med J 26:672–676, 1983.

144. McClain EJ, Boyes JH: Missed fracture of the greater multangular. J Bone Joint Surg 48A:1525–1528, 1966.

145. McLaughlin HL, Parkes JC: Fracture of the carpal navicular (scaphoid) bone: Gradations in therapy based upon pathology. J Trauma 9:311–319, 1969.

146. McNamara MG, Corley FG: Dislocation of the carpal scaphoid: An 8-year follow-up. J Hand Surg 17A:496–498, 1992.

147. Meyers MH, Wells, R, Harvey JP Jr: Naviculocapitate fracture syndrome: Review of the literature and a case report. J Bone Joint Surg 53A:1383–1386, 1971.

148. Meyn MA Jr, Roth AM: Isolated dislocation of the trapezoid bone. J Hand Surg 5:602–604, 1980.

149. Milch H: Fracture of the hamate bone. J Bone Joint Surg 16:459–462, 1934.

149A. Milek MA, Boulas HJ: Flexor tendon ruptures secondary to hamate hook fractures. J Hand Surg 15A:740–744, 1990.

150. Minami M, Yamazaki J, Ishii S: Isolated dislocation of the pisiform: A case report and review of the literature. J Hand Surg 9A:125–127, 1984.

151. Minami M, Yamazaki J, Chisaka N, et al: Nonunion of the capitate. J Hand Surg 12A:1089–1091, 1987.

152. Mintzer C, Waters PM: Acute open reduction of a displaced scaphoid fracture in a child. J Hand Surg 19A:760–761, 1994.

153. Moody BS, Belliappa PP, Dias JJ, Barton NJ: Nonunion of fractures of the scaphoid tuberosity. J Bone Joint Surg 75B:423–425, 1993.

154. Monahan PRW, Galaski CSB: The scaphocapitate fracture syndrome: A mechanism of injury. J Bone Joint Surg 54B:122–124, 1972.

155. Moneim MS: The tangential posteroanterior radiographs to demonstrate scapholunate dissociation. J Bone Joint Surg 63A:1324–1326, 1981.

156. Moneim MS, Hofammans KE III, Omer GE: Trans-scaphoid perilunate fracture-dislocation: Results of open reduction and pin fixation. Clin Orthop 190:227–235, 1984.

157. Morawa LG, Ross PM, Schock CC: Fracture and dislocation involving the navicular-lunate axis. Clin Orthop 118:48–53, 1976.

158. Morgan DAF, Walters JW: A perspective study of 100 consecutive carpal scaphoid fractures. Aust N Z J Surg 54:233–241, 1984.

159. Munck JT, Andersen JH, Thommasen P, et al: Scanning and radiology of the carpal scaphoid bone. Acta Orthop Scand 50:663–665, 1979.

160. Murakami Y: Dislocation of the carpal scaphoid. Hand 9:79–81, 1977.

161. Murahami S, Nakajima H: Aseptic necrosis of the capitate bone in two gymnasts. Am J Sports Med 12:170–173, 1984.

162. Mussbichler H: Injuries of the carpal scaphoid in children. Acta Radiol (Stockh) 56:316–368, 1961.

163. Naam NH, Smith DK, Gilula LA: Transtriquetral perihamate ulnar axial dislocation and palmar lunate dislocation. J Hand Surg 17A:762–766, 1992.

164. Nafie SA: Fractures of the carpal bones in children. Injury 18:117–119, 1987.

164A. Nelson DL, Manske PR, Pruitt DL, et al: Lunotriquetral arthrodesis. J Hand Surg 18A:1113–1120, 1993.

165. Neviaser RJ: Proximal row carpectomy for post-traumatic disorders of the carpus. J Hand Surg 8:301–305, 1983.

166. Newman JH, Watts I: Avascular necrosis of the capitate and dorsiflexion instability. Hand 12:176–178, 1980.

167. Nielsen PT, Hedeboe J, Thommasen P: Bone scintigraphy in the evaluation of fracture of the carpal scaphoid bone. Acta Orthop Scand 54:303–306, 1983.

168. O'Brien ET: Acute fractures and dislocations of the carpus. In Lichtman DM (ed): The Wrist and Its Disorders. Philadelphia, WB Saunders, 1985.

169. O'Carroll PF, Gallagher JE: Irreducible trans-scaphoid-perilunate dislocation. Irish J Med Sci 152:424–437, 1983.

170. Okuhara T, Matsui T, Sugimoto Y: Spontaneous rupture of flexor tendons of little finger due to projection of the hook of the hamate. Hand 14:71–74, 1982.

171. Oshio I, Ogino T, Miyake A: Dislocation of the hamate associated with fracture of the trapezial ridge. J Hand Surg 11A:658–660, 1986.

172. Palmer A, Dobyns JH, Linscheid RL: Management of post-traumatic instability of the wrist secondary to ligament rupture. J Hand Surg 3:507–532, 1978.

173. Palmer AK: Trapezial ridge fractures. J Hand Surg 6:561–564, 1981.

174. Peiro A, Martos F, Mut T, et al: Trans-scaphoid perilunate dislocation in a child: A case report. Acta Orthop Scand 52:31–34, 1981.

175. Pellegrino EA, Peterson ED: Trans-scaphoid perilunate dislocation of the wrist. J Bone Joint Surg 55A:1319, 1973.

176. Peterson CL: Dislocation of the multangulum majus or trapezium and its treatment in two cases with extirpation. Arch Chir Neurol 2:369–376, 1950.

177. Pick RY, Segal D: Carpal scaphoid fracture and nonunion in an eight-year child. J Bone Joint Surg 65A:1188–1189, 1983.

177A. Pin PG, Nowak M, Logan SE, et al: Coincident rupture of the scapholunate and lunotriquetral ligaments without perilunate dislocation: Pathomechanics and management. J Hand Surg 15A:110–119, 1990.

177B. Pin PG, Young VL, Gilula LA, Weeks PM: Management of chronic lunotriquetral ligament tears. J Hand Surg 14A:77–83, 1989.

178. Polivy KD, Millender LH, Newberg A, et al: Fractures of the hook of the hamate: A failure of clinical diagnosis. J Hand Surg 10A:101–104, 1985.

179. Porter ML, Seehra K: Fracture-dislocation of the triquetrum, treated with a Herbert screw. J Bone Joint Surg 73B:347–348, 1991.

180. Pournaras J, Kapas A: Volar perilunate dislocation: A case report. J Bone Joint Surg 61A:625–626, 1979.

181. Primiano GA, Reef TC: Disruption of the proximal carpal arch of the hand. J Bone Joint Surg 56A:328–332, 1974.

182. Rahme H: Idiopathic avascular necrosis of the capitate bone: A case report. Hand 15:274–275, 1983.

183. Rand J, Linscheid RL, Dobyns JH: Capitate fractures: A long term follow-up. Clin Orthop 165:209–216, 1982.

184. Reagan DS, Linscheid RL, Dobyns JH: Lunotriquetral sprains. J Hand Surg 9A:502–514, 1984.

185. Resnik CS, Gilberman RH, Resnick D: Trans-scaphoid-trans-capitate, perilunate fracture dislocation (scaphocapitate syndrome). Skeletal Radiol 9:192–194, 1983.

186. Rhoades CE, Reckling FW: Palmar dislocation of the trapezoid: A case report. J Hand Surg 8:85–88, 1983.

187. Richards RR, Bell RS: Internal fixation of a capitate fracture with Herbert screws. J Hand Surg 15A:885–887, 1990.

188. Roth Jr, deLorenzi C: Displaced intra-articular coronal fracture of the body of the hamate treated with a Herbert screw. J Hand Surg 13A:619–621, 1988.

189. Ruby LK: Fractures and dislocations of the carpus. In Browner RB, Jupiter, JB, Levine AM, Trafton PG (eds): Skeletal Trauma. Philadelphia, WB Saunders, 1992, pp 1025–1062.

190. Ruby LK, Stinson J, Belsky MR: The natural history of scaphoid nonunion. J Bone Joint Surg 67:428–432, 1985.

191. Russe O: Fracture of the carpal navicular. J Bone Joint Surg 42A:759–768, 1960.

192. Russell TB: Intercarpal dislocations and fracture-dislocations: A review of fifty-nine cases. J Bone Joint Surg 31B:524–531, 1949.

193. Saunier J, Chamay A: Volar perilunate dislocation of the wrist. Clin Orthop 157:139–142, 1981.

194. Schlosser H, Murray JF: Fracture of the hook of the hamate. Can J Surg 27:587–589, 1984.

195. Seidenstein H: Two unusual dislocations of the wrist. J Bone Joint Surg 38A:1137–1141, 1956.

196. Seimon LP: Compound dislocation of the trapezium. J Bone Joint Surg 54A:1297–1300, 1972.

197. Shands AR Jr: Analysis of more important orthopaedic information. Surgery 16:584–586, 1944.

198. Siegel MW, Hertzberg H: Complete dislocation of greater multangular (trapezium): A case report. J Bone Joint Surg 51A:769–772, 1969.

199. Skelly WJ, Nahigian SH, Hidvegi EB: Palmar lunate transtriquetral fracture dislocation. J Hand Surg 16A:536–539, 1991.

200. Soto-Hall R: Recent fractures of the carpal scaphoid. JAMA 129:335–338, 1945.

201. Soucacos PN, Hartofilakidis-Garafalidis GC: Dislocation of the triangular bone: Report of a case. J Bone Joint Surg 63A:1012–1013, 1981.

202. Southcott R, Rosman MA: Non-union of carpal scaphoid fracture in children. J Bone Joint Surg 59B:20–23, 1977.

203. Speed K: Traumatic Injuries of the Carpus. New York, D Appleton and Co, 1929.

204. Squire M: Carpal mechanics and trauma. J Bone Joint Surg 41B:210, 1959.

205. Stahl F: On lunatomalacia (Kienböck's disease): A clinical and roentgenological study, especially on its pathogenesis and the late results of immobilization treatment. Acta Chir Scand 95(suppl 126):133, 1947.

206. Stark A, Brostrom LA, Svartengren G: Scaphoid nonunion treated with the Matti-Russe technique: Long-term results. Clin Orthop 214:175–180, 1987.

207. Stark HH, Jobe FW, Boyes JH, et al: Fracture of the hook of the hamate in athletes. J Bone Joint Surg 59A:575–582, 1977.

208. Stein AH: Dorsal dislocation of the lesser multangular. J Bone Joint Surg 53A:377–379, 1971.

209. Stein F, Miale A, Stein A: Enhanced diagnosis of hand and wrist disorders by triple phase radionucleide bone imaging. Bull Hosp J Dis 44:477–484, 1984.

210. Stein F, Seigel MW: Naviculo-capitate fracture syndrome: A case report. J Bone Joint Surg 51A:391–395, 1969.

210A. Steinberg BD, Plancher KD, Idler RS: Percutaneous Kirschner wire fixation through the snuffbox: An anatomic study. J Hand Surg 20A:57–62, 1995.

211. Stern PJ: Trans-scaphoid-lunate dislocation: A report of two cases. J Hand Surg 9A:370–373, 1984.

212. Stevanovic MV, Stark HH, Filler BC: Scaphotrapezial dislocation: A case report. J Bone Joint Surg 72A:449–452, 1990.

213. Stewart MJ: Fractures of the carpal navicular (scaphoid): A report of 436 cases. J Bone Joint Surg 36A:998–1006, 1954.

214. Stewart MJ, Cross H: The management of injuries in the carpal lunate with a review of sixty cases. J Bone Joint Surg 50A:1489, 1968.

215. Stordahl A, Schjoth A, Woxholt G, et al: Bone scanning of fractures of the scaphoid. J Hand Surg 9B:189–190, 1984.

216. Sukul DMK, Johannes EJ: Transcapho-transcapitate fracture dislocation of the carpus. J Hand Surg 17A:348–353, 1992.

217. Suzuki K, Herbert TJ: Spontaneous correction of dorsal intercalated segment instability deformity with scaphoid nonunion in the skeletally immature. J. Hand Surg 18A:1012–1015, 1993.

218. Tachakara SS: A case of trapezio-scaphoid subluxation. Br J Clin Pract 31:162, 1977.

219. Takami H, Takahashi S, Ando M: Rupture of flexor tendon associated with previous fracture of the hook of the hamate. Hand 15:73–76, 1983.

220. Taleisnik J: The ligaments of the wrist. J Hand Surg 1:110–118, 1976.

221. Taleisnik J: Wrist: Anatomy, function and injury. American Academy of Orthopaedic Surgeons Instructional Course Lectures 27:61–87, 1978.

222. Taleisnik J, Kelly PJ: The extraosseous and intraosseous blood supply of the scaphoid bone. J Bone Joint Surg 48A:1125–1137, 1966.

223. Taleisnik J, Malerich M, Prietto M: Palmar carpal instability secondary to dislocation of scaphoid and lunate: Report of a case and review of the literature. J Hand Surg 7:606–612, 1982.

224. Tanz SS: Rotation effect in lunar and perilunar dislocations. Clin Orthop 57:147–152, 1968.

225. Teisen H, Hjarbaek J: Lunate fractures. J Hand Surg 13B:458–462, 1988.

226. Tiel-Van Buul MMC, Van Beek EJR, Broekuizen AH, et al: Radiography and scintigraphy of suspected scaphoid fracture. J Bone Joint Surg 75B:61–65, 1993.

227. Terry DW Jr, Ramin JE: The navicular fat stripe: A useful roentgen feature for evaluating wrist trauma. Am J Roentgenol Radium Ther Nucl Med 124:25–28, 1975.

228. Thomaidis VT: Elbow-wrist-thumb immobilization in the treatment of fractures of the carpal scaphoid. Acta Orthop Scand 44:679–689, 1973.

229. Thomas AP, Birch R: An unusual hamate fracture. Hand 15:281–286, 1983.

230. Thomas HO: Isolated dislocation of the carpal scaphoid. Acta Orthop Scand 48:369–372, 1977.

231. Trumble TE, Glisson RR, Seaber AV, Urbaniak IR: A biomechanical comparison of the methods for treating Kienböck's disease. J Hand Surg 11A:88–93, 1986.

231A. Trumble TE, Irving J: Histologic and magnetic resonance imaging correlations in Kienböck's disease. J Hand Surg 15A:879–884, 1990.

231B. Uhl RL, Williamson SC, Bowman MW, et al: Dorsal capsulodesis using suture anchors [abstract]. Presented at 62nd Annual Meeting of American Academy of Orthopaedic Surgeons, Orlando, FL, February 16–21, 1995.

232. Vahvanen V, Westerlund M: Fracture of the carpal scaphoid in children. Acta Orthop Scand 51:909–913, 1980.

233. Vance RM, Gelberman RH, Evans EF: Scaphocapitate fractures. J Bone Joint Surg 62A:271–276, 1980.

234. Van Duyvenbode JFFH, Keijser LCM, Hauet EJ, et al: Pseudarthrosis of the scaphoid treated by Matti-Russe Operation. J Bone Joint Surg 73B:603–606, 1991.

235. Vander Grend R, Dell PC, Glowczewskie BS, et al: Intraosseous blood supply of the capitate and its correlation with aseptic necrosis. J Hand Surg 9A:677–680, 1984.

236. Vasilas A, Grieco RV, Bartone NF: Roentgen aspects of injuries to the pisiform bone and piso-triquetral joint. J Bone Joint Surg 42A:1317–1328, 1960.

237. Vender MI, Watson HK, Wienner BD, Black DM: Degenerative change in symptomatic scaphoid nonunion. J Hand Surg 12A:514–519, 1987.

238. Verdan C: Fractures of the scaphoid. Surg Clin North Am 40:461–464, 1960.

239. Verdan C, Narakas A: Fractures and pseudo-arthrosis of the scaphoid. Surg Clin North Am 48:1083–1095, 1968.

240. Vichick DA, Dehne E: Fractures of the carpal scaphoid: An akinetic approach. Presented at Society of Military Orthopaedic Surgeons Meeting, San Antonio, TX, November, 1977.
241. Viegas SF, Bean JW, Schram RA: Trans-scaphoid fracture-dislocation treated with open reduction Herbert screw internal fixation. J Hand Surg 12A:992–999, 1987.
242. Viegas SF, Patterson RM, Peterson PD, et al: Ulnar-sided perilunate instability: An anatomic and biomechanic study. J Hand Surg 15A:268–278, 1990.
243. Viegas SF: Carpal Instabilities. In Manske PR (ed): Hand Surgery Update. Englewood, NJ, American Society for Surgery of the Hand, 1994, pp 10.1–10.13.
244. Wagner CJ: Perilunar dislocations. J Bone Joint Surg 38A:1198–1230, 1956.
245. Walker GBW: Dislocation of the carpal scaphoid reduced by open operation. Br J Surg 30:380–381, 1943.
245A. Watson HK, Ashmead D IV, Makhlouf MV: Examination of the scaphoid. J Hand Surg 13A:657–660, 1988.
246. Watson, HK, Hempton RF: Limited wrist arthrodesis. I: The triscaphoid joint. J Hand Surg 5:320–327, 1980.
247. Watson HK, Ballet FL: The SLAC wrist: Scapholunate advanced collapse pattern of degenerative arthritis. J Hand Surg 9A:358–365, 1984.
248. Watson HK, Pitts EC, Ashmead D IV, et al: Dorsal approach to scaphoid non-union. J Hand Surg 18A:359–365, 1993.
249. Watson-Jones R: Fractures and Joint Injuries, ed 3. Edinburgh, E & S Livingstone, 1943.
250. Weber ER: Biomechanical implications of scaphoid waist fracture. Clin Orthop 149:83–89, 1980.
251. Weber ER, Chao EYS: An experimental approach to the mechanism of scaphoid waist fractures. J Hand Surg 3:142–148, 1978.
252. Weil C, Ruby LK: The dorsal approach to the wrist revised. J Hand Surg 11A:911–912, 1986.
253. Weiss C, Laskin RS, Spinner M: Irreducible trans-scaphoid perilunate dislocation: A case report. J Bone Joint Surg 52A:565–568, 1970.
254. Weseley MS, Barenfield PA: Trans-scaphoid trans-capitate, transtriquetral, perilunate fracture-dislocation of the wrist: A case report. J Bone Joint Surg 54A:1073–1078, 1972.
255. Whalen JL, Bishop AT, Lindscheid RL: Non-operative treatment of acute hamate hook fractures. J Hand Surg 17A:507–511, 1992.
256. White RE, Omer GE: Transient vascular compromise of the lunate after fracture-dislocation or dislocation of the carpus. J Hand Surg 9A:181–184, 1984.
257. Woodward AH, Neviaser RJ, Nisefeld F: Radial and volar perilunate trans-scaphoid fracture-dislocation: A case report. South Med J 68:926–928, 1975.
258. Worland RL, Dick HM: Trans-navicular perilunate dislocation. J Trauma 15:407–412, 1975.
259. Yanni D, Lieppinz P, Laurence M: Fractures of the carpal scaphoid: A critical study of the standard splint. J Bone Joint Surg 73B:600–602, 1991.
259A. Youm Y, Flatt A: Kinematics of the wrist. Clin Orthop 149:21–32, 1980.
260. Zichner L: Repair of non-unions by electrically pulsed current stimulation. Clin Orthop 161:115–121, 1981.

CHAPTER 14

Scaphoid Non-Union

Gregory R. Mack, MD, Jon Pembroke Kelly, MD, and David M. Lichtman, MD

A scaphoid fracture becomes a non-union when it fails to unite, for any reason, within 6 months of injury. Radiographs demonstrate no bony trabeculae across the fracture site. The challenge to the surgeon is to achieve union and relieve symptoms. Management is difficult because treatment does not ensure union, the time required to obtain union may be long, and union alone does not always ensure a good result.[95, 143] Because most non-unions occur in young men in their second or third decade,[49, 124] prolonged treatment may also create significant economic hardship.[32, 143]

The criterion for successful treatment is a functional outcome superior to the natural history of scaphoid non-union. Symptomatic non-unions have a high probability of degenerative change,[82, 91, 111] and even asymptomatic non-unions are likely to develop degenerative change and eventual symptoms.[78] We advise all patients with non-unions that degenerative changes are probable, although symptoms vary. For symptomatic non-unions, we recommend surgery before such changes occur. The procedure of choice for most non-unions consists of reduction, bone grafting, and fixation, which usually achieve both union and a functional outcome.[128] If wrist instability or significant arthritis is present, simple bone grafting may not address the true source of symptoms. Malunion after grafting is likely to be symptomatic.[5, 65] Failure to achieve union prolongs disability and may require regrafting or a salvage procedure.[28] The outcome of surgery may also fall short of patient expectations and occupational demands. To assess the risks and benefits of surgery, the physician must (1) clearly understand the causes and natural history of scaphoid non-union and (2) develop a working knowledge of appropriate surgical procedures for each type of non-union.

ETIOLOGY

Most treated scaphoid fractures are undisplaced and heal within 12 weeks.[4, 19, 41, 80, 93] The rate of non-union, however, may be as high as 12 percent.[38] Many factors may contribute to non-union: severity of the initial injury, fracture pattern and location, displacement of fracture fragments, associated ligamentous injury, dorsal intercalated segment instability (DISI),

loss of blood supply to the proximal fragment, delayed diagnosis, and ineffective immobilization. Both extrinsic factors relating to treatment and intrinsic factors peculiar to the pathologic anatomy are involved.

Extrinsic Factors

Barr and colleagues[9] and London[80] stated that late diagnosis and inadequate immobilization are the most common causes of non-union. Early diagnosis of scaphoid fracture requires a high index of suspicion and adequate radiographs. Patients with anatomic snuffbox tenderness and negative initial radiographs may require repeat films at 2 to 3 weeks, when bone resorption at the fracture site facilitates diagnosis.[85, 123] (Imaging techniques are discussed in Chapters 7, 8, and 9.) Primary health care providers for susceptible populations, including athletic trainers, team physicians, and emergency room physicians, need to be aware of the relative ease of treating the acute scaphoid fracture compared with the difficulty of managing a non-union thought to be a sprain.

Adequate immobilization of the acute fracture controls fragment position until bony union occurs. We immobilize the undisplaced acute fracture in a long-arm thumb spica cast for 6 weeks and then a short-arm thumb spica cast until union is documented radiographically. Treatment is likely to fail if the patient is noncompliant. Non-union may also occur if the physician discontinues immobilization before radiographs demonstrate adequate trabeculation across the fracture site. The need to confirm union of the acute fractures before releasing the patient cannot be overemphasized. It is not rare for a patient with established non-union to give a history of prior fracture that a physician said was healed.

Intrinsic Factors

In order to heal, a scaphoid fracture requires coaptation of the fracture fragments, adequate blood supply, and immobilization until union is established. Factors that interfere with these requirements delay or prevent union. They are displacement, carpal instability, avascular necrosis, and fracture location.

DISPLACEMENT

Displacement is defined as cortical offset of the fracture surfaces by 1 mm or more as seen in radiographs taken in any plane (Fig. 14–1).[32, 33, 41, 82] Leslie and Dickson[74] observed that fractures that displaced under treatment had a lower rate of union. Displacement alone, however, does not preclude union. When performing delayed open reduction and internal fixation of displaced fractures, we have seen healing as early as 3 weeks after injury in some middle to distal third fractures. We have not seen this with proximal third fractures, fractures with DISI deformity, or fractures with a dorsal gap on the lateral radiograph. This experience is consistent with the view that displacement contributes to non-union through loss of coaptation of the fracture surfaces.

INSTABILITY

Instability represents a collapse deformity between the proximal and distal carpal rows, with abnormal increases of the scapholunate angle (SLA), radiolunate angle (RLA), and/or capitolunate angle (CLA) (Fig. 14–2). Gilford and associates[52] characterized the scaphoid as the stabilizing link between the proximal and distal carpal rows. Fisk,[45] Johnson,[66] and Mayfield[87] suggested that displaced acute fractures have associated perilunar ligamentous damage, which predisposes the wrist to collapse into a DISI pattern.[16, 92] The pathomechanics of carpal instability have been well described by Linscheid and coworkers,[79] and the reader is referred to Chapters 4, 5, and 12 for a contemporary update. Normally, the intact loaded scaphoid provides a flexion moment on the proximal row that is well balanced by an extension moment on the ulnar side of the proximal row. Fracture of the scaphoid releases the potential energy between the two sides of the proximal row, which are free to rotate. The triquetrum, lunate, and proximal fragment

of the scaphoid, no longer restrained by the distal fragment, slide volarly into extension. This position of lowest potential energy is characteristic of unstable scaphoid fractures and non-unions (see Fig. 14–2). The kinetic changes that occur with carpal collapse due to scaphoid fracture are similar to those that occur with scapholunate dissociation, because both represent stage I perilunar instability. In stable, undisplaced fractures, the axis of the scaphoid remains unbroken, collapse deformity is not present, and the fracture surfaces are still in contact with each other.

Clinically, the DISI pattern may occur at the time of injury or may develop over time.[82] Smith and associates[119] produced the DISI pattern in cadaver scaphoids by osteotomy alone. In established non-union, motion may erode trabeculae and produce a volar defect at the fracture site. Belsole and associates[13] compared computerized tomographic (CT) images of un-united scaphoids with those of opposite normal scaphoids to calculate the size and shape of the defect caused by resorption. They characterized the defect as prismatic in shape with a quadrilateral base that faced palmarly. They also observed that the proximal fragment was most likely to be extended, supinated, and radially deviated in relation to the distal pole.[13] Because the prismatic volar defect allows the scaphoid to angulate, the fracture site may have a cystic appearance on the posteroanterior (PA) radiograph (Fig. 14–3), which should be distinguished from true cyst formation.[86] The shape of the scaphoid non-union with volar resorption and DISI is analagous to the so-called humpback deformity of scaphoid malunion,[5, 46] which describes the apex-dorsal angulation seen in the lateral radiograph. Because the distal pole abuts the dorsal lip of the radius, osteophytic change that develops with time on the dorsal ridge of the scaphoid accentuates the humpback appearance.

AVASCULAR NECROSIS

When fracture interrupts the blood supply to the proximal pole, avascular necrosis (AVN) may occur. Obletz and Halbstein[101] found no arterial foramina proximal to the waist of the scaphoid in 13 percent of 297 cadaver specimens. An additional 20 percent of specimens had only one foramen proximal to the waist. Gelberman and Menon[51] also showed that the proximal pole of the scaphoid was dependent on blood supply from vessels entering the distal half of the bone in 14 percent of specimens. The proximal pole does not receive significant blood supply from the scapholunate ligaments. Berger and Kauer[15] noted small vessels within the radioscapholunate ligament that arborize to supply the fibrous portion of the scapholunate interosseous ligament, but they demonstrated that none of these vessels penetrates the scaphoid cortex. Interruption of the distally based blood supply would therefore account for the increased radiographic density of the proximal pole seen in some scaphoid fractures.[86] Fragmentation and

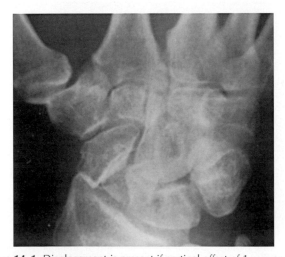

Figure 14–1. Displacement is present if cortical offset of 1 mm or more is demonstrated in any roentgenographic view.

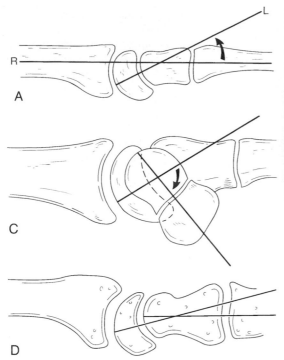

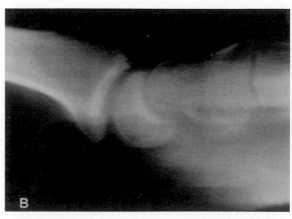

Figure 14–2. *A,* Lunate dorsiflexion is a characteristic finding with the DISI deformity and may be determined by measuring the radiolunate angle. Normally, the angle formed by the axes of the radius and the lunate should be less than 10°.[114] Note that the third metacarpal is parallel to the radius. *B,* Lateral tomogram of wrist shown in Figure 14–3*A* and *B* demonstrates abnormal lunate dorsiflexion consistent with the rotated proximal scaphoid fragment and indicative of collapse deformity at the midcarpal joint. *C,* Scapholunate angle. The scapholunate relationship should be less than 70°.[79] For scaphoid non-union, we measure this as the angle formed by the axis of the lunate and the axis of the distal scaphoid fragment. *D,* The capitolunate angle should be less than 10°.[16] Lunate dorsiflexion indicates rotation of the proximal scaphoid fragment, which reflects the amount of angulation at the fracture site. This may be associated with dorsal gapping in the acute fracture and volar resorption in a non-union.

collapse of the proximal pole, such as occurs in AVN of the femoral head, are less common in scaphoid AVN and usually represent a late phenomenon (Fig. 14–4).

Avascularity may be apparent on plain radiographs as a relative increase in the density of the proximal pole of the scaphoid compared with the remainder of the carpus, which may develop osteopenia due to immobilization and hyperemia. In promptly treated fractures, radiographic AVN is a potentially reversible

phenomenon,[112] and radiographic resolution may be a useful indicator of fracture healing (Fig. 14–5). Green,[55] however, has reported that increased density seen on the radiographs of scaphoid non-unions does not necessarily correlate with the true vascular integrity of the proximal pole. He observed and recorded the number and quality of punctate bleeding points in the cancellous portion of the bone while performing Russe's volar inlay bone grafting, and found the extent of cancellous bleeding to be a reliable

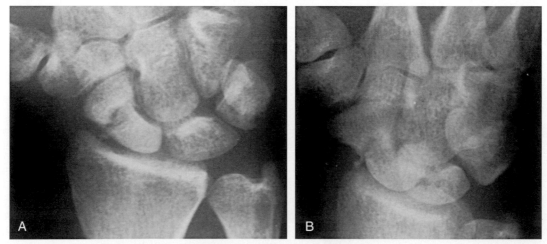

Figure 14–3. *A,* Anteroposterior radiograph of wrist in radial deviation shows apparent cystic change at the fracture site. *B,* Oblique view shows rotation of the proximal fragment, consistent with dorsiflexion instability pattern. Cortical offset of the fracture surfaces is also apparent. This is a type II non-union.

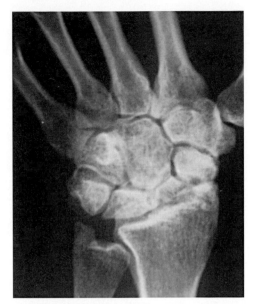

Figure 14–4. Old scaphoid non-union shows a relative "collapse" of the proximal pole. Note arthritic change between capitate and proximal scaphoid fragment and cystic degenerative changes in the capitate and lunate, consistent with a type IV non-union. This non-union is 27 years old. The radiolunate articulation is still intact.

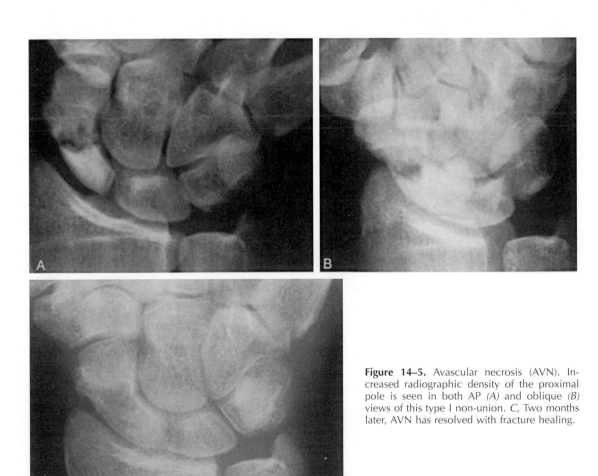

Figure 14–5. Avascular necrosis (AVN). Increased radiographic density of the proximal pole is seen in both AP *(A)* and oblique *(B)* views of this type I non-union. *C,* Two months later, AVN has resolved with fracture healing.

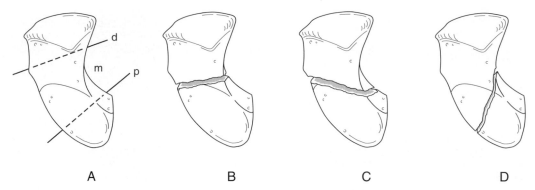

| | | | |
| A | B | C | D |

Figure 14–6. Fracture pattern and location as described by Russe: *A,* Non-union may be located in the proximal, middle, or distal third of the scaphoid. *B,* Transverse fracture pattern. Fracture line in this plane is perpendicular to the longitudinal axis of the scaphoid. *C,* Horizontal oblique pattern. Fracture line is oblique with respect to the scaphoid axis but horizontal with respect to the long axis of the radius. *D,* Vertical oblique pattern. Line of non-union is oblique with respect to the scaphoid axis but somewhat vertical in comparison with the axis of the radius.

prognostic indicator for the success of bone grafting. He also concluded that radiographs did not accurately predict avascularity found at surgery. Histologic studies have shown, however, that some viable bone may be present despite clinical evidence of complete necrosis.[140] The most sensitive evaluation for AVN is magnetic resonance (MR) imaging.

FRACTURE PATTERN AND LOCATION

The pattern and location of a scaphoid fracture (Fig. 14–6) may affect its ability to heal. In a prospective study of 100 consecutive fractures, Morgan and Walters[93] concluded that a fracture of the proximal third or a vertical oblique fracture of the middle third has a greater risk of non-union. A proximal third injury takes longer to heal, whether treated as an acute fracture[39, 64] or grafted as a non-union.[32, 139] This feature may be related to the smaller diameter of the proximal pole, to interruption of its blood supply, or both.

NATURAL HISTORY

The outcomes of untreated non-unions provide the baseline for assessing the results of surgical treatment. Since 1984, several studies have documented key features of untreated non-unions, including changes with time, the sequence in which they occur, and the relation of degenerative changes to symptoms. Mack and associates[82] studied the outcomes of 47 untreated non-unions 5 to 53 years after fracture and observed that the extent of arthritis correlated with the amount of time elapsed since fracture. Between 5 and 10 years after fracture, degenerative change tended to be confined to the scaphoid (Fig. 14–7).[82] Between 10 and 19 years, there was a significant incidence of radioscaphoid arthritis, including pointing of the radial styloid, joint space narrowing, and/or sclerosis (Fig. 14–8). In the third decade, arthritis was more extensive (Fig. 14–9), and after 30

years, arthritis was present throughout the wrist (see Fig. 14–15). The incidence of fracture displacement and wrist instability also increased with time, and both correlated with the presence of arthritic change. The rising incidence of displacement and instability suggested that even nondisplaced non-unions could displace or angulate with time.

Ruby and colleagues[111] studied 56 untreated non-unions and found an overall incidence for arthritis of 55 percent in their series, and a 97 percent incidence in those non-unions 5 years old or older. The observed sequence of degenerative change involved first the radioscaphoid joint and then the scaphocapitate and capitolunate joints; degenerative change in undisplaced non-unions was confined to the radioscaphoid joint.

Vender and associates[142] reported the findings in 64 symptomatic non-unions and also noted that degenerative change occurred first in the radioscaphoid joint and then skipped to the capitolunate joint, exhibiting the same sequential patterns of degenerative change as seen with rotary subluxation of the scaph-

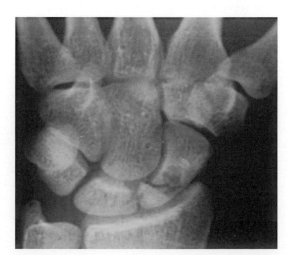

Figure 14–7. Scaphoid non-union with degenerative changes confined to the scaphoid. This non-union is 29 months old.

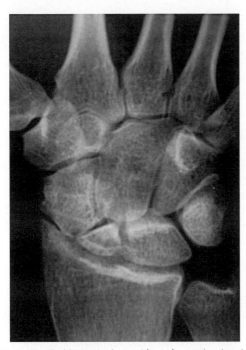

Figure 14–8. Scaphoid non-union with radioscaphoid arthritis. The radial styloid is pointed, and there is a relative loss of height of the joint space between the styloid and the distal fragment of the scaphoid. Displacement is also apparent. This type III scaphoid non-union is 11 years old.

oid. A key observation was sparing of the radiolunate joint even with degenerative change in the midcarpal joint.[142] Watson and Ballet[146] noted that osteoarthritis of the wrist begins at the radioscaphoid joint (which they attributed to abnormal "nesting" of the scaphoid in the lateral elliptical fossa of the distal radius) before progressing to the capitolunate joint. They coined the term *SLAC* (scapholunate advanced collapse) *wrist* to characterize the wrist with DISI and advanced degenerative change. It is not surprising that the sequence and patterns of degenerative change that occur in scaphoid non-union are similar to those seen in scapholunate dissociation. Both have the kinetic changes of stage I perilunar instability (see Chapters 5, 12, and 15), with one being a greater arc injury (scaphoid non-union) and the other a lesser arc injury (scapholunate dissociation). Because of this similarity, we characterize late degenerative change due to scaphoid non-union as "Scaphoid Non-union Advanced Collapse", or SNAC wrist.

Kerluke and McCabe[69] challenged the validity of published natural history studies and suggested that possible observer error in interpreting radiographs, selective referral to tertiary centers, and the lack of inception cohorts of non-unions (to allow longitudinal analysis of asymptomatic non-unions that would not otherwise come to medical attention) biased the results of these studies. Reported data nonetheless demonstrate that symptomatic non-unions undergo progressive degenerative change with time in a sequence that is predictable, and that even nondis-

placed non-unions may displace with time. Asymptomatic, nondisplaced non-unions may have a better prognosis than displaced non-unions, but identifying a significant population of these non-unions for longitudinal follow-up is difficult. Scott[116] in 1956 attributed the symptoms of 19 out of 20 previously undiagnosed non-unions to re-injury.[116] He noted that symptoms were paradoxically less in those with heavier occupational demands and suggested that, in addition to symptom tolerance, those with greater symptoms naturally selected less strenuous occupations. Ruby and colleagues[111] noted that 46 percent of their patients had few or no symptoms until after a second injury, but 89 percent were ultimately symptomatic. Milliez and associates[91] reported that 20 of 52 patients with non-unions had a latent period with few or no symptoms after injury, but only 46 percent of their patients had received no treatment prior to evaluation of the non-unions. Lindstrom and Nystrom[78] studied 33 patients with non-unions, 16 of which were diagnosed as incidental radiographic findings. Initially, 30 percent were asymptomatic and the rest of the patients were relatively symptom free except for certain activities, but longitudinal follow-up 10 to 17 years after the initial diagnosis showed increased symptoms and progressive degenerative change in all cases.[78]

Additional changes in the carpal architecture may occur after the appearance of capitolunate and scaphocapitate arthritis. These changes include radial migration of the distal carpal row, collapse of the proximal pole, and loss of carpal height. The changes

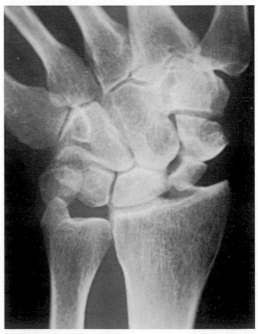

Figure 14–9. Scaphoid non-union with degenerative arthritis. Note significant involvement of both the radioscaphoid and capitolunate joints. Involvement of the midcarpal joint is consistent with a type IV non-union. Note the relative sparing of the radiolunate joint. This non-union is 20 years old.

occur more commonly in non-unions of more than 20 years' duration.[82] The distal radius may take on a triple-scalloped appearance in the PA radiograph. The styloid remodels and may appear to develop a third articular fossa adjacent to the distal pole of the scaphoid (Fig. 14–10).

SYMPTOMS

The symptoms of scaphoid non-union are wrist pain, weakness of grip, and loss of motion, especially dorsiflexion. Symptoms may occur any time after a scaphoid fracture has become a non-union. Many non-unions are continuously symptomatic from the time of the initial injury; others remain asymptomatic for an indefinite period[80, 81] and then become symptomatic either when degenerative changes begin to appear or when the wrist is re-injured.[70, 80, 116] Occasionally, a non-union is discovered as an incidental radiographic finding in a patient who presents with another problem in the hand. We advise the asymptomatic patient that most scaphoid non-unions develop degenerative changes with time but that the onset and severity of eventual symptoms cannot be accurately predicted. Displaced non-unions, in our experience, are likely to have more severe symptoms

than nondisplaced non-unions. The symptoms of any scaphoid non-union may be aggravated by re-injury, including even minor trauma and exertional stress of a repetitive nature. Intensity of symptoms varies with the patient's use of the wrist, occupation, hand dominance, age, and pain tolerance.

CLASSIFICATION

According to the presence or absence of displacement and carpal instability and to the extent of degenerative change, there are five distinct types of scaphoid non-union (Table 14–1). Understanding each type facilitates therapeutic and surgical decision-making.

Type I: Simple Non-Union

Simple non-union is stable, is nondisplaced, and has no degenerative change. There is no separation or shift of the fragments in any radiographic view, including the ulnar deviation view (Fig. 14–11). The relationship of the lunate to the radius and the distal carpal row is normal. The criterion for this relationship is the absence of significant lunate dorsiflexion in the neutral lateral radiograph. For this view, the third metacarpal must be parallel to the radius in both the coronal and sagittal planes. The scapholunate angle is less than 70°, the radiolunate angle is less than 10°, and the capitolunate angle is less than 10°.[16]

Type II: Unstable Non-Union

Unstable non-union is characterized by significant displacement or instability (DISI) but no degenerative change. Displacement of a non-union predisposes the wrist to instability (Fig. 14–12).[32, 33] *Displacement* is defined as offset of the fracture fragments by 1 mm or more (see Fig. 14–12).[32, 33, 41, 82] If there is no displacement in standard views, yet the fragments can be separated or shifted by stress views, the non-union should be considered unstable. If the scapholunate

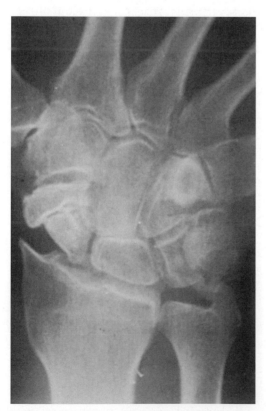

Figure 14–10. "Triple-scallop" appearance of the distal radial articular surface, due to remodeling of the styloid as a result of chronic degenerative change, that seems to form a third articular fossa for the distal fragment in this type V scaphoid non-union. There are early degenerative changes at the radiolunate joint. This non-union is 35 years old.

Table 14–1. TYPES OF SCAPHOID NON-UNION

Type	Name	Characteristics
I	Simple	No displacement No degenerative change
II	Unstable	Displacement > 1 mm or scapholunate angle > 70°
III	Early arthritic	Radioscaphoid arthritis present
IV	Scaphoid non-union–advanced collapse ("SNAC wrist")	Radioscaphoid arthritis and midcarpal arthritis
V	Scaphoid non-union–advanced collapse–plus ("SNAC-plus")	Arthritis throughout wrist

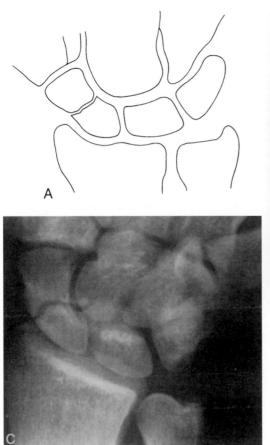

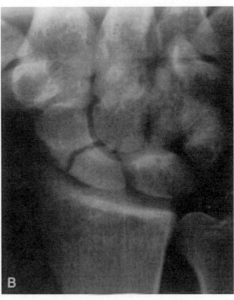

Figure 14–11. *A,* Type I non-union. There is no displacement, carpal instability, or degenerative change. *B,* Standard posteroanterior (PA) radiograph. *C,* Ulnar deviation (PA view) fails to displace the non-union.

Figure 14–12. *A,* Type II non-union. If displacement of the nonunion is present, the midcarpal joint is potentially unstable. Traction views are unnecessary. *B,* Posteroanterior radiograph demonstrates displacement. Cortical displacement need not be apparent, however, if a DISI pattern is seen in the lateral radiograph.

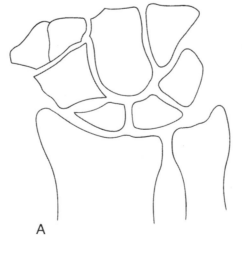

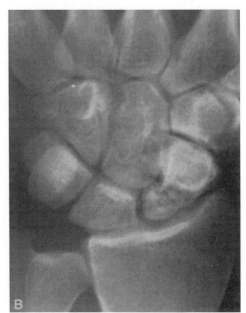

angle[79] is greater than 70°, the radiolunate angle is greater than or equal to 10°,[82, 114] and/or the capitolunate angle is greater than 10°,[16] the non-union is unstable.

Type III: Non-Union with Early Degenerative Change

Radioscaphoid arthritis is present in type III non-union, with joint space narrowing, subchondral sclerosis and/or pointing of the radial styloid (Fig. 14–13). Displacement or carpal instability or both are usually present.

Type IV: Scaphoid Non-Union–Advanced Collapse ("SNAC Wrist")

Arthritis is present not only in the radioscaphoid joint but also in the midcarpal joint. This is the key distinction between type III and type IV non-unions. Midcarpal involvement is usually seen in the capitolunate and scaphocapitate joints. The radiolunate joint is not involved (Fig. 14–14).

Type V: Scaphoid Non-Union–Advanced Collapse–Plus ("SNAC Plus")

With advanced degenerative change, arthritis is generalized and the radiolunate joint is affected (Figs. 14–10 and 14–15).

CLINICAL EVALUATION

The essential elements of a complete evaluation of a scaphoid non-union are an accurate history, an appropriate but thorough physical examination, a detailed analysis of radiographs, and a determination of the character and prognosis of non-union. Most important, a thorough understanding of the patient's functional requirements is necessary to make a rational choice of treatment options.

History

The physician documents the chronologic events leading to non-union, including all prior injuries to the wrist and their treatment. Failure to identify prior injury may lead to the misdiagnosis of a non-union as a new fracture. When we question each patient about prior injury, we specifically inquire about wrist "sprains," participation in organized athletics, any history of wrist soreness, and "normal" radiographs obtained in emergency rooms.

The patient's complaints are reviewed to determine functional and objective needs. Most patients describe some pain, weakness, or loss of motion. The patient's hand dominance, occupation, and work status since injury are recorded along with the relationship of symptoms to work.

Physical Examination

Thorough examination helps substantiate subjective complaints with objective findings, assesses the severity of impairment, and provides data to compare with the outcome of treatment. Key elements to re-

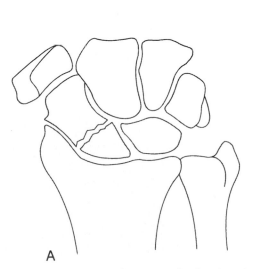
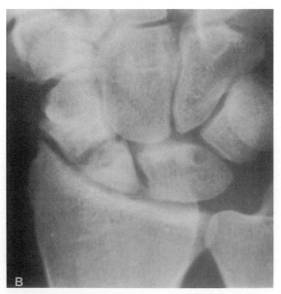

Figure 14–13. *A,* Type III non-union. Arthritis is confined to the radioscaphoid joint. *B,* Posteroanterior radiograph. Note absence of arthritis in the capitolunate joint.

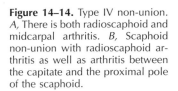
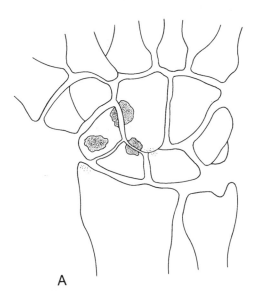
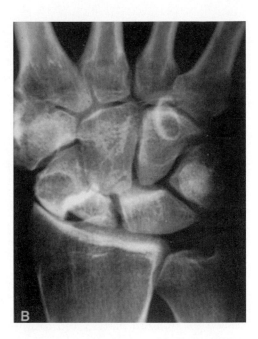

Figure 14–14. Type IV non-union. *A,* There is both radioscaphoid and midcarpal arthritis. *B,* Scaphoid non-union with radioscaphoid arthritis as well as arthritis between the capitate and the proximal pole of the scaphoid.

cord are grip strength, range of motion, crepitus, swelling, and localized tenderness.

The size and location of scars, neuromata, arthritic findings in other joints, and motion of the shoulder, elbow, and forearm should be documented. All measurements are compared with those of the opposite, normal limb. Wrist dorsiflexion, palmar flexion, radial deviation, and ulnar deviation are recorded.

The anatomic snuffbox, the scaphoid tuberosity, the radial styloid, the radiocarpal joint, and the first dorsal compartment are palpated. Both wrists are inspected and palpated to identify swelling or fullness. Ganglia may occur volar, dorsal, or radial to an arthritic radioscaphoid joint.

The physician should move the wrist carefully to identify maneuvers or positions that cause pain or reproduce symptoms. Pain with radial deviation may correlate with radioscaphoid arthritis. Dorsiflexing the wrist in the plane of the so-called dart-thrower's motion, i.e., from volarflexion–ulnar deviation to dorsiflexion–radial deviation, may reproduce symptoms as the arthritic scaphoid impinges on the styloid and lip of the radius dorsally. This clinical finding may occur in non-union or malunion before degenerative change is apparent on standard radiographs. Pain with simple dorsiflexion or palmar flexion is less specific but is a more consistent finding in a type IV non-union with midcarpal arthritis.

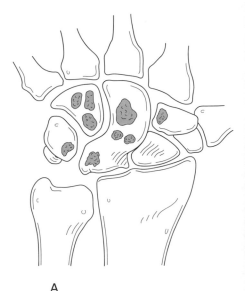
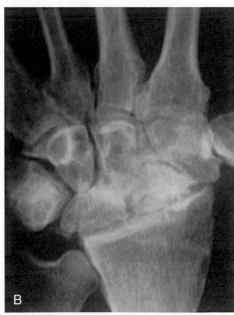

Figure 14–15. *A* and *B,* Advanced degenerative change in scaphoid non-union is generalized. This is a Type V non-union. In addition to extensive radiocarpal and midcarpal arthritis, the radiolunate joint has degenerative change.

RADIOGRAPHIC ANALYSIS

Radiographic studies for the management of scaphoid fractures and non-unions include standard radiographs, special views, tomography, computed tomography, magnetic resonance (MR) imaging. The value of each study is the information it provides in four basic steps of radiographic evaluation: classification, assessment of healing, evaluation for AVN, and preoperative assessment of the size, shape, and orientation of both scaphoid fragments.

Plain Radiographs

We use plain radiographs to classify scaphoid nonunion. We obtain a standard PA view, a lateral view with the third metacarpal parallel to the radius, and oblique views of the wrist with the forearm in 45° pronation and 45° supination. These views are assessed for fracture pattern and location (see Fig. 14–6), displacement (see Fig. 14–1), carpal instability (see Fig. 14–2), and arthritic change. The criteria for displacement, instability, and degenerative change have been described previously. If the scapholunate angle is less than 70° but we still suspect instability,

e.g., if there is degenerative change, we also obtain grip-compression and PA–ulnar deviation views. If the PA–ulnar deviation view demonstrates separation of the fragments, we suspect that the non-union is not only unstable[4] but also a pseudarthrosis.

Assessment of Healing

For the assessment of scaphoid fracture healing, plain radiographs are usually adequate. Care must be taken not to mistake overlap of the fragments for healing (Fig. 14–16). When doubt persists about healing, special radiographic views, such as PA–ulnar deviation and grip-compression views, may be helpful.[10] Traction views are not necessary. Views that demonstrate healing most clearly direct the beam through the plane of the fracture. Elongating the radiographic image of the scaphoid by placing the film cassette at various planes of obliquity to the x-ray beam (rather than perpendicular to it) may enhance visualization of the extent of trabeculation at the fracture site.[133]

Plain radiographs may also be adequate for the assessment of union after bone grafting. Care should be taken in the assessment of sequential sets of films to identify any change in technique. Films taken with

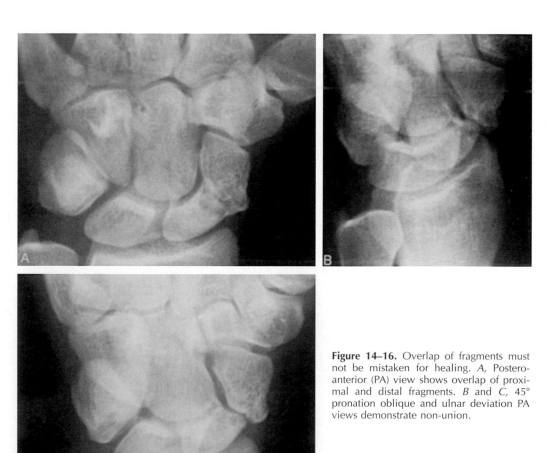

Figure 14–16. Overlap of fragments must not be mistaken for healing. *A,* Posteroanterior (PA) view shows overlap of proximal and distal fragments. *B* and *C,* 45° pronation oblique and ulnar deviation PA views demonstrate non-union.

slightly lower voltage or amperage than the previous set may suggest an increase in the bony density at the graft site, which could be misconstrued as healing. If doubt exists after an adequate period of immobilization, we obtain tomograms or a CT scan. Tomography to assess union is taken in two planes (PA and lateral) with 2-mm cuts. Positioning the thumb parallel to the axis of the forearm facilitates visualization of the full length of the scaphoid and the alignment of its fragments.[43] A CT scan with 1.0-mm to 1.5-mm cuts of the longitudinal axis of the scaphoid serves the same purpose.[113] Trispiral tomography, if available, provides a sharper image than standard (linear) tomography. The cost of a CT scan is now more comparable to that of tomography, imparts 25 to 50 percent less radiation, and is more readily available, because tomography is an older technology for which replacement hardware may be difficult to obtain.

MR imaging may also demonstrate union (proximal and distal poles have identical signal on T_1- and T_2-weighted images) or non-union of a scaphoid frac-ture[61]; however, we do not routinely use it to assess healing after bone grafting because of the expense.

Evaluation for Avascular Necrosis

If we plan to bone-graft a non-union but suspect AVN, we may obtain an MR image. AVN is more likely when the fracture is in the proximal third, when plain radiographs show increased proximal pole density, or when pseudarthrosis is present. MR imaging has been shown to be highly sensitive for AVN compared with plain radiography (Fig. 14–17).[107, 109, 136] Decrease in the marrow signal intensity in T_1-weighted images suggests AVN. The specificity of MR imaging for AVN has been reported to be both high[107, 136] and low.[109] False-positive image results in the assessment of scaphoid fractures may represent abnormal signal due to hyperemia, hematoma, or edema when the study is performed too early after injury. We believe that the importance of a positive

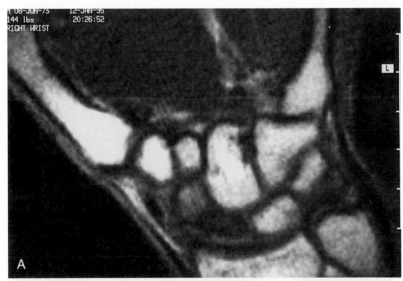
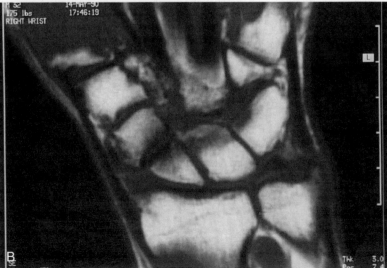

Figure 14–17. *A,* Magnetic resonance (MR) image of scaphoid non-union shows decreased signal intensity of the proximal pole on T_1-weighted image consistent with avascular necrosis. *B,* A T_1-weighted image of a 10-year-old scaphoid non-union shows equal signal intensity of both scaphoid fragments and of the adjacent carpal bones.

MR image in scaphoid non-union is its implication of diminished healing capacity for bone grafting. As will be discussed later in the surgical techniques section, this finding may alter our choice of fixation; if AVN is present with other risk factors, such as small fragment size or arthritis, we may consider a procedure other than bone grafting.

Assessment of Scaphoid Size and Shape

Radiographic studies that demonstrate the size and shape of a non-union and its defect facilitate surgical planning. For a type I non-union, which has relatively normal external contours and can be treated by in situ grafting, standard radiographs are usually adequate. A type II non-union, however, is more difficult to graft and fix because it requires a wedge or interposition bone graft to bridge the volar defect. We try to estimate the required graft size and the degree of angulation to be corrected from the lateral radiograph. If these features are not easily visualized in the lateral radiograph, we obtain tomograms or a CT scan in the longitudinal axis of the scaphoid.[43, 113]

Several radiographic studies may provide preoperative estimates of the size and shape of the bone graft required. They include measurement of the scaphoid length, three-dimensional reconstruction of the non-union with a CT scan,[99] and lateral comparison radiographs.[44] In our experience, tomograms or CT cuts made in the longitudinal axis of the scaphoid are adequate for tracing the fragment outlines and demonstrating the defect that is likely to be created when fracture angulation and any DISI deformity are corrected. These preoperative measurements provide estimates of the graft size and shape, however, and we generally do not obtain special studies to delineate the scaphoid shape unless it cannot be easily visualized with the plain radiographs—e.g., if the fracture line is oblique, if the proximal pole is less than a third of the scaphoid, and/or if density changes within the scaphoid make it difficult to distinguish from other carpal bones in the lateral radiograph. With or without special studies, we make the final determination of the defect by direct observation and measurement at surgery, after resection of the non-union and alignment of the fragments through the volar approach.

Although MR imaging may also be useful for preoperative assessment of fracture orientation, the shape of the scaphoid,[118] and the size of defect,[13] we currently do not use it for this assessment because of expense.

Belsole and coworkers[13] have demonstrated that the size and shape of a volar defect can be calculated with comparative three-dimensional CT scans of both wrists.[13] Although this modality may give the clearest nonoperative visualization of a non-union, it is not yet cost-effective as a clinical tool.

PRINCIPLES OF TREATMENT

Treatment of Delayed Unions

Undisplaced fractures less than 6 months old may be treated by immobilization. In our experience, the majority of middle or distal third fractures less than 6 months old will heal if immobilization is adequate and is continued until healing is clearly demonstrated radiographically. The time for union of a neglected or subacute fracture will be prolonged, however, and increases with the age of the fracture.[7] It is important to clearly establish the original date of injury, to rule out the possibility that the presumed fracture may be a re-injury of an old non-union, and to be certain that neither displacement nor carpal instability is present. If there is any doubt about the position of the fracture, additional views or tomograms may be appropriate before the patient is subjected to a long period of closed treatment.

NONOPERATIVE TREATMENT

Because scaphoid non-union occurs most commonly in the active young adult male, two issues should be addressed: whether symptoms impair the patient's ability to work and, if so, whether treatment will allow the patient to return to work. Symptomatic non-union in a young patient is usually best managed surgically. Non-union in the older patient with infrequent symptoms may respond to activity modification, temporary splinting, and limited use of a nonsteroidal anti-inflammatory agent. If degenerative change is present, conservative management may defer the need for a salvage procedure.

Electrical Stimulation

Electrical stimulation is a useful alternative to bone grafting for the undisplaced scaphoid non-union. Electrical stimulation of scaphoid non-union has achieved union rates of 67 to 95 percent.* Electricity may be delivered to the site of non-union either directly or indirectly while it is immobilized in a long-arm cast.

One direct and two indirect methods of electrical stimulation have been used. The direct method uses three or four stainless steel pins inserted percutaneously through the tuberosity under radiographic control.[6, 19, 20, 25, 90] The pins are sheathed in polytetrafluoroethylene (Teflon) for insulation except for their tips. Maximum electrical activity occurs at the metal-sheath junction. This method has provided union rates of 71 to 95 percent,[6, 19, 25, 91] but is infrequently used because of problems with the pins, including placement difficulty, breakage, premature removal, and infection.[102]

Indirect methods are pulsating electromagnetic fields (PEMFs)[11, 12, 48] and capacitive coupling.[117] The

---

*References 2, 6, 11, 12, 19, 20, 25, 48, 90.

PEMF or inductive technique uses a pair of external coils supplied by a pulse generator to produce time-varying magnetic fields that induce weak electric currents in bone.[11] The coils are centered over the non-union and may be incorporated into the cast. Beckenbaugh[12] reported that union after PEMF stimulation was more likely with a long-arm cast than with a short-arm cast and that treatment may last 4 to 6 months. Union rates with PEMF stimulation range from 67 to 87 percent.[2, 11, 12, 48, 102] One research team's follow-up of patients from a previous study suggests that pulsed electromagnetic fields may be less effective in the treatment of scaphoid non-unions than the original study indicated; it was most helpful in non-unions of less than 2 years' duration.[2]

The reported union rate for capacitative coupling is 77 percent.[102] A prospective double-blind study of long bone non-unions found capacitative coupling to be effective.[117] No prospective study has directly compared electrical stimulation with bone grafting. Electrical stimulation has a low risk of complication, but the rates of union are higher for bone grafting. Electrical stimulation may be most useful for early, nondisplaced non-unions in patients who decline surgery.

SURGICAL MANAGEMENT

For the treatment of scaphoid non-union, a variety of surgical procedures have been described. No single procedure, however, is appropriate for all non-unions. To choose the best procedure, the surgeon must understand treatment principles, the type and characteristics of the non-union, and the advantage or disadvantage of each procedure that may be appropriate. The following guidelines for treatment of scaphoid non-union are summarized in Table 14–2.

Type I Scaphoid Non-Union

Treatment options for type I scaphoid non-union include bone grafting and electrical stimulation, but in situ bone grafting is the treatment of choice. We rarely use electrical stimulation, because bone grafting has a higher union rate.[32] The surgeons who first described in situ grafting did not use supplemental pin fixation.[83, 96, 97, 98, 112] When Cooney and associates[32] made the clear distinction between the stable nondisplaced and the unstable displaced scaphoid non-union, they advocated use of pin fixation in bone grafting of either type. Stark and colleagues[128] demonstrated a 97 percent rate of union with iliac bone grafting and Kirschner wire fixation. Although we have obtained union in nondisplaced non-unions without fixation, we now use fixation to supplement most bone grafts. Pins improve the probability of union[32] and may prevent angulation, displacement, and micromotion at the fracture site, without adding significant morbidity to the surgical procedure.

Type II Scaphoid Non-Union

Type II non-union usually requires wedge or interposition bone grafting and internal fixation. Treatment of a type II non-union should not only obtain union but also restore the proper length, position, and alignment of the scaphoid. Angulation may be due to initial displacement or chronic resorption at the fracture site anteriorly. Interposition of bone graft in the anterior wedge-shaped defect is necessary to restore length and correct carpal instability.[34, 45] By correcting the associated DISI deformity, interposition bone grafting may also improve wrist dorsiflexion. Stable internal fixation of both fragments and the interposed bone graft is mandatory.

Proximal third bone grafts take longer to heal and are technically challenging. It is well established that grafted non-unions of the proximal third of the scaphoid take longer to heal than grafted non-unions of the middle or distal thirds.[32, 143] A small proximal fragment is more likely to be avascular and is more difficult to stabilize. Screw fixation of the small proximal fragment, if larger than 20 percent of the scaphoid,

Table 14–2. TREATMENT OF SCAPHOID NON-UNION*

		Treatment	
Stage	Type	*Our Preference*	*Alternative(s) Treatment*
I	Simple	Inlay bone graft (volar approach)	Inlay graft (dorsal)[148] Electrical stimulation
II	Unstable	Volar wedge graft: Use pins if AVN present Compression screw if no AVN	
III	Early	Wedge graft, ORIF, and styloidectomy	Proximal row carpectomy
IV	SNAC wrist	Four-bone midcarpal fusion with scaphoid excision	Distraction-resection arthroplasty[47] Wrist arthrodesis
V	"SNAC–plus"	Arthrodesis with AO/ASIF plate and distal radius graft	Arthrodesis with inlay graft

AO/ASIF = Arbeitsgemeinschaft fur Osteosynthesfragen/Association for the Study of Internal Fixation; AVN = avascular necrosis; ORIF = open reduction, internal fixation.

may be appropriate through the dorsal approach but requires adequate bone for thread purchase. If the length of the proximal pole is less than 4 mm after the non-union is resected or constitutes less than 20 percent of the scaphoid on the preoperative radiograph, fixation and grafting will be difficult, and alternative treatment should be considered. Other treatment options are scaphoid excision with midcarpal arthrodesis, and proximal row carpectomy. Vascularized bone grafting may also be considered.[150]

Type III Scaphoid Non-Union

Surgical options for type III non-unions are interposition bone grafting with radial styloidectomy, and proximal row carpectomy.* Radioscaphoid arthritis alone is not a contraindication to interpositional bone grafting but is one of several risk factors that may compromise the outcome of grafting. Other risk factors are avascular necrosis, a large volar defect, location of non-union in the proximal third of the scaphoid, and osteophytes of the dorsal ridge of the scaphoid and the dorsal lip of the distal radius. We generally prefer interpositional grafting for scaphoid non-union because we believe that restoring normal anatomy is most likely to give the longest-lasting functional result.

If radioscaphoid arthritis plus one of these risk factors is present, however, we perform a proximal row carpectomy, for the following reasons: Avascular necrosis, though not a contraindication to bone grafting, may reduce the probability of union and is likely to increase the time to union. Prolonged immobilization of a wrist with symptomatic arthritic change may lead to greater postoperative stiffness. A large volar defect also requires more time for graft incorporation. If the non-union is in the proximal third, there is not only a higher risk of AVN but also greater difficulty obtaining stable fixation and the need to resect a much larger portion of the arthritic styloid, which may disturb the origin of the radiocapitate ligament. If radioscaphoid arthritis is visible not only on the PA but also on the lateral radiograph, the functional outcome of grafting plus styloidectomy may not fully relieve pain or restore dorsiflexion. If the patient has signs of dorsal radioscaphoid impingement, including pain with dorsiflexion activities and/or local tenderness and fullness, yet does not appear to have dorsal spurring on the plain lateral radiograph, we obtain tomograms or a CT scan in the longitudinal axis of the scaphoid. If these demonstrate dorsal osteophytes, we perform a proximal row carpectomy.

Radial styloidectomy alone may be considered for the older patient whose symptoms are localized to the radioscaphoid joint. Once the styloid is removed, however, relief is only temporary if the distal carpal row continues to shift radially as degenerative change continues. We do not perform limited intercarpal

arthrodesis for type III non-union, because the midcarpal joint is not involved.

Type IV Scaphoid Non-Union

Surgical options for type IV non-union are scaphoid excision with midcarpal arthrodesis ("SNAC wrist" procedure) and wrist arthrodesis. Proximal row carpectomy is generally not indicated for type IV non-union because the head of the capitate in such cases is also affected by arthritic change. Fitzgerald and colleagues,[47] however, have modified the procedure for this situation and characterized it as a "fibrous distraction arthroplasty."[47]

Type V Scaphoid Non-Union

Wrist arthrodesis is the surgical treatment of choice for type V non-union of the scaphoid.

SURGICAL TECHNIQUES

Anatomy

The scaphoid receives its Greek name from its unique boatlike shape. Its major convexity articulates with the distal radius, and its major concavity contains and helps stabilize the head of the capitate. Volarly, the concavity of the middle third rests on the radiocapitate ligament. The volar side of the distal third is palpable as the tuberosity. Except for the tuberosity, the dorsal ridge, and proximal ligamentous attachments to the radius and lunate, most of the scaphoid's surface is articular. Proximally, the scapholunate interosseous ligament connects the opposing surfaces of those two bones. The radioscapholunate ligament, which has more vincular than ligamentous properties, links the interosseous ligament with the radius. Distally, the palmar ligaments secure the scaphoid tightly to the trapezium, trapezoid, and capitate. The radial collateral ligament extends from the radial styloid to the distal scaphoid.[132] The scaphoid nests obliquely in the lateral articular fossa of the distal radius, with its longitudinal axis tilted approximately 45° toward the palm and 40° to 45° radially.[146]

Blood supply from the radial artery enters the scaphoid dorsally and volarly. Dorsal vessels enter foramina on the dorsal ridge between the scaphoid's radial and trapezial articular surfaces. Volar vessels enter the volar and radial sides of the tuberosity.[51] Immediately proximal to the tuberosity, on the palmar surface, is a small, rough triangular area in which vascular perforations may be identified.[131] Small vessels entering here are reflected when the tuberosity is exposed through the extended volar approach. A denser network of small vessels perforates the lateral cortex of the distal end of the scaphoid and may appear as small punctate bleeding points during surgical exposure of the tuberosity subperiosteally (appearance of these bleeding points indicates that the

---

*References 35, 63, 100, 125–127, 134, 141.

exposure has gone too far radially). Dorsal vessels supply the proximal 70 to 80 percent of the scaphoid, and volar vessels supply its distal 20 to 30 percent. In approximately 14 percent of scaphoids, the dorsal vessels enter just distal to the waist.[51] (The reader is referred to Chapter 3 for details.)

Volarly, the flexor carpi radialis crosses the scaphoid. The first dorsal compartment is radial to the scaphoid and volar to its proximal two thirds. The tendons of the second compartment, the extensor carpi radialis (ECR) longus and ECR brevis, are directly dorsal to the scaphoid (Fig. 14–18).

The scaphoid tuberosity is palpable at the base of the palm, just beyond the volar wrist flexion crease, in line with and just radial to the flexor carpi radialis. Deviating the wrist radially and ulnarly helps differentiate the scaphoid tuberosity from the trapezial ridge, which lies just distal to it. The tuberosity is more prominent in radial deviation but disappears in ulnar deviation, whereas wrist motion does not affect the prominence of the trapezial ridge. The midportion of the scaphoid is palpable in the anatomic snuffbox.

Surgical Approaches

There are three surgical approaches to the scaphoid: volar, immediately radial to or through the sheath of the flexor carpi radialis (FCR); dorsal, beneath the extensor carpi radialis brevis (ECRB) and extensor carpi radialis longus (ECRL); and radial, through the anatomic snuffbox, just dorsal to the extensor pollicis brevis (EPB).

VOLAR APPROACH

The volar approach is simplest and safest because it is least likely to disrupt the scaphoid blood supply or to injure the superficial sensory branch of the radial nerve (SBRN).[51, 112] It also provides a good view for fragment reduction during inlay or interposition grafting. Extending this approach distally facilitates placement of the compression jig for a headless scaphoid screw on the tuberosity. The chief disadvantage of the volar approach is that it requires division and repair of the strong, inelastic volar wrist capsule and the radiocapitate ligament, which may contribute to excessive scarring and decrease wrist dorsiflexion. The volar approach is made as follows:

Begin the incision directly over the center of the scaphoid tuberosity in the palm, and continue proximally 1.5 inches directly over the FCR (Fig. 14–19A). Alternatively, a zigzag incision may produce less scarring (Fig. 14–19B). Expose the scaphoid proximal to the tuberosity by dividing longitudinally both the roof and floor of the FCR sheath, and retract the tendon ulnarly; this keeps the plane of dissection away from the radial artery and out of the carpal tunnel. Alternatively, dissection radial to the sheath of the FCR may decrease scarring of that tendon that might otherwise limit dorsiflexion. Expose and incise

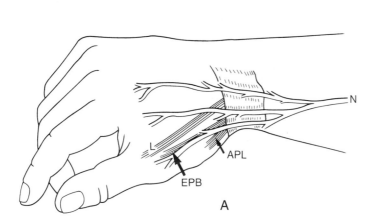
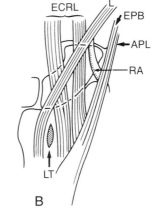
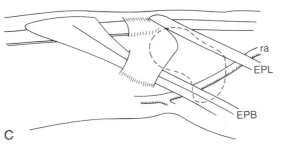

Figure 14–18. Anatomic structures of the dorsoradial aspect of the wrist are the superficial branch of the radial nerve *(N)*, extensor pollicis longus *(L)*, extensor carpi radialis brevis *(ECRB)*, extensor carpi radialis longus *(ECRL)*, radial artery *(RA)*, extensor pollicis brevis *(EPB)*, and abductor pollicis longus *(APL)*. *A,* The terminal sensory branches of the radial nerve cross the tendons of the first three extensor compartments. The radial wrist extensors, which the EPL crosses, are not shown. *B,* Location of the scaphoid, as seen from its dorsal aspect, with respect to the tendons of the first three extensor compartments, Lister's tubercle *(LT)*, and the radial artery. *C,* Lateral diagram shows location of the scaphoid and radial styloid with respect to extensor tendons and radial artery *(ra)*.

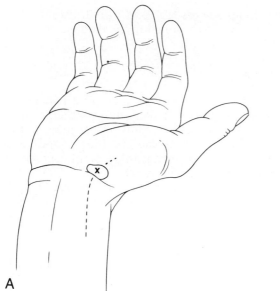

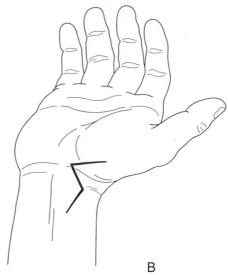

Figure 14–19. Skin incision for volar approach to the scaphoid. *A,* The standard skin incision *(dashed line)* begins at the scaphoid tuberosity *(X).* Dorsiflexion and radial deviation facilitate identification of the tuberosity. To expose the tuberosity and scaphotrapezial joint, the incision is extended distally along the metacarpal axis *(dotted line).* *B,* A zigzag skin incision with a radially based flap at the wrist crease may be more cosmetic than the standard incision.

the volar wrist capsule in line with the skin incision. Reflect continuous capsuloperiosteal flaps radially and ulnarly by sharp dissection of Sharpey's fibers off the distal radius with an end-cutting knife blade. This relaxes the interval for better exposure. Divide the distal fibers of the pronator quadratus if necessary. To manipulate the scaphoid and its non-union in the fossa of the distal radius, gently insert a curved blunt instrument such as a narrow Langenbeck elevator. To prevent cartilage injury when inserting the elevator, have an assistant apply manual traction to the thumb or index and long fingers to distract the radiocarpal joint. If carpal collapse is present, it may be necessary to release attachments between the scaphoid and capitate, and between the capitate and lunate, in order to obtain correction.

For applying a compression jig, extend the skin incision distally from the tuberosity to the middle of the trapezium in a line that parallels the axis of the thumb. Divide the superficial fascia of the thenar muscles and reflect the muscle ulnarly. The superficial branch of the radial artery, whose size is variable, is likely to cross the distal portion of the operative field. Retract it radially. Continue the capsular incision distally onto the tuberosity and trapezium. Take care not to damage the cartilage on either side of the scaphotrapezial joint. Reflect capsuloperiosteal flaps radially and ulnarly to expose this joint, but avoid excessive lateral exposure of the scaphoid tuberosity so as not to interfere with vascularity. It is possible to perform radial styloidectomy through this approach by extending the lateral subperiosteal dissection of the proximal incision.

DORSAL APPROACH

The advantage of the dorsal approach is that it does not disrupt the strong volar wrist capsule. It is the preferred approach for fixation of a non-union with a small proximal pole. Take care not to injure the superficial sensory branch of the radial nerve or the vessels that enter the dorsal ridge of the scaphoid (Fig. 14–18*A*). Mobilize and retract the tendons of the second and third dorsal compartments for exposure (Fig. 14–18*B*).

Landmarks include Lister's tubercule, the radiocarpal joint, and the extensor pollicis longus (EPL). Make the distal part of the skin incision parallel to the EPL, from the level of the thumb carpometacarpal joint to the radiocarpal joint. For retrograde screw fixation of the proximal pole of the scaphoid, continue the incision in the same line 0.25 inch proximal to the radiocarpal joint. Otherwise, curve it toward the ulna proximally at the level of the radiocarpal joint, just distal to Lister's tubercle (Fig. 14–20*A*). Extension of the ulnar limb of the skin incision affords more exposure if needed. The sensory branch of the radial nerve and the accompanying vein cross the radial half of the operative field within their surrounding fat. Because this nerve is vulnerable to injury, protect it by mobilizing and gently retracting it to either side of the operative field. Identify the EPL, ECRL, and ECRB, and free them from investing fascia and synovial tissue to facilitate gentle retraction (Fig. 14–20*B* and *C*). Retract the EPL radially. Retract the wrist extensor tendons radially to visualize the proximal pole; retract the ECRB ulnarly to view the middle third of the scaphoid. Division of the extensor retinaculum proximal to Lister's tubercle is usually not necessary.

Identify the radioscaphoid joint by palpation with a blunt instrument while gently moving the wrist. Incise the wrist capsule transversely over the proximal third of the scaphoid. Extend the capsular incision distally along the axis of the scaphoid, but visualize the dorsal ridge vessels and protect them from

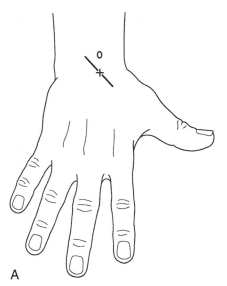
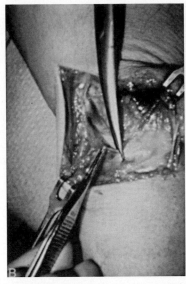
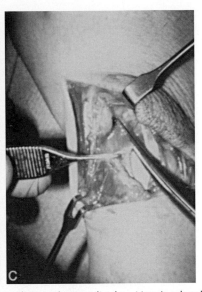

Figure 14–20. *A,* Skin incision for dorsal approach to the scaphoid. *X* indicates the level of the radiocarpal joint, distal to Lister's tubercle. *B,* Tendovaginotomy of the extensor pollicis longus. Branches of the superficial branch of the radial nerve have been mobilized and retracted with their fat to prevent retraction injury. The tendon should be mobilized *from distal to proximal* by dividing the extensor retinaculum as far as but not past Lister's tubercle. The tendon is more vulnerable to injury where it "turns the corner" around the tubercle. *C,* With the extensor pollicis longus retracted, the two radial wrist extensor tendons are mobilized.

injury. For removal of the scaphoid, take care distally not to injure the deep branch of the radial artery, which crosses the distal third laterally before it lies dorsoradial to the scaphotrapezial joint. For proximal row carpectomy, continue the skin and capsular incisions over the lunate and triquetrum toward the ulnar styloid.

Watson and colleagues[148] have described a dorsal approach to the waist of the scaphoid through a transverse incision over the scaphoid just distal to the radial styloid for dorsal cancellous bone grafting. Incise the skin just distal to the level of the radial styloid, and approach the scaphoid between the ECRL and ECRB tendons.

RADIAL APPROACH

The radial approach exposes the scaphoid directly through the anatomic snuffbox in the interval between the EPL and the EPB (Fig. 14–21). It is the preferred approach for simple radial styloidectomy,[8] and some have employed it for dorsoradial inlay bone grafting when using the styloid as bone graft[32] and for wrist arthrodesis.[57] The radial approach also exposes a small portion of the scaphoid for dorsal fixation from distal to proximal with pins or a headless screw. Its advantage over the dorsal approach is protection of the sensory branch of the radial nerve under its dorsal flap. Without concomitant styloidectomy, however, performing bone grafting through the radial approach is not practical. Because the radial artery crosses the distal third of the scaphoid, it is important to identify and protect this artery when using the radial approach. Zaidemberg and associates[150] have used an extension of the radial approach to expose

the dorsal irrigating branch of the radial artery and to rotate a vascularized bone graft to the scaphoid.

The incision is curvilinear but parallels the EPB distally over the proximal quarter of the thumb metacarpal; it courses through the snuffbox, curves ulnarly at the level of the radial styloid, and extends as far as the EPL (Fig. 14–21*A*).[50] Gently retract branches of the SBRN within the dorsal flap. Expose the capsule between the EPL and the EPB. Protect the radial artery, which lies distally in the wound beneath the EPB. Make a transverse capsular incision with the wrist in ulnar deviation; continue it proximally and ulnarly if more exposure is needed.

To perform radial styloidectomy through this approach, make the skin incision longitudinally, directly over the radial styloid (see Fig. 14–21*B*).[8]

Bone Grafting

The literature describes three basic types of bone grafting for scaphoid non-union: in situ grafts, interposition grafts, and vascularized grafts. In situ grafts are most appropriate for nondisplaced type I nonunions, which do not have cortical resorption, whereas type II non-unions require interposition grafts to correct angulation secondary to volar resorption. Vascularized grafts may be most appropriate for special circumstances in which conventional grafting is likely to fail or has already done so.

The primary goal of every scaphoid bone graft procedure is to establish bony continuity between the proximal and distal fragments. To achieve it, the surgeon must (1) resect pseudarthrotic and fibrous tissue back to healthy bone, (2) accurately bridge the non-

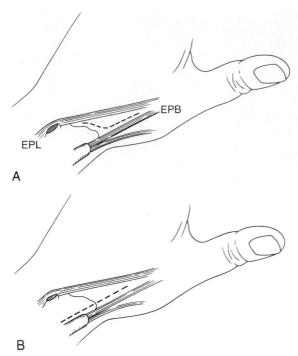

Figure 14–21. Radial approach to the scaphoid. *A,* Skin incision for exposure of the scaphoid in the anatomic snuffbox. The incision is centered distally between the extensor pollicis longus *(EPL)* and the extensor pollicis brevis *(EPB)* and parallels the EPB before curving dorsally and ulnarly at the radiocarpal joint. Dorsally, the incision may extend to the EPL. *B,* Skin incision for radial styloidectomy is centered over the styloid and parallels the EPB.

union with autogenous, corticocancellous bone, (3) not disturb the blood supply or viability of the fragments, either by surgical dissection or by excessive heat from power instruments, and (4) be certain the bone fragments are stable at the conclusion of the procedure.

In Situ Grafts

There are four in situ graft techniques: volar inlay bone grafting (Russe),[112] dorsal inlay bone grafting,[83, 148] dorsoradial grafting through the radial approach,[32] and dorsal peg grafting with cortical bone.[96–98] Of these, the Russe procedure has long been the standard of care, because many surgeons have obtained favorable results with its use.*

VOLAR INLAY GRAFT TECHNIQUE

Russe[112] modified the procedure that he published in 1960 and described the modification to Green,[55] who reported his own experience with the modified technique, which is performed as follows:

Expose the scaphoid through the volar approach between the FCR and radial artery. Do not disturb its dorsal or lateral surfaces. Resect pseudarthrotic tissue

---

*References 32, 40, 42, 53, 60, 88, 94, 95, 115, 122, 138, 139

with a fine curette and an end-cutting knife blade to expose the opposing bone surfaces of the proximal and distal fragments. Cut a 3 × 12 mm cortical window in the volar aspect of the scaphoid with small, sharp osteotomes. Curette the bone by hand until cancellous bleeding appears on either side of the nonunion, and create a trough to accept the bone graft. Small punctate bleeding points within the medullary cavity, which may appear during curettage of either fragment even with the tourniquet inflated, indicate that the fragment has viable bone.[55] Thoroughly excavate all avascular cancellous bone from the proximal fragment.

Obtain two corticocancellous bone grafts from the ilium or the distal radius. They should measure slightly more than 2 mm in width. Green[55] uses bone graft from the distal radius because its cortex is thinner, and inserts them into the cavity with the cortical sides outward (Fig. 14–22). Fill the remainder of the cavity with small chips of cancellous bone graft. We use iliac crest grafts and insert them with their cancellous surfaces outward (DML) or use a single rectangular corticocancellous graft and thin its cortex with fine-tipped bone biters or rongeurs (GRM and JPK). Immobilize the wrist in a well-fitting long-arm thumb spica cast in slight flexion and slight radial deviation. Change the cast every 6 to 8 weeks until healing occurs. After the first 6 weeks, apply a short-arm thumb spica cast. All fingers should be freely mobile throughout the postoperative period.

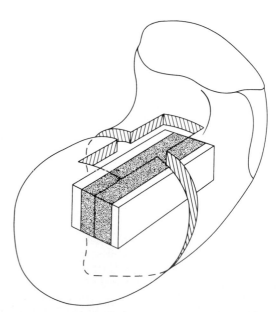

Figure 14–22. Russe[112] technique of volar inlay bone grafting, as described by Green.[55] Two struts of corticocancellous graft are countersunk within the bone, cortical sides outward, and multiple 1-mm to 2-mm "chips" of cancellous bone (not shown) fill the remainder of the cavity prepared for the strut grafts. Green prefers graft obtained from the distal radius, because its cortex is thinner than the cortex of iliac graft. Alternative volar inlay techniques include placing the cancellous sides outward and using a single corticocancellous iliac graft with its thinned cortex facing anteriorly.

DORSORADIAL INLAY GRAFT TECHNIQUE

Matti[83] introduced the excavation concept for bone grafting of the scaphoid in 1936. He performed his procedure through a dorsal approach. We do not perform inlay grafting of the distal two thirds of the scaphoid through the dorsal approach because of the possibility of disrupting the dorsal ridge vessels. Watson and colleagues[148] reported 89 percent union in 36 cases with dorsal cancellous grafting and pin fixation. This technique is performed as follows:

Resect the non-union and fashion a 4-mm to 7-mm concavity to accept cancellous bone graft from the ipsilateral radius. Insert fixation pins retrograde from proximal to distal into the distal fragment and out the skin prior to reduction, cancellous graft placement, and fixation of the proximal fragment. When using this approach, take care not to injure the dorsal ridge vessels.

DORSAL GRAFT THROUGH THE RADIAL APPROACH

Barnard and Stubbins[8] and Dobyns and Lipscomb (see Cooney[32]) modified the Matti[63] technique by using a radial approach between the tendons of the first and second extensor compartments. Whereas Matti bridged the curetted defect with cancellous bone from the ilium, Dobyns and Lipscomb resected the radial styloid, used it to make a corticocancellous bone graft, and inlayed it on the dorsoradial aspect of the scaphoid. They resected the styloid proximal to the level of the non-union, and used a 5 × 20 mm graft. Pins enter and stabilize the fragments through the distal fragment. This technique requires care to protect the radial artery, its intercarpal branch, and the dorsal ridge vessels.

Cooney and associates[32] compared the results of dorsal inlay grafting through the radial approach with the results of volar inlay grafting and reported union in 91 percent and 87 percent of the cases, respectively. Their series included both stable and unstable non-unions treated both with and without internal fixation.

DORSAL BONE PEG TECHNIQUE (MURRAY)

Murray[96] published the first description of his procedure in 1934. He used a radial approach and inserted cortical bone graft from the tibia into a 5/16-inch drill hole made through the dorsal distal aspect of the scaphoid. He reported that 96 of 100 non-unions he treated by dorsal peg grafting healed in an average time of 3.3 months. Palmer and Widen[103] obtained comparable results with his technique, but other surgeons have not.[32, 49, 135] This technique is chiefly of historical interest.

STABILIZATION OPTIONS FOR GRAFTED NON-UNIONS

Internal fixation should stabilize a grafted non-union well enough to maintain fragment position and prevent angulation. Ideally, internal fixation of the carefully selected, low-risk non-union may allow light use of the wrist during healing, which may result in an earlier and greater range of motion.[18, 44, 58, 89] Internal fixation *without bone graft,* however, is not reliable, with union rates varying from 0 to 80 percent.[50, 53, 75, 84, 89]

A variety of fixation choices are available to supplement grafting but basically consist of Kirschner wire or screw fixation. Kirschner wire fixation is much simpler and has been highly effective with iliac bone grafting,[128] such that it is an acceptable choice of fixation for all interposition grafting. We use three pins and insert them through the tuberosity. Each pin engages the subchondral bone of the proximal pole without penetrating it, and at least one of the pins should stabilize the graft. We bend the distal (tuberosity) end of each pin beneath the skin to avoid discomfort and ulceration. Pins require removal after union occurs. We perform most of our scaphoid pin removals 3 to 4 months after grafting.

Screw fixation may provide greater stability and compression than pins, and may thereby shorten the duration of immobilization after bone grafting. Headless screws do not require removal. Scaphoid fixation screws include the AO/ASIF,* cannulated screw, the Herbert screw, the Herbert-Whipple cannulated screw, and the Accutrak screw. Fernandez[44] emphasized that case selection and precise technique are more critical to surgical outcome than the type of screw, and has successfully used the AO/ASIF 2.7-mm cortical screw for scaphoid non-unions. We prefer the headless scaphoid screws, each of which uses a compression device and has special threads that further compress the fracture.

The choice between pins and a screw may be difficult. Three factors that affect this choice are AVN, fracture obliquity, and the skill and experience of the surgeon. We do not use a screw if AVN is present, because after we curette nonviable bone from the proximal pole, it cannot hold the thread of a compression screw securely. Obliquity of the fracture line can make screw placement difficult, because the less perpendicular a fracture is to the axis of fixation, the more the jig and screw will tend to shift the fragments as it compresses them. A precompression Kirschner wire to stabilize the fragments helps this situation but may also impair compression if it is not parallel to the screw axis. This in turn may weaken the thread-bone interface as the screw is tightened. Skill and experience with a compression jig-and-screw system help the surgeon visualize preoperatively how to apply the jig and obtain sound screw purchase. We

---

*AO stands for Arbeitsgemeinschaft fur Osteosynthesfragen, and ASIF stands for Association for the Study of Internal Fixation.

recommend practicing with one of these systems on a fresh anatomic specimen or an anatomic model, and carefully selecting a transverse non-union of the middle third without arthritic change as one's first case. Technical considerations for screw fixation are discussed in the section on interposition bone grafting.

Herbert and Fisher[58] have demonstrated that a small proximal fragment can be secured with the Herbert screw through a dorsal approach. Curettage and iliac cancellous graft are still required. Dorsal freehand insertion of a noncannulated screw may carry a slight risk of distal cortical penetration.

We check the position of fixation hardware intraoperatively with at least three radiographs—PA, lateral, 45° pronation oblique—to ensure adequate fixation without cortical penetration. As with femoral head fixation, it is possible to have cortical penetration despite radiographs that do not show it, especially when the dorsal approach is used. If the screw threads appear close to the scaphocapitate joint, we visualize that joint directly.

INTERPOSITION GRAFTING

Type II non-unions require interposition grafting to bridge the volar defect caused by chronic resorption of volar cortex. An interposition graft not only makes intimate contact with medullary bone on either side of the non-union but also helps to correct angulation by providing a volar wedge between the proximal and distal fragments.

Technique of Interposition Grafting

Use the volar approach and extend the incision distally to expose the scaphotrapezial joint. Reflect capsuloperiosteal flaps off the proximal ridge of the trapezium, the scaphoid tuberosity, and the distal radius. Resect the non-union with a small, sharp osteotome or 6400 (end-cutting) Beaver knife blade. Make the osteotomy cuts through trabecular bone to remove the sclerotic faces of the non-union, which would impair healing (Fig. 14–23). Do not disturb viable articular cartilage or the soft tissue adherent to the dorsal aspect of the non-union. Reduce any carpal instability by applying pressure on the palmar pole of

the lunate with a blunt instrument such as a narrow Langenbeck periosteal elevator; this helps to demonstrate the size and shape of the scaphoid defect. Gentle dorsiflexion of the wrist over a bump achieves the same result.

Measure the scaphoid defect in all its dimensions to determine the size of bone graft required. The shape of the graft is basically a corticocancellous wedge that corrects angulation between the proximal and distal poles. Its cortical side is anterior to maintain the proper distance between the volar cortices of the proximal and distal fragments. Its cancellous surface should make intimate contact with the medullary bone of the proximal and distal poles; to do so, it may need to protrude proximally and distally beyond the margins of the wedge to fill any additional defect of the medullary cavities left by curettage. The cancellous part of the graft should be slightly larger than the defect it will fill, to allow slight collapse and interdigitation with both the proximal and distal fragments when compression is applied. With the wrist gently dorsiflexed and the proximal pole reduced to a neutral position, measure the distance between the anterior cortices of the proximal and distal fragments, the depth of the defect from anterior to posterior, the width of the scaphoid from medial to lateral, and the maximum endosteal length of the defect. We sketch a diagram of these measurements intraoperatively, and obtain a block of corticocancellous iliac graft whose dimensions are slightly larger than those of the defect.

Expose the iliac crest at its most lateral aspect, where the thickness of the ilium beneath the crest is greatest. Studying the shape of the crest and ilium preoperatively on an accurate skeletal model is helpful. Make two parallel cuts in the periosteum on the top of the crest 3 cm apart. Connect these cuts with a third periosteal incision along the lateral margin of the crest (Fig. 14–24A) that corresponds to the interval between the insertion of the most distal fibers of the external oblique and the most proximal fibers of the gluteal muscles. It is not necessary to elevate the periosteum from the top of the crest itself, except for the very limited area where the osteotomy cuts are made. The cortex of the crest is then osteotomized to create a 3.0 × 1.5 cm "lid," which is hinged medially (Fig. 14–24B). The outer table of the ilium is exposed

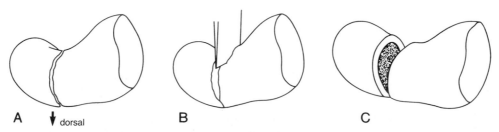

A ↓ dorsal   **B**   **C**

Figure 14–23. Osteotomy of the scaphoid for block or wedge bone grafting. *A,* Non-union of right scaphoid viewed from radial aspect. *B,* Resection of non-union with sharp 5/16-inch small osteotome. *C,* A volar wedge-shaped defect is usually demonstrated by realignment of the non-union fragments to their proper anatomic position.

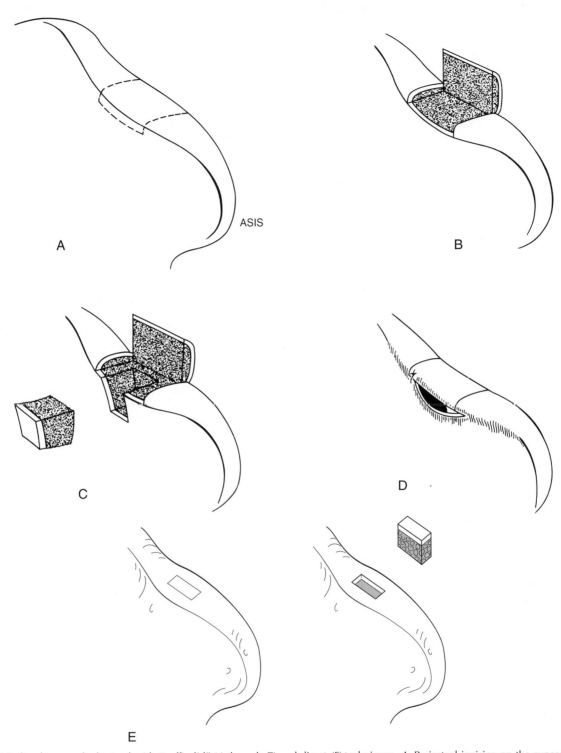

Figure 14–24. Iliac bone graft obtained with "coffin-lid" (*A* through *D*) and direct *(E)* techniques. *A,* Periosteal incision on the superolateral aspect of the crest. Palpable landmarks are the superolateral margin of the crest itself and the anterior superior iliac spine (ASIS). *B,* The periosteal cuts are deepened with very sharp osteotomes to create a medially hinged cortical lid. *C,* Corticocancellous block is removed by sharp cuts on all sides using osteotomes. The medial vertical cut is made along the medullary face of the inner table of the ilium. *D,* Closure of the cortical "lid" and its attached periosteum. *E,* Corticocancellous graft obtained directly through the dorsal aspect of the widest portion of the crest. Iliac grafts with cortices from the outer table or crest require cortical thinning with fine rongeurs or bone biters.

distal to this area by reflecting the gluteal muscle inferiorly with a Cobb elevator.

From the exposed area, obtain a corticocancellous block of bone large enough to fill the scaphoid defect (Fig. 14–24C). Make all bone cuts precisely, with sharp hand instruments, rather than power tools, which may burn and devitalize the periphery of the graft. Trim the graft and shape it to fit the previously measured defect. Thin the cortex as much as possible with fine-pointed bone biters.

Techniques for obtaining the iliac graft vary. In addition to using the technique just described, we have obtained corticocancellous graft from the lateral aspect of the ilium without elevating the crest, but exposure is more difficult and the depth of the graft may be difficult to predict. Another alternative for a small graft is to obtain a block directly from the dorsum of the crest (Fig. 14–24E).

To insert the graft, open the defect anteriorly by dorsiflexing the wrist as much as possible, dorsiflexing the proximal pole as much as possible with a Freer elevator, and deviating the wrist ulnarly. Firmly seat the graft with a bone tamp until its thinned anterior cortical surface is level with the cortices on either side of the non-union (Fig. 14–25). The larger cancellous portion of the graft will distract the fragments about 1 mm beyond the desired final position.

Inspect the articular surfaces of the proximal and distal poles to check the reduction. Their arcs should be congruous. Compress the scaphoid, but take care to avoid angulation of the fragments and displacement of the graft. We use any of four means to maintain reduction while compressing the fracture; they are: (1) positioning the wrist to align the distal fragment, using dorsiflexion to match the position of a dorsiflexed proximal fragment and/or radial deviation to help align or compress the fracture site; (2) direct stabilization of the proximal pole, either with a narrow Langenbeck periosteal elevator carefully po-

sitioned on the dorsoradial aspect of the proximal pole or by a temporary transfixion pin to secure either the lunate or the proximal pole to the radius; (3) stabilization of the graft and fracture fragments with a Kirschner wire before compression is applied; and (4) use of a scaphoid compression jig.

Placement of a scaphoid compression jig may be the most critical and most difficult part of this procedure. In addition to considering the mechanical effect of the jig on the reduction, the surgeon needs to plan the screw path carefully. The screw must pass through both fracture fragments and the graft from distal to proximal. If the hook of the jig is too far in the ulnar direction, the screw will miss the proximal pole; if the hook is too radial, it will slip and score the cartilage; if the hook is too volar, the screw will tend to "bowstring" volar to the graft; and if the hook is too dorsal, placement of the barrel distally will be difficult. For accurate barrel placement, it will be necessary to lever the distal pole of the scaphoid palmarly and to position the barrel against the distal articular surface. Place the barrel as distal as possible on the scaphoid tuberosity. Sectioning anterior capsular fibers of the scaphotrapezial joint and resecting a small portion of the trapezial ridge may facilitate placement of the barrel but should not be necessary if scaphoid angulation is adequately corrected.

As compression is applied, the cancellous portion of the graft will collapse slightly to make intimate contact with the fracture surfaces on either side. This should occur just before the cortex of the graft engages the anterior cortices of the proximal and distal pole. If the graft is fragmented, of poor quality, or too small, or if the distal (barrel) end of the compression jig is applied too anteriorly, the fracture will collapse and re-angulate as compression is applied. If the osteotomy cuts are not parallel, a purely wedge-shaped graft may tend to extrude; if it does so, re-reduce the fragments and stabilize the construct with a single

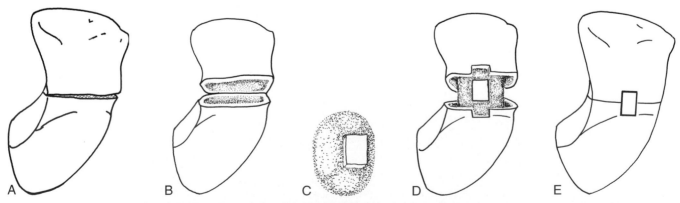

Figure 14–25. Diagrammatic representation of interposition block graft bridging a volar scaphoid defect, with its cortical side abutting the volar cortices of the proximal and distal fragments. The cancellous edges of the graft extend beyond its cortex and are tapered to achieve a "lozenge" shape. A, Anterior aspect of non-union. B, Nonbony tissue has been resected from non-union site, which is "booked" open to allow curettage to the level of healthy cancellous bone. C, Corticocancellous graft shaped to the intramedullary defect. The cancellous portion exceeds the length of its cortex. D, Insertion of the graft into the proximal and distal halves of the scaphoid. Notching of the cortices of the scaphoid positions the graft's cortex outside the medullary cavity. If the scaphoid cortices are not notched, the graft can function as an interposition graft by distracting the scaphoid anteriorly. E, The scaphoid is reduced over the graft.

0.035-inch or 0.045-inch wire inserted parallel to the path for screw placement (Fig. 14–26). This also provides some rotational control and may give a small amount of leverage for manipulating the scaphoid while applying the jig. If there is any question of jig position at this point, confirm it radiographically.[21] For a noncannulated system, drive a single 0.028-inch wire through the barrel of the jig and down the intended screw path. For a cannulated system, the guide wire serves this purpose. Confirm the reduction and final screw placement radiographically, and trim the periphery of the graft flush with the margins of the proximal and distal fragments with fine-tipped rongeurs.

If interposition bone grafting fails to correct a DISI deformity, the bone graft may be too short anteriorly. It is also possible that there may be associated scapholunate ligament damage[92] or long-standing capsular contracture that prevents full correction of lunate dorsiflexion. Correction of lunate dorsiflexion in the course of bone grafting may be facilitated by pinning it to the radius in its neutral position.

INTERPOSITION BONE GRAFTING WITH RADIAL STYLOIDECTOMY

Both the volar and radial approaches to the scaphoid allow resection of the radial styloid when one is grafting the scaphoid. We prefer the volar approach because it makes interposition bone grafting and correction of angular deformity easier. In the radial approach, the styloid is resected and a part of it is used for in situ dorsoradial inlay bone grafting.[32]

To perform styloidectomy with interposition bone grafting through the volar approach, extend the longitudinal capsular incision sufficiently proximal to allow reflection of the radial capsuloperiosteal flap off the volar and radial side of the radial styloid. Retract this flap and the tendons of the first dorsal compartment, and osteotomize the styloid with a 5/16-inch osteotome just proximal to the level of the non-union. Grasp the styloid fragment with a narrow instrument such as an Alliss clamp, and rotate it to put tension on the styloid's uncut capsular and periosteal fibers. One of the authors (GRM) uses a 0.25-inch sharp curette to dissect the last dorsal fibers off the styloid. It is safer to use a second incision, 2 cm in length and immediately dorsal to the first compartment and parallel to it, to visualize reflection of the dorsal capsule from the styloid.

REVASCULARIZATION PROCEDURES

In persistent scaphoid non-union, avascularity of the proximal pole may be the primary deterrent to suc-

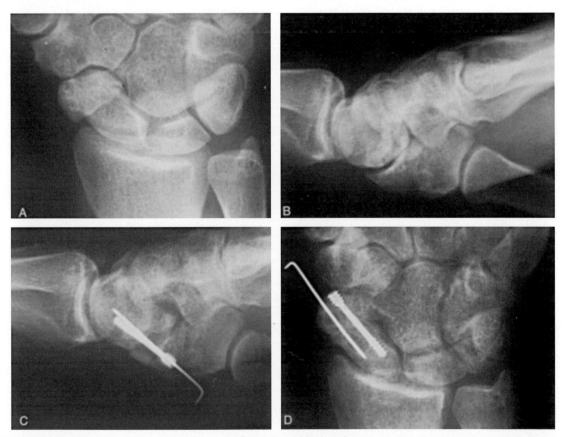

Figure 14–26. Type II scaphoid non-union treated by interposition bone block technique. A, Preoperative posteroanterior view demonstrates displacement. B, Preoperative lateral view suggests dorsiflexion of lunate and proximal scaphoid fragment. C, Postoperative lateral view demonstrates Herbert screw and a 0.035-inch pin transfixing both the scaphoid fragments and the interposition graft. D, At 6 weeks, the graft appears to be incorporated. The wide end of the screw is somewhat proud but not symptomatic.

cessful osteosynthesis. Whereas conventional grafting depends on creeping substitution both to incorporate the graft and to revascularize the proximal pole, revascularization procedures augment circulation directly. Most scaphoid revascularization procedures use pedicled grafts. The exceptions are Hori and colleagues'[59] implantation of the second dorsal metacarpal vascular bundle into the scaphoid, and Pechlaner and associates'[104] use of a free vascularized iliac crest graft. Other surgeons utilize a vascular bone graft from the ulna[56] or radius.[24, 68, 73, 150]

The cases selected for these procedures have ranged from delayed unions of 4 or 5 months[68, 150] to chronic non-unions for which previous procedures have failed,[56, 59, 68, 73, 150] and results appear promising. Researchers report union for all procedures, with a shorter time to union than conventional grafting.

No large prospective study confirms these preliminary reports. Because revascularization procedures require more surgical dissection, we see their best use as a viable alternative to a salvage procedure for patients who do not have midcarpal arthritis (type II and III scaphoid non-unions) for whom previous conventional bone grafting has failed.

For a vascularized bone graft, we prefer to use a corticocancellous distal radius graft pedicled on the dorsal irrigating branch of the radial artery.[150] We use a long chevron incision, which begins at the radial artery about 1.5 inches above the wrist, extends dorsally and distally to the proximal end of the scaphoid (about 1.5 cm distal to Lister's tubercle), and then extends distally and radially along the axis of the extensor pollicis longus (EPL). We mobilize and retract the superficial neurovascular structures, including any branches of the radial nerve, and try to take these volarly with the volar flap if possible. The surgical interval is between the first and second extensor compartments.[150]

Open the first compartment to retract its tendons radially, and free up the tendons of the second compartment to retract them dorsally and ulnarly. We also mobilize the EPL before incising the capsule of the radioscaphoid joint. Make the capsular incision parallel to the dorsal lip of the radius. Resect pseudarthrotic tissue from the non-union, and prepare a slot for the bone graft along the dorsal edge of the

articular surface. We insert 0.035-inch pins retrograde into the distal fragment before bone grafting. Select the donor site beneath the pedicle along the dorsal edge of the distal radius (Fig. 14–27). Incise the periosteum, and remove the graft with small sharp osteotomes. Incise the capsule beneath the pedicle if necessary to avoid kinking or constriction when rotating it into place. Reduce the non-union, inset the graft, and secure the non-union with the pre-positioned pins.

Arthroplasty for Scaphoid Non-Union

Arthroplasty procedures for scaphoid non-union include excision of the proximal pole, with or without interposition of a rolled fascial or tendon graft; soft tissue interposition arthroplasty; proximal row carpectomy[35, 63, 67, 100, 125–127]; and radial styloidectomy (Fig. 14–28).[8, 26, 49, 76, 85, 124]

Proximal pole excision is a simple procedure, but it resects the nonarthritic portion of the radioscaphoid joint and does not address arthritic change between the styloid and the distal pole. Although it is intended to relieve pain at the non-union site, we do not recommend it because it may destabilize the scapholunate interval.

Bentzon and Randlov-Madsen[14] described soft tissue interposition arthroplasty for painful pseudarthrosis of the scaphoid. This procedure interposes a fat-fascia flap between the proximal and the distal scaphoid fragments. These researchers did not recommend this procedure in cases with a small proximal fragment.[14] Perey[106] and Agner[3] reported favorably on this procedure. Boeckstyns and Busch[17] combined radial styloidectomy with the Bentzon technique and reported satisfactory clinical results. We do not use either technique, however, because soft tissue procedures for non-union will not stabilize the carpus or prevent degenerative change.

The indications for prosthetic replacement of the scaphoid with a molded silicone implant no longer exist. The role of this implant was prevention or treatment of degenerative change due to scaphoid non-union.[130] Most non-unions with degenerative changes are displaced and have associated carpal in-

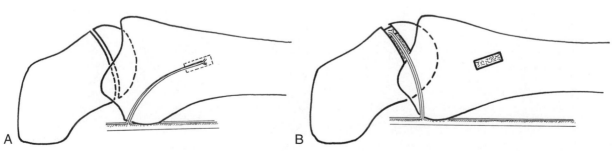

Figure 14–27. Vascularized pedicle bone graft from the distal radius (modified from description by Zaidemberg and colleagues[150]). *A,* Dorsal irrigating branch of the radial artery. *B,* Graft site on dorsoradial cortex of distal radius has been rotated on its vascular pedicle into the curetted non-union site of the scaphoid.

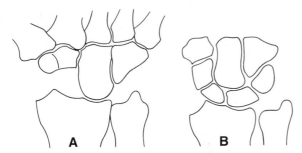

Figure 14–28. Arthroplasty for scaphoid non-union includes proximal row carpectomy (A) and radial styloidectomy (B).

stability,[82] which may lead to excessive shear stress and compressive loading, microfibrillation of its surface, and, in many cases, a late foreign body synovitis of the wrist.[29, 105, 121] Use of the silicone implant in combination with a midcarpal arthrodesis was thought to "stress shield" the implant, but Viegas[144] demonstrated significant residual load-bearing by the implant following simulated midcarpal fusion.

PROXIMAL ROW CARPECTOMY

Proximal row carpectomy (PRC) is a well-recognized procedure for scaphoid non-union,[35, 100] with favorable results as long as 20 years after surgery.[63] Removal of the proximal row repositions the head of the capitate on the distal radius and converts the wrist from a double-hinged system with an intercalated segment to a single nonconstrained joint. Ideally, intact articular cartilage on the dome of the capitate and lunate fossa of the distal radius would appear to favor smooth articulation, but modification of this procedure in patients with capitolunate arthritis suggests that it may also function as a fibrous arthroplasty.[47] Clinical results are comparable to those of scaphoid excision and midcarpal arthrodesis.[134]

Because proximal row carpectomy is a salvage procedure, it is appropriate for established non-unions not suitable for bone grafting. It may be best suited for the type III non-union, in which arthritic change is already present but confined to the radioscaphoid articulation. Good results have also been reported, however, when minimal capitolunate arthritis is present.[100, 141] This procedure is also indicated for type II non-unions not suitable for bone grafting, e.g., those with small or fragmented proximal poles, or failed prior bone grafting. It requires a shorter period of immobilization than bone grafting, and its results are more predictable for high-risk, difficult non-unions, such as those with AVN, small proximal poles, extensive resorption, and long-standing fixed DISI deformity. Two modifications of this procedure may extend its indications to non-unions with midcarpal arthritis (type IV). Fitzgerald and coworkers[47] reported proximal row resection arthroplasty with proximal capitate resection, capsular interposition, and distraction. Tomaino and associates[134] obtained good results from proximal row carpectomy combined with fascial interposition.[134]

Proximal row carpectomy preserves an arc of wrist motion that is functional despite a change in the center of rotation and the juxtaposition of two articular surfaces of different radii.[62] Grip strength is initially diminished but tends to improve over the course of a year.[37, 100, 134] Initial weakness probably reflects the effect that shortening of the wrist has on the length-tension (Blix) curve of the musculotendinous units crossing the wrist, which may improve with time.[23] Grip strengths at 1 year may range from 58 to 90 percent of that in the opposite normal hand.[37, 62, 100] Motion is often greater than the preoperative condition, and may reach 53 to 64 percent of the normal arc.[35, 36] If proximal row carpectomy fails to relieve pain, it may be converted to a wrist arthrodesis.

We perform proximal row carpectomy through either a longitudinal, transverse, or oblique incision. The longitudinal incision provides more exposure, facilitates mobilization of the SBRN, and is also preferred for arthrodesis at a later date if PRC fails. We center it at, or just ulnar to, Lister's tubercle. The transverse incision is more cosmetic than the longitudinal. It extends from the ulnar styloid to the radial styloid, and requires subcutaneous mobilization of longitudinal structures to facilitate exposure. We recommend curving the radial third of the incision slightly distally to facilitate exposure and removal of the scaphoid. The oblique incision is also a modification of the transverse incision to facilitate scaphoid removal. It follows a straight line just ulnar and parallel to the extensor pollicis longus and is centered over the lunate.

After making the skin incision, identify and protect the dorsal cutaneous branches of the radial and ulnar nerves. Open the distal half of the extensor retinaculum with a step-cut to facilitate later reapproximation. Mobilize the tendons of the second and third dorsal compartments radially, and those of the fourth ulnarly. Incise the wrist capsule transversely over the proximal row, and "T" it centrally and distally if necessary.[100] Separate the dorsal capsule from the bones of the proximal row. Take care not to damage the radial artery when exposing the scaphoid. Do not violate the volar capsule.

The orientation of capsular exposure may determine the order of carpal bone resection. It is usually easiest to remove the scaphoid last. If exposure is centered over the lunate, remove it first. Grasp the lunate with a towel clamp and transect the lunotriquetral and scapholunate ligaments. Rotation of the lunate into a volar-flexed position facilitates this step and also "tents" the volar capsule, which is then reflected off the lunate. If a defect is left in the volar capsule, repair it. Neviaser[100] recommends leaving a volar shell fragment of lunate to prevent a capsular defect. Resect the triquetrum next, and then the scaphoid. The scaphoid is the most difficult to remove because of its distal and volar ligamentous attachments. We sometimes find it helpful to insert a 0.062-inch pin into the distal fragment to manipulate it for exposure. Leaving a portion of the distal pole or tuberosity may create a source of impingement,[141] although clinical results may still be good.[47, 134]

Removal of the radial styloid as part of proximal row carpectomy is controversial. Although intraoperative radiographs may suggest impingement, the styloid actually lies volar to the trapezium.[62] Nevertheless, Tomaino and colleagues[134] and Culp and associates[36] showed improved radial deviation following PRC with styloidectomy. We recommend styloid resection if there is intraoperative impingement either in neutral or in radial deviation. Do not resect the origin of the radiocapitate ligament. Van Heest and House[141] resect no more than 5 to 7 mm of styloid.

After removing the proximal row, release the tourniquet and establish hemostasis. Position the capitate in the lunate fossa of the distal radius, and obtain intraoperative radiographs to confirm correct seating. It is usually not necessary to use pin fixation to hold the capitate in the lunate fossa of the radius. At this point, if arthritic change involves the capitate, Fitzgerald and coworkers[47] use pins to *prevent* seating of the capitate in the lunate fossa, and characterize the modified procedure as a "fibrous distraction arthroplasty."

Repair the dorsal capsule, close the skin, and apply a sterile dressing with splints to immobilize the wrist in a neutral position. Remove the sutures at 10 to 12 days, and apply a well-molded short-arm cast. Continue immobilization for a total of approximately 4 weeks. Follow this for the next month with a removable volar wrist splint carefully molded to the new contour of the wrist, and prescribe a graduated program of exercises to mobilize and strengthen the wrist. Strength may increase slowly for up to 12 months postoperatively.

RADIAL STYLOIDECTOMY

Styloidectomy is essentially a hemiresection arthroplasty that relieves painful impingement of the distal scaphoid fragment on the radial styloid. Impingement occurs secondary to volar and radial displacement of the distal pole of the scaphoid, resulting in joint space narrowing, sclerosis, and pointing of the radial styloid. Styloidectomy can be done alone or in combination with bone grafting.[85] As an isolated procedure for type III non-union, it is a simple procedure that does not require prolonged immobilization. Relief may be only temporary, however, because the procedure does not prevent further radial migration of the distal carpal row (Fig. 14–29).[26]

Barnard and Stubbins[8] and Smith and Friedman[120] described the technique of radial styloidectomy. The skin incision may be longitudinal or transverse. The transverse incision is more cosmetic, but the longitudinal incision is safer, because injury to the fine terminal sensory branches of the radial nerve is less likely.

Make a 4-cm incision directly over the radial styloid (see Fig. 14–21). Retract the cephalic vein dorsally. Identify the sensory nerves and gently retract them with their fat. Incise the first dorsal compartment and retract tendons dorsally. Incise and reflect the periosteum over the styloid. To be effective, resection need include only that part of the articular surface upon which the distal pole of the scaphoid impinges and the non-union articulates. Excessive styloid resection may destabilize the carpus radially by transecting the origin of the radiocapitate ligament. We do not resect more than 1 cm in the adult. This procedure therefore may be contraindicated in proximal pole fractures. After repair of the capsule and periosteum, splint the wrist for 7 to 10 days, and then begin a graduated exercise program to restore wrist motion.

Limited Intercarpal Arthrodesis for Scaphoid Non-Union

Limited intercarpal arthrodesis[147] is indicated in scaphoid non-union when degenerative change involves the midcarpal joint (type IV). It is also appropriate for the type III non-union with a small proximal pole, in lieu of proximal row carpectomy.

For type IV non-union, we resect the scaphoid and fuse the midcarpal joint. Midcarpal arthrodesis and scaphoid excision, with or without fascial interposition, provides stability and a predictable range of motion through the unaffected radiolunate joint. We prefer the so-called four-bone arthrodesis[137] of the capitate, lunate, hamate, and triquetrum, because it provides greater surface area than capitolunate arthrodesis alone. We do not recommend scaphocapitate arthrodesis[108] for type IV non-union, because it may not relieve radioscaphoid or capitolunate symptoms. Viegas[144] recommends removal of the distal pole of the scaphoid and incorporation of the proximal pole into an adjacent capitolunate arthrodesis,[144] because the radius–proximal pole articulation, like the radiolunate joint, is frequently spared from degenerative change.

Other surgeons have reported problems with midcarpal fusions, including a non-union rate as high as 33 percent,[110] limited dorsiflexion,[71] and incomplete pain relief.[72] In our experience, it is more difficult to obtain union when the fusion is confined to the capitolunate joint. Midcarpal fusion decreases the size of the dorsiflexion-palmarflexion arc, but capitolunate positioning allows the surgeon to include more dorsiflexion and less palmarflexion in that arc. It is important to correct the DISI deformity and fuse at a capitolunate angle of 0.[134, 144]

For the type III non-union with a small or ungraftable proximal pole, we prefer proximal row carpectomy to limited wrist arthrodesis.

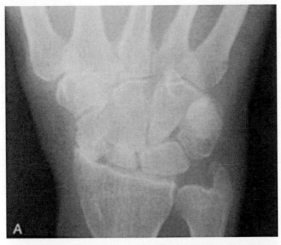

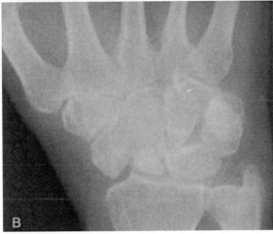

Figure 14–29. Type IV scaphoid non-union treated by radial styloidectomy for symptoms localized to the radioscaphoid joint. *A,* Preoperative view of 24-year-old scaphoid non-union shows arthritis. *B,* Seven months later, radial migration of the distal carpal row has occurred, with the distal scaphoid fragment filling the defect left by the styloidectomy. *C,* Ten years later, radial shift is still apparent, and the proximal scaphoid fragment has collapsed.

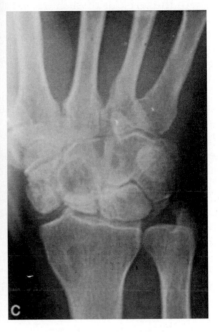

Our current technique for limited arthrodesis excises the scaphoid, exposes and resects the midcarpal and intercarpal surfaces of the capitate-hamate-lunate-triquetrum, interposes cancellous bone graft from the iliac crest, and stabilizes the arthrodesis with 0.062-inch pins. It is easiest to pre-position the pins in the distal bones, reduce and compress the carpal bones to the position desired for fusion, and then drive the pins retrograde into the two proximal bones. Direct visualization of the arthrodesis site is difficult during reduction. Because the lunate is already dorsiflexed, we dorsiflex the wrist, radially deviate it slightly, compress it axially, and then drive the pins retrograde into the lunate and triquetrum. An alternative modification of this technique is to correct lunate dorsiflexion and temporarily transfix the lunate to the radius prior to reduction and pinning at the midcarpal level. In addition to restoring an optimal flexion-extension relationship between the proximal and distal carpal bones, it is also important not to translocate them. Because the proximal row in DISI is dorsiflexed, the distal row tends to maintain a dorsally translocated position with respect to it.

Gordon and King[54] reported favorable results with adequate follow-up in five scaphoid non-unions treated by partial wrist arthrodesis, including four with arthrodesis of the radius to the scaphoid and the lunate. The types and techniques of intercarpal arthrodeses and their indications are also discussed in Chapters 32 and 37.

Wrist Arthrodesis

Wrist arthrodesis is the surgical treatment of choice for scaphoid non-union with advanced degenerative arthritis (type V). Conservative treatment, such as rest, short periods of splinting, and nonsteroidal anti-inflammatory medication, may control arthritic symptoms in some patients. Arthrodesis is also an alternative for a type IV non-union. Arthrodesis is the most definitive treatment for arthritic wrist pain. Its disadvantage is permanent loss of radiocarpal and midcarpal motion.

There are three basic techniques: inlay grafting through the dorsal approach,[1, 27, 31, 77, 129] dorsal arthrodesis with plate fixation,[149] and arthrodesis with inlay bone grafting through a radial approach.[57] Each technique decorticates and grafts the intercarpal joints from the radius to the base of the index and long metacarpals. Failure to fuse the index and long carpometacarpal joints may lead to late symptoms at that level. Inlay grafting techniques require postoperative immobilization in a long-arm cast for 8 to 12 weeks or until union occurs. Arthrodesis with plate fixation requires distal extension of the dorsal approach, but lessens the extent and duration of immobilization, can be performed with local rather than iliac bone graft, and has a high union rate.[149] Arthrodesis through the radial approach is more difficult, because exposure is limited. This technique does not add bulk to the wrist or disturb the extensor retinaculum.

WRIST ARTHRODESIS THROUGH A DORSAL APPROACH

Abbott and colleagues[1] described the basic technique for wrist arthrodesis. Variations of the dorsal technique differ chiefly in the source and shape of the bone graft and the extent of the fusion.[27, 31, 77, 129] The following technique is based on our own experience and incorporates the key principles of dorsal arthrodesis of the wrist.

Use a longitudinal incision and center it over Lister's tubercle (see Fig. 14–30). Make the incision slightly curvilinear to facilitate exposure. The incision should extend from 1.5 inches proximal to the radiocarpal joint to the base of the index and long metacarpals.

Incise the extensor retinaculum between the third and fourth extensor compartments. It is safest to do so by incising over the jaws of a slightly opened hemostat that is positioned radially within the fourth

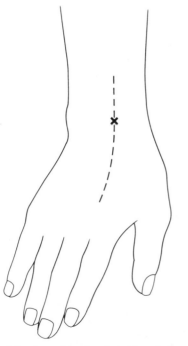

Figure 14–30. Incision for wrist arthrodesis through dorsal approach is centered over Lister's tubercle *(X)*.

compartment. Repair the extensor retinaculum to prevent bow-stringing of the extensor tendons. This may be difficult because the ligament is inelastic and its fibers are transverse. If the ligament is thin, open it with a step-cut to facilitate closure. Carry the incision between the third and fourth compartments down to the bone to facilitate elevation of the second, third, and fourth compartments subperiosteally.

The extent of fusion should include all the affected joints but should exclude the distal radioulnar joint and the fourth and fifth carpometacarpal joints to preserve their mobility for grasp (Fig. 14–31). The triquetrohamate, lunotriquetral, and capitohamate joints are unlikely to be symptomatic if not fused and therefore are excluded from the arthrodesis unless they have arthritic involvement. Incise the capsule to its distal insertion on the base of the second and third metacarpals. "T" the capsule at the radiocarpal joint if necessary to increase exposure. Divide the radial wrist extensor tendons if they impair exposure. Excise proliferative synovium, if present, but preserve the margins of the incised dorsal capsule to present a smooth gliding surface to the underside of the extensor tendons and to help contain the bone graft. If the capsule is insufficient, interpose a portion of the extensor retinaculum between the exposed portion of the fusion mass and the extensor tendons.

Denude the radiocarpal and intercarpal joints to be fused, including the scaphoid non-union or pseudarthrosis, of their cartilage, subchondral bone, and fibrous tissue. Do not disturb the attachments of the palmar capsule to the carpal bones, and do not injure the triangular fibrocartilage.

Inlay a corticocancellous iliac bone graft from the radius to the base of the index and the long metacarpals. The graft should be long enough to bridge the fusion area, approximately 2 cm wide, 6.5 cm long, and 0.5 cm thick. Countersink the graft into slots in the distal radius and in the base of the index and the long metacarpals. Use an oscillating saw to make the slots, and resect the dorsal aspects of the carpal bones to accommodate the graft and make good contact with its undersurface (Fig. 14–31*C*).

Fill the interstices of the denuded intercarpal, radiocarpal, and second and third carpometacarpal joints with small cancellous chips of iliac bone graft.

Countersink the graft into the distal radius and the second and third metacarpals by dorsiflexing the wrist. Position the wrist in 5° to 10° ulnar deviation and approximately 15° dorsiflexion. These angles are formed by the axes of the radius and the long metacarpal; in this position, a line extended from the axis of the radial shaft should roughly bisect the web between the opposed thumb and digits.[22] If stability is not achieved with the graft in place and the wrist slightly dorsiflexed, insert a nonthreaded pin through the distal radius and across the carpus into the base of the third metacarpal.

Apply a sterile dressing and long-arm splint to maintain rigid immobilization of the elbow at 90°, the forearm in neutral rotation, and the wrist in slight

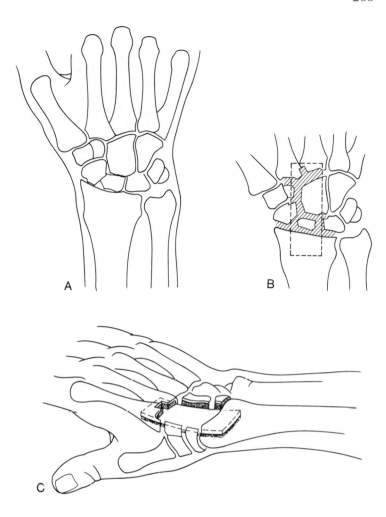

Figure 14–31. *A,* Diagrammatic representation of a type IV scaphoid non-union prior to wrist arthrodesis. *B,* Cartilage and subchondral bone resected from the radiocarpal, midcarpal, and carpometacarpal joints, denoted by shaded area. Note that the articulations of the trapezium, hamate, triquetrum, fourth and fifth metacarpals, and distal ulna are not disturbed. (If plate fixation is to be used, the second carpometacarpal joint is also not disturbed.) *Dashed line* denotes rectangular bed for inlaid corticocancellous iliac graft technique. *C,* Arthrodesis technique, which uses corticocancellous iliac bone graft, extends it from the medullary cavity of the distal radius into base of index and long metacarpals. In this illustration, the ends of the graft are countersunk beneath the cortices of the distal radius and the index and long metacarpals.

dorsiflexion and ulnar deviation. At 10 days, remove the sutures and apply a long-arm cast in the same position. We routinely change the cast and obtain radiographs at the sixth and twelfth weeks after surgery, but more frequent cast changes and repairs are sometimes necessary in active patients.

WRIST ARTHRODESIS WITH PLATE FIXATION

Plate fixation simplifies the stabilization of a dorsal wrist arthrodesis. Without a plate, the arthrodesis depends on a countersunk graft, external immobilization, and/or pins to maintain position until union occurs. It may be difficult to obtain stable pin fixation. Historically, conventional compression plates have been inadequate, because they limit the wrist position to neutral, they are bulky and difficult to contour, and neither they nor their screws fit the metacarpals well. A dynamic compression plate large enough for the radius will be too large for the third metacarpal, and may cause extensor tendonitis.[149]

The AO/ASIF wrist arthrodesis plate avoids these problems. Secure plate fixation allows less restrictive immobilization after surgery. It has a low profile, is precontoured in 10° of dorsiflexion, and has a smaller distal plate width and screw size (2.7 mm) to facilitate metacarpal fixation. The dorsiflexion contour saves intraoperative time otherwise spent adjusting an inlay graft. Because the plate is also made of titanium, which has a modulus of elasticity closer than stainless steel's to that of bone, stress risers adjacent to the plate are less likely.

Arthrodesis with dorsal plate fixation does not use an inlaid block graft but still requires decortication and grafting of the joints being fused. Weiss and Hastings[149] cite the use of bone graft from the distal radius as a distinct advantage over traditional inlay grafting. In addition to these advantages, we are enthusiastic about this technique because it has not been associated with the high incidence of complications associated with wrist arthrodesis.[30]

Extend the dorsal approach for wrist arthrodesis distally onto the third metacarpal. Expose the dorsal aspect of the distal radius, and resect Lister's tubercle. Resect the dorsal fourth of the carpus, and decorticate the intercarpal joints between the distal radius and the third metacarpal. Do not disturb the triquetrohamate or ulnocarpal joints. Do not include the second,[149] fourth, or fifth carpometacarpal joints. Obtain cancellous bone graft from the distal radius with a large curette, and fill the denuded intercarpal joints.

The AO/ASIF plate comes in three sizes. Choose the appropriate plate, and secure it first to the third metacarpal with 2.7-mm screws. Adjust the position of the wrist in the anteroposterior plane, and secure the plate to the radius with 3.5-mm screws. Immobilize the wrist postoperatively with splints until suture removal at 10 to 14 days, and then place the limb in a short-arm molded plastic orthosis.[149] Discontinue immobilization when radiographs demonstrate consolidation of the fusion at all levels.

WRIST ARTHRODESIS THROUGH A RADIAL APPROACH (HADDAD AND RIORDAN)[39]

Make the skin incision on the lateral side of the distal forearm, 1.5 inches proximal to the radial styloid. Follow the radius distally to the radial styloid, and then curve the incision gently upward to the base of the index metacarpal (Fig. 14–32A). Identify the superficial sensory branch of the radial nerve, and mobilize it from the deep structures. Reflect and retract it gently with the volar skin flap. This exposes the extensor tendons of the first, second, and third compartments.

Incise the extensor retinaculum and the periosteum of the distal radius between the first and second dorsal compartments. Elevate periosteal flaps dorsally and volarly. Retract the tendons of the first compartment with the volar periosteal flap. Clear identification and incision of the interval between the first and second compartments make it unnecessary to open the first compartment. Identify the extensor carpi radialis longus at the base of the index metacarpal, and transect it 1 cm proximal to its insertion. It is helpful

to first secure the proximal end of the tendon with a 2-0 suture for later retrieval and repair. Expose the dorsal and radial aspects of the carpus by reflecting the capsular flaps in continuity with the periosteal flaps reflected off the radius. Expose the dorsal and radial aspects of the scaphoid, the trapezoid, the capitate, and the lunate, and the base of the index and long metacarpals.

Throughout the dissection, great care must be taken to avoid injury to the radial artery in the anatomic snuffbox (see Fig. 14–18C). The intercarpal branch of this artery may be ligated and divided, but the radial artery itself should be gently retracted palmarly with the volar flap.

Denude the articular surfaces of the radius, scaphoid, lunate, capitate, trapezoid, and proximal ends of the index and long metacarpals with rongeurs. Do not disturb the hamate, triquetrum, ulnar two metacarpals, or triangular fibrocartilage. Position the wrist in 5° to 10° ulnar deviation and approximately 15° dorsiflexion. These angles are formed by the axes of the radius and the long metacarpal; in this position, a line extended from the axis of the radial shaft should roughly bisect the web between the opposed thumb and digits.[22]

Cut a slot in the lateral cortex of the distal radius, and extend it distally through the carpus to the base of the index and long metacarpals. This is done by using a sharp oscillating saw with a 1-inch blade, while one assistant secures the position of the wrist and a second assistant retracts the soft tissue flaps. The slot should be large enough to accept a corticocancellous graft approximately 2.5 cm wide, 5 cm long, and 5 mm thick (Fig. 14–32B). The graft is obtained from the inner table of the ilium, near the

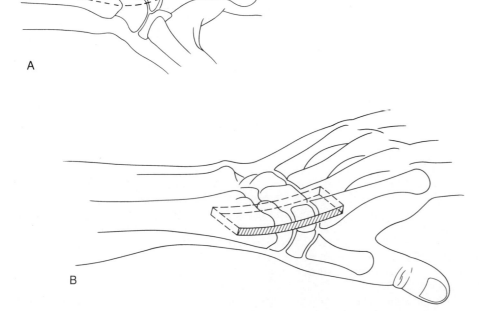

Figure 14–32. *A*, Incision for wrist arthrodesis through radial approach. *B*, Radial slot extending from distal radius to base of index and long metacarpals.

iliac crest. The inner table is recommended because its cortical surface is concave and its cancellous surface is convex. We also use cancellous bone chips for the arthrodesis. The bone graft is keyed into the rectangular slot, and the spaces of the denuded joints are filled with cancellous bone chips.

With the graft in place, the wrist should be stable with slight upward pressure on the palm during application of the postoperative dressing and subsequent casts. Because the inner table of the ilium is thin, the graft may break when the wrist is dorsiflexed. If this occurs or if the wrist is unstable, or both, pass a nonthreaded Kirschner wire obliquely across the arthrodesis to maintain position. Close the capsuloperiosteal flaps, repair the extensor carpi radialis longus, and close the skin.

Postoperative care is the same as that described for arthrodesis with inlay grafting through the dorsal approach.

References

1. Abbott LC, Saunders JB, Bost FC: Arthrodesis of the wrist with the use of grafts of cancellous bone. J Bone Joint Surg 24:883–898, 1942.
2. Adams BD, Frykman GK, Taleisnik J: Treatment of scaphoid nonunion with casting and pulsed electromagnetic fields: A study continuation. J Hand Surg 17A:910–914, 1992.
3. Agner O: Treatment of ununited fractures of the carpal scaphoid by Bentzon's operation. Acta Orthop Scand 33:56–65, 1962.
4. Alho A, Kankaanpaa U: Management of fractured scaphoid bone: A prospective study of 100 fractures. Acta Orthop Scand 46:737–743, 1965.
5. Amadio PC, Berquist TH, Smith DK, et al: Scaphoid malunion. J Hand Surg 14A:679–687, 1989.
6. Aversa JM: Electrical treatment of scaphoid nonunions. Presented at the 50th Annual Meeting of the American Academy of Orthopaedic Surgeons, Anaheim, CA, 1983.
7. Bannerman MM: Fractures of the carpal scaphoid bone: An analysis of sixty-six cases. Arch Surg 53:164–168, 1946.
8. Barnard L, Stubbins SG: Styloidectomy of the radius in the surgical treatment of nonunion of the carpal navicular. J Bone Joint Surg 30A:98–102, 1948.
9. Barr JS, Elliston WA, Musnick H, et al: Fracture of the carpal navicular (scaphoid) bone: An end-result study in military personnel. J Bone Joint Surg 35A:609–625, 1953.
10. Barton NJ: Twenty questions about scaphoid fractures. J Hand Surg 17B:289–310, 1992.
11. Bassett CA, Mitchell SN, Gaston SR: Pulsing electromagnetic field treatment in ununited fractures and failed arthrodeses. JAMA 247:623–628, 1982.
12. Beckenbaugh RD: Noninvasive pulsed electromagnetic stimulation in the treatment of scaphoid nonunion. Presented at the 52nd Annual Meeting of the American Academy of Orthopaedic Surgeons, Las Vegas, 1985.
13. Belsole RJ, Hilbelink DR, Llewellyn JA, et al: Computed analyses of the pathomechanics of scaphoid waist nonunions. J Hand Surg 16A:899–906, 1991.
14. Bentzon PGK, Randlov-Madsen A: On fracture of the carpal scaphoid: A method for operative treatment of inveterate fractures. Acta Orthop Scand 16:30–39, 1946.
15. Berger RA, Kauer JMG: Radioscapholunate ligament: A gross anatomic and histologic study of fetal and adult wrists. J Hand Surg 16A:350–355, 1991.
16. Black DM, Watson HK, Vender MI: Scapholunate gap with scaphoid nonunion. Clin Orthop 224:205–209, 1987.
17. Boeckstyns ME, Busch P: Surgical treatment of scaphoid pseudarthrosis: Evaluation of the results after soft tissue arthroplasty and inlay bone grafting. J Hand Surg 9A:378–382, 1984.
18. Bongers KJ, Ponsen RJ: Operative and nonoperative management of fractures of the carpal scaphoid: Five years' experience. Neth J Surg 32:142–145, 1980.
19. Bora FW, Osterman AL, Brighton CT: The electrical treatment of scaphoid nonunion. Clin Orthop 161:33–38, 1981.
20. Bora FW, Osterman AL, Woodbury DF, et al: Treatment of nonunion of the scaphoid by direct current. Orthop Clin North Am 15:107–112, 1984.
21. Botte MJ, Gelberman RH: Modified technique for Herbert screw insertion in fractures of the scaphoid. J Hand Surg 12A:149–150, 1987.
22. Boyes JW: Surgical Repair of Joints. In Bunnell S: Bunnell's Surgery of the Hand, ed 5. Philadelphia, JB Lippincott, 1970, p 297.
23. Brand PW: Biomechanics of tendon transfer. Hand Clin 4:137–154, 1988.
24. Braun RM: Pronator pedicle bone grafting in the forearm and proximal carpal row. Orthop Trans 7:35, 1983.
25. Brighton CT, Black J, Friedenberg ZB, et al: A multicenter study of the treatment of the non-union with constant direct current. J Bone Joint Surg 63A:2–13, 1981.
26. Brown PE, Dameron TB: Surgical treatment for nonunion of the scaphoid. South Med J 68:415–421, 1975.
27. Butler AA: Arthrodesis of the wrist joint: Graft from the inner table of the ilium. Am J Surg 78:625–630, 1949.
28. Carrozzella JC, Stern PJ, Murdock PA: The fate of failed bone graft surgery for scaphoid nonunions. J Hand Surg 14A:800–806, 1989.
29. Carter PR, Benton LJ: Late osseous complications of the carpal Silastic implants. Presented at the 40th Annual Meeting of the American Society for Surgery of the Hand, Las Vegas, 1985.
30. Clendenin MB, Green DP: Arthrodesis of the wrist: Complications and their management. J Hand Surg 6:253–257, 1981.
31. Colonna PC: A method for fusion of the wrist. South Med J 37:195–199, 1944.
32. Cooney WP, Dobyns JH, Linscheid RL: Nonunion of the scaphoid: Analysis of the results from bone grafting. J Hand Surg 5:343–354, 1980.
33. Cooney WP, Linscheid RL, Dobyns JH: Scaphoid fractures: Problems associated with nonunion and avascular necrosis. Orthop Clin North Am 15:381–391, 1984.
34. Cooney WP, Linscheid RL, Dobyns JH, et al: Scaphoid nonunion: Role of anterior interpositional bone grafts. J Hand Surg 13A:635–650, 1988.
35. Crabbe WA: Excision of the proximal row of the carpus. J Hand Surg 46B:708–711, 1964.
36. Culp RW, McGuigan FX, Turner MA, et al: Proximal row carpectomy: A multicenter study. J Hand Surg 18A:19–25, 1993.
37. De Smet L, Aerts P, Fabry G: Avascular necrosis of the scaphoid: Report of three cases treated with a proximal row carpectomy. J Hand Surg 17A:907–909, 1992.
38. Dias JJ, Brenkel IJ, Finlay DBL: Patterns of union in fractures of the waist of the scaphoid. J Bone Joint Surg 71B:307–310, 1989.
39. Dickison JC, Shannon JG: Fractures of the carpal scaphoid in the Canadian Army: A review and commentary. Surg Gynecol Obstet 79:225–239, 1944.
40. Dooley BJ: Inlay bone-grafting for nonunion of the scaphoid bone by the anterior approach. J Bone Joint Surg 50B:102–109, 1968.
41. Eddeland AE, Eiken O, Hellgren E, et al: Fractures of the scaphoid. Scand J Plast Reconstr Surg 9:234–239, 1975.
42. Eitenmuller JP, Haas HG: Behandlungsergebnisse bei 258 Kahnbeinverletzungen an der Hand. Arch Orthop Trauma Surg 91:45–51, 1978.
43. Engdahl DE, Schacherer TG: A new method of evaluating angulation of scaphoid nonunions. J Hand Surg 14A:1033–1034, 1989.
44. Fernandez DL: A technique for anterior wedge-shaped grafts

for scaphoid nonunions with carpal instability. J Hand Surg 9A:733–737, 1984.

45. Fisk GR: Carpal instability and the fractured scaphoid. Ann R Coll Surg Engl 46:63–76, 1970.

46. Fisk GR: An overview of injuries of the wrist. Clin Orthop 149:137–144, 1980.

47. Fitzgerald JP, Peimer CA, Smith RJ: Distraction resection arthroplasty of the wrist. J Hand Surg 14A:774–782, 1989.

48. Frykman GK, Helal B, Kaufman R, et al: Pulsing electromagnetic field treatment of nonunions of the scaphoid. Presented at the 37th Annual Meeting of the American Society for Surgery of the Hand, New Orleans, 1982.

49. Gartland JJ: Evaluation of treatment for non-union of the carpal navicular. J Bone Joint Surg 44A:169–174, 1962.

50. Gasser H: Delayed union and pseudarthosis of the carpal navicular: Treatment by compression screw osteosynthesis. J Bone Joint Surg 47A:249–266, 1965.

51. Gelberman RH, Menon J: The vascularity of the scaphoid bone. J Hand Surg 5:508–514, 1980.

52. Gilford WW, Bolton BM, Lambrinudi C: The mechanism of the wrist joint: With special reference to fractures of the scaphoid. Guy's Hosp Rep 92:52–59, 1943.

53. Glass KS, Hochberg F: Nonunion of the carpal navicular bone: Comparison of two methods of treatment. Bull N Y Acad Med 54:865–868, 1978.

54. Gordon LH, King D: Partial wrist arthrodesis for old ununited fractures of the carpal navicular. Am J Surg 102:460–464, 1961.

55. Green DP: The effect of avascular necrosis on Russe bone grafting for scaphoid nonunion. J Hand Surg 10A:597–605, 1985.

56. Guimberteau JC, Panconi B: Recalcitrant non-union of the scaphoid treated with a vascularized bone graft based on the ulnar artery. J Bone Joint Surg 72A:88–97, 1990.

57. Haddad RJ, Riordan DC: Arthrodesis of the wrist: A surgical technique. J Bone Joint Surg 49A:950–954, 1947.

58. Herbert TJ, Fisher WE: Management of the fractured scaphoid using a new bone screw. J Bone Joint Surg 66B:114–123, 1984.

59. Hori Y, Tamai S, Okuda H, et al: Blood vessel transplantation to bone. J Hand Surg 4A:23–33, 1979.

60. Hull WJ, House JH, Gustillo RB, et al: The surgical approach and source of bone graft for symptomatic nonunion of the scaphoid. Clin Orthop 115:241–247, 1976.

61. Imaeda T, Nakamura R, Miura T, et al: Magnetic resonance imaging in scaphoid fractures. J Hand Surg 17B:20–27, 1992.

62. Imbriglia JE, Broudy AS, Hagberg WC, et al: Proximal row carpectomy: Clinical evaluation. J Hand Surg 15A:426–430, 1990.

63. Inglis AE, Jones EC: Proximal-row carpectomy for diseases of the proximal row. J Bone Joint Surg 59A:460–463, 1977.

64. Jahna H: Die konservative Behandlung des veralteten Kahnbeinbruchs der Hand. Verh Dtsch Ges Orthop 43:156–160, 1955.

65. Jiranek WA, Ruby LK, Millender LB, et al: Long-term results after Russe bone-grafting: The effect of malunion of the scaphoid. J Bone Joint Surg 74A:1217–1227, 1992.

66. Johnson RP: The acutely injured wrist and its residuals. Clin Orthop 149:33–44, 1980.

67. Jorgensen EC: Proximal-row carpectomy: An end-result study of twenty-two cases. J Bone Joint Surg 51A:1104–1111, 1969.

68. Kawai H, Yamamoto K: Pronator quadratus pedicle bone graft for old scaphoid fractures. J Bone Joint Surg 70B:829–831, 1988.

69. Kerluke L, McCabe SJ: Nonunion of the scaphoid: A critical analysis of recent natural history studies. J Hand Surg 18A:1–3, 1993.

70. Kessler I, Heller J, Silberman Z, et al: Some aspects in non-union of fractures of the carpal scaphoid. J Trauma 3:442–452, 1963.

71. Kirschenbaum D, Schneider LH, Kirkpatrick WH, et al: Scaphoid excision and capitolunate arthrodesis for radioscaphoid arthritis. J Hand Surg 18A:780–785, 1993.

72. Krimmer VH, Sauerbier M, Vispo-Seara JL, et al: Advanced carpal collapse in scaphoid nonunion: Partial mediocarpal fusion as a therapeutic concept. Handchir Mikrochir Plast Chir 24:191–198, 1992.

73. Kuhlmann JN, Mimoun M, Boabighi A, et al: Vascularized bone graft pedicled on the volar carpal artery for non-union of the scaphoid. J Hand Surg 12B:203–210, 1987.

74. Leslie IJ, Dickson RA: The fractured carpal scaphoid: Natural history and factors influencing outcome. J Bone Joint Surg 63B:225–230, 1981.

75. Leyshon A, Ireland J, Trickey EL: The treatment of delayed union and nonunion of the carpal scaphoid by screw fixation. J Bone Joint Surg 66B:124–127, 1984.

76. Lichtman DM, Alexander CE: Decision-making in scaphoid nonunion. Orthop Rev 11:55–67, 1982.

77. Liebolt FL: Surgical fusion of the wrist. Surg Gynecol Obstet 66:1008–1023, 1938.

78. Lindstrom G, Nystrom A: Natural history of scaphoid non-union, with special reference to "asymptomatic" cases. J Hand Surg 17B:697–700, 1992.

79. Linscheid RL, Dobyns JH, Beabout JW, et al: Traumatic instability of the wrist. J Bone Joint Surg 54A:1612–1632, 1972.

80. London PS: The broken scaphoid bone: The case against pessimism. J Bone Joint Surg 43B:237–243, 1961.

81. Louis DF, Calhoun TP, Garn SM, et al: Congenital bipartite scaphoid—fact or fiction? J Bone Joint Surg 58A:1108–1112, 1976.

82. Mack GR, Bosse MJ, Gelberman RH, et al: The natural history of scaphoid nonunion. J Bone Joint Surg 66A:504–509, 1984.

83. Matti H: Technik und Resultate meiner Pseudarthrosenoperation. Zentralblatt Chir 63:1442–1453, 1936.

84. Maudsley RH, Chen SC: Screw fixation in the management of the fractured carpal scaphoid. J Bone Joint Surg 54B:432–441, 1972.

85. Mazet R, Hohl M: Radial styloidectomy and styloidectomy plus bone graft in the treatment of old ununited carpal scaphoid fractures. Ann Surg 152:296–302, 1960.

86. Mazet R, Hohl M: Fractures of the carpal navicular. J Bone Joint Surg 45A:82–111, 1963.

87. Mayfield JK: Mechanism of carpal injuries. Clin Orthop 149:45–54, 1980.

88. McDonald G, Petrie D: Un-united fracture of the saphoid. Clin Orthop 108:110–114, 1975.

89. McLaughlin HL: Fracture of the carpal navicular (scaphoid) bone: Some observations based on treatment by open reduction and internal fixation. J Bone Joint Surg 36A:765–774, 1954.

90. Meyer RD, Sherill J, Daniel W: Electrical stimulation for treatment of nonunion of navicular fractures. Presented at the 50th Annual Meeting of the America Academy of Orthopaedic Surgeons, Anaheim, CA, 1983.

91. Milliez PY, Courandier JM, Thomine JM, et al: The natural history of scaphoid non-union: A review of fifty-two cases. Ann Chir Main 6:195–202, 1987.

92. Monsivais JJ, Nitz PA, Scully TJ: The role of carpal instability in scaphoid nonunion: Casual or causal? J Hand Surg 11B:201–206, 1986.

93. Morgan DA, Walters JW: A prospective study of 100 consecutive carpal scaphoid fractures. Aust N Z J Surg 54:233–241, 1984.

94. Mulder JD: Pseudarthrosis of the scaphoid bone. J Bone Joint Surg 45B:621, 1963.

95. Mulder JD: The results of 100 cases of pseudarthrosis in the scaphoid bone treated by the Matti-Russe operation. J Bone Joint Surg 50B:110–115, 1968.

96. Murray G: Bone graft for nonunion of the carpal scaphoid. Br J Surg 22:63–68, 1934.

97. Murray G: Bone graft for nonunion of the carpal scaphoid. Surg Gynecol Obstet 60:540–541, 1935.

98. Murray G: End results of bone-grafting for nonunion of the carpal navicular. J Bone Joint Surg 28:749–756, 1946.

99. Nakamura R, Imaeda T, Horii E, et al: Analysis of scaphoid fracture displacement by three-dimensional computed tomography. J Hand Surg 16:485–492, 1991.

100. Neviaser RJ: Proximal row carpectomy for post-traumatic disorders of the carpus. J Hand Surg 8:301–305, 1983.

101. Obletz BE, Halbstein BM: Nonunion of fractures of the carpal navicular. J Bone Joint Surg 20:424–428, 1938.

102. Osterman AL, Bora FW Jr: Electrical stimulation applied to bone and nerve injuries in the upper extremity. Orthop Clin North Am 17:353–364, 1986.

103. Palmer I, Widen A: Treatment of fractures and pseudarthrosis of the scaphoid with central grafting (autogenous bonepeg). Acta Chir Scand 110:206–212, 1955.

104. Pechlaner S, Hussl H, Kunzel KH: Alternative Operationsmethode bei Kahnbeinpseudarthrosen: Prospektive Studie. Handchirurgie, Microchirurgie, Plastische Chirurgie 19:302–305, 1987.

105. Peimer CA, Medige J, Eckert BS, et al: Invasive silicone synovitis of the wrist. Presented at the 40th Annual Meeting of the American Society for Surgery of the Hand, Las Vegas, 1985.

106. Perey O: A re-examination of cases of pseudarthrosis of the navicular bone operated on according to Bentzon's technique. Acta Orthop Scand 23:26–33, 1952.

107. Perlik PC, Guilford WB: Magnetic resonance imaging to assess vascularity of scaphoid non-unions. J Hand Surg 16A:479–484, 1991.

108. Pisano SM, Peimer CA, Wheeler DR, et al: Scaphocapitate intercarpal arthrodesis. J Hand Surg 16A:328–333, 1991.

109. Reinus WR, Conway WF, Totty WG, et al: Carpal avascular necrosis: MR imaging. Radiology 160:689–693, 1986.

110. Rotman MB, Manske PR, Pruitt DL, et al: Scaphocapitolunate arthrodesis. J Hand Surg 18A:26–33, 1993.

111. Ruby LK, Stinson J, Belsky MR: The natural history of nonunion of the scaphoid: A review of fifty-five cases. J Bone Joint Surg 67A:428–432, 1985.

112. Russe O: Fracture of the carpal navicular: Diagnosis, nonoperative treatment, and operative treatment. J Bone Joint Surg 42A:759–768, 1960.

113. Sanders WE: Evaluation of the humpback scaphoid by computed tomography in the longitudinal axial plane of the scaphoid. J Hand Surg 13A:182–187, 1988.

114. Sarrafian SK, Melamed JL, Goshgarian GM: Study of wrist motion in flexion and extension. Clin Orthop 126:153–159, 1977.

115. Schneider LH, Aulicino P: Nonunion of the carpal scaphoid: The Russe procedure. J Trauma 22:315–319, 1982.

116. Scott JH: Assessment of ununited fractures of the carpal scaphoid. Proc R Soc Med 49:961–962, 1961.

117. Scott G, King JB: A prospective, double-blind trial of electrical capacitive coupling in the treatment of non-union of long bones. J Bone Joint Surg 76A:820–825, 1994.

118. Smith DK: Anatomic features of the carpal scaphoid: Validation of biometric measurements and symmetry with three-dimensional MR imaging. Radiology 187:187–191, 1993.

119. Smith DK, Cooney W III, An KN, et al: The effects of simulated unstable scaphoid fractures on carpal motion. J Hand Surg 14A(Pt 1):283–289, 1989.

120. Smith L, Friedman B: Treatment of ununited fracture of the carpal navicular by styloidectomy of the radius. J Bone Joint Surg 38A:368–375, 1956.

121. Smith RJ, Atkinson RE, Jupiter JB: Silicone synovitis of the wrist. J Hand Surg 10A:47–60, 1985.

122. Southcott R, Rosman MA: Nonunion of carpal scaphoid fractures in children. J Bone Joint Surg 59B:20–23, 1977.

123. Speed K: The fate of the fracatured navicular. Ann Surg 80:532–535, 1924.

124. Sprague B, Justis EJ: Nonunion of the carpal navicular. Arch Surg 108:692–697, 1974.

125. Stack JK: End results of excision of the carpal bones. Arch Surg 57:245–252, 1948.

126. Stamm TT: Excision of the proximal row of the carpus. Proc R Soc Med 38:74–75, 1944.

127. Stamm TT: Developments in orthopaedic operative procedures. Guy's Hosp Rep 112:1–114, 1963.

128. Stark HH, Rickard TA, Zemel NP, et al: Treatment of ununited fractures of the scaphoid by iliac bone grafts and Kirschner-wire fixation. J Bone Joint Surg 70A:982–991, 1988.

129. Stein I: Gill turnabout radial graft for wrist arthrodesis. Surg Gynecol Obstet 106:231–232, 1958.

130. Swanson AB: Silicone rubber implants for the replacement of the carpal scaphoid and lunate bones. Orthop Clin North Am 1:299–309, 1970.

131. Taleisnik J, Kelly PJ: The extraosseous and intraosseous blood supply of the scaphoid bone. J Bone Joint Surg 48A:1125–1137, 1966.

132. Taleisnik J: The ligaments of the wrist. J Hand Surg 1:110–118, 1976.

133. Tiel-van Buul MMC, van Beek EJR, Dijkstra TF, et al: Radiography of the carpal scaphoid: Experimental evaluation of "the carpal box" and first clinical results. Invest Radiol 27:954–959, 1992.

134. Tomaino MM, Miller RJ, Cole I, et al: Scapholunate advanced collapse wrist: Proximal row carpectomy or limited wrist arthrodesis with scaphoid excision? J Hand Surg 19A:134–142, 1994.

135. Torngren S, Sandqvist S: Pseudarthrosis in the scaphoid bone treated by grafting with autogeneous bone-peg. Acta Orthop Scand 45:82 88, 1974.

136. Trumble TE: Avascular necrosis after scaphoid fracture: A correlation of magnetic resonance imaging and histology. J Hand Surg 15A:557–564, 1990.

137. Trumble T, Bour CJ, Smith RJ, et al: Intercarpal arthrodesis for static and dynamic volar intercalated segment instability. J Hand Surg 13A:396–402, 1988.

138. Trojan E: Grafting of ununited fractures of the scaphoid. Proc R Soc Med 67:1078–1080, 1974.

139. Unger HS, Stryker WC: Nonunion of the carpal navicular: Analysis of 42 cases treated by the Russe procedure. South Med J 02.020–622, 1960.

140. Urban MA, Green DP, Aufdemorte TB: The patchy configuration of scaphoid avascular necrosis. J Hand Surg 18A:669–674, 1993.

141. Van Heest AE, House JH: Proximal row carpectomy. In Gelberman RH (ed): Master Techniques in Orthopaedic Surgery: The Wrist. New York, Raven Press, 1994.

142. Vender MI, Watson HK, Weiner BD, et al: Degenerative change in symptomatic scaphoid non-union. J Hand Surg 12A:514–519, 1987.

143. Verdan C, Narakas A: Fractures and pseudarthrosis of the scaphoid. Surg Clin North Am 48:1083–1095, 1968.

144. Viegas SF: Limited arthrodesis for scaphoid nonunion. J Hand Surg 19A:127–133, 1994.

145. Viegas SF, Patterson RM, Peterson PD, et al: The silicone scaphoid: A biomechanical study. J Hand Surg 16A:91–97, 1991.

146. Watson HK, Ballet FL: The SLAC wrist: Scapholunate advanced collapse pattern of degenerative arthritis. J Hand Surg 9:358–365, 1984.

147. Watson HK, Goodman ML, Johnson TR: Limited wrist arthrodesis. Part II: Intercarpal and radiocarpal combinations. J Hand Surg 6:223–233, 1981.

148. Watson HK, Pitts EC, Ashmead D, et al: Dorsal approach to scaphoid nonunion. J Hand Surg 18A:359–365, 1993.

149. Weiss A-PC, Hastings H: Wrist arthrodesis for traumatic conditions: A study of plate and local bone graft application. J Hand Surg 20A:50–56, 1995.

150. Zaidemberg C, Siebert JW, Angrigiani C: A new vascularizaed bone graft for scaphoid nonunion. J Hand Surg 16A:474–478, 1991.

CHAPTER 15

Scapholunate Injuries

Gerald Blatt, MD, Brian Tobias, DO, and David M. Lichtman, MD

When first popularized, *carpal instability*[52, 248] was essentially synonymous with *scapholunate instability*.[190, 293] In 1976, Mayfield and associates[198, 199] described a continuum of "progressive perilunate instabilities," with scapholunate instability representing the first stage. Since then, several additional patterns of carpal instability have been identified,[4, 63, 84, 132, 180, 185, 274, 304] although scapholunate instability remains the most common type.[245, 278, 306] Scapholunate instability can occur as an isolated clinical entity[185, 245, 275] or as a residual of a perilunate injury[16, 48, 49] and is also commonly seen in association with scaphoid[102, 213, 262] and distal radial[114, 156, 167, 209, 241] fractures.

Despite the frequency of scapholunate instability, several characteristics of this injury remain poorly understood, and therefore, the classification and treatment have been incomplete. As defined by Kleinman,[158] scapholunate instability requires a "disruption of the mechanical linkage between the scaphoid and lunate bones." However, although the anatomic structure of the scapholunate articulation has been more accurately defined,* the specific cascade of ligament failure leading to progressive instability remains undetermined.[137, 149, 185, 201, 246, 260] In addition, some authorities have reported that injury to the scaphotrapeziotrapezoid (STT) articulation may be required for more advanced scapholunate instability patterns.[149, 271]

Multiple investigators have also suggested that some clinically significant scapholunate injuries are not associated with intercarpal instability and that a spectrum of severity of ligament injury exists that ranges from minor sprains, which may be stable, to complete ligament disruptions, which are progressively unstable.[125, 150, 182, 186, 277, 306, 310] Furthermore, the acute scapholunate injury possesses a unique potential for ligament healing, whereas in the chronic injury, the opportunity for ligament repair has often passed, and "secondary changes" may be present. These secondary changes, which significantly alter the prognosis and treatment of chronic scapholunate injuries, include capsular contractures, intercarpal collapse deformities, scaphoid and midcarpal fixation, degenerative arthritis, and scapholunate advanced collapse.†

As the appreciation of these sometimes subtle but critical characteristics of scapholunate injuries has evolved, so has the clinical approach. This chapter reviews the current understanding of the normal periscaphoid anatomy and biomechanics as well as the etiology, pathomechanics, and natural history of scapholunate injuries. In addition, we introduce a new classification system for scapholunate injuries, review the diagnostic and therapeutic options available, and present a treatment approach to guide in the management of these common, yet often therapeutically challenging injuries.

ANATOMY

Many investigators have contributed to the current understanding of the anatomy of the wrist and its nomenclature.* A thorough discussion of their work is contained in Chapter 2. However, a short review of carpal anatomy as it pertains to the scapholunate articulation is pertinent.

The scaphoid and lunate carpal bones form the primary osseous contributors to the scapholunate articulation, although the interarticular surface area is small and does not provide inherent osseous stability. As identified by Kauer,[154] the scaphoid and lunate proximal articular curvatures are not symmetric. The greater lunate arc results in a scapholunate intercarpal shift with wrist motion (Fig. 15–1). The lunate proximal-to-distal length is greater palmarly than it is dorsally; thus, the lunate has an inherent tendency to dorsiflex.[153]

As originally reported by Mayfield and associates[198] and Talesnik,[272] the major ligaments stabilizing the wrist are intracapsular. The integrity of these ligaments at both the scapholunate and scaphotrapezotrapezoid articulations profoundly affects scapholunate stability.[84, 88, 161, 185, 271, 309] Berger and colleagues[23–27] have more accurately defined the scapholunate ligament complex, and Drewniany and coworkers[89] have clarified the original description by Crosby and associates[66] of the scaphotrapezial ligament complex.

The scapholunate ligament complex is divided into two major groups, intrinsic and extrinsic (Table 15–1). The intrinsic scapholunate ligament complex consists of the three components of the scapholunate

---

*References 16, 23–27, 33, 62, 140, 154, 155, 185, 295, 296.
†References 62, 94, 127, 150, 185, 277, 304, 307, 311.

*References 6, 16, 23–27, 33, 36, 62, 140, 154–155, 185, 196, 272, 295, 296.

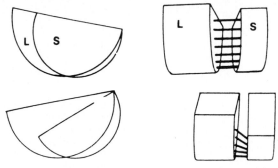

Figure 15–1. As identified by Kauer,[154] the scaphoid *(S)* and lunate *(L)* proximal articular curvatures are asymmetrical, resulting in a scapholunate intercarpal shift during wrist motion. (From Kauer JMB: Functional anatomy of the wrist. Clin Orthop 149:73, 1980.)

interosseous ligament (SLI), dorsal, palmar and proximal. The extrinsic scapholunate ligament complex has four components: the radioscaphocapitate ligament (RSC), the long radiolunate ligament (LRL), the short radiolunate ligament (SRL), and the radioscapholunate ligament (RSL) or ligament of Testut.[202] The extrinsic ligaments tend to be stiffer, whereas the intrinsic ligaments are stronger and more elastic, and may elongate significantly before permanent deformation occurs.[189]

The scaphotrapeziotrapezoid (STT) ligament complex (Table 15–2) also has four components: the scaphotrapezial ligament (STL), the fibrous floor of the flexor carpi radialis tendon sheath, the scaphocapitate ligament (SCL), and the dorsal capsule (DC). The anatomic restraints of the STT articulation are structurally more significant anteriorly, and although the primary ligamentous stabilizer(s) remain undefined, the scaphotrapezial ligament and palmar capsule/flexor carpi radialis (PC/FCR) tendon sheath appear predominant.[89]

The Scapholunate Ligament Complex

The intrinsic scapholunate interosseous ligament is a C-shaped structure that connects the scaphoid and lunate along the periphery of their adjacent dorsal, proximal, and palmar articular margins. The articulation remains open distally at the midcarpal joint (Fig.

Table 15–1. THE SCAPHOLUNATE LIGAMENT COMPLEX

Intrinsic scapholunate ligament complex	Extrinsic scapholunate ligament complex
Scapholunate interosseous ligament	Radioscaphocapitate ligament
Dorsal component	Radiocollateral component
Proximal component	Radioscaphoid component
Palmar component	Radiocapitate component
	Long radiolunate ligament
	Short radiolunate ligament
	Radioscapholunate ligament (ligament of Testut)

Table 15–2. THE SCAPHOTRAPEZIOTRAPEZOID LIGAMENT COMPLEX

Scaphotrapezial ligament
Palmar capsule/flexor carpi radialis tendon sheath
Scaphocapitate ligament
Dorsal capsule

15–2). The scapholunate interosseous ligament increases in length from dorsal to palmar to accommodate the different articular curvatures of these carpals[155]; it has been shown to stretch by 50 to 100 percent of its original length before failure.[198]

The dorsal component is trapezoidal, being more narrow proximally, and averages 5 mm in proximal-to-distal length and 3 mm in thickness. Histologically, it consists of transversely oriented collagen fibers. The dorsal radiocarpal joint capsule inserts into this dorsal component proximally and isolates its distal three quarters from the radiocarpal joint space. Distally, the dorsal component blends with the scaphotriquetral ligament, and proximally, it merges with the proximal component of the scapholunate ligament.[23, 26]

The proximal component is avascular and histologically consists of thin, pliable fibrocartilage.[140] Occasionally, a wedge-shaped distal protrusion is seen that extends into the scapholunate articulation, analogous to a knee meniscus.[179] Palmarly, the proximal component merges with the palmar component and the extrinsic radioscapholunate ligament.[24]

The palmar component is relatively thin compared with its dorsal counterpart, averaging 1 mm in thickness. It also consists of collagen fibers; here, however, the fibers are oriented slightly obliquely, from proximal-ulnar to distal-radial.[23] The long radiolunate ligament passes anteriorly across the palmar component before the palmar component blends with the radioscaphocapitate ligament distally. The radioscapholunate ligament inserts into the palmar component, effectively isolating it from the radiocarpal joint.[25, 26]

This regional structural differentiation of the intrinsic scapholunate interosseous ligament may reflect the functional contribution of each component to proximal scapholunate stability. The dorsal and, to a lesser extent, palmar components may provide the intrinsic strength of the scapholunate articulation, and the proximal membranous portion may function as a pliable axis about which the palmar and dorsal components rotate and translate with wrist motion.

The extrinsic radioscaphocapitate ligament is a broad, strong ligament that also consists of three major components, identified according to their insertional locations: the radial collateral, the radioscaphoid, and the radiocapitate[24] (Fig. 15–3). The radial collateral component inserts onto the distal pole of the scaphoid before blending distally with the scaphotrapezial ligament. The radioscaphoid component inserts onto the scaphoid wrist before merging dis-

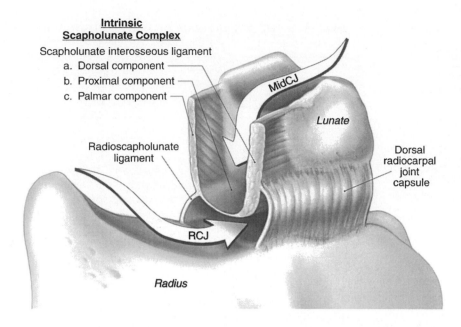

Intrinsic
Scapholunate Complex

Scapholunate interosseous ligament
    a. Dorsal component
    b. Proximal component
    c. Palmar component

Radioscapholunate
ligament

MidCJ

Lunate

Dorsal
radiocarpal
joint
capsule

RCJ

Radius

Figure 15–2. As defined by Berger and colleagues,[23–27] the intrinsic scapholunate interosseous ligament is a C-shaped complex open distally at the midcarpal joint *(mid CJ)* that connects the scaphoid and lunate along the periphery of their adjacent articular surfaces and is subdivided into anatomically and histiologically distinct dorsal, proximal, and palmar components. However, the scapholunate interosseous ligament is not completely visible from the radiocarpal joint space, because the dorsal radiocarpal joint *(RCJ)* capsule inserts proximally into the dorsal component, isolating its distal three quarters from the radiocarpal joint, and palmarly, the extrinsic radioscapholunate ligament inserts at the junction of the proximal and palmar components, effectively isolating the palmar component from the radiocarpal joint. (See text for complete description.)

tally with the scaphocapitate ligament. The radiocapitate component arches across the proximal pole of the scaphoid toward the capitate, blending slightly with the scaphocapitate ligament before the bulk of the fibers continue across the head of the capitate to form a ligamentous "sling" as they interdigitate with the ulna-based ulnocarpal ligament.[26] The radial collateral and radioscaphoid components of the radioscaphocapitate ligament are primary scaphoid stabilizers, providing the only ligamentous link between the radius and the scaphoid.

The adjacent extrinsic long radiolunate ligament also arises from the anterior lip of the radius contiguous with the radioscaphocapitate ligament to form

the central palmar radiocarpal ligamentous link of the extrinsic scapholunate ligament complex (see Fig. 15–3). Separated from the radioscaphocapitate ligament by an interligamentous sulcus, it continues distal-ulnarly, superficial to the palmar component of the scapholunate interosseous ligament and the radioscapholunate ligament, to insert along the radial palmar surface of the lunate.[23] The long radiolunate ligament resists ulnar translation and dorsiflexion of the lunate with respect to the radius.

The extrinsic short radiolunate ligament is a flat sheet of collagen fibers that originates from the palmar margin of the radius lunate facet to insert distally into the palmar edge of the lunate, adjacent to the

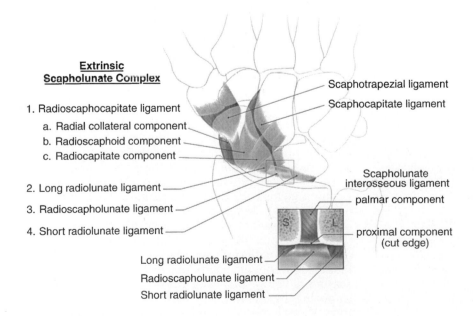

Extrinsic
Scapholunate Complex

1. Radioscaphocapitate ligament
    a. Radial collateral component
    b. Radioscaphoid component
    c. Radiocapitate component

2. Long radiolunate ligament
3. Radioscapholunate ligament
4. Short radiolunate ligament

Scaphotrapezial ligament
Scaphocapitate ligament

Scapholunate
interosseous ligament
    palmar component
    proximal component
    (cut edge)

S   L

Long radiolunate ligament
Radioscapholunate ligament
Short radiolunate ligament

Figure 15–3. As further defined by Berger and colleagues,[23–27] the extrinsic scapholunate ligaments form a broad volar complex connecting the radius, scaphoid *(S)*, and lunate *(L)* that consists of four anatomically distinct structures: including the radioscaphocapitate, long radiolunate, short radiolunate, and radioscapholunate ligaments. (See text for complete description.)

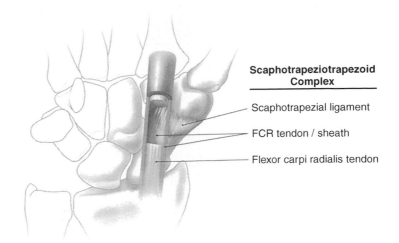

Figure 15–4. As originally described by Crosby and associates[66] and clarified by Drewniany and coworkers,[89] the scaphotrapeziotrapezoid *(STT)* ligament complex consists of four anatomically distinct components: the scaphotrapezial ligament, palmar capsule/flexor carpi radialis *(FCR)* tendon sheath, the scaphocapitate ligament, and the dorsal capsule. (See text for complete description.)

Scaphotrapeziotrapezoid Complex

- Scaphotrapezial ligament
- FCR tendon / sheath
- Flexor carpi radialis tendon

palmar extent of the proximal lunate articular cartilage[26] (see Fig. 15–3). The short radiolunate ligament is a key stabilizer of the lunate, providing the primary checkrein to lunate extension.

The final component of the scapholunate extrinsic ligament complex is the radioscapholunate ligament or ligament of Testut[282] (see Fig. 15–3, *inset*). This structure, found overlying the interval between the long radiolunate and short radiolunate ligaments, defines the division between the proximal and palmar components of the scapholunate interosseous ligament.[23] The radioscapholunate ligament is a relatively weak, predominantly synovial structure that provides for passage of the branches of the anterior interosseous and radial arteries, as well as the anterior interosseous nerve, to the scapholunate interosseous ligament.[26, 140]

The Scaphotrapeziotrapezoid Ligament Complex

The scaphotrapezial ligament is located along the radiopalmar surface of the STT articulation just radial to the flexor carpi radialis tendon sheath (Fig. 15–4). It originates from the scaphoid tubercle, where terminal fibers of the radial collateral component of the radioscaphocapitate ligament blend with it, and it inserts distally along the trapezial ridge. The underlying scaphotrapeziotrapezoid palmar capsule is a relatively thin structure that is reinforced volar ulnarly by the thick fibrous floor of the FCR tendon sheath.

The scaphocapitate capsular ligament originates from the scaphoid tubercle to insert along the capitate neck, separate from the adjacent radioscaphoid component of the radioscaphocapitate ligament. A distinct interval is often difficult to identify, because the fibers of the two components merge imperceptibly. The final component of the STT ligament complex, the dorsal capsular ligament, is often insufficient and appears to contribute little to stability.[89]

CARPAL KINETICS AND PATHOKINEMATICS

The major links for mobility in the carpus, as defined by Alexander and Lichtman[4] in their "oval ring" concept, are at the STT and triquetrohamate (TH) articulations (Fig. 15–5). In the normal, uninjured wrist, the proximal carpal row dorsiflexes in ulnar deviation and palmar-flexes in radial deviation[38, 155, 172, 196, 252, 314] (Fig. 15–6*A* and *B*). These movements occur because the flexion and extension moments generated

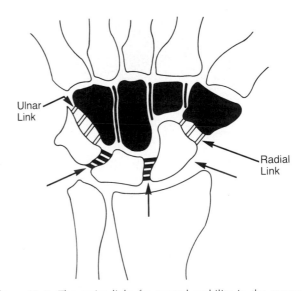

Figure 15–5. The major links for normal mobility in the carpus, as defined by Alexander and Lichtman[4] in their "oval ring" concept, are at the scaphotrapeziotrapezoid (STT) and the triquetrohamate (TH) articulations. The proximal and distal carpal row links in this carpal ring are not rigid, and intercarpal motion does occur within the proximal and distal carpal rows to promote smooth, intercalated wrist motion. However, any disruption in the "oval ring," either osseous or ligamentous, leads to abnormal intercarpal motion in the affected carpal link and may result in instability. (From Lichtman DM, Schneider JR, Swafford AR, et al: Ulnar midcarpal instability: Clinical and laboratory analysis. J Hand Surg 6:515, 1981.)

Ulnar Link

Radial Link

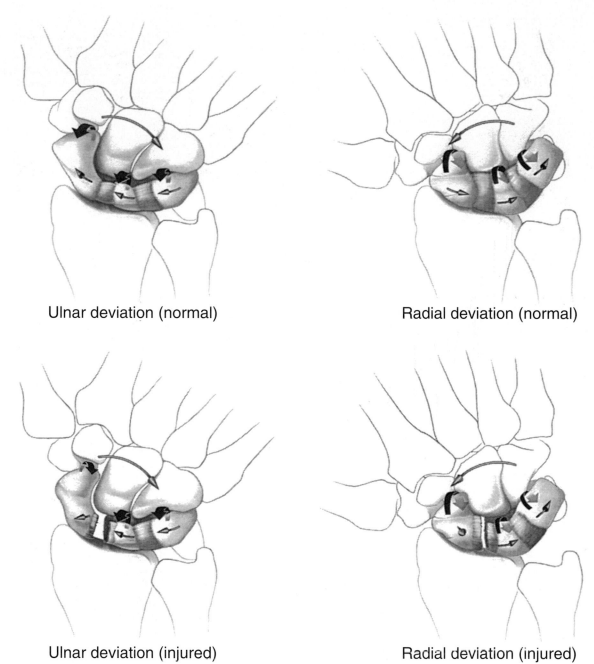

Ulnar deviation (normal)   Radial deviation (normal)

Ulnar deviation (injured)   Radial deviation (injured)

Figure 15–6. *A* and *B,* In the normal, uninjured wrist, the flexion moment generated at the scaphotrapeziotrapezoid (STT) articulation in radial deviation results in proximal carpal row palmar-flexion. In addition, the extension moment generated at the triquetrohamate (TH) articulation in ulnar deviation results in proximal carpal row dorsiflexion. This occurs because the respective moments are balanced across the intact proximal carpal row link. *C* and *D,* In the injured wrist, after the scapholunate articulation has been disrupted, an imbalance across the proximal carpal row link is created. Thus, the normal proximal carpal row flexion moment produced at the STT articulation cannot be counterbalanced ulnarly, and the scaphoid flexes independent of the lunate and triquetrum (which are released into extension). Similarly, the proximal carpal row extension moment produced at the TH articulation is not counterbalanced radially, and the lunate and triquetrum extend independent of the scaphoid (which is released into palmar-flexion).

at the STT and TH articular links, respectively, are balanced across the intact proximal carpal row.

However, these intercarpal ligament links of the proximal (and distal) carpal rows are not rigid, and intercarpal motion does occur within these carpal rows to promote smooth intercalated wrist motion. This physiologic intercarpal motion is influenced by several factors, including the individual carpal bone

geometry and ligament restraints, the position of the adjacent carpal bones, and the direction and velocity of wrist motion.[20, 21, 247, 252, 260, 299] Normal scapholunate intercarpal motion is approximately 10° (±3°) during wrist radial and ulnar deviation and 25° (±15°) in wrist flexion and extension.[245, 247]

After an injury (Fig. 15–6C and D), when the scapholunate link is disrupted, an imbalance across the

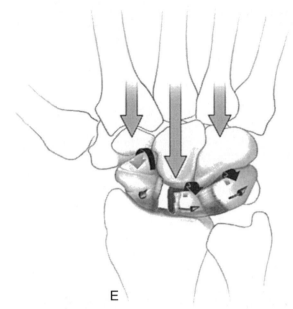

E

Grip stress neutral deviation (injury)

Figure 15–6. *Continued E,* In "power grip" stress loading of the injured wrist with a scapholunate disruption, the capitate is driven like a battering ram into the scapholunate articulation, further potentiating the intercarpal disruption and highlighting any occult intercarpal instability.

proximal carpal row is created. Therefore, the normal proximal carpal row flexion moment produced at the STT articulation is not counterbalanced ulnarly, and the scaphoid flexes independent of the lunate and triquetrum (which are released into extension). Similarly, the proximal carpal row extension moment produced at the TH articulation is not counterbalanced radially, and the lunate and triquetrum extend independent of the scaphoid (which is released into palmar-flexion). In addition, during power grip loading of the wrist (Fig. 15–6E), the capitate is driven like a battering ram into the scapholunate articulation, further aggravating the ligament disruption and potentiating progressive intercarpal instability.

Although the specific anatomic cascade of ligament failure leading to this progressive scapholunate injury is not completely understood, the long-term consequences of abnormal intercarpal motion secondary to disruption of the scapholunate linkage include altered articular cartilage contact pressures[32, 43, 298, 299] and progressive secondary changes (capsular contractures, intercarpal collapse deformities, scaphoid and/or midcarpal fixation, degenerative arthritis, and scapholunate advanced collapse [SLAC wrist]).* More complete discussions of the current appreciation of wrist mechanics and pathomechanics are contained in Chapters 4, 5, and 12.

MECHANISM OF INJURY

Many patients describe the mechanism of their scapholunate injury as a fall forward onto an outstretched

hand, which results in an axial compression force at the base of the palm. Others state that they fell backward onto a pronated hand, so the direction of the axial compression force was to the ulnar side of the wrist or hypothenar eminence.[171, 191, 211, 283, 306]

Although a variety of clinical injury patterns can occur, it appears that the consistent factors in scapholunate injury are axial compression, wrist hyperextension, intercarpal supination, and ulnar deviation, as described by Mayfield and colleagues.[196, 198, 199] This mechanism alone however, does not explain all scapholunate injuries.[29, 45, 52, 84, 88, 102, 141, 254] Partial carpal fixation, allowing unbalanced injury force transmission, may also contribute. In light of the detailed scapholunate ligamentous anatomy described by Berger and coworkers[23–27] and the potential contributions of STT joint injury as identified by Szabo and associates,[271] further investigation into the specific cascade of ligament injury leading to progressive periscaphoid instability is warranted.

Short and colleagues[260] have shown that sectioning the scapholunate interosseous ligament alone leads to increased scaphoid flexion and pronation, without concomitant lunate flexion or pathologic extension, during physiologic cyclic passive motion of the wrist. After sectioning the scapholunate interosseous ligament, they also demonstrated a redistribution of radiocarpal articular pressure from the radioscaphoid fossa to the radiolunate fossa. Hankin and coworkers[131] have reported that an STT disruption can also lead to a similar scaphoid palmar flexion deformity. However, Ruby and colleagues[246] and others[185, 201] have shown that disruption of the scapholunate interosseous ligament alone does not produce a visible scapholunate diastasis. A radiographically demonstrable scapholunate dissociation requires "significant" ligament injury and may be absent even with disruption of both the scapholunate interosseous and radioscaphocapitate ligaments.[201]

Szabo and associates[271] found that the ligament injuries seen in scaphoid dislocation support a progressive sequence of periscaphoid ligament failure that begins at the proximal pole of the scaphoid and scapholunate articulation and progresses distally to the STT articulation. Inoue and Maeda[149] also suggest that significant scapholunate and STT injury overlap exists.

Even though our understanding of the specific anatomic cascade of ligament failure is incomplete, the clinical spectrum of scapholunate injury probably varies with the magnitude, duration, and direction of the force vectors as well as the position and direction of wrist motion. Only very slight alterations in this alignment-force mechanism are required to change the spectrum of periscaphoid injury from sprain[151] to scaphoid dislocation,* to perilunate dislocation,[2, 28, 52, 103, 186, 199, 254] to scaphoid fractures[102, 116, 268, 294] or ulnar translocation of the carpus.[84, 232]

---

*References 1, 12, 94, 99, 132, 160, 186, 259, 273, 304, 310, 312.

*References 8, 45, 58, 69, 102, 104, 139, 149, 171, 226, 255, 281, 283, 284.

Table 15–3. THE DEFINING CHARACTERISTICS OF SCAPHOLUNATE INJURIES

Chronicity	Time since injury
	Presence of secondary changes
Severity	Extent of intercarpal instability

CLASSIFICATION OF SCAPHOLUNATE INJURIES

Scapholunate injuries have been described and categorized on the basis of their clinical, radiographic, and arthroscopic features, as well as a variety of etiologic factors.* At this time, there is no universally accepted classification system for these injuries.[6, 127, 207] However, certain characteristics of scapholunate injuries—*chronicity*, as determined by the time since injury and the presence of secondary changes, and *severity*, as evidenced by the extent of intercarpal instability—play a critical role in determining the prognosis and treatment of these injuries (Table 15–3).

The time from injury to diagnosis and treatment is a strong indicator of the potential for ligament repair.[6, 84, 174, 182, 245, 278, 306, 313] Following the *acute* scapholunate injury, there is a limited time during which the injured ligaments maintain their potential for healing and thus are surgically repairable.[84, 108, 125, 184, 207, 275, 306] The duration of this acute period has not been clearly determined, and empiric suggestions range from 3 to 20 or more weeks.[184, 275]

Although consistent in their absence of ligament healing potential, *chronic* scapholunate injuries are not always otherwise equal, and they may be associated with various secondary changes.[12, 61, 132, 150, 175, 185, 259, 304] As previously discussed, these secondary changes uniquely define many chronic scapholunate injuries. They include capsular contracture, fixed scaphoid and intercarpal collapse deformities, scapholunate advanced collapse (SLAC) wrist, and pancarpal degenerative arthritis.

The SLAC wrist, probably the most significant of the secondary changes, was first described by Watson and colleagues.[304, 308] They identified the association of progressive proximal capitate migration and radioscaphoid and/or capitolunate arthrosis with untreated chronic scapholunate dissociation (Figs. 15–7 and 15–8). Watson and Ryu[311] later subdivided SLAC wrist into three stages according to the location of the secondary arthrosis: In *stage I* SLAC wrist, arthrosis is limited to the radial styloid-scaphoid articulation; in *stage II*, arthrosis involves the entire radioscaphoid articulation; and in *stage III*, there is capitolunate arthrosis. Watson and colleagues[309, 313] have also described isolated scaphotrapeziotrapezoid arthrosis in

untreated chronic scapholunate injuries. In these cases, the scapholunate instability is concentrated at the distal scaphoid articulation, leading to progressive degeneration.

The presence of intercarpal instability is a major factor in the determination of the severity of both acute and chronic scapholunate injuries. Watson and colleagues[274, 303, 306, 310] have incorporated many of the specific clinical and radiographic findings of scapholunate instability to classify these injuries as predynamic, dynamic, or static. According to these investigators, *predynamic scapholunate instability* is associated with a positive clinical examination and

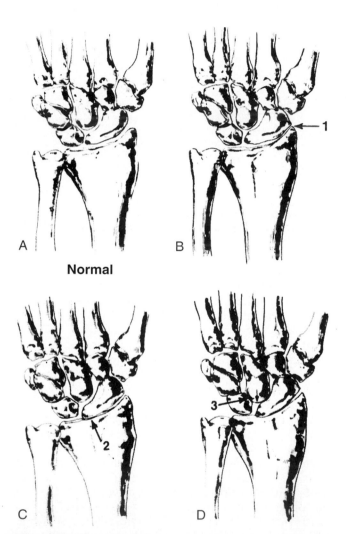

Figure 15–7. The most common pattern of degenerative arthritis seen in untreated chronic scapholunate instability is termed SLAC wrist, or scapholunate advanced collapse deformity. This predictably progressive sequence of degenerative changes associated with chronic scapholunate injuries is subdivided into three stages according to the location of the secondary arthrosis. *A,* Normal wrist for comparison. *B, Stage I* SLAC wrist manifests as arthrosis limited to the radial styloid-scaphoid articulation *(1). C,* In *Stage II,* arthrosis involves the entire radioscaphoid articulation *(2). D, Stage III* is signified by the presence of capitolunate arthrosis *(3).* (From Watson KH, Ryu J: Degenerative disorders of the carpus. Orthop Clin North Am 15:337–354, 1984.)

*References 1, 34, 62, 85, 114, 125, 142, 163, 175, 185, 197, 243, 245, 278, 310.

normal radiographic findings whereas in *dynamic scapholunate instability*, carpal alignment is abnormal on wrist "grip stress" radiographic views[118] and/or with stress cineradiography.[125] In contrast, *static instability* manifests as abnormal carpal alignment, including scaphoid malrotation, scapholunate diastasis, and often a dorsal intercalary segment instability (DISI) collapse pattern on standard non-stress wrist radiographs.[84, 117]

To highlight the presence of "occult" scapholunate injuries, Geissler and associates[113, 114] developed an arthroscopic classification of intercarpal instability on the basis of the severity of intra-articular ligament injuries seen arthroscopically. In grade I and grade II injuries, there is attenuation and/or hemorrhage of the interosseous ligament. The carpus is stable in grade I, but in grade II injury, midcarpal scapholunate incongruity can be seen, representing occult instability. In grade III and grade IV injuries, there is a complete disruption of the interosseous ligament in association with midcarpal and radiocarpal scapholunate incongruity and progressive intercarpal instability.

Although both of these descriptive classifications

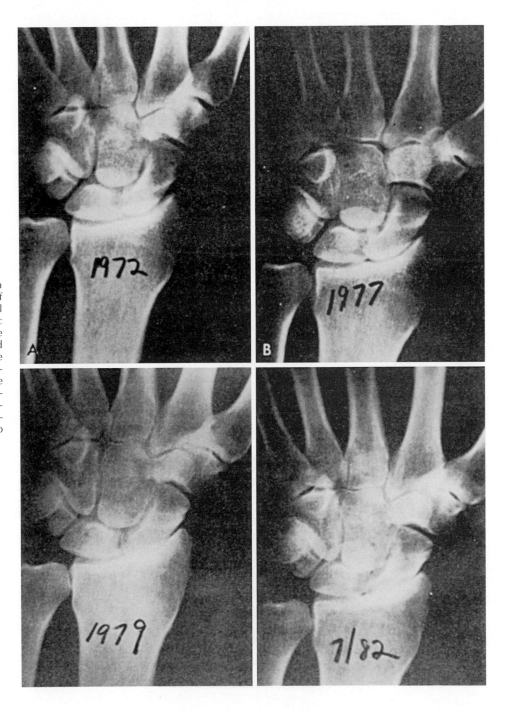

Figure 15–8. A 10-year case observation demonstrates the progressive sequence of SLAC wrist degeneration. *A*, The initial wrist radiographs demonstrate a chronic scapholunate injury with early osteophyte formation at the radial styloid-scaphoid articulation. *B* and *C*, Degenerative changes progress to involve the radioscaphoid articulation. *D*, Subsequently, the capitolunate articulation is involved, although the radiolunate articulation is preserved. (From Watson KH, Ryu J: Degenerative disorders of the carpus. Orthop Clin North Am 15:337–354, 1984.)

(Watson and Geissler) are useful in estimating the severity of ligament disruption and the degree of intercarpal instability, neither addresses the presence of secondary fixed deformities or end-stage pancarpal arthrosis seen in association with chronic injuries.[12, 132]

We therefore propose a more comprehensive classification for scapholunate injuries that blends both chronicity, as determined by time since injury and the presence of secondary changes, and severity, as evidenced by the extent of intercarpal instability. We believe that this classification system, presented in Table 15–4, is straightforward and easy to understand, but most important, it provides practical guidelines for treatment and prognostic determinations of scapholunate injuries.

Initially, we divide all scapholunate injuries into two major groups, *acute* and *chronic*, according to the time elapsed from injury to diagnosis and initial treatment. Although great variation is possible, we have selected up to 6 weeks after injury to define the acute scapholunate injury period, during which we believe that ligament repair is feasible. We classify any scapholunate injury diagnosed and/or treated thereafter as chronic.

Next, we subclassify both acute and chronic scapholunate injuries as either *stable* or *unstable*. We believe that scapholunate injuries occur secondary to a yet unknown, but predictably progressive anatomic cascade of ligament failures. This progressive severity of injury continuum includes those symptomatic scapholunate injuries that are associated with an incomplete ligament disruption, but no clinical, radiographic, or arthroscopically demonstrable intercarpal instability (*stable* injuries) as well as the more complete ligament disruptions that are associated with intercarpal instability (*unstable* injuries).

We incorporate progressive degrees of intercarpal instability in the unstable category by additionally subdividing both acute and chronic unstable scapholunate injuries into *dynamic* and *static* groups similar to those described by Watson and colleagues. A dynamic instability requires clinical induction to be appreciated, whereas a static instability is present at rest, as demonstrated on nonstress radiographs and/or arthroscopic examination.

In addition to appreciating these differences in ligament healing potential and the presence of a progressive severity of injury continuum, we believe that the occurrence of secondary changes uniquely defines certain chronic scapholunate injuries. Specifically, we find that capsular contracture resulting in a fixed, clinically unreducible scaphoid (palmar-flexion) or midcarpal collapse (DISI) deformity, SLAC wrist, and pancarpal arthrosis are the most clinically significant. Therefore, we have further subclassified chronic scapholunate injuries into *fixed* (clinically unreducible) deformities, *SLAC wrist*, and *pancarpal arthrosis* categories to emphasize these often underappreciated but otherwise critical characteristics. In addition, we have modified the SLAC wrist classification to include the occurrence of isolated STT arthrosis seen with some chronic scapholunate injuries.

Although not integral to our classification system and treatment approach, the etiologic determination of scapholunate injuries can provide additional insight into the pathologic cascade and natural history of the disorder. Scapholunate instability has been reported in association with distal radius fractures,[114, 126, 156, 185, 209, 241, 262] scaphoid fractures,[102, 138, 163, 213, 294] lunate dislocation,[103, 254] rheumatoid arthritis,[67, 133, 162, 181, 187] calcium pyrophosphate dihydrate crystal deposition disease,[86, 234, 235] Kienböck's disease,[34] degenerative arthritis,[134, 138, 307, 329] and infections[307] as well as iatrogenic conditions, including excision of dorsal wrist ganglions.[54, 65, 91].

DIAGNOSIS

Patients with a potential scapholunate injury can present with a variety of different clinical scenarios and/or coexistent conditions.* The most successful results of treating scapholunate injuries are obtained following the prompt diagnosis of the acute injury.[177, 184, 219, 278] Therefore, a vigilant history, thorough physical examination, and accurate radiographic evaluation are required to determine the correct diagnosis.

History

Patients with an isolated acute scapholunate injury usually present with a recent history of wrist trauma, but occasionally, they may describe a less severe initiating event, such as forcefully power-gripping a tool or performing a pushup. Despite the potential for

Table 15–4. CLASSIFICATION OF SCAPHOLUNATE INJURIES

Acute
1 Stable
2 Unstable
  a Dynamic
  b Static

Chronic
1 Stable
2 Unstable
  a Dynamic
  b Static
3 Fixed
  a Scaphoid "irreducible" *but* midcarpal joint reducible
  b Scaphoid "irreducible" *and* midcarpal joint irreducible
4 With scapholunate advanced collapse (SLAC wrist)
  a Radial styloid–scaphoid arthrosis
  b Radioscaphoid arthrosis
  c Capitolunate arthrosis
  d Scaphotrapeziotrapezoid arthrosis
5 With pancarpal arthrosis

---

*References 14, 49, 76, 81, 128, 135, 163, 183, 235, 253, 328.

significant ligament disruption, many patients present nonemergently with only subtle complaints of wrist stiffness, motion-related "clicking" or "snapping," and/or weakness with pinch or grip.[275] A history of a painful snap over the dorsoradial aspect of the wrist at the time of injury that was associated with localized soft tissue swelling and increased pain with motion is helpful, although not diagnostic.[193, 313] When multiple acute injuries are present, the acute scapholunate injury can easily be overlooked, and many patients with such injuries are initially treated for a wrist sprain or occult scaphoid fracture.

Patients with chronic scapholunate injuries often may not recall any specific etiologic traumatic event, although a history of multiple wrist "sprains" is not unusual. Those patients who do recall a specific injury usually also describe a variable period after the injury when their symptoms abated and they returned to significant pain-free use of the wrist and hand.[151] Over time, however, their wrist pain, swelling, and stiffness usually recur and are often associated with progressive functional limitations.[53]

Physical Examination

The initial examination of an acute or chronic scapholunate injury often reveals only diffuse nonspecific pain and soft tissue swelling, which are common to many wrist injuries,[125, 185, 199] although intercarpal instability, fixed contractures, and a positive finger extension test, as described in Chapter 6, are occasionally present.

When instability is present, a palpable and sometimes audible "click" may be elicited at the scapholunate interval with wrist motion. The scaphoid shift test, as described by Watson and colleagues[303, 306, 313] (Fig. 15–9), can be used to reproduce and evaluate this "click"; the technique for performing this test is described in Chapter 6. The scaphoid shift test is a subjective provocative maneuver that requires considerable experience to perform and interpret accurately.[173, 327] Easterling and Wolfe[92] have shown that 14 percent of normal patients demonstrate bilateral asymmetry with the scaphoid shift test and that there is a 32 percent prevalence of painless scaphoid shift in the uninjured population. Wolfe and Crisco[327] reported a 25 percent incidence of bilateral scaphoid shift in the uninjured population, a finding that may indicate generalized ligament laxity, especially when the patient is asymptomatic.

To further evaluate increased scaphoid mobility at the STT articulation, we perform the STT shuck test (Fig. 15–10). This test is performed while the patient is positioned as for the scaphoid shift test. The examiner then stabilizes the patient's scaphoid between the examiner's ipsilateral thumb, index, and middle fingers while using his or her contralateral hand to

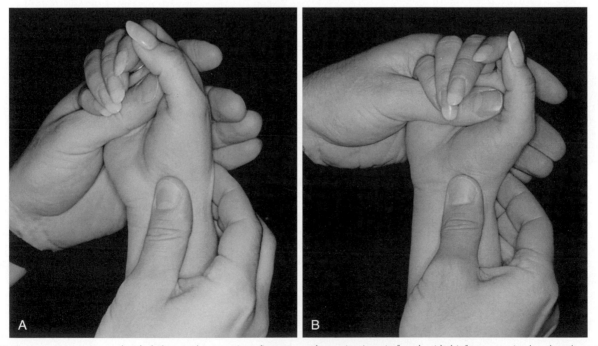

Figure 15–9. *A,* In Watson's scaphoid shift test, the examiner first grasps the patient's wrist/hand with his/her opposite hand and gently ulnar-deviates the patient's wrist. The examiner then places his/her ipsilateral thumb on the patient's scaphoid tubercle (volar) and his/her corresponding index and middle fingertips over the dorsal aspect of the patient's scapholunate articulation. *B,* The patient's wrist is then gently brought into radial deviation (by the examiner's opposite hand), and the scaphoid palmar flexion is resisted with the examiner's (ipsilateral) thumb on the scaphoid tubercle while the examiner palpates the dorsum of the scapholunate articulation. Significant findings include asymmetric increased or decreased scaphoid mobility pain and/or crepitance.

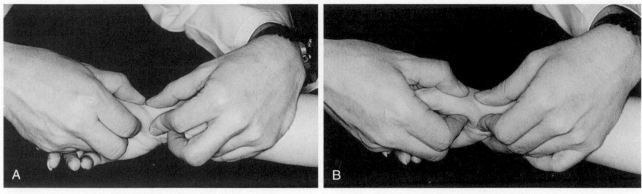

Figure 15–10. The "STT shuck" test is used to further evaluate increased scaphoid mobility at the scaphotrapeziotrapezoid (STT) articulation. *A*, The examiner stabilizes the patient's scaphoid between his/her opposite thumb, index, and middle fingers while using his/her ipsilateral hand to hold the patient's thumb metacarpal base and trapezium as a unit. *B*, The STT articulation is then passively subluxed dorsally and volarly. The examiner is careful to note any hypermobility, pain, or crepitance. This maneuver is performed several times to "precondition" the wrist and bilaterally to establish asymmetry.

hold the patient's thumb metacarpal base and trapezium as a unit. The examiner then passively subluxes the STT articulation dorsally and volarly, being careful to note any hypermobility, pain, or crepitance. This maneuver is performed several times to "precondition" the wrist, and bilaterally to establish asymmetry. In the patient with advanced secondary changes, including a fixed scaphoid deformity, the results of both the STT shuck test and Watson's scaphoid shift test are inconsistent and unreliable.

The physical examination of a scapholunate injury does not offer a simple positive or negative diagnosis, but instead yields a spectrum of findings.[173, 303] To accurately diagnose a scapholunate injury and deter-

mine its chronicity and severity, the examiner must correlate these findings with additional information obtained from appropriate imaging* and other special[61, 212, 218, 277, 306, 310] studies.

Radiology

Plain radiographs of the wrist are the single most important imaging studies to be performed in patients with a possible scapholunate injury.† However, the

---

*References 10, 18, 110, 117, 118, 194, 195, 210, 285, 290.
†References 19, 47, 80, 84, 110, 117, 118, 141, 144, 145, 151, 185, 194, 195, 241, 256.

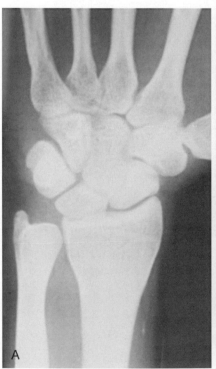

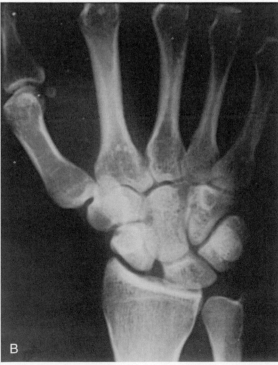

Figure 15–11. *A*, Routine PA projection with the wrist in pronation reveals apparent normal carpal alignment. *B*, The same wrist in supination on AP projection demonstrates scapholunate dissociation, or "Terry-Thomas" sign.

standard wrist posteroanterior (PA) projection can be misleading. Even in the presence of a static scapholunate instability, it may give the false impression of normal carpal alignment[19, 46, 51, 110, 118, 290, 306, 310] (Fig. 15–11).

Many "standard" radiographic specialty views, positions, and techniques have been described to minimize the frequency of undiagnosed scapholunate injuries.[73, 79, 110, 117, 176, 201, 206] Specifically, Gilula and Weeks[117] report that the wrist supination view (anteroposterior [AP] projection) highlights the scapholunate articulation and is an excellent view on which to appreciate a subtle static scapholunate dissociation. In addition, Dobyns and coworkers[84] have reported that a compression stress load applied across the wrist accentuates any carpal malalignment when ligament laxity or dynamic instability is present. To further maximize the diagnosis of scapholunate injuries, Gilula and coworkers[118, 290] have described a static wrist instability "motion series," consisting of 18 views, that provides a comprehensive evaluation of the carpus. We have found this extensive series to be impractical for routine clinical screening and prefer to use a modified series that consists of bilateral, unstressed wrist AP and lateral views in neutral, wrist PA views in radial and ulnar deviation, and bilateral wrist supination (AP) "grip" stress views (Table 15–5). When additional visualization of the scaphoid is desired, an oblique wrist ulnar deviation view can be added.[206]

Once adequate bilateral wrist radiographs have been obtained,[151, 257] examination includes inspection of the individual carpal bone architecture, intercarpal alignment,[125, 186] greater and lesser carpal arc congruity,[117, 118] carpal height ratio,[214, 331] ulnar variance,[98, 223] and soft tissue changes.[72] Specific key diagnostic radiographic features of a scapholunate injury are lack or loss of scapholunate articular parallelism,[125] scapholunate diastasis,[109, 117, 186, 274] decreased scaphoid cortical ring-to-proximal-pole interval,[30, 51, 125] asymmetric radioscaphoid interval,[201] increased radioscaphoid, capitolunate, and/or scapholunate angle,[117, 176] lunate extension,[47] and DISI pattern.[172, 186] Progressive degenerative changes consistent with SLAC wrist may also be present[304] (Table 15–6).

The *lack or loss of interarticular parallelism* between the opposing surfaces of the scaphoid and lunate on the AP nonstress view is a subtle sign of scapholunate incongruity that may represent an im-

Table 15–5. MODIFIED WRIST INSTABILITY "MOTION" SERIES OF RADIOGRAPHS

AP wrist in neutral
Lateral wrist in neutral
PA wrist in radial deviation
PA wrist in ulnar deviation
AP wrist (supination) "grip" stress view

Table 15–6. KEY RADIOGRAPHIC CHARACTERISTICS OF UNSTABLE SCAPHOLUNATE INJURIES

Anteroposterior view	Loss of scapholunate articular parallelism
	Scapholunate diastasis > 3 mm
	Decreased scaphoid cortical ring-to-pole interval, (> 4 mm asymmetry) or absolute value < 7 mm)
	Asymmetric radioscaphoid interval (normal = 0.4 mm)
	Lunate extension
	Degenerative arthritis
Lateral view	Radioscaphoid angle > 80°
	Capitolunate angle > 20°
	Scapholunate angle > 70°
	DISI deformity
	Degenerative arthritis

portant supportive finding for occult instability.[125] The presence of a *scapholunate diastasis*, or a widened space between the scaphoid and lunate, is a more obvious sign of significant scapholunate injury, especially when it is present unilaterally and the gap is greater than 3 mm.[117, 186, 222, 274] This has been referred to, among more timely descriptions, as the "Terry-Thomas" sign[109] (Fig. 15–12).

The scaphoid cortical *ring-to-proximal-pole inter-*

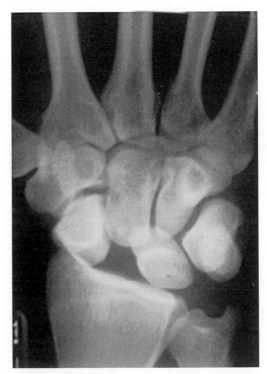

Figure 15–12. Scapholunate diastasis, or a widened space between the scaphoid and lunate (unstressed), is a more obvious sign of significant scapholunate injury, especially when it occurs unilaterally and the gap is greater than 3 mm. In addition, when the scaphoid is foreshortened and the cortical "ring" shadow is present, a rotatory scaphoid subluxation is confirmed.

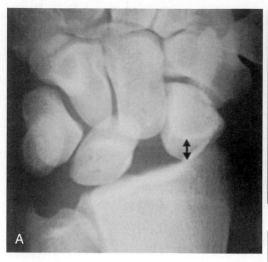

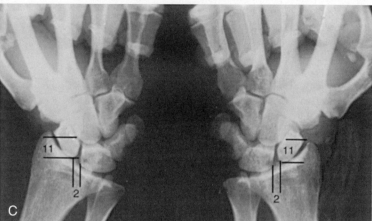

Pre-operative

One Year Postoperative

Figure 15–13. *A,* The scaphoid cortical ring-to-proximal-pole interval is measured from the proximal border of the scaphoid cortical ring to the proximal pole of the scaphoid. When abnormal scaphoid rotation (palmar flexion) is present, the ring-to-proximal-pole distance is reduced by at least 4 mm compared with the opposite, uninjured side, and/or is no greater than 7 mm. *B,* Before operation, the ring-to-proximal-pole distance in this deformity is 6 mm, compared with 11 mm on the normal side. *C,* Postoperatively, derotation of the scaphoid and restoration of axial length are confirmed.

val, originally described by Blatt[30] as a simple, objective measurement of abnormal scaphoid rotation, is obtained from the frontal (AP projection) radiograph. The interval is measured from the proximal border of the scaphoid cortical ring to the proximal pole of the scaphoid. When abnormal scaphoid rotation (palmar-flexion) is present, the ring-to-proximal-pole distance is reduced by at least 4 mm compared with the other, uninjured side, and/or is no greater than 7 mm (Fig. 15–13*A*).[30] Furthermore, when the abnormal scaphoid rotation is corrected, the ring-to-proximal-pole distance is restored to equal that of the uninjured side (Fig. 15–13*B* and *C*).

The *radioscaphoid interval,* described by Meade and associates,[201] is another relatively straightforward measurement that reflects scaphoid palmar-flexion on the AP view (Fig. 15–14). The radioscaphoid interval is determined by drawing a line connecting the most radial and ulnar margins of the scaphoid fossa of the radius, and then measuring along a perpendicular bisecting this line, the distance between the scaphoid facet of the radius and the proximal scaphoid articular surface. The average change in this interval with radial and ulnar deviation in the normal wrist is 0.4 mm. When the radioscaphocapitate ligament is

sectioned, the average radioscaphoid interval is increased almost eight times. Thus, the radioscaphoid interval appears to be an important indicator of significant ligament injury[201] seen with scaphoid rotation as well as ulnar translocation.[232]

To further assess the degree of scaphoid instability, the lateral radiographic projection of the wrist in neutral deviation is closely reviewed.[97, 186] Three important reference angles to be determined and compared bilaterally[117, 176, 257] are the *radioscaphoid, capitolunate* and *scapholunate angles.* Complete descriptions of the tangent and axial techniques[111, 176] used to obtain these angle measurements are given in Chapter 7.

The *radioscaphoid angle* measures an average of 58°, with ranges between 33° and 73°.[273] The *capitolunate angle* is considered normal within a +15° to −20° degree range; when this angle exceeds +20°, significant lunate dorsiflexion instability is present.[186] The *scapholunate angle* normally averages 47°, although any angle between 30° and 60° is acceptable when bilaterally symmetric.[185] The scapholunate angle is not sensitive for less severe forms of scapholunate injury.[201] When the scapholunate angle is greater than 70°, however, excessive scaphoid flexion is present, and significant ligament disruption should be suspected.[84]

Another radiographic sign of an unstable static scapholunate injury seen in the lateral view is the *DISI deformity.*[117, 172, 186] Linscheid and associates[186] originally coined this term to describe the findings of lunate extension and scaphoid flexion often seen in association with a static scapholunate instability. A DISI deformity is now characterized by (1) a scapholunate angle greater than 70°, (2) a capitolunate angle greater than 20°, and (3) a dorsiflexed and palmarly displaced lunate[84, 184, 222] (Fig. 15–15). The DISI deformity is not pathognomonic for scapholunate instability, however, and can be seen in association with unstable scaphoid fractures[103, 262] *("bony" DISI),* distal radius fractures[163, 279] *("compensatory" DISI),* radius malunion[279, 314] *("adaptive" DISI),* and other capsular wrist problems[83, 125, 186] as well as scapholunate instability[185] *("ligamentous" DISI).*

Cantor and Braunstein[47] described a technique to distinguish lunate extension and flexion on the frontal (AP) radiograph and allow the diagnosis of intercalary instabilities without the use of the lateral radiograph. In DISI, the distal lunate contour is rounded (distally prominent palmar horn), and the distal contour width is wider than the lunate "ridge line," confirming lunate extension (Fig. 15–16A). Conversely, in the volar intercalary instability (VISI), the distal lunate contour is angular (distally prominent dorsal horn), and the distal contour width is

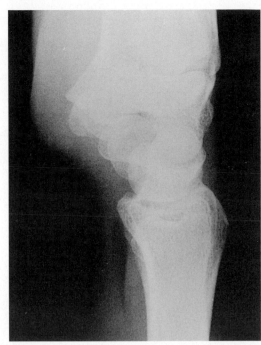

Figure 15–15. The DISI (dorsiflexed intercalary instability) deformity is another radiographic sign of an unstable static scapholunate injury. It is characterized by a scapholunate angle greater than 70°, a capitolunate angle greater than 20°, and a dorsiflexed and palmarly displaced lunate. However, the DISI deformity is not pathognomonic for a scapholunate injury.

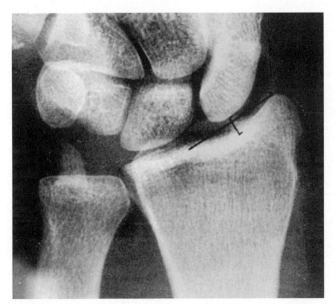

Figure 15–14. The radioscaphoid interval is determined by drawing a line connecting the most radial and ulnar margins of the scaphoid fossa of the radius, and then measuring along a perpendicular bisecting this line, the distance between the scaphoid facet of the radius and the proximal scaphoid articular surface. When the radioscaphoid interval is abnormal, significant scaphoid rotation and/or ulnar translocation is present. (From Meade TD, Schneider LH, Cherny K: Radiographic analysis of selective ligament sectioning at the carpal scaphoid: A cadaveric study. J Hand Surg 15A:855–862, 1990.)

narrower than the lunate "ridge line," indicating lunate flexion (Fig. 15–16C and D).

The *SLAC deformity* is a late sign of chronic scapholunate instability.[12, 99, 184, 309] Although its onset is variable, the classic SLAC pattern consists of (1) rotatory scaphoid subluxation, (2) ulnar translocation of the lunate, and (3) proximal capitate migration associated with (4) periscaphoid and/or capitolunate arthrosis.[304, 306, 309] The carpal height ratio may also be altered in SLAC wrist.[214, 331]

Lastly, the incidence of ulnar-negative variance[98, 146, 223, 300] has been reported to be higher in patients with post-traumatic scapholunate dissociation.[73, 79] However, the clinical and therapeutic implications of this observation are undetermined at present.[278]

Special Studies

Although many of the radiographic features already discussed are characteristically present in unstable scapholunate injuries, there can be significant scapholunate ligament complex damage without clinical or plain radiographic evidence of intercarpal instability.[201, 306] Therefore, the diagnosis of scapholunate injury can often require more advanced diagnostic techniques, such as triple-injection wrist arthrography,* arthroscopy,[3, 33, 61, 62, 114, 164, 212, 253, 322] videofluo-

*References 22, 37, 48, 61, 119, 137, 192, 202, 224, 316, 332.

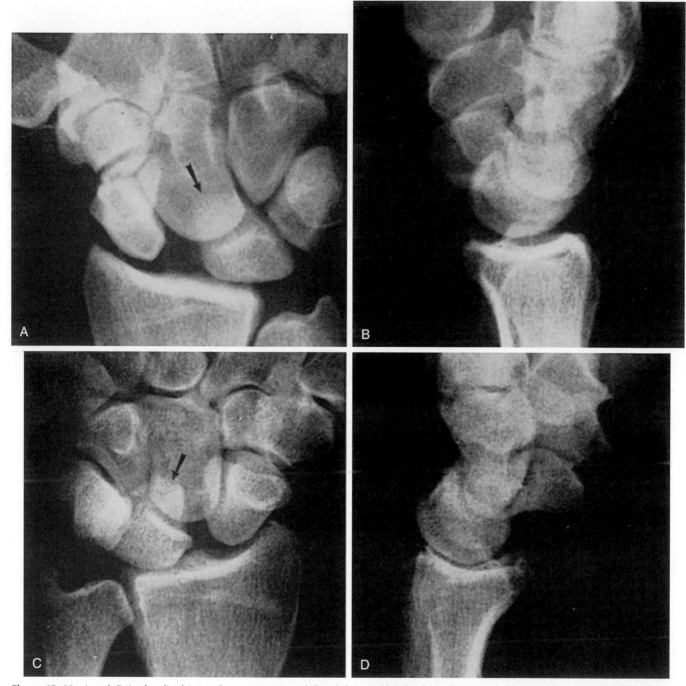

Figure 15–16. *A* and *B,* In the distal intercalary segment instability deformity, the distal lunate contour is rounded *(arrow),* corresponding to a distally prominant palmar horn, and the distal contour width is wider than the lunate "ridge line," confirming lunate extension: *C* and *D,* Conversely, in the volar intercalary segment instability deformity, the distal lunate contour is angular *(arrow),* corresponding to a distally prominent dorsal horn, and the distal contour width is narrower than the lunate "ridge line," indicating lunate flexion. (From Cantor RM, Braunstein EM: Diagnosis of dorsal and palmar rotation of the lunate on a frontal radiograph. J Hand Surg 13A:187–193, 1988.)

roscopy,[10, 37, 125, 252] and magnetic resonance (MR) imaging.[16, 129, 210, 285, 317, 318, 333]

ARTHROGRAPHY

Traditionally, triple-injection wrist arthrography has been the "next step" after plain radiographs are in-

conclusive to further evaluate for a scapholunate injury, because it is very helpful in identifying subtle intercarpal communications.* The passage of arthrographic dye through the scapholunate interval in a patient clinically suspected of having a scapholunate

---

*References 22, 37, 48, 61, 119, 192, 202, 224, 245, 332.

injury can be diagnostically very reassuring. However, the correlation of these arthrographic communications with the site of symptomatic wrist pathology is inconsistent.[48, 61, 137, 192, 202] Furthermore, Cantor and associates[48] have identified a high prevalence of bilaterally symmetric, asymptomatic, arthrographic lesions, including a 57 percent prevalence of bilateral scapholunate defects. Herbert and colleagues[137] found that 74 percent of their patients in whom bilateral arthrograms were obtained also had abnormal findings in the asymptomatic wrist.

Although wrist arthrography still holds a place in the evaluation of acute and chronic wrist pain, it does not reliably demonstrate ligament laxity, mild cases of synovitis, associated osteochondral injuries, or the extent of ligament injury.[117, 119] Therefore, we rarely order wrist arthrograms now, and we recommend MR imaging and/or wrist arthroscopy, unless contraindicated, as the procedure of choice to further evaluate suspected scapholunate injuries.

ARTHROSCOPY

Wrist arthroscopy is more specific and dependable than wrist arthrography and allows direct determination of the size, severity, and exact location of ligament injury.[3, 61, 62, 114, 164, 212, 218, 253, 322] The surgeon can also concomitantly evaluate the extent of intercarpal instability and identify any associated osteochondral injuries or synovitis. Nagle and Benson[212] reported that a pathologic diagnosis was established in 98 percent of their patients undergoing wrist arthroscopy for the evaluation of wrist pain of undetermined etiology, and that the information obtained from wrist arthroscopy assisted in the determination of definitive surgical treatment.

Wrist arthroscopy is an invasive procedure. Although the incidence of complications is low, they can be functionally significant.[164, 243, 302] The diagnostically limiting factor in wrist arthroscopy is the surgeon's ability to detect the intra-articular abnormalities.[163, 212, 243, 253] Therefore, the surgeon must be proficient to maximize the benefit-to-risk ratio of diagnostic wrist arthroscopy. A detailed discussion of the setup, technique, and indications for wrist arthroscopy is presented in Chapter 10.

VIDEOFLUOROSCOPY

Videofluoroscopy of the wrist is a noninvasive procedure that can provide valuable information regarding wrist pathomechanics if routine radiographs and special views do not demonstrate the site of pathology.[10, 37, 125] We find it to be especially useful in distinguishing a scapholunate "click" from a midcarpal "clunk." Our standard videofluoroscopy series includes bilateral AP active radial and ulnar deviation views as well as lateral active flexion and extension and radial and ulnar deviation views. Careful and repeated examination of the film is often required to accurately determine the correct diagnosis.

MR IMAGING

There has been much interest regarding the application of MR imaging to the diagnosis of carpal instabilities.[16, 129, 210, 285, 317, 318, 333] This modality has been shown to clearly identify the intrinsic and extrinsic scapholunate ligaments of the wrist[27, 285, 317, 318] (Fig. 15–17). However, detection of abnormal findings is radiologist dependent, and the role of MR imaging in the diagnosis of carpal instabilities remains controversial.[210, 285, 333]

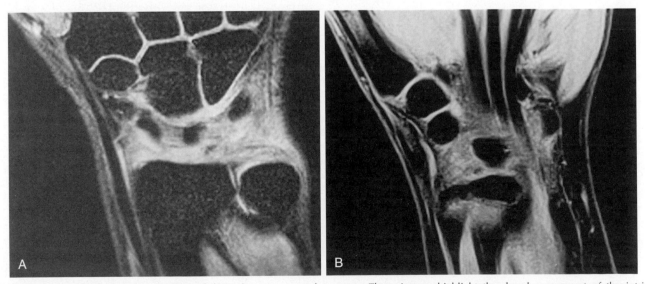

Figure 15–17. Magnetic resonance images of the right wrist, normal anatomy. These images highlight the dorsal component of the intrinsic scapholunate interosseous ligament *(A)* and the volar radioscaphocapitate, long and short radiolunate, and the radioscapholunate ligaments *(B)* of the extrinsic scapholunate complex.

COMPUTED TOMOGRAPHY

Computed tomography (CT) may also be very helpful in the evaluation of scapholunate injuries when a primary or coexistent scaphoid fracture or other occult osseous injuries is being considered.[20, 21, 44, 145, 186, 251] As shown by Sanders[251] and Bush and associates,[44] a CT scan oriented along the true axis of the scaphoid highlights any scaphoid injury or deformity.

BONE SCAN

The triple-phase bone scan continues to be useful in the localization of obscure wrist pain because of its sensitivity for acute osseous injuries and inflammatory conditions.[83, 118, 183, 194] Because of this modality's poor specificity, however, other studies are often indicated to clarify the etiology, and the use of bone scanning in scapholunate injury diagnosis is limited.

Differential Diagnosis

The differential diagnosis of scapholunate injuries can be challenging, because of the often ambiguous presentation and the multiple adjacent sites of potential pathology. The common causes of wrist pain that can be confused or can coexist with scapholunate injuries are listed in Table 15–7. Awareness of these potentially coexistent and/or differential diagnoses combined with a thorough clinical evaluation most often leads to the correct diagnosis.

TREATMENT

Acute Scapholunate Injuries

The natural history of an untreated scapholunate injury comprises progressive ligament disruption,

Table 15–7. DIFFERENTIAL DIAGNOSIS FOR SCAPHOLUNATE INJURIES*

Dorsal wrist ganglion[9, 91, 130, 250]
Anterior interosseous nerve syndrome[77]
Posterior interosseous nerve syndrome[49, 78]
Gymnast's wrist[83, 193]
Carpometacarpal boss[71, 125]
Extensor pollicis longus tenosynovitis or rupture[90, 135]
Extensor indicis proprius syndrome[237, 264]
de Quervain's stenosing tenosynovitis[81, 125]
Intersection syndrome[128, 328]
Cheiralgia paresthetica[75, 76, 95]
Scaphoid fracture[102, 183, 219, 294]
Scaphoid non-union[29, 208]
Radius fracture[209]
Osteochondral fracture[61, 163, 243, 253]
Avascular necrosis of the scaphoid or lunate[49, 53]
Other carpal instabilities[182, 199]
Vascular thrombus[14, 165]

*Superscript numbers indicate end-of-chapter references.

scapholunate instability, and intercarpal collapse followed by the variable onset of secondary changes, including fixed deformities and degenerative arthritis.* Because there are no reconstructive procedures to restore normal function[57] in a chronic injury, prompt diagnosis and treatment of an acute scapholunate injury constitute the most effective method of maintaining function and preventing progressive degeneration.

The treatment goals in acute scapholunate injuries are (1) relief of the patient's functionally limiting symptoms and (2) prevention of progressive instability and chronic secondary changes through (3) restoration of scapholunate reduction and (4) maintenance of physiologic stabilization. Many alternative techniques have been suggested to treat the acute scapholunate injury, such as cast immobilization,[156, 183] closed reduction with internal fixation,[183, 222, 245] arthroscopic débridement of torn ligaments,[230] arthroscopically assisted reduction and internal fixation,[219, 321, 322] open reduction with primary ligament repair and internal fixation,[18, 59, 63, 177, 188, 204, 248, 274] open reduction with tendon graft reconstruction,[5, 13, 84, 184, 222, 273] and scapholunate autograft or allograft reconstruction.[57, 270]

CAST IMMOBILIZATION

Linscheid and Dobyns[183] have recommended immobilization of the acute reduced scapholunate injury in a short-arm splint with the wrist in neutral that extends distally to include the fingers. This splint is changed to a short-arm cast once the soft tissue swelling has resolved. If the scapholunate reduction is maintained as determined by serial radiographs, short-arm cast immobilization is continued for a total of 6 weeks, followed by application of a removable splint for 3 to 6 months.

King[156] has suggested closed reduction and cast immobilization for the "displaced" acute scapholunate injury; however, wrist cineradiographs indicate that no single wrist position consistently reduces the scapholunate complex.[125] Palmar and colleagues[222] reported poor results in their series of acute scapholunate injuries treated with this technique, presumably secondary to inadequate reduction and stabilization.

CLOSED REDUCTION AND INTERNAL FIXATION

In an attempt to improve scapholunate reduction and obtain more adequate stabilization, various closed reduction techniques with percutaneous internal fixation stabilization have been recommended.[183, 222, 231] When these closed reduction techniques are performed and the scaphoid is reduced (dorsiflexed), however, the torn *intrinsic* scapholunate ligaments are approximated, but the injured *extrinsic* scapholu-

*References 17, 132, 150, 199, 259, 275, 304, 311, 329

nate ligaments are distracted. When the wrist is flexed to reduce the torn *extrinsic* scapholunate ligaments, the injured *intrinsic* scapholunate ligaments are distracted.[196, 198]

Crawford and Taleisnik[65] described a technique to "neutralize" this paradox of closed scapholunate reduction. This technique involves initial scapholunate reduction and stabilization to approximate the intrinsic scapholunate ligaments before midcarpal reduction and stabilization under fluoroscopic control to approximate any injured extrinsic scapholunate ligaments. The wrist is immobilized in a short-arm cast for 8 to 10 weeks, at which time the cast and pins are removed, and the wrist is placed in a removable splint for an additional 4 weeks.

Despite the benefits of this neutralizing technique, the assessment of a closed scapholunate reduction still requires meticulous inspection of detailed, sometimes difficult to interpret, radiographic parameters and subjective estimations of stability. Furthermore, closed techniques do not allow for diagnosis of other potentially injured structures or complicating factors, such as ligament interposition. Therefore, the risks of an incomplete diagnosis and/or malreduction remain significant, and many authorities now recommend more direct scapholunate injury diagnosis and instability determination before proceeding with treatment.*

ARTHROSCOPICALLY ASSISTED TECHNIQUES

The advantages of arthroscopically assisted techniques in the treatment of acute scapholunate injuries include direct visualization of all damaged structures and the severity of injury combined with visual and manual determination of intercarpal instability and direct confirmation of reduction accuracy and stabilization.[3, 62, 114, 212, 218, 253] In addition, arthroscopy provides the opportunity to treat many other associated intra-articular injuries, such as occult osteochondral fractures.[243, 253]

Whipple[321, 322] proposed arthroscopically assisted scapholunate reduction and internal fixation (AASRIF) combined with limited scapholunate ankylosis for the treatment of acute scapholunate injuries. This technique combines the advantages of arthroscopy with the benefits of multiple transarticular pin fixation. Follow-up of 40 patients over 2 to 7 years who were treated with this technique revealed that in 85 percent of patients with less than 3 months of preoperative symptoms and less than 3 mm of initial scapholunate diastasis, the procedure obtained symptomatic relief and maintained the reduction and functional stability. However, only 53 percent of patients with more than 3 months of preoperative symptoms and greater than 3 mm of scapholunate diastasis had a successful outcome..[322]

Ruby[245] also recommended arthroscopic and fluoroscopically assisted scapholunate reduction with multiple pin fixation for the treatment of acute scapholunate injuries; however, he restricted the use of this technique to patients with acute incomplete tears of the scapholunate interosseous ligament. Poehling[230] recommended arthroscopic débridement of the acute scapholunate interosseous ligament injury without stabilization; however, follow-up evaluations reveal progressive recurrence of the patient's functionally limiting symptoms.

OPEN REDUCTION, PRIMARY LIGAMENT REPAIR, AND INTERNAL FIXATION

Several authorities have recommended open reduction and primary scapholunate interosseous ligament repair with internal fixation for the acute scapholunate injury.* The advantages of the open techniques parallel those reported for the arthroscopically assisted techniques, except that direct primary ligament repair is possible with the open technique. Both palmar[59, 103] and dorsal[177, 219, 274] approaches have been described.

The palmar approach was first suggested by Fisk[103] to address the volar scapholunate ligament complex, which was then thought to be the primary stabilizing structure. Subsequently, Conyers[59] also recommended a volar approach and combined it with imbrication of the palmar ligaments to restore stability. Taleisnik[274] recommended a dorsal approach for the open treatment of acute scapholunate injuries. In this technique, the avulsed dorsal component of the scapholunate interosseous ligament is directly reattached to the bone with the use of intraosseous sutures[274] (Fig. 15–18) or bone suture anchors.[40, 233, 265] Retrospective review of the dorsal technique by Minami and Kaneda[204] revealed a significant reduction in posttraumatic scapholunate instability with maintenance of good range of motion. When an acute extrinsic and intrinsic scapholunate ligament injury with instability is present, some surgeons recommend a combined volar and dorsal approach with primary extrinsic and intrinsic ligament repair.[125, 184, 204, 278]

OPEN REDUCTION WITH SCAPHOLUNATE TENDON GRAFT RECONSTRUCTION

The predominant limiting factor in primary ligament repair using the open technique is that ligament damage may preclude primary repair, thus compromising long-term stabilization. Although this factor is more common in the chronic scapholunate injury, several authorities have suggested primary tendon graft re-

---

construction of the acute scapholunate injury when inadequate ligament is available for repair.[5, 13, 84, 184, 222, 273] Multiple techniques using various donor tendons passed through drill holes in selected bones, including the scaphoid, lunate, capitate, and distal radius, have been described.[5, 84, 184, 204] Although some limited success has been reported,[5, 84] a series of troublesome complications have become associated with these procedures, including incomplete or lost reduction, debilitating motion restriction, intercarpal collapse, and recurrent instability, as well as infection, carpal fractures, and progressive arthrosis.[84, 120, 121, 305]

SCAPHOLUNATE ALLOGRAFT OR AUTOGRAFT RECONSTRUCTION

The use of scapholunate allografts[57] and autografts[270] for reconstruction of acute scapholunate injuries has also been considered. Using fresh cadaver specimens, Coe and associates[57] evaluated the biomechanical feasibility of scapholunate allograft reconstruction. They found that there were no significant differences, in wrist range of motion, radiocarpal articular surface contact area or pressure, or relative scapholunate intercarpal motion during passive radioulnar deviation,

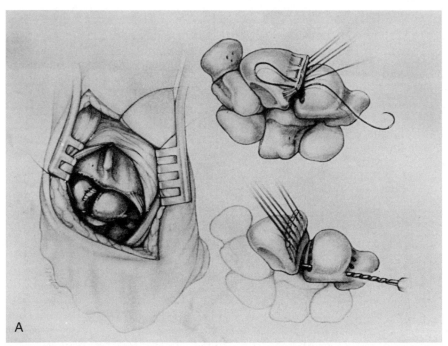

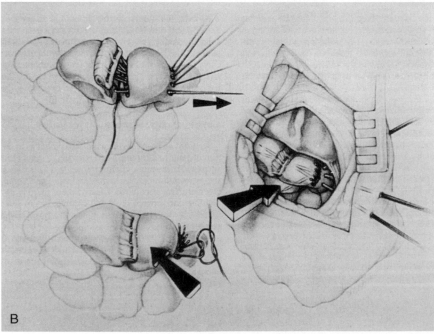

Figure 15–18. Taleisnik's technique for repair of the dorsal component of the scapholunate interosseous ligament. *A,* A standard dorsal approach is used. The scapholunate interosseous ligament still attached to the lunate is identified, and multiple sutures are placed within the dorsal component. The proposed site of ligament reattachment to the scaphoid is then débrided, and drill holes are placed in the scaphoid from the waist to emerge along the attachment site. *B,* With straight needles, the sutures are then passed through the drill holes toward the scaphoid waist. The scapholunate is reduced and stabilized with Kirschner-wires, after which the sutures are tied over the scaphoid. (From Taleisnik J: Post-traumatic carpal instability. Clin Orthop 149:73–82, 1980.)

Table 15–8. CHRONIC SCAPHOLUNATE INJURIES: POSTOPERATIVE RANGE OF MOTION AND GRIP STRENGTH BY PROCEDURE

Procedure	Range of Motion (Degrees)				Grip Strength (% of Normal Side)
	Extension	Flexion	Radial Deviation	Ulnas Deviation	
Blatt dorsal capsulodesis (Wintman et al[325])	68	51	19	39	87
Four-bone ligament reconstruction (Almquist et al[5])	52	37	*N	*N	73
Scaphotrapeziotrapezoid (STT) arthrodesis (Eckenrode et al[94])	45	40	14	25	74
Scaphocapitate (SC) arthrodesis (Pisano et al[229])	42	32	10	24	74
Scaphocapitolunate (SCL) arthrodesis (Rotman et al[244])	35	30	10	20	70
Radioscapholunate (RSL) arthrodesis (Bach et al[15])	31	17	8	13	75
SLAC wrist reconstruction					
Ashmead et al[12]	36	35	18	20	72
Krakauer et al[169]	27	27	14	16	79
Wyrick et al[330]	36	31	4	22	75
Proximal row carpectomy					
Tomaino et al[287]	37	37	8	19	79
Wyrick et al[330]	47	38	4	27	94
Krakauer et al[169]	39	33	14	18	66

*Normal

between the intact and the allografted cadaver wrists.

Svoboda and coworkers[270] evaluated the mechanical properties of three potential bone-tendon-bone autografts for scapholunate interosseous ligament reconstruction—the dorsal metatarsal ligament of the fourth and fifth metatarsals, the dorsal tarsometatarsal ligament between the lateral cuneiform and the third metatarsal, and the dorsal calcaneocuboid ligament. Although the dorsal tarsometatarsal ligament autograft was biomechanically the most similar to the intact scapholunate interosseous ligament, its strength was inadequate.

Certainly, before either of these techniques can be widely accepted, many physiologic variables remain to be addressed, such as graft healing, the effect of graft mismatch and subtle articular incongruities, graft donor site morbidity, and in vivo functional graft stability and durability.

Chronic Scapholunate Injuries

The treatment of the chronic scapholunate injury can be challenging and unpredictable. Although the goals of treatment in chronic scapholunate injuries parallel those in acute injuries, the absence of ligament healing potential and the inevitability of secondary changes dictate some significant modifications in the treatment approach.

As in the treatment of the acute injury, the goals of treatment in the chronic scapholunate injury are (1) relief of the patient's functionally limiting symptoms and (2) prevention of progressive instability and chronic secondary changes (which are not already present) by (3) restoring scapholunate reduction and (4) maintaining "physiologic" stabilization whenever possible. Additional goals for chronic injury treatment are (5) neutralization of any deforming forces (caspular contractures), (6) restoration of stable midcarpal reduction, (7) treatment of localized arthrosis, and (8) maintenance of as much asymptomatic "functional" range of motion as possible.

A variety of alternative techniques have been suggested to treat the symptomatic chronic scapholunate injury: arthroscopic débridement of partial ligament injuries,[230] arthroscopically assisted reduction and internal fixation with scapholunate ankylosis,[321, 322] open reduction and dorsal scapholunate ligament repair,[122, 177, 184, 204, 222, 275] open reduction with imbrication of the palmar ligaments,[59, 60] Blatt dorsal capsulodesis,[30, 31, 177, 325] open reduction with tendon graft ligament reconstruction,[5, 13, 39, 84, 120, 121, 184, 222, 273] scapholunate autograft or allograft reconstruction,[57, 270] a variety of limited intercarpal arthrodeses* involving the scapholunate,[11, 60, 144, 248] scaphotrapezotrapezoid,† scaphocapitate,[229] or scaphocapitolunate[134, 143, 205, 244] articulations, radioscapholunate arthrodesis,[15, 308] radial styloidectomy,[17, 239] scaphoidectomy with four-corner arthrodesis,[12, 105, 157, 169, 288, 304, 330] proximal row carpectomy,‡ total wrist arthrodesis,[1, 15, 36, 55, 56, 125, 236, 278, 307] and wrist denervation.[41, 42, 74, 77, 96, 324] Table 15–8 summarizes the postoperative range of motion and strength results for the procedures recommended to treat chronic scapholunate injury.

*References 123, 134, 205, 258, 276, 289, 291, 308, 326.
†References 13, 66, 94, 106, 158–161, 227, 305, 309, 313.
‡References 64, 70, 93, 100, 124, 147, 148, 152, 215, 216, 236, 266, 287, 323, 330.

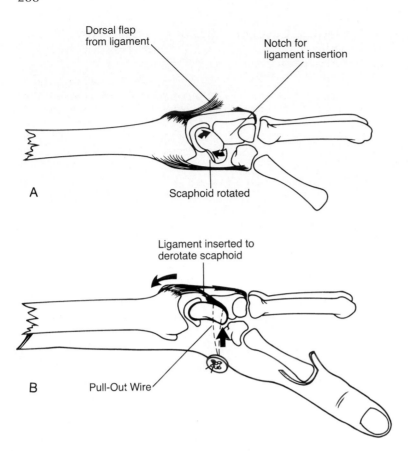

Dorsal flap
from ligament

Notch for
ligament insertion

A

Scaphoid rotated

Ligament inserted to
derotate scaphoid

B   Pull-Out Wire

Figure 15–19. A graphic representation of the technique of dorsal capsulodesis. *A,* A proximally based ligamentous flap is developed from the dorsal wrist capsule. A notch for the ligament insertion is created in the dorsal cortex of the distal pole of the scaphoid, distal to the midaxis of rotation. *B,* The scaphoid has been derotated, and the ligament inserted with a pullout wire suture.

OPEN REDUCTION AND DIRECT SCAPHOLUNATE LIGAMENT RECONSTRUCTION

For the chronic scapholunate injury in which the scaphoid is reducible, adequate ligament is available for repair, and no secondary changes have occurred, several authorities have recommended open reduction and direct repair of the dorsal component of the scapholunate interosseous ligament.[122, 177, 204, 222, 274] However, retrospective reviews of this technique for the treatment of chronic scapholunate injuries are inconsistent with respect to long-term stabilization and prevention of progressive secondary changes.[30, 177, 204, 205, 275, 305] When a potentially insufficient direct scapholunate repair is identified primarily, most investigators suggest augmentation with or selection of an alternative treatment technique.[5, 30, 39, 122, 134, 177, 184, 227, 276, 289, 308]

BLATT CAPSULODESIS

In 1986, Blatt[30] introduced a technique of dorsal capsulodesis for stabilization of chronic static scapholunate instability when the scaphoid is reducible. Since then, the Blatt capsulodesis has also been recommended for treatment of acute dynamic and static scapholunate instabilities.[30, 177, 325] The principle of the dorsal capsulodesis is to neutralize the forceful palmar-flexion deformity of the unstable scaphoid with a dorsal, proximally based checkrein mecha-

nism created from the dorsal wrist capsule (Fig. 15–19). The scapholunate diastasis is essentially ignored, although a significant feature of this procedure is its ability to indirectly reduce the scapholunate relation at the time of surgery.

Wintman and associates[325] found, in 17 patients with symptomatic chronic dynamic scapholunate instability treated with Blatt capsulodesis, an 89 percent rate of reported pain relief and a 94 percent stabilization rate (as determined by postoperative scaphoid shift testing). Furthermore, significant wrist motion was preserved, consisting of 68° of extension, 51° of flexion, 19° of radial deviation, and 39° of ulnar deviation, as well as 87 percent of contralateral grip strength. Lavernia and associates[177] reported a similar experience in 21 patients with chronic scapholunate instability treated with Blatt capsulodesis, although a consistent loss of wrist flexion (average 17°) was identified postoperatively in their review.

OPEN REDUCTION AND LIGAMENT RECONSTRUCTION WITH TENDON GRAFTS

As already discussed, scapholunate ligament reconstruction with tendon grafts is technically demanding and has been unreliable.* Glickel and Millender[120, 121]

_____

*References 5, 13, 84, 107, 108, 168, 170, 184, 189, 222, 238, 265, 269, 273.

reviewed 21 patients with chronic scapholunate instability who underwent various "tendoligament" reconstructions and found that although pain decreased in 86 percent of the patients, only 2 patients were pain free. Furthermore, the wrist range of motion generally decreased to approximately 75 percent of that in the noninjured side, and grip strength improved only slightly with these procedures. A 9 percent failure rate and a 14 percent complication rate were also identified, which excluded the incidence of malreductions, lost reductions, recurrent instability, and progressive arthrosis.

Conversely, Almquist and colleagues[5] reported on 36 patients with chronic "complete" scapholunate injuries who were treated with four-bone ligament reconstruction using a combined volar and dorsal approach, scapholunate interosseous wiring, and an extensor carpi radialis brevis tendon graft (Fig. 15–20). They reported "good" results in 86 percent of patients, without progressive arthrosis but with preservation of wrist motion and maintenance of 73 percent of grip strength. The failure rate was 8 percent, although these investigators believed that the failures

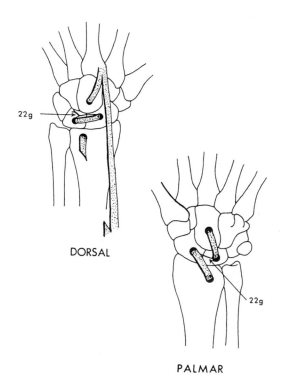

DORSAL

PALMAR

Figure 15–20. The "four-bone ligament reconstruction" (Almquist) requires a combined volar and dorsal approach. The ulnar half of the extensor carpi radialis brevis (ECRB) tendon is harvested through the dorsal incision (maintaining its distal attachment), and the scapholunate articulation is reduced. Appropriate drill holes are then placed in the capitate, scaphoid, lunate, and radius. The scapholunate dissociation is then stabilized with a 22-gauge wire loop, followed by passage of the ECRB tendon slip through the capitate (dorsal to volar), the lunate (palmar to dorsal), the scaphoid (dorsal to palmar), and then the radius (palmar to dorsal) to exit in the fourth dorsal compartment. (From Almquist EE, Bach AW, Sack JT, et al: Four bone ligament reconstruction for treatment of chronic complete scapholunate separation. J Hand Surg 16A:322–327, 1991.)

were secondary to "technical difficulties" and considered them correctable with improved surgical "expertise."

Brunelli[39] also suggested an alternative method of ligament reconstruction using the flexor carpi radialis tendon to treat chronic scapholunate instability. In this technique, the scaphoid is reduced and stabilized, at both the STT and scapholunate articulations, with a combination checkrein and tendon sling created by passing a slip of the flexor carpi radialis tendon through a distal scaphoid bone tunnel (directed from volar to dorsal) and securing it to the dorsum of the radius. A "reducible" scaphoid and supple midcarpal joint appear to be prerequisites for this procedure. However, Brunelli[39] reported "very satisfactory" results with this technique in the treatment of 13 patients with chronic scapholunate injuries.

LIMITED INTERCARPAL ARTHRODESIS

Limited intercarpal arthrodeses have been recommended by many surgeons to treat the chronic scapholunate injury,* because fusion can reliably restore durable scaphoid stability while neutralizing any resistant malreduction contractures and prevent progressive degenerative changes.[134, 205, 258, 276, 289, 308] Although all limited intercarpal arthrodeses are associated with some loss of wrist motion, the amount of motion lost varies with the joints fused.[87, 112, 115, 203, 297] Furthermore, it is the pain-free range of motion a patient requires to perform functionally significant tasks[38, 225, 244, 249] that is critical when one is considering limited intercarpal arthrodesis.

Scapholunate Arthrodesis. A scapholunate arthrodesis can be quite difficult to achieve because of the limited opposing articular surface area and the tremendous forces generated across this articulation.[134, 143, 189, 308] Hom and Ruby[143] reported only a 14 percent arthrodesis rate and a 42 percent failure rate (requiring further surgical treatment) in their review of seven patients who had chronic scapholunate dissociation and were treated with scapholunate arthrodesis using a dorsal approach. However, Conyers[60] has reported that scapholunate arthrodesis occurred incidentally in 60 percent of his patients after palmar scapholunate ligament imbrication and now suggests that this may be a reasonable alternative technique in the treatment of chronic scapholunate instability.

Scaphotrapeziotrapezoid Arthrodesis. Scaphotrapezial-trapezoid intercarpal arthrodesis was first proposed by Peterson and Lipscomb[227] and later popularized by Watson and Hempton,[309] among others,[13, 66, 94, 106, 158–161, 305, 313] to treat chronic scapholunate instability (Fig. 15–21). However, an STT arthrodesis is associated with increased load transmission through the scaphoid fossa, which may theoretically lead to progressive degenerative radioscaphoid arthrosis.[112, 297]

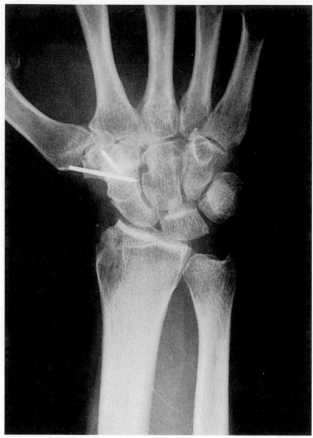

Figure 15–21. Scaphotrapeziotrapezoidal (STT) intercarpal arthrodesis for treatment of chronic scapholunate injury with STT arthrosis and fixed scaphoid deformity.

Kleinman and associates[159–161] in their comprehensive review of STT arthrodesis, did not identify any progressive radiocarpal arthrosis, but they did report a significant complication rate with this procedure. They concluded that although STT arthrodesis remains an effective treatment for chronic scapholunate instability, careful patient screening and attention to surgical detail are required to minimize complications. Further discussion of the indications for, technique of, and outcomes of STT arthrodesis are presented in Chapter 37.

Scaphocapitate Arthrodesis. Arthrodesis of the scaphocapitate articulation, although initially described for treatment of scaphoid non-union,[136, 268] has also been recommended for the treatment of chronic scapholunate injuries.[229] In addition to the advantages of lateral column height restoration and a broad bone interface for arthrodesis, scaphocapitate arthrodesis is technically easier than some of the other limited intercarpal arthrodeses and provides predictable scaphoid stabilization in the treatment of chronic scapholunate instability.[229] The indications for and outcomes of scaphocapitate arthrodesis are presented in Chapter 37.

Scaphocapitolunate Arthrodesis. Scaphocapitolunate (SCL) intercarpal arthrodesis[134, 143, 205, 244, 291, 308] is

another treatment for chronic scapholunate instability that also addresses any fixed midcarpal collapse deformities and/or localized midcarpal degenerative changes that may be present (Fig. 15–22). Although SCL arthrodesis results in slightly greater loss of wrist motion than SC or STT fusions,[87, 112, 115, 203] Viegas and coworkers[297] have shown that after SCL arthrodesis, the radiocarpal articular contact patterns more closely resemble those in the normal wrist and, thus, that the radiocarpal load is transmitted more proportionately through both the scaphoid and lunate fossae, in contrast to the disproportionate scaphoid fossa load transmission seen with SC or STT fusion.

RADIAL STYLOIDECTOMY

In an attempt to treat the limited arthrosis present in stage I SLAC wrist or to prevent radial styloid impingement after STT arthrodesis, radial styloidectomy has been recommended to augment the treatment of chronic scapholunate injuries.[17, 239] However, radial styloidectomy may itself result in instability and secondary ulnar translocation if the extrinsic scapholunate ligaments are disrupted (Fig. 15–23),[82, 232, 261] and careful attention to surgical detail is imperative.[261]

RADIOSCAPHOLUNATE ARTHRODESIS

Radioscapholunate (RSL) arthrodesis has been proposed for treatment of stage II SLAC wrist with symptomatic radioscaphoid arthrosis.[15, 308] A prerequisite for this procedure is a stable, well-aligned midcarpal joint without arthritic involvement. The advantages of RSL arthrodesis are scapholunate stabilization in combination with eradication of the painful radioscaphoid arthrosis and maintenance of a functional range of wrist motion through the midcarpal articulation.

Bach and colleagues[15] reviewed 36 patients, 21 of whom had scapholunate dissociation, who were treated with radioscapholunate arthrodesis. They observed an 81 percent rate of pain relief with preservation of 31° of extension, 17° of flexion, 8° of radial deviation, and 13° of ulnar deviation. In addition, 75 percent of grip strength was preserved compared with the uninjured side. However, a 19 percent rate of failure, requiring conversion to total wrist arthrodesis, was identified as secondary to progressive midcarpal arthrosis.

SCAPHOIDECTOMY WITH FOUR-CORNER ARTHRODESIS

In 1984, Watson and Ballet[304] recommended scaphoid excision and four-corner limited arthrodesis for the treatment of all stages of SLAC wrist. Although initially they suggested concomitant Silastic scaphoid implant arthroplasty, persistent reports of particulate synovitis[50, 228, 263, 286] have led to the abandonment of this aspect of the procedure (Fig. 15–24). The advan-

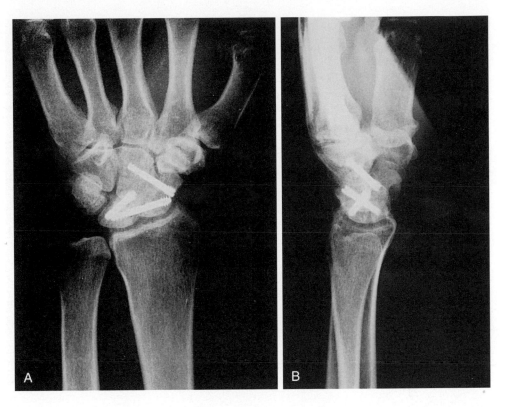

Figure 15–22. *A* and *B*, Scaphocapitolunate (SCL) intercarpal arthrodesis for treatment of chronic scapholunate injury with fixed scaphoid and midcarpal instability.

tages of the SLAC wrist reconstruction are neutralization of capsular contractures, restoration of midcarpal stability, elimination of symptomatic midcarpal arthrosis, and preservation of radiocarpal motion through the uninvolved radiolunate joint. Contraindications to the SLAC wrist reconstruction include radiolunate arthrosis and ulnar translocation instability.[12]

Watson and Ryu[311] have reported excellent results in 20 patients with SLAC wrist reconstruction, consisting of preservation of 57 percent of wrist extension/flexion and 77 percent of grip strength. Ashmead and coworkers[12] also noted a significant incidence of pain relief in patients with SLAC wrist reconstruction, along with preservation of 53 percent of wrist extension/flexion (36° of extension, 35° of flexion), 59 percent of radial and ulnar deviation (18° of radial deviation, 20° of ulnar deviation), and 72 percent of grip strength.

Conversely, Krakauer and associates[169] found, in their review of 31 patients with SLAC reconstruction (average follow-up 50 months), that only 70 percent

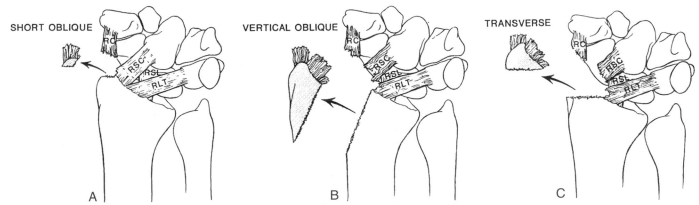

Figure 15–23. These three radial styloid osteotomies—short oblique *(A)*, verticle oblique *(B)*, and transverse *(C)* demonstrate the potential for significant extrinsic scapholunate ligament disruption that may occur with this procedure and lead to greater instability. The extent of ligament disruption may be predicted by correlating the amount of styloid removed with the consistent anatomy of the extrinsic scapholunate ligament complex. RC = radiocollateral ligament; RLT = radiolunotriquetral ligament; RSL = radioscapholunate ligament. (*From* Siegel DB, Gelberman RH: Radial styloidectomy: An anatomical study with special reference to radiocarpal intracapsular ligamentous morphology. J Hand Surg 16A:40–44, 1991.)

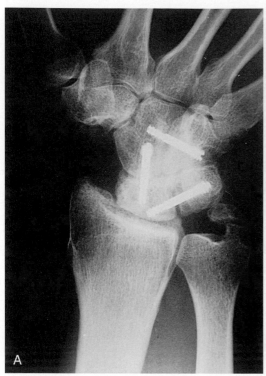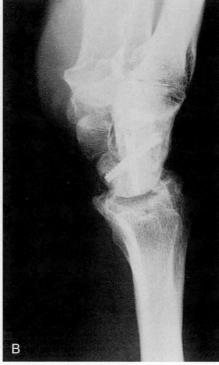

Figure 15–24. *A* and *B,* Scaphoidectomy with "four-corner" limited arthrodesis for the treatment of stage II SLAC wrist in a young laborer.

reported pain relief and that postoperative wrist motion was significantly decreased, to 27° of extension, 27° of flexion, 14° of radial deviation, and 16° of ulnar deviation, although 79 percent of grip strength was maintained. Wyrick and coworkers[330] found a similar 70 percent incidence of pain relief in their 17 patients with SLAC reconstruction (average follow-up 27 months), but they reported slightly better preservation of wrist motion—36° of extension, 31° of flexion, 4° of radial deviation, and 22° of ulnar deviation—and maintenance of 75 percent of grip strength. In addition, a significant complication rate has been identified with SLAC wrist reconstruction, including a 17 percent incidence of non-union and a 30 percent "failure rate" requiring further surgical treatment.[12, 169, 288, 330]

PROXIMAL ROW CARPECTOMY

Proximal row carpectomy has also been recommended for the treatment of SLAC wrist when the radiolunate and capitolunate articulations are free of degenerative arthritis.* This procedure addresses both the underlying carpal instability and the secondary changes (including intercarpal collapse deformities, capsular contractures, scaphoid and/or midcarpal fixation, and radiocarpal arthritis) that may be associated with chronic scapholunate injuries, by converting the complex carpal link system into a hinge joint with "rolling motion" (translation plus rotation [Fig. 15–25]).[124, 147, 148, 152, 216] The advantages of proximal row carpectomy include its technical simplicity, low morbidity, short postoperative course, and preservation of significant wrist motion and grip strength.*

A review of 23 patients who underwent proximal row carpectomy for the treatment of SLAC wrist by Tomaino and colleagues[287] revealed that 87 percent of patients had long-term pain relief with preservation of 67 percent of wrist motion (37° of extension, 37° of flexion, 8° of radial deviation, and 19° of ulnar deviation) and 79 percent of grip strength. Wyrick and coworkers[330] also noted significant patient satisfaction after proximal row carpectomy, with maintenance of 64 percent of wrist motion (47° of extension, 38° of flexion, 4° of radial deviation, and 27° of ulnar deviation) and 94 percent of grip strength. However, Krakauer and associates[169] reported only a 42 percent rate of pain relief in their patients who underwent this procedure for the treatment of SLAC wrist.

The complication rate associated with proximal row carpectomy is generally relatively low, and functional work capacity evaluations after the procedure indicate that performance is equal to that after scaphoidectomy and four-corner arthrodesis.[124, 147, 330] However, radiocapitate arthrosis and restricted radial

---

*References 64, 70, 93, 100, 124, 147, 148, 152, 215, 216, 236, 266, 287, 323, 330.

*References 64, 70, 124, 147, 148, 152, 215, 216, 266, 287, 288, 323, 330.

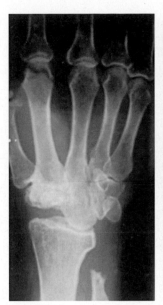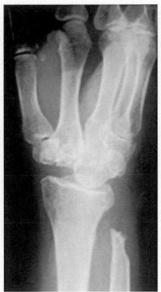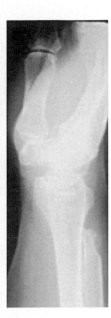

Figure 15–25. Radiographs of wrist 8 years after proximal row carpectomy and distal ulna resection. Note well-maintained radiocapitate joint space.

deviation may affect functional outcome.* Minimal radiocarpal joint space narrowing is rarely of any clinical consequence[216, 287] although uncommonly, symptomatic radiocapitate arthrosis may dictate conversion to a total wrist arthrodesis.[169, 216, 287, 330] In addition, restricted radial deviation after proximal row carpectomy[147, 216, 330] probably reflects elimination of the intercalary segment and is not altered by radial styloidectomy.[331]

Eaton and colleagues[93] have suggested proximal row carpectomy combined with dorsal capsule "interposition" arthroplasty as an alternative treatment of stage III SLAC wrist. Although early reports are encouraging, the efficacy of capsular interposition has not been proven, and the risk of incomplete pain relief that may require further surgical treatment is a concern.[287] Currently, the extent of capitolunate arthrosis that would preclude proximal row carpectomy combined with dorsal capsule "interposition" arthroplasty is unknown.[124, 287]

TOTAL WRIST ARTHRODESIS

Total wrist arthrodesis has been the gold standard for treatment of many degenerative disorders of the wrist because it provides predictable pain relief, stability, and durability.[1, 15, 36, 55, 56, 125, 236, 278, 307] Total wrist arthrodesis is also often the salvage option of choice when other treatments for chronic scapholunate injuries have failed.[12, 36, 56, 125, 169, 236, 307] The postoperative functional adjustment after total wrist arthrodesis requires adequate shoulder and elbow function and may take up to a year to occur.[319] Additional indica-

tions and the surgical techniques for total wrist arthrodesis are discussed in Chapter 38.

Richards and Roth[236] have suggested simultaneous proximal row carpectomy and total wrist arthrodesis for the treatment of end-stage wrist arthrosis, citing the theoretical advantages of sclerotic proximal carpal row excision (that would otherwise incorporate slowly), decreased number of articulations to be fused (enhancing the union rate), simplified correction of fixed midcarpal deformities and ulnar translocation instability, and avoidance of the ulnocarpal impingement occasionally seen with conventional total wrist arthrodesis. Richards and Roth[236] reported a 100 percent rate of union, a 78 percent rate of pain relief, and maintenance of 79 percent of contralateral grip strength. They also identified a 44 percent complication rate, although 53 percent of the complications were plate related and deemed correctable with modifications of fixation.

WRIST DENERVATION

Total wrist denervation has been suggested as a motion-preserving procedure for the treatment of painful, functionally limiting wrist conditions, especially when irreversible articular damage is present and no alternative treatment option other than total wrist arthrodesis is available.[41, 42, 74, 77, 96, 324] Buck-Gramko[41] reported a 65 percent rate of good to excellent pain relief with total wrist denervation; however, when an underlying symptomatic osseous lesion was present, the success rate was significantly less.

Subsequently, Dellon and colleagues[74, 77] suggested limited wrist denervation as an adjunct to the treatment of acute and chronic scapholunate injuries, after their anatomic and clinical experiences indicated

*References 64, 70, 124, 147, 148, 152, 215, 216, 266, 287, 288, 323, 330.

that coexistent injury to the terminal branches of either the anterior or posterior interosseous nerve was relatively common and may provide an additional source of pain. These investigators recommended preoperative diagnostic nerve blocks preceded and followed by functional testing to maximally evaluate the potential effect of neurogenic pain relief.

Extensive anatomic dissections of the posterior interosseous nerve by McCarthy and Breen[200] indicate that the terminal innervation of this nerve may include the radiocarpal and midcarpal joints, the dorsal wrist capsule, the adjacent carpometacarpal joint and metacarpal periosteum, as well as the second or third interossei. However, the theoretical complications of a Charcot joint or intrinsic contractures have not been reported in long-term follow-up of patients undergoing total or partial wrist dennervation.[41, 42, 74, 77, 96, 324]

Authors' Preferred Treatment Approach

Although many alternative techniques have been suggested for the treatment of the scapholunate injuries, we recommend the following treatment approach based on the previously discussed classification, the goals of treatment, and the prognosis for each scapholunate injury. Tables 15–9 and 15–10 summarize this approach.

Table 15–9. ACUTE SCAPHOLUNATE INJURY: TREATMENT APPROACH

Diagnosis	Treatment
Stable	Immobilize with short-arm thumb spica splint; reexamine @ 2 weeks.
	If normal: Discontinue splint, and allow activity as tolerated.
	If abnormal: Continue short-arm thumb spica cast. Reexamine @ 2 weeks. (Total of 4 weeks)
	If normal: discontinue cast. Apply removable forearm-based thumb spica splint (leaving interphalangeal joints free). Begin a progressive hand program. (Discontinue splint over the next 4 weeks).
	If abnormal: Obtain wrist MR imaging. if MR imaging is normal but patient is symptomatic, or if MRI is positive for scapholunate injury, perform wrist arthroscopy.
Unstable Dynamic	Arthroscopically assisted scapholunate reduction and internal (multiple K-wire) scapholunate stabilization under fluoroscopic guidance. If reduction is lost or patient remains symptomatic, treat as *chronic* dynamically unstable scapholunate injury (see Table 15–10).
Static	Open reduction and primary ligament repair with internal (K-wire) fixation/stabilization. If reduction is lost or patient remains symptomatic, treat as *chronic,* statically unstable, scapholunate injury (see Table 15–10).

ACUTE SCAPHOLUNATE INJURIES

Acute Stable Scapholunate Injury

An acutely painful wrist following trauma is a common presentation. When the physical findings are compatible with a scapholunate injury but the results of the radiographic evaluation, including a modified wrist instability motion series, (see Table 15–5), are negative, we prefer to immobilize the wrist in a short-arm thumb spica splint for 2 weeks and then reevaluate it. If the repeat clinical and radiographic examinations are unchanged, we recommend continued immobilization in a short-arm thumb spica cast for 2 more weeks (total 4 weeks) to allow time for any occult ligament injury to heal. At 4 weeks after injury, if the examinations are normal, we discontinue cast immobilization, apply a removable forearm-based thumb spica splint (leaving the interphalangeal joints [IPJs] free), and begin a progressive hand therapy program. Activity is increased as tolerated, and the removable splint is usually discontinued over the next 4 weeks.

When signs of occult scaphoid fracture or scapholunate injury persist or progress after 4 weeks of immobilization, we recommend additional diagnostic studies of the wrist, usually MR imaging. If a scaphoid fracture is identified, we proceed with treatment as outlined in Chapter 13. If MR imaging is normal or suggestive of scapholunate injury, we proceed with wrist arthroscopy, as follows:

At arthroscopy, carefully inspect for any scapholunate ligament complex injury or other associated intraarticular pathology. If a scapholunate injury is identified, assess scapholunate stability, using intraarticular and extra-articular techniques, while observing from both the radiocarpal and midcarpal portals. When the scapholunate articulation is stable, débride any incomplete intrinsic and/or extrinsic scapholunate ligament flap tears, being careful to preserve the adjacent intact ligament(s).

Postoperatively, immobilize the wrist in a short-arm thumb spica splint for 2 weeks, and replace it with a removable forearm-based thumb spica splint (IPJ free), which is used for 4 weeks. Initiate a progressive hand therapy program as tolerated.

Acute Unstable Scapholunate Injury Dynamic

We treat patients with a clinically and/or arthroscopically diagnosed acute scapholunate injury that is dynamically unstable with an arthroscopically assisted scapholunate reduction and scapholunate stabilization under fluoroscopic guidance using multiple Kirschner (K) wire internal fixation.[307, 308]

Technique. Under general or regional anesthesia, with tourniquet control, and with standard wrist arthroscopy equipment, setup, and techniques (as described in Chapter 10, perform a systematic visual and manual arthroscopic examination of the wrist.

Table 15–10. CHRONIC SCAPHOLUNATE INJURY: APPROACH

Diagnosis	Treatment
Stable	Arthroscopic débridement of damaged ligament(s) edges, with caretaker to preserve the intact ligament(s) with multiple K-wire internal fixation stabilization. If patient is persistently symptomatic, suspect occult instability, and treat as chronic dynamically unstable scapholunate injury (see below).
Unstable	Blatt capsulodesis. If patient is persistently symptomatic, treat as chronic statically unstable scapholunate injury with *irreducible* scaphoid.
Static	Blatt capsulodesis, but if dorsal capsule is inadequate, proceed to limited intercarpal arthrodesis. If reduction is lost or patient is persistently symptomatic, treat as chronic scapholunate injury with *fixed* scaphoid.
With fixed scaphoid	Scaphotrapeziotrapezoid or scaphocapitate arthrodesis with radial styloidectomy. If reduction is lost or patient is persistently symptomatic, treat as chronic scapholunate injury with *fixed* midcarpal joint.
With scapholunate advanced collapse (SLAC wrist)	
Stage I	Radial styloidectomy combined treatment of the chronic scapholunate injury as determined by scaphoid and midcarpal reducibility. (If degree of radial styloidectomy is potentially destabilizing, proceed to treatment as for stage II SLAC.)
Stage II	For young, active patient, scaphoidectomy with four-corner arthrodesis. For older, less active patient, proximal row carpectomy.
Stage III	For young, active patient, scaphoidectomy with four-corner arthrodesis. For older, less active patient, proximal row carpectomy combined with dorsal capsular interposition arthroplasty.
Stage IV	Scaphotrapeziotrapezoid arthrodesis combined with radial styloidectomy
With pancarpal arthrosis	Total wrist arthrodesis.

After confirming a dynamic scapholunate instability, identify and débride any incompletely torn intrinsic or extrinsic scapholunate ligament(s), being careful to preserve the adjacent intact ligament(s). Débride the scapholunate articulation through the rent in the intrinsic scapholunate ligament complex. Prepare for scapholunate stabilization by presetting the scapholunate and scaphocapitate K wires (0.045-inch) in the scaphoid using a limited open technique through the anatomic snuffbox. Gently reduce the scapholunate articulation with external volar scaphoid tubercle digital pressure while inspecting the scapholunate articulation from the ulnar midcarpal portal. Take care to align the volar scapholunate articular edges, and ensure that no intercarpal stepoff is present. If needed, place percutaneous K-wire "joysticks" dorsally in the scaphoid and/or lunate to assist with an occasionally difficult reduction. Once the scapholunate articulation is reduced, advance the multiple preset 0.045-inch K wires across the scapholunate articulation under fluoroscopic guidance. Evaluate the midcarpal joint for capitolunate reduction. When capitolunate reduction is required, translate the capitate (and distal carpal row) volarly with respect to the lunate. Stabilize the reduced midcarpal joint by advancing the two preset 0.045-inch K wires across the scaphocapitate joint. Arthroscopically confirm the scapholunate and midcarpal reductions, and reassess intercarpal stability while gently moving the wrist through a full range of motion. After satisfactory stable reduction is confirmed by arthroscopic and fluoroscopic examination, obtain intraoperative non-stress AP and lateral wrist radiographs.

Postoperatively, immobilize the wrist in a sugar tong thumb spica splint for 2 weeks, followed by a short-arm thumb spica cast with interosseous mold for 8 more weeks. At 10 weeks postoperatively, remove the K-wire fixation and obtain a modified wrist instability motion series of radiographs. If the scapholunate reduction is maintained, place the wrist in a removable forearm-based thumb spica splint for 4 weeks, and begin a progressive hand therapy program. If the scapholunate reduction has been lost or the patient remains symptomatic during rehabilitation, treat the injury as a *chronic* scapholunate injury that is dynamically unstable (see later).

Acute Unstable Scapholunate Injury: Static

The acute scapholunate injury that is statically unstable represents a severe ligament disruption, and we recommend open reduction, primary ligament repair, and Kirschner-wire stabilization.

Technique. Expose the wrist through a standard dorsal longitudinal approach, and confirm the extent of ligament injury and intercarpal instability. Consider a posterior interosseous neurectomy. Place threaded 0.045-inch K wires in the scaphoid and lunate, being careful to avoid any sites of potential fixation, for use as joysticks to assist in a traumatic carpal manipulation. Débride the scapholunate articulation, and create a dorsal proximal scaphoid bone trough, exposing raw cancellous bone at the proposed re-insertion site for the dorsal component of the scapholunate ligament. Two different methods of ligament fixation are available, and they appear to be equally efficient and durable: Either (1) place drill holes into the proximal scaphoid bone trough perpendicular to the scapholunate articulation to emerge along the dorsal surface of the scaphoid waist for later suture passage or (2) place two suture bone anchors in the scaphoid trough using standard manufacturer's technique. Preset two scapholunate and two scaphocapitate 0.045-inch K wires in the scaphoid using a limited open technique through the anatomic snuffbox.

Reduce the scapholunate articulation with external volar scaphoid tubercle digital pressure, and scapholunate intercarpal compression, created by manually clamping the previously placed scaphoid and lunate joysticks together under direct vision. Stabilize the scapholunate reduction by advancing the two preset 0.045-inch scapholunate K wires, under fluoroscopic guidance. Gently reduce and stabilize the capitolunate joint with the two preset 0.045-inch scaphocapitate K wires. Advance the dorsal component of the intrinsic scapholunate interosseous ligament into the scaphoid bone trough, and secure with preset sutures. Use heavy nonabsorbable (2–0 or 3–0) Ticron suture. When a potentially inadequate primary ligament repair is suspected, we augment our repair with a Blatt dorsal capsulodesis. Fluoroscopically assess the carpal reduction and manually evaluate intercarpal stability before obtaining intraoperative AP and lateral wrist radiographs.

Postoperatively, immobilize the wrist in a sugar tong thumb spica splint, which is replaced by a short-arm thumb spica cast with interosseous mold at the first postoperative visit. After a total of 8 weeks of postoperative immobilization, remove the K-wire fixation, and obtain a modified wrist instability motion series. If the scapholunate reduction has been maintained, place the wrist in a removable forearm-based thumb spica splint for 8 weeks, and initiate a progressive hand therapy program. If the scapholunate reduction has been lost or the patient remains symptomatic during rehabilitation, treat the injury as a *chronic* scapholunate injury that is statically unstable but reducible (see later).

CHRONIC SCAPHOLUNATE INJURIES

Chronic Stable Scapholunate Injury

The chronic stable scapholunate injury is most often diagnosed arthroscopically. As in the acute stable scapholunate injury, arthroscopic examination often reveals an incomplete intrinsic and/or extrinsic scapholunate ligament injury without demonstrable instability. In such cases, we recommend arthroscopic débridement of any torn ligament(s) edges, with care taken to preserve the intact ligament(s) and internal fixation with multiple K wires, as for the acute scapholunate injury that is dynamically unstable. If a patient remains persistently symptomatic, we recom-

mend treatment as for a chronic scapholunate injury with dynamic instability (see later).

Chronic Unstable Scapholunate Injury: Dynamic

Although the procedure was initially designed for the patient who presented with a statically unstable chronic scapholunate injury, we recommend the Blatt capsulodesis[30, 31] for patients with dynamically unstable chronic scapholunate injuries as well. If a patient remains persistently symptomatic postoperatively, we recommend treatment as for a chronic scapholunate injury with fixed scaphoid deformity (see later).

Chronic Unstable Scapholunate Injury: Static

The classic indication for a Blatt dorsal capsulodesis[30] is the static unstable chronic scapholunate injury. If the dorsal capsule is inadequate, we proceed with limited intercarpal fusion as described for chronic scapholunate injury with fixed scaphoid deformity. When a potentially significant but reducible midcarpal collapse deformity persists despite Blatt dorsal capsulodesis stabilization, a four-bone ligament reconstruction, as suggested by Almquist and colleagues,[5] may be a reasonable alternative.

Technique. Expose the dorsal wrist capsule through a standard dorsal longitudinal approach. Perform a posterior interosseous neurectomy as described by Dellon[74] to address any potential coexistent neurogenic pain. Create a proximally based wide dorsal capsular flap, 1.0 to 1.5 cm, originating from the dorsal aspect of the distal radius proximal to the lunate facet. Explore the wrist, and determine the extent of ligament injury and intercarpal instability as well as any associated injuries. Explore and débride the scapholunate to facilitate reduction. Place threaded 0.045-inch K wires in the dorsum of the scaphoid and lunate, being careful to avoid any sites of potential fixation, to use as joysticks and to assist in atraumatic carpal manipulation.

Confirm scaphoid reducibility by manually over-reducing (dorsiflexing) the scaphoid to allow exposure of the dorsal half of the distal scaphoid articular surface at the STT joint. If the dorsal half of the distal scaphoid articular surface cannot be exposed, the scaphoid is fixed, and a volar STT capsular contracture is present. Attempt to release the volar STT contracture from the dorsum with a Freer elevator passed through the joint. If the scaphoid resists reduction, proceed as for a chronic scapholunate injury with fixed scaphoid deformity (see later).

If the scaphoid is reducible, make a notch in the dorsum of the distal pole of the scaphoid, distal to the palmar-flexion dorsiflexion axis of scaphoid at the proposed site of capsulodesis flap insertion. Two different methods of capsulodesis attachment are available and appear to be equally efficient and durable. Either (1) place drill holes into the distal scaphoid bone trough parallel to the STT articulation to emerge along the volar surface of the scaphoid tubercle for later suture passage (Fig. 15–26) or (2) place two bone suture anchors in the distal scaphoid trough using standard manufacturer technique. Decorticate the dorsal ridge of the scaphoid, exposing a raw cancellous bone surface to promote subsequent flap ad-

herence. Preset two scapholunate and two scaphocapitate 0.045-inch K wires in the scaphoid using a limited open technique through the anatomic snuffbox. Manually reduce and stabilize the scaphoid by advancing the preset scapholunate and scaphocapitate K wires under fluoroscopic guidance.

Advance and secure the dorsal capsular flap to the distal scaphoid bone trough with heavy nonabsorba-

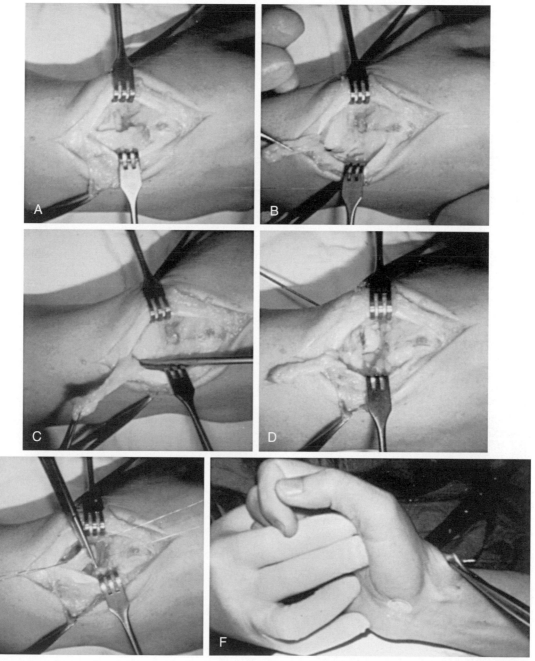

Figure 15–26. A sequence of surgical exposures to demonstrate the technique of dorsal ligament capsulodesis. *A,* A longitudinal dorsoradial incision through the wrist capsule provides exposure of the scaphoid. *B,* A 1-cm-wide flap of the dorsal capsule has been developed and hinged back on its intact origin from the dorsum of the distal radius. The proximal pole of the rotated scaphoid is noted. *C,* A probe is placed into the visible scapholunate gap, confirming disruption of the interosseous and dorsal scapholunate ligaments. *D,* The scaphoid has been reduced and maintained with a 0.045-inch Kirschner wire. A cortical notch is created in the distal pole of the scaphoid, proximal to the articular surface but distal to the midaxis of rotation. *E,* Trimmed to the appropriate length, the dorsal ligament is inserted into the fresh bony notch with a wire pull-out suture. The proximal checkrein mechanism has been established. *F,* The wire suture is tied over a button on the radiovolar aspect of the wrist.

ble (2-0 or 3-0 Ticron) suture. Confirm the carpal reduction fluoroscopically, and reassess intercarpal stability by gently moving the wrist through a full range of motion while carefully inspecting the carpus for persistent instability. When a satisfactory stable reduction is confirmed, obtain intraoperative AP and lateral wrist radiographs (Fig. 15–27).

Postoperatively, immobilize the wrists in a sugar tong thumb spica splint with the wrist in 20° of extension and neutral radial/ulnar deviation. Ten to 14 days postoperatively, replace the splint with a short-arm thumb spica cast with interosseous mold. At the eighth postoperative week, remove the cast, place the wrist in a removable forearm-based thumb spica splint, and begin progressive radiocarpal motion. At the 12th postoperative week, remove the K-wire fixation, and obtain a modified wrist instability motion series. If the periscaphoid reduction has been maintained, continue splint immobilization and progress the hand therapy (Fig. 15–28). If the peri-

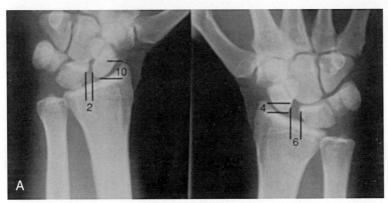

Preoperative

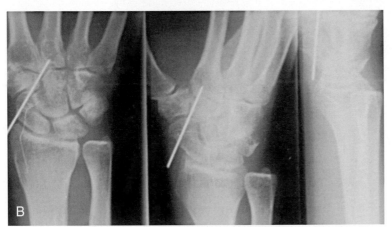

Postoperative

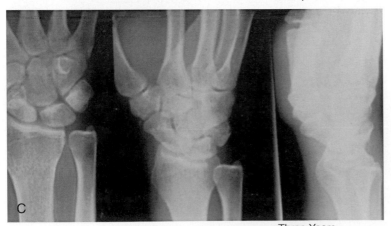

Three Years
Postoperative

Figure 15–27. *A,* Preoperative radiograph demonstrating scapholunate dissociation, rotatory subluxation of the scaphoid, and shortened ring-to-proximal-pole distance. *B,* Following surgical procedure of dorsal capsulodesis, the reduced scaphoid is maintained by K-wire fixation, and the wire suture keeps the ligament in place. *C,* Long-term follow-up demonstrates continued alignment and stability.

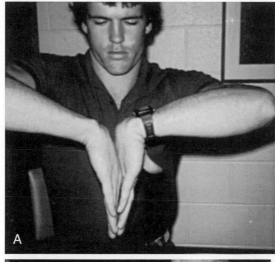
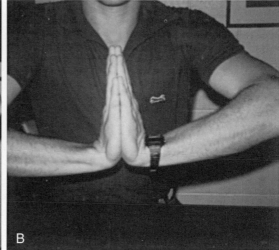
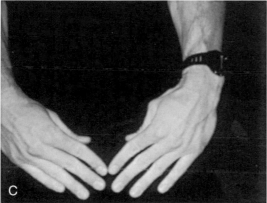

Figure 15–28. *A, B,* and *C,* Postoperative range of motion study reveals full recovery of wrist extension with some loss of wrist flexion.

scaphoid reduction has been lost, treat the injury as a statically unstable chronic scapholunate injury.

Chronic Scapholunate Injury with Fixed Scaphoid Deformity

The chronic scapholunate injury that is associated with an irreducible scaphoid is very resistant to soft tissue stabilization techniques despite adequate release of soft tissue contracture. We therefore recommend limited intercarpal arthrodesis to neutralize the deforming forces and maintain a physiologic and durable reduction. Both STT and scaphocapitate arthrodeses with radial styloidectomy have proved to be effective methods to accomplish this goal, and a detailed discussion of these techniques of intercarpal arthrodesis is contained in Chapter 37.

Chronic Scapholunate Injury with Fixed Scaphoid and Midcarpal Deformities

When a chronic scapholunate injury is associated with fixed, irreducible scaphoid and midcarpal joints, we prefer to proceed with a scaphocapitolunate arthrodesis. Although slightly greater motion loss occurs with SCL arthrodesis, we believe that

this disadvantage is outweighed by the midcarpal stabilizing effect and more physiologic radiocarpal wear.[87, 115, 203, 297] When an intercarpal arthrodesis is contraindicated, proximal row carpectomy is a reasonable alternative.

Chronic Scapholunate Injury with Stage I SLAC Wrist

Radial styloid–scaphoid arthrosis can be seen in association with a statically unstable or fixed chronic scapholunate injury. Therefore, we recommend radial styloidectomy combined with treatment of the chronic scapholunate injury as determined by scaphoid and midcarpal reducibility. However, if a potentially destabilizing radial styloidectomy is anticipated to adequately resect the area of arthrosis, we recommend proceeding to treatment as described for stage II SLAC wrist (see later) rather than risk further iatrogenic destabilization and/or ulnar translocation.

Chronic Scapholunate Injury with Stage II SLAC Wrist

In the young, high demand patient with stage II SLAC wrist, we recommend a scaphoidectomy with four-corner arthrodesis; in the older, low demand patient, we perform a proximal row carpectomy. We believe that proximal row carpectomy is a time-tested primary treatment for stage II SLAC wrist whose indications continue to expand.* The surgical technique for SLAC reconstruction and proximal row carpectomy are discussed in Chapters 34 and 37. If carpal ulnar translocation coexists with stage II SLAC, a radio-scapholunate arthrodesis is a more appropriate initial treatment, despite the small risk of late-onset midcarpal arthrosis that may require further surgical treatment.

Chronic Scapholunate Injury with Stage III SLAC Wrist

In the young high demand patient with stage III SLAC wrist, we perform a scaphoidectomy with four-corner arthrodesis; in the older, low demand patient, we now offer a proximal row carpectomy combined with dorsal capsular interposition arthroplasty as described by Eaton and coworkers.[93] In our experience, this latter procedure has provided excellent pain relief while maintaining significant wrist motion in these "low-demand" patients. The surgical technique for proximal row carpectomy with dorsal capsular interposition arthroplasty is discussed in Chapter 34.

Chronic Scapholunate Injury with Stage IV SLAC Wrist

For the patient with our modified stage IV SLAC wrist and STT arthrosis, we recommend STT arthrodesis combined with radial styloidectomy. The surgical technique for STT arthrodesis is discussed in Chapter 37.

Chronic Scapholunate Injury with Pancarpal Arthrosis

Total wrist arthrodesis is our treatment of choice for the chronic scapholunate injury with pancarpal destruction. The surgical technique for total wrist arthrodesis is discussed in Chapter 38.

SUMMARY

Although our understanding of the anatomy and pathomechanics of scapholunate injuries has improved, our knowledge is still incomplete, and the diagnosis and management of acute and chronic scapholunate injuries remain a significant challenge. Certainly, the diagnosis of "wrist sprain" is not ap-

propriate, and a vigilant history, thorough physical examination, and accurate radiographic evaluation are required to determine the correct diagnosis and avoid late-onset instability and secondary degeneration.

In an attempt to provide a straightforward, comprehensive, and practical guideline for the treatment and prognosis of scapholunate injuries, we present our classification system based on chronicity and severity. However, the optimal treatment for all scapholunate injuries is undetermined, and the surgeon must rely on injury classification and the goals of treatment to dictate the applicability of each available option. In addition, the treating surgeon must take into account the many other medical, social, and economic factors, as well as the patient's anticipated postoperative functional demand on the wrist and tolerance for motion loss and/or staged procedures, before determining the appropriate course of treatment.

References

1. Adelaar RS: Traumatic wrist instabilities. Contemp Orthop 4:309–324, 1982.
2. Adkinson JW, Chapman MW: Treatment of acute lunate and perilunate dislocations. Clin Orthop 164:199, 1982.
3. Adolfsson L: Arthroscopy for the diagnosis of post traumatic wrist pain. J Hand Surg 17B:46–50, 1992.
4. Alexander CE, Lichtman DM: Ulnar carpal instabilities. Orthop Clin North Am 15:307–320, 1984.
5. Almquist EE, Bach AW, Sack JT, et al: Four bone ligament reconstruction for treatment of chronic complete scapholunate separation. J Hand Surg 16A:322–327, 1991.
6. Amadio PC: Carpal kinematics and instability: A clinical and anatomic primer. Clin Anat 4:1–12, 1991.
7. Amadio PC: Pyridoxine as an adjunct in the treatment of carpal tunnel syndrome. J Hand Surg 10A:237–241, 1985.
8. Amalio SC, Uppal R, Samuel AW: Isolated dislocation of the carpal scaphoid. J Hand Surg 10B:385–388, 1985.
9. Angelides AC, Wallace PF: The dorsal ganglion of the wrist: Its pathogenesis, gross and microscopic anatomy and surgical treatment. J Hand Surg 1:228–235, 1976.
10. Arkless R: Cineradiography in normal and abnormal wrists. Am J Roentgenol 96:837, 1966.
11. Armstrong GWD: Rotational subluxation of the scaphoid. Can J Surg 11:306, 1968.
12. Ashmead DIV, Watson HK, Daman C, et al: Scapholunate advanced collapse wrist salvage. J Hand Surg 19A:741–750, 1994.
13. Augsberger S, Necking L, Horton J, et al: A comparison of scaphoid-trapezium-trapezoid fusion and four bone tendon weave for scapholunate dissociation. J Hand Surg 17A:360–369, 1992.
14. Aulicino PL: Neurovascular injuries in the hands of athletes. Hand Clin 3:455–466, 1990.
15. Bach AW, Almquist EE, Neuman DM: Proximal row fusion as a solution for radiocarpal arthritis. J Hand Surg 6:253–257, 1981.
16. Baker LL, et al: High resolution magnetic resonance imaging of the wrist: Normal anatomy. Skeletal Radiol 16:128–132, 1987.
17. Barnard L, Stubbins S: Styloidectomy of the radius in the surgical treatment of nonunion of the carpal navicular. J Bone Joint Surg 30A:98–102, 1948.
18. Beckenbaugh RD: Accurate evaluation and management of the painful wrist following injury: An approach to carpal instability, Orthop Clin North Am 15:289–306, 1984.

*References 70, 93, 124, 147, 152, 215, 216, 287, 323, 330.

19. Belsole RJ: Radiography of the wrist. Clin Orthop 202:50–56, 1986.

20. Belsole RJ, Hilbelink D, Llewellyn JA, et al: Scaphoid orientation and location from computed three dimensional carpal models. Orthop Clin North Am 17:505–510, 1986.

21. Belsole RJ, Hilbelink D, Llewellyn JA, et al: Carpal orientation from computed reference axis. J Hand Surg 16A:82–90, 1991.

22. Belsole RJ, Quinn SF, Greene TL, et al: Digital subtraction arthrography of the wrist. J Bone Joint Surg 72A:846–851, 1990.

23. Berger RA: The gross and histologic anatomy of the scapholunate interosseous ligament. J Hand Surg 21A:170–178, 1996.

24. Berger RA, Blair WF: The radioscapholunate ligament: A gross and histologic description. Anat Rec 210:393–405, 1984.

25. Berger RA, Kauer JMG, Landsmeer JMG: Radioscapholunate ligament: A gross anatomic and histologic study of fetal and adult wrist. J Hand Surg 16A:350–355, 1991.

26. Berger RA, Landsmeer JMF: The palmar radiocarpal ligaments: A study of adult and fetal human wrist joints. J Hand Surg 15A:847–854, 1990.

27. Berger RA, Linscheid RL, Berquist TH: Magnetic resource imaging of anterior radiocarpal ligaments. J Hand Surg 19A:295–303, 1994.

28. Bjelland JC, Bush JC: Secondary rotational subluxation of the carpal navicular. Ariz Med 34:267, 1977.

29. Black DM, Watson HK, Vender MI: Scapholunate gap with scaphoid nonunion. Clin Orthop 224:205–209, 1987.

30. Blatt G: Capsulodesis in reconstructive hand surgery: Dorsal capsulodesis for unstable scaphoid and volar capsulodesis following excision of the distal ulna. Hand Clin 3:81–102, 1987.

31. Blatt G: Dorsal capsulodesis for rotary subluxation of the carpal scaphoid. Presented at the annual meeting of the American Society for Surgery of the Hand, New Orleans, 1986.

32. Blevens AD, Light TR, Jablonsky WS, et al: Radiocarpal articular contact characteristics with scapholunate instability. J Hand Surg 14A:781–790, 1989.

33. Botte MJ, Cooney WP, Linscheid RL: Arthroscopy of the wrist: Anatomy and technique. J Hand Surg 14A:313–316, 1989.

34. Bourne MH, Linscheid RL, Dobyns JH: Concomitant scapholunate dissociation and Kienböck's disease. J Hand Surg 16A:460–464, 1991.

35. Boyes JG: Subluxation of the carpal navicular bone. South Med J 69:141, 1976.

36. Boyes JH: Bunnell's Surgery of the Hand, ed 5. Philadelphia, JB Lippincott, 1970.

37. Braunstein EM, Louis DS, Greene TL, Hamkin FM: Fluoroscopic and arthrographic evaluation of carpal instability. Am J Roentgenol 144:1259–1262, 1985.

38. Brumfield RH, Champoux JA: A biomechanical study of normal functional wrist motion. Clin Orthop 187:23–25, 1984.

39. Brunelli G: American Society for Surgery of the Hand Correspondence letter #63–1995.

40. Buch BD, Innis P, McClinton MA, Kotami Y: The Mitek Mini G2 suture anchor: Biomechanical analysis of use in the hand. J Hand Surg 20A:877–881, 1995.

41. Buck-Gramcko D: Denervation of the wrist joint. J Hand Surg 2:54–61, 1977.

42. Buck-Gramcko D: Wrist denervation procedures in the treatment of Kienböck's disease. Hand Clinics 3:517–520, 1993.

43. Burgess RC: The effect of rotatory subluxation of the scaphoid and radioscaphoid contact. J Hand Surg 12A:771–774, 1987.

44. Bush CH, Gillespy T III, Dell PC: High resolution CT of the wrist: Initial experience with scaphoid disorders and surgical fusions. Am J Roentgenol 149:757–760, 1987.

45. Buzby BF: Isolated radial dislocation of carpal scaphoid. Ann Surg 100:553, 1934.

46. Campbell RD JR, Thompson TC, Lance EM, et al: Indications for open reduction of the lunate and perilunate dislocations of the carpal bones. J Bone Joint Surg 47A:915, 1965.

47. Cantor RM, Braunstein EM: Diagnosis of dorsal and palmar rotation of the lunate on a frontal radiograph. J Hand Surg 13A:187–193, 1988.

48. Cantor RM, Stern PJ, Wyrick JD, Michaels SE: The relevance of ligament tears or perforations in the diagnosis of wrist pain: An arthrographic study. J Hand Surg 19A:945–953, 1994.

49. Carr D, David P: Distal posterior interosseous nerve syndrome. J Hand Surg 10A:873–878, 1985.

50. Carter PR, Benton LJ, Dysert PA: Silicone rubber carpal implants: A study of the incidence of late osseous complications. J Hand Surg 11A:639–644, 1986.

51. Cautilli GP, Wehbe MA: Scapholunate distance and cortical ring sign. J Hand Surg 16A:501–503, 1991.

52. Cave EF: Retrolunar dislocation of the capitate with fracture or subluxation of the navicular bone. J Bone Joint Surg 23:830, 1941.

53. Chidgey LK: Chronic wrist pain. Orthop Clin North Am 23:49–64, 1992.

54. Clay NR, Clement DA: The treatment of dorsal wrist ganglion by radical excision. J Hand Surg 13A:187–191, 1988.

55. Clayton MC, Ferlic DC: Arthrodesis of the arthritic wrist. Clin Orthop 187:89–93, 1984.

56. Clenedin MB, Green DP: Arthrodesis of the wrist: Complications and their management. J Hand Surg 6:253–257, 1981.

57. Coe M, Spitellie P, Trumble TE, et al: The scapholunate allograft: A biomechanical feasibility study. J Hand Surg 20A:590–596, 1995.

58. Connell MC, Dyson RP: Dislocation of the carpal scaphoid: Report of a case. J Bone Joint Surg 37B:252, 1955.

59. Conyers DJ: Scapholunate interosseous reconstruction and imbrication of palmar ligaments. J Hand Surg 15A:690–700, 1990.

60. Conyers DJ: Scapholunate arthrodesis as a treatment for scapholunate ligament rupture. Presented at forty-fifth annual meeting of the American Society for Surgery of the Hand, Toronto, Sept, 1990.

61. Cooney WP: Evaluation of chronic wrist pain by arthrography, arthroscopy and arthrotomy. J Hand Surg 18A:15–22, 1993.

62. Cooney WP, Dobyns JH, Linsheid RL: Arthroscopy of the wrist: Anatomy and classification of carpal instability. Arthroscopy 6:133–140, 1990.

63. Cooney WP III, Linscheid RL, Dobyns JH: Carpal instability treatment of ligament injuries of the wrist. Instr Course Lect 41:33–44, 1992.

64. Crabbe WA: Excision of the proximal row of the carpus. J Bone Joint Surg 46B:708–711, 1964.

65. Crawford GP, Taleisnik J: Rotary subluxation of the scaphoid after excision of a dorsal carpal ganglion and wrist manipulation. J Hand Surg 8:921–925, 1983.

66. Crosby EB, Linscheid RC, Dobyns JH: Scaphotrapezial trapezoidal arthrodesis. J Hand Surg 3:223–234, 1978.

67. Cowan-Collins L, Lidsky MD, Sharp JT, Moreland L: Malposition of the carpal bones in rheumatoid arthritis. Radiology 103:95–98, 1972.

68. Crisco JJ, Wolfe SW: The biomechanical properties of the periscaphoid ligament complex. In Schuind F (ed): Advances in the Biomechanics of the Hand and Wrist. New York, Plenum Press, 1994, pp 681–687.

69. Crittenden JJ, Jones DM, Santerelli AG: Bilateral rotational dislocation of the carpal navicular: Case report. Radiology 94:629, 1970.

70. Culp RW, McGuigan FX, Turner MA, et al: Proximal row carpectomy: A multicenter study. J Hand Surg 18A:19–25, 1993.

71. Cuono CB, Watson HK: The carpal boss: Surgical treatment and etiologic considerations. Plast Reconstr Surg 63:88–93, 1979.

72. Curtis DJ, Downey EF Jr, Bromer AC, et al: Importance of soft tissue evaluation in hand and wrist trauma: Statistical evaluation. AJR 142:781–788, 1984.

73. Czitrom AA, Dobyns JH, Linscheid RL: Ulnar variance in carpal instability. J Hand Surg 12A:205–212, 1987.

74. Dellon AL: Partial dorsal wrist denervation: Resection of the

distal posterior interosseous nerve. J Hand Surg 10A:527–533, 1985.

75. Dellon AL, MacKinnon SE: Susceptibility of the superficial sensory branch of the radial nerve to form painful neuromas. J Hand Surg 9B:42–45, 1984.

76. Dellon AL, MacKinnon SE: Radial sensory nerve entrapment in the forearm. J Hand Surg 11A:191–205, 1986.

77. Dellon AL, MacKinnon SE, Daneshaur A: Terminal branch of the anterior interosseous nerve as a source of wrist pain. J Hand Surg 9B:316–322, 1984.

78. Dellon AL, Seif SS: Anatomic dissection relating the posterior interosseous nerve to the carpus and etiology of dorsal wrist ganglion pain. J Hand Surg 3:326–332, 1978.

79. Demos TC: Radiologic case study: Painful wrist. Orthopedics 1:151, 1978.

80. Destot E: Traumatismes du Poignet et Rayons x. Paris, Masson, 1923.

81. DeQuervain F: Ueber eine Form von chronischer Tendovaginitis. Correspondenz-Blatt für Schweizer Aerzte 25:389–394, 1895.

82. Dibeneditto MR, Lubbers LM, Coleman CR: A standardized measurement of ulnar carpal translocation. J Hand Surg 15A:1009–1010, 1990.

83. Dobyns JH, Gabel GT: Gymnast's wrist. Hand Clin 3:493–505, 1990.

84. Dobyns JH, Linscheid RL, Chao EYS, et al: Traumatic instability of the wrist. Instruct Course Lect 24:182, 1975.

85. Dobyns JH, Linscheid RL, Macksound NS: Carpal instability—nondissociative. J Hand Surg 19B:763–773, 1994.

86. Doherty W, Lovallo JL: Scapholunate advanced collapse pattern of arthritis in calcium pyrophosphate deposition disease of the wrist. J Hand Surg 18A:1095–1098, 1993.

87. Douglas DP, Peimer CA, Koniuch MP: Motion of the wrist after simulated limited intercarpal arthrodesis: An experimental study. J Bone Joint Surg 69A:1413–1418, 1987.

88. Drewniany JJ, Palmar AK: Isolated complete radial dislocation of the scaphoid. J Bone Joint Surg 65A:871–872, 1983.

89. Drewniany JJ, Palmar AK, Flatt AE: The scaphotrapezial ligament complex: An anatomic and biomechanical study. J Hand Surg 10A:492–498, 1985.

90. Dumms F: Über trommlerlähmungen. Deutsch Militärztliche Zeitschrift 25:145–155, 1896.

91. Duncan KH, Lewis RC Jr: Scapholunate instability following ganglion cyst excision: A case report. Clin Orthop 228:250–253, 1988.

92. Easterling KJ, Wolfe SW: Scaphoid shift in the uninjured wrist. J Hand Surg 19A:604–606, 1994.

93. Eaton RG, Akleman E, Eaton BH: Fascial implant arthroplasty for treatment of radioscaphoid degenerative disease. J Hand Surg 14A:766–774, 1989.

94. Eckenrode JF, Lewis DS, Greene TL: Scaphoid-trapezium-trapezoid fusion in the treatment of chronic scapholunate instability. J Hand Surg 11A:497–502, 1986.

95. Ehrlich W, Dellon AL, MacKinnon SE: Cheiralgia paresthetica (entrapment of the radial sensory nerve) J Hand Surg 11A:205–206, 1986.

96. Ekerot L, Holmberg J: Denervation of the wrist joint. J Hand Surg 7:312, 1982.

97. England JPS: Subluxation of the carpal scaphoid. Proc R Soc Med 63:581, 1970.

98. Epner RA, Bowers WH, Guilford WB: Ulnar variance: The effect of wrist positioning and roentgen filming technique. J Hand Surg 7A:298–305, 1982.

99. Fassler PR, Stern PJ, Kiefhaber TR: Asymptomatic SLAC wrist: Does it exist? J Hand Surg 18A:682–686, 1993.

100. Ferlic DC, Clayton MC, Mills MF: Proximal row carpectomy: A review of rheumatoid and nonrheumatoid wrist. J Hand Surg 16A:420–424, 1991.

101. Finkelstein H: Stenosing tenovaginitis of the radial styloid process. J Bone Joint Surg 12:509, 1930.

102. Fisk GR: Carpal instability and the fractured scaphoid. Ann R Coll Surg Engl 46:63, 1970.

103. Fisk GR: Malalignment of the scaphoid after lunate dislocation. Am Chir Main 3:353–356, 1984.

104. Fitton JM: Rotational dislocation of the scaphoid. In Stack GH, Bolton H (eds): Proceedings of the Second Hand Club, British Society of Surgery of the Hand. Brentwood, Essex, The Westway Press, 1962.

105. Fitzgerald JP, Piemer CA, Smith RJ: Distraction resection arthroplasty of the wrist. J Hand Surg 14A:774–781, 1989.

106. Fortin PT, Louis DS: Long term follow-up of scaphoid-trapezium-trapezoid arthrodesis. J Hand Surg 18A:675–681, 1993.

107. Forward AD, Cowan RJ: Tendon suture to bone: An experimental investigation in rabbits. J Bone Joint Surg 45A:807–823, 1963.

108. Frank C, Amiel D, Woo SLY, Akeson W: Normal ligament properties and ligament healing. Clin Orthop 196:15–25, 1985.

109. Frankel VH: The Terry-Thomas sign. Clin Orthop 129:321, 1977.

110. Frot B, Alnot JY, Folinais D, Benacerraf R: Visualization of the scapholunate joint: Description of a simple roentgenographic view. Ann Chir Main 5:335–338, 1986.

111. Garcia-Ellias M, An K, Cooney WP, Linscheid RL: Reliability of carpal angle determinations. J Hand Surg 14A:1017–1021, 1989.

112. Garcia-Elias M, An K, Cooney WP, et al: Wrist kinematics after limited intercarpal arthrodesis. J Hand Surg 14A:791–799, 1989.

113. Geissler WB: Arthroscopically assisted reduction of intraarticular fractures of the distal radius. Hand Clin 11:19–29, 1995.

114. Geissler WB, Freeland AE, Savoie FH, et al: Intracarpal soft tissue lesions associated with an intraarticular fracture of the distal end of the radius. 78A:357–365, 1996.

115. Gellman H, Kauffman D, Lenihan M, et al: An in vitro analysis of wrist motion: The effect of limited intercarpal arthrodesis and the contributions of the radiocarpal and midcarpal joints. J Hand Surg 13A:378–383, 1988.

116. Gilford WW, Bolton RH, Lambrinudi C: The mechanism of the wrist joint: With special reference to fractures of the scaphoid. Guy's Hosp Rep 92:52, 1943.

117. Gilula LA, Weeks PM: Post-traumatic ligamentous instability of the wrist. Radiology 129:641, 1978.

118. Gilula LA, Destout JM, Weeks PM, et al: Roentgenographic diagnosis of the painful wrist. Clin Orthop 187:52–64, 1984.

119. Gilula LA, Totty WG, Weeks PM: Wrist arthrography: The value of fluoroscopic spot viewing. Radiology 146:555–556, 1983.

120. Glickel SZ, Millender L: Results of ligamentous reconstruction for chronic intercarpal instability. Orthop Trans 6:167, 1982.

121. Glickel SZ, Millender L: Ligamentous reconstruction for chronic intercarpal instability. J Hand Surg 9A:514–527, 1984.

122. Goldner JL: Treatment of carpal instability without joint fusion—current assessment. J Hand Surg 7:325, 1982.

123. Graner O, Lopoes El, Carralko BC, Atlas S: Arthrodesis of the carpal bones in Kienböck's disease: Painful ununited fractures of the navicular and lunate bones with avascular necrosis and old fracture dislocation of the carpal bones. J Bone Joint Surg 48A:767–774, 1966.

124. Green DP: Proximal row carpectomy. Hand Clin 3:163–168, 1987.

125. Green DP: Carpal dislocation and instabilities. In Green DP (ed): Operative Hand Surgery, vol 1. New York, Churchill Livingstone, 1992.

126. Green DP, O'Brien ET: Open reduction of carpal dislocations: Indications and operative techniques. J Hand Surg 3:250, 1978.

127. Green DP, O'Brien ET: Classification and management of carpal dislocations. Clin Orthop 149:55–72, 1980.

128. Grundberg AB, Reagan DS: Pathologic anatomy of the forearm: Intersection syndrome. J Hand Surg 10A:299–302, 1985.

129. Gundry CR, Kursunoglu-Brahme S, Schwaighoter B, et al: Is MR better than arthrography for evaluating the ligaments of the wrist? AJR 154:337–341, 1990.

130. Gunther SF: Dorsal wrist pain and occult scapholunate ganglion. J Hand Surg 10A:697–703, 1985.

131. Hankin FM, Amadio PC, Woyjtys EM, Braunstein EM: Carpal instability with volar flexion of the proximal carpal row associated with injury to the scaphotrapezial ligament: Report of two cases. J Hand Surg 13B:298–302, 1988.

132. Harrington RH, Lichtman DM, Brockmole DM: Common pathways of degenerative arthritis of the wrist. Hand Clin 3:507–527, 1987.

133. Hastings DE, Evans JA: Rheumatoid wrist deformities and their relationship to ulnar drift. J Bone Joint Surg 57A:930, 1975.

134. Hastings DE, Silver RL: Intercarpal arthrodesis in the management of chronic carpal instability after trauma. J Hand Surg 9A:834–840, 1984.

135. Helal B, Chen SC, Iwegbu G: Rupture of the extensor pollicis longis tendon in undisplaced colles fracture. Hand 14:41–47, 1983.

136. Helfet AJ: A new operation for ununited fracture of the scaphoid. J Bone Joint Surg 34B:329, 1952.

137. Herbert TL, Faithfull RG, McCann DJ, Ireland J: Bilateral arthrography of the wrist. J Hand Surg 15B:233–235, 1990.

138. Hergenroeder PT, Penix AR: Bilateral scapholunate dissociation with degenerative arthritis. J Hand Surg 6:620, 1981.

139. Higgs SL: Two cases of dislocation of carpal scaphoid. Proc R Soc Med 23:61, 1930.

140. Hixon ML, Stewart C: Microvascular anatomy of the radioscapholunate ligament of the wrist. J Hand Surg 15A:279–282, 1990.

141. Hockley BJ: Carpal instability and carpal injuries. Aust Radiol 23:158, 1979.

142. Hodge JC, Gilula LA, Larsen CF, Amadio PC: Analysis of carpal instability. II: Clinical applications. J Hand Surg 20A:765–776, 1995.

143. Hom S, Ruby LK: Attempted scapholunate arthrodesis for chronic scapholunate dissociation. J Hand Surg 16A:334–339, 1991.

144. Howard FM, Fahey T, Wojcik E: Rotatory subluxation of the navicular. Clin Orthop 104:134, 1974.

145. Hudson RM, Caragol WJ, Faye JJ: Isolated rotatory subluxation of the carpal navicular. Am J Roentgenol 126:601, 1976.

146. Hulton V: Über anatomische Variationen der homdglenkknochen. Acta Radiol 9:155–165, 1928.

147. Imbriglia JE, Broudy AS, Hagburg WC, McKernan D: Proximal row carpectomy: Clinical evaluation. J Hand Surg 15A:426–430, 1990.

148. Inglis AE, Jones EC: Proximal row carpectomy for diseases of the proximal row. J Bone Joint Surg 59A:400–403, 1977.

149. Inoue G, Maeda N: Isolated dorsal dislocation of the scaphoid. J Hand Surg 15B:368–369, 1990.

150. Johnson RP: The acutely injured wrist and its residuals. Clin Orthop 149:33–44, 1980.

151. Jones WA: Beware of the sprained wrist: The incidence and diagnosis of scapholunate instability. J Bone Joint Surg 70B:293–297, 1988.

152. Jorgensen EC: Proximal row carpectomy: An end result of twenty-two cases. J Bone Joint Surg 51A:1104–1111, 1969.

153. Kauer JMG: The interdependence of carpal articular chains. Acta Anat (Basel) 88:481–501, 1974.

154. Kauer JMG: Functional anatomy of the wrist. Clin Orthop 149:73, 1980.

155. Kauer JMG, deLange A: The carpal joint anatomy and function. Hand Clin 3:23–29, 1987.

156. King RJ: Scapholunate diastasis associated with a Barton fracture treated by manipulation, or Terry Thomas and the wine waiter. J R Soc Med 76:421–423, 1983.

157. Kirschenbaum O, Schneider LH, Kirkpatrick WH: Scaphoid excision and capitolunate arthrodesis for radioscaphoid arthritis. J Hand Surg 18A:780–785, 1993.

158. Kleinman WB: Management of chronic rotatory subluxation of the scaphoid by scapho-trapezio-trapezoid arthrodesis: Rationale for technique, postoperative changes in biomechanics and results. Hand Clin 3:113–133, 1987.

159. Kleinman WB: Long term study of chronic scapholunate instability treated by scapho-trapezio-trapezoid arthrodesis. J Hand Surg 14A:429–495, 1989.

160. Kleinman WB, Carroll C IV: Scapho-trapezio-trapezoid arthrodesis for treatment of chronic static and dynamic scapholunate instability: A 10 year perspective on pitfalls and complications. J Hand Surg 15A:408–414, 1990.

161. Kleinman WB, Steichen JB, Strickland JW: Management of chronic rotary subluxation of the scaphoid by scaphotrapezio-trapezoid arthrodesis. J Hand Surg 7:125, 1982.

162. Koka R, D'arcy C: Stabilization of the wrist in rheumatoid disease. J Hand Surg 14B:288–290, 1989.

163. Koman LA, Mooney JF III, Poehling GG: Fractures and ligament injuries of the wrist. Hand Clin 3:477–491, 1990.

164. Koman LA, Poehling GG, Toby EB, et al: Chronic wrist pain: Indications for wrist arthroscopy. Arthroscopy 6:116–119, 1990.

165. Kornberg M, Aulicino DL, DuPuy TE: Ulnar arterial aneurysms and thrombosis in the hand and forearm. Orthop Rev 12:25–33, 1983.

166. Kovalkovits I, Ficzere O: Habituelle scapholunare dissoziatin. Chirurg 48:428, 1977.

167. Kozin SH, Wood MB: Early soft tissue complications after fractures of the distal part of the radius. AAOS Instructional Course Lecture. J Bone Joint Surg 75A:144–153, 1993.

168. Krackow KA, Thomas SC, Jones LC: Ligament-tendon fixation: Analysis of a new stitch and comparison with standard techniques. Orthopedics 11:909–917, 1988.

169. Krakauer JD, Bishop AT, Cooney WP: Surgical treatment of scapholunate advanced collapse. J Hand Surg 19A:751–759, 1994.

170. Kuhlman JN, Luboinski J, Laudet C, et al: Properties of fibrous structures of the wrist. J Hand Surg 15B:335–341, 1990.

171. Kuth JR: Isolated dislocation of the carpal navicular: A case report. J Bone Joint Surg 21:479, 1939.

172. Landsmeer JM: Studies in the anatomy of articulation. I: The equilibrium of the "intercalated" bone. Acta Morphol Neerl Scand 3:287, 1961.

173. Lane LB: The scaphoid shift test. J Hand Surg 18A:366–368, 1993.

174. Larsen CF, Amadio PC, Gilula LA, Hodge JC: Analysis of carpal instability. I: Description of the scheme. J Hand Surg 20A:757–764, 1995.

175. Larsen CF, Brondum V: Posttraumatic carpal instability: A 9 year followup of 18 patients. Acta Orthop Scand 64:465–468, 1993.

176. Larsen CF, Mathiesen FK, Lindquist S: Measurement at carpal bone angles on lateral wrist radiographs. J Hand Surg 16A:888–893, 1991.

177. Lavernia CJ, Cohen MS, Taleisnik J: The treatment of scapholunate dissociation by ligamentous repair and capsulodesis. J Hand Surg 17A:354–359, 1992.

178. Leslie BM: Rheumatoid extensor tendon ruptures. Hand Clinics 5:191–202, 1989.

179. Lewis OJ, Hamshere RJ, Bucknill TM: The anatomy of the wrist joint. J Anat 106:539, 1970.

180. Lichtman DM, Schneider JR, Swafford AR, et al: Ulnar midcarpal instability: Clinical and laboratory analysis. J Hand Surg 6:515, 1981.

181. Linscheid RL: Mechanical forces affecting the deformity of the rheumatoid wrist. J Bone Joint Surg 51A:790, 1969.

182. Linscheid RL: Scapholunate ligamentous instabilities (dissociations, subdislocations, dislocations). Ann Chir Main 3:323–330, 1984.

183. Linscheid RL, Dobyns JH: Athletic injuries of the wrist. J Hand Surg 10A:821–829, 1985.

184. Linscheid RL, Dobyns JH: The treatment of scapholunate dissociation. Hand Clin 4:645–652, 1992.

185. Linscheid RL, Dobyns JH, Beabout JW, Bryan RS: Traumatic carpal instability of the wrist: Diagnosis, classification, and pathomechanics. J Bone Joint Surg 54A:1612–1632, 1972.

186. Linscheid RL, Dobyns JH, Beckenbaugh RD, et al: Instability patterns of the wrist. J Hand Surg 8:682–686, 1983.

187. Lister G: Rheumatoid arthritis. In The Hand: Diagnosis and Indications, ed 3. Edinburgh, Churchill Livingstone, 1990.

188. Loeb TM, Urbaniak JR, Goldner JL: Traumatic carpal instability: Putting the pieces together. Orthop Trans 1:163, 1977.

189. Logan SE, Nowak MD, Gould PL, Weeks PM: Biomechanical behavior of the scapholunate ligament. Biomed Sci Instrum 22:81–85, 1986.
190. MacConaill MD: Mechanical anatomy of the carpus and its bearing on some surgical problems. J Anat 75:166, 1941.
191. Maki NJ, Chuinard RG, D'Ambrosia R: Isolated complete radial dislocation of the scaphoid: A case report and review of the literature. J Bone Joint Surg 64A:615, 1982.
192. Manaster BJ, Mann RJ, Rubenstein S: Wrist pain: Correlation of clinical and plain film findings with arthrographic results. J Hand Surg 14:466–473, 1989.
193. Mandelbaum BR, Bartolozzi AR, Davis CA, et al: Wrist pain syndrome in the gymnast: Pathogenic, diagnostic, and therapeutic considerations. Am J Sports Med 17:305, 1989.
194. Mann FA, Wilson AJ, Linn MR, Gilula LA: Wrist disorders: radio-clinical algorithms. In Brunelli G, Saffar P (eds): Wrist Imaging. New York, Springer, 1992, pp 203–212.
195. Mann FA, Wilson AJ, Gilula LA: Radiographic evaluation of the wrist: What does the hand surgeon want to know? Radiology 184:15–24, 1992.
196. Mayfield JK: Carpal injuries—an experimental approach—anatomy, kinematics and perilunate injuries. J Bone Joint Surg 57A:725, 1975.
197. Mayfield JK: Patterns of injury to the carpal ligaments: A spectrum. Clin Orthop 187:36–42, 1984.
198. Mayfield JK, Johnson RP, Kilcoyne RF: The ligaments of the human wrist and their functional significance. Anat Rec 186:417, 1976.
199. Mayfield JK, Johnson RP, Kilcoyne RF: Carpal dislocation: Pathomechanics and progressive perilunar instability. J Hand Surg 5:226, 1980.
200. McCarthy CK, Breen TF: Arborization of the distal posterior interosseous nerve. J Hand Surg 20A:218–220, 1995.
201. Meade TD, Schneider LH, Cherry K: Radiographic analysis of selective ligament sectioning at the carpal scaphoid: A cadaveric study. J Hand Surg 15A:855–862, 1990
202. Metz VM, Mann FA, Gilula LA: Three compartment wrist arthrography: Correlation of pain site with location of unidirectional and bidirectional communications. Am J Roentgenol 160:819–822, 1993.
203. Meyerdierks EM, Mosher JF, Werner FW: Limited wrist arthrodesis: A laboratory study. J Hand Surg 12A:526–529, 1987.
204. Minami A, Kaneda K: Repair and/or reconstruction of the scapholunate interosseous ligament in lunate and perilunate dissociations. J Hand Surg 18:1099–1106, 1993.
205. Minami A, Ogino T, Minami M: Limited wrist fusion. J Hand Surg 13A:660–667, 1988.
206. Moneim MS: The tangential posteroanterior radiograph to demonstrate scapholunate dissociation. J Bone Joint Surg 63A:1324, 1984.
207. Moneim MS, Bolger JT, Omer GE: Radiocarpal dislocation: Classification and rationale for treatment. Clin Orthop 192:199–209, 1985.
208. Monsivais JJ, Nitz PA, Scully TJ: The role of carpal instability in scaphoid nonunion: Casual or causal? J Hand Surg 11B:201–206, 1986.
209. Mudgal CS, Jones WA: Scapholunate diastasis: A component of fractures of the digital radius. J Hand Surg 15B:503–505, 1990.
210. Munk PL, Vellet AD, Levin MF, et al: Current status of magnetic resonance imaging of the wrist. Can Assoc Radiol J 43:8–18, 1992.
211. Murakami Y: Dislocation of the carpal scaphoid. Hand 9:79, 1977.
212. Nagle DJ, Benson LS: Wrist arthroscopy: Indications and results. Arthroscopy 8:198–203, 1992.
213. Nakamura R, Imaeda T, Tsuge S, Watanabe K: Scaphoid nonunion with DISI deformity: A survey of clinical cases with special reference to ligamentous injury. J Hand Surg 16B:156–161, 1991.
214. Natress GR, King JW, McMurtry RY, Brant RE: An alternative method for determination of the carpal height ratio. J Bone Joint Surg 76A:88–94, 1994.
215. Neviaser RJ: Proximal row carpectomy for post traumatic disorders of the carpus. J Hand Surg 8:301–305, 1983.
216. Neviaser RJ: On resection of the proximal row. Clin Orthop 202:12–15, 1986.
217. Nigst H: Luxations et subluxations du scaphoide. Ann Chir 27:519, 1973.
218. North ER, Meyer S: Wrist injuries: Correlation of clinical and arthroscopic findings. J Hand Surg 15A:915–920, 1990.
219. O'Brien ET: Acute fractures and dislocations of the carpus. Orthop Clin North Am 15:237–258, 1984.
220. O'Driscoll SW, Horii E, Ness R, et al: The relationship between wrist position, grasp size and grip strength. J Hand Surg 17A:169–177, 1992.
221. Oreck SL, Gillespie T, Youm Y: Patterns of injury in experimentally induced ulnar sided wrist injuries. Orthop Trans 10:201–202, 1986.
222. Palmer AK, Dobyns JH, Linscheid RL: Management of post-traumatic instability of the wrist secondary to ligament rupture. J Hand Surg 3:507, 1978.
223. Palmar AK, Glisson RR, Werner FW: Ulnar variance determination. J Hand Surg 7A:376–379, 1982.
224. Palmer AK, Levinsohn EM, Kuzma GR: Arthrography of the wrist. J Hand Surg 8:15, 1983.
225. Palmar AK, Werner FW, Murphy D, Glisson R: Functional wrist motion: A biomechanical study. J Hand Surg 10A:39–46, 1985.
226. Parkes JC, Stovell PB: Dislocation of the carpal scaphoid: A report of two cases. J Trauma 13:384, 1973.
227. Peterson HA, Lipscomb PR: Intercarpal arthrodesis. Arch Surg 95:127, 1967.
228. Piemer CA, Medige J, Eckert BS, et al: Invasive silicone synovitis at the wrist. Orthop Trans 9:193–194, 1985.
229. Pisano PM, Piemer CA, Wheeler DR, Sherwin F: Scaphocapitate intercarpal arthrodesis. J Hand Surg 16A:328–333, 1991.
230. Poehling GG: Treatment of intraarticular fractures of the wrist. Course Lect 1992.
231. Rask MR: Carponavicular subluxation: Report of a case treated with percutaneous pins. Orthopedics 2:134, 1979.
232. Rayhack JM, Linscheid RL, Dobyns JH, Smith JH: Post traumatic ulnar translocation of the carpus. J Hand Surg 12A:180–189, 1987.
233. Rehak DC, Sotereanous DG, Bowman MW, Herndon JH: The Mitek bone anchor: Application to the hand wrist and elbow. J Hand Surg 19:853–860, 1994.
234. Resnick CS, Miller BW, Gelberman RH, Resnick D: Hand and wrist involvement in calcium pyrophosphate dihydrate crystal deposition disease. J Hand Surg 8:856–863, 1983.
235. Resnick D, Niwayama G, Goergen TL, et al: Clinical radiographic and pathologic abnormalities in calcium pyrophosphate dihydrate deposition disease (CPPD) pseudogout. Radiology 122:1–15, 1977.
236. Richards RS, Roth JH: Simultaneous proximal row carpectomy and radius to distal carpal row arthrodesis. J Hand Surg 19A:728–732, 1994.
237. Ritter MA, Inglis AE: The extensor indicis proprius syndrome. J Bone Joint Surg 51A:1645, 1969.
238. Rodeo SA, Arnoczky SP, Torzilli PA, et al: Tendon healing in a bone tunnel: A biomechanical and histiological study in dogs. J Bone Joint Surg 75A:1795–1803, 1993.
239. Rogers WD, Watson HK: Radical styloid impingement after triscaphe arthrodesis. J Hand Surg 14A:297–301, 1989.
240. Rosenfeld N, Rascoff JH: Tendon ruptures of the hand associated with renal dialysis. Plast Reconstr Surg 65:77–79, 1980.
241. Rosenthal DI, Schwartz M, Phillips WC, et al: Fracture of the radius with instability of the wrist. Am J Roentgenol 141:113, 1983.
242. Roth JH, Haddad RG: Radiocarpal arthroscopy and arthrography in the diagnosis of ulnar wrist pain. Arthroscopy 2:234–243, 1986.
243. Roth JH, Poehling GG, Whipple TL: Arthroscopic surgery of the wrist. Instr Course Lect 37:183–194, 1988.
244. Rotman MB, Manske PR, Pruitt DL, Szerzinski J: Scaphocapitolunate arthrodesis. J Hand Surg 18A:26–33, 1993.
245. Ruby LK: Carpal instability. (Instructional Course Lectures AAOS.) J Bone Joint Surg 77A:476–487, 1995.

246. Ruby LK, An KN, Linscheid RL, et al: The effect of scapholunate ligament section on scapholunate motion. J Hand Surg 12A:767–771, 1987.

247. Ruby LK, Cooney WP III, An KN, et al: Relative motion of selected carpal bones: A kinematic analysis of the human wrist. J Hand Surg 13A:1–10, 1988.

248. Russell TB: Intercarpal dislocations and fracture-dislocations: A review of fifty nine cases. J Bone Joint Surg 31B:521–531, 1949.

249. Ryu J, Cooney WP, Askew LJ, et al: Functional ranges of motion of the wrist joint. J Hand Surg 16A:409–419, 1991.

250. Sanders WE: The occult dorsal carpal ganglion. J Hand Surg 10B:257–260, 1985.

251. Sanders WE: Evaluation of the humpback scaphoid by computed tomography in the longitudinal axial plane of the scaphoid. J Hand Surg 13A:182–187, 1988.

252. Sarrafian SK, Melamed JL, Goshgarian GM: Study of wrist motion in flexion and extension. Clin Orthop 126:153–159, 1977.

253. Savoie FH: The role of arthroscopy in the diagnosis and management of cartilaginous lesions of the wrist. Hand Clin 1:1–5, 1995.

254. Schakel M, Dell PC: Transscaphoid palmar lunate dislocation with concurrent scapholunate ligament disruption. J Hand Surg 11A:653–656, 1986.

255. Schlossbach T: Dislocation of the carpal navicular bone not associated with fracture. J Med Soc NJ 51:533, 1954.

256. Schuhl JF, Leroy D, Comtet JJ: Biodynamics of the wrist: Radiographic approach to scapholunate instability. J Hand Surg 10:1006–1008, 1985.

257. Schuind F, Stallenberg B, Franz B: Does the normal contralateral wrist provide the best reference for x-ray film measurements of the pathologic wrist? J Hand Surg 21A:24–30, 1996.

258. Schwartz S: Localized fusion at the wrist joint. J Bone Joint Surg 49A:1591–1596, 1967.

259. Sebald JR, Dobyns JH, Linscheid RL: The natural history of collapse deformities of the wrist. Clin Orthop 104:140–148, 1974.

260. Short WH, Werner FW, Fortino MD, et al: A dynamic biomechanical study of scapholunate ligament sectioning. J Hand Surg 20A:986–999, 1995.

261. Siegel DB, Gelberman RH: Radial styloidectomy: An anatomical study with special reference to radiocarpal intracapsular ligamentous morphology. J Hand Surg 16A:40–44, 1991.

262. Smith DK, Gilula LA, Amadio PC: Dorsal lunate tilt (DISI configuration) sign of scaphoid fracture dislocation. Radiology 176:497–499, 1990.

263. Smith RJ, Atkinson RE, Jupiter JB: Silicon synovitis of the wrist. J Hand Surg 10A:47–60, 1985.

264. Spinner M, Olshansky K: The extensor indicis proprius syndrome: A clinical test. Plast Reconstr Surg 51:134–138, 1973.

265. St. Pierre P, Olsen EJ, Elliott JJ, et al: Tendon-healing to cortical bone compared with healing to a cancellous trough. J Bone Joint Surg 77A:1858–1866, 1995.

266. Stamm TT: Excising the proximal row of the carpus. Guys Hosp Rep 112:6–8, 1963.

267. Steinberg BD, Plancher KD, Idler RS: Percutaneous Kirschner wire fixation through the snuff box: An anatomic study. J Hand Surg 20A:57–62, 1995.

268. Sutro CJ: Treatment of nonunion of the carpal navicular bone. Surgery 20:536–540, 1946.

269. Sutro CJ: Hypermobility of bones due to "overlengthened" capsular and ligamentous tissue. Surgery 21:67, 1947.

270. Svoboda SJ, Eglseder WA Jr, Belkoff SM: Autografts from the foot for reconstruction of the scapholunate interosseous ligament. J Hand Surg 20A:980–985, 1995.

271. Szabo RM, Newland CC, Johnson PG, et al: Spectrum of injury and treatment options for isolated dislocation of the scaphoid. J Bone Joint Surg 77A:608–615, 1995.

272. Taleisnik J: The ligaments of the wrist. J Hand Surg 1:110, 1976.

273. Taleisnik J: Wrist: anatomy, functions and injury. Am Acad Orthop Surg Instr Course Lect 27:61, 1978.

274. Taleisnik J: Post-traumatic carpal instability. Clin Orthop 149:73–82, 1980.

275. Taleisnik J: Scapholunate dissociation. In Strickland JW, Steichen JB (eds): Difficult Problems in Hand Surgery. St Louis, CV Mosby, 1982.

276. Taleisnik J: Subtotal arthrodesis of the wrist. Clin Orthop 187:81–88, 1984.

277. Taleisnik J: The Wrist. New York, Churchill Livingstone, 1985.

278. Taleisnik J: Current concepts review: Carpal instability. J Bone Joint Surg 70A:1262–1268, 1988.

279. Taleisnik J, Watson HK: Midcarpal instability caused by malunited fractures of the distal radius. J Hand Surg 9A:350–357, 1984.

280. Tanz SS: Rotation effect in lunar and perilunar dislocations. Clin Orthop 57:147, 1968.

281. Taylor AR: Dislocation of the scaphoid. Postgrad Med J 45:186, 1969.

282. Testut L, Latarjet A: Traite d'anatomie humaine. Paris, Gaston Doin, 1928, pp 628–630.

283. Thomas HO: Isolated dislocation of the carpal scaphoid. Acta Orthop Scand 48:369, 1977.

284. Thompson TC, Campbell RD Jr, Arnold WD: Primary and secondary dislocation of the scaphoid bone. J Bone Joint Surg 46B:73, 1964.

285. Timins ME, Jahnke JP, Krah SF, et al: MR imaging of the major carpal stabilizing ligaments: Normal anatomy and clinical examples. Radiographics 15:575–587, 1995.

286. Toby EB, Glisson RR, Seaber AR, Urbaniak JR: Prosthetic silicone scaphoid strains: Effects of intercarpal fusions. J Hand Surg 16A:469–473, 1991.

287. Tomaino MM, Delsignore J, Burton RI: Long term results following proximal row carpectomy. J Hand Surg 19A:694–703, 1994.

288. Tomaino MM, Miller RJ, Cole I, Burton RI: Scapholunate advanced collapse wrist: Proximal row carpectomy or limited wrist arthrodesis with scaphoid excision? J Hand Surg 19A:358–365, 1994.

289. Trumble T, Bour CJ, Smith RJ, Edwards GS: Intercarpal arthrodesis for static and dynamic volar intercalated segmental instability. J Hand Surg 13A:384–390, 1988.

290. Truong NP, Mann FA, Gilula LA, Kang GW: Wrist instability series: Increased yield with clinical radiographic screening criteria. Radiology 192:481–484, 1994

291. Uematsu A: Intercarpal fusion for treatment of carpal instability: A preliminary report. Clin Orthop 144:159–165, 1979.

292. Vance R, Gelberman R, Braun R: Chronic bilateral scapholunate dissociation without symptoms. J Hand Surg 4:178, 1979.

293. Vaughan-Jackson OJ: A case of recurrent subluxation of the carpal scaphoid. J Bone Joint Surg 31B:532, 1949.

294. Vender MI, Watson HK, Black DM, Strickland JW: Acute scaphoid fracture with scapholunate gap. J Hand Surg 14A:1004–1007, 1989.

295. Viegas SF: Midcarpal arthroscopy: Anatomy and techniques. Arthroscopy 8:385–390, 1992.

296. Viegas SF, Patterson RM, Hokanson JA, Davis J: Wrist anatomy: Incidence, distribution and correlation of anatomic variations tears and arthrosis. J Hand Surg 18A:463–475, 1993.

297. Viegas SF, Patterson RM, Peterson PD, et al: Evaluation of the biomechanical efficacy of limited intercarpal fusion for treatment of scapholunate dissociation. J Hand Surg 15A:120–128, 1990.

298. Viegas SF, Trencer AF, Cantrell J, et al: Load transfer characteristics of the wrist. Part I: The normal wrist. J Hand Surg 12A:971–978, 1987.

299. Viegas SF, Trencer AF, Cantrell J, et al: Load transfer characteristics of the wrist. Part II: Perilunate instability. J Hand Surg 12A:978–985, 1987.

300. Voorhees DE, Daffner RH, Nunley JA, Gilula LA: Carpal ligamentous disruptions and negative ulnar variance. Skeletal Radiol 13:257–262, 1985.

301. Walker GBW: Dislocation of the carpal scaphoid reduced by open operation. Br J Surg 30:380, 1943.

302. Warhold LG, Ruth RM: Complications of wrist arthroscopy and how to prevent them. Hand Clin 2:81–89, 1995.

303. Watson HK, Ashmead D, Makhoulf MV: Examination of the scaphoid. J Hand Surg 13A:657–660, 1988.

304. Watson HK, Ballet FL: The SLAC wrist: Scapholunate advanced collapse pattern of degenerative arthritis. J Hand Surg 9A:358, 1984.

305. Watson HK, Belniak R, Garcia-Elias M: Treatment of scapholunate dissociation: Preferred treatment STT fusion vs. other methods. Orthopedics 14:365–370, 1991.

306. Watson HK, Black DM: Instability of the wrist. Hand Clin 3:103–111, 1987.

307. Watson HK, Brenner LH: Degenerative disorders of the wrist. J Hand Surg 10A:1002–1006, 1985.

308. Watson HK, Goodman ML, Johnson TR: Limited wrist arthrodesis. Part II: Intercarpal and radio-carpal combination. J Hand Surg 6:223, 1981.

309. Watson HK, Hempton RF: Limited wrist arthrodesis. Part I: The triscaphoid joint. J Hand Surg 5:320–327, 1980.

310. Watson HK, Ottoni L, Pitts EL, Handel AG: Rotary subluxation of the scaphoid: A spectrum of instability. J Hand Surg 18B:62–64, 1993.

311. Watson KH, Ryu J: Degenerative disorders of the carpus. Orthop Clin North Am 15:337–354, 1984.

312. Watson HK, Ryu J: Evolution of arthritis of the wrist. Clin Orthop 202:157–167, 1986.

313. Watson HK, Ryu J, Akelman E: Limited triscaphoid intercarpal arthrodesis for rotary subluxation of the scaphoid. J Bone Joint Surg 68A:345–349, 1986.

314. Weber ER: Concepts governing rotational shift of the intercalated segment of the carpus. Orthop Clin North Am 15:193–207, 1984.

315. Weil C, Ruby LK: The dorsal approach to the wrist revisited. J Hand Surg 11A:911–912, 1986.

316. Weiss AP, Akelman E, Lambiase R: Comparison of the findings of triple injection cinearthrography of the wrist with those of arthroscopy. J Bone Joint Surg 78A:348–356, 1996.

317. Weiss KC, Beltran J, Lubbers LM: High field MR surface coil imaging of the hand and wrist. Part II: Pathologic correlations and clinical relevance. Radiology 160:147–152, 1986.

318. Weiss KC, Beltran J, Shamam OM, et al: High field MR surface coil imaging of the hand and wrist. Part I: Normal anatomy. Radiology 160:143–146, 1986.

319. Weiss APC, Wiedman GJr, Quenzer D, et al: Upper extremity function after wrist arthrodesis. J Hand Surg 20A:813–817, 1995.

320. Whipple TL: Powered instruments for wrist arthroscopy. Arthroscopy 4:290–294, 1988.

321. Whipple TL: Arthroscopic surgery: The Wrist. Philadelphia, JB Lippincott, 1992.

322. Whipple TL: The role of arthroscopy in the treatment of scapholunate instability. Hand Clin 2:37–40, 1995.

323. White GM, Clark GL, Elias LS: Proximal row carpectomy for post traumatic disorders of the wrist. J Hand Surg 13A:310–315, 1987.

324. Wilhelm A: Die gelenkdenervation und ihre anatomischen grundlagen. Einneves behandlungsprinzip in der handchirivrgie zur behandlungen der lunatummalazie und navicularepseudoarthrise. Hefte Unfallheilkund. New York, Springer Verlag, 86:1–109, 1966.

325. Wintman BI, Gelberman RH, Katz JN: Dynamic scapholunate instability: Results of operative treatment with dorsal capsulodesis. J Hand Surg 20A:971–979, 1995.

326. Witt JD, McCollough CJ: Bilateral spontaneous scapholunate subluxation treated with limited intercarpal fusion. J Hand Surg 15B:460–462, 1990.

327. Wolfe SW, Crisco JJ: Mechanical evaluation of the scaphoid shift test. J Hand Surg 19A:762–768, 1994.

328. Wood MB, Dobyns JH: Sports related extraarticular wrist syndromes. Clin Orthop 202:93–102, 1986.

329. Wright TW, Del Charco M, Wheeler D: Incidence of ligament lesions and associated degenerative changes in the elderly wrist. J Hand Surg 19A:313–318, 1994.

330. Wyrick JD, Stern PJ, Kiefthaber TR: Motion preserving procedures in the treatment of scapholunate advanced collapse wrist: Proximal row carpectomy versus four corner arthrodesis. J Hand Surg 20A:965–970, 1995.

331. Youm Y, McMurtry RY, Flatt AE, Gillespe TE: Kinematics of the wrist. J Bone Joint Surg 60A:423–431, 1978.

332. Zinberg EM, Palmar AK, Coren AB, Levinsohn EM: The triple injection wrist arthrogram. J Hand Surg 13A:803–809, 1988.

333. Zlatkin MB, Chao PC, Osterman AL, et al: Chronic wrist pain: Evaluation with high resolution MR imaging. Radiology 173:723–729, 1989.

CHAPTER 16

Triquetrolunate Instability

Charlotte E. Alexander, MD, and David M. Lichtman, MD

Carpal instability represents a spectrum of bony and ligamentous damage. There is an abundance of information in the literature dealing primarily with various types of radial carpal instabilities, scapholunate dissociation, rotatory subluxation of the scaphoid, and perilunate instability.[10–12, 27, 28, 30, 32, 35, 41, 44] Over the past decade, carpal instabilities involving the ulnar aspect of the wrist have become better recognized. These instabilities are several forms of midcarpal instability and triquetrolunate instability. In light of a greater appreciation of the pathology and clinical nature of the carpal instabilities, triquetrolunate instability has been classified with the perilunate group.

Because wrist mechanics are extremely complex, numerous investigators have devoted much effort to the study of carpal kinematics.[10–12, 14, 15, 21, 25–33, 35, 40, 45, 48, 49] Kinematic models have been devised in order to increase understanding of wrist mechanics, principally the modified columnar model of Taleisnik and the "ring" model proposed by Lichtman (Figs. 16–1 and 16–2). In the ring model, the proximal carpal and distal carpal rows move basically as semirigid units and are connected by two physiologic mobile links, the rotatory triquetrohamate joint and the mobile scaphotrapezial joint. A break in the ring on the ulnar side of the wrist could occur at the triquetrohamate joint, resulting in midcarpal instability, or through the triquetrolunate joint, leading to triquetrolunate dissociation. Although the proximal carpal row acts as a semirigid unit in the ring model, there is significantly more motion between the scaphoid and lunate than between the lunate and triquetrum. This feature explains why the majority of triquetrolunate coalitions are asymptomatic.

As a unit, the proximal carpal row volar flexes with radial deviation as the scaphoid is forced into a palmar-flexed position between the trapezium and the radius. The lunate and triquetrum move dorsally and volar-flex because of the helicoid shape of the hamate articular surface. Conversely, with ulnar deviation, the proximal carpal row dorsiflexes. Magnetic resonance imaging (MRI) studies have shown that, along with dorsiflexion, the lunate and triquetrum translate volarly on the radius during ulnar deviation, maintaining a colinear relationship between the radius and the capitate.[39]

Reagan and coworkers[38] were the first to present a series of patients with injuries to the triquetrolunate articulation. Taleisnik and coworkers[43] attributed the patterns of volar flexion instability to disruption of the triquetrolunate ligaments. With a break in the ring through the triquetrolunate joint, the proximal carpal row no longer moves as a unit. The lunate palmar flexes with the scaphoid in response to dynamic forces on the radial side of the carpus, whereas the triquetrum tends to dorsiflex as it is forced ulnarly by the head of the capitate and assumes a dorsiflexed position in relation to the hamate. Thus, a static volar intercalary segment instability (VISI) deformity (palmar flexion of the lunate) may be seen on routine lateral radiographs.

The ligamentous anatomy on the ulnar side of the wrist has been described by numerous authorities with various interpretations and names for the complex ligamentous structures.[13, 18, 20, 26, 44, 45] The lunate and triquetrum are stabilized as a single mechanical unit by several intrinsic and extrinsic carpal ligamentous structures. The interosseous ligament is a short, stout membrane that connects the lunate and triquetral articular surfaces. The extrinsic ligamentous support consists of dorsal and palmar radiotriquetrolunate ligaments, the dorsal scaphotriquetral ligament, and the ulnotriquetral, ulnolunate, and ulnar carpal ligamentous complex. The ulnotriquetral and ulnolu-

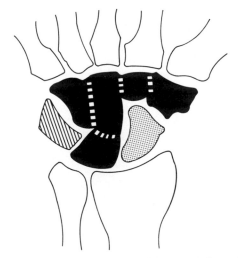

Figure 16–1. Taleisnik's[45a] modification of the central (flexion/extension) column. The central column consists of the entire distal row and lunate, the scaphoid is the lateral column, and the triquetrum is the rotatory medial column. (From Lichtman DM, Schneider JR, Swafford AR, et al: Ulnar midcarpal instability: Clinical and laboratory analysis. J Hand Surg 6:515–523, 1981.)

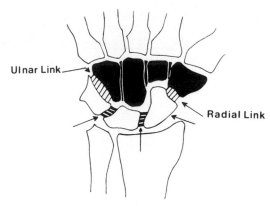

Figure 16–2. Ring concept of carpal kinematics as proposed by Lichtman.[26] The proximal and distal rows are rigid posts stabilized by interosseous ligaments. Normal controlled mobility occurs at the scaphotrapezial joint and the triquetrohamate joint. Any break in the ring, either bony or ligamentous (arrows), can produce a DISI or VISI deformity. (From Lichtman DM, Schneider JR, Swafford AR, et al: Ulnar midcarpal instability: Clinical and laboratory analysis. J Hand Surg 6:515–523, 1981.)

nate ligaments may actually be part of the ulnar carpal ligamentous complex rather than distinct entities. Two groups have demonstrated that with sectioning of the triquetrolunate membrane and of the palmar and dorsal triquetrolunate ligaments, subtle abnormal motion occurs between the lunate and triquetrum but is not detectable on plain radiographs.[20, 46] However, sectioning of the dorsal radiotriquetral and scaphotriquetral ligaments, in conjunction with the interosseous membrane and the palmar and dorsal triquetrolunate ligaments, leads to a static VISI deformity on radiography.

In this chapter, we discuss the pathomechanics, clinical presentation, diagnosis, and various types of treatment options for triquetrolunate instability.

PATHOGENESIS

In 1980, Mayfield and colleagues[30] presented a study dealing with the pathomechanics of perilunar instability. They demonstrated that loading in maximal extension, ulnar deviation, and intercarpal supination would produce progressive perilunar instability, beginning with fracture of the radial styloid or scaphoid, or disruption of the scapholunate joint. It has been subsequently proposed that triquetrolunate instability represents a "forme fruste" of grade III perilunar instability, in which the scapholunate or transscaphoid component has healed, leaving only the triquetrolunate disruption at clinical presentation.[24] It has also been argued that triquetrolunate instability occurs as a result of loading in maximal extension, radial deviation, and, possibly, pronation.[12, 38] Reagan and coworkers[38] suggested that this mechanism may cause perilunar instability in reverse order. They found partial scapholunate tears in two cases of triquetrolunate dissociation.[38] Radial deviation places

more tension on the ulnar portion of the arcuate ligament and possibly the triquetrolunate ligaments. Consequently, this force causes disruption of the triquetrolunate ligaments prior to rupture of the radiocapitate or scapholunate ligament. Forced pronation of the wrist, which increases the length of the ulna in relation to the radius and consequently the load on the ulnar aspect of the wrist, should logically lead to disruption of the triquetrolunate ligament prior to disruption of the scapholunate ligament. Elsewhere in this text the ulnocarpal abutment syndrome is discussed (see Chapters 21 and 22). Triquetrolunate ligament injuries may be caused by increased load transmission across the ulnar side of the wrist, in conjunction with an ulnar-positive variant (an excessively long ulna). Ulnar and triquetral chondromalacia as well as triangular fibrocartilage complex (TFCC) tears, may commonly accompany triquetrolunate instability when the ulna is longer than the radius.

CLINICAL FINDINGS

Reagan and coworkers[38] divided triquetrolunate instability into two groups, triquetrolunate tears (sprains) and triquetrolunate dissociation. Patients with partial disruption of the triquetrolunate interosseous ligaments are in the first group, and those with complete triquetrolunate ligamentous disruptions in the second group. Patients with triquetrolunate tears should not have discernible changes on plain radiographs, whereas those with triquetrolunate dissociation may have a static VISI deformity on lateral radiographs.

The primary presenting complaint in all of the patients is pain on the ulnar aspect of the wrist. The pain may or may not be associated with a wrist click in radial or ulnar deviation. Some patients complain of stiffness, weakness, or instability. The onset of symptoms is usually related to a traumatic event described as a fall on the outstretched hand or a twisting or rotatory injury.

On physical examination, there is tenderness over the ulnar aspect of the wrist, particularly the triquetrolunate joint. Occasionally, a click can be reproduced at the time of examination. Reagan and coworkers[38] have described a triquetrolunate ballottement test, a positive result of which can be helpful in diagnosing triquetrolunate instability (Fig. 16–3). To perform this test, the examiner stabilizes the lunate with the thumb and index finger of one hand and attempts to displace the triquetrum and pisiform dorsally, then palmarly, with the other hand. A positive test result indicates excessive laxity associated with pain and crepitus. Ambrose and Posner[1] have described another screening test, the ulnar snuffbox test. In this test, the examiner applies lateral pressure in the sulcus between the extensor carpi ulnaris (ECU) and flexor carpi ulnaris (FCU) distal to the ulna. A test that reproduces the patient's pain

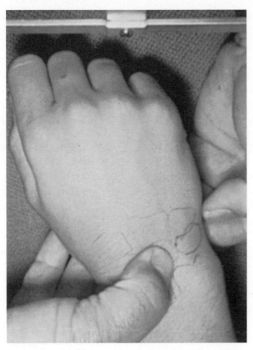

Figure 16–3. The triquetrolunate ballottement test, as described by Reagan and colleagues,[38] is used to detect abnormal motion and pain at the triquetrolunate joint. (From Reagan DS, Linscheid RL, Dobyns JH: Lunotriquetral sprains. J Hand Surg 9:502–513, 1984.)

be obtained for all patients with suspected instability. This series consists of a posteroanterior (PA) view in neutral, ulnar, and radial deviation; a clenched-fist anteroposterior (AP) view; an oblique view; a 30° off lateral oblique view to show the pisotriquetral joint; a lateral view with the wrist in neutral and at both extremes of flexion and extension; and a lateral clenched-fist view. A PA view with the forearm in neutral rotation to determine ulnar variance is also valuable to help identify patients with ulnar impaction syndrome. Standard static radiographs are normal in patients with triquetrolunate tears or sprains and may also be normal in those with triquetrolunate dissociation and dynamic instability. Stress radiographs, i.e., clenched-fist AP view in pronation or ulnar deviation or the clenched-fist lateral view, may be necessary to elicit the abnormality in patients with dynamic instability. These abnormalities include disruption of the normal smooth convexity of the proximal carpal row with the triquetrum displaced proximally on the anteroposterior radiograph. Disruption of the normal arc is particularly pronounced with ulnar deviation, producing overlapping of the lunate and triquetrum (Fig. 16–5).[38] In

strongly suggests triquetrolunate injury. Injection of a small amount of lidocaine (approximately 0.5 ml) into the triquetrolunate joint may also be helpful in localizing the pathology, i.e., intra-articular versus extra-articular. Grip strength and range of motion may or may not be altered.

Triquetrolunate instability may be difficult, in some cases, to differentiate clinically from many other disease entities affecting the ulnar aspect of the wrist. Differential diagnosis should include TFCC tears, subluxation or dislocation of the distal radioulnar joint, subluxation of the ECU, midcarpal instability, ulnar impaction syndrome, and ulnar head chondromalacia.

Although complete triquetrolunate coalition is usually asymptomatic, partial triquetrolunate coalition can produce ulnar wrist pain usually in association with minor trauma.[18, 42] Gross and colleagues[18] reported on eight symptomatic synostoses in five patients. Six of the wrists were treated successfully with triquetrolunate arthrodesis. All of the patients had radiographically normal-appearing joints distally and narrowing of the joints proximally. The common observation at surgery was very thin cartilage in the proximal aspect of the joint with partial synostosis. This partial synostosis with resultant degenerative change in the proximal aspect of the joint was believed to be the etiology of the symptoms (Fig. 16–4).

RADIOGRAPHIC EVALUATION

Some or all of the carpal instability series of radiographs recommended by Gilula and Weeks[15] should

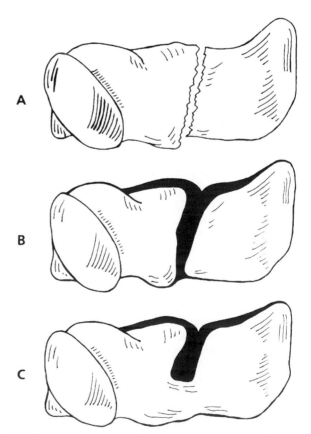

Figure 16–4. A, In degenerative or post-traumatic arthritis, there is uniform narrowing and osteophyte formation. B, In partial coalition, the proximal aspect of the joint is narrow, and the distal portion is normal. C, Incomplete joint formation, usually seen as failure of joint development proximally. (From Gross SC, Watson HK, Strickland JW, et al: Triquetrolunate arthritis secondary to synostosis. J Hand Surg 14:95–102, 1989.)

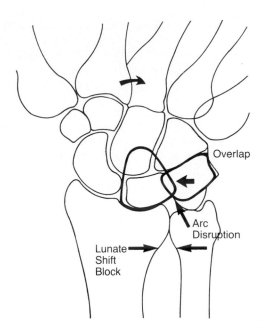

Figure 16–5. Disruption of the smooth convexity of the proximal carpal row is more pronounced with ulnar deviation. Note the overlapping of the lunate and triquetrum. (From Reagan DS, Linscheid RL, Dobyns JH: Lunotriquetral sprains. J Hand Surg 9:502–513, 1984.)

some instances, there may be increased distance between the lunate and triquetrum.[17] On lateral films, the triquetrum may be dorsiflexed in relation to the lunate compared with the other wrist. The average normal triquetrolunate angle measurement has been reported by Reagan and coworkers[38] to be $+14°$. They found that in triquetrolunate dissociation, this angle is less than 0 with an average of $-16°$. The triquetrolunate angle is the angle between the longitudinal axis of the triquetrum and the longitudinal axis of the lunate (Fig. 16–6). A VISI deformity may or may not be present on the lateral radiograph.

Arthrography has been advocated by various authorities to better evaluate the anatomic abnormalities in patients with instability symptoms.[16, 24, 36] It is important to obtain serial films or to use fluoroscopy immediately after injection to detect the location of the leak between the radiocarpal and midcarpal rows. Arthrograms are probably the most helpful diagnostic aids in the evaluation of triquetrolunate tears (sprains). Sequential injections of the midcarpal and radiocarpal spaces decrease the false-negative rate, because some tears may leak in only one direction. Levinsohn and coworkers[23] found that midcarpal injections were more sensitive for demonstrating scapholunate or triquetrolunate perforations than radiocarpal injections. A positive study demonstrates a communication between the midcarpal and radiocarpal joints through the triquetrolunate space (Fig. 16–7). Reagan and coworkers[38] found that all of 11 surgically treated patients with positive arthrograms had significant triquetrolunate ligament tears. Arthrography cannot identify all triquetrolunate tears, how-

ever. The Levinsohn study had a 14 percent false-negative rate for triquetrolunate perforations.[23] Even with positive studies, the presence of a tear may not be clinically significant. All arthrographic findings must be carefully correlated with the history and the physical and other diagnostic findings.

Patients with isolated triquetrolunate tears need to be differentiated from those with ulnar impaction syndrome. In addition to standard views for determining ulnar variance, Pin and associates[37] recommend obtaining a bone scan, which is often positive in ulnar impaction syndrome. In a patient with an ulnar-positive variant and cystic changes in the proximal and adjacent surfaces of the lunate and triquetrum, ulnar impaction should be suspected. Ulnar impaction is discussed more extensively elsewhere in the text. In general, treatment for ulnar impaction is focused on ulnar shortening procedures.

Cineradiographs are usually normal and are therefore helpful in distinguishing between midcarpal instability and triquetrolunate instability.

Partial triquetrolunate coalition is diagnosed with standard radiographs alone. Classically, there is proximal triquetrolunate joint narrowing with a normal-appearing distal portion of the joint or the "champagne glass" appearance as described by Watson and colleagues[18, 47] (Fig. 16–8).

MR imaging, which is now highly reliable for diagnosing avascular necrosis of the lunate or the scaphoid, can occasionally detect a triquetrolunate ligament tear. At this point, however, MR imaging is more reliable for TFCC tears and occasionally for scapholunate ligament disruptions than for triquetrolunate tears.[7, 50] The interosseous membrane, if visualized, demonstrates a low signal intensity on T_1-weighted images.[7] Arthrography should still be considered the standard radiographic modality for diagnosing triquetrolunate tears.

TREATMENT

All patients with a diagnosis of partial triquetrolunate tears (sprains) with acute injuries should have a trial of immobilization. Immobilization and anti-inflammatory agents may also be used for patients with chronic triquetrolunate dissociation. For treatment of acute sprains, Ambrose and Posner[1] advocate use of a wrist splint with a lateral supracondylar extension to prevent pronation for 6 to 8 weeks, followed by gradual weaning. Surgical treatment should be reserved for patients with chronic symptoms that have not responded to immobilization or anti-inflammatory agents and for those with acute triquetrolunate dissociation and significant changes on standard radiographs.

It may be beneficial to aspirate the wrist and perform arthrography as part of the initial evaluation of a patient who presents within 2 to 3 weeks of injury with a significant history of trauma and a wrist effusion but for whom carpal instability series is normal.

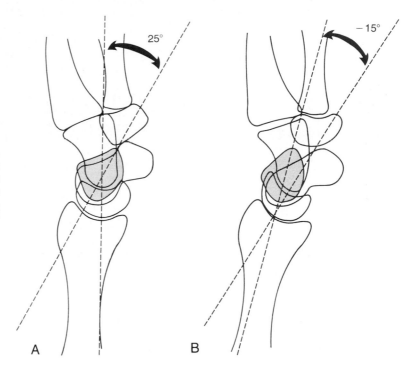

Figure 16–6. Triquetrolunate angle determination on diagram of lateral radiograph. *A*, Normal triquetrolunate angle. *B*, In triquetrolunate dissociation, the triquetrolunate angle is less than 0 secondary to volar flexion of the lunate in relationship to the triquetrum. (After Reagan DS, Linscheid RL, Dobyns JH: Lunotriquetral sprains. J Hand Surg 9:502–513, 1984.)

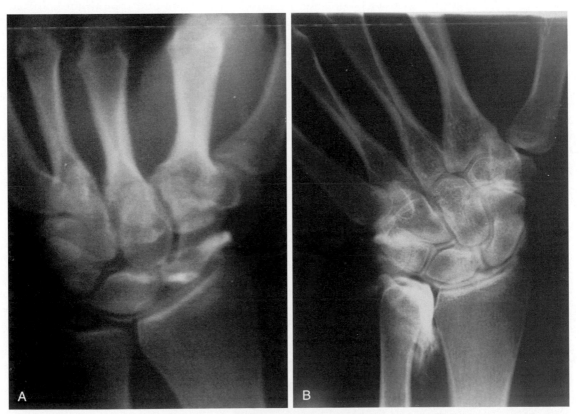

Figure 16–7. Sequential views after radiocarpal injection. *A*, Leak into the midcarpal row is demonstrated by a small wisp of dye seen in the triquetrolunate space. *B*, Post-exercise view shows communication between radiocarpal and midcarpal joint as well as distal radioulnar joints. Note that the intact scapholunate interosseous ligament is outlined with contrast material.

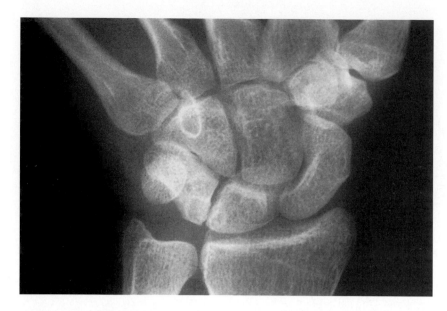

Figure 16–8. Preoperative radiograph demonstrates the classic "champagne goblet" narrowing of the proximal triquetrolunate joint space seen in partial coalition. (From Gross SC, Watson HK, Strickland JW, et al: Triquetrolunate arthritis secondary to synostosis. J Hand Surg 14:95–102, 1989.)

If the arthrogram demonstrates a major leak through the triquetrolunate joint, arthroscopy should be performed early to evaluate the extent of the triquetrolunate joint disruption. Patients who have acute triquetrolunate dissociation with wide diastasis should undergo arthroscopic or open reduction with pin fixation (preferably within the first 8 weeks). If a flap tear is present but no dissociation occurs, then the tear can be débrided and pinned, but immobilization is still the cornerstone of treatment.

Arthroscopy has become a valuable adjunct to the hand surgeon's armamentarium and undoubtedly enhances our ability to diagnose and treat ulnocarpal disorders. Compared with arthrography, arthroscopy is much more helpful in delineating the location and extent of triquetrolunate ligament disruptions.[5] Triquetrolunate tears associated with degenerative TFCC tears can be differentiated from traumatic triquetrolunate tears. Concomitant chondral changes of the lunate and triquetrum associated with ulnar impaction syndrome can also be identified.

With arthroscopic visualization, the surgeon should probe the triquetrolunate joint, applying pressure to the lunate and triquetrum (assistant can perform a ballottement test) to determine the amount of instability present (Fig. 16–9). From the midcarpal joint, visualization of the triquetrolunate joint while the same manuever is performed also demonstrates instability, if present. In our experience and that of others, patients with chronic triquetrolunate tears or dissociation that is of less than 6 months' duration and refractory to conservative management who are undergoing arthroscopic evaluation can benefit from débridement of the interosseous membrane edges and

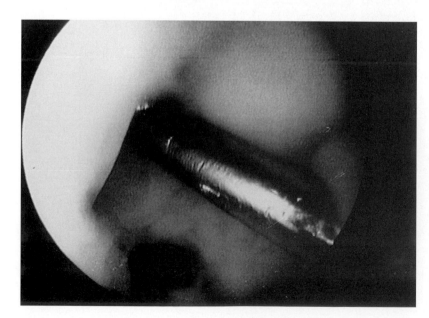

Figure 16–9. A probe is placed in a tear in the interosseous membrane. The lunate is on the left and the triquetrum on the right.

arthroscopically controlled percutaneous pinning of the triquetrolunate joint.[1] If pinning is performed, the wrist is immobilized in a short-arm cast, and the pins are removed at 8 weeks. Percutaneous triquetrolunate pinning may diminish a patient's symptoms, obviating more aggressive procedures such as ligament reconstruction and triquetrolunate arthrodesis.

In addition to arthroscopic débridement and pinning, surgical treatment options for chronic tears and chronic triquetrolunate dissociation are repair of the interosseous ligament, reconstruction of the triquetrolunate ligaments using a free tendon graft, and triquetrolunate arthrodesis. When surgical exploration is undertaken, a dorsal ulnar approach should be used, exposing the wrist capsule between the fourth and fifth dorsal compartments. A second volar incision may be required for ligament repairs and reconstructions. For ligament reconstruction, a portion of the ECU tendon can be passed through drill holes in the lunate and triquetrum and sutured to itself.[6, 38] This procedure is technically difficult, and care must be taken to avoid damage to the ulnar neurovascular bundle.

Ligament repairs are best performed by nonabsorbable horizontal mattress sutures through the torn flap of ligament passed into drill holes over the dorsal ulnar aspect of the triquetrum, as recommended by Linscheid.[6] The triquetrolunate joint is reduced, and the repair or reconstruction is protected with Kirschner (K) wire fixation between the lunate and triquetrum for 6 to 8 weeks. Splint immobilization is continued for 4 to 6 weeks longer. Despite the technical difficulty of ligament reconstruction, Favero and others[8] from the Mayo Clinic reported an 89 percent satisfaction rate in 30 patients undergoing ligament reconstruction or repair, and prefer it to triquetrolunate arthrodesis.

Triquetrolunate arthrodesis has been advocated by numerous authorities for the treatment of chronic disruptions of the triquetrolunate joint.[22, 34, 37, 47] Various success rates and methods of fixation have been reported.[22, 34, 37, 47] Pin and associates[37] reported a 100 percent fusion rate in 11 patients using cancellous bone graft and a compression screw. Kirschenbaum and coworkers[22] attained fusion in 12 of 14 patients undergoing triquetrolunate arthrodesis using cancellous bone chips and multiple Kirschner wires. Nelson and colleagues[34] stressed the importance of immobilization longer than 6 weeks and using fluoroscopic spot views to assess the fusion. They advocated using a Herbert screw and a single Kirschner wire for fixation and immobilization for at least 8 weeks. Although varying results have been obtained with all methods of surgical treatment, we prefer arthrodesis to ligament reconstruction.

When performing an arthrodesis, maintain the normal external dimensions of the triquetrum and lunate. We prefer using a corticocancellous iliac crest strut graft rather than cancellous graft alone to provide additional stability. Create a trough in the dorsal surface of the triquetrum and the lunate after stabiliz-

ing the two bones with a Kirschner wire. Deepen this slot almost to the palmar cortical surface of both bones. Place the strut graft in this trough so that it fits snugly. Thoroughly denude the cartilaginous surfaces of the triquetrolunate joint, but maintain the space with sufficient cancellous bone graft chips (Fig. 16–10). Use two or three 0.045-inch Kirschner wires for internal fixation, and immobilize the wrist for 10 to 12 weeks or until radiographic fusion has occurred. Arthrodesis should probably be the surgical treatment of choice in patients who have significant triquetrolunate dissociation or who perform strenous activities with their wrist.

Triquetrolunate fusion is also indicated for the treatment of symptomatic partial triquetrolunate coalition. Ulnar impaction syndrome with associated triquetrolunate joint tear can often be treated by addressing the length of the ulna alone. If a TFCC tear is present, symptoms may be improved by a wafer distal ulnar resection as described by Feldon and associates[9] or by arthroscopic débridement of the TFCC and recession of the ulna head using a bur. Chun and Palmer[4] recommend ulnar shortening as the primary treatment for patients with ulnar-positive variance and symptoms and a history (no significant history of trauma) compatible with ulnar impaction syndrome.

OUR PREFERRED METHOD OF TREATMENT

Acute Injuries

Patients presenting with acute ulnar wrist pain, a history of trauma, physical findings compatible with

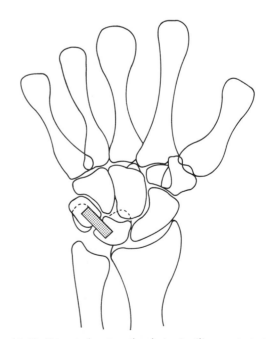

Figure 16–10. Triquetrolunate arthrodesis. An iliac crest strut graft is used and stabilization is attained with Kirschner wires. After denuding of the articular surfaces between the lunate and triquetrum, the space is maintained using cancellous bone chips.

a triquetrolunate joint injury, and normal radiographs (with or without ulnar-positive variance) are treated with splinting and an anti-inflammatory agent for 1 to 2 months. If symptoms persist, arthroscopy is performed. If a significant triquetrolunate ligament disruption is present, the injury is less than 6 months old, and there is no TFCC tear or ulnar-positive variance, we débride the ligament edges and percutaneously pin the triquetrolunate joint with two to three K wires for 8 weeks. The K wires and cast are removed after 8 weeks, and the patient is started on a rehabilitation program. Patients who continue to have disabling symptoms ultimately undergo open triquetrolunate arthrodesis.

Arthroscopic evaluation and percutaneous pinning are performed early in patients who present with acute dissociation as seen on radiographs.

Chronic Injuries

The initial treatment for chronic tears or dissociation is splinting and anti-inflammatory agents. Operative intervention is indicated if symptoms persist. If dissociation is noted on radiography, then an open triquetrolunate arthrodesis is performed. If the ulnar variance is positive, the ulna is also shortened. Patients with persistent symptoms and negative radiographs (no dissociation or impaction) undergo arthrography. If the arthrogram is positive (or the symptoms are clearly mechanical), then arthroscopy is performed, and the triquetrolunate ligament is débrided or repaired, if torn.

Patients with triquetrolunate tear (no radiographic evidence of dissociation) and ulnar impaction syndrome (i.e., ulnar-positive variance) are treated differently. We usually perform arthroscopy first, and the triquetrolunate tear and TFCC tear (if present) are débrided. If the triquetrolunate joint is stable, there is no need to pin or fuse it. Next, the ulna must be shortened. If the TFCC has been débrided, we remove a wafer of the ulnar head arthroscopically (see Chapters 10 and 11). If the TFCC is intact, an open Feldon wafer procedure[9] or a formal ulnar shortening is performed during the same anesthesia period or at a later date.

References

1. Ambrose L, Posner MA: Lunate-triquetral and midcarpal joint instability. Hand Clin 8:653–668, 1992.
2. Arkless R: A detailed study of movement of the wrist joint. Am J Roentgenol 96:839–844, 1966.
3. Brumfield RH, Champoux JA: A biomechanical study of normal functional wrist motion. Clin Orthop 187:23–25, 1984.
4. Chun S, Palmer AK: The ulnar impaction syndrome: Followup of ulnar shortening osteotomy. J Hand Surg 18A:46–53, 1993.
5. Cooney WP: Evaluation of chronic wrist pain by arthrography, arthroscopy, and arthrotomy. J Hand Surg 18A:815–822, 1993.
6. Cooney WP, Linscheid RL, Dobyns JH: Carpal instability: Treatment of ligament injuries of the wrist. Instructional Course Lectures 41:33–44, 1992.
7. Dalinka MS, Meyer S, Kricun ME, et al: Magnetic resonance imaging of the wrist. Hand Clin 7:87–98, 1991.
8. Favero KJ, Bishop AT, Linscheid RL: Luno-triquetral ligament disruption: A comparative study of treatment methods (abstract SS-80). In Proceedings of the American Society for Surgery of the Hand, 46th Annual Meeting, Orlando, FL, 1991.
9. Feldon P, Terrono AL, Belsky MR: Wafer distal ulna resection for posttraumatic disorders of the distal radioulnar joint. J Hand Surg 17A:731–737, 1992.
10. Fisk G: An overview of injuries of the wrist. Clin Orthop 149:137–144, 1980.
11. Fisk G: Carpal instability and the fractured scaphoid. Ann Roy Coll Surg Eng 46:63–76, 1970.
12. Fisk G: The wrist. J Bone Joint Surg 66B:396–407, 1984.
13. Garcia-Elias M, Domenech-Mateu JM: Anatomy of the ulnocarpal ligaments (abstract RS-12). In Proceedings of the American Society for Surgery of the Hand, 46th Annual Meeting, Orlando, FL, 1991.
14. Gilford W, Bolton R, Lambrinudi C: The mechanism of the wrist joint. Guy's Hosp Rep 92:52–59, 1943.
15. Gilula LA, Weeks PM: Post-traumatic ligamentous instabilities of the wrist. Radiology 129:641–651, 1978.
16. Gilula LA, Totty WG, Weeks PM: Wrist arthrography. Radiology 146:555–556, 1983.
17. Gilula LA: Carpal injuries: Analytic approach and case exercises. Am J Radiol 133:503–517, 1979.
18. Gross SC, Watson HK, Strickland JW, et al: Triquetrolunate arthritis secondary to synostosis. J Hand Surg 14A:95–102, 1989.
19. Hogikyan JV, Louis DS: Embryologic development and variations in the anatomy of the ulnocarpal ligamentous complex. J Hand Surg 17A:719–723, 1992.
20. Horii E, Garcia-Elias M, An KN, et al: A kinematic study of triquetrolunate dissociations. J Hand Surg 16A:355–362, 1991.
21. Kauer JMG: Functional anatomy of the wrist. Clinical Orthop 149:9–20, 1980.
22. Kirschenbaum D, Coyle MP, Leddy JP: Chronic lunotriquetral instability: Diagnosis and treatment. J Hand Surg 18A:1107–1112, 1993.
23. Levinsohn EM, Rosen ID, Palmer AK: Wrist arthrography: Value of the three-compartment injection method. Radiology 179:231–238, 1991.
24. Levinsohn EM, Palmer AK: Arthrography of the traumatized wrist. Radiology 146:647–651, 1983.
25. Lichtman DM, Noble WH, Alexander CE: Dynamic triquetrolunate instability: Case report. J Hand Surg 9:185–187, 1984.
26. Lichtman DM, Schneider JR, Swafford AR, et al: Ulnar midcarpal instability: Clinical and laboratory analysis. J Hand Surg 6:515–523, 1981.
27. Linscheid RL, Dobyns JH, Beckenbaugh RD, et al: Instability patterns of the wrist. J Hand Surg 8:682–686, 1983.
28. Linscheid RL, Dobyns JH, Chao EYS, et al: Traumatic instability of the wrist: Diagnosis, classification, and pathomechanics. J Bone Joint Surg 54A:1612–1632, 1972.
29. MacConaill MA: The mechanical anatomy of the carpus and its bearings on some surgical problems. J Anat 75:166–175, 1941.
30. Mayfield JK, Johnson RP, Kilcoyne RK: Carpal dislocations: Pathomechanics and progressive perilunar instability. J Hand Surg 5:226–241, 1980.
31. Mayfield JK, Johnson RP, Kilcoyne RF: The ligaments of the human wrist and their functional significance. Anat Rec 186:417–428, 1976.
32. Mayfield JK: Patterns of injury to carpal ligaments. Clin Orthop 187:36–42, 1984.
33. McMurtry RY, Youm Y, Flatt AE, Gillespie TE: Kinematics of the wrist: Clinical applications. J Bone Joint Surg 60A:955–961, 1978.
34. Nelson DL, Manske PR, Pruitt DL, et al: Lunotriquetral arthrodesis. J Hand Surg 18A:1113–1120, 1993.
35. Palmer AK, Dobyns JH, Linscheid RL: Management of posttraumatic instability of the wrist secondary to ligament rupture. J Hand Surg 3:507–532, 1978.
36. Palmer AK, Levinsohn EM, Kuzma GR: Arthrography of the wrist. J Hand Surg 8:15–23, 1983.

37. Pin PG, Young VL, Gilula LA, et al: Management of chronic triquetrolunate ligament tears. J Hand Surg 14A:77–83, 1989.

38. Reagan DS, Linscheid RL, Dobyns JH: Lunotriquetral sprains. J Hand Surg 9:502–513, 1984.

39. Reicher MA, Kellerhouse LE: MRI of the Wrist and Hand. New York, Raven Press, 1990, pp 69–85.

40. Sarrafian S, Melamed J, Goshgarian G: Study of wrist motion of flexion and extension. Clin Orthop 126:153–159, 1977.

41. Sebald JR, Dobyns JH, Linscheid RL: The natural history of collapse deformities of the wrist. Clin Orthop 104:140–148, 1974.

42. Simmons BP, McKenzie WD: Symptomatic carpal coalition. J Hand Surg 10A:190–193, 1985.

43. Taleisnik J, Malerich M, Prietto M: Palmar carpal instability secondary to dislocation of the scaphoid and lunate: Report of case and review of the literature. J Hand Surg 7:606–612, 1982.

44. Taleisnik J: Post-traumatic carpal instability. Clin Orthop 149:73–82, 1980.

45. Taleisnik J: The ligaments of the wrist. J Hand Surg 1:110–118, 1976.

45a. Taleisnik J: Classification of carpal instability. Bull Hosp Joint Dis 44:511–531, 1984.

46. Viegas SF, Patterson RM, Peterson PD, et al: Ulnar-sided perilunate instability: An anatomic and biomechanic study. J Hand Surg 15A:268–278, 1990.

47. Watson HK, Guidera PM, Zeppieri J, et al: Lunate-triquetral arthrodesis. Presented at American Society for Surgery of the Hand Annual Meeting, San Francisco, September, 1995.

48. Wright R: A detailed study of movement of the wrist joint. J Anat 70:137–143, 1933.

49. Youm Y, McMurtry RY, Flatt AE, Gillespie TE: Kinematics of the wrist. I: An experimental study of radial-ulnar deviation and flexion-extension. J Bone Joint Surg 60A:423–431, 1978.

50. Zlatkin MB, Chao PC, Osterman AL, et al: Chronic wrist pain: Evaluation with high-resolution MR imaging. Radiology 173:723–729, 1989.

CHAPTER 17

Midcarpal and Proximal Carpal Instabilities

David M. Lichtman, MD, Eric S. Gaenslen, MD,
and Garry R. Pollock, MD, PharmD

MIDCARPAL INSTABILITY

Although primary laxity of the midcarpal joint was first demonstrated in 1934 by Mouchet and Bélot,[21] it was not until 1980 that midcarpal instability (MCI) was recognized as a source of clinical symptoms.[12] At that time, the senior author of this chapter (DML) described a series of patients who presented with a volar sag on the ulnar side of the wrist and a history of a painful "clunk" at the midcarpal joint with ulnar deviation. Since then, the pathogenesis of what has been termed *midcarpal instability* has been further defined. We believe that laxity of certain carpal ligaments results in lack of support for the proximal carpal row and midcarpal joint, which in turn leads to a loss of the normal joint reactive forces between the proximal and distal carpal rows. A dynamic flexion deformity (volar intercalated segmental instability, or VISI) occurs in the proximal row as the distal row translates palmarly owing to the lax ligaments. As the wrist moves from radial to ulnar deviation, there is no longer the coupled rotation of the carpus with the smooth transition in the proximal row from the physiologic VISI (flexion) to the dorsal intercalated segmental instability, or DISI (extension), configuration. Instead, the proximal row remains flexed and the distal row remains palmarly subluxed for a prolonged period, until the extreme of ulnar deviation is reached, at which point the distal row abruptly reduces, and the proximal row snaps into extension.

Since 1980, there has been an increasing interest in and recognition of instabilities on the ulnar side of the wrist and midcarpal joint.* Along with this attention has come a proliferation of nomenclature (Table 17–1). We now refer to the clinical pattern described previously as *palmar midcarpal instability (PMCI)* because of the palmar translation of the distal row. In earlier reports, we had termed this entity "ulnar midcarpal instability."[1, 13] PMCI is the most common pattern of MCI. A much less common variant of midcarpal instability, in which the proximal carpal row is extended (DISI) and the distal carpal

row is subluxed dorsally when the wrist is in neutral, is termed *dorsal midcarpal instability (DMCI)*.

Louis and associates[17] have described the capitolunate instability pattern (CLIP wrist) in a series of 11 patients in whom dorsal subluxation of the capitate on the lunate and the scaphoid on the scaphoid fossa of the radius could be demonstrated. These patients have a different clinical and radiographic picture from that characteristic of patients with PMCI, but may have features similar to those of patients with the less common DMCI. Johnson and Carrera[9] used the term "chronic capitolunate instability (CCI)" to describe the picture in a series of 12 patients with post-traumatic wrist clicking and weakness in whom plain and videofluoroscopic features were normal and in whom a dorsal capitate–displacement apprehension test reproduced the symptoms. These post-traumatic findings represent another potential variation of DMCI.

Wright and colleagues[42] have described a group of patients with clinical characteristics identical to those of patients with PMCI. They have used the term "carpal instability–nondissociative" (CIND) to describe this condition and to distinguish it from the perilunate forms of dissociative instability.

Table 17–1 presents a classification scheme of midcarpal instabilities based on a compendium of these authors' findings. Extrinsic MCI is discussed more extensively later in this chapter.

Anatomy and Pathogenesis

Several models have been proposed to help explain wrist mechanics, including Taleisnik's columnar model and the senior author's ring model (see Chapter 12). Although the columnar model (Fig. 17–1) is useful in considering load distribution across the wrist, we believe that the ring model better characterizes carpal motion and the link mechanism of the proximal and distal carpal rows (Fig. 17–2). The proximal and distal carpal rows move in relative synchrony during flexion and extension, but their relative motion during radial and ulnar deviation is more complex. In radial deviation, the proximal row moves

---

*References 1–4, 6, 8, 9, 14, 17, 18, 26, 31–34, 36, 41, 42.

316

Table 17–1. CLASSIFICATION OF MIDCARPAL INSTABILITY (MCI)

Suggested Terminology	Original Terminology and Chapter Reference(s)	Proposed Etiology	Direction of Subluxation	Suggested Surgical Treatment
Palmar MCI	Ulnar midcarpal instability[12, 13] Carpal instability–nondissociative (CIND)[43]	Laxity of ulnar arm of the ulnar arcuate ligament and the dorsal radiolunatotriquetral ligament	Palmar	Limited carpal arthrodesis
		As above, or ulnar-minus variant	Palmar*	Limited carpal arthrodesis or ulnar lengthening (depending on etiology)
Dorsal MCI	Capitolunate instability pattern (CLIP)[17, 42] Chronic capitolunate instability[9]	Laxity of the palmar radioscaphocapitate or ligament	Dorsal	Palmar capsular reefing (radioscaphocapitate to radiolunatotriquetral)
Extrinsic MCI	MCI secondary to distal radius malunion[32]	Dorsal displacement and angulation of distal radius; adaptive Z-deformity of carpus	Dorsal	Corrective distal radius osteotomy

*Majority of cases presented represented palmar MCI, although a few were dorsal.

dorsally and flexes, and the distal row translates palmarly in relation to the proximal row. As the wrist moves to neutral and then into ulnar deviation, the proximal row rotates into neutral flexion/extension, and then into a low extended position. The motion of each row relative to the other depends on intimate midcarpal joint contact and the resultant joint contact forces generated—particularly at the radial midcarpal link (scaphotrapezotrapezoid joint) and ulnar midcarpal link (triquetrohamate joint). Intimate midcarpal joint contact depends, in turn, on the integrity of the ligaments spanning the midcarpal joint as well as of those that limit rotation of the proximal row.

Ligament sectioning studies have been performed to help identify the pathologic anatomy of MCI.[13, 26, 33, 34] Although patients with MCI demonstrate gross instability at the triquetrohamate joint, triquetrohamate capsule sectioning in fresh cadaver specimens fails to create a MCI pattern of joint motion. It is not until the volar arm of the arcuate ligament is cut that carpal kinematics similar to those seen in patients with MCI can be demonstrated. The volar arcuate ligament complex, and specifically its ulnar arm, is a major palmar stabilizer of the midcarpal joint (Fig. 17–3). The ulnar arm of the arcuate ligament is the palmar triquetrohamatocapitate ligament. The proximal attachment of this ligament is at the palmar sur-

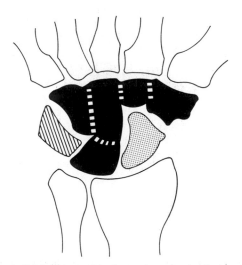

Figure 17–1. Taleisnik's model of carpal mechanics involves a central flexion/extension column made up of the lunate and the entire distal row; a lateral mobile column made up of the scaphoid; and a rotatory medial column made up of the triquetrum. (*From* Lichtman DM, Schneider JR, Swafford AR, et al: Ulnar midcarpal instability. Clinical and laboratory analysis. J Hand Surg 6:515–523, 1981.)

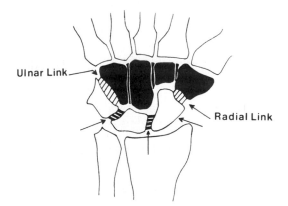

Figure 17–2. In the "ring" model, the proximal and distal rows are firmly stabilized by interosseous ligaments (dark shading) and are linked together at the radial and ulnar aspects. Motion between the two rows occurs in a controlled manner through the motion radially of the scaphoid and ulnarly at the triquetrohamate joint. Any bony or ligamentous disruption of the ring (*arrows*) can produce an uncontrolled dorsal or volar intercalated segmental instability (DISI or VISI) pattern. (*From* Lichtman DM, Schneider JR, Swafford AR, et al: Ulnar midcarpal instability. Clinical and laboratory analysis. J Hand Surg 6:515–523, 1981.)

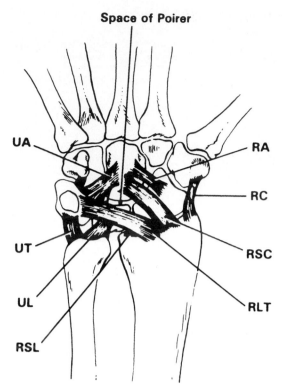

Space of Poirer

Figure 17–3. The palmar arcuate ligament complex is a major stabilizer of the midcarpal joint. The triquetrohamatocapitate ligament makes up the ulnar arm, and the radial arm is confluent with and distal to the radioscaphocapitate *(RSC)* ligament. The space of Poirer is the relatively weak area between the capitate and lunate in which few ligamentous structures are present. *RC* = radial collateral ligament; *RA* = radial arm of arcuate ligament; *RSL* = radioscapholunate ligament; *UA* = ulnar arm of arcuate ligament; *UL* = ulnolunate ligament; *UT* = ulnotriquetral ligament.

face of the triquetrum, the palmar triquetrolunate ligament, and the ulnar corner of the palmar lunate. The ulnar arm of this ligament then attaches to the proximal corner of the hamate and inserts distally into the palmar neck of the capitate. The radial arm of the arcuate ligament is confluent with and distal to the palmar radioscaphocapitate ligament. The functional significance of these radial fibers has not yet been determined.

Dorsally, the capitolunate and triquetrohamate ligaments provide minimal stability to the midcarpal joint.[13] The dorsal radiolunotriquetral (RLT) ligament, however, acts as a checkrein to prevent flexion of the proximal row.[36] Because a static VISI is always a component of PMCI, we believe that laxity of the RLT ligament also contributes to palmar midcarpal instability.

In several of our patients with midcarpal instability, we have had the opportunity to directly observe the contribution of the dorsal RLT ligament to midcarpal stability at the time of surgery. When the RLT is excessively lax, the proximal row assumes a VISI position in the unsupported wrist. The midcarpal shift test (described in the next section) is markedly

positive. However, temporarily tightening this ligament (e.g., crimping the RLT ligament in a clamp) corrects the VISI deformity and stabilizes the midcarpal joint, eliminating the previously observed midcarpal shift.

With laxity of the midpalmar ligaments (palmar arcuate, dorsal radiolunotriquetral), specifically in the face of a palmar flexed proximal row (VISI), the normal reactive forces at the midcarpal joint no longer control the smooth intercalary motion of the proximal row. Instead of the smooth glide from flexion to extension as the wrist deviates ulnarward, the entire proximal row stays in its palmar-flexed position relative to the distal row. As ulnar deviation is completed, the triquetrohamate joint is now compressed, and the normal joint reactive forces are suddenly reactivated. Thus, the proximal row rapidly rotates into extension, moving palmarly while the distal row translates dorsally. The final resting position in ulnar deviation is physiologic, but a "catch-up clunk" occurs, which is the source of the patient's symptoms.

Clinical Findings

Patients with PMCI present with a characteristic history of a painful "clunk" on the ulnar side of the wrist during activities involving active ulnar deviation with the forearm in pronation. There may or may not be a history of significant trauma. Asymptomatic wrist clunking may have occurred for many years prior to the current painful presentation. The condition is often bilateral, especially in patients with generalized ligament laxity. Females seem to be as equally affected as males.

On physical examination, a palmar sag of the ulnar side of the carpus is commonly noted, along with a prominent-appearing ulnar head with the wrist in neutral deviation (Fig. 17–4). A localized synovitis may be present, and if so, the sag and relative prominence of the ulnar head may be less dramatic. In the presence of synovitis, there is tenderness over the ulnar carpus, particularly at the triquetrohamate joint. The patient can often reproduce the clunk with active ulnar deviation of the pronated wrist, and the examiner can easily visualize and palpate the sudden change in carpal position that accompanies the clunk. At the extreme of ulnar deviation (after the clunk), the volar sag of the ulnar carpus is gone.

MIDCARPAL SHIFT TEST

If the patient is unable to actively reproduce the clunk, it may be reproduced passively by the examiner with the midcarpal shift test.[11] To perform this test on the right wrist, the examiner stabilizes the forearm with the left hand and holds it in a pronated position (Fig. 17–5). With the patient's wrist in about 15° of ulnar deviation, the examiner's right hand grasps the patient's right hand and, with the thumb,

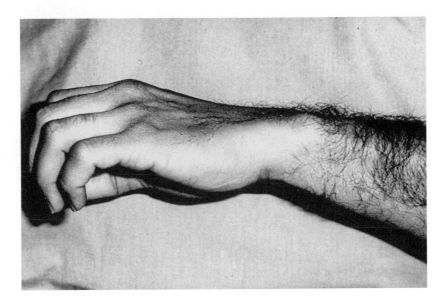

Figure 17–4. Lateral view of the wrist in neutral deviation in a patient with palmar midcarpal instability. A palmar sag of the ulnar side of the carpus is noted, along with a prominent-appearing ulnar head.

exerts palmarly directed pressure at the level of the distal capitate (Fig. 17–6). The ease and extent of palmar translation are noted. The wrist is then simultaneously axially loaded and ulnarly deviated (Fig. 17–7). The test is positive if a painful clunk occurs with passive ulnar deviation that *reproduces the patient's symptoms*. Palmar translation and the production of a clunk alone are not significant, because these findings can be elicited in patients with lax ligaments who do not have PMCI. They are also often found in the asymptomatic contralateral wrist of a patient with PMCI.

The midcarpal shift test is one of several provocative wrist maneuvers that are subjective and difficult to quantify. Therefore, we proposed a grading system for the test that is based on three criteria: the force required to produce palmar translation, the quality of wrist clunk, and whether or not the patient can reproduce the clunk spontaneously (Table 17–2). The midcarpal shift test result is graded from I to V according to the ease and extent of palmar translation along with the severity of the clunk. Grades I through IV are considered to be increasing degrees of "normal" midcarpal laxity and can be produced only passively by the examiner. Grade V is reserved for those wrists in which the patient can reproduce the clunk spontaneously, and it represents the pathologic condition of midcarpal instability.

To test the validity of the midcarpal shift test, we performed a double-blind study on volunteer subjects to compare experimentally determined midcarpal laxity/stiffness with the clinical grading scheme just

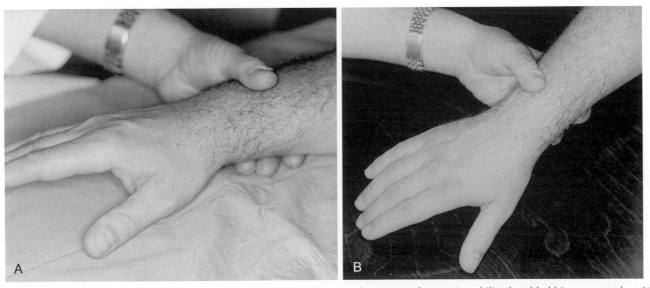

Figure 17–5. The midcarpal shift test (MST) being performed on a right wrist. The patient's forearm is stabilized and held in a pronated position by the examiner's left hand. *A,* side view; *B,* top view.

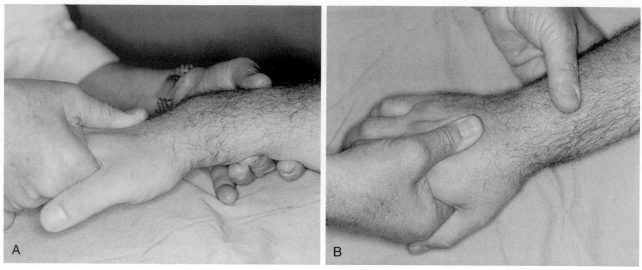

Figure 17–6. Midcarpal shift test continued: With the patient's wrist in neutral deviation, the examiner's right hand grasps the patient's right hand and, with the thumb, exerts pressure in a palmar direction on the dorsal wrist at the level of the distal capitate. *A*, side view; *B*, top view.

described for midcarpal instability and as performed by the senior author (DML). The initial results indicate a strong correlation between the clinical grade and the measured mechanical force required for palmar translation. Specifically, we observed two types of midcarpal curve patterns, one for stiff wrists and one for lax wrists. For those wrists whose clinical translation grades were higher (grades III and IV), the lax midcarpal curve pattern was predominant, which we believe is a signature marker for the biomechanical behavior of midcarpal instability (Fig. 17–8). Three patients with clinical grade V midcarpal instability were also biomechanically tested. Each patient

demonstrated the classic instability signature curve already described for the symptomatic wrist.

It is difficult to predict when (and whether) a painless, excessively lax midcarpal joint will become symptomatic PMCI. Generally, when the ligaments become lax enough so that the wrist clunks spontaneously (grade V), the patient will become symptomatic. Three potential sources of pain may each make a relative contribution to the patient's symptoms. First, a localized synovitis can occur; second, long-term instability may result in midcarpal articular wear and chondromalacia; and third, pain fibers from the ligaments themselves may become activated as

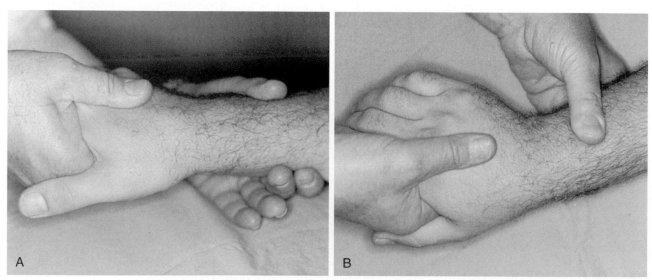

Figure 17–7. Midcarpal shift test continued: The wrist is then simultaneously axially loaded and ulnarly deviated to recreate the relevant forces that cause the symptoms to occur. *A*, side view; *B*, top view.

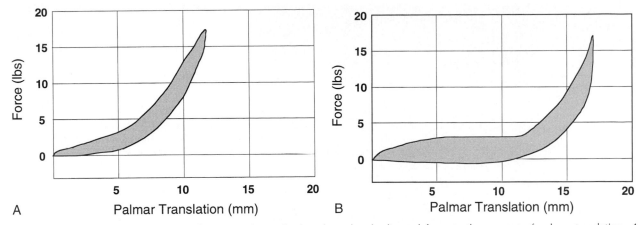

Figure 17–8. The midcarpal curve patterns that were observed relate the palmarly directed force to the amount of palmar translation. *A,* stiff midcarpal curve; *B,* lax midcarpal curve. Each curve is similar, with loading in the initial and terminal phases; but in the lax wrist curve, rapid palmar displacement occurred upon loading after only minimal application of force. This is the biomechanical signature marker for midcarpal instability. This phenomenon was not observed in the stiff wrist curve pattern.

the ligaments become further stretched with time. Pain and tenderness are often concentrated on the ulnar side of the wrist at the triquetrohamate joint, because of concentration of forces at this site with ulnar deviation and as the "catch-up clunk" occurs.

Diagnostic Studies

Plain radiographs of the wrist may be unremarkable, because PMCI is a dynamic condition and static films cannot capture the pathologic motion of the carpus. However, the lateral view in neutral radioulnar deviation usually shows a VISI configuration with slight palmar translocation of the distal carpal row (Fig. 17–9). If the wrist is resting on the x-ray plate, however, the VISI configuration may inadvertently be reduced. The imaging study of choice is videofluoroscopy in the posteroanterior (PA) and lateral planes as the patient moves the wrist from radial to ulnar deviation. Close and repeated inspection enables direct visualization of the pathologic carpal motion as previously described. In the PA plane, one can see the entire proximal row jump from flexion to extension as a single unit when the wrist deviates ulnarly. It is particularly important on this view to rule out any dissociative lesions, such as scapholunate or triquetrolunate instability. On the lateral view, using

Table 17–2. MIDCARPAL SHIFT TEST

Grade	Palmar Midcarpal Translation	Clunk
I	None	None
II	Minimal	Minimal
III	Moderate	Moderate
IV	Maximal	Significant
V	Self-induced	Self-induced

the lunate as the marker, one can readily confirm that the sudden motion is from flexion to extension as the wrist deviates ulnarly. This is primarily a dynamic phenomenon, occurring instantaneously, so sequential still radiographs cannot capture the essence of the event.

Wrist arthrography in patients with PMCI is usually normal, because the pathologic process is characteristically one of ligamentous attenuation rather than tear. Occasionally, a positive arthrogram with dye flow through the scapholunate or lunotriquetral joint is seen coexistent with midcarpal instability. In such cases, the clinical picture of PMCI usually predominates over that of any dissociative instability.

Diagnostic arthroscopy can now define areas of laxity or pathology in the supporting ligaments (T. Whipple, MD, personal communication, 1994).[39] Arthroscopy can also be utilized to rule out definitively a concurrent dissociative lesion. The role of magnetic resonance (MR) imaging in the evaluation of the PMCI has yet to be defined. Presumably, ligament pathology will become better defined as the technique is improved.

Differential Diagnosis

Because the characteristic clunking of PMCI commonly is present in asymptomatic wrists, it is important to rule out other causes of ulnar-sided wrist pain in persons with both pain and wrist clunk. Other diagnoses to consider are lunotriquetral instability, distal radioulnar joint instability, triangular fibrocartilage complex (TFCC) tears, ulnocarpal impaction syndrome, and extensor carpi ulnaris tendon (ECU) subluxation. Each of these entities is discussed elsewhere in this text.

Nonoperative Treatment

Many cases of PMCI, especially the milder variety, respond well to nonoperative management. This pro-

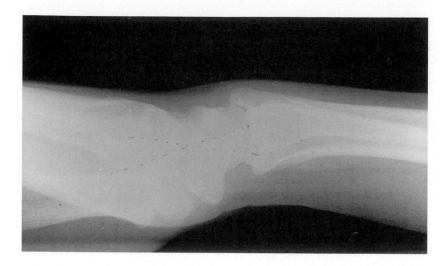

Figure 17–9. Lateral wrist radiograph in neutral deviation of a patient with palmar midcarpal instability. There is a volar intercalated segmental instability (VISI) deformity and a zigzag pattern to the axes of the radius, lunate, and capitate.

cess begins with educating the patient about the nature of the problem and the necessity to avoid offending activities, and the use of nonsteroidal anti-inflammatory medications to address any synovitic or arthritic component of the patient's symptoms. Steroid injections may also be used, although we use them infrequently. A trial of wrist immobilization in a standard cock-up splint is indicated for acute synovitis.

We have had much success for milder cases using a three-point splint that pushes dorsally on the pisiform bone (Fig. 17–10). Dorsally directed pressure on the pisiform reduces the ulnar carpal sag along with the VISI position of the proximal row. In this supported position, midcarpal dynamics are corrected, and the wrist does not clunk. Wrist range of motion is not significantly obstructed, and the painful clunk is eliminated, while the splint is in use. When the splint is not in use, patients should be instructed on strengthening exercises that may help control their symptoms.

The pathomechanics of the midcarpal joint can also be corrected by dynamic muscle action. Activating the hypothenar muscles along with the ECU, and possibly the flexor carpi ulnaris (FCU), can "reset" the midcarpal joint into its physiologic position. In this case, physiologic joint contact forces are reproduced by dynamic muscle compression rather than normal ligament support. If dynamic muscle action is used to stabilize the midcarpal joint, upon activation of ulnar deviation, the instability will be eliminated.

Dynamic stabilization can be demonstrated to the patient by pushing dorsally on the pisiform. In this position, the wrist does not clunk with ulnar deviation. The patient can then be instructed to maintain this position by activation of the ECU and hypothenar muscles. If this muscle activation is habituated during ulnar deviation then the painful clunk may be eliminated. Combinations of dynamic and passive measures can adequately control symptoms in most patients. In those for whom nonoperative treatment

fails to achieve satisfactory symptom control, surgical treatment is recommended.

Operative Treatment

Surgical treatment aims to prevent the pathologic motion at the midcarpal joint. This aim can be achieved by ligament reconstruction, capsular tightening, or a limited midcarpal arthrodesis. Initially, tendon grafts were utilized to reconstruct the functional break in the ring at the triquetrohamate joint.[1] These were not uniformly successful, however, as the grafts tended to stretch out over time and symptoms recurred.

SOFT TISSUE RECONSTRUCTION

We have performed several combinations of soft tissue reefing procedures,[11] including (1) distal advancement of the palmar ulnar arm of the arcuate ligament, (2) dorsal radiocarpal capsulodesis, and (3) sewing the palmar radioscaphocapitate ligament to the palmar radiolunotriquetral ligament to close the space of Poirier.

Our initial approach involving soft tissue procedures primarily focused on advancement of the palmar ulnar arm of the arcuate ligament (Fig. 17–11A). In this procedure, the ulnar arm of the arcuate ligament is dissected free from the palmar capsule through a palmar approach, as follows: Detach the arcuate ligament from its insertion on the capitate, and free it proximally to its origins on the triquetrum and ulnar border of the lunate. Avoid injury to the palmar triquetrolunate interosseous ligament. Weave a Bunnell suture through the arcuate ligament, exiting on its distal surface. Advance the ligament distally on the capitate, and create a bony trough for its insertion. Distal traction on the arcuate ligament will pull on the triquetrum and lunate and correct the VISI configuration of the proximal row. Pass the Bun-

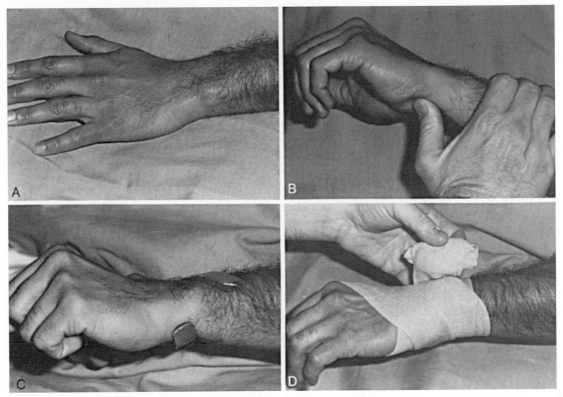

Figure 17–10. A splint for palmar midcarpal instability is indicated for those whose symptoms primarily occur during athletic or other strenuous activities. *A*, The characteristic midcarpal sag. *B*, This can be reduced by dorsally directed pressure on the pisiform. *C* and *D*, A splint that applies a continuous dorsal pressure on the pisiform is held in place by an elastic wrap or taping.

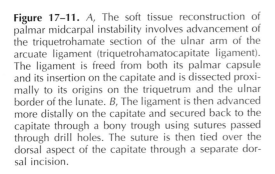

Figure 17–11. *A*, The soft tissue reconstruction of palmar midcarpal instability involves advancement of the triquetrohamate section of the ulnar arm of the arcuate ligament (triquetrohamatocapitate ligament). The ligament is freed from both its palmar capsule and its insertion on the capitate and is dissected proximally to its origins on the triquetrum and the ulnar border of the lunate. *B*, The ligament is then advanced more distally on the capitate and secured back to the capitate through a bony trough using sutures passed through drill holes. The suture is then tied over the dorsal aspect of the capitate through a separate dorsal incision.

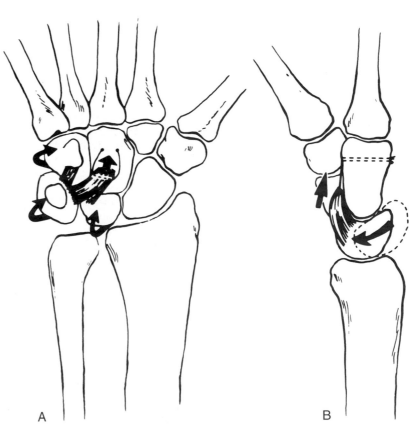

A   B

nell suture dorsally through drill holes in the capitate. Obtain the reduced (neutral) position of the proximal and distal carpal rows prior to tying the suture. Double-check to make sure the VISI deformity is completely corrected. Tie the suture over the capitate through a separate dorsal incision (Fig. 17–11B). Maintain the position with Kirschner wires passed from the triquetrum and the hamate to the capitate and from the capitate to the lunate. Immobilize the wrist in a short-arm cast for 10 weeks.

In the series just cited, nine patients underwent soft tissue reconstruction, with five undergoing advancement of the ulnar arm of the arcuate ligament as a solitary procedure.[11] Two of the five had a return of the clunk postoperatively. Therefore, we now always perform a dorsal capsulodesis along with the palmar reefing.

In a few later patients, we have perfomed a dorsal capsulodesis as the only soft tissue reconstructive procedure, as follows: Expose the dorsal capsule through a longitudinal incision between the third and fourth dorsal compartments. Make a 2.5-cm transverse incision in the dorsal radiolunotriquetral ligament between the radius and the proximal carpal row. Imbricate the dorsal RLT ligament in a "pants-over-vest" suture technique, eliminating any redundancy. The VISI deformity should be corrected by this imbrication. Intraoperative examination by performing the midcarpal shift test should demonstrate increased ligamentous tightness and elimination of the clunk. Restoration of normal intracarpal alignment is verified intraoperatively on a lateral radiograph. Immobilize the wrist in neutral position for 8 to 10 weeks with a sugar-tong splint for 2 weeks, followed by a short-arm cast. No pin fixation is required when the dorsal capsulodesis is performed, either as a solitary procedure or when combined with advancement of palmar ligaments.

It is too early to accurately evaluate the clinical outcome for this selective procedure compared with those previously described, but our early findings are promising.

LIMITED WRIST ARTHRODESIS

Limited wrist arthrodesis consists of either a triquetrohamate (ulnar column) fusion or a triquetrohamate-capitolunate (four-quadrant) fusion. We have noted that fusion of the triquetrohamate joint alone may result in radial-sided wrist symptoms, perhaps owing to increased mobility at the radial side of the midcarpal joint. Since this observation was made, we have utilized only four-quadrant fusions.[11]

The four-quadrant fusion is performed as follows: Approach the wrist through a longitudinal dorsal incision, and expose the carpus between the fourth and fifth extensor compartments. Perform the midcarpal shift test as an added step to confirm the preoperative diagnosis. Inspect the triquetrohamate joint closely, because it is the likely site of maximal instability and articular wear. Drive a Kirschner wire across the triquetrohamate joint, and repeat the midcarpal shift test. The clunk should be eliminated (if it is not, reconsider the preoperative diagnosis). Remove the wire, and denude the appropriate articular surfaces. Pack the spaces with cancellous bone graft. Take care to maintain the normal carpal/intercarpal spatial relationships. Fuse the lunate in a colinear relationship with the capitate. Use Kirschner wires and a short-arm cast to maintain wrist position in neutral flexion/extension and neutral radioulnar deviation. Remove the Kirschner wires at 8 weeks, and the cast at 10 weeks or with radiographic confirmation that bony union is achieved.

Limited intercarpal arthrodesis has provided predictable satisfactory result.[11] Of six patients who underwent limited midcarpal arthrodesis (three triquetrohamate fusions and three four-quadrant fusions), all had a successful result at an average of 51 months postoperatively. Average loss of wrist range of motion was 28 percent, but grip strength increased 10 percent.

SURGICAL RESULTS

Limited wrist arthrodesis (four-quadrant fusion) and soft tissue reefing procedures, when successful, result in comparable limitations of wrist motion and comparable increases in grip strength.[11] Limited wrist arthrodesis appears to offer more predictable relief of PMCI symptoms in the short to intermediate term than do the soft tissue reefing procedures. Our recommended treatment for palmar midcarpal instability is limited wrist arthrodesis (four-quadrant fusion) as the surgical procedure of choice. We believe, however, that the clinical evaluation of soft tissue reefing procedures should be continued. Although results in the short to intermediate term are better following four-quadrant fusion, we are concerned that the loss of the load-sharing and load-dispersing functions of the intercarpal joints may result in a higher incidence of ulnocarpal or radiocarpal arthritis. In capsular reconstruction, the load-sharing and load-dispersing functions of the intercarpal joints are preserved.

EXTRINSIC MIDCARPAL INSTABILITY

Extrinsic midcarpal instability can occur secondary to malunion of fractures of the distal radius. This disorder was first described by Linscheid and colleagues,[16] and a subsequent series of patients has been reported by Taleisnik and Watson.[32] Patients with this condition develop pain and clunking at the midcarpal joint several months after cast immobilization is discontinued. Findings on physical examination include synovitis and tenderness over the triquetrohamate joint, and a demonstrable clunk with active ulnar deviation of the pronated wrist. Radiographically, the major change in the architecture of the distal radius is a dramatic reversal of palmar tilt. On the lateral view with the wrist in neutral deviation, the lunate and capitate remain colinear, but with an axis parallel and dorsal to that of the shaft of the radius. On the lateral view with the wrist in ulnar deviation, the lunate assumes a dorsiflexed position, but without the normal palmar translation typically seen. In this position, the axis of the capitate is no longer colinear with the lunate, but remains dorsal and parallel to the axis of the shaft of the radius (Fig. 17–12A). It is believed that the painful subluxation is compensatory and secondary to the inability of the lunate to translate palmarly with ulnar deviation of the wrist because of the excessive dorsal tilt of the articular surface of the distal radius. Corrective osteotomy of the distal radius with restoration of radiocarpal alignment relieves the symptoms of extrinsic MCI (Fig. 17–12B). (See Chapter 20 for details of this operation.)

PROXIMAL CARPAL INSTABILITIES

Proximal carpal instabilities are quite uncommon. These conditions are characterized by subluxation or dislocation of the entire carpus relative to the distal radius. This group of instabilities has been classified by Taleisnik[29, 30] according to the direction of carpal translocation: dorsal, palmar, and ulnar. Radial translocation of the carpus has not been described.

Dorsal carpal translocation can be manifest in a variety of forms. The most common presentation of dorsal carpal translocation in the acute setting is in conjunction with a dorsal Barton's fracture of the distal radius. This entity is discussed in greater detail in Chapter 19. Subacute or chronic dorsal carpal translocation is usually seen in association with malunited fractures of the distal radius in which the dorsal lip is displaced or in which there is excessive dorsal tilt of the distal radius (Fig. 17–13A). The carpus may remain subluxed dorsally throughout the radiocarpal range of motion, or the subluxation may occur suddenly with ulnar deviation of the wrist[29, 30]—essentially, the clinical picture of extrinsic midcarpal instability. Management consists of corrective osteotomy of the distal radius (Fig. 17–13B).

Palmar carpal translocation is less common than its dorsal variant. Most often, it occurs following a palmar Barton's fracture of the distal radius (Fig. 17–14). Management of this acute injury is discussed in Chapter 19. Chronic subluxation secondary to malunion of Barton's fracture is managed with osteotomy of the distal radius.

Ulnocarpal translocation, unlike its dorsal and palmar counterparts, is rarely an acute post-traumatic finding. Evidence indicates that loss of most of the radiocarpal stabilizers is necessary in order for acute ulnar translation to occur.[35] Open repair of the torn ligaments with pinning of the carpus in the reduced position is recommended.[23] More commonly, ulnar carpal instability results from loss of ligamentous support of the ulnocarpal and radiocarpal joints secondary to long-standing rheumatoid arthritis or other forms of chronic synovitis. With loss of ligamentous support, particularly the palmar radiolunate and dorsal radiotriquetral ligaments, the carpus translates ul-

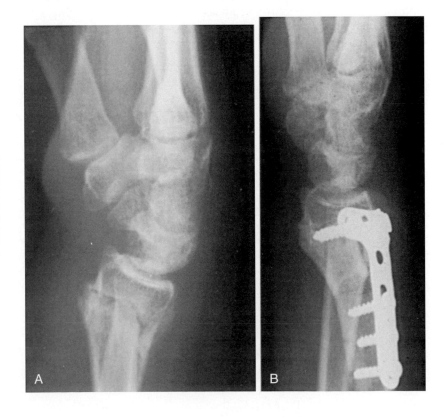

Figure 17–12. A, Extrinsic midcarpal instability secondary to malunion of a distal radius fracture. This lateral view in ulnar deviation shows the expected dorsiflexed position of the lunate. The longitudinal axis of the capitate remains parallel but is dorsal to the longitudinal axis of the radius. B, Postoperative lateral radiograph of the wrist shown in A. Osteotomy has corrected the excessive dorsal tilt of the distal radius and has restored the normal intercarpal alignment. The patient is no longer symptomatic.

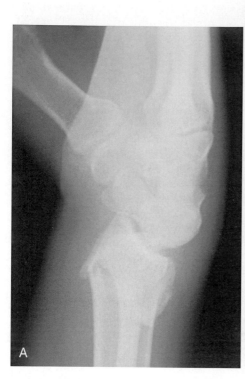

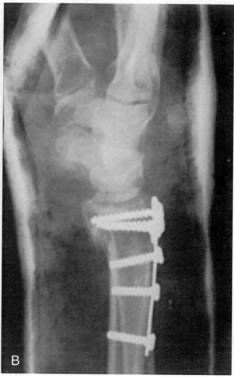

Figure 17–13. *A,* Chronic dorsal carpal translocation following malunion of a dorsal Barton's fracture. Note that the intercarpal alignment is normal. *B,* Post-operative lateral radiograph of the wrist shown in *A.* Osteotomy has corrected the excessive dorsal carpal translocation.

narly because of the slope of the articular surface of the radius (Fig. 17–15). Other intracarpal instabilities may coexist. Because of the complexity of the soft tissue compromise, soft tissue reconstructive procedures are not likely to be successful. A localized fusion of the radius to the reduced lunate is recommended.[38] Otherwise, radiocarpal arthrodesis can be performed if symptoms warrant it.

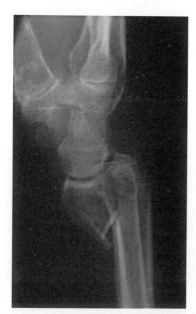

Figure 17–14. Chronic volar carpal translocation following malunion of a volar Barton's fracture.

Ulnocarpal translocation can also be iatrogenic. Such a scenario is most commonly seen following a Darrach procedure in patients with compromised radiocarpal ligament support. In rheumatoid patients with an excessive radial inclination (more than 30°) or early signs of ulnar lunate migration (more than 50 percent of the lunate subluxed over the ulnar radius), a prophylactic radiolunate arthrodesis should be performed along with the Darrach procedure. Following distal radius fracture, if the lunate has migrated ulnarward, a standard Darrach procedure should also be avoided. In questionable cases, a Sauve-Kapandji procedure (see Chapter 24) is a better option to support the ulnar carpus.

CONCLUSION

Over the past 15 years, palmar midcarpal instability has become an increasingly recognized source of wrist impairment. Patients with this condition have a fairly characteristic presentation of symptoms, physical signs, and radiographic findings. The mid-carpal shift test described in this chapter, as well as the findings on videofluoroscopy, are diagnostic. Unlike for most other forms of wrist instability, non-operative treatment as described here is often successful for midcarpal instability. If nonoperative treatment fails, four-quadrant fusion is indicated. Capsular reconstructive procedures are still under investigation. Dorsal capsulodesis alone is commonly successful; if not, a four-quadrant fusion can be done as a later procedure.

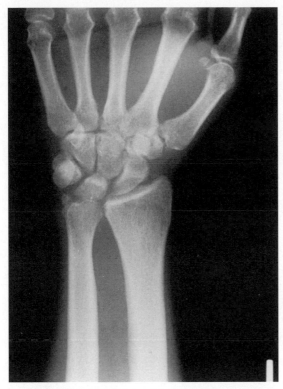

Figure 17–15. Ulnar translocation of the entire carpus due to insufficiency of the ulnocarpal and radiocarpal ligaments. The lunate is seen ulnar to the radius, and the space between the radial styloid and the scaphoid is increased.

Proximal carpal instabilities are unusual but must be recognized and treated appropriately when encountered. Iatrogenic forms are obviously preventable. As we gain more experience, treatment options will become more standardized.

References

1. Alexander CE, Lichtman DM: Ulnar carpal instabilities. Orthop Clin North Am 15:307–320, 1984.
2. Alexander CE, Lichtman DM: Triquetrolunate and midcarpal instability. In Lichtman DM (ed): The Wrist and Its Disorders. Philadelphia, WB Saunders, 1988, pp 274–285.
3. Ambrose L, Posner MA: Lunate-triquetral and midcarpal joint instability. Hand Clin 8:653–668, 1992.
4. Braunstein EM, Louis DS, Greene TL, Hankin FM: Fluoroscopic and arthrographic evaluation of carpal instability. AJR 144:1259–262, 1985.
5. Brown DE, Lichtman DM: Midcarpal instability. Hand Clin 3:135–140, 1987.
6. Dobyns JH, Linscheid RL, Wadih SM, et al: Carpal instability, nondissociative (CIND). Presented at the Annual Meeting of the American Academy of Orthopedic Surgeons, San Francisco, Jan 1987.
7. Goldner L: Treatment of carpal instability without joint fusion: Current assessment. J Hand Surg 7:325–326, 1982.
8. Green DP: Carpal dislocations and instabilities. In Green DP (ed): Operative Hand Surgery. New York, Churchill Livingstone, 1994, pp 861–928.
9. Johnson RP, Carrera GF: Chronic capitolunate instability. J Bone Joint Surg 68A:1164–1176, 1980.
10. Lichtman DM: Midcarpal instability. In McGinty JB (ed): Operative Arthroscopy. New York, Raven Press, 1991, pp 647–650.
11. Lichtman DM, Bruckner JD, Culp RW, Alexander CE: Palmar midcarpal instability: Results of surgical reconstruction. J Hand Surg 18:307–315, 1993.
12. Lichtman DM, Schneider JR, Swafford AR: Midcarpal instability. Presented at the 35th Annual Meeting of the American Society for Surgery of the Hand, Atlanta, Feb 4–6, 1980.
13. Lichtman DM, Schneider JR, Swafford AR, Mack GR: Ulnar midcarpal instability: Clinical and laboratory analysis. J Hand Surg 6:515–523, 1981.
14. Lichtman DM, Niccolai TM: The ulnar arcuate ligament complex: Its anatomy and functional significance. Presented at the 43rd Annual Meeting of the American Society For Surgery of the Hand, Baltimore, Sept 14–17, 1988.
15. Lichtman DM, Martin RA: Introduction to the carpal instabilities. In Lichtman DM (ed): The Wrist and Its Disorders. Philadelphia, WB Saunders, 1988, pp 244–250.
16. Linscheid RL, Dobyns JH, Beabout JW, Bryan RS: Traumatic instability of the wrist: Diagnosis, classification, and pathomechanics. J Bone Joint Surg 54A:1612, 1972.
17. Louis DS, Hankin FM, Greene TL, et al: Central carpal instability–capitate lunate instability pattern: Diagnosis by dynamic displacement. Orthopedics 7:1693–1696, 1984.
18. Mayfield JK: Patterns of injury to carpal ligaments. Clin Orthop 187:36–42, 1984.
19. Mayfield JK, Johnson RP, Kilcoyne RF: The ligaments of the human wrist and their functional significance. Anat Rec 186:417–428, 1976.
20. Mayfield JK, Honnson RP, Kilcoyne RF: Carpal dislocations: Pathomechanics and progressive perilunar instability. J Hand Surg 5:226–241, 1980.
21. Mouchet A, Bélot J: Poignet à résult (subluxation médiocarpiènne en avant). Bull Mém Soc Nat Chir 60:1243–1244, 1934.
22. Pournaras J, Kappas A: Volar perilunar dislocation. J Bone Joint Surg 61:625, 1979.
23. Rayhack JM, Linscheid RL, Dobyns JH, Smith JH: Post-traumatic ulnar translocation of the carpus. J Hand Surg 12A:180–189, 1987.
24. Ruby K, Cooney WP III, An KN, et al: Relative motion of selected carpal bones: A kinematic analysis of the normal wrist. J Hand Surg 13A:1–10, 1988.
25. Ruby LK, An KN, Cooney WP III, et al: The effect of scapholunate ligament section on scapholunate motion. J Hand Surg 12A:767–771, 1987.
26. Saffar P: Midcarpal instability. In Carpal Injuries: Anatomy, Radiology, Current Treatment. Paris, Springer-Verlag, 1990, pp 83–87.
27. Sennwald GR, Zdravkovic V, Kern HP, Jacob HAC: Kinematics of the wrist and its ligaments. J Hand Surg 18:805–814, 1993.
28. Taleisnik J: The ligaments of the wrist. J Hand Surg 1:110–118, 1976.
29. Taleisnik J: Post-traumatic carpal instability. Clin Orthop 149:73–82, 1980.
30. Taleisnik J: The Wrist. New York, Churchill Livingstone, 1985, pp 305–326.
31. Taleisnik J: Pain on the ulnar side of the wrist. Hand Clin 3:51–68, 1987.
32. Taleisnik JH, Watson HK: Midcarpal instability caused by malunited fractures of the distal radius. J Hand Surg 9A:350–357, 1984.
33. Trumble T, Bour CJ, Smith RJ, Glisson RR: Kinematics of the ulnar carpus related to the volar intercalated segment instability pattern. J Hand Surg 15A:384–392, 1990.
34. Trumble T, Bour CH, Smith RJ, Edwards GS: Intercarpal arthrodesis for static and dynamic volar intercalated instability. J Hand Surg 13A:384–390, 1988.
35. Viegas SF, Patterson RM, Ward K: Extrinsic wrist ligaments in the pathomechanics of ulnar translocation instability. J Hand Surg 20A:312–318, 1995.
36. Viegas SF, Pogue DJ, Hokanson JA: Ulnar sided perilunate instability: An anatomic and biomechanic study. J Hand Surg 15A:268–277, 1990.
37. Watson HK, Goodman ML, Johnson TR: Limited wrist

arthrodesis. Part II: Intercarpal and radiocarpal combinations. J Hand Surg 6:223–233, 1981.

38. Watson HK, Johnson TR, Hemptom RF, Jones DS: Limited wrist arthrodesis. Presented at 34th Annual Meeting of the American Society for Surgery of the Hand (abstract). J Hand Surg 4:286, 1979.

39. Whipple T: Arthroscopic Surgery: The Wrist. Philadelphia, JB Lippincott, 1992, pp 119–129.

40. Whipple T: Wrist Investigators Workshop. Rochester, MN, June, 1994.

41. White SJ, Louis DS, Braunstein FM, et al: Capitate-lunate instability: Recognition by manipulation under fluoroscopy. AJR 143:361–364, 1984.

42. Wright TW, Dobyns JH, Linscheid RL: Carpal instability, nondissociative. Presented at the 45th Annual Meeting of the American Society for Surgery of the Hand, Toronto, Sept 1990.

CHAPTER 18

Kienböck's Disease and Idiopathic Necrosis of Carpal Bones

Charlotte E. Alexander, MD, A. Herbert Alexander, MD, and David M. Lichtman, MD

Kienböck's disease (avascular necrosis of the carpal lunate bone) should be considered in any patient presenting with wrist pain of uncertain origin. Often, the early stages of the disease are clinically and roentgenographically indistinguishable from other causes of wrist pain. The patient is usually young, 20 to 40 years of age,[2, 60, 61] and may complain of pain and stiffness in the wrist. The male-to-female ratio is 2 to 1.[60, 61] The lesion, though not rare, is uncommon, and the average orthopedist can expect to see a case every 1 or 2 years. The incidence of bilateral Kienböck's disease is extremely low, there being few reports of this occurrence.[62, 69]

Clinically, the patient notes tenderness dorsally about the lunate, sometimes in association with synovial swelling consistent with localized synovitis. Early on, however, the patient may appear to simply have a wrist sprain. With progression, symptoms of synovitis predominate, and in the late stage, arthritis is the predominant clinical condition.

Invariably, the grip strength is significantly decreased compared with that of the normal hand,[60, 61] and the range of motion of the wrist may be somewhat reduced. The diagnosis is established through radiographs, particularly in the later stages of the disease, when the sclerotic appearance of the lunate is so characteristic. Early in the course of Kienböck's disease, the radiographs may actually be normal; however, magnetic resonance (MR) imaging can be valuable in making the diagnosis at an early stage (Fig. 18–1). Because of the varying appearance of the radiographs of a patient with Kienböck's disease, at least two classifications have been devised.[60, 61, 94] Figures 18–2 through 18–5 represent our classification system, which is useful for determining the extent of involvement and choosing appropriate treatment.

ETIOLOGY

The various names (lunatomalacia, aseptic necrosis, osteochondritis, traumatic osteoporosis, osteitis) used synonymously for Kienböck's disease are an indication that its exact etiology remains in dispute. Peste,[82] in 1843, first described collapse of the carpal lunate. His discovery, before the advent of radiography, was based on anatomic specimens. He believed the lesion to be a fracture with a traumatic etiology. Kienböck,[51, 52] in 1910, also thought this lesion to be the result of trauma. Kienböck believed that repeated sprains, contusions, or subluxations lead to ligamentous and vascular injury resulting in loss of blood supply to the lunate.[51, 52] Since then, numerous authorities have described the pathologic changes as avascular necrosis.[3, 6, 9, 13, 32, 33, 62–62, 71, 99]

In 1928, Hùlten[40] noted that a short ulna was present in 78 percent of his patients with Kienböck's disease, whereas only 23 percent of normals had a short ulna. He called this condition ulna minus vari-

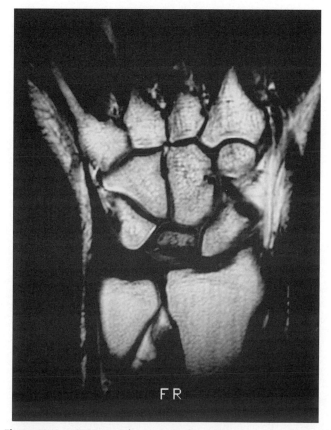

Figure 18–1. MR imaging demonstrates heterogenous decreased signal intensity in T_1-weighted image indicative of Kienböck's disease.

ant (Fig. 18–2). Since the condition was first discovered, many others have confirmed negative ulnar variance in their patients with Kienböck's disease.[9, 33, 34, 58, 60, 61, 64, 95, 110] Theoretically, a short ulna relative to the distal articular surface of the radius causes increased shear forces on the ulnar side of wrist and particularly on the lunate. This is thought to be a contributing factor in the development of avascular necrosis.

Other studies, however, have not found this strong correlation between ulnar variance and Kienböck's disease.[24, 57, 102] Nakamura and associates[72] noted that most Japanese patients with Kienböck's disease have neutral or positive ulnar variance. In one study, 33 percent of their patients with Kienböck's disease had positive ulnar variance. They also noted that there is no significant difference in the incidence of negative ulnar variance in Kienböck's patients and that of the general population in Japan, 25 percent compared with 27 percent, respectively.[74]

Gelberman and coworkers[34] described a method for establishing the degree of ulnar variance (Fig. 18–3). It consists of extending a line from the distal radial articular surface toward the ulna and measuring the distance between this line and the carpal surface of the ulna.

Palmer and associates[77] further standardized the method for determining ulnar variance. They found that the position of the distal ulna in relation to the distal radial surface changes with varying degrees of forearm rotation and that the change in variance was least with the elbow flexed 90°. The standard view recommended is a posteroanterior wrist radiograph obtained with the patient's shoulder abducted 90°,

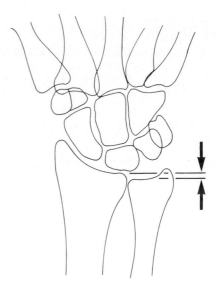

Figure 18–3. Measurement of ulnar variance. Ulnar variance may be determined by extending a line from the radius's articular surface ulnarward and measuring in millimeters the distance between this line and the carpal surface of the ulna. (After Gelberman RH, Salamon PB, Jurist JM, Posch JL: Ulnar variance in Kienböck's disease. J Bone Joint Surg 57A:674–676, 1975.)

the elbow flexed 90°, and the forearm in neutral rotation. They then utilized a template of concentric circles (similar to the one used in establishing sphericity in Legg-Perthes disease).[70] The concentric circle that best approximates the distal surface of the radius is selected as a reference and compared in millimeters with the carpal surface of the ulna. The importance of accurate measurement of ulnar variance is highlighted by the recent gain in popularity of ulnar lengthening and radial shortening techniques to treat Kienböck's disease.

Acute fracture or trauma as an etiology has been implicated in many series, as the majority of patients report a history of injury predating the exacerbation of symptoms.[9, 49, 58, 61, 94] Beckenbaugh and coworkers[8] found lines suggestive of fracture on radiographs of 82 percent of their patients. More and more investigators are documenting the presence of these fractures in Kienböck's disease, particularly with tomography; however, it remains unclear whether these fractures are the cause or the result of the avascular necrosis. Stahl[94] believed that in a lunate with an already tenuous blood supply, traumatic compression fractures lead to avascular necrosis. Lee[59] found three vascular patterns in lunates from cadavers: (1) a single, either volar or dorsal vessel supplying the entire bone; (2) several vessels at both volar and dorsal surfaces of the lunate without central anastomosis; and (3) several vessels at both volar and dorsal surfaces of the lunate with central anastomosis. Therefore, according to Lee,[59] patients with the first two patterns are at greater risk for developing Kienböck's disease. Injection studies by Panagis and coworkers[78] support this contention, as they found a single palmar nutrient vessel

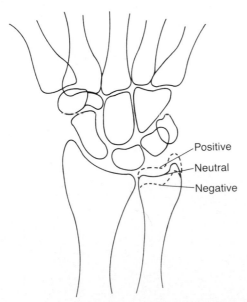

Figure 18–2. Schematic representation of the roentgenographic appearance of ulnar variance. *Neutral* variance occurs when the carpal surfaces of the radius and ulna are equal. If the ulna is "shorter" relative to the radius, *negative* ulnar variance exists; if the ulna is "longer" than the radius, the relationship is described as *positive* variance.

in 20 percent of fresh lunate specimens. Using fresh specimens, Gelberman and associates[33, 35] also studied the extraosseous and intraosseous blood supply of the lunate. They found the extraosseous supply to be extensive, with branches of the radial and anterior interosseous arteries forming a dorsal lunate plexus. Branches of the radial, ulnar, anterior interosseous, and recurrent deep palmar arch arteries form a volar plexus. In most specimens, vascularity reached the lunate through one or two foramina from the volar plexus and one or two foramina from the dorsal plexus. In only 7 percent of specimens was there only a volar contribution. These lunates with a single volar contribution theoretically would be at greatest risk for a single traumatic event (e.g., fracture or dislocation of the carpus) resulting in avascular necrosis. However, seldom is this history present in a patient with Kienböck's disease. Gelberman and coworkers[33] found that the intraosseous blood supply consisted of three patterns: Y in 59 percent of specimens, I in 31 percent, and X in 10 percent with the dorsal and volar anastomosis just distal to the center of the lunate (Fig. 18–4).

Evaluation of the terminal vessels in the lunate enabled Gelberman and coworkers[33] to conclude that the proximal subchondral bone, adjacent to the radial articular surface, was least vascular. Because of the rich extraosseous blood supply, these researchers discounted the theory held by some that interruption of vessels entering a single pole of the lunate caused avascularity. On the basis of this work, Gelberman and coworkers[33] suggest that it is intraosseous disruption of vascularity due to repeated trauma with compression fracture that causes Kienböck's disease.

Researchers have looked at other anatomic features for possible etiologic factors. Tsuge and Nakamura,[102] in a study comparing 41 Kienböck's wrists with 66 normal wrists, found that radial inclination tended to be flatter in patients with Kienböck's disease. Extrapolation of these results to explain the etiology of Kienböck's disease is risky. All of these specimens were from patients with normal lunates. The patient with Kienböck's disease may have an altogether different, yet compromised, vascular pattern, putting it at risk for avascular necrosis.

In a study that questions the current concept that Kienböck's disease is caused by arterial insufficiency,

Jensen[47] measured the intraosseous pressures in 10 patients with Kienböck's disease. Pressures in the lunate were found to be significantly higher than pressures in the radial styloid and capitate. These results suggest an interruption of the blood flow due to venous congestion, rather than arterial insufficiency, as the primary cause of avascular necrosis.

To summarize current thinking on the etiology of Kienböck's disease: Acute trauma or repeated minor trauma due to excessive shear force leads to interruption of the blood supply to the susceptible or "at-risk" lunate. Avascular necrosis results. The susceptible lunate is one that has a single nutrient vessel supplying the entire bone or a compromised intraosseous blood supply.

DIAGNOSIS

Kienböck's disease is an isolated disorder of the lunate diagnosed from characteristic radiographic density changes, often accompanied by fracture lines, fragmentation, and progressive collapse. It should be distinguished from other causes of wrist pain and swelling, particularly in the early stages, when the radiographs may be negative. Disorders to be ruled out include rheumatoid arthritis, post-traumatic arthritis, synovial-based inflammatory disease, acute fracture, carpal instability, and ulnar abutment syndromes. The radiographic hallmark of increased density typically seen in Kienböck's disease should be distinguished from transient vascular compromise. White and Omer[113] described this radiographic condition as seen following fracture-dislocation or dislocation of the carpus. In 3 of 24 patients sustaining this injury, there was a postinjury transient increase in lunate radiodensity that could have been confused with Kienböck's disease. This radiodensity lasted from 5 to 32 months, and it should be treated expectantly.

In more severe Kienböck's disease, as the lunate collapses, there is proximal migration of the capitate, widening of the proximal carpal row, and, frequently, rotation of the scaphoid, which causes it to appear foreshortened on anteroposterior (AP) radiographs. This foreshortening has been referred to as the "ring" sign (Fig. 18–5). Tomograms or computed tomography (CT) scans may be helpful to identify linear fractures or localized areas of sclerosis not readily apparent on plain radiographs. Scintigraphic imaging and MR imaging may be of benefit in patients who have otherwise negative radiographs.[5, 26, 43, 55, 75, 85] MR imaging has the distinct advantage of requiring no radiation and being more specific for effects of vascular changes. Low signal intensity on T1-weighted images is indicative of a vascular change. The severity of the disease can be further evaluated by the intensity of the T2-weighted signal.[43] Increased T2 signal or decreased signal with a high spot is believed to be indicative of revascularization and a good prognostic indicator.[43, 93] MR imaging is probably also helpful in following the outcome of surgical intervention such as radial shortening. Nakamura and associates[75]

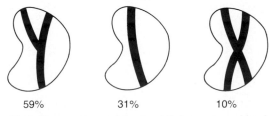

Figure 18–4. Three patterns of the lunate's intraosseous blood supply. (After Gelberman RH, Bauman TD, Menon J, Akeson WH: The vascularity of the lunate bone and Kienböck's disease. J Hand Surg 5:272–278, 1980.)

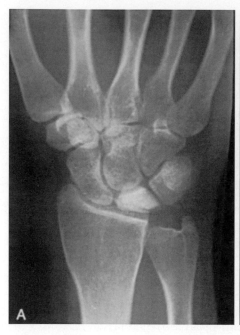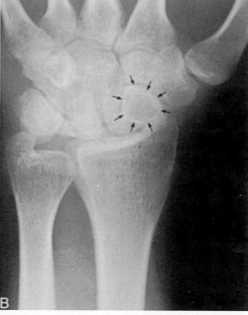

Figure 18–5. *A*, Anteroposterior view of early stage of Kienböck's disease demonstrating a normal relationship of the scaphoid to the remaining carpus. *B*, Late-stage Kienböck's disease, in which scaphoid rotation has led to a characteristic appearance referred to as the "ring sign" on an anteroposterior view.

looked at MR imaging changes after radial shortening. They found that both T1-weighted and T2-weighted signal increased within 1 year postoperatively. There was good correlation between increasing T1 signal and radiographic improvement in the appearance of the lunate. T2 signal increased earlier and appeared to be a more sensitive indicator of revascularization.

On rare occasions, Kienböck's disease has been reported in association with other conditions. There are case reports of Kienböck's disease in sickle cell disease,[58] carpal coalition,[63] and gout.[18] One article identified streptococcal infection in several cases and attempted to cite this organism as the causative factor.[83] Rooker and Goodfellow[87] found five cases of Kienböck's disease in a group of 53 adults with cerebral palsy. An abnormally flexed wrist posture was the common feature in all five cases. This finding suggested to the researchers that the extreme posture compromised the blood supply to the lunate. We have seen a few cases of bilateral Kienböck's disease and two cases of the disease associated with Madelung's deformity.

Once the diagnosis of Kienböck's disease is established, determination of the extent of involvement should be determined to use as a guide through the maze of treatment options. As an alternative to MR imaging, casting for 2 to 3 weeks in early cases usually brings out the diagnosis by demonstrating the relative disuse osteoporosis of the adjacent carpal bones.

STAGING

Stahl's[94] original classification, modified by Lichtman and coworkers,[60, 61] consists of four stages of Kienböck's disease as follows:

Stage I. Radiographs are normal except for the possibility of either a linear or compression fracture (Fig. 18–6). Scintigraphic imaging is positive because of a reactive synovitis, and MR imaging changes are diagnostic. Unless a compression fracture is visible, this stage is clinically indistinguishable from a wrist sprain.

Stage II. Definite density changes are apparent in the lunate relative to the other carpal bones; however, the size, shape, and anatomic relationship of the bones are not significantly altered. Fracture lines may be noted. Later in this stage, AP radiographs show loss of height on the radial side of the lunate (Fig. 18–7). Symptoms are recurrent pain, swelling, and tenderness in the wrist.

Acute

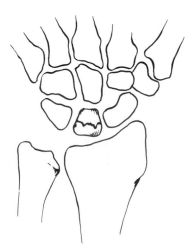

Figure 18–6. Schematic representation of the roentgenographic appearance of stage I Kienböck's disease. (From Lichtman DM, Alexander AH, Mack GR, Gunther SF: Kienböck's disease—update on silicone replacement arthroplasty. J Hand Surg 7:343–347, 1982.)

Density Changes

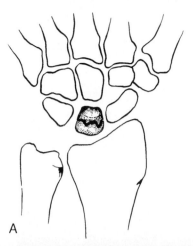

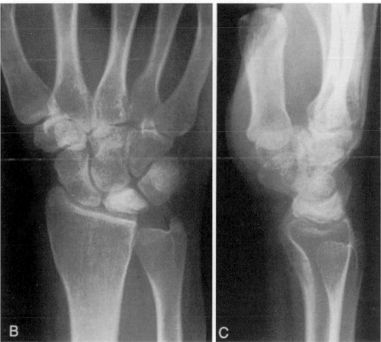

Figure 18–7. *A,* Schematic representation of the roentgenographic appearance of stage II Kienböck's disease. *B* and *C,* Anteroposterior and lateral views of a patient with stage II Kienböck's disease. Note the obvious density change and slight amount of collapse of the lunate on the radial border. The overall shape of the lunate, however, remains intact, and there is no proximal migration of the capitate. This patient also has negative ulnar variance. (From Lichtman DM, Alexander AH, Mack GR, Gunther SF: Kienböck's disease—update on silicone replacement arthroplasty. J Hand Surg 7:343–347, 1982.)

Stage III. The entire lunate has collapsed in the frontal plane and is elongated in the sagittal plane (Fig. 18–8). The capitate migrates proximally. Scapholunate dissociation, flexion of the scaphoid (ring sign), or ulnar migration of the triquetrum may be seen on AP radiographs.

To better assess the extent of collapse in stage III, it is helpful to establish the carpal height ratio.[116] *Carpal height* is the distance between the base of the third metacarpal and the distal radial articular surface (Fig. 18–9) as determined on a posteroanterior (PA) radiograph of the wrist. The *carpal height ratio* is the carpal height divided by the length of the third metacarpal. In normals, this ratio is 0.54 ± 0.03. Carpal height ratio is becoming more important, because the factors determining results of treatment in

stage III Kienböck's disease appear to be tied to the extent of collapse. We now divide stage III into stage IIIA (lunate collapse without fixed rotation of the scaphoid) and stage IIIB (lunate collapse with fixed scaphoid rotation and other secondary derangements). Clinically, patients with these disease stages have the same symptoms as those with stage II disease, but with greater wrist stiffness.

Stage IV. All findings characteristic of stage III are present as well as generalized degenerative changes in the carpus (Fig. 18–10).

TREATMENT

A great deal of controversy still exists regarding the appropriate treatment of Kienböck's disease. Current

Collapse of Lunate

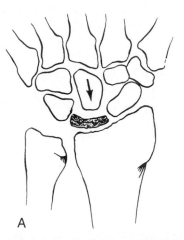

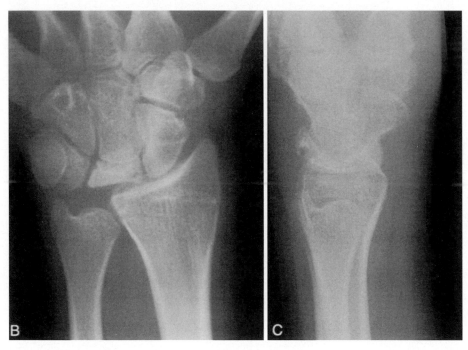

Figure 18–8. *A*, Schematic representation of the roentgenographic appearance of stage III Kienböck's disease. *B* and *C*, Anteroposterior and lateral views of a patient with stage III Kienböck's disease. The lunate is collapsed, the capitate displaced proximalward, and the scaphoid rotated, and there is negative ulnar variance. (*A* from Lichtman DM, Alexander AH, Mack GR, Gunther SF: Kienböck's disease—update on silicone replacement arthroplasty. J Hand Surg 7:343–347, 1982.)

treatment options include immobilization, lunate excision, revascularization, ulnar lengthening or radial shortening, radial wedge osteotomy (lateral closing), limited intercarpal fusion such as scaphocapitate or scaphotrapeziotrapezoid (STT) fusion, and salvage procedures. Silicone replacement arthroplasty was advocated for stage II and stage IIIA disease at one time[28, 96–98] but we no longer perform it because of particulate synovitis.[1, 7, 17, 79] Table 18–1 lists several of the many treatment options for Kienböck's disease, along with the stage for which we recommend the procedure.

Immobilization

Prolonged immobilization of the wrist has been tried in all stages of Kienböck's disease. Stahl[94] advocated

immobilization, yet in some series, this treatment has been shown to lead to continued collapse of the lunate or to otherwise unsatisfactory results owing to the need for prolonged treatment.[61, 88, 107] Lichtman and colleagues[61] reported on 22 patients with unstaged disease who were treated with cast or splint immobilization, of whom 17 had progressive collapse during immobilization and 19 had unsatisfactory results. For stage I disease, however, immobilization may be indicated to try to keep the vascular insult to a minimum and to give the lunate a chance to heal. Transient ischemia of the lunate, which is followed by spontaneous revascularization, may also give use to changes on MR imaging. Therefore, a trial of conservative treatment is indicated to differentiate transient ischemia from Kienböck's disease.

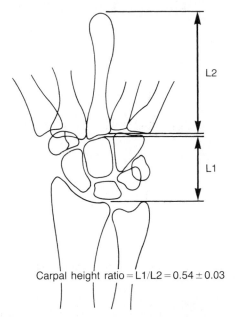

Carpal height ratio = L1/L2 = 0.54 ± 0.03

Figure 18–9. Carpal height ratio is defined as the carpal height *(L1)* divided by the length of the third metacarpal *(L2).* In normals, this ratio is 0.54 ± 0.03. (After Youm Y, McMurtry RY, Flatt AE, Posch JL: Ulnar variance in Kienböck's disease. J Bone Joint Surg 60A:423–431, 1978.)

Revascularization

In stage II Kienböck's disease, before the lunate has collapsed, it is possible for the lunate to regain blood supply without significant alteration of wrist anatomy. Braun[14] has described a method by which a small piece of volar radial bone, still attached to the pronator quadratus muscle, is grafted to the avascular lunate (Fig. 18–11) (RM Braun, MD, personal communications, July 1989). A similar revascularization procedure uses the pisiform. Pisiform transfer on its vascular pedicle was reported by Erbs and Böhm[30] in 32 patients. They found uniformly good results at 5-year follow-up. Presumably, most of these patients had stage II disease. Of the 14 patients with "advanced" Kienböck's disease, however, 50 percent became symptom free or had pain only under stressful conditions. Eckardt[27] reported on the same technique with

Table 18–1. AUTHORS' RECOMMENDED TREATMENTS FOR KIENBÖCK'S DISEASE

Treatment(s)	Stage of Disease
Immobilization	I
Revascularization	II with ulnar-positive variance
Radial wedge osteotomy	II, IIIA with ulnar-positive variance
Radial shortening	II, IIIA with ulnar neutral or with ulnar-negative variance
Scaphoid-trapezium-trapezoid or scaphocapitate fusion	IIIB
Salvage (proximal row carpectomy, wrist arthrodesis)	IV

good results in 2 patients with 4-year follow-up and stage I disease.

Direct transplantation of a vascular bundle into the avascular lunate was described by Hori and coworkers.[42] They had successful results in 8 of 9 patients. Uchida and Sugioka,[106] from their experimental studies, advocate direct transplantation of vessels rather than vascularized bone pedicles. In a rabbit model, they found that the bone grafts were gradually resorbed. In our own experimental study using amputated and transplanted rat femoral heads isolated with silicone, we found that blood supply could be restored with direct vessel transfer.[90] Because of the progressive postoperative decrease in vertical height of the lunate after revascularization, some surgeons have added the use of an external fixator and even combined revascularization with other unloading procedures, such as STT fusion.[114] Tamai and coworkers[100] reported 67 percent good results in 51 patients in all stages of Kienböck's disease treated with vascular bundle implantation with or without bone grafting. On the basis of their results, they advocate vascular bundle implantation alone in stage I and stage II; vascular bundle implantation, bone grafting (to reconstitute lunate height) and STT pinning in stage IIIA; and vascular bundle implantation, bone grafting, and STT fusion in stage IIIB disease.

Authors' Operative Technique for Revascularization

Expose the wrist capsule through a curvilinear dorsal approach between the second and third metacarpals and over the ulnar aspect of Lister's tubercle (Fig. 18–12). After splitting the extensor retinaculum between the second and third compartments, retract the extensor pollicis and wrist extensors radially and the extensor digitorum communis ulnarly. Next, create a proximally based rectangular capsular flap centered over the lunate. If necessary, use fluoroscopy and Kirschner (K) wires to localize the lunate. Dissect out the second intermetacarpal artery and vein as far distally as possible, and doubly ligate the bundle using 4-0 nylon suture. Leave the suture long and the needle in place on the proximal vessel, and cut between the ligatures with microscissors. Now, obtain a corticocancellous graft 1.0 × 0.5 cm from the dorsal aspect of the distal radius. Using a 0.045-inch K wire, drill a hole in the center of the graft. Make a window in the dorsal nonarticular portion of the lunate, and curette out the devascularized bone. Pass the needle from the 4–0 nylon suture tied to the vascular bundle through the hole in the 1.0 × 0.5 cm block, and tie the suture to pull the vascular bundle into the bone graft and secure it (Fig. 18–13). Place the bone block and bundle into the defect in the lunate, and pack cancellous bone graft from the radius around the block, taking care not to compress the bundle (Fig. 18–14). Deflate the tourniquet and observe the bundle for pulsation. If pulsation is not visible to the point of entry of the bundle into the lunate, relieve any

Pan Carpal Arthrosis

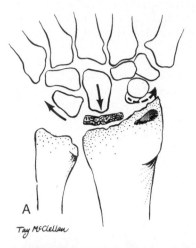

Tay McClellan

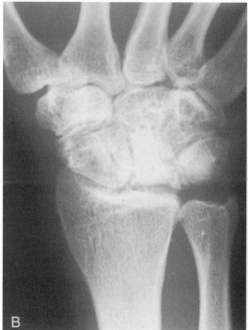

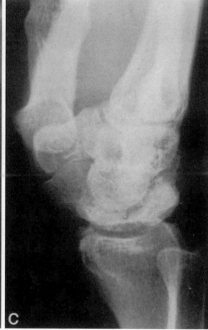

Figure 18–10. *A,* Schematic representation of the roentgenographic appearance of stage IV Kienböck's disease. *B* and *C,* Anteroposterior and lateral views of a patient with early stage IV Kienböck's disease. Note that besides the severe collapse of the lunate, there is sclerosis and osteophyte formation in the remaining carpus. (*A* from Lichtman DM, Alexander AH, Mack GR, Gunther SF: Kienböck's disease—update on silicone replacement arthroplasty. J Hand Surg 7:343–347, 1982.)

constriction—e.g., perform a Z lengthening of the extensor carpi radialis brevis (ECRB). After adequate hemostasis has been obtained, close the capsular flap, extensor retinaculum, and skin.

We occasionally use an external fixator for immobilization for 3 months. It is important not to distract through the fixator, as distraction can create a scapholunate dissociation because of preexisting compromise of the bony insertion of the scapholunate ligament.

Lunate Decompressive Procedures

Radial shortening and ulnar lengthening, STT and scaphocapitate (SC) fusions, capitate shortening, cap-

itohamate fusion, and, most recently, radial wedge osteotomy fall into the category of lunate decompressive procedures. The theoretical purpose of all of these procedures is to unload the lunate and allow it to revascularize. Numerous biomechanical studies using computerized models, strain-gauge testing, and pressure-sensitive film have been performed to better quantify the effects of the various unloading procedures.[42, 65, 92, 101, 109, 112] In a biomechanical study, Trumble and colleagues[101] demonstrated that both STT fusion and radial shortening decrease the load on the radiolunate joint, with 90 percent of the decrease in load occurring with 2 mm of shortening. Horii and associates[42] found that STT fusion decreased the load by only 5 percent. The difference in these two studies could be explained by the fact that Trumble's group

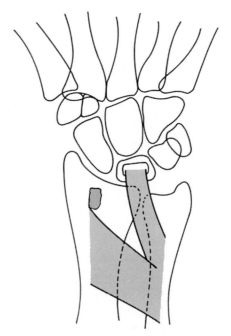

Figure 18–11. Pronator quadratus muscle pedicle revascularization procedure.

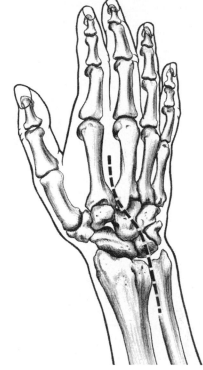

Figure 18–12. A dorsal curvilinear incision begins between the second and thrid metacarpals distally and extends 4 cm proximal to Lister's tubercle. (From Lichtman DM, Ross G: Revascularization of the lunate in Kienböck's disease. In Gelberman RH (ed): Master Techniques in Orthopaedic Surgery: The Wrist. New York, Raven Press, 1994, p 363.)

fused the scaphoid in extension, whereas Horii's group fused the scaphoid in flexion. Werner and Palmer[112] demonstrated that STT and SC fusions in neutral or extension redirect load entirely to the radioscaphoid fossa, whereas radial shortening and ulnar lengthening redirect load both medially and laterally.

ULNAR LENGTHENING AND RADIAL SHORTENING

On the basis of the assumption that ulnar minus variance is a causative factor in Kienböck's disease, many authorities have advocated equalization of the distal articular surfaces by either ulnar lengthening[6, 8, 39, 80, 81, 95] or radial shortening.* Good results have

*References 3, 16, 29, 39, 52–54, 62, 76, 88, 107.

been reported in both of these procedures. Almquist[4] reported good results in 11 of 12 of their own patients and in 69 of 79 patients in the literature regardless of stage. In 1990, Nakamura and associates[72] reported satisfactory results in 19 of 23 patients. However, patients with more than 4 mm of radial shortening and age greater than 30 years were more likely to have poor results. Weiss and coworkers[111] reported

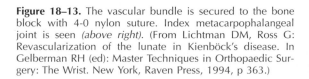

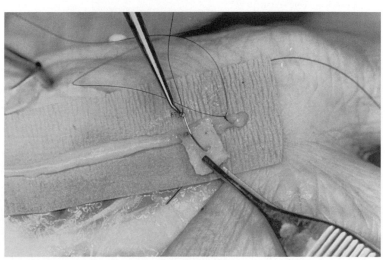

Figure 18–13. The vascular bundle is secured to the bone block with 4-0 nylon suture. Index metacarpophalangeal joint is seen *(above right)*. (From Lichtman DM, Ross G: Revascularization of the lunate in Kienböck's disease. In Gelberman RH (ed): Master Techniques in Orthopaedic Surgery: The Wrist. New York, Raven Press, 1994, p 363.)

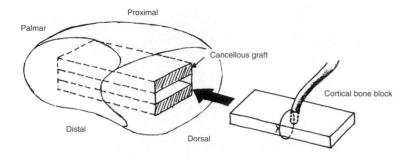

Figure 18–14. Placement of bone graft into the lunate. (Redrawn from Lichtman DM, Ross G: Revascularization of the lunate in Kienböck's disease. In Gelberman RH (ed): Master Techniques in Orthopaedic Surgery: The Wrist. New York, Raven Press, 1994, p 363.)

excellent results in 29 patients, including 4 patients with stage IIIB disease.

Even those authorities who do not consider negative ulnar variance a causative factor believe that good results from radial shortening are due to redistribution of load in the wrist.[24] Neither procedure, however, can restore an already collapsed lunate; therefore, these procedures remain questionable in advanced Kienböck's disease.

Both radial shortening and ulnar lengthening require osteotomy. After either, fixation is usually accomplished with a compression plate. It is generally recommended that the ulnar variance be changed to a 1-mm positive variance either with radial shortening or by placing an appropriately sized interpositional graft in ulnar lengthening. Sundberg and Linscheid[95] found ulnar lengthening to be successful in all but 1 of 19 patients followed for an average of 8.2 months. They reported no non-unions. Biomechanically, ulnar lengthening has essentially the same affect as radial shortening. Ulnar lengthening has the slight disadvantage of requiring a second surgical incision for a bone graft and theoretically a slightly higher risk of non-union. Ulnar lengthening or radial

shortening per se "burns no bridges," i.e., does not preclude further treatment in the event of failure.

Authors' Operative Technique for Radial Shortening

We prefer radial shortening with an oblique osteotomy using a 7- or 8-hole 3.5-mm direct compression (DC) plate with an interfragmentary screw through the plate. This method probably has less potential for non-union than a transverse osteotomy. Our method is performed as follows.

Use a standard volar approach to the distal radius. Prior to osteotomy of the radius, mark two parallel oblique lines for the proposed osteotomy on the radial aspect of the radius with a marking pen, electrocautery tip, or saw. Determine the amount of shortening to be performed by measuring the ulnar variance on a preoperative posteroanterior (PA) view of the wrist in neutral rotation and adding 1 mm (no more than 4 mm of shortening). Draw a line parallel to the longitudinal axis of the radius at the osteotomy site to prevent rotation. Contour the DC plate and secure it to the radius proximal to the proposed osteotomy.

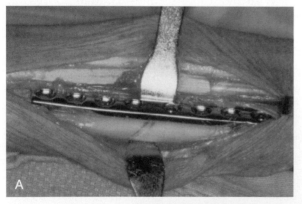

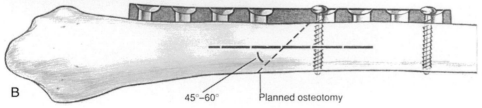

Figure 18–15. *A* and *B*, A seven- or eight-hole, 3.5-mm dynamic compression plate (DCP) is contoured and secured to the radius with two proximal screws prior to marking of the osteotomy on the radial border of the radius. Two parallel lines are drawn for the predetermined amount of shortening. (From Alexander CE, Alexander AH, Lichtman DM: Radial shortening in Kienböck's disease. In Gelberman RH (ed): Master Techniques in Orthopaedic Surgery: The Wrist. New York, Raven Press, 1994, p 373.)

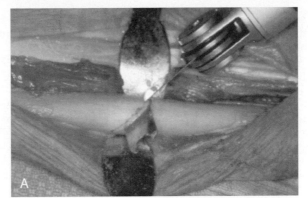

Figure 18–16. *A* and *B*, Parallel oblique osteotomies are performed using a microsagittal saw with a 9-mm blade. The first osteotomy is performed leaving the dorsal cortex intact, and a saw blade is left in the osteotomy to serve as an alignment guide for the second osteotomy. (From Alexander CE, Alexander AH, Lichtman DM. Radial shortening in Kienböck's disease. In Gelberman RH (ed): Master Techniques in Orthopaedic Surgery: The Wrist. New York, Raven Press, 1994, p 373.)

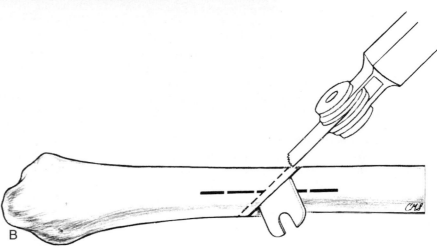

Drill, tap, and place the screws in the hole just adjacent to the osteotomy site and the most proximal screw hole prior to performing the osteotomy (Fig. 18–15). Then remove the plate and perform the osteotomy. Begin but do not complete the first oblique cut 45° to 60° to the longitudinal axis of the radius, leaving the dorsal radial cortex intact. Place a free saw blade in this osteotomy to use as a guide for making the second osteotomy parallel to the first (Fig. 18–16). After the second osteotomy is completed, finish the first one. Then reattach the plate to the proximal portion of the radius, and secure it distally to the radius with a bone clamp, with the radial osteotomy anatomically reduced. Next, drill the 3.5-mm gliding hole for a 3.5-mm interfragmentary screw. Then place a screw in compression just distal to the gliding hole on the plate. In some instances, it is necessary to place another screw in compression in order to obtain adequate compression. This must be done prior to drilling the dorsal cortex and securing

the interfragmentary screw. Place the second compression screw in the second hole on the proximal radius, opposite the first compression screw. Prior to tightening this screw loosen the other screws on the same side of the osteotomy one quarter turn to allow the plate to slide. Next, place the interfragmentary screw, and then insert alternating screws using standard AO technique (Fig. 18–17).

Immobilize the affected extremity in a short-arm cast for 8 weeks. Immobilization is used to "rest" the lunate rather than to protect the internal fixation.

RADIAL WEDGE OSTEOTOMY

The development of another decompressive procedure, radial wedge osteotomy, was prompted by the significant number of Kienböck's disease cases in the Japanese population with neutral or positive ulnar variance. Kojima and associates[56] and Tsumura and coworkers[103, 104] proposed lateral closing wedge oste-

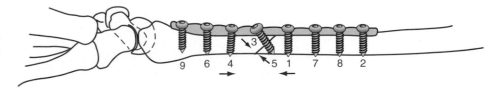

Figure 18–17. This diagram demonstrates the order in which the screws are applied.

otomy for Kienböck's disease. In their biomechanical studies, they demonstrated unloading of the lunate with decreasing radial inclination. In another experimental study, however, Werner and Palmer[112] found that medial closing and lateral opening wedge osteotomy decreased force at the radiolunate joint and that lateral closing wedge osteotomy actually increased force at the radiolunate joint.

Despite contradictory findings in experimental studies, Nakamura and colleagues[73] have reported satisfactory results in 25 of 27 patients with lateral closing wedge osteotomy with decreasing radial inclination by 5° to 15° using a step-cut osteotomy. Disadvantages of the procedure include technical difficulty and risk of decreasing forearm rotation. Twelve patients in their study had decreases in rotation of 10° to 35°.[73] These clinical results have been supported by the group's own biomechanical studies as well. Using a two-dimensional mathematical model, Watanabe and colleagues[109] reported that with an average osteotomy angle of 9.6° load was decreased by 23 percent at the lunocapitate joint, 10 percent at the radiolunate joint, and 36 percent at the ulnolunate joint. Nakamura also contends that the closing wedge osteotomy shifts the lunate radially, thereby increasing the total radiolunate contact area and decreasing the unit load.[105]

Clinical improvement after radial shortening or radial wedge osteotomy does not necessarily correlate with radiographic evidence of revascularization, such as increase in T1 or T2 signal on MR imaging or decreased sclerosis on standard radiographs. MR imaging does seem to be helpful in demonstrating evidence of revascularization postoperatively. Nakamura and associates[75] found increase in signal intensity postoperatively in all 19 of their patients treated with radial shortening or radial wedge osteotomy. Eight of the 9 patients who had normal or near-normal T1

signal intensity also had improvement in the radiographic appearance of the lunate.

INTERCARPAL FUSIONS

Limited Intercarpal Fusion

Graner and associates[38] described arthrodesis of the lunate to adjacent carpal bones for advanced Kienböck's disease—presumably stage III or stage IV. They considered it as appropriate treatment only if conventional methods failed to provide relief of symptoms. The most important advantage of arthrodesis is that some radiocarpal motion is maintained, unlike in complete wrist arthrodesis. In their series, 18 patients with an average of 22 months of follow-up underwent limited intercarpal arthrodesis; all had satisfactory results. Patients with severe fragmentation of the lunate undergo resection of the necrotic bone, osteotomy of the capitate in its midportion, and proximal displacement of the proximal capitate fragment (Fig. 18–18), which is secured to the scaphoid and triquetrum with bone pegs. Essentially, the space vacated by excision of the lunate is filled by the proximal half of the capitate, and the space left by osteotomy of the capitate is filled by autogenous bone graft. The procedure is then completed by arthrodesis of contiguous surfaces of the hamate, capitate, scaphoid, and triquetrum, by first denuding articular surfaces and securing the bones with small cortical bone pegs. When the lunate remains suitably intact, osteotomy of the capitate is omitted, as is lunate excision, and the contiguous surfaces of the lunate, scaphoid, triquetrum, hamate, and capitate undergo arthrodesis (Fig. 18–19).

Capitohamate Fusion

Chuinard and Zeman[20] advocated capitohamate fusion as a method of preventing proximal capitate

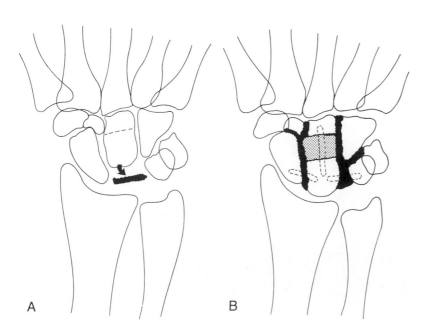

A   B

Figure 18–18. A and B, Limited intercarpal fusion in the presence of severe collapse and fragmentation of the lunate. The fragmented lunate is excised, the capitate osteotomized in its midportion, the proximal pole of the capitate displaced proximalward, and the gap in the capitate filled with bone graft. The contiguous surfaces of the capitate, scaphoid, triquetrum, and hamate are arthrodesed. (After Graner O, Lopes EI, Carrallo BC, Atlas S: Arthrodesis of the carpal bones in the treatment of Kienböck's disease, painful ununited fractures of the navicular and lunate bones with avascular necrosis, and old fracture dislocations of carpal bones. J Bone Joint Surg 48:767–774, 1966.)

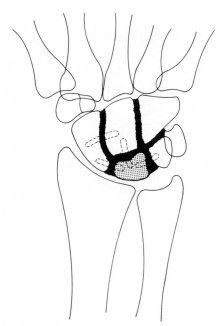

Figure 18–19. Limited intercarpal fusion in the face of a relatively intact lunate. Arthrodesis of the contiguous surfaces of the lunate, scaphoid, capitate, hamate, and triquetrum is done. When the lunate is intact, capitate osteotomy and excision of the lunate are omitted. (After Graner O, Lopes El, Carrallo BC, Atlas S: Arthrodesis of the carpal bones in the treatment of Kienböck's disease, painful ununited fractures of the navicular and lunate bones with avascular necrosis, and old fracture-dislocations of carpal bones. J Bone Joint Surg 48:767–774, 1966.)

migration in the presence of a collapsed lunate. Biomechanical studies have shown that capitohamate fusion is ineffective in changing the load on the lunate.[101] Trumble and colleagues[101] found no change in load using uniaxial strain gauges. Werner and Palmer[112] also demonstrated no alteration of load either on the ulnar aspect of the wrist on the radiocarpal joint. We do not currently recommend capitohamate fusion alone, because the hamate is already bound to the capitate by strong ligaments; furthermore, collapse of the capitate is accompanied by proximal migration of the entire distal carpal row (including the hamate) and widening of the proximal carpal row. Thus, it seems unlikely that capitohamate fusion alone can prevent proximal migration of the distal carpal row.

Triscaphe and Scaphocapitate Fusion

Watson and colleagues[110] described triscaphe arthrodesis with and without silicone replacement arthroplasty (SRA). Their patients underwent fusion of the scaphoid, trapezium, and trapezoid (STT fusion) and half underwent concomitant SRA. These researchers graphically demonstrate clenched-fist radiographs of a patient with SRA showing a 22 percent reduction (compression of the implant) in capitoradial space compared with the relaxed position. They suggested that triscaphe arthrodesis is capable of sup-

porting the remaining carpus either with a collapsed lunate or for SRA. Ten of 16 patients (average followup 20 months) had complete relief of symptoms, with 6 reporting aching in the affected wrist only after activity. Since the original report, the same group has reported a significant problem with radial styloid impingement, and they recommend radial styloidectomy in conjunction with STT arthrodesis.[86] Voche and associates[108] reported good pain relief in 16 patients with STT arthrodesis for Kienböck's disease, however, 9 patients developed postoperative radioscaphoid arthritis, either of the distal radial scaphoid or the proximal pole. This was attributed to either error in selection of patients (early stage IV) or error in technique (fusion in an extended position). All patients in their series had significant limitation of motion. Minami and associates[68] reported similar findings in 15 patients who underwent STT fusion combined with excision of the lunate and 57 months of followup. Five patients had progression of osteoarthritis postoperatively. These researchers concluded that STT fusion is best indicated for stage IIIB disease. STT fusion is a technically demanding procedure. The recommended angle for fusing the scaphoid is 45°, as more extension usually results in radioscaphoid arthritis. Drawbacks of STT fusion are the consequent restriction of motion, particularly radial deviation and the possibility of progressive degenerative arthritis.

Scaphocapitate (SC) fusion is biomechanically similar to STT arthrodesis in unloading the lunate and is technically somewhat simpler (Fig. 18–20). Limitation of motion is also a consequence of the procedure, as in STT arthrodesis, and one study noted a 12 percent non-union rate.[84]

We currently reserve STT or SC fusion as a treatment for stage IIIB disease in which the scaphoid is in marked flexion. In this instance, the treatment is directed more at correcting the carpal instability than decompressing an already collapsed lunate. A good STT or SC fusion will realign the scaphoid in its radial fossa and, it is hoped, prevent scapholunate advanced collapse (SLAC) wrist deformity (see Chapters 32 and 37).

Excision of the Lunate

Lunate excision was one of the first surgical procedures for Kienböck's disease. The rationale of this procedure is to remove sequestered bone that is provoking painful synovitis. Some have reported good results from simple excision.[19, 25, 37, 63] Others criticize the operation,[11, 63, 94] predicting late proximal migration of the capitate. There is at least one report of the same results with both excision and immobilization.[99] Nahigian and associates[71] combined simple excision with dorsal capsular flap arthroplasty to prevent migration of the capitate and reported good results in four patients. Schmitt and coworkers[91] described a similar technique of capsuloplasty using

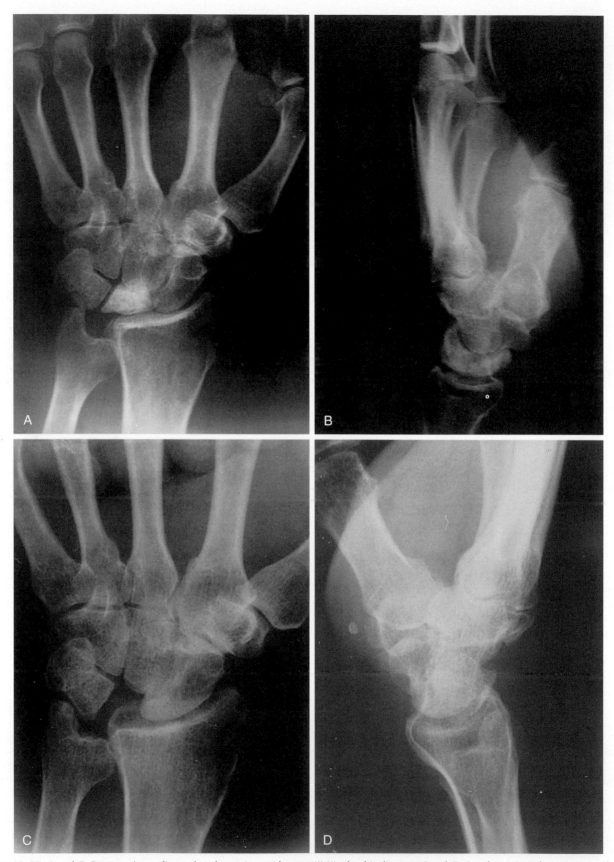

Figure 18–20. *A* and *B*, Preoperative radiographs of a patient with stage III Kienböck's disease. *C* and *D*, Scaphocapitate fusion was performed.

"epitendinous" tissue from the flexor tendons to fill the gap. They reported 80 percent satisfactory results in 42 cases. Another similar technique is excisional arthroplasty and replacement with a rolled tendon graft (palmaris longus tendon). This is performed much like the procedure of metacarpotrapezial joint arthroplasty described by Froimson.[31] Ishiguro[46] also reported on the use of autogenous tendon graft (generally the palmaris longus, the plantaris, or a portion of the flexor carpi radialis tendon) placed in the bed of the excised lunate. Twenty-four of the 26 patients with average follow-up of 2.5 years, were satisfied with their result. Using the criteria of Lichtman and associates,[61] Ishiguro[46] further noted that 6 of 10 patients with stage III and 11 of 16 patients with stage IV Kienböck's disease had satisfactory results. Kato and associates[50] originally treated patients with either silicone replacement arthroplasty or a "coiled palmaris longus tendon" and had disappointing results. They have since abandoned excisional arthroplasty as an isolated procedure as well as silicone replacement arthroplasty. In 1994, the same group reported on excisional arthroplasty combined with STT fusion with satisfactory results in 12 of 15 patients.[68]

Because in stage I and stage II Kienböck's disease, there still exists a chance for lunate revascularization, soft tissue (palmaris longus tendon) replacement arthroplasty with or without STT fusion is best reserved for stage III disease. We currently use soft tissue replacement arthroplasty as a salvage for a failed implant (particulate synovitis).

Salvage Procedures

For severe Kienböck's disease (stage IV), good results have been reported from proximal row carpectomy[10, 22, 45, 48] and wrist arthrodesis.[60, 61, 99] There is some controversy as to whether intact proximal capitate cartilage is a prerequisite to good results from proximal row carpectomy.[23, 24] Begley and Engber[9] noted that 10 of their 14 patients had partial-thickness articular cartilage degeneration on the proximal capitate, which did not preclude a satisfactory result. Patients who develop further degenerative changes can still have a good result from radiocarpal fusion.[23] As noted previously, limited intercarpal arthrodesis using the method of Graner and associates[38] is another option. Denervation of the wrist joint has been described by several authorities to be successful in relieving pain without impairing function or mobility.[15, 36, 89, 114] For details on proximal row carpectomy, see Chapter 34. Techniques of wrist arthrodesis are discussed in Chapter 38.

PITFALLS AND COMPLICATIONS OF TREATMENT

Because of the varied treatments advocated for Kienböck's disease, it is apparent that no single treatment stands out as the best. Choice of treatment must be predicated on the experience of the surgeon, the desires, activity level, and goals of the patient, and the stage of the disease. Finally, consideration of the risks involved with each treatment, including pitfalls and complications, may help one to select the optimal treatment for an individual patient.

Silicone replacement arthroplasty, once a widely accepted procedure, has been abandoned owing to deterioration of results with time[1] and the development of particulate arthritis. Revascularization procedures show promising results in stage I and stage II disease and have been used in stage III disease in conjunction with bone grafting.[12] However, because of the prolonged structural instability of the lunate during the revascularization process, ongoing carpal collapse cannot be prevented. Although carpal height and lunate height can be restored with bone grafting and application of an external fixator, carpal height diminishes rapidly after the external fixator is removed.[12] Bochud and Büchler[12] noted maximum collapse at 6 to 9 months. Yajima and colleagues[115] have advocated STT fusion in stage IIIB disease and STT pinning in stage IIIA disease in conjunction with revascularization to avoid this collapse.

Radial shortening and ulnar lengthening are relatively simple procedures that have yielded good results in stage II and stage III disease. Although some authorities have reported good results in stage IIIB disease,[72, 111] radial shortening and ulnar lengthening are probably more effective in stage IIIA disease, because carpal instability is uncorrected. Condit and colleagues[21] found no good or excellent results with radial shortening if the radioscaphoid angle was greater than 60°.

Radial shortening and ulnar lengthening are not without inherent risks. With both procedures, nonunion is possible. A second operation may be required for plate removal, particularly after ulnar lengthening because of the more subcutaneous location of the plate. Care must be taken not to overlengthen the ulna or overshorten the radius. The surgeon should aim for no more than a 1+ ulnar variance to prevent ulnocarpal abutment. For the same reason, ulnar deviation may also be restricted by these procedures. Their application in patients with neutral and positive ulnar variance is not advised, though good results have been reported even in these patients.[39, 72] Radial wedge osteotomy should be considered as an alternative.

Both STT and scaphocapitate (SC) arthrodesis unload the lunate but create a significant decrease in range of motion and may result in progressive arthrosis secondary to load transfer exclusively to the radioscaphoid joint. STT arthrodesis in Condit and colleagues'[21] series resulted in a significant number of wrist arthrodeses. However, they judged that STT intercarpal arthrodesis may be indicated in stage IIIB disease with ulnar-positive variance. We concur and perform STT or SC arthrodesis exclusively in stage IIIB disease regardless of variance.

AUTHORS' PREFERRED METHOD OF TREATMENT (see Table 18–1)

Stage I Disease. Until the diagnosis is established with certainty, we prefer immobilization. Transient ischemia can imitate stage I Kienböck's disease clinically and on MR imaging. If the patient's symptoms are unimproved after 3 to 6 months or progression to stage II disease is noted, revascularization with ulnar-positive variance or radial shortening in neutral or negative variance is performed.

Stage II and IIIA Disease. Radial shortening is the procedure of choice in patients with negative or neutral ulnar variance. Our goal is to achieve 1 mm of ulnar-positive variance after osteotomy. If the patient has positive ulnar variance, revascularization using direct implantation of the second dorsal metacarpal artery and vein is performed with concomitant external fixation. As an alternative, lateral closing wedge osteomy may be considered.

Stage IIIB Disease. To stabilize the carpus, we recommend scaphocapitate or STT fusion for stage IIIB Kienböck's disease. If significant synovitis is present, we excise the lunate and interpose an autogenous palmaris longus tendon graft. Radial shortening may be a viable alternative in patients with early stage IIIB disease. If the patient has no improvement with radial shortening, STT arthrodesis and lunate excision can still be performed.

Stage IV Disease. In stage IV, we are no longer treating Kienböck's disease per se. The patient clinically and radiographically has degenerative wrist disease. Depending on the patient's desires and the condition of the proximal capitate and radial articulation, proximal row carpectomy or wrist arthrodesis is our treatment of choice.

SUMMARY

Kienböck's disease is an isolated disorder of the lunate resulting from vascular compromise exacerbated or initiated by excessive load on the bone. The symptoms include wrist pain, limited range of motion, and decreased grip strength. The diagnosis is made from characteristic changes seen in the lunate on radiographs of the wrist. The severity of the disease can be categorized by staging the extent of involvement. This is helpful in guiding the practitioner through the maze of treatment options. The treatment of Kienböck's disease begins with conservative measures such as immobilization and analgesics or anti-inflammatory medication. If symptoms are not relieved, the degree of involvement determines which of several surgical options exist to choose for a successful result.

References

1. Alexander AH, Turner MA, Alexander CE, Lichtman DM: Lunate silicone replacement arthroplasty in Kienböck's disease—a long term followup. J Hand Surg 15A:401–407, 1990.
2. Alexander AH, Lichtman DM: The Kienböck's dilemma—how to cope. In Nakamura R, Linscheid RL, Miura T (eds): Wrist Disorders: Current Concepts and Challenges. Tokyo, Springer-Verlag, 1992, pp 79–87.
3. Almquist EE, Burns JF: Radial shortening for the treatment of Kienböck's disease—a 5- to 10-year follow-up. J Hand Surg 7:348–352, 1982.
4. Almquist EE: Kienböck's disease. Hand Clin 3:141–148, 1987.
5. Amadio PC, Hanssen AD, Berquist TH: The genesis of Kienböck's disease: Evaluation of a case by magnetic resonance imaging. J Hand Surg 12A:1044–1049, 1987.
6. Armistead RB, Linscheid RL, Dobyns JH, Beckenbaugh RD: Ulnar lengthening in the treatment of Kienböck's disease. J Bone Joint Surg 6rA:170–178, 1982.
7. Atkinson RE, Smith RJ, Jupiter JB: Silicone synovitis of the wrist. Presented at the 40th Annual Meeting of the American Society for Surgery of the Hand, Las Vegas, Jan 1985.
8. Axelsson R: Niveauoperationen bei mondbeinnekrose. Handchirurgie 5:187–196, 1973.
9. Beckenbaugh RD, Shives TC, Dobyns JH, Linscheid RL: Kienböck's disease: The natural history of Kienböck's disease and consideration of lunate fractures. Clin Orthop 149:98–106, 1980.
10. Begley BW, Engber WD: Proximal row carpectomy in advanced Kienböck's disease. J Hand Surg 19A:1016–1018, 1994.
11. Blaine ES: Lunate osteomalacia. JAMA 96:492, 1931.
12. Bochud RC, Büchler U: Kienböck's disease, early stage III—height reconstrucution and core revascularization of the lunate. J Hand Surg 19B:466–478, 1994.
13. Bolhofner B, Belsole RJ: Kienböck's disease: Current concepts in diagnosis and management. Contemp Orthop 3:713–720, 1981.
14. Braun R: The pronator pedicle bone grafting in the forearm and proximal carpal row. Presented at the 38th Annual Meeting of the American Society for Surgery of the Hand, March 1983.
15. Buck-Gramcko D: Denervation of the wrist joint. J Hand Surg 2:54–61, 1977.
16. Calandriello B, Palandri C: Die behandlung der lunatum malazie durch speichenverkurzung. Z Orthop 101:531–534, 1966.
17. Carter PR, Benton LJ: Late osseous complications of carpal Silastic implants. Presented at the 40th Annual Meeting of the American Society for Surgery of the Hand, Las Vegas, Jan 1985.
18. Castagnoli M, Giacomello A, Argentina RS, Zoppini A: Kienböck's disease in gout. Arthritis Rheum 24:974–975, 1981.
19. Cave EF: Kienböck's disease of the lunate. J Bone Joint Surg 21:858–866, 1939.
20. Chuinard RG, Zeman SC: Kienböck's disease: An analysis and rationale for treatment by capitate-hamate fusion. Orthop Trans 4:18, 1980.
21. Condit DP, Idler RS, Fischer TJ, et al: Preoperative factors and outcome after lunate decompression for Kienböck's disease. J Hand Surg 18A:691–696, 1993.
22. Crabbe WA: Excision of the proximal row of the carpus. J Bone Joint Surg 46B:708–711, 1964.
23. Culp RW, McGuigan FX, Turner MA, et al: Proximal row carpectomy: A multicenter study. J Hand Surg 18A:19–25, 1993.
24. D'Hoore K, De Smet L, Verellen K, et al: Negative ulnar variance is not a risk factor for Kienböck's disease. J Hand Surg 19A:229–231, 1994.
25. Dornan A: The results of treatment in Kienböck's disease. J Bone Joint Surg 31B:518–520, 1949.
26. Duong RB, Nishiyama H, Mantil JC, et al: Kienböck's disease: Scintigraphic demonstration in correlation with clinical, radiographic, and pathologic findings. Clin Nucl Med 7:418–420, 1982.
27. Eckardt K: Spätergebnisse nach pisiforme-verpflanzung bei lunatum-malazie. Handchirurgie 16:90–92, 1984.

28. Eiken O, Necking LE: Lunate implant arthroplasty, evaluation of 19 patients. Scand J Plast Reconstr Surg 18:247–252, 1984.

29. Eiken O, Niechajev I: Radius shortening in malacia of the lunate. Scand J Plast Reconstr Surg 14:191–196, 1980.

30. Erbs G, Böhm E: Langzeitergebnisse der os pisiforme-verlagerung bei mondbeinnekrose. Handchirurgie 16:85–89, 1984.

31. Froimson AI: Tendon arthroplasty of the trapeziometacarpal joint. Clin Orthop 70:191–199, 1970.

32. Fu FH, Imbriglia JF: An anatomical study of the lunate bone in Kienböck's disease. Orthopedics 8:483–487, 1985.

33. Gelberman RH, Bauman TD, Menon J, Akeson WH: The vascularity of the lunate bone and Kienböck's disease. J Hand Surg 5:272–278, 1980.

34. Gelberman RH, Salamon PB, Jurist JM, Posch JL: Ulnar variance in Kienböck's disease. J Bone Joint Surg 57A:674–676, 1975.

35. Gelberman RH, Szabo RM: Kienböck's disease. Orthop Clin North Am 15:355–367, 1984.

36. Geldmacher J, Legal HR, Brug E: Results of denervation of the wrist and wrist joint by Wilhelm method. Hand 4:57, 1972.

37. Gillespie HS: Excision of the lunate bone in Kienböck's disease. J Bone Joint Surg 43B:245–249, 1961.

38. Graner O, Lopes EI, Carvalho BC, Atlas S: Arthrodesis of the carpal bones in the treatment of Kienböck's disease, painful ununited fractures of the navicular and lunate bones with avascular necrosis, and old fracture-dislocations of carpal bones. J Bone Joint Surg 48B:767–774, 1966.

39. Grassi G, Santoro D, Coli G, Cianciulli M: The surgical treatment of Kienböck's disease. Ital J Orthop Traumatol 4:149–154, 1978.

40. Hülten O: Uber anatomische variationen der handgelenkknochen. Acta Radiol Scand 9:155, 1928.

41. Hori Y, Tamai S, Okuda H, et al: Blood vessel transplantation to bone. J Hand Surg 4:23–33, 1979.

42. Horii E, Garcia-Elias M, Cooney WP, et al: Effect on force transmission across the carpus in procedures used to treat Kienböck's disaese. J Hand Surg 15A:393–400, 1990.

43. Imaeda T, Nakamura R, Miura T, et al: Magnetic resonance imaging on Kienböck's disease. J Hand Surg 17B:12–19, 1992.

44. Imbriglia JE, Broudy AS, Hagberg WC, et al: Proximal row carpectomy: Clinical evaluation. J Hand Surg 15A:426–430, 1990.

45. Inglis AE, Jones EC: Proximal-row carpectomy for diseases of the proximal row. J Bone Joint Surg 59A:460–463, 1977.

46. Ishiguro T: Experimental and clinical studies of Kienböck's disease—excision of the lunate followed by packing of the free tendon. J Jpn Orthop Ass 58:509–522, 1984.

47. Jensen CH: Intraosseous pressure in Kienböck's disease. J Hand Surg 18A:355–359, 1993.

48. Jorgensen EC: Proximal-row carpectomy: An end result study of 22 cases. J Bone Joint Surg 51A:1104–1111, 1969.

49. Kashiwagi D, Fukiwara A, Inoue T, et al: An experimental and clinical study on lunatomalacia. Orthop Trans 1:7, 1977.

50. Kato H, Usui M, Minami A: Long-term result of Kienböck's disease treated by excisional arthroplasty with a silicone implant or coiled palmaris longus tendon. J Hand Surg 11A:645–653, 1986.

51. Kienböck R: Concerning traumatic malacia of the lunate and its consequences: Degeneration and compression fractures. Clin Orthop 149:4–8, 1980.

52. Kienböck R: Uber traumatische Malazie des Mondbeins und ihre Folgezustande: Entartungsformen und Kompressionsfrakturen. Fortsch Roentgenstrahlen 16:78–103, 1910.

53. Kinnard P, Tricoire JL, Basora J: Radial shortening for Kienböck's disease. Can J Surg 3:261–262, 1983.

54. Kleven H: The treatment of lunatomalacia. Tidsskr Nor Laegeforen 91:1944–1946, 1971.

55. Koenig H, Lucas D, Meissner R: The wrist: A preliminary report on high-resolution MR imaging. Radiology 160:463–467, 1986.

56. Kojima T, Kido M, Tsura H, et al: Wedge osteotomy of radius for Kienböck's disease. J Jpn Soc Surg Hand 1:431–434, 1984.

57. Kristensen S, Thomassen E, Christensen F: Ulnar variance and Kienböck's disease. J Hand Surg 11B:255–260, 1986.

58. Lanzer W, Szabo R, Gelberman R: Avascular necrosis of the lunate and sickle cell anemia. Clin Orthop 187:168–171, 1984.

59. Lee M: The intraosseous arterial pattern of the carpal lunate bone and its relation to avascular necrosis. Acta Orthop Scand 33:43–55, 1963.

60. Lichtman DM, Alexander AH, Mack GR, Gunther SF: Kienböck's disease—update on silicone replacement arthroplasty. J Hand Surg 7:343–347, 1982.

61. Lichtman DM, Mack GR, MacDonald RI, et al: Kienböck's disease: The role of silicone replacement arthroplasty. J Bone Joint Surg 59A:899–908, 1977.

62. Lin E, Engel J, Marganitt B: Surgery in Kienböck's disease. Orthop Rev 12:51–57, 1983.

63. Macnicol MF: Kienböck's disease in association with carpal coalition. Hand 14:185–187, 1982.

64. Marek RM: Avascular necrosis of the carpal lunate. Clin Orthop 10:96–107, 1957.

65. Masear VR, Zook EG, Pichora DR, et al: Strain-gauge evaluation of lunate unloading procedures. J Hand Surg 17A:437–443, 1992.

66. Matsushita K, Firrell JC, Tsai T: X-ray evaluation of radial shortening for Kienböck's disease. J Hand Surg 17A:450–455, 1992.

67. McMurtry RY, Youm Y, Flatt AE, Gillespie TE: Kinematics of the wrist. II: Clinical applications. J Bone Joint Surg 60A:955–961, 1978.

68. Minami A, Kimura T, Suzuki K: Long term results of Kienböck's disease treated by triscaphe arthrodesis and excisional arthroplasty with a coiled palmaris longus tendon. J Hand Surg 19A:219–228, 1994.

69. Morgan RF, McCue FC III: Bilateral Kienböck's disease. J Hand Surg 8:928–932, 1983.

70. Mose K: Methods of measuring in Legg-Calvé-Perthes disease with special regard to prognosis. Clin Orthop 150:103–109, 1980.

71. Nahigian SH, Li CS, Richey DG, Shaw DT: The dorsal flap arthroplasty in the treatment of Kienböck's disease. J Bone Joint Surg 52A:245–251, 1970.

72. Nakamura R, Imaeda T, Miura T: Radial shortening for Kienböck's disease: Factors affecting the operative result. J Hand Surg 15B:40–45, 1990.

73. Nakamura R, Tsuge S, Watanabe K, et al: Radial wedge osteotomy for Kienböck's disease. J Bone Joint Surg (Am) 73:1391–1396, 1991.

74. Nakamura R, Tsuge S, Watanabe K, et al: Kienböck's disease and ulnar variance. In Nakamura R, Linscheid RL, Miura T (eds): Wrist Disorders: Current Concepts and Challenges. Tokyo, Springer-Verlag, 1992, pp 89–93.

75. Nakamura R, Watanabe K, Tsunoda K, et al: Radial osteotomy for Kienböck's disease evaluated by magnetic resonance imaging: 24 cases followed for 1–3 years. Acta Orthop Scand 64:207–211, 1993.

76. Ovesen J: Shortening of the radius in the treatment of lunatomalacia. J Bone Joint Surg 63B:231–235, 1981.

77. Palmer AK, Glisson RR, Werner FW: Ulnar variance determination. J Hand Surg 7:376–379, 1982.

78. Panagis JS, Gelberman RH, Taleisnik J, Baumgaertner M: The arterial anatomy of the human carpus. Part II: The intraosseous vascularity. J Hand Surg 8:375–382, 1983.

79. Peimer CA, Medige J, Ecker BS, et al: Reactive synovitis after arthroplasty. J Hand Surg 11A:624–638, 1986.

80. Persson M: Causal treatment of lunatomalacia: Further experiences of operative ulna lengthening. Acta Chir Scand 100:531–544, 1950.

81. Persson M: Pathogenese und behandlund der Kienböckschen lunatummalazie: der frakturtheorie im lichte der erfolge operativer radiusverkurzung (Hulte'n) und einer neuen operationsmethode-ulnaverlangerung. Acta Chir Scand Suppl 98, 1945.

82. Peste: [Discussion]. Bull Soc anat Paris 18:169–170, 1843.

83. Phemister DB, Day L: Streptococcal infections of the epiphyses and short bones, their relation to Kohler's disease of the tarsal navicular, Legg-Perthes' disease and Kienböck's disease of the os lunatum. JAMA 95:995–1002, 1930.

84. Pisano SM, Peimer CA, Wheeler DR, et al: Scaphocapitate intercarpal arthrodesis. J Hand Surg 16A:328–333, 1991.

85. Reinus WR, Conway WF, Totty WG, et al: Carpal avascular necrosis: MR imaging. Radiology 160:689–693, 1986.

86. Rogers WD, Watson HK: Radial styloid impingement after triscaphe arthrodesis. J Hand Surg 14A:297–301, 1989.

87. Rooker GD, Goodfellow JW: Kienböck's disease in cerebral palsy. J Bone Joint Surg 59B:363–365, 1977.

88. Rosemeyer B, Artmann M, Viernstein K: Lunatummalacie nachuntersuchungsergebnisse und therapeutische erwagungne. Arch Orthop Unfallchir 85:119–127, 1976.

89. Rostlund T, Somnier F, Axelsson R: Denervation of the wrist joint—an alternative in conditions of chronic pain. Orthop Scand 51:609–616, 1980.

90. Saldana MJ, Niebauer JJ, Brown R, et al: Microsurgical revascularization of ischemic rat femoral heads. J Hand Surg 15A:309–315, 1990.

91. Schmitt E, Hassinger M, Mittelmeier H: Die lunatummalazie und ihre behandlung mit lunatumexstirpation. Z Orthop 122:643–650, 1984.

92. Short WH, Werner FW, Fortino MD, et al: Distribution of pressures and forces on the wrist after simulated intercarpal fusion and Kienböck's disease. J Hand Surg 17A:443–449, 1992.

93. Sowa DT, Holder LE, Patt PG, et al: Application of magnetic resonance imaging to ischemic necrosis of the lunate. J Hand Surg 14A:1008–1016, 1989.

94. Stahl F: On lunatomalacia (Kienböck's disease), a clinical and roentgenological study, especially on its pathogenesis and the late results of immobilization treatment. Acta Chir Scand [Suppl] 126:1–133, 1947.

95. Sundberg SB, Linscheid RL: Kienböck's disease—results of treatment with ulnar lengthening. Clin Orthop 187:43–51, 1984.

96. Swanson AB, Wilson KM, Mayhew DE, et al: Long-term bone response around carpal bone implants. Presented at the 40th Annual Meeting of the American Society for Surgery of the Hand, Las Vegas, Jan 1985.

97. Swanson AB: Flexible Implant Resection Arthroplasty in the Hand and Extremities. St Louis, CV Mosby, 1973.

98. Swanson AB: Silicone rubber implants for the replacement of the carpal scaphoid and lunate bones. Orthop Clin North Am 1:299–309, 1970.

99. Tajima T: An investigation of the treatment of Kienböck's disease. J Bone Joint Surg 48A:1649–1655, 1966.

100. Tamai S, Yajima H, Ono H: Revascularization procedures in the treatment of Kienböck's disease. Hand Clin 9:455–466, 1993.

101. Trumble TE, Glisson RR, Seaber AV, et al: A biomechanical comparison of the methods for treating Kienböck's disease. J Hand Surg 11A:88–93, 1986.

102. Tsuge S, Nakamura R: Anatomical risk factors for Kienböck's disease. J Hand Surg 18B:70–75, 1993.

103. Tsumura H, Himeno S, An KN, et al: Biomechanical analysis of Kienböck's disease. Orthop Trans 11:327, 1987.

104. Tsumura H, Himeno S, Morita H, et al: The optimum correcting angle of wedge osteotomy at the distal end of the radius for Kienböck's disease. J Jpn Soc Surg Hand 1:435–439, 1987.

105. Tsunoda K, Nakamura R, Watanabe K, et al: Changes in carpal alignment following radial osteotomy for Kienböck's disease. J Hand Surg 18B:289–293, 1993.

106. Uchida Y, Sugioka Y: Effects of vascularized bone graft on surrounding necrotic bone: An experimental study. J Reconstr Microsurg 6:101–107, 1990.

107. Viernstein K, Weigert M: Die radiusverkurzungsosteotomie bei der lunatummalzie. Munch Med Wochenschr 109:1992, 1967.

108. Voche P, Bour C, Merle M: Scapho-trapezio-trapezoid arthrodesis in the treatment of Kienböck's disease. J Hand Surg 17B:5–11, 1992.

109. Watanabe K, Nakamura R, Horii E, et al: Biomechanical analysis of radial wedge osteotomy for the treatment of Kienböck's disease. J Hand Surg 18A:686–690, 1993.

110. Watson HK, Ryu J, Dibella A: An approach to Kienböck's disease: Triscaphe arthrodesis. J Hand Surg 10A:179–187, 1985.

111. Weiss AP, Weiland AJ, Moore R, et al: Radial shortening for Kienböck's disease. J Bone Joint Surg (Am) 73:384–391, 1991.

112. Werner FW, Palmer AK: Biomechanical evaluation of operative procedures to treat Kienböck's disease. Hand Clin 9:431–443, 1993.

113. White RE, Omer GE: Transient vascular compromise of the lunate after fracture-dislocation or dislocation of the carpus. J Hand Surg 9A:181–184, 1984.

114. Wilhelm A: Die gelenkdenervation und ihre anatomischen grundlagen: Ein neues behandlungsprinzip in der handchirurgie. Hefte Unfallheilkd 86:1–109, 1966.

115. Yajima H, Tamai S, Mizumoto S, et al: Treatment of Kienböck's disease with vascular bundle implantation and triscaphe arthrodesis. In Nakamura R, Linscheid RL, Miura T (eds): Wrist Disorders, Current Concepts and Challenges, Tokyo, Springer-Verlag, 1992, pp 101–118.

116. Youm Y, McMurtry RY, Flatt AE, Gillepsie TE: Kinematics of the wrist. Part I: An experimental study of radial-ulnar deviation and flexion-extension. J Bone Joint Surg 60A:423–431, 1978.

PART IV
Distal Radius and Ulna

CHAPTER 19

Fractures of the Distal Radius

Michael E. Rettig, MD, Keith B. Raskin, MD, and
Charles P. Melone, Jr, MD

Fractures of the distal radius constitute one of the most common skeletal injuries treated by orthopedic surgeons. These injuries account for one sixth of all fractures evaluated in emergency rooms and have often been considered primarily stable extra-articular fractures in the elderly. However, increasing experience has revealed that the vast majority of distal radius fractures are articular injuries that result in disruption of both the radiocarpal and distal radioulnar joints. Better understanding of the spectrum of distal radial fractures has led to changing concepts of treatment. Prominent among the concepts is that optimal management of distal radial fractures requires differentiation of the relatively low-energy metaphyseal injuries, traditionally termed Colles' fractures, from the more violent injuries that disrupt the articular surfaces. The articular injuries are more frequently comminuted and unstable, and therefore less suitable for more traditional methods of closed reduction and cast immobilization. Without supplemental skeletal fixation, re-displacement of the fracture—commonly to its pre-reduction position—is inevitable. Resultant malunion then predictably leads to pain, limited range of motion, weakness, and post-traumatic arthritis.

The optimal method of obtaining and maintaining an accurate restoration of distal radial anatomy remains a topic of considerable controversy. A wide array of techniques, including closed, percutaneous, and open methods of reduction and stabilization, have been increasingly advocated as successful treatment. Although these methods have been eloquently described, the fracture per se is less commonly defined with precision. It must be recognized that articular fractures constitute a diverse spectrum of injuries for which optimal management requires differing methods of treatment. Employment of a single technique for dissimilar injuries predictably yields a variable and often disappointing quality of recovery.

Much of the confusion can be eliminated by recognition of specific, key fracture characteristics: (1) consistent patterns of articular fracture anatomy, (2) articular fracture stability, and (3) articular fracture reducibility. With prompt detection of these features, an accurate diagnosis can be established, and a ratio-

nal plan of management based on precise fracture configurations can be formulated for the vast majority of distal radius injuries.

CLASSIFICATION

The classifications commonly employed for distal radius fractures reflect the extent of articular surface involvement (Table 19–1). Persistent distortion of articular contours is the major factor predisposing to an unfavorable outcome. In their evaluation of healed fractures, Gartland and Werley[22] observed that 88 percent of the fractures involved the articular surface. Moreover, these researchers emphasized that residual displacement consistently led to an unsatisfactory result. All Colles' fractures were not equivalent; some were extra-articular and others were intra-articular. Gartland and Werley[22] concluded that closed reduc-

Table 19–1. CLASSIFICATIONS OF DISTAL RADIUS FRACTURES

Reference	Type	Fracture
Gartland and Werley (1951)[22]	I	Extra-articular
	II*	Articular—undisplaced radiocarpal joint
	III*	Articular—displaced radiocarpal joint
Thomas (1957)[47]	I	Extra-articular—oblique
	II*	Articular
	III	Extra-articular—transverse
Frykman (1967)[21]	I	Extra-articular
	II	Extra-articular—distal ulna
	III*	Articular—radiocarpal
	IV*	Articular—radiocarpal, distal ulna
	V*	Articular—radioulnar
	VI*	Articular—radioulnar, distal ulna
	VII*	Articular—radiocarpal, radioulnar
	VII*	Articular—radiocarpal, radioulnar, distal ulna

*Articular fractures.

347

348

tion with cast immobilization was inadequate treatment for displaced articular fractures.

Frykman,[21] like Gartland and Werley,[22] devised a classification system based on the differentiation of extra-articular from intra-articular injuries. In a comprehensive analysis of 516 fractures, he reported a 64 percent incidence of articular disruption and, compared with extra-articular injuries, an inferior extent of recovery for the articular group. He also emphasized the frequency of distal radioulnar joint disruption and distal ulnar fractures and the serious impairment that can result from radioulnar malalignment. However, Frykman[21] did not emphasize fracture stability, comminution, and displacement.

Thomas,[47] acknowledging frequent difficulties in management of volarly displaced fractures, categorized Smith's fractures into three types. The most unstable injury is the Smith's type II fracture—an injury identical to Barton's fracture-dislocation. Typically, the plane of injury traverses the distal end of the radius, displacing its palmar articular surface anteriorly with the carpus. Because of the uniformly poor results with closed reduction and manipulation, open treatment has often been recommended for these unstable articular fractures.

The classification system developed by the AO group was organized to aid in identifying more severe injuries of the distal radius.[37] The classification divides distal radius fractures into extra-articular (type A), partial articular (type B), and complete articular (type C). Each type is then subdivided into three subgroups. Type B, for example, can be divided into B1 (sagittal plane fracture), B2 (dorsal rim fracture), and B3 (volar rim fracture). These subdivisions can be further divided according to fracture complexity and difficulty in treatment.

Fernandez[19] has suggested a classification based on the mechanism of injury. Knowledge of the mechanism facilitates treatment through the application of a force opposite to the one that produced the injury. Furthermore, associated ligamentous lesions and subluxations and fractures of the neighboring carpal bones, as well as concomitant soft tissue damage, are directly related to the type and degree of violence sustained. Treatment recommendations for each subcategory (bending, shearing, compression, avulsion, and high velocity) are based on the mechanism and displacement pattern.

Classifications identifying unstable and irreducible fractures and thereby facilitating treatment options based on the fracture pattern have also been formulated. In 1990, at a symposium conference on fractures of the distal radius, a new treatment-related "Universal" classification of distal radius fractures was proposed (Fig. 19–1). This treatment-directed scheme is based on fracture location, displacement, stability, and reducibility. Modeled after the Gartland and Werley[22] approach, this classification subdivides extra-articular and intra-articular fractures into nondisplaced and displaced fractures. Further subdivision is based on radiographic hallmarks of instability

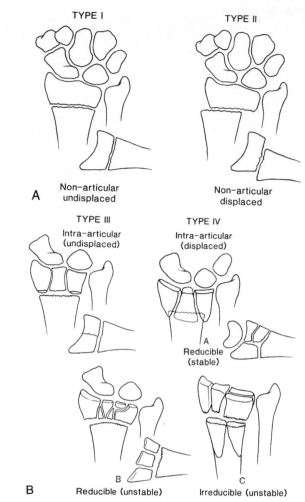

Figure 19–1. Universal classification of distal radius fractures. *A,* Type I: nonarticular; type II: nonarticular, displaced. *B,* Type III: intraarticular; type IV: intraarticular, displaced. (See Table 19–1.) (From Cooney WP, Agee JM, Hastings H, et al: Symposium: Management of intraarticular fractures of the distal radius. Contemp Orthop 21:71–104, 1990.)

and reducibility. The merit of this classification is that it incorporates the parameters requiring recognition for comprehensive management.

The intra-articular fracture is further categorized in the Mayo Clinic classification system. After studying the radiographic presentation of more than 60 intra-articular fractures, Missakian and colleagues[36] found that the majority belonged to one of four joint involvement types. Type I is intra-articular, but nondisplaced; type II involves only the scaphoid articular surface; type III involves the lunate and sigmoid notch articular surfaces; and type IV involves two or more articular surfaces (scaphoid, lunate, or sigmoid notch of the radius). The goal of the Mayo Clinic system is primarily to call attention to the intra-articular fracture components that require treatment beyond the fracture involving the radial metaphysis and the radial shaft.

As with the Mayo Clinic system, our experience with distal radius fractures has shown that radio-

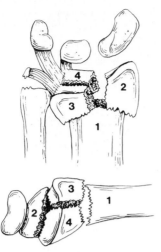

Figure 19–2. Articular fractures, despite variable and often extensive comminution, comprise four basic components: *1* = metaphyseal or shaft; *2* = radial styloid; *3* = dorsal medial; and *4* = palmar medial. (From Melone CP Jr: Distal radius fractures: Patterns of articular fragmentation. Orthop Clin North Am 24:221, 1993.)

graphic evidence of articular disruption is present in the majority of cases.[32–34, 40] Consistent radiographic observations have led to the formulation of a classification subset of articular injuries that has considerably facilitated their treatment. Stability and reducibility can be determined, and a treatment plan can be formulated, on the basis of an analysis of the fracture pattern. Rather than a global classification

system, these categories should be considered a subset of more complex articular injuries.

Despite frequent comminution, articular fractures comprise four basic components: (1) the radial shaft, (2) the radial styloid, (3) a dorsal medial fragment, and (4) a palmar medial fragment (Fig. 19–2). To underscore their pivotal position as the cornerstone of both the radiocarpal and distal radioulnar joints, the two medial fragments, along with their strong ligamentous attachments to the carpus and the ulnar styloid, have been termed the medial complex (Fig. 19–3). Because even minimal displacement of the key medial fragments is likely to cause a major biarticular disruption with a serious compromise of articular function, anatomic preservation of this complex must be recognized as an absolute requirement for optimal fracture management. Displacement of these strategically positioned medial fragments also forms the basis for an increasingly comprehensive system of categorizing articular injuries into precise patterns of fragmentation (Fig. 19–4).

Type I fractures are minimally displaced, are stable after closed reduction, and are effectively treated by a short period of continuous cast immobilization. Progressive remobilization and strengthening supplement splint immobilization until rehabilitation is complete.

The most common articular fracture is the dorsally displaced type II fracture, the die-punch fracture (Fig. 19–5). In such a fracture, the lunate selectively impacts the dorsal medial component, resulting in an unstable fracture characterized by greater comminution of the dorsal metaphysis with marked dorsal

Figure 19–3. The skeletal and soft tissue components of the medial complex are demonstrated *(shaded area)*. The successful use of traction for articular fractures depends on the strength of the ligament component, which remains intact regardless of the severity of the fracture. Maintenance of the critical soft tissues under constant tension affords stability to the attached articular fragments.

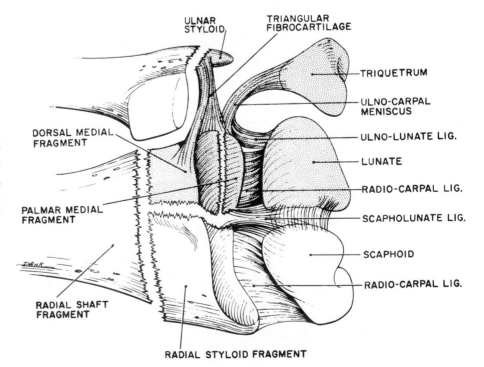

THE MEDIAL COMPLEX

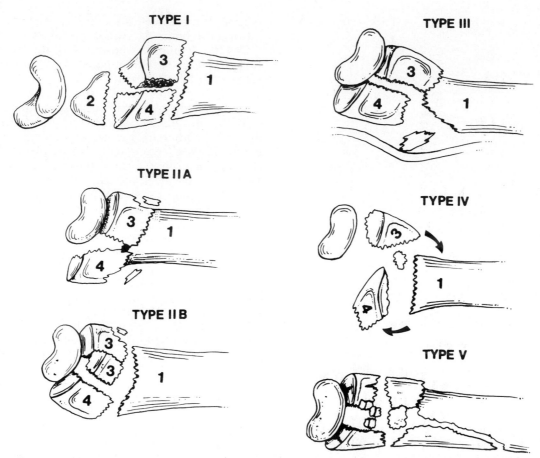

Figure 19–4. Displacement of the key medial fragments disrupts both the radiocarpal and distal radioulnar joints and is the basis for an increasingly comprehensive system of categorizing distal radius articular fractures. Compared with the type IIA injury, the type IIB fracture is characterized by greater comminution and displacement of the medial fragments with articular disruption that is refractory to closed methods of reduction. The type V fracture results from a severe force comprising both compression and crush that causes extensive comminution, often extending from the articular surface to the diaphysis. (From Melone CP Jr: Distal radius fractures: Patterns of articular fragmentation. Orthop Clin North Am 24:221, 1993.)

tilting and considerable shortening of the radius. Less commonly, greater lunate compression is applied to the palmar medial fragment, resulting in displacement of the medial complex along with the carpus. In the majority of type II fractures, the medial complex

components are neither widely separated nor rotated, and are generally amenable to closed reduction and skeletal fixation (type IIA).

In contrast, radiographic evaluation of these fractures has revealed a recurring variation in the charac-

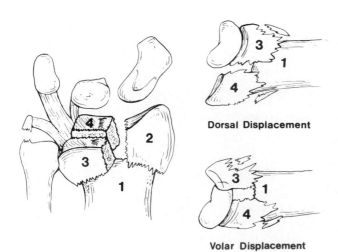

Figure 19–5. The unstable type II fracture resulting from the die-punch mechanism of injury. In most cases, the lunate selectively impacts the dorsal medial fragment, resulting in dorsal displacement of the articular surfaces. Less commonly, the palmar medial fragment and the carpus demonstrate volar displacement. Regardless of the direction of displacement, these fractures are reducible by closed techniques. (From Melone CP Jr: Distal radius fractures: Patterns of articular fragmentation. Orthop Clin North Am 24:221, 1993.)

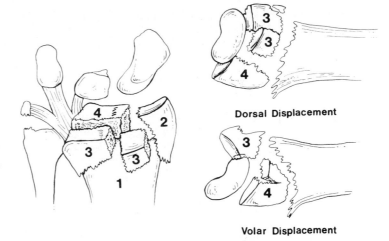

Figure 19–6. The unstable type IIB fracture results from a violent compression force, termed the double die-punch mechanism of injury, and demonstrates greater comminution and displacement of the medial fragments, usually in a dorsal direction. This fracture type consistently has proved irreducible by closed methods of reduction. With greater compression and fragmentation of the palmar medial fragment, the less commonly encountered irreducible type IIB fracture with volar displacement occurs. (From Melone CP Jr: Distal radius fractures: Patterns of articular fragmentation. Orthop Clin North Am 24:221, 1993.)

teristic die-punch pattern that has consistently proved to be irreducible by closed methods (type IIB). The distinctive pattern of fragmentation is characterized by greater comminution and displacement of the medial fragments, usually in a dorsal direction, with the scaphoid and lunate seen impacting the articular surface (double die-punch), and with an offset of the radiocarpal joint exceeding 2 mm (Fig. 19–6).

Radiographic signs of a greater magnitude of injury similarly are observed for the irreducible die-punch fracture with volar displacement. The hallmarks of this fracture pattern are greater comminution and displacement of the palmar medial fragment, resulting in a radiocarpal stepoff exceeding 5 mm as viewed in the sagittal plane.

The type III spike fracture demonstrates articular disruption similar to that in type II injuries as well as displacement of an additional and substantial fracture component, the spike fragment, from the volar metaphysis (Fig. 19–7). Displacement of the fragment may occur at the time of injury or during fracture manipulation and causes not only injury to adjacent nerves and tendons but also a further compromise of fracture stability.

The type IV fracture pattern is characterized by wide separation or rotation of the dorsal and palmar

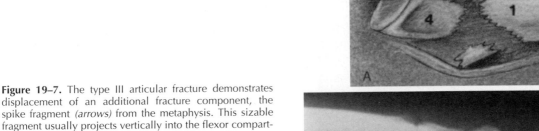

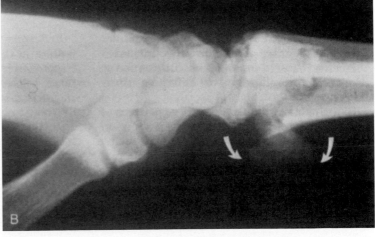

Figure 19–7. The type III articular fracture demonstrates displacement of an additional fracture component, the spike fragment (arrows) from the metaphysis. This sizable fragment usually projects vertically into the flexor compartment of the wrist, causing injury to the median nerve and adjacent tendons. (From Melone CP Jr: Distal radius fractures: Patterns of articular fragmentation. Orthop Clin North Am 24:221, 1993.)

medial fragments with severe disruption of the distal radius articulations (Fig. 19–8). Not infrequently, the palmar medial fragment is rotated 180°, causing its articular surface to face proximally, toward the radial shaft. This injury also results in extensive concomitant soft tissue and skeletal damage.

An increasingly violent magnitude of injury accounts for the occurrence of an additional pattern of articular disruption called the type V explosion fracture (Fig. 19–9). This severe lesion results from an enormous force, comprising both axial compression and direct crush, that causes profound comminution commonly extending from the articular surfaces to the diaphysis. This major skeletal injury usually occurs in association with massive soft tissue trauma that is likely to disrupt skin, nerves, or vascular structures.

For purposes of clarity, this classification can be correlated with those previously described. The type I injuries in this classification of articular fractures are analogous to the group II fractures of Gartland and Werley,[22] the type II to type VI fractures of Frykman,[21] the Universal types III and IVA, and the AO type C1.[37] The unstable type IIA articular fractures in this classification are analogous to the group III fractures of Gartland and Werley,[22] the type VII and type VIII fractures of Frykman,[21] the Universal type IVB, the Mayo Clinic system type II,[36] and the AO type C2.[37] The unstable and irreducible type IIB fracture in this classification are similar to the Universal type IVC, the Mayo Clinic system types III and IV,[36] and the AO type C3.[37] Type III and type IV articular fractures in this classification system have not been previously defined.

PRINCIPLES OF MANAGEMENT

The fundamental goal of treatment for distal radius fractures is an accurate and stable reduction. It is

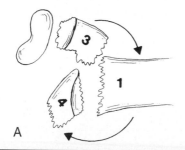
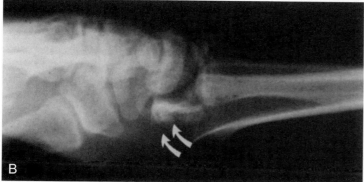
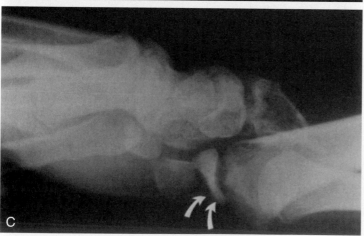

Figure 19–8. *A,* The type IV fracture pattern is characterized by wide separation of the dorsal and palmar medial fragments with severe disruption of the distal radius articulations. This injury results in a major biarticular disruption, as well as frequent concomitant soft tissue injury, and always requires open reduction with internal fixation for restoration of articular congruity. The type IV injury shown in *B* demonstrates 90° rotation of the palmar medial fragment *(arrows),* whereas in that shown in *C,* the palmar medial fragment has rotated 180°, causing a complete reversal of its articular surface toward the radial shaft. (From Melone CP Jr: Distal radius fractures: Patterns of articular fragmentation. Orthop Clin North Am 24:221, 1993.)

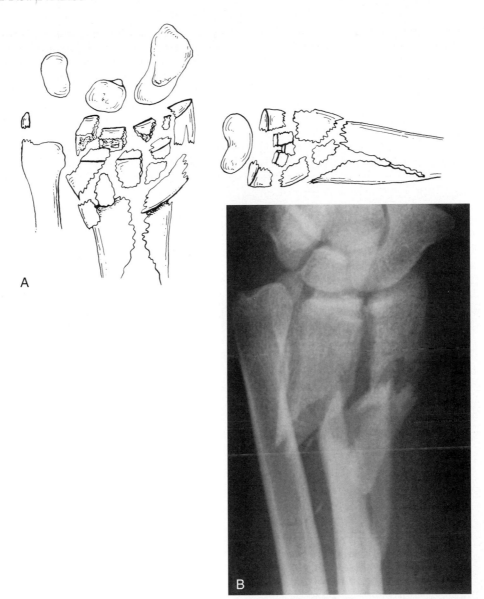

Figure 19–9. The type V explosion fracture, demonstrating profound comminution extending from the articular surfaces to the diaphysis. This severe injury often occurs in association with massive soft tissue trauma, requiring revascularization or resurfacing procedures prior to definitive articular restoration. (From Melone CP Jr: Distal radius fractures: Patterns of articular fragmentation. Orthop Clin North Am 24:221, 1993.)

generally acknowledged that the reduction may be easily achieved but difficult to maintain.[1] Successful treatment requires a method of reduction that restores anatomic relationships between the fractured radius and adjacent ulna and carpus and maintains this alignment until the healing process is complete. It has also become increasingly acknowledged that a suboptimal outcome is likely to result if seemingly minor alterations of fracture anatomy persist. For example, only 2 mm of articular offset, 10° of dorsal tilt, or 3 to 5 mm of radial shortening is apt to compromise recovery.[3, 7–9, 25, 28, 31, 48] Although a good functional result can be achieved despite a poor radiographic result, excellent function is more likely to be attained when normal anatomy has been restored. For articular fractures, precise restitution of the medial

complex is essential for the preservation of the distal radius articulations, and such restitution occasionally requires open treatment. Also, because the unstable fractures are commonly complicated by serious concomitant soft tissue and skeletal damage, optimal treatment requires prompt recognition of these associated injuries.

Fracture Stability

Understanding the stability of an articular fracture is paramount in selecting the appropriate treatment. Although stable fractures can often be reduced and maintained in a cast, closed techniques are doomed to failure for the unstable fracture. Reduction of the unstable fracture may be possible, but maintenance of the reduction until fracture healing is unlikely. As Gartland and Werley[22] observed in their classic review of articular fractures managed by closed reduction, re-displacement of the unstable fracture, commonly to its pre-reduction position, is inevitable. The quandary is considerably lessened by recognition of those characteristics of articular fragmentation and displacement that render the fracture unstable and thus not suitable for treatment solely by manipulation and immobilization. The obvious hallmarks of articular fracture instability are excessive comminution and severity of displacement. Other signs less obvious yet highly suggestive of a fracture prone to re-displacement, however, usually can be identified.

Clearly identifiable radiographic features should be considered markers of fracture instability (Fig. 19–10). First, radial shortening in excess of 10 mm predisposes to further collapse, resulting in both disabling distal radioulnar instability and ulnocarpal joint impaction. Lindstrom has indicated that residual shortening of only 6 mm can seriously compromise wrist function.[11] Palmer and colleagues[38] have demonstrated that even a lesser discrepancy in radioulnar length is likely to cause deleterious alterations in load-bearing that lead to articular deterioration. Because even relatively stable articular fractures tend to collapse several millimeters owing to impaction of comminuted metaphyseal fragments, a successful reduction should secure the pre-injury level of the medial complex and its critical relationships with the radial styloid, the proximal carpus, and the ulnar head. In all fractures, comparison radiographs of the patient's other wrist should be assessed to determine normal length and to avoid misinterpretation due to anatomic variation. Second, angulation or tilting of the radial articular surface exceeding 20° in the sagittal plane causes a serious disturbance of radiocarpal colinear alignment as well as incongruity of the distal radioulnar joint. Like radial shortening, this typical feature of the unstable articular fracture is exceedingly difficult to correct by casting. Finally, metaphyseal comminution involving both the volar and dorsal radial cortices eliminates an intact bony buttress upon which a stable reduction must hinge (Fig. 19–11). Lateral radiographs obtained at the time of

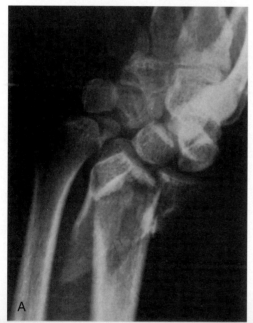

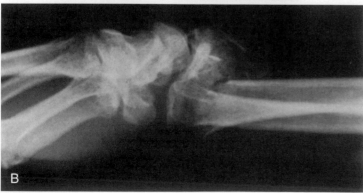

Figure 19–10. The radiographic hallmarks of the unstable articular fracture. *A,* The posteroanterior view demonstrates extensive medial component fragmentation with severe radiocarpal incongruity as well as excessive radial shortening with distal radioulnar joint subluxation. *B,* The lateral projection demonstrates impaction and dorsal tilting of the articular surfaces exceeding 20° with loss of the normal radiocarpal colinear relationship as well as comminution of both the dorsal and volar metaphyseal cortices. (From Melone CP Jr: Distal radius fractures: Patterns of articular fragmentation. Orthop Clin North Am 24:221, 1993.)

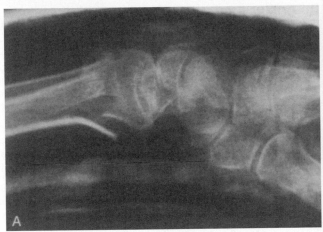

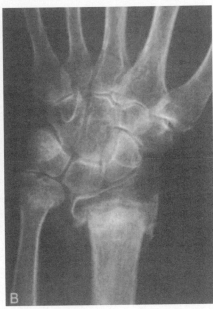

Figure 19–11. *A*, Extensive comminution of both posterior and anterior cortices renders distal radius fractures unstable. *B*, Without supplementary fixation, collapse with loss of reduction is inevitable.

injury clearly demonstrate this bicortical comminution, whereas frontal projections taken after attempts at reduction often display an articular surface bereft of a sturdy osseous support because of extensive metaphyseal cavitation. Recognition of these radiographic signs of instability is essential for satisfactory management of these injuries.

Reducibility of Articular Fragments

Obtaining a stable anatomic reduction of disrupted articular surfaces is the optimal means of ensuring a favorable result for displaced articular fractures. Recognition that subtle alterations in articular contours are prone to profound disturbances in wrist mechanics and function has led to more stringent but increasingly accepted standards for a successful reduction. The prevailing key criteria are a radiocarpal stepoff less than 2 mm, dorsal tilting less than 10°, and radial shortening less than 5 mm. If methods of closed treatment fail to secure restoration of articular anatomy, alternative and increasingly invasive methods must be attempted. If all methods of closed technique, including those employing supplementary external fixation or percutaneous pinning, are unsuccessful, the fracture is defined as "irreducible" and requires open treatment for restoration of the articular surfaces.

Fracture fragment irreducibility can usually be predicted with a high degree of accuracy using preoperative high-quality radiographs. Occasionally, computed tomographic scans and trispiral tomograms add additional information concerning the displaced fracture fragments.[27, 35, 39] Basic to this concept is the need to differentiate the frequently encountered, dorsally displaced die-punch fracture that is unstable but reducible by closed techniques (type IIA) from the frac-

ture that is irreducible and requires open reduction for preservation of articular congruity. The irreducible die-punch fracture with dorsal displacement (type IIB) is readily identified because of the double die-punch mechanism, whereby the scaphoid as well as the lunate is seen impacting the distal radius, causing greater involvement of the scaphoid articular facet and further displacement of articular fragments (Fig. 19–12). There is extensive dorsal medial comminution, often resulting in five basic fracture components, and an offset of the radiocarpal joint exceeding 2 mm.[41]

Similarly, a radiocarpal stepoff exceeding 5 mm as viewed on the lateral radiograph is the cardinal sign of the less common but also irreducible type IIB fracture with volar displacement (Fig. 19–13). A palmar medial fragment excessively displaced in the sagittal plane is strongly suggestive of a fracture likely to require open reduction and internal fixation.

Open treatment, of course, is also necessary for reduction of the widely separated and irreducible fragments characterizing type III spike and type IV split fractures as well as for repair of concomitant soft tissue and skeletal damage, frequently occurring with these skeletal injuries.

Methods of Reduction and Stabilization

A prevalent misconception has been that distal radius articular fractures, regardless of their extent, usually can be managed with equal success by similar techniques. Rational management, however, is contingent on recognition of the variable magnitude of articular disruption, and on skillful treatment based on specific fracture configurations. Each fracture should be distinguished by its extent of articular displacement, its sta-

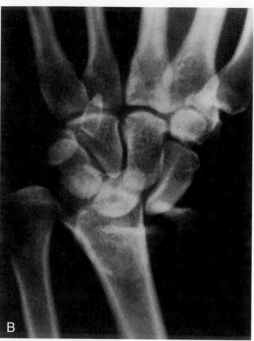

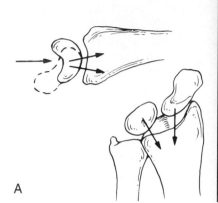

A

B

Figure 19–12. *A,* The double die-punch mechanism of injury, whereby the scaphoid as well as the lunate impacts and disrupts the distal radius articular surfaces, causing *(B)* greater involvement of the scaphoid facet, excessive displacement of the articular fragments, and the highly unstable and irreducible type IIB fracture pattern. Other key radiographic signs of this irreducible die-punch fracture are demonstrated: extensive dorsal medial comminution with radiocarpal incongruity exceeding 2 mm and radial shortening greater than 5 mm. (From Melone CP Jr: Distal radius fractures: Patterns of articular fragmentation. Orthop Clin North Am 24:221, 1993.)

bility, and its reducibility. After the fracture is thoroughly evaluated, optimal treatment can be instituted.

Minimally displaced distal radius fractures can be reduced by closed manipulation. The reduction is performed after aspiration of the fracture hematoma under sterile conditions and local infiltration of lidocaine. The reduction is essentially a reversal of the mechanism of injury. Usually a hyperextension-compression force applied to the pronated wrist results in posterior displacement with relative supination of the distal fragments; thus, the reduction is achieved by axial traction of the wrist, followed by pronation of the displaced fracture fragments, palmar flexion, ulnar deviation, and cast immobilization.

A satisfactory reduction requires restoration of normal radial length (usually neutral ulnar variance) and stability provided by accurate apposition of the anterior cortices of the radius. Invariably, the dorsal cortex is comminuted, and stability of the reduction hinges on the buttress of a relatively intact anterior cortex. If both cortices are extensively comminuted, the fracture is unstable, and collapse with loss of reduction is inevitable.

If the fracture is unstable, the commonly encountered, dorsally displaced fracture that is unstable and reducible but requires some form of skeletal fixation must be distinguished from the irreducible die-punch fracture. Compared with the reducible type II fracture, the irreducible articular pattern demonstrates greater comminution and displacement of the medial fragments, usually in the dorsal direction, with persistent articular stepoff or gapping greater than 2 mm.

Specific fracture patterns also facilitate a rational choice of operative techniques from the ever-expanding list of methods advocated for the treatment of distal radius fractures. Whereas the unstable type II fracture with relatively mild displacement and comminution can be managed successfully by pins and plaster,[10, 29, 34] or percutaneous Kirschner wires,[11, 12, 23] type II injuries with greater articular fragmentation and instability are preferentially stabilized by external fixators.[14, 16, 18, 26, 40, 42, 46, 49] Although the underlying principles of ligamentotaxis for pins and plaster and external fixators are the same, the external fixator affords the distinct advantages of superior mechanical efficiency, the capacity for secondary adjustment in fracture position, and unobstructed access for wound care. For those complex fractures requiring open reduction and internal fixation, use of the external fixator is an excellent means of providing both supplemental stabilization and secure immobilization during the period of fracture healing.

Awareness that closed reduction in conjunction with external fixation or percutaneous internal fixation cannot always restore articular anatomy has led to increasing employment of open treatment for the more complex articular disruptions.* For the irreducible medial fragments of the type IIB fracture with dorsal displacement, a limited exposure of the articular surfaces permits an accurate articular restoration yet minimizes additional soft tissue and skeletal trauma. Type III, type IV, and type V injuries, in contrast, require a far more extensive exposure, occasionally combining dorsal and volar approaches, for comprehensive repair of the severe skeletal and soft tissue damage.

Recognizing a substantive contribution of metaphyseal comminution to articular fracture instability

---

*References 4, 5, 7, 9, 20, 25, 28, 33, 36, 41, 48.

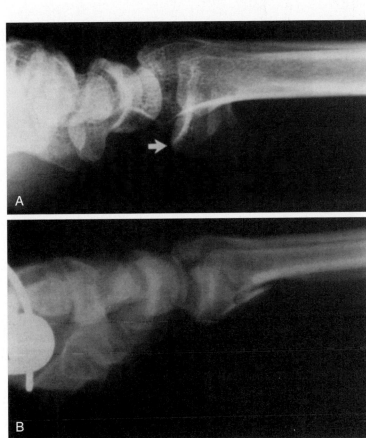

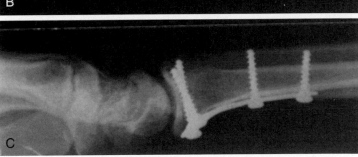

Figure 19–13. The type IIB fracture with volar displacement. *A,* The radiographic hallmark of this irreducible injury is palmar medial displacement exceeding 5 mm as viewed in the sagittal plane *(arrow). B,* Not surprisingly, this injury proved refractory to reduction by closed manipulation and continuous distraction. *C,* Restoration of articular congruity is achieved by open reduction with plate and screw fixation. (From Melone CP Jr: Distal radius fractures: Patterns of articular fragmentation. Orthop Clin North Am 24:221, 1993.)

and irreducibility, Leung and associates[30] have emphasized the efficacy of bone grafting in serious injuries requiring open treatment. In such fractures, it has been increasingly realized that reconstitution of subchondral metaphyseal defects with an abundance of cancellous bone provides structural support for the articular surfaces, enhances skeletal stability, and accelerates fracture union. Metaphyseal comminution with osseous cavitation is a characteristic feature of unstable and irreducible fractures for which bone grafting should be acknowledged as a key component of primary treatment.

Concomitant Injuries

A force that is great enough to cause distal radius articular disruption is also likely to result in injury to the adjacent nerves and tendons as well as to the distal ulna and carpus.[33] In such cases, maximum

recovery requires both precise treatment of the fracture and prompt recognition and repair of concomitant soft tissue and skeletal damage.

SOFT TISSUE INJURIES

Careful examination at the time of injury, prior to the administration of an anesthetic, is necessary to detect nerve injury, which should be suspected with all displaced fractures. Median or ulnar neuropathy (or, in many cases, both) has occurred in 55 percent of the unstable articular injuries. In all but one case, nerve contusion by a displaced bone fragment resulted in a neurapraxia with loss of sensibility immediately after injury. The one exception was a complete transection of the median nerve occurring with a type IV fracture.

Treatment of nerve injury is guided by the concurrent type of fracture. For type II fractures with neuropathy, an accurate closed reduction maintained by

358

traction has invariably been followed by complete recovery of nerve function over a period of several months. Nerve transection did not occur with type II fractures, and no case required primary or secondary nerve surgery. Thus, one can expect type II fracture neuropathy to improve spontaneously with successful fracture treatment.

In contrast, neuropathy associated with type III, IV, and V fractures required a prompt neurolysis and possibly even nerve suturing, in conjunction with open reduction and internal fixation of the fracture. The nerve must be thoroughly decompressed from the distal forearm to the palm in order to prevent the occurrence of a secondary compression neuropathy.

It is important to recognize that every structure traversing the wrist is vulnerable to disruption with displaced articular fractures. Obviously, repair of these critical soft tissues is essential to optimal man-

agement. One must also realize that the excessive trauma causing these fractures is apt to result in profound edema within the flexor compartment of the wrist. Like neuropathy, compartmental ischemia must always be suspected and, if present, alleviated promptly by fasciotomy. Unstable articular fractures should not be considered simple Colles' fractures; they are violent injuries that can seriously threaten survival of the damaged tissues.

SKELETAL INJURIES

Unstable scaphoid fractures occurring with type II articular fractures create a dilemma: Traction may be necessary for stability of the articular fracture but detrimental to healing of the scaphoid fracture. The problem is solved by open reduction and internal fixation of the scaphoid with a compression screw (Fig. 19–14). The operation stabilizes the scaphoid so

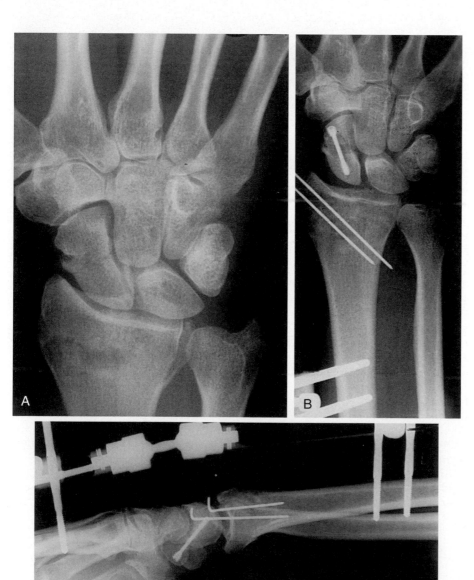

Figure 19–14. *A,* Type IIA unstable articular fracture with concomitant scaphoid waist fracture. *B* and *C,* Fracture has been stabilized by the combined techniques of external fixation, internal fixation with Kirschner wires of the radius fracture, and compression screw fixation of the scaphoid fracture.

that traction can be continued. Displaced scaphoid fractures associated with type III or type IV fractures require open reduction and internal fixation in conjunction with open treatment of the articular fractures.

Scapholunate ligament disruption has occurred with severely displaced articular fractures. Because of the strong soft tissue attachments, the lunate displaces along with the medial complex, whereas the scaphoid remains with the radial styloid. Restoration of the medial complex corrects the carpal diastasis; open ligament repair with Kirschner pin fixation of the scapholunate articulation permits successful ligament healing and preservation of carpal stability.

The most frequent concomitant skeletal injury is fracture of the ulnar styloid. Distal avulsion fractures must be differentiated from displaced fractures at the base with concomitant distal radioulnar joint instability. Neither the ulnar styloid fracture nor its common failure to unite appreciably influences recovery, provided that the radial articular surfaces are successfully restored. Displaced ulnar styloid fractures with resultant distal ulnar instability require open repair to reestablish distal radioulnar joint relationships.

REHABILITATION

Attainment of maximum recovery after fracture depends largely on a carefully planned and executed program of therapy. Patients should be cautioned that a perfect reduction does not ensure a satisfactory recovery; they should also be reassured that a motivated patient working with a skilled therapist can often turn a fair anatomic result into an excellent functional result.

Rehabilitation starts immediately after fracture reduction and stabilization; digital, elbow, and shoulder motion is encouraged and must not be impaired by faulty techniques of immobilization (Fig. 19–15). Mobilization of the uninjured finger joints can be enhanced by static and dynamic splinting, massage, anti-inflammatory medication, and a variety of other therapeutic modalities commonly used by the hand therapist. With early, aggressive therapy, the disastrous complications of digital joint contractures and reflex sympathetic dystrophy rarely develop.

In an effort to improve functional recovery, dynamic external fixators that allow wrist range of motion with loss of reduction have been developed.[13, 44] In our experience, early motion does not enhance the final results of unstable distal radius fractures.

After the fracture is healed, the pins are removed in the physician's office, a protective splint is provided, and mobilization of the wrist is begun. Over several months, the patient progresses from active exercises to increasingly resistive activities with weights. Steady improvement is expected for at least 8 months after injury.

ASSESSMENT OF RESULTS

A thorough evaluation of treatment should include a review of surgical complications; measurement of recovery of wrist motion, of grip and pinch strength, and of preservation of nerve, tendon, and adjacent joint function; radiographic analysis of articular restoration; consideration of the duration of impaired activity; and the patient's appraisal of function. The Gartland and Werley[22] system of demerits and the Lindstrom[31] classification of radiographic results incorporate these parameters (Tables 19–2 and 19–3). The modified system of Green-O'Brien provides a score based only on subjective and objective clinical information;[36] it is a very stringent system, in that normal or near-normal function, strength, and motion are required for an excellent result.

AUTHORS' PREFERRED METHODS OF SURGICAL TREATMENT

Closed Reduction and External Fixation: Type IIA Fractures

A consensus exists that although minimally displaced stable fractures usually can be managed with success by closed methods of treatment, unstable articular fractures commonly require more invasive techniques to maintain an accurate reduction during the healing process. Foremost among these techniques is continuous skeletal traction, in the form of pins and plaster and external fixation, employing the concept of ligamentotaxis. Traction maintains the critical soft tissue attachments to the displaced fracture fragments under constant tension, aligning and stabilizing the attached articular fragments.

Modifications of external fixation pins and frames have resulted in balanced systems combining efficient skeletal support with an unobtrusive construct. Pins are safely inserted by limited open techniques, thus avoiding injury to susceptible nerves and other vulnerable soft tissues while permitting precision placement within the metacarpals and radial shaft. In our experience, 3-mm blunt-tip self-tapping half-pins manually placed after pre-drilling are consistently effective in providing stabilization. This procedure is performed as follows:

Approach the distal pin site through a 2-cm longitudinal incision along the dorsal-radial border of the index metacarpal. Protect the terminal dorsal-radial sensory nerve, and reflect the first dorsal interosseous muscle volarly. Prepare the pin sites by pre-drilling with a low-speed power drill. Take care to avoid unicortical pin placement, which can lead to subsequent loosening or infection. Direct the pin placement in a slight dorsal-to-volar alignment to avoid impingement upon thumb extension, as well as to facilitate access to the lateral wrist for both radiographic evaluation and percutaneous Kirschner wire insertion (Fig. 19–16).

Next, approach the proximal pin site through a 2-cm longitudinal incision over the dorsal-radial aspect of the radius shaft approximately 3 to 5 cm proximal

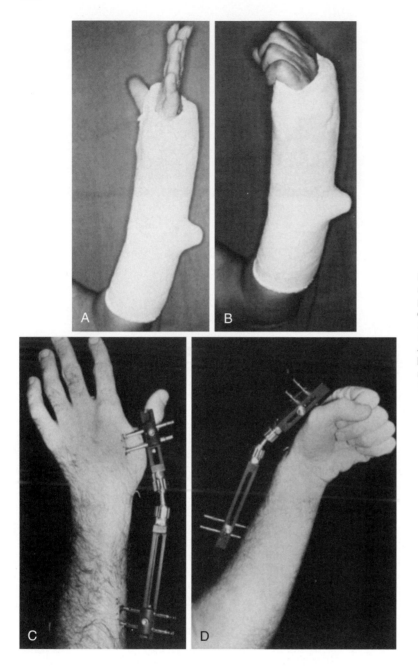

Figure 19–15. *A* and *B,* Early unimpeded active range of motion of fingers and thumb demonstrated with pins and plaster. *C* and *D,* Equally successful early digital motion demonstrated with external fixator technique. (*A* and *B* from Isani A, Melone CP Jr: Classification and management of intra-articular fractures of the distal radius. Hand Clinics 4:353, 1988. *C* and *D* from Raskin KB, Melone CP Jr: Unstable articular fractures of the distal radius: Comparative techniques of ligamentotaxis. Orthop Clin North Am 24:239, 1993.)

to the fracture site. The gap between the extensor carpi radialis longus and extensor carpi radialis brevis leads to direct protection of the underlying superficial radial nerve. Bicortical pin placement in the radius is again essential (Fig. 19–17). Insert two pins at the distal and proximal sites. After the fixator frame is secured to the pins, manual traction of the digits with countertraction equally applied to the flexed elbow affords initial ligamentotaxis across the fracture site as the reduction is achieved by manipulation. Newer frames permit further distraction by devices incorporated within adjustable components. Some frames, including the Agee WristJack, require gross reduction by manipulation or traction prior to placement of the pins. The external fixator then applies "fine tuning" and maintenance of position via ligamentotaxis.

Traditionally, pins and plaster have been the preferred method of traction for comminuted articular fractures (Fig. 19–18). Adequate anesthesia and muscle relaxation are achieved by regional anesthesia with axillary block. Necessary equipment includes a variable-speed power drill, 3/32 smooth Steinmann pins, a sterile traction bow, a 5-lb counterweight, and 4-inch plaster rolls. Detailed attention is directed toward pin placement using low-speed constant pressure. Unicortical eccentric pin placement, high-speed bone necrosis, and the reaming effect of multiple passes with the Steinmann pin can all increase the likelihood of pin loosening, infection, and iatrogenic fractures. The procedure is performed as follows:

Carefully drive the distal pin through the base of the second and third metacarpals, avoiding tension

Table 19–2. MODIFIED McBRIDE DEMERIT POINT SYSTEM FOR EVALUATING TREATMENT OF UNSTABLE DISTAL RADIUS FRACTURES

Parameter and Point Range	Points
Residual deformity (0 to 3)	
Prominent ulnar styloid	1
Residual dorsal tilt	2
Radial deviation of hand	2 to 3
Subjective evaluation (0 to 6)	
Excellent: no pain, disability, or limitation of motion	0
Good: occasional pain, slight limitation of motion, no disability	2
Fair: occasional pain, some limitation of motion, feeling of weakness in wrist, no particular disability if careful, activities slightly restricted	4
Poor: pain, limitation of motion, disability, activities more or less markedly restricted	6
Objective evaluation (0 to 5)*	
Loss of:	
Dorsiflexion	5
Ulnar deviation	3
Pronation	2
Supination	2
Palmar flexion	2
Radial deviation	1
Circumduction	1
Pain in distal radioulnar joint	1
Grip strength—60% or less of that of other side	1
Complications (0 to 5)	
Arthritic change:	
Minimum	1
Minimum with pain	3
Moderate	2
Moderate with pain	4
Severe	3
Severe with pain	5
Nerve complications (median)	1 to 3
Poor finger function due to cast	1 to 2
End-result total scores:	
Excellent	0 to 2
Good	3 to 8
Fair	9 to 20
Poor	21 and above

*Points are deducted for ranges of motion less than 45° dorsiflexion, 30° palmar flexion, 15° radial deviation, 15° ulnar deviation, 50° pronation, 50° supination. In this system, these are the minimum motions considered consistent with normal functions.

Modified from Sarmiento A, Pratt GW, Berry NC, et al: J Bone Joint Surg 57A:313, 1975.

Table 19–3. LINDSTROM RADIOGRAPHIC CLASSIFICATION FOR EVALUATING UNSTABLE DISTAL RADIUS FRACTURES

Grade	Definition
1*	No deformity No dorsal angulation beyond neutral Shortening 3 mm or less
2*	Slight deformity Dorsal angulation 1° to 11° Shortening 3 to 6 mm
3	Mild to moderate deformity Dorsal angulation 11° to 15° Shortening 6 to 12 mm
4	Severe deformity Dorsal angulation greater than 15° Shortening greater than 12 mm

*Grades 1 and 2 are considered consistent with satisfactory (good to excellent) function.
Data from Lindstrom.

well as the long axis of the radius. The "bare area" of the dorsal shaft surface is optimally suited and easily located between the first and second compartments at the musculotendinous junction. Engage both cortices with precision placement of the pin. Apply a traction bow to the metacarpal pin, suspend the hand, and apply a 5-lb counterweight to the well-padded upper arm with the elbow flexed. After several minutes of continuous traction, palpate and reduce the fracture by gentle manipulation. In most patients, use supplementary percutaneous 0.045-inch smooth Kirschner (K) wires to enhance the fracture component stability and to provide a sturdy buttress for the reconstituted radiocarpal articular surface. Place the wires obliquely from the styloid fragment to the metaphysis, always avoiding the radioulnar joint. Preoperative radiographs and intraoperative fluoroscopy help to determine the need for additional percutaneous stabilization before cast application.

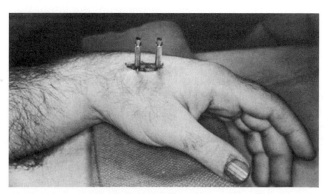

Figure 19–16. Distal pin insertion for external fixator in a dorsal-to-volar orientation, allowing unimpaired thumb extension while enhancing access to the lateral surface of the forearm to facilitate Kirschner wire placement and radiographic evaluation. (From Raskin KB, Melone CP Jr: Unstable articular fractures of the distal radius: Comparative techniques of ligamentotaxis. Orthop Clin North Am 24:239, 1993.)

across the dorsal skin when the pin exits over the fourth metacarpal. During this maneuver, maintain the metacarpal transverse arch, and hold the thumb in full palmar abduction to avoid disabling web space contractures. Pin placement in the ulnar metacarpal increases the risk for iatrogenic fracture because of the narrow diameter of these structures and should thus be avoided. Place the proximal pin in the radial shaft for direct control of the fracture site. Further stability is afforded by perpendicular placement of this proximal pin with respect to the distal pin as

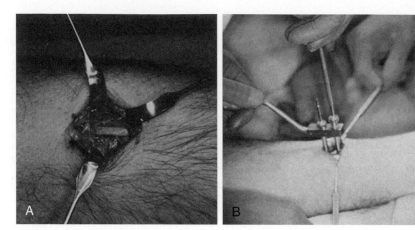

Figure 19–17. *A,* Proximal dissection between the brachialis and extensor carpi radialis longus, isolating the radial sensory nerve prior to pin placement. *B,* Protection of radial nerve and surrounding soft tissue during manual placement of proximal external fixation pins. (From Raskin KB, Melone CP Jr: Unstable articular fractures of the distal radius: Comparative techniques of ligamentotaxis. Orthop Clin North Am 24:239, 1993.)

Confirm restoration of radial alignment as well as articular congruity by intraoperative radiography. Precisely fashion the cast to secure the Steinmann pins, and leave the fingers and thumb free for immediate and unimpeded motion.

Owing to its distinct versatility, the external fixator has now supplanted pins and plaster as our primary choice for fracture stabilization.[40] The particular advantages of the external fixator are its superior mechanical efficiency, its capacity for secondary fracture adjustment during the healing process, and the fact that it ensures unimpeded access to wounds. Like Seitz and colleagues,[42] we routinely supplement external fixators with percutaneous pin fixation as a way to improve reduction and stabilization of articular components (Fig. 19–19). Nonetheless, pins and plaster remain a viable secondary option for treatment. Regardless of the technique of ligamentotaxis, surgical restoration of articular congruity along with attention to key technical details has resulted in a reproducibly successful recovery.

In most fractures, ligamentotaxis alone successfully restores articular congruity and radial length and inclination. The stout volar radiocarpal ligaments are credited for this unique capacity of fracture reduction. However, the restoration of normal volar tilt is less successful, owing to the lack of distractive force from the longer and poorly defined dorsal radiocarpal ligaments.[6] External fixators incorporating multiplanar ligamentotaxis (Agee WristJack, Hand Biomechanics Lab, Sacramento, CA) have been developed in an effort to restore volar tilt.[2] Fracture reduction is obtained by dorsal-palmar fragment alignment using a dorsal-palmar fixator adjustment mechanism. Palmar translation of the hand restores palmar tilt to the distal fragment. Anatomic volar tilt can be achieved with a uniplanar external fixator by closed manipulation of the distal fragment, in conjunction with multiple Kirschner wires inserted from the volar aspect of the styloid fragment to the dorsal cortex of the intact radial shaft (Fig. 19–20),[40] as follows:

Immediately postoperatively, we elevate the hand and encourage active digital motion. In fractures treated by pins and plaster, the cast remains undisturbed for 8 weeks postoperatively. The external fixator frame is covered with sterile gauze at the skin contact interface, avoiding the need for daily treatment. The pins are exposed only during dressing changes in the office, which are done approximately four times during the 8-week healing phase. We use a supplemental volar Orthoplast splint to improve patient comfort and limit soft tissue disturbance. On removal of the frame and pins in the office, we perform an irrigation and curettage of the pin tract sites in a sterile fashion. We then institute wrist rehabilitation.

Open Reduction and Internal Fixation

TYPE IIB FRACTURES

Compared with the reducible type IIA fracture, the irreducible articular pattern demonstrates greater comminution and displacement of the medial complex, usually in a dorsal direction, persistent articular stepoff or gapping greater than 2 mm, irreversible articular tilting in excess of 20°, and uncorrectable radial shortening exceeding 5 mm (Fig. 19–21). Restoration of articular congruity can be accomplished only by open treatment—usually requiring a limited dorsal exposure for articular reduction. After primary ligamentotaxis with an external fixator, use K-wires to derotate and reduce articular fragments to each other, and then to the radial metaphysis. If larger fragments are present, plates and screws may be used for fixation. It is essential to use iliac crest bone graft for restitution of skeletal integrity and support of the articular fragments. Even in the presence of extensive comminution, meticulous fracture reduction can successfully preserve articular contours.

Similarly, the volarly displaced type IIB fracture

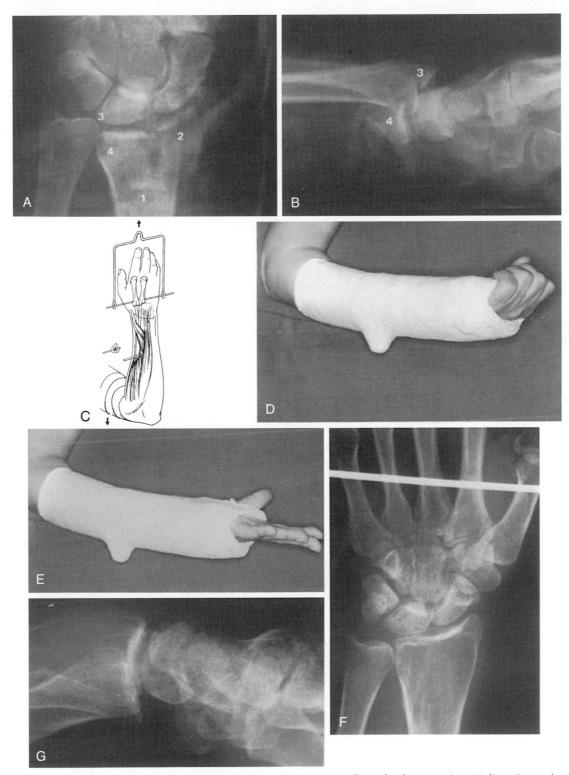

Figure 19–18. Type II articular fracture treated with pins and plaster. Preoperative radiographs demonstrating *(A)* disruption and collapse of the articular surface and *(B)* anterior displacement of the palmar medial fragment. *1* = radial shaft; *2* = radial styloid; *3* = dorsal medial fragment; *4* = palmar medial fragment. *C,* The distal pin passes through the base of the index and middle metacarpals, and the proximal pin passes through the radius at the "bare bone interval." The wrist is suspended by a traction bow, and a countertraction weight is applied to the padded arm. *Inset,* the radial pin must achieve bicortical purchase but avoid the critical soft tissue of the forearm. *D* and *E,* After an accurate reduction, the pins are incorporated in a short arm cast that permits immediate active motion of the fingers and thumb. *F* and *G,* Postoperative radiographs illustrating uncomplicated fracture union with excellent preservation of the joint surfaces.

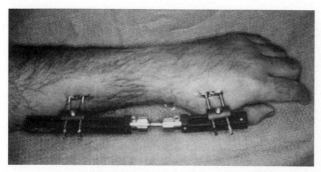

Figure 19–19. Completed external fixation apparatus with applied ligamentotaxis and supplemental percutaneous Kirschner wire insertion. (From Raskin KB, Melone CP Jr: Unstable articular fractures of the distal radius: Comparative techniques of ligamentotaxis. Orthop Clin North Am 24:239, 1993.)

requires open treatment to restore articular congruity. It is this fracture pattern that is best suited to plate-and-screw fixation,[17, 45] which is performed as follows:

Through an extended carpal tunnel approach, expose the displaced fracture fragments by reflecting the pronator quadratus. Then manipulate and reduce the medial fragments. Once anatomic reduction is achieved, contour a straight or oblique T plate to the distal radius. In the lesser comminuted fractures, employ the buttress concept to avoid inserting screws into the distal fragment. In contrast, for substantially comminuted fractures, use adjunctive techniques such as supplementary external fixation, bone grafting, and concomitant soft tissue repairs (Fig. 19–22).

TYPE III FRACTURES

The type III fracture is characterized by displacement of the medial complex as a unit, and of an additional volar spike fragment from the comminuted radial metaphysis. Typically, this bony spike projects anteriorly, contusing the median nerve and adjacent tendons (Fig. 19–23). Although the medial fragment can be successfully managed by external fixation, the spike fragment is irreducible by closed methods and must be accurately reduced and stabilized (or occasionally excised).

TYPE IV FRACTURES

Techniques of ligamentotaxis cannot correct the severe articular disruption of type IV fractures. The type IV fracture constitutes a severe disruption of the distal radius articulations and is always associated with extensive periarticular damage. The key step in articular restoration is precise reduction of the medial fragments (Fig. 19–24). Usually, the palmar medial fragment is displaced most severely and must be derotated, reduced, and stabilized with Kirschner wires to the dorsal medial fragment. These fragments, as a unit, are then reduced and fixed to the radial shaft,

restoring radioulnar joint congruity, and to the radial styloid, reconstituting the radiocarpal joint.

Inasmuch as the major fracture displacement of both type III and type IV injuries usually is volar, and the soft tissue injury occurs within the flexor compartment of the wrist, the volar approach extending from the carpal tunnel to the ulnar aspect of the wrist is the preferential means of surgical exposure. In cases with widely displaced radial styloid fragments, irreducible dorsal medial fragments, displaced scaphoid fractures, carpal dissociation, or extensor tendon injuries, extensile exposure often requires a second incision over the dorsum of the wrist. Although the small, comminuted fracture fragments generally are not suitable for techniques of rigid fixation, secure stabilization can be achieved with multiple Kirschner wires. In patients with severe comminution, supplementary external fixation and primary bone grafting augment fracture stability and enhance security against collapse of the articular surfaces.

TYPE V FRACTURES

For the type V explosion injury, preparatory stabilization with an external fixation device provides a sturdy framework for critical revascularization or resurfacing procedures and serves to maintain skeletal alignment before definitive articular reconstruction. Contingent on fragment size and comminution, internal fixation is achieved with wires, plates and screws, or a combination of devices.

EXTRA-ARTICULAR FRACTURES

In contrast to articular fractures, extra-articular fractures principally result from tension forces and tend to be stable after closed reduction and cast immobilization. Facilitated by a regional anesthetic, manipulation of Colles'-type fractures is accomplished by axial traction followed by palmar flexion, ulnar deviation, and pronation of the wrist. Volarly displaced fractures are reduced by traction and supination. As for all distal radius fractures, a stable reduction hinges on the restoration of an intact cortical buttress, either posterior or anterior. Thus, if both radial cortices are extensively comminuted, the injury is inherently unstable, and without supplementary fixation, loss of reduction is inevitable. Unlike their articular counterparts, these fractures are well suited to closed reduction coupled with methods of percutaneous pin stabilization (Fig. 19–25).[12, 23] The lesser comminuted and larger radial styloid fragment affords an accessible and strategically located purchase point for precise placement of percutaneous pins.

SUMMARY

Distal radius articular fractures principally result from the die-punch mechanism of injury that leads

Text continued on page 371

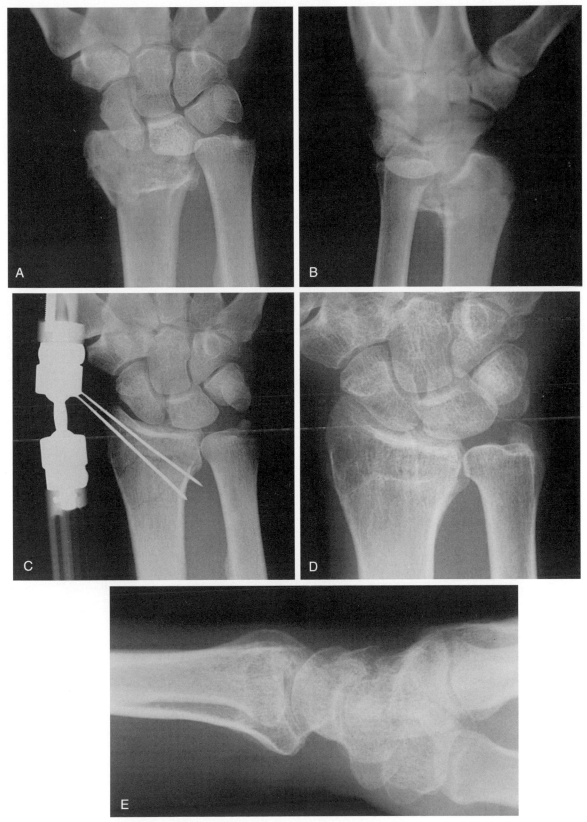

Figure 19–20. *A* and *B,* Type IIA unstable articular fracture. *C,* Fracture has been stabilized by the combined method of external fixation and adjunctive internal fixation with Kirschner wires. After successful closed reduction, the external fixator maintains radial length, whereas the percutaneous Kirschner wires secure articular congruity and volar tilt. *D* and *E,* Postoperatively, an accurate restoration of the disrupted articular surface is demonstrated.

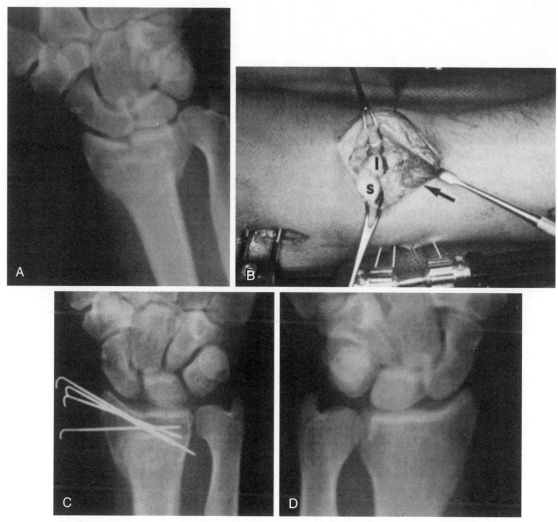

Figure 19–21. *A,* An irreducible type IIB die-punch fracture with severe radiocarpal and distal radioulnar joint disruption. *B,* Treatment comprised open reduction and internal fixation of the articular surfaces through a limited dorsal exposure, supplementary stabilization with an external fixator, and subchondral iliac bone grafting *(arrow). s* = scaphoid; *l* = lunate. *C,* Postoperative radiograph at time of external and internal pin removal demonstrates restoration of radiocarpal and radioulnar joint congruity as well as radial length, comparable to those in *(D)* the uninjured, contralateral wrist. (From Melone CP Jr: Distal radius fractures: Patterns of articular fragmentation. Orthop Clin North Am 24:221, 1993.)

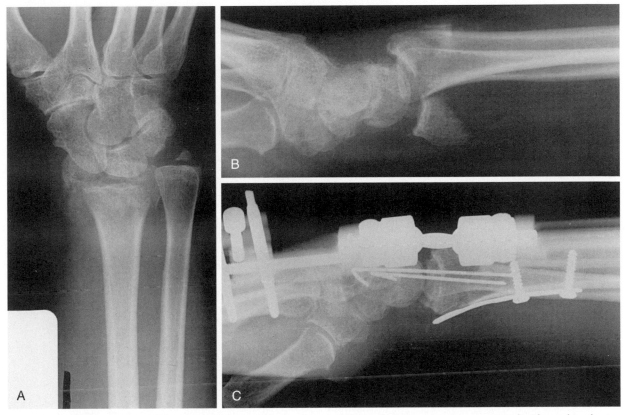

Figure 19–22. *A* and *B,* Type IIB unstable articular fracture with dorsal comminution. *C,* Fracture has been managed with combined external and volar buttress plate fixation. Additional Kirschner wires for the radial styloid fragments.

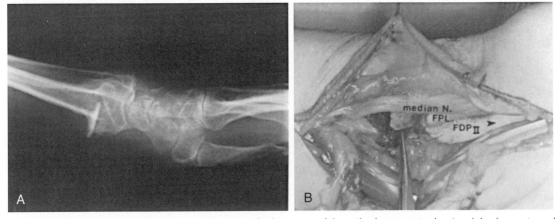

Figure 19–23. *A,* Malunited type III articular fracture. *B,* Persistent displacement of the spike fragment (at the tip of the forceps) resulted in chronic median neuropathy and attrition ruptures of the flexor pollicis longus tendon (FPL) and flexor digitorum profundus tendon of the index finger (FDP II). These soft tissue injuries could have been prevented by an accurate reduction at the time of injury.

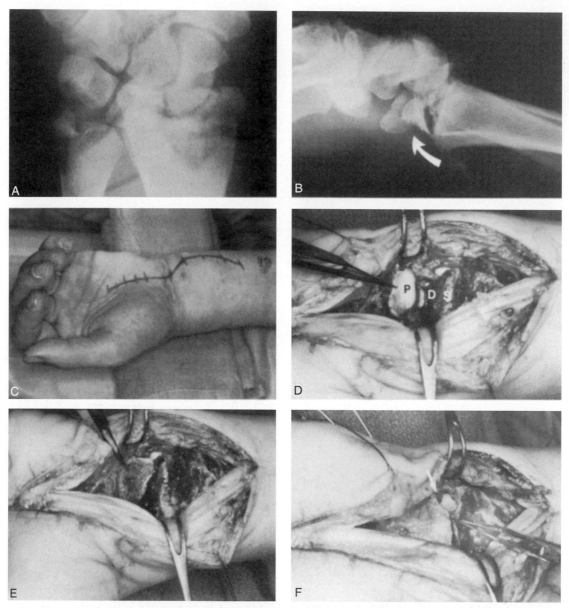

Figure 19–24. Type IV articular fracture demonstrating severe biarticular disruption *(A)* with the palmar medial fragment (at the tip of the *arrow*) rotated 180° *(B)*. An additional small spike fragment (at the base of the *arrow*) is displaced into the flexor compartment. *C*, Open reduction is required for accurate restoration of the articular surfaces and is best achieved through a volar approach that affords direct access to the displaced fragments as well as any damaged soft tissues. *D*, Exposure of the wrist demonstrates wide separation of the medial complex; *(D)*, dorsal medial fragment with the articular surface of the palmar fragment *(P)* facing the radial shaft *(S)* rather than the lunate). *E* and *F*, Precise reduction, achieved by derotation of the palmar medial fragment (at the tip of the forceps), is the key step in restitution of radiocarpal and radioulnar joint congruity. Note the anatomically repositioned ulnar head *(arrow)* within the reconstituted sigmoid notch.

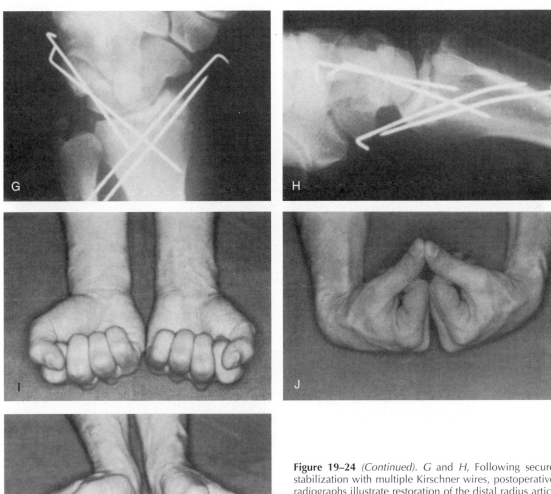

Figure 19–24 *(Continued). G* and *H,* Following secure stabilization with multiple Kirschner wires, postoperative radiographs illustrate restoration of the distal radius articulations. *I,* Seven months after surgery, the injured wrist *(right)* displays minimal deformity with a highly functional recovery of palmar flexion *(J)* and dorsiflexion *(K).*

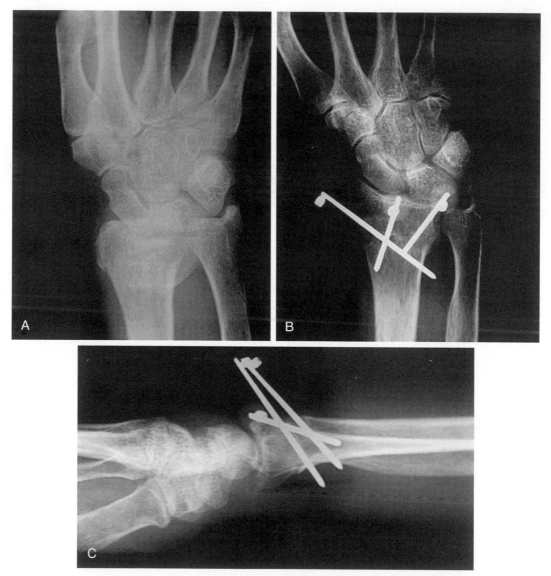

Figure 19–25. *A,* Displaced extra-articular fracture. *B* and *C,* Alignment has been restored with intrafocal Kirschner wires.

to consistent patterns of articular disruption with readily identified radiographic signs of instability and reducibility. Treatment-oriented classifications have replaced the once popular eponymic grouping of these diverse injuries. Recognition of fracture instability and irreducibility based on the radiographic evaluation of fragment comminution and displacement as well as articular congruity is the focus of current classifications. A clear consensus exists that malunion, especially with articular incongruity, is likely to result in a severe compromise in functional recovery. Although closed reduction with cast immobilization remains a reliable standard of treatment for stable and minimally displaced articular fractures, similar management for unstable articular disruption is prone to failure. Prompt awareness of fracture displacement, instability, and reducibility coupled with precision treatment tailored to each fracture pattern undoubtedly can lessen the multitude of complications so commonly associated with distal radius fractures.

The most commonly encountered type II unstable die-punch fracture requires stabilization, provided by external fixation frequently coupled with percutaneous internal fixation, to maintain an accurate reduction. Restoration of articular congruity in an irreducible type IIB dorsal die-punch fracture, in contrast, can be accomplished only by open treatment, usually consisting of a limited exposure for reduction and internal fixation of the radiocarpal articular surface, supplementary external fixation, and adjunctive iliac bone grafting. The irreducible type IIB articular fracture with volar displacement is most suitable for stabilization by plate-and-screw fixation; however, in patients with excessive comminution, Kirschner wires provide a satisfactory alternative method of fixation. The type III fracture spike fragment is secured with either small screws or wires in conjunction with closed or limited open articular restitution and appropriate nerve and tendon surgery. The irreducible type IV fracture demonstrating wide separation of articular components always requires extensive open treatment for restoration of articular congruity as well as repair of associated skeletal and soft tissue injuries. In the type V explosion injury, provisional stabilization employing external fixation provides a sturdy framework for critical revascularization or resurfacing procedures and serves to maintain radial alignment before definitive articular reconstruction.

In more severe injuries, early detection and repair of the frequently occurring periarticular injuries are essential for a favorable recovery. In those fractures requiring open reduction with internal fixation, supplementary external fixation and iliac crest bone grafting have proved to be increasingly beneficial adjuncts to management. In all cases, preservation of articular congruity with precise restoration of key articular fragments is the principal prerequisite for a successful outcome.

References

1. Abbaszadegan H, Jonsson U, vonSivers K: Prediction of instability of Colles' fractures. Acta Orthop Scand 60:646, 1989.
2. Agee JM: External fixation: Technical advances based upon multiplanar ligamentotaxis. Orthop Clin North Am 24:265, 1993.
3. Aro HT, Koivunen T: Minor axial shortening of the radius affects outcome of Colles' fracture treatment. J Hand Surg 16A:392, 1991.
4. Axelrod TS, McMurtry RY: Open reduction and internal fixation of comminuted, intraarticular fractures of the distal radius. J Hand Surg 15A:1, 1990.
5. Axelrod T, Paley D, Green J, et al: Limited open reduction of the lunate facet in comminuted intraarticular fractures of the distal radius. J Hand Surg 13A:38, 1988.
6. Bartosh RA, Saldana MJ: Intraarticular fractures of the distal radius: A cadaveric study to determine if ligamentotaxis restores radiopalmar tilt. J Hand Surg 15A:18, 1990.
7. Bass RL, Blair WF, Hubbard PP: Results of combined internal and external fixation for the treatment of severe AO-C3 fractures of the distal radius. J Hand Surg 20A:373, 1995.
8. Bassett RL: Displaced intraarticular fractures of the distal radius. Clin Orthop 214:148, 1987.
9. Bradway JK, Amadio PC, Cooney WP: Open reduction and internal fixation of displaced, comminuted intra-articular fractures of the distal end of the radius. J Bone Joint Surg 71A:839, 1989.
10. Carrozzella J, Stern PJ: Treatment of comminuted distal radius fractures with pins and plaster. Hand Clin 4:391, 1988.
11. Chapman DR, Bennett JB, Bryan WJ, et al: Complications of distal radius fractures: Pins and plaster treatment. J Hand Surg 7:509, 1982.
12. Clancey GJ: Percutaneous Kirschner-wire fixation of Colles fractures. J Bone Joint Surg 66A:1008, 1984.
13. Clyburn TA: Dynamic external fixation for comminuted intra-articular fractures of the distal end of the radius. J Bone Joint Surg 69A:248, 1987.
14. Cooney WP: External fixation of distal radius fractures. Clin Orthop 214:148, 1987.
15. Cooney WP, Agee JM, Hastings H, et al: Symposium: Management of intraarticular fractures of the distal radius. Contemp Orthop 21:71, 1990.
16. Cooney WP, Linscheid RL, Dobyns JH: External pin fixation for unstable Colles' fractures. J Bone Joint Surg 61A:840, 1979.
17. DeOliveira JC: Barton's fractures. J Bone Joint Surg 55A:586, 1973.
18. Edwards G: Intraarticular fractures of the distal part of the radius treated with the small AO external fixator. J Bone Joint Surg 73A:1241, 1991.
19. Fernandez DL: A practical, simplified, comprehensive and treatment oriented classification of fractures of the distal radius. Presented at the 4th International Federation of Societies for Surgery of the Hand, Bone and Joint Injuries Committee, Paris, May, 1992.
20. Fernandez DL, Geissler WB: Treatment of displaced articular fractures of the radius. J Hand Surg 16A:375, 1991.
21. Frykman G: Fractures of the distal radius, including sequelae of shoulder-hand syndrome: Disturbance of the distal radioulnar joint and impairment of nerve function: A clinical and experimental study. Acta Orthop Scand Suppl 108:1, 1973.
22. Gartland JJ JR, Werley CW: Evaluation of healed Colles' fractures. J Bone Joint Surg 33A:895, 1951.
23. Greatting MD, Bishop AT: Intrafocal (Kapandji) pinning of unstable fractures of the distal radius. Orthop Clin North Am 24:301, 1993.
24. Green DP: Pins and plaster treatment of comminuted fractures of the distal end of the radius. J Bone Joint Surg 57A:304, 1975.
25. Hastings H, Leibovic S: Indications and techniques of open reduction and internal fixation of distal radius fractures. Orthop Clin North Am 24:309, 1993.
26. Jenkins NH: The unstable Colles' fracture. J Hand Surg 14B:149, 1989.
27. Johnston GHF, Friedman L, Kriegler JC: Computerized tomographic evaluation of acute distal radial fractures. J Hand Surg 17A:738, 1992.
28. Knirk JL, Jupiter JB: Intra-articular fractures of the distal end of the radius in young adults. J Bone Joint Surg 68A:647, 1986.

29. Leibovic SJ, Geissler WB: Treatment of complex intra-articular distal radius fractures. Orthop Clin North Am 25:685, 1994.

30. Leung KS, Shen WY, Leung PC, et al: Ligamentotaxis and bone grafting for comminuted fractures of the distal radius. J Bone Joint Surg 71B:838, 1989.

31. Lindstrom A: Fractures of the distal end of the radius: A clinical and statistical study of end results. Acta Orthop Scand Suppl 41:1, 1959.

32. Melone CP Jr: Articular fractures of the distal radius. Orthop Clin North Am 15:217, 1984.

33. Melone CP Jr: Open treatment for displaced articular fractures of the distal radius. Clin Orthop 202:103, 1986.

34. Melone CP Jr: Distal radius fractures: Patterns of articular fragmentation. Orthop Clin North Am 24:239, 1993.

35. Metz VM, Gilula LA: Imaging techniques for distal radius fractures and related injuries. Orthop Clin North Am 24:217, 1993.

36. Missakian ML, Cooney WP, Amadio PC, et al: Open reduction and internal fixation for distal radius fractures. J Hand Surg 17A:745, 1992.

37. Muller ME, Nazarian S, Koch P: Classification AO der Fracturen. Berlin, Springer, 1987.

38. Palmer AK, Short WH, Werner FW, et al: A biomechanical study of distal radius fractures. J Hand Surg 12A:529, 1987.

39. Pruitt DL, Gilula LA, Manske PR, et al: Computed tomography scanning with image reconstruction in evaluation of distal radius fractures. J Hand Surg 19A:720, 1994.

40. Raskin KB, Melone CP Jr: Unstable articular fractures of the distal radius: Comparative techniques of ligamentotaxis. Orthop Clin North Am 24:275, 1993.

41. Scheck M: Long-term follow-up treatment of comminuted fractures of the distal end of the radius by transfixation with Kirschner wires and cast. J Bone Joint Surg 44A:337, 1962.

42. Seitz WH, Froimson AI, Leb R, et al: Augmented external fixation of unstable distal radius fractures. J Hand Surg 16A:1010, 1991.

43. Seitz WH, Putnam MD, Dick HM: Limited open surgical approach for external fixation of distal radius fractures. J Hand Surg 15A:288, 1990.

44. Sommerkamp TG, Seeman M, Silliman J: Dynamic external fixation of unstable fractures of the distal part of the radius. J Bone Joint Surg 76A:1149, 1994.

45. Sprenger TR: Anterior margin articular fractures of the distal radius. J Orthop Trauma 7:6, 1993.

46. Szabo RM, Weber SC: Comminuted intraarticular fractures of the distal radius. Clin Orthop 230:39, 1988.

47. Thomas FB: Reduction of Smith's fracture. J Bone Joint Surg 39B:463, 1957.

48. Trumble TE, Schmitt SR, Vedder NB: Factors affecting functional outcome of displaced intra-articular distal radius fractures. J Hand Surg 19A:325, 1994.

49. Weber SC, Szabo RM: Severely comminuted distal radius fractures as an unsolved problem: Complications associated with external fixation and pins and plaster techniques. J Hand Surg 11A:157, 1986.

CHAPTER 20

Distal Radius Malunion

Steven R. Novotny, MD and David M. Lichtman, MD

Of distal radius malunion, Colles[1] stated "the deformity will remain undiminished throughout life, the limb will at some remote period again enjoy perfect freedom in all its motions and be completely exempt from pain." It may be true that a number of patients will obtain acceptable function and limited discomfort despite residual deformity; these patients often represent an older population with fewer functional demands. Bacorn and Kurtzke,[2] in reviewing more than 2100 distal radius fractures, showed only 3 percent without permanent disability and a significant correlation between an increasing residual deformity and subsequent disability. In their review of the literature, Amadio and Botte[3] found a malunion rate ranging from 12 to 70 percent for immobilization alone. In the 4056 cases reported in the review, the aggregate malunion rate was 23.5 percent. The malunion rate for the patients undergoing operative intervention ranged from 0 to 33 percent, averaging 10.1 percent of the 417 cases reported.

Three radiographic measurements are commonly used to assess the anatomy of the distal radius.[4–7] The palmar tilt is measured in the sagittal view and is approximately 11° (Fig. 20–1).[5] Radial inclination is measured on posterior to anterior radiographs and averages 22° (Fig. 20–2).[4, 5, 7, 8] Radial length can be measured along the longitudinal axis of the radius. It is the distance between the tip of the radial styloid and the ulnar head articular surface. Radial length averages 11 to 12 mm (Fig. 20–3).[5, 8, 9] Radial width can be an important measurement in assessing malunion. Van der Linden[10] measured the distance between the radius's longitudinal axis and the lateral aspect of the radial styloid. This distance can indicate the amount of radial translation requiring correction (Fig. 20–4).

Distal radius fractures not only change the radiocarpal relationships but also affect the distal radioulnar joint (DRUJ) and the ulnocarpal articulation. The DRUJ's stability is dependent on the triangular fibrocartilage complex (TFCC) and the geometry of the radioulnar articulation.[11] This can be severely affected by radial malunion. Palmer and Werner[12] defined the TFCC and showed that it is a major stabilizer of the DRUJ. Experimental data showed that approximately 80 percent of the axial load is borne by the distal radius and 20 percent by the distal ulna.[13] Ulnar variance did not affect the force transmitted through the ulna, but radial shortening or ulnar lengthening dramatically altered the ulnocarpal load.[14]

There is no agreed-upon definition of distal radius malunion to guide the treating surgeon. This situation is probably fostered by the observation that not all nonanatomically aligned fractures result in a poor functioning outcome and, conversely, not all anatomically realigned fractures obtain a good result.[4, 5, 8, 9, 15] The patient's symptoms, not the malunion itself, become the indications for treatment. Pain can be from the radiocarpal joint, DRUJ, ulnocarpal joint, or midcarpal articulations. Restricted motions result from radiocarpal malalignment and DRUJ disruption. Malunion after a Colles' fracture is usually multidirectional. In dorsally displaced fractures, the distal fragment is usually shortened and supinated; in palmarly displaced fractures, the distal structures are also proximally displaced and pronated. Radial short-

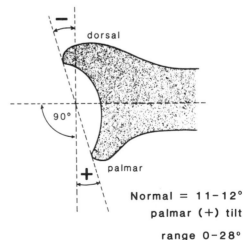

PALMAR TILT

Normal = 11–12°

palmar (+) tilt

range 0–28°

RADIAL LENGTH

Figure 20–1. The palmar tilt is measured in the sagittal plane and averages 11 to 12 degrees. (From Jupiter JB, Masem M: Reconstruction of post-traumatic deformity of the distal radius and ulna. Hand Clinics 4:377–390, 1988.)

RADIAL INCLINATION

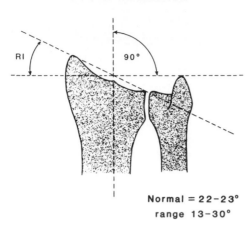

Normal = 22-23°
range 13-30°

Figure 20–2. The radial inclination *(RI)*, measured in the frontal plane is 22° to 23°. (From Jupiter JB, Masem M: Reconstruction of post-traumatic deformity of the distal radius and ulna. Hand Clinics 4:377–390, 1988.)

RADIAL SHIFT

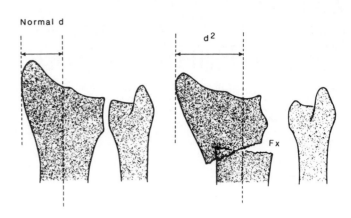

Figure 20–4. Radial shift measures the translation of the radius in the frontal plane. d = distance from radius longitudinal axis to radial styloid; d^2 = postinjury distance from radius longitudinal axis to radial styloid; Fx = fracture. (From Jupiter JB, Masem M: Reconstruction of post-traumatic deformity of the distal radius and ulna. Hand Clinics 4:377–390, 1988.)

ening leads to distal radioulnar joint instability. Significant alterations in grip strength are also reported besides restricted motion and deformity.

Villar and associates[16] followed 90 consecutive Colles' fracture patients for 3 years. Persistent dorsal tilt after 1 week was associated with late loss of flexion and supination. The most significant parameter to affect grip strength was radial shortening, which also affected the final range of motion. Jenkins and Mintowt-Czyz[17] came to a different conclusion after analysis of their 61 patients with 1 to 3 years of follow-up. They concluded that recovery of grip strength is related to residual radial inclination and dorsal angulation deformity, not to radial shortening

as previously proposed.[16] They did identify radial shortening as an important determinant of long-term pain.

Reduced grip strength is commonly reported as a complication of distal radius fracture. O'Driscoll and associates[18] measured grip strength in various wrist positions. In their subjects, the self-selected position of maximum grip strength was 35° of extension and 7° of ulnar deviation. Grip strength was significantly less in any position that deviated from this self-selected position. These researchers also showed that the position for maximal grip is influenced by the object size. The wrist would tend toward flexion if grasping large objects and extension for smaller objects. Lamoreaux and Hoffer[19] studied the effect of

RADIAL LENGTH

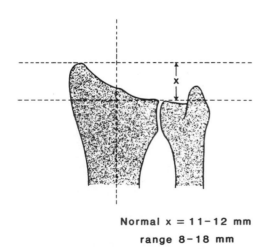

Normal x = 11-12 mm
range 8-18 mm

Figure 20–3. The radial length *(x)* is measured in the frontal plane, and it averages 11 to 12 mm. (From Jupiter JB, Masem M: Reconstruction of post-traumatic deformity of the distal radius and ulna. Hand Clinics 4:377–390, 1988.)

AXIAL LOAD

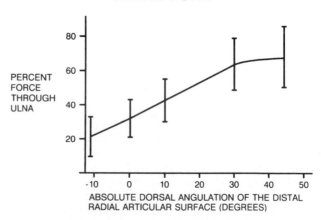

Figure 20–5. Measurement of load transmission across the ulnocarpal joint with increasing dorsal angulation of the distal radius. (From Short WH, Palmer AK, Werner FW, Murphy DJ: A biomechanical study of distal radial fractures. J Hand Surg 12A:529–534, 1987.)

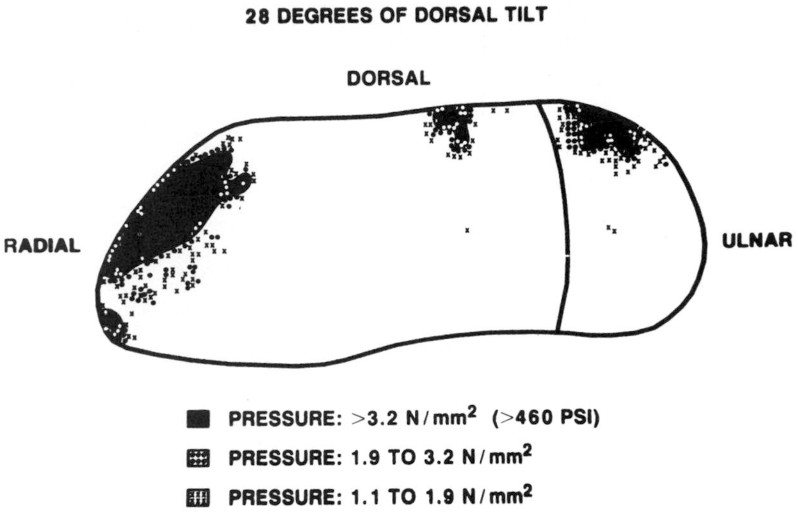

28 DEGREES OF DORSAL TILT

Figure 20–6. Computerized plot of pressure-sensitive film readings of the radial articular surface with the radius in the anatomic position. (From Short WH, Palmer AK, Werner FW, Murphy DJ: A biomechanical study of distal radial fractures. J Hand Surg 12A:529–534, 1987.)

■ PRESSURE: >3.2 N/mm² (>460 PSI)

▦ PRESSURE: 1.9 TO 3.2 N/mm²

▦ PRESSURE: 1.1 TO 1.9 N/mm²

maximal radial and ulnar deviations on grip strength and reported that these positions significantly diminish grip strength compared with the neutral position. Their work supports the use of realignment procedures to increase grip strength for maladies that result in wrist deviation deformities.

Mechanical studies in cadaver specimens using pressure-sensitive film have provided great insight into the changes in force transmission that occur across the radiocarpal and ulnocarpal joints with distal radius angulation. Short and coworkers[20] demonstrated that the pressure across the radioscaphoid and ulnocarpal joints was located more dorsally, and the radiolunate pressure decreased, with a 20° dorsal radius angulation from the original palmar tilt position (Figs. 20–5 to 20–8). With further dorsal angulation, the pressure centrum moves further dorsally, and the pressure area concentrates. With a 30° change in dorsal angulation, 50 percent of the load is borne by the ulna, which reaches a maximum of 65 percent at a 50° change in dorsal radius angulation. These findings were corroborated by Pogue and associates,[21] who simulated distal radius malunions and also varied radial inclination and radial shortening in their experimental model. They showed that with a reduction in radial inclination to 0, the scaphoid fossa contact area significantly decreased. Radial inclination measured at 10° and 0° showed an increased contact area in the lunate fossa. Radial shortening did not affect the scaphoid pressure contact area, but all tested positions of radial shortening showed a larger lunate pressure contact area. Shortening of 6 to 8 mm resulted in ulnar impingement of the lunate. A very interesting observation was that shortening beyond 4 mm, 0° radial inclination, 30° palmar inclination, or 15° dorsal inclination were not obtainable without an ulna styloid fracture or a complete TFCC disruption. Miyake and colleagues,[22] using pressure-sensitive film and finite element analysis, confirmed that the pressure shifts dorsally and the pressure area concentrates when 30° of dorsal angulation is reached. These three studies suggest that the load

Figure 20–7. Computerized pressure-sensitive film readings plotted with the distal radius articular surface tilted 39° dorsally from the anatomic position. The pressure areas concentrate and shift dorsally. (From Short WH: Palmer AK, Werner FW, Murphy DJ: A biomechanical study of distal radial fractures. J Hand Surg 12A:529–534, 1987.)

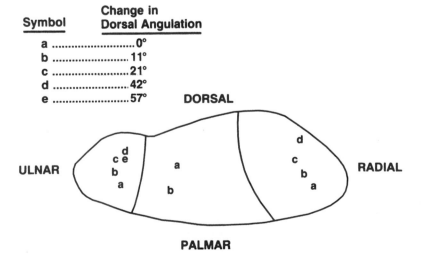

Symbol	Change in Dorsal Angulation
a	0°
b	11°
c	21°
d	42°
e	57°

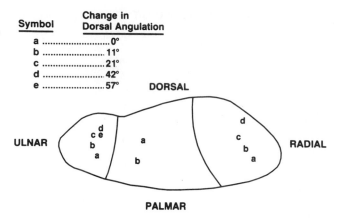

Symbol	Change in Dorsal Angulation
a	0°
b	11°
c	21°
d	42°
e	57°

Figure 20–8. Pressure centrums of the ulnocarpal, radioscaphoid, and radiolunate joints are diagramed and illustrated through a varying range of distal radius angulation. (From Short WH, Palmer AK, Werner FW, Murphy DJ: A biomechanical study of distal radial fractures. J Hand Surg 12A:529–534, 1987.)

shift and the load concentration changes may account for the symptoms seen in distal radius malunion.[20–22]

Taleisnik and Watson[7] described another cause of wrist pain after malunion of the distal radius. Their younger, more active patients developed a midcarpal instability pattern after their fractures had healed in malposition. These researchers believe that loss of the distal articular surface palmar tilt predisposes the carpus to a dorsal collapse pattern. This instability led in their study to a mechanical synovitis in the midcarpal joint, subsequent pain, and a weak grip.[7] Bickenstaff and Bell[23] prospectively followed 32 Colles' fracture patients for 1 to 3 years for evidence of carpal malalignment. They found significant correlation with respect to carpal alignment measurement and clinical outcome. They showed the most significant indication of a poor result to be the extent of carpal malalignment as measured by the radial tilt and radiolunate, lunatocapitate, and scapholunate angles. As the distal radial articular surface angulates dorsally, the lunate contact area translates dorsally. The angular relationship between the radial articular surface and the longitudinal axis of the lunate remains essentially unchanged. To rebalance the radiocarpal mechanical alignment, the capitate will flex on the lunate. This functionally produces a dorsal intercalary segment instability (DISI) pattern in the carpus, though not a true DISI, because the lunate has not rotated dorsally on the distal radius articular surface. Taleisnik and Watson[7] suggest that dorsal instability is the cause of morbidity after Colles' fracture, not an association. The instability develops as a response to the gradual loss of radial tilt during plaster immobilization and subsequent remodeling, and it is much more common than identified by others.[7]

TREATMENT CONSIDERATIONS

Throughout the years, a number of procedures and variations of the procedures have been proposed to correct the symptoms or the deformity of a malunited distal radius fracture. The surgical options include osteotomy aimed at restoring normal anatomic relationships. Another option is one of the ulnar carpal unloading procedures, such as the Darrach distal radius resection or Milch ulnar cuff resection. Arthrodesis can be employed in a limited or total fashion. A combination of these procedures can be used, depending on the patient's pathoanatomy and symptoms.

Darrach,[24] in 1913, described the treatment of a malpositioned Colles' fracture by distal ulnar resection. Darrach[24] held that the operation was indicated in old cases of fractures of the distal radius when the range of motion of the wrist and forearm was impeded secondary to the relative lengthening of the ulnar from radial shortening and angulations. Milch[25] proposed the ulnar cuff resection as a means of reducing the residual wrist deformity and symptoms. Dingman[26] reported on the long-term evaluation of 24 patients after a Darrach procedure. Seventy-five percent of the patients obtained a good or excellent result. Dingman[26] did note that excessive resection of the ulna could lead to a poor result, and he recommended that only the amount of bone that would allow the distal ulna to lie adjacent to the sigmoid notch should be removed. He also recommended that the ulnar styloid process and the ulnar collateral ligament be left attached. Af Ekenstam and colleagues[27] were able to follow 24 of 27 patients treated for distal radius malunion by a distal ulnar resection. They found that 50 percent of the patients had no improvement from the procedure. A subset of the patients with DRUJ arthrosis was identified who did obtain relief. Osteophyte formation and a reduction of the articular cartilage joint space were the radiographic parameters used to diagnose arthrosis. Eight of the 11 patients with radiographic evidence of DRUJ degenerative changes were helped by the operation. Only 4 of the 13 without degenerative change on radiography experienced relief. Af Ekenstam and colleagues[27] suggest that resection of the distal end of the ulna is probably indicated only when the distal radioulnar joint shows signs of arthrosis.

Corrective osteotomy of the distal radius for malunion and its sequelae has been described in case reports and in small series since the early 1900s.[28–30] Durman[31] in 1935 reported four cases of corrective osteotomy using a dorsoradial approach and an appropriately shaped wedge bone graft obtained from the distal radius to maintain the reduction. Campbell[32] in 1937 reported that he had performed 19 osteotomies of the distal radius. He used a lateral incision and an opening wedge osteotomy. A longitudinal wedge of prominent distal ulna was harvested and placed into the osteotomy defect. Eleven of the 19 patients were followed, all of whom had excellent results. Speed and Knight[33] continued Campbell's work. They reported on 60 malunited Colles' fractures that underwent surgical correction. Though they did not report on the results, they did use a variety of surgical procedures and concluded that no single type of corrective procedure was applicable in all instances.

Fernandez[34] described an opening wedge metaphyseal osteotomy that combines the use of a bone graft and rigid internal fixation to allow early unrestricted range of motion. The operation was contraindicated in the presence of advanced degenerative radiocarpal or intracarpal changes, fixed carpal malalignment, or disabling trophic residuals. A Darrach procedure also was employed if radial shortening exceeded 12 mm, if degenerative changes were identified in the DRUJ, and if the distal ulna was unstable.

Fernandez[34] reported on 20 patients with malunited distal radius fractures treated with his technique. Seventy-five percent of the 20 patients had a good or excellent result. Three of the 5 patients with resection of the distal ulna had unsatisfactory results. Fernandez[34] noted that 9 of 10 patients in whom preoperative radial shortening was less than 6 mm had normal preoperative supination and pronation. Ten of the 20 patients whose average preoperative radial shortening was 12.6 mm had significant preoperative reduction in supination and pronation. Nine of the 10 had restoration of normal forearm rotation with correction of the radial length. Fernandez[34] judged that the deformity became symptomatic with 25° to 30° of sagittal or frontal plane angulation and with a radial length discrepancy of 6 mm or greater. He recommended these parameters as guidelines for selecting surgical candidates, who usually are young, manually active patients.

Af Ekenstam and colleagues[35] reviewed 39 symptomatic patients treated by distal radius osteotomy. All patients demonstrated DRUJ instability clinically, and all patients related some improvement in their symptoms. Thirty-six of the 39 were judged as having a good or an excellent result at follow-up. Thirty-five patients had pain referable to the DRUJ preoperatively. Twenty-four patients underwent a concurrent stabilization procedure for an unstable DRUJ. This included reattachment of the TFCC to the fovea, osteosynthesis of the ulnar styloid, or a combination of the two. Six patients treated with a TFCC reconstruction had a persistently unstable DRUJ, but 5 of these had a residual radial malangulation of 10° to 15°. Af Ekenstam and colleagues[34] make the case that correction of radial malangulation was particularly important to give satisfactory clinical results. The inclination of the sigmoid notch should be approximately 20°, corresponding to the ulnar head inclination. TFCC stabilization is reserved for persistent instability after correction of the malangulation and is not a prerequisite if normal DRUJ geometry is restored.

Fernandez[36] in 1988 reported on 15 patients with distal radius malunion and predominantly DRUJ symptoms, including limited forearm rotation. All patients underwent distal radius osteotomy[34] with the addition of a Bower's hemiresection interposition arthroplasty.[37] He believed this was indicated as a primary procedure on the basis of review of cases treated by osteotomy alone. Approximately 50 percent of the patients subsequently required an additional ulnar-sided procedure. All of the 15 patients treated by osteotomy and partial ulnar resection demonstrated improved rotation and stability of the DRUJ as well as satisfactory relief of pain. On the basis of this experience, Fernandez[36] believed that partial ulnar head resection should be performed primarily in combination with a radial osteotomy when either limited forearm rotation secondary to pain or degenerative DRUJ changes exist preoperatively.

Watson and Castle[38] reported on a series of osteotomies using distal radius trapezoidal bone graft and Kirschner (K) wire fixation. The K wires "cage" the graft in place. These results are comparable to those in patients treated with rigid internal fixation and iliac crest bone graft. The technique has the advantages of avoiding disruption of extensor retinaculum, enabling the removal of hardware in the office, and treating the patients on an outpatient basis. Roesgen and Hierholzen[39] followed 70 of 82 patients treated with osteotomies. Eighty percent of the patients underwent corrective surgery within 6 months of the initial fracture. Early correction of the deformity did not impair the result. The surgeon must be prepared to perform an ulnar shortening or equivalent procedure if the radial length cannot be restored by osteotomy and interposition bone graft.[40, 41] Posner and Ambrose[42] proposed a biplanar closing wedge osteotomy without bone graft. Resection of the ulna head and decompression of the median nerve were done to eliminate the potential for further surgical intervention. Kwasny and associates[43] showed successful resolution of median neuropathy in 12 of 13 patients by correcting the malunion alone. One patient required carpal ligament release 6 months after the osteotomy because of persistent symptoms.

Fernandez,[34] among others, has advocated preoperative planning with three-dimensional models of the bone graft. Most surgeons recognize that this can be a difficult and inexact exercise at times. Jupiter and associates[44] have used computer-assisted design and manufacturing technology to create solid models of the malunited and normal radius in complex, multidirectional malunions. They believed that, besides providing a "hands-on" exercise, use of this technology enables the size and shape of the bone graft to be predetermined and the internal fixation to be templated preoperatively. This can, however, be an expensive and time-consuming process; it may best be saved for complex deformities or for the generation of an educational series of saw bones for laboratory training. Jupiter and associates[44] report having treated five patients with such techniques. Bilic and colleagues[45] developed a computer-aided preoperative planning method that provides a three-dimensional "wire" model. From these models, the graft size and shape can be predetermined. These researchers reported good results in 27 patients treated with this method.

TECHNIQUES

Fernandez Technique

To perform an opening wedge osteotomy of the distal radius for malunion, make the incision volar if the distal fragment is volarly angulated or dorsal if the fragment is dorsally angulated. The volar approach is the distal limb of Henry's extensile exposure.[46] Make the skin incision radial to the flexor carpi radialis (FCR). Start a 10-cm longitudinal incision at the level of the radial styloid and bring it proximally. Retract the radial artery radially and the FCR ulnarly. Dissect the radial attachment of the pronator quadratus subperiosteally and reflect it ulnarly. Once the radius is exposed, the planning of the osteotomy, the bone grafting, and the internal fixation are the same as for the dorsal approach.

For the dorsal approach, make a 10-cm longitudinal incision in line with Lister's tubercle, extending 2 cm distal to it. Either release the extensor pollicis longus tendon from its compartment or reflect it subperiosteally radially by sharp dissection. Reflect the fourth dorsal compartment ulnarly to expose the distal radius. Identify the posterior interosseous nerve either in the fourth compartment or on the interosseous membrane proximally, and resect it if indicated. Remove Lister's tubercle to provide a flat surface for the plate.

To control the planes of the osteotomy and monitor the plane of correction, use intraoperative guides to provide for reproducible articulation realignment (Fig. 20–9). Place a 0.045-inch K wire perpendicularly through the radius 4 cm proximal to the planned osteotomy site. Hand place a free K wire in the radiocarpal joint to reference the angulation of that joint. Drive a second K wire into the distal radius, deviating 5° to 10° from the intra-articular wire. Then transect the radius 1.5 to 2.5 cm proximal to the radiocarpal joint parallel to the distal radius K wire. Manipulate the distal K wire parallel to the proximal K wire to correct the radiocarpal sagittal plane tilt. If radial length or radial inclination needs correction, use a cervical lamina spreader or a small AO distractor to distract the osteotomy site. Obtain posteroanterior and lateral radiographs to confirm the radiocarpal and DRUJ alignment. Fashion a tricortical iliac crest bone graft to hold the reduction. Use cancellous graft to fill in the remaining defect. Contour a T-shaped buttress plate to fit the radius, maintaining the corrected alignment and holding the bone graft in place (Fig. 20–10).

The options of internal fixation have been expanded with the introduction of a low-profile, countersunk distal radius plate. The plate design includes recessed screw holes that eliminate protruding screw heads and potential tendon irritation. The templating system allows the plate's countersunk screw-hole design to lie flush on the dorsal cortex. This feature may decrease the frequency of symptoms that necessitate removal of hardware.

Watson Technique

Watson's technique corrects distal radial malangulation through a dorsal osteotomy. We utilize the longitudinal dorsal incision, though Watson describes a different approach. In the Watson technique, make a transverse skin incision 3 cm proximal to the radial styloid. Next, elevate the periosteum around the radius proximal to the retinaculum. Place two K wires perpendicular to each other, one proximal and one distal to the osteotomy site. Make an osteotomy 1 to 1.5 cm proximal to the radiocarpal joint. Manipulate the distal K wire until it subtends the desired 10° angle of palmar tilt. If greater radial inclination is required, open the osteotomy more on the radial side.

Harvest a trapezoidal unicortical wedge graft longitudinally from the center of the distal radius. Radial length cannot be restored unless another source of structural graft is used. Lock the bone graft in place by one or two longitudinal K wires (Fig. 20–11). The K wires "cage" the graft in place by passing volar to the dorsal radius cortex in the proximal and distal radial fragments. The K wires pass dorsally to the cortex of the bone graft, thus "caging" it in place (Fig. 20–12). At 6 weeks, remove the K wires in the office. Use long-arm immobilization for 4 weeks; then apply a short-arm cast for 2 weeks, until K-wire removal. Start range-of-motion exercises at this time.

Authors' Considerations

The algorithms (shown in Fig. 20–13) provide a framework by which to evaluate logically a problem and recommend treatment. The algorithms' limita-

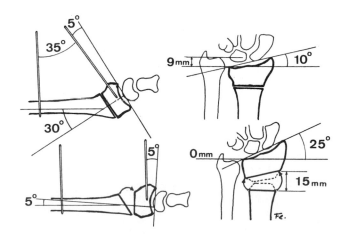

Figure 20–9. *Top left* view demonstrates the K-wire placement to intraoperatively reference the correction of the dorsal tilt. *Bottom left* view shows the sagittal correction after the osteotomy with resultant dorsal bone gap. *Top right,* Precorrection loss of radial inclination and radial shortening. *Bottom right,* Postcorrection alignment demonstrates that the cortex is opened more on the dorsal radial than the dorsal ulnar side. (From Fernandez DL: Correction of post-traumatic wrist deformity in adults by osteotomy, bone grafting, and internal fixation. J Bone Joint Surg 64A:1164–1178, 1982.)

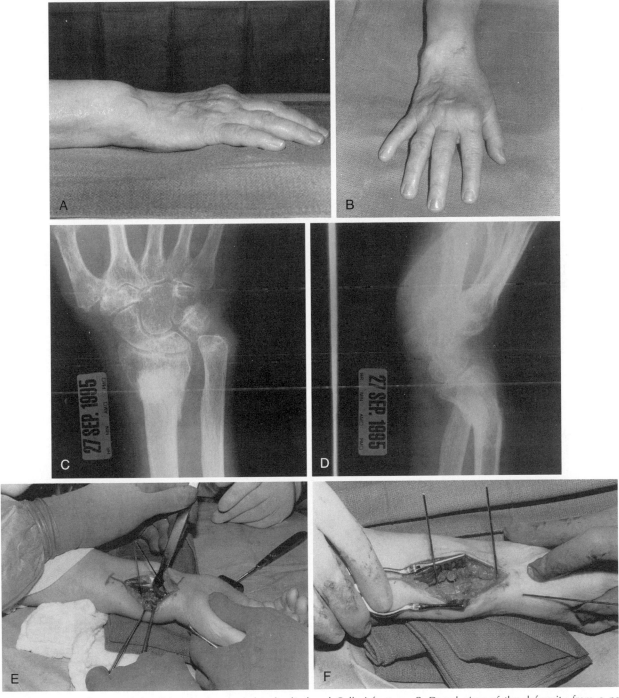

Figure 20–10. *A,* Lateral view of the deformity from a palmarly displaced Colles' fracture. *B,* Dorsal view of the deformity from a palmarly displaced Colles' fracture. *C* and *D,* Preoperative PA and lateral radiographs of the palmarly displaced Colle's fracture. *E,* Intraoperative view of the volar approach with the guide wires in place; proximally, perpendicular to the radius shaft; distally, 5° off parallel to the distal radius articular surface. *F,* Correction of the malposition with tricortical iliac crest graft in place. Notice the K wires are now parallel.

Illustration continued on following page

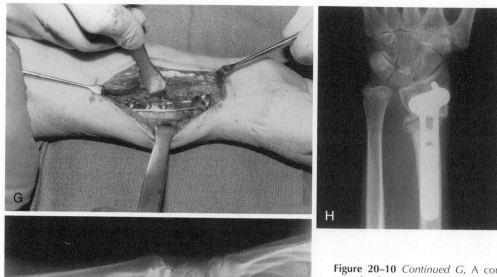

Figure 20–10 *Continued G,* A contoured volar AO buttress plate is applied. *H* and *I,* Postoperative PA and lateral radiographs with the volar plate applied.

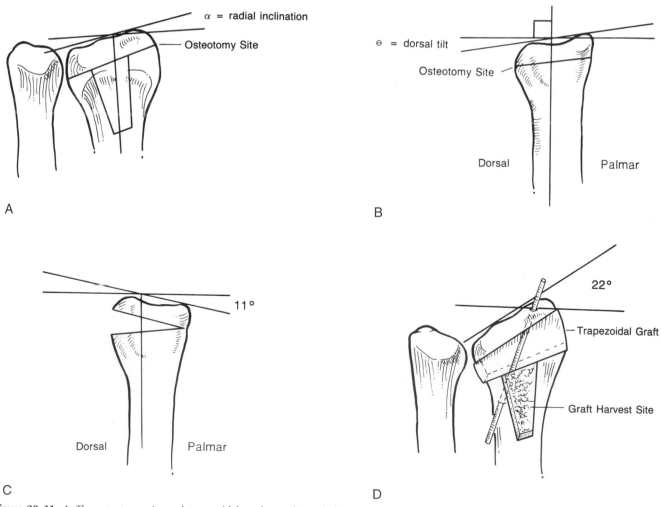

Figure 20–11. *A,* The osteotomy site and trapezoidal wedge graft needed to restore radial inclination. *B,* Sagittal view showing the dorsal tilt of the distal radius articular surface. *C,* After the osteotomy, the dorsal cortex has a trapezoidal wedge defect. *D,* Radial inclination is corrected with the trapezoidal wedge graft obtained from the distal radius, and is fixed by a caging pin. (From Watson HK, Castle TH: Trapezoidal osteotomy of the distal radius for unacceptable articular angulation after Colles' fracture. J Hand Surg 13A:837–843, 1988.)

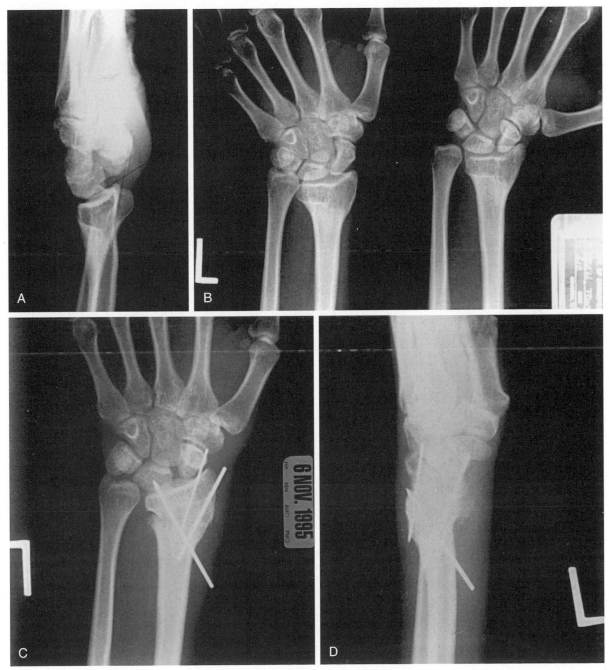

Figure 20–12. *A* and *B*, Preoperative radiographs of a 17-year-old slender female with a symptomatic nonunion of the left distal radius. *C* and *D*, Postoperative radiographs of the same patient. A "caging" technique was used because her subcutaneous tissue would not hide a dorsal plate. Extra K wires were used to provide increased stability for the tricortical iliac crest graft in an attempt to allow protected range of motion before 6 weeks postoperatively. In this case, the caging pin migrated proximally and had to be removed from the dorsal forearm.

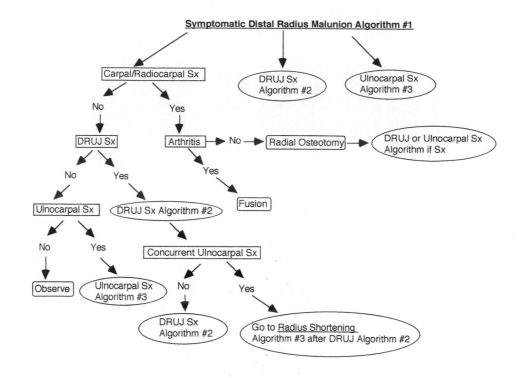

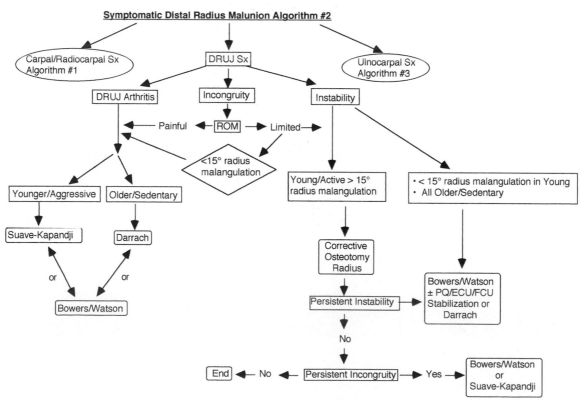

Figure 20–13. *See legend on opposite page*

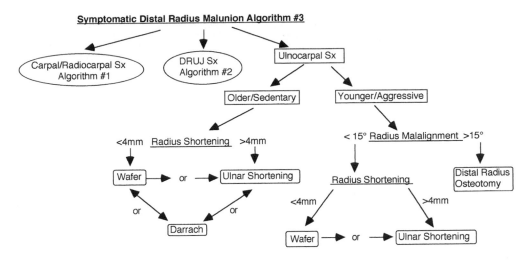

Figure 20–13 *Continued.* Surgical algorithms for patients with carpal or radiocarpal symptoms (Algorithm #1), distal radial-ulnar joint symptoms (Algorithm #2), and ulnocarpal symptoms (Algorithm #3). *DRUJ* = distal radial-ulnar joint; PQ = pronator quadratus; ECU = extensor carpi ulnaris; FCU = flexor carpi ulnaris; ROM = range of motion.

tions are the clinician's ability to localize the area of pathology and the algorithms' inability to account for every unique patient characteristic. Clinical evaluation and surgeon experience combined with patient goals and realistic expectations ultimately guide the treatment plan.

A thorough evaluation includes comparison radiographs of the asymptomatic extremity to help determine normal architecture and relationships. Carpal instability, degenerative changes, and ulnar length variations are easily recognized. Dynamic radiographs or videofluoroscopy occasionally may be employed when dynamic instability is suspected. In selected cases, advanced imaging, such as a computed tomography scan of the DRUJ, may be necessary to determine whether degenerative changes or instability exists. Bone scans can be helpful to isolate areas of increased osseous stress when symptoms are non-localized.

Selective anesthetic blocks often localize the source of the patient's complaints. Lidocaine injection into the DRUJ can differentiate ulnocarpal pain from DRUJ symptoms. A radiocarpal injection can (1) help detect early degenerative arthritis symptoms after an intra-articular fracture and (2) differentiate it from midcarpal synovitis secondary to instability in patients with vague pain complaints.

The age of the patient and the age of the fracture are variables that influence the decision-making process. A more vigorous attempt to restore the anatomy is undertaken in physiologically younger patients with early symptoms than in physiologically older patients with long-standing symptoms or a long-standing malunion with recent complaints. The functional demands of the individual also temper the treatment plans.

Currently, we are using the Fernandez technique to correct palmarly displaced distal radius malunions. In patients with dorsally displaced distal fragments, we employ a variety of techniques. We have used both the Watson and Fernandez techniques, and we usually obtain our bone graft from the iliac crest. The use of iliac crest bone graft enables radial length to be restored if necessary by either technique. In thin people in whom we would expect problems of prominent hardware, we use K-wire fixation (cage technique). If the patient is not expected to have prominent hardware, we fix the osteotomy with a plate. The newer low-profile, minimal-contact dorsal plate may offer a good solution as this plate probably will not need to be removed.

DRUJ malalignment usually responds to corrective osteotomy of the distal radius, as described previously. Radial shortening without other significant malalignment is best treated by ulnar shortening to level the distal radial and ulnar articular surfaces. In elderly patients, a resection arthroplasty of the DRUJ (Darrach procedure) is often the most expedient choice.

If a corrective radial osteotomy fails to restore congruent stability to the DRUJ, most patients require a concurrent hemiresection arthroplasty of the ulna. In the young patient and in patients with high functional demands, such as construction workers, a Suave-Kapandji[47] procedure may be indicated to give the carpus additional support.

Extrinsic midcarpal instability (a painful midcarpal clunk caused by dorsal radius malalignment) can be treated with corrective osteotomy at the fracture site. Symptomatic radiocarpal arthritis secondary to articular step-off may require a proximal row–distal radius fusion. With this procedure, an associated midcarpal malalignment can be corrected by sculpting the distal radial articular surfaces appropriately. If arthritic changes are extensive throughout the carpus, consideration should be given to total wrist fusion.

References

1. Colles A: On the fracture of the carpal extremity of the radius. Edin Med Surg J 10:182–186, 1814.

2. Bacorn RW, Kurtzke JF: Colles' fracture: A study of two thousand cases from the New York State Workmen's Compensation Board. J Bone Joint Surg 35A:643–658, 1953.
3. Amadio PC, Botte MJ: Treatment of malunion of the distal radius. Hand Clinics 3:541–549, 1987.
4. Dowling JJ, Sawyer B: Comminuted Colles' fractures: Evaluation of a method of treatment. J Bone Joint Surg 43A:657–668, 1961.
5. Friberg S, Lundstrom B: Radiographic measurements of the radiocarpal joint in normal adults. Acta Radiol [Diagn] (Stockh) 17:249, 1976.
6. Gartland JJ, Werley CW: Evaluation of healed Colles' fractures. J Bone Joint Surg 33A:895–907, 1951.
7. Taleisnik J, Watson HK: Midcarpal instability caused by malunited fractures of the distal radius. J Hand Surg 9A:350–357, 1984.
8. Scheck M: Long-term follow-up of treatment of comminuted fractures of the distal end of the radius by transfixation with Kirschner wires and cast. J Bone Joint Surg 44A:337–351, 1962.
9. Sarmiento A, Pratt GW, Berry NC, et al: Colles' fractures: Functional bracing in supination. J Bone Joint Surg 57A:311–317, 1975.
10. Van der Linden W, Ericson R: Colles' fracture: How should its displacement be measured and how should it be immobilized? J Bone Joint Surg 63A:1285–1288, 1981.
11. Af Ekenstam FW, Hagert CG: Anatomical studies on the geometry and stability of the distal radioulnar joint. Scand J Plast Reconstr Surg 19:17–25, 1985.
12. Palmer AK, Werner FW: The triangular fibrocartilage complex of the wrist—anatomy and function. J Hand Surg 6A:153–162, 1981.
13. Palmer AK, Werner FW: Biomechanics of the distal radioulnar joint. Clin Orthop 187:26–35, 1984.
14. Werner FW, Palmer AK, Fortino MD, et al: Force transmission through the distal ulna: Effect of ulnar variance, lunate fossa angulation, and radial and palmar tilt of the distal radius. J Hand Surg 17A:423–428, 1992.
15. Lindstrom A: Fractures of the distal end of the radius. Acta Orthop Scand Suppl 41:1–159, 1959.
16. Villar RN, Marsh D, Ruston N, Greatorex RA: Three years after Colles' fracture: A prospective review. J Bone Joint Surg 69B:635–638, 1987.
17. Jenkins NH, Mintowt-Czyz WJ: Mal-union and dysfunction in Colles' fracture. J Hand Surg 13B:291–293, 1988.
18. O'Driscoll SW, Horii E, Ness R, et al: The relationship between wrist position, grasp size, and grip strength. J Hand Surg 17A:169–177, 1992.
19. Lamoreaux L, Hoffer MM: The effect of wrist deviation on grip and pinch strength. Clin Orthop 314:1252–1255, 1995.
20. Short WH, Palmer AK, Werner FW, Murphy DJ: A biomechanical study of distal radial fractures. J Hand Surg 12A:529–534, 1987.
21. Pogue DJ, Viegas SF, Patterson RM, et al: Effects of distal radius fracture malunion on wrist joint mechanics. J Hand Surg 15A:721–727, 1990.
22. Miyake T, Hashizume H, Inoue QS, Nagayama N: Malunited Colles' fracture: Analysis of stress distribution. J Hand Surg 19B:737–742, 1994.
23. Bickenstaff DR, Bell MJ: Carpal malalignment in Colles' fractures. J Hand Surg 14B:155–160, 1989.
24. Darrach W: Partial excision of lower shaft of ulna for deformity following Colles' fracture. Ann Surg 57:764–765, 1913.

25. Milch H: Cuff resection of the ulna for malunited Colles' fracture. J Bone Joint Surg 23:311–313, 1941.
26. Dingman P: Resection of the distal end of the ulna (Darrach operation): An end-result study of twenty-four cases. J Bone Joint Surg 34A:893–900, 1952.
27. Af Ekenstam F, Engkvist O, Wadin K: Results from resection of the distal end of the ulna after fractures of the lower end of the radius. Scand J Plast Reconstr Surg 16:177–181, 1982.
28. Meyerding UW: Malunion of the radius and ulna preventing closing of the hand and flexion of the wrist. Surg Clin North Am 12:874, 1932.
29. Thorton L: A plastic operation for reduction of old transverse fractures of the distal end of the radius, healed with displacement and deformity. Surg Gynecol Obstet 42:844, 1926.
30. Ghormley RK, Mroz RJ: Fractures of the wrist: A review of one hundred and seventy-six cases. Surg Gynecol Obstet 55:377, 1932.
31. Durman DC: An operation for correction of deformities of the wrist following fracture. J Bone Joint Surg 17:1014–1016, 1935.
32. Campbell WC: Malunited Colles' fractures. JAMA 109:1105–1107, 1937.
33. Speed JS, Knight RA: The treatment of malunited Colles' fractures. J Bone Joint Surg 27:261–367, 1945.
34. Fernandez DL: Correction of post-traumatic wrist deformity in adults by osteotomy, bone grafting, and internal fixation. J Bone Joint Surg 64A:1164–1178, 1982.
35. Af Ekenstam F, Hagert CG, Engkvist O, et al: Corrective osteotomy of malunited fracture of the distal end of the radius. Scand J Plast Reconstr Surg 19:175–187, 1985.
36. Fernandez DL: Radial osteotomy and Bower's arthroplasty for malunited fractures of the distal end of the radius. J Bone Joint Surg 70A:1538–1551, 1988.
37. Bowers WH: Distal radioulnar joint arthroplasty: The hemiresection-interposition technique. J Hand Surg 10A:169–178, 1985.
38. Watson HK, Castle TH: Trapezoidal osteotomy of the distal radius for unacceptable articular angulation after Colles' fracture. J Hand Surg 13A:837–843, 1988.
39. Roesgen M, Hierholzen G: Corrective osteotomy of the distal radius after fracture to restore the function of wrist joint, forearm, and hand. Arch Orthop Trauma Surg 107:301–308, 1988.
40. Brown JN, Bill MJ: Distal radial osteotomy for malunion of wrist fractures in young patients. J Hand Surg 19B:589–593, 1994.
41. Hove LM, Mölster AO: Surgery for posttraumatic wrist deformity: Radial osteotomy and/or ulnar shortening in 16 Colles' fractures. Acta Orthop Scand 65:434–438, 1994.
42. Posner MA, Ambrose L: Malunited Colles' fractures: Correction with a biplanar closing wedge osteotomy. J Hand Surg 16A:1017–1021, 1991.
43. Kwasny O, Fuch M, Schabus R: Opening wedge osteotomy for malunion of the distal radius with neuropathy. Acta Orthop Scand 65:207–593, 1994.
44. Jupiter JB, Ruder J, Roth DA: Computer-generated bone models in the planning of osteotomy of multidirectional distal radius malunions. J Hand Surg 17A:106–115, 1992.
45. Bilic R, Zdravkovic V, Boljevic Z: Osteotomy for deformity of the radius: Computer-assisted three-dimensional modeling. J Bone Joint Surg 76B:150–154, 1994.
46. Henry AK: Extensile Exposure, ed 2. Edinburgh, Churchill Livingstone, 1970, pp 100–106.
47. Suave et Kapandji: Nouvelle techniques de traitement chirurgique des luxations recidivantes isolées de l'extremité inferieure du cubitus. J Chir 47:589, 1936.

CHAPTER 21

Disorders of the Distal Radioulnar Joint and Triangular Fibrocartilage Complex: An Overview

Jon B. Loftus, MD, and Andrew K. Palmer, MD

The distal radioulnar joint (DRUJ) and triangular fibrocartilage complex (TFCC) constitute the core of a tremendously complicated area of the wrist. Dr. William Darrach, at the beginning of this century, described an excision of the ulnar head in his classic article, "Anterior Dislocation of the Head of the Ulna."[30, 92] He described the resection being performed to treat chronic dislocation of the distal ulna. The following year, he published a description of partial excision of the lower shaft of the ulna for deformity following Colles' fracture.[32] This latter operation has withstood the test of time and is still often used to treat ulnar impaction due to shortening of the radius following a Colles' fracture. Despite this early work on the DRUJ, the poor understanding of the anatomy and biomechanics of the ulnar side of the wrist has often led to less than satisfactory outcomes in patients with ulnar-sided wrist pain. Yet over the last 10 to 15 years, a surge in research on the distal radioulnar joint and triangular fibrocartilage complex has led to a greater understanding of the biomechanics and pathomechanics of this area of the wrist. From this basic science research have come advances in the diagnostic and therapeutic abilities of the hand surgeon in treating patients with ulnar-sided wrist pain.

The fact that the distal radioulnar joint and the triangular fibrocartilage complex are such complicated structures should not be a surprise, considering that this structure is one of the features that separates the family of Hominoidea, which we belong to, from the lesser-developed animals. The evolutionary demand placed on our ancestors focused on two highly specialized areas, the brain and the hand, with the hand itself having two unique properties—the opposable thumb and the forearm that can prosupinate. Our brains obviously are the most intricate and complex (some, more than others) of all living animals. So, too, has hand development paralleled brain development, and together they allowed humans to "rise above the rest."[3] Deciding whether the evolution of the brain allowed higher development of the hand or vice versa is like arguing about who should be doing hand surgery—plastic or orthopedic surgeons. Unfortu-

nately, we cannot supply the answer here, although it has been debated in the past. Galen had this insight: "Thus, man is the most intelligent of the animals and so also hands are the instruments most suitable for an intelligent animal. For it is not because he has hands that he is the most intelligent as Anaxagoras says but because he is the most intelligent that he has hands as Aristotle says, judging him most correctly."[3, 39] (Obviously, most hand surgeons probably side with Anaxagoras.) Thus, evolutionary and teleologic perspectives offer some insight into the complexity of the distal radioulnar joint and the triangular fibrocartilage complex.

The remaining chapters in this section attempt to elucidate many of the latest advances that have been made in studying the ulnar side of the wrist. This chapter is entitled "An Overview," because we want to stress the importance of studying the distal radioulnar joint and triangular fibrocartilage complex within the context of prosupination. For the purpose of organization, the DRUJ and TFCC are often investigated by authorities in this field as separate entities. We cannot stress too strongly, though, that to truly understand the pathomechanics behind an ulnar-sided wrist problem, one must have an understanding not only of the separate entities in question but also of how the entities interact. As discussed later, this thought includes not only the relationship between the distal radioulnar joint and the triangular fibrocartilage complex but also their relationship to the ulnar carpal joint, the lunotriquetral articulation, the midcarpal joint, the interosseous membrane, and the proximal radioulnar joint. Thus, we urge the reader not only to read each scientific paper but also to treat each clinical problem involving the distal radioulnar joint and triangular fibrocartilage complex within the context of "prosupination." Doing so enhances understanding of this somewhat perplexing area of the body.

ANATOMY AND BIOMECHANICS

As is true in most aspects of surgery, an appreciation of the anatomy of the structure being investigated clinically is the only basis upon which one can build an understanding of the pathomechanics that affect that structure. Knowledge of the distal radioulnar joint and the triangular fibrocartilage complex is no exception to this rule. Furthermore, the DRUJ and the TFCC must be studied as a unit. Anatomically, they are closely associated with each other, and biomechanically, they cannot be studied independently.

Distal Radioulnar Joint

In terms of the entire picture of prosupination, the distal radioulnar joint is very much related to not only the interosseous membrane but also the proximal radioulnar joint. The proximal ulna is the structure that is fixed to the humerus; therefore, in principle, the ulna is the foundation around which the radius and carpus move or prosupinate. It is an actual misnomer to refer to the ulnar head as dislocating or subluxing, because it is the radius that is dislocating or subluxing relative to the ulna. We are all guilty of this error, so we will not belabor the point here. The articulating surfaces of the distal radius and the ulnar head constitute the DRUJ (Fig. 21–1).

The articulating surface of the radius is referred to as the sigmoid notch (Fig. 21–2). It is concave such that it articulates with the convexity of the ulnar head's articulating surface. The ridge separating the lunate facet from the sigmoid notch serves as the origin of the triangular fibrocartilage, with the distinct dorsal and palmar radioulnar ligaments arising from the respective dorsal and palmar aspects of this ridge. The sigmoid notch also has distinct dorsal and palmar borders. Proximally, there is a less distinct margin as it becomes a component of the metaphysis of the radius. Actually, at this level, the sigmoid notch becomes convex compared with the more prominent concavity distally. The portion of the ulnar head that articulates with the sigmoid notch is

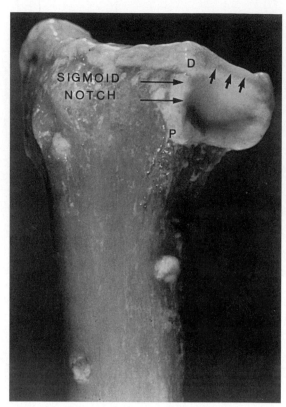

Figure 21–2. Sigmoid notch *(large arrows)* of the radius. The triangular fibrocartilage complex originates from the distal margin *(small arrows)* of the sigmoid notch. *D* = distal; *P* = proximal.

referred to as the "seat," and the articular surface in juxtaposition to the proximal (undersurface) of the TFCC is the "pole." The seat of the ulnar head has approximately 130° of articular convexity.

Articular cartilage covers the ulnar head dorsally, volarly, and radially with respect to its articulation with the sigmoid notch of the radius. The pole of the ulnar head is covered with articular cartilage as well. The ulnar head seat has a radius of curvature of approximately 10 mm. The radius of curvature of the sigmoid notch is approximately 15 mm. The arcs subtend angles of approximately 60° and 105° of the sigmoid notch and ulnar seat, respectively (Fig. 21–3).[35] Thus, the ulnar head and the sigmoid notch obviously are not congruent. These articulating surfaces allow 150° of motion in prosupination by permitting, not only rotation of the radius about the ulnar head, but also a guiding or translational motion of the distal radioulnar joint. Bowers[16] and Pirela-Cruz and colleagues[109] analyzed the translational motion of the DRUJ with computed tomography (CT) analysis. They documented a mean palmar and dorsal translational motion of 2.2 mm in their study of 16 DRUJs in eight normal volunteers. They also documented a motion of the distal radioulnar joint in addition to rotational and translational motion: one of abduction and adduction, referred to as "diastatic motion."[109] The translational motion also has an ef-

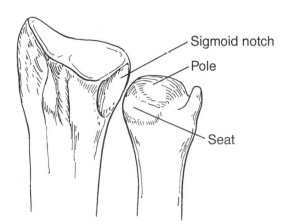

Figure 21–1. The distal radioulnar joint: articulating surfaces of the radius (sigmoid notch) and ulnar head (seat). The pole of the ulnar head is covered with articular cartilage and is juxtaposed to the undersurface of the triangular fibrocartilage complex.

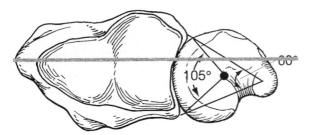

Figure 21–3. The radius of curvature of the seat of the ulna is 10 mm, with the arcs subtending an angle of 105°. The radius of curvature of the sigmoid notch is approximately 15 mm, and the arcs subtend an angle of approximately 60°. Thus, the distal radioulnar joint is not purely congruent. This anatomic feature allows for the translational motion of the ulna within the sigmoid notch during prosupination.

fect on the articulation between the sigmoid notch and the seat of the ulnar head. In the neutral position, approximately 70° of the 130° articular surface of the ulnar head articulates with the sigmoid notch. This articulation decreases significantly with prosupination, at the extremes of which there is less than 10 percent contact of the articular surfaces,[35] with only 2 to 3 mm of articular surfaces contacting each other. Upon stressing of the distal radioulnar joint in a dorsal volar direction, this translational motion increased to 5.4 mm for palmar motion and 2.8 mm for dorsal motion.[109] The translational motion is dorsal in pronation and palmar in supination. A helpful hint to remind one of this fact is to look at one's own wrist: With prosupination, the distal ulna becomes prominent with pronation.

One other motion of the distal radioulnar joint is the pistoning-type effect that is seen with application of a load along the longitudinal axis of this joint. The ulna moves in a longitudinal fashion as well with prosupination. Relative to the radius, the ulna moves distally with pronation and proximally with supination. With stress loading of the wrist, the ulna moves distally relative to the radius (see Fig. 21–18).

Ishii and associates[56] measured the pressure distribution within the distal radioulnar joint with axial loads applied to the wrist in varying degrees of forearm rotation. They used a thin, malleable pressure sensor that allowed for dynamic pressure measurements instead of static data collection. They showed that with the increasing application of an axial load across the wrist, the average area of the sigmoid notch in contact with the ulnar head also increased. Their work also showed that in pronation, there is compressive loading between the dorsal sigmoid notch and the ulnar head, and in supination, there is compressive loading between the palmar sigmoid notch and the ulnar head. These data supported the concept, initially presented by Bowers,[13] that in part, the stability of the distal radioulnar joint is maintained by the compression between the dorsal lip of the sigmoid notch and the ulnar head in pronation and by the palmar lip of the sigmoid notch and the ulnar head in supination.

With respect to the longitudinal axis of the forearm, the ulnar head has an average inclination of 20° (Fig. 21–4). It follows that the sigmoid notch, being parallel to the seat of the ulnar head, would have the same inclination.[35, 71] Sagerman and coworkers[119] noted, in fact, that the average ulnar seat inclination was 21°, yet the range was from a reverse angle of −13.8° up to a very sharp positive angle of 40.5°. Whether by coincidence or through evolutionary development, this average 20° inclination also roughly parallels the rotational axis of the forearm. Although this is an oversimplification, one can think of the rotational axis of the forearm as running from the radial head at the proximal radioulnar joint to the ulnar head at the distal radioulnar joint. Obviously, the rotational axis changes with prosupination; for more detailed information on this very complex topic, the reader is referred to excellent work published by Ekenstam and Hagert[35] as well as others.[26, 45, 62, 105, 115]

It seems evident that from the anatomy of the ulnar seat and sigmoid notch and the inherent mobility of the DRUJ, including translational motion, and aside from the compressive load between the ulna and dorsal and palmar rims of the sigmoid notch, the distal radioulnar joint without the soft tissue envelope is inherently unstable. The primary constraint to the distal radioulnar joint has generally been accepted to be the triangular fibrocartilage complex, with the palmar and dorsal radioulnar ligament components of the TFCC being the principal stabilizers of the joint. Other stabilizers of the distal radioulnar joint are the interosseous membrane (with the pronator quadratus), the joint capsule, and the extensor carpi ulnaris tendon subsheath.

Triangular Fibrocartilage Complex

Before examining the biomechanics of the triangular fibrocartilage complex, let us take a step back and

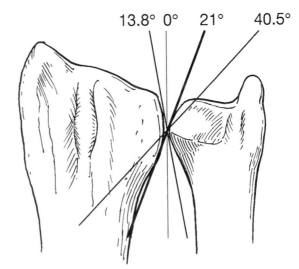

Figure 21–4. The ulnar seat inclination averages 21°, but as noted by Sagerman and colleagues,[120] the range is from a reverse angle of negative 13.8° up to a positive angle of 40.5°.

define exactly what it is. The senior author (AKP) coined the term *triangular fibrocartilage complex,*[106] but the area has been referred to by other names. Taleisnik[130] called it the "ulnar carpal complex (UCC)" and Bowers[15] has referred to it as the "ulnar carpal ligament complex (UCLC)." The individual components are the central portion of the triangular fibrocartilage (TFC) or articular disk, the dorsal and palmar radioulnar ligaments, the meniscus homolog (ulnocarpal meniscus), the ulnar collateral ligament,

the sheaths of the extensor carpi ulnaris, and the ulnolunate and ulnotriquetral ligaments (Fig. 21–5). (When we use the term "TFC" or "triangular fibrocartilage," we are referring to the central horizontal articular disk as well as the adjoining palmar and dorsal radioulnar ligaments. When the other structures are included, the word "complex" is added.)

It would be incorrect to assume that each of these single components can be anatomically identified; rather, they are distinct areas within the TFCC. As

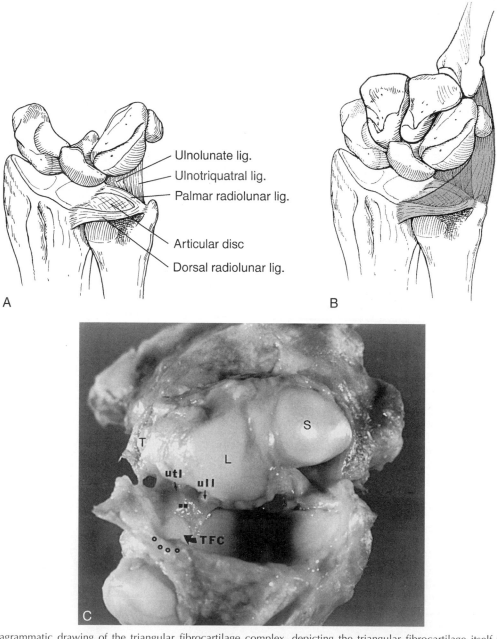

Figure 21–5. *A,* Diagrammatic drawing of the triangular fibrocartilage complex, depicting the triangular fibrocartilage itself with its dorsal and palmar radioulnar ligaments. The ulnolunate and ulnotriquetral ligaments run from the fovea of the ulna to the carpus. *B,* Same view as in *A* with the addition of the meniscal reflection. *C,* Anatomic dissection of the triangular fibrocartilage complex. Of note is that the meniscus homolog, the ulnar collateral ligament, and the subsheath of the extensor carpi ulnaris tendon are not depicted in this anatomic dissection. *TFC* = articular disc of triangular fibrocartilage; *open circles* = dorsal radioulnar ligament; *squares* = palmar radioulnar ligament; *utl* = ulnotriquetral ligament; *ull* = ulnolunate ligament; *T* = triquetrum; *L* = lunate; *S* = scaphoid.

stated previously, the TFCC arises from the junction of the sigmoid and lunate fossae of the radius. The palmar and dorsal thickenings are the origins of the palmar and dorsal radioulnar ligaments, respectively. From the origin, this structure courses ulnarward to insert at the base of the ulnar styloid and the fovea. From the ulnar aspect of the palmar radioulnar ligament and the ulnar styloid arise the ulnocarpal ligaments. Extending distally in a fan-shaped manner, they insert on the lunate and triquetrum as the ulnolunate and ulnotriquetral ligaments, respectively. The strongest attachment is to the lunotriquetral interosseous ligament itself and the triquetrum, with weaker attachments to the lunate. Although the senior chapter author coined the term "triangular fibrocartilage complex," it should be acknowledged that identification of the ulnolunate and ulnotriquetral ligaments as distinct ligaments was not made in his original work. It is our view that Bowers[16] should be credited with the description of these ulnocarpal ligaments and that they are an important part of the triangular fibrocartilage complex.

Further ulnarly, the TFCC becomes thickened again into the meniscus homolog (4 mm in average thickness) and inserts distally into the triquetrum hamate and the base of the fifth metacarpal. The prestyloid recess is a constant perforation found just distal to the ulnar styloid but proximal to the thickened meniscus homolog. The prime stabilizers of the distal radioulnar joint, the dorsal and palmar radioulnar ligaments, are thickened areas of the TFC, averaging 4 to 5 mm. The central horizontal portion of the TFC, the articular disk, is thickened near its origin on the radius (average 2 mm); it thins out centrally, where it abuts the lunate, and frequently is found to be perforated in this area. This central thin portion of the TFC was found to be perforated in 53% of specimens in one of the early studies on the TFCC.[106] All these specimens with perforated TFCCs revealed erosive lesions on the cartilage of the ulnar head and lunate, leading to the conclusion that a central degenerative perforation of the TFCC is secondary to ulnar impaction syndrome. Mikic's[82] earlier work supported this conclusion, and he found no central perforations in individuals less than 20 years of age in whom the wrist was untraumatized. It follows that ulnar impaction syndrome is more prevalent in individuals with ulnar-positive variance, and this reasoning is supported by Palmer and Werner's[106] original work, which revealed an association of ulnar-positive variance with an increased incidence of TFCC perforation as well as ulnolunate erosion. Dorsolaterally, the TFCC incorporates the floor of the sheath of the extensor carpi ulnaris, forming a strong attachment.

It must be stressed, again, that although each structure of the triangular fibrocartilage complex is morphologically unique as studied in the laboratory, all structures act as a unit from a clinical and functional perspective. In essence, the TFCC unites the distal radioulnar joint to the ulnar carpus. Via the TFC and the ulnar carpal ligaments, the volar ulnar carpus is suspended from the dorsal ulnar radius.[16] When the ulnocarpal ligaments are attenuated in conditions such as rheumatoid arthritis, this suspension becomes lax, leading to caput ulnae (see Fig. 21–15).

Stabilizing Forces on DRUJ

Now let us turn our attention back to the stabilizing forces acting on the distal radioulnar joint. Numerous studies have been presented and published in attempts to clarify this very complex concept. Suffice it to say that there is a tremendous divergence of opinions as to what is the prime stabilizer of the DRUJ. Virtually every structure associated with the distal radioulnar joint has been identified as its prime stabilizer in various articles. The list obviously includes the triangular fibrocartilage complex itself,[41, 82, 83, 86, 116, 136] the dorsal and palmar distal radioulnar ligaments (part of the TFC) and ulnar collateral ligament,[46, 51, 73, 116, 136] the extensor carpi ulnaris and its fibroosseous canal,[126] the subsheath of the extensor carpi ulnaris,[63] and the pronator quadratus muscle with the interosseous membrane.[106, 136]

With respect to the dorsal and palmar radioulnar ligaments, there are two opposing theories. One theory, as supported by Ekenstam and Hagert,[35] holds that the dorsal radioulnar ligament becomes tight with supination and the palmar radioulnar ligament becomes tight in pronation. Schuind and associates[122] have shown the exact opposite; they believe that the dorsal radioulnar ligament prevents separation of the radius and ulna during loading, that this ligament is tight in pronation, and that the palmar radioulnar ligament is tight in supination. Adams and Holley[2] came to a very similar conclusion. They did not actually measure the dorsal and palmar radioulnar ligaments, but instead measured the strain on the dorsal and palmar borders of the articular disk itself; their findings supported the conclusion of Schuind and associates[122] in that strains along the palmar margins of the articular disk increased or were unchanged and the strain on the dorsal margin of the disk decreased during supination, with the opposite pattern occurring in pronation.

Schuind and associates[122] tried to explain the relative merits of both the dorsal and palmar radioulnar ligaments in prosupination. Their objective data clearly support the concept that the dorsal radioulnar ligament is taut in pronation and the palmar radioulnar ligament is taut in supination; that arrangement, however, would inherently create instability in the distal radioulnar joint, such that in supination, there would be instability in a palmar direction, and the instability would be in a dorsal direction with pronation. Thus, these findings led to the conclusion that the inherent instability of the distal radioulnar joint in a dorsal direction with pronation would be counteracted by progressive tension in the palmar radioulnar ligament, and vice versa in supination.

Interestingly enough, work in our laboratory by

Kihara and colleagues[60] showed that it was difficult to determine the roles of the dorsal and palmar radioulnar ligaments in stabilizing the DRUJ with the interosseous membrane intact. With the interosseous membrane disrupted, however, the results once again supported the conclusions reached by Schuind and associates[123] and Adams and Holley.[2] Possibly the most important finding in this study was that the four structures studied—the dorsal radioulnar ligament, the palmar radioulnar ligament, the distal interosseous membrane including the pronator quadratus muscle, and the entire interosseous membrane—all contribute to distal radioulnar joint stability in dorsal, palmar, and lateral directions. Clearly, more work needs to be done to elucidate the stabilizing forces acting upon the distal radioulnar joint.

Ulnar Variance and the TFCC

Another function of the triangular fibrocartilage complex that needs to be addressed is that it also serves as a load-bearing cushion for the transmission of axial loads between the ulnar carpus and the forearm. Whenever one discusses load transmission through the ulnar side of the wrist, inevitably that load is related to ulnar variance.[105] Thus, to begin with, we would like to present a definition of ulnar variance, at the same time acknowledging that a universal definition does not exist. Simply speaking, an arm in which the ulna is relatively longer than the radius has an *ulnar-positive* variance, and one in which the ulna is shorter than the radius has an *ulnar-negative* variance.

In 1928, Hultén[54] noted the association of ulnar-negative variance with Keinböck's disease. This association was subsequently confirmed by other authorities.[22, 40] Founded upon these observations, ulnar-lengthening or radial-shortening procedures became accepted modes of treatment for Kienböck's disease. Ulnar shortening also became an accepted form of treating ulnar impaction syndrome secondary to a relatively long ulna. Obviously, a reproducible and precise means of measuring ulnar variance was needed, because diagnoses and surgical treatments were being based on the ulnar variance.

It has been found that a standard position for radiographs is necessary to predictably reproduce results for determining ulnar variance. The generally accepted standard is for a posteroanterior (PA) radiograph to be taken with the wrist in neutral forearm rotation, the elbow flexed 90°, and the shoulder ab-

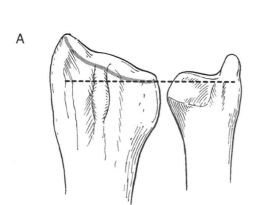

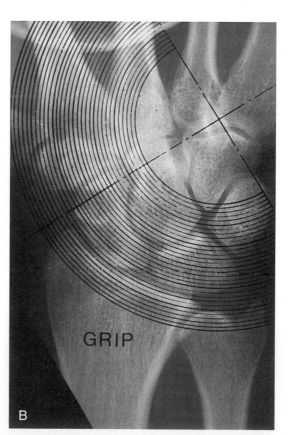

GRIP

Figure 21–6. Two methods of determining ulnar variance. *A,* As a perpendicular to the long axis of the radius, the tangent is drawn off the most proximal aspect of the lunate fossa. *B,* A template of concentric semicircles is matched to the curve of the distal radius. In both methods, the ulnar variance is determined by measuring in millimeters the most distal aspect of the ulnar head in either a positive or negative direction from the corresponding line drawn from the distal radius as a tangent or concentric semicircle.

Table 21–1. Axial Load Borne by the Radius and Ulna as a Percentage of the Total Load (100%)

	Percentage of Axial Load		
	Intact	*TFCC Excised*	*Distal Ulna Excised*
Radius	81.6	93.8	100
Ulna	18.4	6.2	0

From Palmer AK, Werner FW: Biomechanics of the distal radial ulnar joint. Clin Orthop 187:26–34, 1984.

ducted 90° (see Fig. 21–16*A*).[101] From here, there are two ways to measure the variance. One way is to draw a line perpendicular to the long axis of the radius off the tangent from the most proximal aspect of the lunate fossa and to measure the corresponding length of the ulna to this reference line (Fig. 21–6*A*). The other way, as described by Palmer,[101] is to use a template of concentric semicircles. First the template is matched to the curve of the distal radius. Then, by following these semicircles, one determines the ulnar variance (Fig. 21–6). Yet, as mentioned previously, different centers have different interpretations of ulnar variance. Clearly, many centers in Japan consider ulnar-neutral variance to be any variance extending from −2 mm to +2 mm.[85]

With respect to load transmission across the wrist joint, the ulnar variance and TFCC play integral parts. It has been documented in our laboratory that removal of the TFCC results in a subtotal unloading of the ulna. In the initial studies on the intact wrists of cadavers, approximately 40 percent of force during axial load was transmitted through the ulna; with the TFCC excised, however, the transmitted force was decreased to 5 percent. Totally excising the distal ulna, such as in a Darrach procedure, transferred the entire load transmission through the wrist to the radiocarpal joint. In response to valid criticism, this work was repeated on 16 specimens using fresh cadaver upper extremities with preserved elbows, and the results were very similar to those of the previous study, in that in the intact wrist, the normal load across the radius was approximately 82 percent, and

that across the ulna was roughly 18 percent (Table 21–1).[105] With the TFCC excised, the axial load borne by the ulna dropped to 6 percent; similarly, with the distal ulna excised, it dropped to 0 percent. Using a similar experimental model, work in our laboratory was directed next at determining changes in force through the ulna as related to ulnar variance.[105] In neutral variance, the axial load borne by the ulna was 18 percent; shortening the ulna 2.5 mm reduced the force to 4 percent. Increasing the ulnar variance by 2.5 mm from neutral increased the load to 42 percent (Fig. 21–7). Similar although less dramatic changes were seen in the same experiment performed with the TFCC excised.[139]

Not only is there a relationship between ulnar variance and load through the ulnar side of the wrist, but there is also a direct relationship between ulnar variance and triangular fibrocartilage complex thickness. Work by Palmer and colleagues[102] revealed that the articular disk portion of the TFCC varied inversely in thickness with respect to the ulnar variance; that is, as the ulnar variance became more positive, the articular disk thickness decreased (Fig. 21–8). This finding supported earlier work by Steinhauser and associates,[127] in 74 uninjured cadaver wrists; they found that wrists with ulnar-negative variance were associated with a thicker articular disk than wrists with ulnar-neutral or ulnar-positive variance.[127]

Surgically Altered Kinetics

One of the well-accepted treatments to date of a triangular fibrocartilage lesion or tear is a débridement of that tear.[1, 95, 100] There is ample biomechanical research to support the surgical rationale.[1] Palmer and associates[107] have shown that excision of less than two thirds of the horizontal portion of the TFCC has no statistically significant effect on forearm axial load transmission in the cadaver model. Conversely, removal of two thirds or more of this central horizontal portion of the TFCC unloads the ulnar aspect of the wrist, with a greater percentage of the load being transmitted to the distal radius. Adams[1] performed a biomechanical study to determine the effects of par-

Figure 21–7. Shortening the ulna by 2.5 mm results in a drop in ulnar load (force through ulna) to 4%. Lengthening of the ulna by 2.5 mm results in an increase in ulnar load to 42%. (*From* Palmer AK, Werner FW: Biomechanics of the distal radial ulnar joint. Clin Orthop 187:26–34, 1984.)

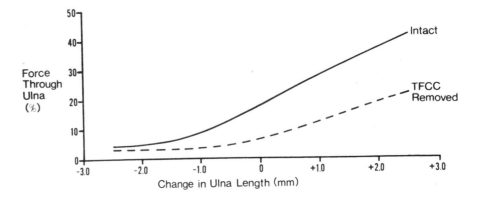

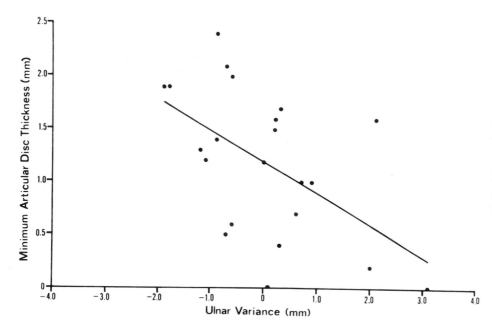

Figure 21–8. Distribution and corresponding regression line for triangular fibrocartilage complex minimum articular disc thickness and ulnar variance. (*From* Palmer AK, Glisson RR, Werner FW, Mech EM: Relationship between ulnar variance and triangular fibrocartilage complex thickness. Reprinted with permission from J Hand Surg 9A:681–683, 1984.)

tial or complete excision of the articular disk of the triangular fibrocartilage complex. He studied both the biomechanics of the DRUJ and the structural integrity of the TFC. Like Palmer and associates,[107] Adams[1] showed that an excision constituting less than two thirds of the articular disk resulted in insignificant biomechanical and structural changes to the DRUJ and the TFC, respectively; however, larger excisions did produce changes.

As noted previously, ulnar variance changes with respect to load on the wrist as well as with respect to prosupination. With pronation and with load on the wrist, the ulna migrates distally relative to the radius (see Fig. 21–18). Through their experiments, Schuind and colleagues[122] concluded that there was an axial laxity of the TFCC that allowed the previously described physiologic changes in ulnar variance without affecting the stability of the DRUJ. From these studies, one can understand why there is often no clinical effect on the stability nor the motion of the distal radioulnar joint when the ulna and radius are surgically lengthened or shortened by a few millimeters. There have been at least two reports, however, of problems of ulnar impingement following ulnar shortening, and the authors of both reports believed that orientation of the sigmoid notch and ulnar seat inclination may be of principal importance in determining distal radioulnar joint congruity following an ulnar-shortening procedure.[119, 132]

Microvascular Anatomy of the Triangular Fibrocartilage Complex

The clinical significance of the microvasculature of the TFCC seems obvious. Where there is blood supply within the triangular fibrocartilage complex, there is the possibility that healing or surgical repair of an injury in a vascularized zone would be successful, whereas any type of reparative process in an avascular zone would seem to be futile. This reasoning not only is intuitive but is also based on previous work, particularly in the knee, where studies on the menisci have shown that the ability to heal an injury is, in fact, related to the blood supply of the menisci.[5, 9, 21, 50, 61]

In an excellent study, Bednar and associates[9] noted two important features of the microvasculature of the triangular fibrocartilage. The first is that the central, horizontal portion of the TFC is avascular. The second is that the vascular supply to the TFC arises from its palmar, dorsal, and ulnar attachments to the joint capsule and then assumes a radial pattern. No vessels supply the TFC from its radial attachment on the radius. The fibrocartilage blends with the articular cartilage of the radius, and the cartilage acts as a barrier, preventing the subchondral bone vessels from penetrating into the TFC (Fig. 21–9).

The work by Bednar and associates[9] confirms an earlier study performed by Thiru-Pathi and coworkers,[131] who noted that the TFCC receives its blood supply in a radial fashion from the major branches supplying the triangular fibrocartilage. These branches are the dorsal and palmar radiocarpal branches of the ulnar artery, the palmar branch of the anterior interosseous artery, and the dorsal branch of the anterior interosseous artery (Fig. 21–10). This study showed a central zone of avascularity of the TFC, with the vascularity limited to the outer 15 to 20 percent of the articular disk. Thiru-Pathi and coworkers[131] also noted that the radial attachment of the TFCC to the radius is avascular.

Chidgey and colleagues,[24] in their study on the TFCC, reported that the palmar and dorsal radioulnar

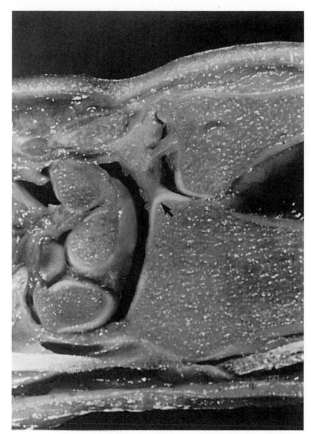

Figure 21–9. Section of the wrist showing the triangular fibrocartilage as it originates from the radius. Note the rim of cartilage *(arrow)* between the subchondral bone of the radius and the triangular fibrocartilage (TFC) itself. This cartilage acts as a barrier between the blood vessels in the bone and the avascular TFC.

ligaments are vascularized, once again showing that the central portion of the articular disk is avascular. In another study, Chidgey[23] noted that in addition to the extrinsic blood supply via the ulnar and anterior interosseous arteries, there is blood supply via the ulnar head at the fovea area. This is the site of the TFC insertion on the ulna.[23]

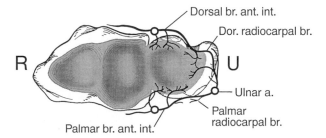

Figure 21–10. Diagrammatic drawing depicting the vascular supply to the triangular fibrocartilage via the following branches (labeled with abbreviated names): Dorsal and palmar radiocarpal branches of the ulnar artery, the palmar branch of the anterior interosseous artery, and the dorsal branch of the anterior interosseous artery. Note the avascularity of the central and radial aspects of the triangular fibrocartilage. *R* = radius; *U* = ulna.

PATHOGENESIS AND PATHOLOGY

Triangular Fibrocartilage Complex

The pathologic conditions affecting the TFCC can be separated into two categories, traumatic and degenerative. Palmer[100] has devised a classification system for TFCC abnormalities (Table 21–2), on the basis of anatomic and biomechanical studies as well as on review of 10 years of clinical experience. The TFCC can be injured at any one of its anatomic locations: horizontal articular disk, peripheral portions, or its attachments. There may also be associated injuries to surrounding structures, such as the cartilage surfaces of the adjacent bones, as well as nearby ligamentous structures, such as the lunotriquetral ligament.

CLASS 1: TRAUMATIC LESIONS

The traumatic lesions of the TFCC usually occur secondary to an acute hyperpronation injury to the forearm or to an axial load-and-distraction injury to the ulnar side of the wrist, as may occur with a fall on an outstretched extremity.[14, 16, 96–98]

Many investigators believe that the most common site for traumatic tear is the *class 1A* tear (Fig. 21–11A). This is a tear of the horizontal portion of the TFCC, usually 2 to 3 mm ulnar to the radial attachment of the TFCC and usually oriented in a palmar dorsal direction.[25, 94, 95, 100, 112] Adams and Holley[2] supported this clinical impression with their biomechanical research. They showed that tension across the articular disk was reduced in supination, whereas tension on the radial aspect of the articular disk was increased in pronation. Also, they found that there was a preferential distribution of the strain to the radial aspect of the articular disk when loads were

Table 21–2. A Classification of TFCC Abnormalities

Class 1 Traumatic
  A Central perforation
  B Ulnar avulsion
      With distal ulnar fracture
      Without distal ulnar fracture
  C Distal avulsion
  D Radial avulsion
      With sigmoid notch fracture
      Without sigmoid notch fracture
Class 2 Degenerative (ulnocarpal abutment syndrome)
  A TFCC wear
  B TFCC wear
      Plus lunate and/or ulnar chondromalacia
  C TFCC perforation
      Plus lunate and/or ulnar chondromalacia
  D TFCC perforation
      Plus lunate and/or ulnar chondromalacia
      Plus lunotriquetral ligament perforation
  E TFCC perforation
      Plus lunate and/or ulnar chondromalacia
      Plus lunotriquetral ligament perforation
      Plus ulnocarpal arthritis

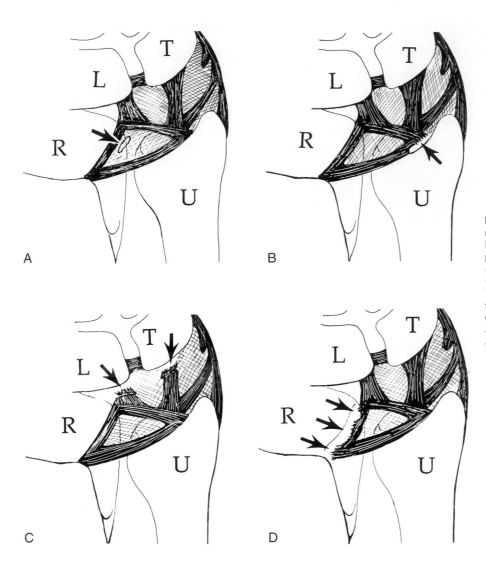

Figure 21–11. Diagrammatic drawing of traumatic, or Class 1, abnormalities of the triangular fibrocartilage complex. *A,* Class 1A, central perforation *(arrow). B,* Class 1B, ulnar avulsion *(arrow),* with or without distal ulnar fracture. *C,* Class 1C, distal avulsion *(arrows). D,* Class 1D, radial avulsion *(arrows),* with or without sigmoid notch fracture. *L* = lunate; *R* = radius; *T* = triquetrum; *U* = ulna. (*From* Palmer AK: Triangular fibrocartilage complex lesions: A classification. J Hand Surg 14A:594–606, 1989.)

applied that simulated the physiologic DRUJ separation that normally occurs with axial loading of the wrist.[71] This biomechanical scheme could also be used to explain *class 1D* lesions, in which a radial avulsion injury is present with or without a sigmoid notch fracture (Fig. 21–11*D*).[2]

Class 1B lesions represent a traumatic avulsion of the TFCC at its insertion at the base of the ulnar styloid, which may or may not be associated with an ulnar styloid fracture (Fig. 21–11*B*). As noted in Palmer's[100] original article, the TFCC is one of the major stabilizers of the distal radioulnar joint, so this lesion would be expected to be associated with DRUJ instability. As elucidated in the biomechanical study by Kihara and associates,[60] for the DRUJ to become unstable after sectioning of the triangular fibrocartilage complex, the interosseous membrane itself must first be disrupted. One might then be able to assume, although this is making a large leap, that class 1B lesions may or may not be associated with instability of the DRUJ, with the instability being determined

by the presence or absence of an intact interosseous membrane.

Class 1C lesions represent tears of the ulnocarpal ligaments as the TFCC attaches to the lunate and triquetrum (Fig. 21–11*C*). This type of injury can be associated with instability of the ulnocarpal joint with palmar translation of the ulnar carpus in relation to the distal ulna.

CLASS 2: DEGENERATIVE LESIONS

Degenerative lesions of the TFCC, however, are thought of as chronic injuries resulting from load on the ulnar side of the wrist. When pain exists from this pathology, the diagnosis of ulnar impaction syndrome is usually made. Palmer[100] has categorized these as class 2 TFCC abnormalities with five subcategories representing a continuum in progression of ulnar impaction syndrome (see Table 21–2).

The ulnar impaction syndrome is thought to occur in a population of people with a tendency toward ulnar-positive variance, and this belief well may be true. It is not, however, uncommon for ulnar impaction syndrome to be present in a patient with ulnar-negative variance. This observation makes sense, because (1) biomechanical studies have shown that the ulna moves distally relative to the radius when a load is placed on the wrist and (2) ulnar variance is inversely related to the thickness of the TFCC.[102] (As the ulnar variance decreases, the TFCC thickness increases.)

Class 2A wear patterns represent degenerative changes of the horizontal portion of the TFCC without perforation (Fig. 21–12*A*). This abnormality of the TFCC is well-documented anatomically and histologically in work by Mikic.[82]

Class 2B lesions represent degenerative changes or chondromalacia of the ulnar aspect of the lunate and/ or the radial aspect of the ulnar head in addition to the degenerative changes of the horizontal portion of the TFCC (Fig. 21–12*B*).

Class 2C lesions represent the previously described chondromalatic lesions on the lunate and ulna as well as a TFCC perforation (Fig. 21–12*C*). This perfo-

ration is located in the avascular portion of the TFCC (ulnar to where a normally located traumatic class 1A tear would be). These tears also tend to be round, compared with the slit-like tears associated with traumatic class 1A injuries.

Class 2D lesions represent further progression, such that the abutment leads to not only the previous changes to the horizontal portion of the TFCC, the lunate, and the ulna but also to a lunotriquetral ligament disruption (Fig. 21–12*D*).

Finally, class 2E lesions represent arthritic changes in the ulnocarpal joint.

Distal Radioulnar Joint

TRAUMATIC LESIONS

Injuries to the DRUJ can be broadly categorized into two groups; those that involve trauma to the bone and those that involve trauma to the soft tissues. The most common fracture involving the DRUJ is a distal radius fracture that extends to include the sigmoid

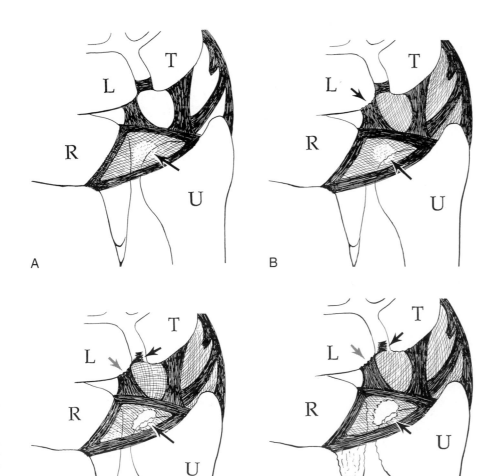

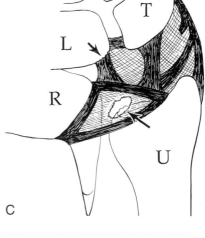

Figure 21–12. Diagrammatic drawing of degenerative, or Class 2, abnormalities of the triangular fibrocartilage complex (TFCC), or ulnocarpal abutment syndrome. *A,* Class 2A, TFCC wear *(arrow)*. *B,* Class 2B, TFCC wear with lunate *(small arrow)* and/or ulnar *(large arrow)* chondromalacia. *C,* Class 2C, TFCC perforation with lunate *(small arrow)* and/or ulnar *(large arrow)* chondromalacia. *D,* Class 2D, TFCC perforation with lunate *(arrow)* and/ or ulnar *(large arrow)* chondromalacia and lunotriquetral ligament perforation *(small arrow)*. *E,* Class 2E, TFCC perforation with lunate *(arrow)* and/or ulnar *(large arrow)* chondromalacia, lunotriquetral ligament perforation *(small arrow)* and ulnocarpal arthritis. *L* = lunate; *R* = radius; *T* = triquetrum; *U* = ulna. *(From Palmer AK: Triangular fibrocartilage complex lesions: A classification. J Hand Surg 14A:594–606, 1989.)*

notch. In his original article on fractures of the distal radius, published in 1814, Colles[27] notes that the DRUJ is involved in distal radius fractures, remarking that "the end of the ulnar admits of being readily moved backwards and forwards." It was Frykman's[38] presentation of a classification scheme for distal radius fractures that eventually brought attention to the importance of the distal radioulnar joint within the context of distal radius fracture. Melone[77, 78] presented his classification scheme for distal radius fractures, identifying four major fracture fragments of the distal radius: the shaft, the radial styloid, the volar medial facet, and the dorsal medial facet. This scheme also drew attention to the dorsal medial and volar medial facets as important fracture fragments, not only in relation to the distal radius articular surface but also to the distal radioulnar joint. Melone[77, 78] referred to these two medial fracture fragments as "the medial complex."

The two sequelae of distal radius fractures with respect to the distal radioulnar joint are ulnar impaction syndrome and loss of forearm rotation. As the fracture settles dorsally, leading to an increase in the dorsal tilt, the ulnar variance progressively increases. This, in turn, often leads to ulnar impaction syndrome.[6] Any incongruity of the distal radioulnar joint, including the above-mentioned settling of the distal radius fracture, can lead to a loss of forearm prosupination.[6, 31, 34, 53, 55]

Knirk and Jupiter[64] studied intraarticular fractures of the distal radius in young adults. Their work seemed to usher in the concept that all distal radius fractures do not, in fact, do well. Their study identified the need to obtain reduction of the articular surface as close to anatomic as possible to ensure the best chance of a good result. They also drew attention to the medial fracture fragments of the distal radius in identifying the need to anatomically reduce the "lunate die-punch" fracture fragment. Of the 43 distal radius fractures they studied, three wrists had posttraumatic changes to the distal radioulnar joint. Again in reference to the DRUJ, but along different lines, 31 of the 43 wrists Knirk and Jupiter[64] studied had an ulnar styloid fracture. They noted that an ulnar styloid non-union was associated with a less favorable final result.[64]

Ulnar styloid fractures can occur as isolated events or, more commonly, in association with distal radius fractures. It is our opinion that there are two biomechanically distinct types of ulnar styloid fractures. The distinction is whether the insertion of the triangular fibrocartilage complex by and large remains with the ulnar head or instead is part of the ulnar styloid fracture fragment. Following a fracture, an ulnar styloid non-union is not uncommon.[7] Hauck and associates[49] described two types of non-unions. Type 1 is a styloid non-union associated with a stable distal radioulnar joint (TFC insertion intact; Fig. 21–13A), and type 2, is a non-union associated with an unstable distal radioulnar joint (TFC insertion disrupted; Fig. 21–13B). These investigators excised the styloid fragment in 11 patients with type 1 stable non-unions, and all had satisfactory relief of pain. Of 9 patients with type 2 non-unions, 3 had large fragments that could be treated by open reduction with internal fixation, and all 3 patients did well. The other 6 patients with type 2 ulnar styloid non-unions underwent excision of the fragment and repair of the triangular fibrocartilage complex, with overall satisfactory results. This supports earlier work presented by Reeves[111] and Burgess and Watson,[19] who treated ulnar styloid non-union and associated ulnar wrist pain by excising the fracture fragment. In both of these studies, however, the patient numbers were quite small, and the results were somewhat mixed.

It should be noted that not a lot has been written about symptomatic ulnar styloid non-unions. Clearly, however, an ulnar styloid fracture is common with a distal radius fracture. It occurs in association with Colles' fracture more than 50 percent of the time.[7, 28, 38, 49, 125] In Frykman's[38] classic article, an ulnar styloid fracture was present in 61 percent of distal radius fractures. It has been reported that 26 percent of ulnar styloid fractures result in non-union.[7] Thus, it is our opinion that symptomatic ulnar styloid non-union is probably under-recognized and/or under-reported in the literature.

Although the ulnar styloid fracture is a fracture, it truly represents an avulsion-type fracture in most instances, and as such, it can in a way be thought of as a soft tissue injury. Consideration of soft tissue injuries about the distal radioulnar joint invariably leads to the discussion of instability of the DRUJ. This topic is covered in detail in Chapters 22 to 24, so we will just make a general comment here regarding DRUJ instability. The gathering body of literature makes it apparent that DRUJ instability is a very complex disorder that should not be thought of as an injury to a single structure. Melone and Nathan[79] noted, in a review of their cases of DRUJ instability in association with TFCC disruption, that the detachment of the TFCC from its insertion on the ulna was the principal cause of the instability. Yet in 67 percent of the cases, they observed associated injuries. They believed that there was a progression of soft tissue injuries on the ulnar side of the wrist that correlated with the severity of the injury. These investigators noted that in all instances, an injury of the TFCC occurred at its insertion on the ulna. In more severe cases, the extensor carpi ulnaris subsheath was also involved. The sequence of soft tissues involved, based on increasing severity of the injury, was as follows: the ulnocarpal ligament, the lunotriquetral ligament, the triquetrocapitate ligament, and the triquetrohamate ligament. This theory of progressive soft tissue involvement with the increasing severity of the injury is not unlike that presented by Mayfield and colleagues[76] with respect to their thoughts concerning progressive perilunate instability. This is indeed an intriguing thought, but obviously one that needs much more work to substantiate and clarify. Along these same lines, Kihara and associates[60] per-

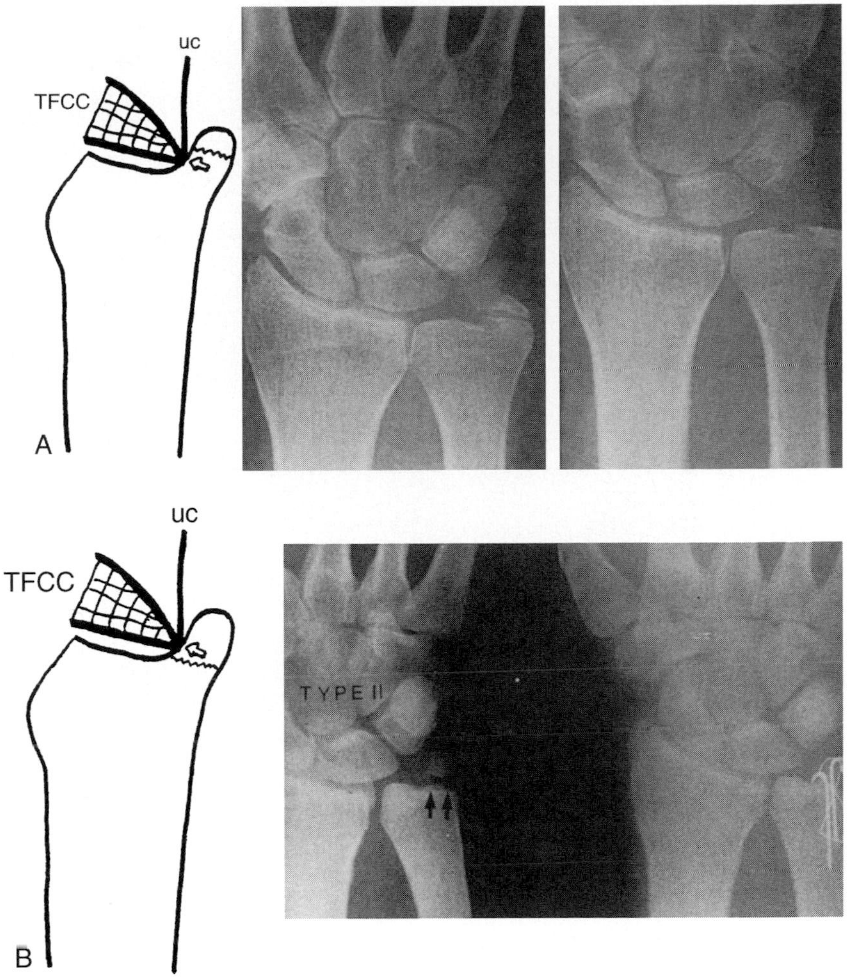

Figure 21–13. Ulnar styloid non-unions. *A,* Type 1: ulnar styloid non-union with the triangular fibrocartilage complex *(TFCC)* and distal radioulnar joint stability intact. *B,* Type 2: ulnar styloid non-union associated with an unstable distal radioulnar joint. *UC* = ulnocarpal ligaments. (*From* Hauck RM, Skahen J III, Palmer AK: Classification and treatment of ulnar styloid non-union. J Hand Surg 21A:418–422, 1996.)

formed a biomechanical cadaver study showing that multiple structures must be sectioned to cause instability of the distal radioulnar joint. The structures examined included the interosseous membrane in its entirety as well as the distal portion of the interosseous membrane with the pronator quadratus muscle, and the palmar and dorsal radioulnar ligaments. Dislocation occurred only with sectioning of all four stabilizing structures.

DEGENERATIVE LESIONS (IMPINGEMENT)

A degenerative process that leads to distal radioulnar joint pathology and pain with prosupination is referred to as *ulnar impingement.* This disorder must be distinguished from ulnar impaction syndrome, which is due to the degenerative changes between the ulnar head and the carpus (Fig. 21–14). Bell and coworkers[10] described a form of impingement that occurs following resection of the distal ulna with a Darrach procedure. They believed that a Darrach procedure is not benign and that with excision of the distal ulna, convergence of the distal radius and ulna can occur, causing degenerative changes and subse-

quent pain from the impingement. Impingement can follow trauma as well. The degenerative changes of the distal radioulnar joint may occur secondary to a malunited sigmoid notch as a sequela of a distal radius fracture. Less commonly, the degenerative changes may follow an ulnar head fracture. Other causes of impingement less common than trauma are chronic instability of the DRUJ, infection, crystalline disease, and, certainly, primary osteoarthritis.[91]

INFLAMMATORY LESIONS

Although trauma is a well-recognized cause of distal radioulnar joint impingement, rheumatoid arthritis certainly is the leading cause of DRUJ arthritis. The disease is not clearly understood from the medical perspective, but we hand surgeons easily recognize the destruction of the articular cartilage wrought by the hypertrophied rheumatoid synovium.[36] Yet the destructive changes to the surrounding soft tissues of the DRUJ can have an even more devastating effect on the function of this joint. As the rheumatoid synovium stretches and invades the supporting soft tissue, the biomechanics of the joint alters, thereby leading to a degenerative wear pattern and secondary

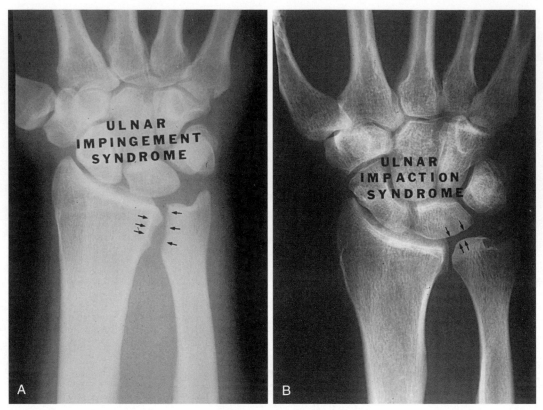

Figure 21–14. *A,* Ulnar impingement syndrome, a degenerative process between the seat of the ulnar head and the sigmoid notch *(arrows)*. *B,* Ulnar impaction syndrome, a degenerative process between the pole of the ulnar head and the ulnar carpus *(arrows)*.

arthritis. Weiler and Bogoch[138] compared the biomechanics of the DRUJ in rheumatoid arthritic patients and that in normal subjects by means of centrode analysis. They used serial CT scans as each patient actively prosupinated the forearm. These investigators noted that the center of rotation of the DRUJ in normal subjects stayed within a well-defined area. In the patients with early rheumatoid arthritis process, they noted that the kinematics were not markedly altered as long as the sigmoid notch joint contour was maintained. When erosions involving the dorsal aspect of the sigmoid notch became evident as the distal ulna dislocated dorsally, however, significant alterations in the kinematics of the DRUJ became obvious.

The soft tissue laxity following the destructive changes of the rheumatoid synovium leads to the caput ulnae syndrome, as described by Bachdahl[8] (Fig. 21–15). With the plethora of synovium involving the ulnar carpal ligaments, the carpus is allowed to supinate on the forearm. In essence, the suspension of the carpus from the dorsoulnar aspect of the radius via the triangular fibrocartilage and the ulnocarpal ligaments is disrupted.[16] The synovitis also affects other surrounding soft tissue structures, including the extensor carpi ulnaris sheath, allowing volar dislocation of the extensor carpi ulnaris tendon. These effects, all taken together, lead not only to the supination of the carpus on the forearm but also to the

dorsal dislocation of the ulnar head. Thus, the classic presentation in caput ulnae syndrome consists of dorsal dislocation of the distal ulna, supination of the carpus on the forearm, and volar dislocation of the extensor carpi ulnaris tendon.[8, 36, 71, 93, 128] This instability of the DRUJ associated with rheumatoid arthritis is caused by three separate mechanisms.[93] First, there is a bony destruction caused by the synovitis.[71] Second, the proliferating synovium weakens the ligaments. Third, the proliferative synovium can cause tendon rupture and/or dislocation.[93, 122] The culmination of this bony, ligamentous, and tendinous involvement is the caput ulnae syndrome. It should be noted that this syndrome is present in up to 30 percent of patients with rheumatoid arthritis.[36]

DIAGNOSIS

Diagnostic Problems

The diagnostic problems associated with identifying distal radioulnar joint and/or triangular fibrocartilage complex lesions are many. The differential diagnosis associated with ulnar-sided wrist pain includes not only DRUJ and/or TFCC problems but also interosseous ligament disorders, such as a lunotriquetral ligament disruption (not associated with impaction), midcarpal nondissociative instability patterns, piso-

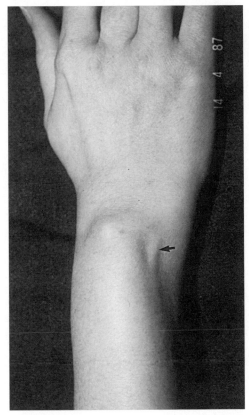

Figure 21–15. Caput ulnar syndrome. Note the classic triad of supination of the carpus on the forearm with dorsal dislocation of the ulnar head and palmar dislocation of the extensor carpi ulnaris tendon (arrow).

each debater truly had belief in the position he was defending.)

Despite the confusion associated with the work-up of ulnar-sided wrist pain, probably no one would disagree that the history and physical examination are of principal importance. Obviously, the history is important as it is in all aspects of medicine. The differential diagnosis of the patient with ulnar-sided wrist pain following a high-speed snowmobile accident is quite different from that of the patient who presents with a long-standing history of progressively deteriorating ulnar-sided wrist pain. Following the history taking, a thorough physical examination is tremendously helpful in arriving at a diagnosis of what is causing the ulnar-sided wrist pain. A good physical examination can often help the clinician at least narrow the differential diagnosis, if not give a fairly good idea of what is causing the patient's problem. In our experience, in the instances in which we side with Dr. Gilula and obtain ancillary radiographic studies, our choice of study often is influenced by the physical findings. We have also found that it is helpful for radiologists to have an idea about where we think the pathology is, so they can focus their attention to this area both technically and in interpretation.

Physical Examination

The physical examination in patients with ulnar-sided wrist pain should include a general upper extremity examination. Range-of-motion measurements should be made of the shoulder, elbow, wrist, and fingers. Grip strength and pinch strength should be measured bilaterally. Inspection of the wrist should be performed to look for areas of swelling, redness, or gross deformities of the wrist. Next, palpation of the wrist is begun. It is not unusual to palpate and visualize extensor carpi ulnaris tendon subluxation with prosupination of the wrist.

The "piano key test" can be helpful in attempting to diagnose DRUJ instability. This test is performed with the hand pronated as one "ballottes" the distal ulna from a dorsal direction, moving it in a volar direction. In a positive "piano key test," there is very little resistance as the ulna moves volarly. As with many aspects of the examination of the hands, one should also examine the other DRUJ, in order to compare the presumed instability of the symptomatic DRUJ with the asymptomatic side. Is the positive "piano key test" isolated to the symptomatic side, or does the patient have a more generalized laxity of distal radioulnar joints, as demonstrated by bilateral, seemingly positive, "piano key tests"?

In addition to the "piano key test," we bimanually examine (shuck) the DRUJ: The examiner holds the radius with one hand and the ulna with the other, and moves the distal radius against the head of the ulna in a volar dorsal direction. This maneuver not only helps identify laxity of the DRUJ; at times, one can feel crepitance or grinding if there is a degenera-

triquetral joint disorders, and extensor carpi ulnaris tendon disorders, to name but a few conditions. In addition, it is not unheard-of for disorders such as Keinböck's disease and even scapholunate ligament disruptions to cause much of the discomfort to be directed to the ulnar side of the wrist.

The greatest problem in the diagnosis, however, is the vast array of ancillary studies available for investigating the ulnar side of the wrist, which often leads to practitioner confusion about how to approach ulnar-sided wrist pain. One needs only to have attended the debate at the 51st annual meeting of the American Society for Surgery of the Hand in Nashville, TN, between Drs. Lee Osterman and Lou Gilula[90] to gain personal insight into the tremendous controversy associated with what type of ancillary studies are best suited to "working up" not only ulnar-sided wrist disorders but global wrist problems in general. In all fairness to the debaters, they were given the topics to debate; Dr. Gilula was given the position to defend that ancillary radiographic studies were helpful in the work-up of wrist disorders, and Dr. Osterman was assigned the position that by and large, extensive radiologic studies are superfluous and wrist arthroscopy should be used as the diagnostic standard for wrist disorders. (Both authors of this chapter, however, had the distinct impression that

tive process present between the radius and the ulna. (Some times, instability of the DRUJ can be found on visualization as well.) In a like manner, we recommend shucking the lunotriquetral joint to assess stability. We stress that the patient's other, asymptomatic wrist be subjected to both shucking tests to look for a difference between the asymptomatic and symptomatic sides with regard to the relative laxity of the joints being examined.

Another examination technique we always use in patients with ulnar-sided wrist pain is to compress the pisotriquetral joint between the examiner's fingers, which are placed on the volar aspect of the pisiform and the dorsal aspect of the triquetrum. We place the thumbs volar, and the index and long fingers dorsal. If pisotriquetral arthritis is present, this test will be positive (i.e., produce pain).

A final aspect of the examination is to listen as the patient moves the wrist. We note two specific sounds with regard to ulnar-sided wrist disorders, a "clunk" and a "click." The "clunk" is the catch-up "clunk" often associated with the midcarpal instability present in a carpal instability–nondissociative (CIND) disease pattern. In this instance, the "clunk" is heard when the pathologically palmar-flexed lunate takes on its normal physiologic dorsiflexed position as the wrist is moved from radial to ulnar deviation. In the normal wrist, there is a smooth transition between the physiologic palmar-flexed lunate in radial deviation and the physiologic dorsiflexed lunate in ulnar deviation. With midcarpal instability, the change in position occurs abruptly. The actual "clunk" is thought to occur secondary to motion between the triquetrum and hamate. The other sound is a "click." This sound, with respect to the ulnar side of the wrist, is often attributed to lunotriquetral ligament or TFCC tears. We believe that the clicking is the catch-

ing of the tear between the articulating surfaces in the ulnocarpal joint as the wrist is put through a range of motion. Of particular importance is that in any aspect of the physical examination, a particular test has significance only if it reproduces the patient's symptoms.[16]

Radiologic Studies

PLAIN RADIOGRAPHS

Upon completion of the physical examination in a patient with ulnar-sided wrist pain, the almost universal practice is to obtain plain films.[74] The technical aspects of obtaining the plain views are of prime importance. At our institution, we have standard positioning for routine radiographs: one lateral, two oblique, and a PA radiograph. The PA radiograph is taken with the shoulder abducted 90°, the elbow flexed 90°, and the forearm in neutral rotation (Fig. 21–16A). This position is strictly adhered to so that a reproducible method of determining ulnar variance can be obtained.[101] Ulnar variance is virtually universally interpreted in patients with ulnar-sided wrist pain. As noted, it is generally accepted that ulnar impaction syndrome is more common in that segment of the population that has ulnar-positive variance.[32, 101] With advanced ulnar impaction syndrome, degenerative changes can often be seen on the plain films on the ulnar side of the proximal lunate and/or the ulnar head (Fig. 21–17). As the disease further progresses and a generalized arthritic pattern develops, greater changes, such as joint narrowing, subchondral sclerosis, and osteophytic spur formation, can be seen.

The lateral view is taken also in neutral forearm rotation with the ulnar side of the wrist flat against

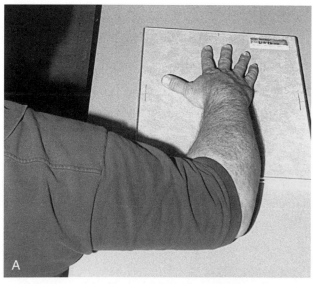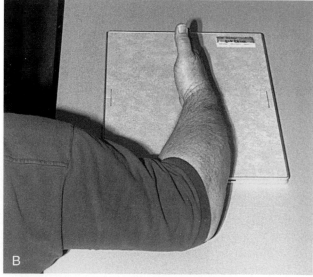

Figure 21–16. A, The standard posteroanterior radiograph of the wrist as taken with the shoulder abducted 90°, the elbow flexed 90°, and the forearm in neutral rotation. B, The lateral radiograph of the wrist as taken also in neutral forearm rotation. The ulnar borders of the hand, the wrist, and the forearm are placed against the x-ray film cassette.

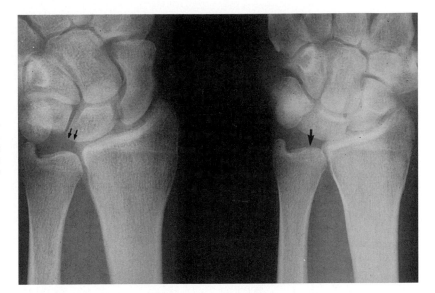

Figure 20–17. Representative radiographs of the destructive changes seen in ulnar impaction syndrome. On the *left,* the degenerative changes are noted on the proximal ulnar aspect of the lunate *(small arrows).* On the *right,* the degenerative changes are noted on the ulnar head *(large arrow).*

the cassette (Fig. 21–16*B*). A word of caution is in order here, however, for interpreting distal radioulnar joint congruency on the lateral view: The radiograph must be a perfect lateral view. A study by Mino and coworkers[84] has shown that minor deviations from neutral forearm rotation cause marked abnormalities on the radiograph, in the relationship of the distal ulna to the distal radius. (To diagnose subluxation of the DRUJ, we recommend a CT scan—see later.) On a lateral view of a normal wrist, the distal ulna is superimposed over the distal radius at its midportion. Obviously, with a suspected DRUJ subluxation or dislocation, this would not be evident, and other clues would be needed to gauge whether the radiographs are true lateral views or not. Mino and coworkers[84] found the following radiographic relationships in all their cadaveric specimens on a perfect lateral view.[84] The lunate, proximal pole of the scaphoid, and triquetrum were all superimposed upon one another, and the radial styloid was uniformly centered over the distal radius. With as little as 10° of pronation or supination, however, the relationships were altered. These investigators noted that with rotation from the neutral forearm position, accurate interpretation from the radiograph of a subluxation or dislocation of the DRUJ was impossible. (Another clue to a true lateral view is that the pisiform projects directly over the dorsal pole of the scaphoid.[67])

One of the oblique views is taken with 45° of supination and the other with 45° of pronation from the standard position of the lateral view.[67] Included in the differential diagnosis of ulnar-sided wrist pain is pisotriquetral joint arthritis, and this joint is seen in the semisupinated oblique view.[42, 67] To see the pisotriquetral joint in most instances, however, it is better to obtain the semisupinated oblique view at approximately 30° of supination from true lateral.

VIDEOFLUOROSCOPY

Videofluoroscopy is a useful adjunct to plain radiographs. It is often used in patients in whom a dy-

namic carpal instability process is suspected. In the distal radioulnar joint, videofluoroscopy can be used to determine whether there truly is an abutment between the distal ulna and the carpus in ulnar impaction syndrome. However, an excellent radiographic study for ulnar impaction syndrome is to obtain a PA view with the fist clenched in addition to the routine PA view. With a load across the wrist, the ulna moves distal relative to the radius, and this change is often quite noticeable on plain radiographs (Fig. 21–18).

Objective data concerning the use of videofluoroscopy in the work-up of wrist pathology are relatively limited. Bond and colleagues[12] reviewed several studies and noted that after normal plain radiographs, videofluoroscopy was most helpful in the diagnosis in 72% of patients. One of the most common dynamic disorders diagnosed in this review was, in fact, lunate-ulnar abutment.[4, 17, 110, 143] Videofluoroscopy should be distinguished from a wrist motion study that has been referred to in the past as "motion views" or a "ligamentous instability series." This latter study is a set of nine radiographic positions in which standard views are supplemented by stress views obtained by having the patient make a clenched fist. We rarely use these static views.

COMPUTED TOMOGRAPHY

The principal use of computed tomography in the work-up of distal radioulnar joint problems is in the investigation of possible DRUJ subluxation. A traumatic subluxation or dislocation of the DRUJ is certainly an accepted pathologic condition, but it is often difficult to prove clinically and with plain radiographs. Under normal circumstances, a true lateral radiograph is not difficult to obtain, but in patients with pain, cast material, or associated other injuries, obtaining a true lateral radiograph may be next to impossible.[84]

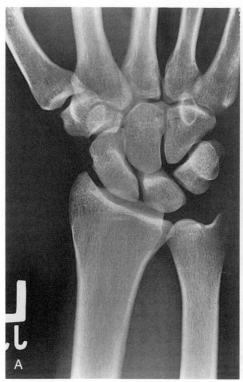
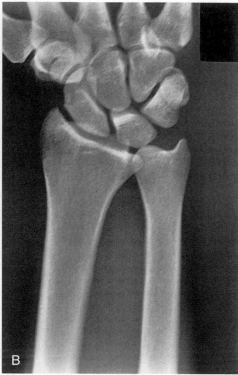

Figure 21–18. *A,* Standard posteroanterior (PA) radiograph of the wrist. *B,* PA radiograph of the same wrist, which has been loaded by having the patient grip the JAMAR Dynamometer. Note the significant increase in ulnar variance with loading of the wrist.

Scalfani[121] was the first to note, in a 1981 study, that DRUJ subluxation could possibly be diagnosed with a CT scan. Mino and colleagues[84] demonstrated that a single CT scan through the DRUJ made the diagnosis of subluxation or dislocation in all positions of forearm rotation. Their study showed that the diagnosis could be made as well with a true lateral plain radiograph, but they noted the inaccuracies associated in the clinical setting with plain radiographs. Furthermore, the position of the forearm with respect to prosupination did not have an effect on the diagnosis of DRUJ subluxation or dislocation in this cadaver model. These investigators also noted that plaster casts did not interfere with the technique. Comparison views can be easily made as well, by including the patient's other, asymptomatic wrist, placed in the same position of prosupination, in the scan (Fig. 21–19).

Mino and colleagues[04] went on to describe objective criteria to document subluxation. If one line is drawn through the dorsoulnar and dorsoradial aspects of the radius and another through the palmoulnar and palmoradial aspects of the radius, the congruent ulnar head should lie between these two divergent lines (Fig. 21–20A). If the ulnar head crosses the respective dorsal or palmar line, subluxation in a dorsal or palmar direction is diagnosed.

There is an inherent flaw, however, in this objective means of measuring the articulation between the distal radius and the distal ulna, namely, that this type of measurement can be made only with the forearm in neutral rotation. The dislocation or, more probable, subluxation often is not diagnosed with the forearm in neutral rotation. With the adherent translational motion of the distal radius about the ulnar head with prosupination, such an objective means of measuring the ulnar head with respect to the distal radius no longer has meaning. It may not be until the patient reaches the extremes of pronation or supination that the subluxation is noted. Therefore, most institutions prefer to study the DRUJ in sequential positions, extending from full pronation through the neutral forearm rotation into full supination. It is when the patient's clinical condition does not permit full forearm prosupination, and possibly only a static view can be obtained, that it is important to include the other, asymptomatic wrist in the same position of prosupination so that comparison views can be used to help in the diagnosis of a subluxation of the DRUJ (see Fig. 21–19). (At our institution, both extremities are routinely studied whenever CT scanning is used to investigate DRUJ stability.)

There are two other objective methods for gauging radioulnar congruency.[20] One is the epicenter method (Fig. 21–20B). In this method, a perpendicular line is drawn from the midpoint between the center of the ulnar head and the ulnar styloid (center of rotation of DRUJ) to the sigmoid notch chord. If this line is in the center of the sigmoid notch, the joint is considered congruous. This helps in assessing the DRUJ in supination. For the second method, with the arm in pronation, the arcs of the sigmoid notch and the ulnar head should be congruous (Fig. 21–20C).[137]

ARTHROGRAPHY

Arthrography is an excellent means of identifying perforations of the TFCC as well as of the scapholu-

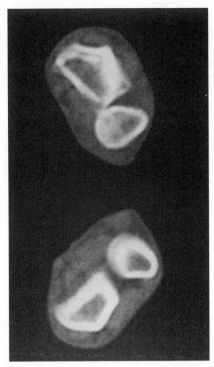

Figure 21–19. Computed tomography scan of bilateral distal radioulnar joints in a semi-supinated position. Note the volar subluxation of the ulna on the right (patient's left wrist).

nate and lunotriquetral interosseous ligaments. In patients with ulnar-sided wrist pain in whom plain radiographs and videofluoroscopy, if used, are normal, the wrist arthrogram often is the next stage of the work-up. Initially, the arthrogram was performed by a single injection of contrast material into the radiocarpal joint, and pathology was documented by leakage of contrast material into either the midcarpal joint or the DRUJ under fluoroscopy.[68, 135]

Levinsohn and coworkers[69, 70] modified the technique by showing that a three-compartment wrist arthrogram was more sensitive in diagnosing abnormalities of the TFCC and interosseous ligaments than the single-compartment injection technique. In the three-compartment technique, the midcarpal, radiocarpal, and distal radioulnar joints are injected separately. These investigators studied 50 consecutive patients with obscure post-traumatic wrist pain, in whom 25 triangular fibrocartilage complex abnormalities were identified, 6 of which (24 percent) were seen only with the DRUJ injection.

With the single-compartment injection technique of arthrography, one must make an assumption that a perforation of the TFCC would be identified with the radiocarpal injection; Levinsohn and coworkers[69, 70] have shown quite nicely that this assumption is erroneous. Eighteen patients were identified radiographically as having central or radially based triangular fibrocartilage complex perforations. In 3 of these patients, the perforations were identified only with injection into the radiocarpal joint, and not with injection into the DRUJ. In the remaining 15 patients, antegrade and retrograde flow was identified across the TFCC. The 6 patients in whom the TFCC abnormality was identified only with the DRUJ injection revealed the leakage to be at the proximal attachment of the TFCC to the base of the ulnar styloid (Fig. 21–21). These would be considered class 1B traumatic lesions in the Palmer[100] classification scheme.

Reinus and associates[112] studied a group of 83 patients using DRUJ arthrography. In 18 percent of patients, identifiable defects were seen on the TFCC's proximal surface, although these investigators noted that further study was needed to appreciate the significance of this finding. They also concluded that a TFCC perforation identified on arthrography was not necessarily associated with a patient's presentation of

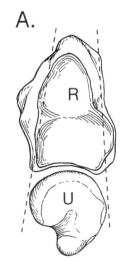
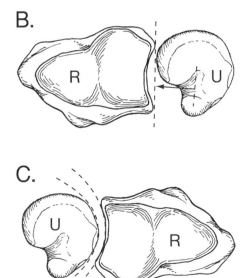

Figure 21–20. Objective methods for evaluating distal radioulnar joint congruency via computed tomography scan assessment. *A,* Method used with the forearm in neutral rotation. *B,* Method used with the forearm in supination. *C,* Method used with the forearm in pronation. *R* = radius; *U* = ulna. See text for description of these measurements.

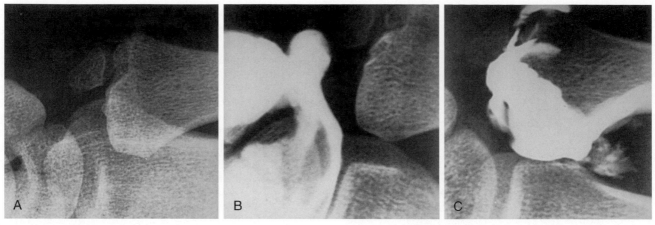

Figure 21–21. Arthrogram of the wrist depicting a class 1B injury to the triangular fibrocartilage complex (TFCC). *A,* Plain radiograph revealing ulnar styloid fracture. *B,* Arthrogram with radiocarpal joint injection, which is normal. *C,* Arthrogram with distal radioulnar joint injection, documenting TFCC injury. Note the contrast leaking out into the soft tissues proximal and ulnar to the ulnar styloid fracture.

pain.[112] It has been documented that 16 percent[48] to 45.8 percent[59] of the normal population is shown to have a TFCC perforation on arthrography.[88] Furthermore, Brown and colleagues[18] studied both wrists arthrographically in patients with unilateral wrist pain. They concluded that asymptomatic perforation of interosseous ligaments and of the TFCC are common and that, therefore, such findings may not be the source of the patient's pain. Nevertheless, Manister and coworkers[75] after adding a digital subtraction to their arthrography, did show a very high correlation (88 percent) between ulnar-sided wrist pain and abnormalities detected arthrographically. Palmer and associates[103] came to the same conclusion, in that they regarded the arthrogram to be an accurate predictor of TFCC pathology in the clinical arena.

In a review of 364 radiocarpal and 123 DRUJ arthrograms, Hardy and colleagues[47] identified an abnormality of the TFCC without a communication between the radiocarpal joint and DRUJ in 12 percent of cases. They divided the abnormalities into two groups, the larger group representing normal variants of the TFCC and the second, smaller group showing partial tears of the TFCC. This division was based on ultimate clinical outcome. Hardy and colleagues[47] stated that partial TFCC tears are most common on the proximal surface of the TFCC (Fig. 21–22). Another study, however, identified 82 patients with noncommunicating defects of both interosseous ligaments and the TFCC using arthrography, but found no statistically significant correlation between arthrographically identified abnormalities and symptoms.[80]

Blair and coworkers[11] concluded that adding the technique of arthrotomography allowed one to identify TFCC abnormalities with respect to the site, orientation, and size of the tear. Arthrography can also be helpful in looking not only at the TFCC but also at surrounding structures. The following is but a partial list of disorders in the wrist that can be identified on arthrography: adhesive capsulitis, cartilage abnor-malities, loose bodies, lymphatic and/or tendon sheath opacification, ganglion filling, and synovial hypertrophy such as seen with inflammatory changes.

Clearly, wrist arthrography does have a place in the armamentarium of the hand surgeon for diagnosing ulnar-sided wrist pain. On the basis of objective studies, it is just as clear that this modality is fraught

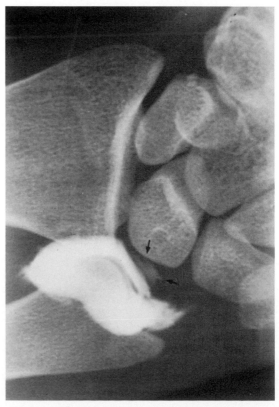

Figure 21–22. Arthrogram of the wrist. Note the abnormality on the proximal surface of the triangular fibrocartilage complex as demonstrated on this distal radioulnar joint injection.

with inconsistencies and can be used only as an adjunct to the history, physical findings, and other ancillary tests employed in the attempt to identify the cause of a patient's ulnar-sided wrist pain. When interpreting a wrist arthrogram that documents a TFCC perforation, the clinician should note that the finding is just that—a perforation or communication that may or may not be a symptomatic degenerative lesion or traumatic tear of the TFCC.

BONE SCAN

The use of nuclear imaging with respect to hand surgery has evolved over the years into what we now refer to as the three-phase bone scan. It allows not only the classic imaging of bone but also the imaging of vascular and soft tissue structures. Phase one is the radionuclide angiogram, which assesses the major vascular supply to the extremity as well as regional profusion. With regard to the upper extremity, the radial and ulnar arteries can be imaged in this phase. The soft tissue blood pool portion of this study is phase two. This phase is normally taken 1 to 2 minutes after injection and reveals "residual blood pool activity." In essence, the positive finding in phase two would represent a soft tissue injury in an area that was hyperemic and where the blood was pooling into the soft tissues. Finally, phase three represents the delayed bone imaging phase of the study. This phase can be equated with the traditional concept of the bone scan, and it is with this phase that disorders within the bones themselves are identified.

There is very little objective data dealing with the work-up of ulnar-sided wrist pain using nuclear imaging. Certainly the bone scan is not the first line of imaging the clinician would use, but it is traditionally employed if the clinical symptoms do not specify an area of the wrist or hand for the clinician to focus on and the plain radiographs are negative. In this situation, bone scans may be helpful in localizing areas of the wrist or hand with pathologic lesions. Pin and associates[108] concluded that a bone scan helped them in the diagnostic evaluation of unclear wrist pain. In essence, the bone scan helped them focus on areas of the wrist where they then used other modalities to arrive at the definitive diagnosis. They also concluded, however, that bone scans become less sensitive with increasing time since the injury.

Probably the most significant use of nuclear imaging in the hand and wrist is to rule out reflex sympathetic dystrophy, osteomyelitis, and occult fractures.[87] Clearly, in patients presenting with ulnar-sided wrist pain, bone scans would not be used very often in the diagnostic evaluation.

MAGNETIC RESONANCE IMAGING

Magnetic resonance (MR) imaging is the newest modality of radiologic examination of the wrist. The first MR imaging study of the hand was performed by Hinshaw and colleagues[52] in 1979. Resolution of the modality has greatly improved over the years with the design of new surface coils and the use of high-field-strength magnets. The technical advances in MR imaging have enhanced our ability as clinicians to view the scapholunate and lunotriquetral interosseous ligaments and, particularly, the triangular fibrocartilage complex. This development follows the large success MR imaging has shown in identifying ligamentous and cartilaginous structures in the larger joints of the body.[20]

Unlike arthrography, which in past years had been considered the standard radiographic study to examine the intrinsic ligaments of the wrist and the TFCC, the MR image is noninvasive and theoretically has the advantage of being able to identify precise locations of tears in these structures as well as to aid in the diagnosis of partial tears. Kang and associates,[58] performing MR imaging on cadaveric wrists, correlated the findings with gross pathologic and histologic analysis. Using spin-echo T_1-weighted and T_2-weighted coronal images, they were able to clearly distinguish degenerative processes occurring particularly in the TFCC from actual perforations. Furthermore, they were able to identify two out of four cases of abnormalities in the lunate and ulna following TFCC perforations.

Schweitzer and coworkers[123] performed an in vivo investigation of MR imaging using arthrography and arthroscopy as the standards. In their study, MR imaging displayed great accuracy in identifying abnormalities of the TFCC and scapholunate and lunotriquetral ligaments. Of particular significance, these investigators noted that the demonstration of fluid within the distal radial ulnar joint correlates with a TFCC tear (Fig. 21–23). This study clearly had weaknesses, however, particularly in that their chosen diagnostic standards, arthroscopy and arthrography, may not be standards at all. Other studies comparing MR imaging with arthroscopy have been carried out. Rhominger and associates[114] showed that 82 percent of triangular fibrocartilage tears identified arthroscopically were also diagnosed via MR imaging. Similarly, only 50 percent of scapholunate ligament tears and 40 percent of lunotriquetral ligament tears diagnosed arthroscopically were detected by MR imaging. Zlatkin and coworkers[146] studied 43 patients with chronic wrist pain and correlated their MR imaging findings with those from arthrography and arthroscopy or arthrotomy. They found that MR imaging had a sensitivity of 1.0 and a specificity of 0.93 in evaluation of triangular fibrocartilage tears. They were able to identify injuries to the intrinsic intercarpal ligaments, particularly the scapholunate ligament, as well with MR imaging, but not with the accuracy with which they identified TFCC injuries. These studies and others have shown that currently, MR imaging of the triangular fibrocartilage complex is better than that of the interosseous ligaments (Fig. 21–24).[113, 114, 146] (The Zlatkin[146] study also showed that subluxation or dis-

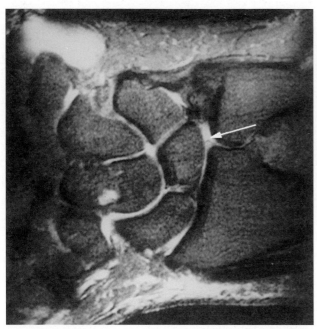

Figure 21–23. Magnetic resonance imaging of the wrist. This T$_2$-weighted image reveals a continuum of fluid from the distal radioulnar joint to the ulnocarpal joint, representing a discontinuity or tear of the triangular fibrocartilage complex. The fluid appears white in this image *(arrow).*

location of the distal radial ulnar joint can be diagnosed with MR imaging.)

An interesting study by Sugimoto and associates[129] confirmed through MR imaging many concepts about the TFCC already documented. They studied 70 asymptomatic volunteers and noted abnormal signal

intensity of the TFCC in 50 percent of the wrists. High signal intensity was associated with ulnar-positive variance and a thin TFCC.

From the preceding studies as well as others, it is evident that TFCC tears and other abnormalities can be diagnosed accurately with MR imaging.[43, 44, 58, 81, 123, 124, 126] Newer advances in MR imaging are allowing precise identification of specific components of the TFCC as well as their abnormalities. Totterman and coworkers[133, 134] used three-dimensional gradient-recalled echo (GRE) sequences and custom-made coils to evaluate triangular fibrocartilage complex anatomy. They studied both cadavers and patients and compared the results with anatomic dissection and surgical exploration, respectively. They identified both the volar and dorsal radioulnar ligaments as well as the classic central portion of the TFC. This study once again confirmed the observation by Palmer and colleagues that TFCC thickness varies inversely with ulnar variance. Totterman and Miller[133] did not have good visualization of the ulnocarpal ligaments. In a later study, Totterman and coworkers[134] used the same three-dimensional GRE sequences to evaluate 31 patients who had subsequent arthroscopy. They showed a high correlation between the results of MR imaging and what was found arthroscopically with respect to identifying specific components of the TFCC that were abnormal. This was true for all areas of the TFCC except the ulnocarpal ligaments. Although their diagnostic standard was arthroscopy, the case can be made that a false-positive MR image showing an abnormality may, in fact, be a true finding that does not appear on arthroscopy (false-negative). This disagreement can be accounted for by recalling that MR imaging reflects changes *within* the tissues

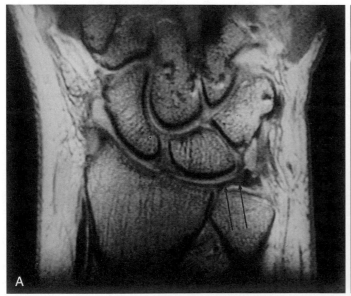
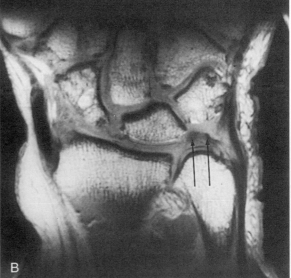

Figure 21–24. T$_1$-weighted imaging of the triangular fibrocartilage complex (TFCC), which appears black *(arrows). A,* Normal TFCC. Note the uniform black image extending from the ulnar aspect of the distal radius ulnarward over the ulnar head. *B,* Abnormal TFCC. Note the bunched appearance of the TFCC over the ulnar head as it appears to have lifted from its origin off the radius.

whereas arthroscopy assesses only the surface structures.

With regard to technique, at our institution, the radiologist's preference is for the patient to be in the prone position with the hands outstretched over the head, so that the wrist and the surrounding coil can be placed in the center of the magnet. It is accepted at our institution and in the literature[29] that this positioning may be less than ideal for patient comfort; patients who cannot tolerate this position are placed in the supine position with the hands at the sides. We also use a flexible coil placed around the wrist, although certainly, manufacturers now make specific wrist coils. At institutions with research interest in MR imaging of the wrist, custom-made coils are often used. MR imaging has multiplanar capabilities, thereby allowing each examination to be tailored to the clinical problem.[29] The axial plane is best used to investigate stability of the distal radioulnar joint and the TFCC. The coronal plain is used to study the TFCC. Multiple sequences are available as well. We use T_1-weighted, T_2-weighted, and GRE sequences. Generally, T_1-weighted images reveal excellent anatomic detail (Fig. 21–24), and T_2-weighted images allow identification of fluid collections in soft tissue structures (Fig. 21–23). Gradient-recalled echo sequencing can distinguish cartilage from fluid and is probably the technique of choice at our institution for examining the TFCC.

The MR imaging technique offers great promise for the evaluation of ulnar-sided wrist pain. At this time, it would be safe to say that MR imaging with the proper surface coil, which is available in the marketplace today, gives excellent resolution of the triangular fibrocartilage complex. In those rare institutions with custom-made coils, the scapholunate and lunotriquetral ligaments can also be identified accurately. With the techniques available generally, however, intrinsic ligament pathology cannot be diagnosed as competently as abnormalities of the TFCC. We believe that MR imaging will replace the arthrogram for investigating ulnar-sided wrist pain. Just as with arthrography, however, the hand surgeon must stop short of calling an identified lesion on MR imaging the source of the patient's wrist pain. As of yet, there is little objective data addressing the correlation of abnormalities identified with MR imaging of the TFCC with symptoms.

Wrist Arthroscopy

There is a significant distinction between radiographic evaluation of the hand and wrist arthroscopy. Wrist arthroscopy is an accepted technique in both the evaluation and treatment of wrist disorders, but as noted previously, when it should be used in the diagnostic work-up of wrist pain is open to some controversy.[90] There are certainly hand surgeons who would prefer wrist arthroscopy to any ancillary radiographic test after history taking, physical examination, and plain radiography.[90] Their point would be that arthroscopy in their hands is the diagnostic standard, and because they will use it sooner or later, it would be a waste of time, effort, and money to perform ancillary radiographic tests that will not change the management of a particular case. This rationale certainly has merit, although from a scientific point of view, we cannot confirm that arthroscopy is the standard, because it just has not been proven to be true. Particularly, as noted previously, Totterman and coworkers[134] comment that compared with arthroscopy, MR imaging of the TFCC may be a truer assessment of the TFCC, because it can diagnose midsubstance lesions.

The more standard use of wrist arthroscopy is for the clinician to obtain various ancillary radiologic tests in the work-up for ulnar-sided wrist pain and then to use the arthroscope, not only as a tool to confirm the diagnosis as made with the radiographic tests but also for treating the pathologic condition. It is in this way that we use wrist arthroscopy. The reader is referred to other texts and articles for general considerations of wrist arthroscopy and its technique.[104, 140–142] We would like, however, to make some specific comments about the technique with regard to distal radial ulnar joint arthroscopy.

At our institution, we have developed a technique for DRUJ arthroscopy that we have found to be reliable in the routine arthroscopy of this joint. In an unpublished study, we prospectively examined 142 patients with wrist arthroscopy (Loftus JB, Palmer AK, Short WH: Unpublished data, 1996). DRUJ arthroscopy was attempted in 87 of 142 patients. In 76 of 87 patients (87 percent), successful DRUJ arthroscopies were performed; in the other 11 patients (13 percent), arthroscopy was attempted but was unsuccessful. The distal radioulnar joint is obviously quite small, and we believe that at times, a 2.7-mm arthroscope is just too big. The rate of documented iatrogenic injuries with the arthroscope in this series was 3.5 percent. Four of the five cases involved injuries to the articular surface of the distal radial ulnar joint, particularly the ulnar head, and the other involved central perforation of the TFCC.

Classically, two portals are described for distal radioulnar joint arthroscopy (Fig. 21–25A).[141] The first portal (DRUJ1) is between the undersurface of the TFCC and the ulnar head or pole of the ulna. The second portal (DRUJ2) is in the axilla proximally, in the space between the sigmoid notch and the seat of the ulna. Our technique is sort of a hybrid between the classic DRUJ1 and DRUJ2 portals (Fig. 21–25B). The arthroscope is placed in the space between the ulnar head and the junction of the triangular fibrocartilage complex with the radius. This location is not just distal to the ulnar pole and is not in the axilla of the sigmoid notch ulnar seat articulation.

Wrist arthroscopy as a diagnostic test has been used only over the last decade or so. Initiation of wrist arthroscopy can be attributed to three individuals, Drs. Gary Polene, Jim Roth, and Terry Whipple.[104] What started out as an informal meeting between the

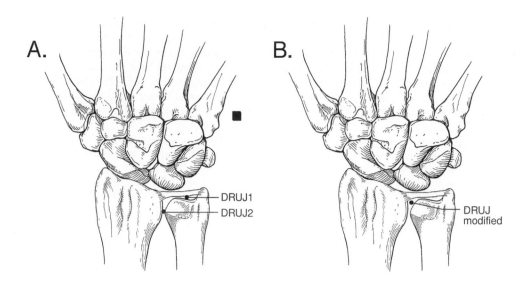

A.

B.

DRUJ1
DRUJ2

DRUJ
modified

Figure 21–25. Distal radioulnar joint (DRUJ) arthroscopy portals. *A,* The standard DRUJ1 and DRUJ2 portals. *B,* Our modification using the single portal for DRUJ arthroscopy.

three turned into a formal means of presenting wrist arthroscopy to the medical community. Obviously, their idea had merit, in that many hand surgeons today consider wrist arthroscopy to be a part of the standard armamentarium for the work-up and treatment of patients with wrist pain. Wrist arthroscopy as a diagnostic tool is an excellent means of assessing the ulnar side of the wrist. It is a relatively benign procedure that also allows the patient to begin motion of the wrist immediately following the procedure (Loftus JB, Palmer AK, Short WH: Unpublished data, 1996).

In deference to hand surgeons who believe that wrist arthroscopy is already the diagnostic standard for the work-up of the patient with wrist pain, there is some data to back their claim. Roth and Haddad[117] performed a prospective study evaluating the role of arthroscopy versus arthrography in the diagnosis of ulnar-sided chronic wrist pain. They used arthrography followed by arthroscopy in the work-up of 37 consecutive patients with undiagnosed ulnar-sided wrist pain. They concluded that "arthroscopy is superior to arthrography in diagnosing intraarticular pathology of the radial carpal articulation."[117] This conclusion can be understood, particularly in light of the fact that arthroscopy is believed to be better than arthrography with respect to the knee joint.[120]

Kulick and associates[66] studied the diagnostic accuracy of wrist arthroscopy by correlating their findings from radiocarpal joint arthroscopy with those from open inspection. They studied 80 wrists and documented good accuracy of radiocarpal arthroscopy. The lesions that were missed by arthroscopy most often involved chondromalacia on the palmar and dorsal surfaces of the various carpal bones as well as partial ligament tears. Koman and coworkers[65] reviewed 54 consecutive wrist arthroscopies in patients with chronic wrist pain. They noted that all patients underwent several state-of-the-art radiologic tests prior to arthroscopy and that after arthroscopy, the

pathologic diagnosis was made in 86 percent of patients. Only 63 percent of these lesions were incompletely diagnosed with a preoperative technique. The majority of the lesions diagnosed with arthroscopy were cartilaginous; the other disorders, in decreasing order of frequency, were: TFCC lesions, ligamentous lesions, synovitis, and fractures. Koman and coworkers[65] concluded that wrist arthroscopy is warranted in an attempt to diagnose TFCC defects, articular cartilage lesions, and chronic wrist pain. In the study by Roth and Haddad[117] of 23 patients in whom diagnosis of TFCC perforation was revealed by arthroscopy, the diagnosis was detected by previous arthrogram in only 16 (70 percent).

It needs to be pointed out, however, that in the Roth and Haddad[117] study, both the arthrogram and the arthroscopy were performed only via the radiocarpal joint. Levinsohn and associates[69, 145] have clearly shown that three-compartment wrist arthrography is superior to the single-compartment technique. Advances made in radiologic techniques over the last several years were not used in the comparison of arthrography with arthroscopy in the studies just described. Specifically, Blair and associates[11] have noted that arthrotomography can aid not only in the identification of a TFCC injury but also in the determination of its location, size, and orientation. With the advent of wrist coils, MR imaging certainly has a place in the diagnostic work-up for a patient with ulnar-sided wrist pain.

Certainly, more work needs to be done in comparing wrist arthrography, arthroscopy, and MR imaging with respect to evaluating the triangular fibrocartilage complex. One cannot say that one technique is far superior to the other from the objective evidence at hand. At this juncture, it seems that this debate could go on for some years, because it is difficult to compare techniques if in one study, one diagnostic test is held as the standard and in another study, another diagnostic test is held as the standard. We therefore suggest that all hand surgeons approach the work-up for the patient with ulnar-sided wrist pain using a rational approach that they can become comfortable with and in order to find a diagnosis for pain.

We generally have used wrist arthrography after history taking, physical examination, and plain radiography and prior to wrist arthroscopy. Now, however, that our institution has obtained the smaller surface coils used on the wrist, and as our radiologists are becoming more comfortable with and confident in interpreting the MR images, we find ourselves using MR imaging in place of arthrography more and more. It should be stressed that this approach applies to ulnar-sided wrist pain only, and not to global wrist pain. Can we envision the day that we will proceed straight to arthroscopy, bypassing arthrograms and MR imaging? Yes. Is it a certainty? No.

In these concluding thoughts concerning the diagnostic work-up for ulnar-sided wrist pain, we have by and large been talking about TFCC pathology. It is virtually universally accepted that a CT scan is the diagnostic tool of choice in those patients in whom distal radioulnar joint instability problems are suspected.

CONCLUSIONS

The treatment of TFCC and DRUJ problems is presented in detail in Chapters 21 to 23. Nevertheless, we present here our approach to the treatment of injuries to the TFCC and DRUJ.

There are two distinct clinical presentations of disorders of the distal radioulnar joint or the TFCC, acute trauma and chronic ulnar-sided wrist pain. With respect to trauma, the injury that is the simplest to conceptualize and understand is a fracture of the distal radius or the ulnar head. Aside from the obvious attention paid to the radiocarpal joint with regard to distal radius fractures, one must keep in mind that these fractures also affect the DRUJ.[6, 31, 34, 55, 64] Malalignment of the medial facet fragments or significant settling of a distal radius fracture can lead to obvious incongruity of the DRUJ. This, in turn, can lead to ulnar impingement with loss of prosupination, pain with prosupination, and/or arthritis. Hence, over the last several years, we have become more aggressive in treating distal radius fractures in attempts to achieve anatomic reduction of the fracture as well as to preserve the length of the distal radius. The effect that ulnar head fractures have on the distal radioulnar joint is obvious, and such fractures are addressed operatively when any significant displacement is present.

Acute soft tissue injuries to the DRUJ and TFCC manifest as acute onset of ulnar-sided wrist pain. If the injury is severe, this presentation most likely is in the emergency room. An acute dislocation is reduced and immobilized for 6 weeks; this treatment may require the use of a regional or general anesthetic. If the acute dislocation is associated with a radius

fracture, either an Essex-Lopresti or Galeazzi fracture, and if this injury is dealt with in the operating room, DRUJ stability is assessed once the fracture is fixed. If the DRUJ is stable, immobilization is all that is warranted, but if it remains unstable, the instability issue needs to be addressed. The joint is pinned after reduction or a more complex repair is undertaken (refer to Chapter 23).

Another clinical scenario that occurs often in our office is the patient who has an acutely injured wrist and now has ulnar-sided wrist pain but in whom radiographs are negative and the DRUJ is stable. Such patients are given the presumptive diagnosis of an injury to the TFCC, and their wrists are immobilized. Immobilization is achieved with a sugar-tong splint, followed by a Muenster cast after the swelling has subsided, and is continued for 6 weeks. In the acute settings in which a DRUJ dislocation or subluxation needs to be ruled out, plain radiographs often are not sufficient, and we rely on the CT scan. In the patient who cannot prosupinate the wrist because of pain, static CT scans are often the only views obtainable. Particularly in this situation, comparison scans showing the other DRUJ are imperative (see Fig. 21–19).

Chronic ulnar-sided wrist pain requires a different approach. Once again, the stability of the distal radioulnar joint must be assessed. If there is any doubt about it, a CT scan is obtained, consisting of views of the involved wrist and the other wrist from full pronation to full supination for comparison. If an instability pattern is identified in a patient with chronic pain, it has to be dealt with operatively (see Chapter 24). In patients in whom DRUJ instability is not an issue and plain radiographs are negative, other ancillary tests are utilized. We usually use wrist arthrography. (Certainly, if the wrist pain is more than ulnar-sided, videofluoroscopy can be very helpful.) However, since our institution has obtained smaller surface coils, we have found ourselves using MR imaging more and more for specific ulnar-sided wrist pain.

If a TFCC injury is noted on the radiologic study, wrist arthroscopy is carried out. If the radiologic studies are negative, a conservative approach to management is taken. This usually includes a course of physical therapy. If the pain remains recalcitrant to the conservative treatment or if a high index of suspicion remains after a negative radiologic study, wrist arthroscopy is used. The procedure not only serves as a diagnostic tool, but if the TFCC is found to be injured, it serves as a therapeutic tool as well. If there is a partial tear of the triangular fibrocartilage complex, it can be débrided. A degenerative tear or a central tear due to trauma can be débrided as well.[94, 99] A peripheral tear from the radial attachment can either be repaired back to the radius[57] or can be débrided. Similarly, a peripheral tear from the ulna can be repaired back to its insertion.

Our approach is a bit different for a patient who presents with chronic ulnar-sided wrist pain that we believe is due not to trauma but rather to ulnar impaction. This diagnosis can often be made from history, physical examination, and plain radiographs. The patient often complains of the insidious onset of ulnar-sided wrist pain. The pain can usually be reproduced in the office by loading the wrist or by ulnar deviation. Plain radiographs may reveal the ulnar head to have degenerative changes or to be abutting the surface of the lunate (see Fig. 21–17). If the standard plain radiographs are unremarkable, a PA clenched-fist view may reveal the impaction (see Fig. 21–18).

Our procedure of choice for ulnar impaction syndrome has become the arthroscopic wafer procedure (Fig. 21–26).[37, 89, 118, 120, 144] Because the DRUJ is so small, the procedure technically is carried out initially from the radiocarpal joint, working through the débrided central perforation of the TFCC. Therefore, this procedure obviously cannot be performed in the early stages of ulnar impaction syndrome, in which a degenerative tear of the TFCC does not exist. If a tear is not present, our procedure of choice is an ulnar-shortening procedure. Obviously, it is of paramount importance to determine whether a TFCC tear is present or not, because this knowledge determines which operation we perform. This information is obtained either via a preoperative arthrogram or MR imaging or, often, by means of diagnostic wrist arthroscopy at the time of surgery. A diagnostic wrist arthroscopy

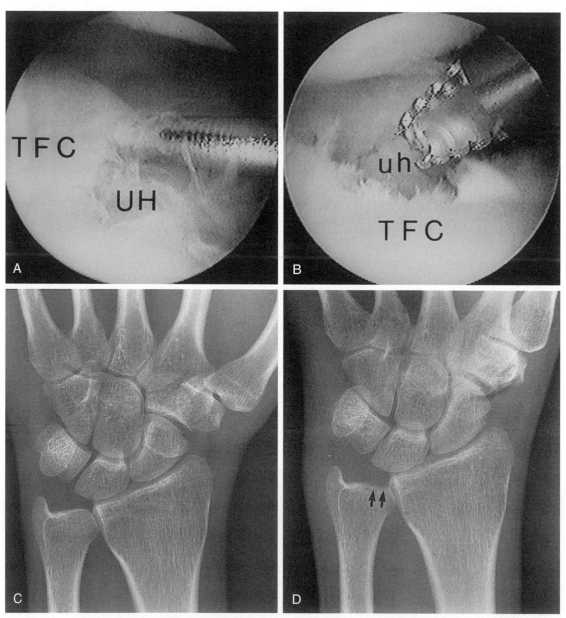

Figure 21–26. Arthroscopic wafer procedure. *A,* Arthroscopic view via the radiocarpal portal. TFC = triangular fibrocartilage; UH = ulnar head. *B,* Note the better visualization of the ulnar head through the débrided central perforation of the TFCC. *C* and *D,* Preoperative and postoperative radiographs of a patient who underwent an arthroscopic wafer procedure as a treatment for ulnar impaction syndrome. Arrows point to resected ulnar head.

would be converted to a therapeutic arthroscopic wafer procedure if a TFCC tear is present, and to an open ulnar-shortening procedure if not. The reader is referred to Chapters 22 to 24 for a more in-depth presentation of the treatment of DRUJ and TFCC disorders.

Our knowledge about the distal radial ulnar joint and triangular fibrocartilage complex has several shortcomings. To begin with, virtually every biomechanical study of the DRUJ and TFCC has of necessity been performed in cadaver models. As such, they are just that—models. Certainly, as technology advances, our ability to study the biomechanics of the wrist in general advances, but it seems we will always be left with this inherent flaw in study design, because we cannot study living tissues biomechanically. Another shortcoming already noted has to do with identifying what is causing a patient's symptoms. Certainly, Mikic's work,[82] which has been supported by the work by Palmer and associates,[106] demonstrates that triangular fibrocartilage complex tears seem to be a normal variant of aging in many instances. It is thus difficult to know when the ulnar-sided wrist pain is related to the objectively documented TFCC perforation. It makes sense that outcome studies are required to eventually answer this question in an indirect manner. We say indirect, because treatments will be instituted for the patient's symptoms. The study of the outcomes of these treatment modalities determining whether or not they are successful will indirectly also determine whether the diagnosis was correct. Finally, there is the issue of which study is best in the work-up for ulnar-sided wrist pain. Clearly, there is as yet no answer. MR imaging has promise, yet one can understand the argument that the most useful diagnostic test is wrist arthroscopy, thereby making radiologic studies, other than plain films, obsolete. Then, of course, there is the standard three-compartment wrist arthrogram, which now and possibly always will have a place in the work-up for ulnar-sided wrist pain.

Despite these shortcomings, some of which may never be satisfactorily eliminated, our understanding of the distal radial ulnar joint and triangular fibrocartilage complex has expanded tremendously in the last 15 years. The enigma of ulnar-sided wrist pain, which at one point was a frustration to both the physician and the patient, now is approached in a sound manner with respect to diagnosis and treatment, on the basis of our expanded knowledge not only of the biomechanics and anatomy of the DRUJ and TFCC but also of their disorders.

References

1. Adams BD: Partial excision of the triangular fibrocartilage complex articular disc: Biomechanical study. J Hand Surg 18A:334–340, 1993.
2. Adams BD, Holley KA: Strains in the articular disk of the triangular fibrocartilage complex: A biomechanical study. J Hand Surg 18A:919–925, 1993.
3. Almquist E: Evolution of the distal radial ulnar joint. Clinical Orthop 275:5–13, 1992.
4. Arkless R: Cineradiography in normal and abnormal wrists. AJR 96:837–844, 1966.
5. Arnoczky SP, Warren RF: The microvasculature of the meniscus and its response to injury: An experimental study in the dog. Am J Sports Med 11:131–141, 1983.
6. Aulicino PL, Siegel JL: Acute injuries of the distal radial ulnar joint. Hand Clin 7:283–293, 1991.
7. Bacorn RW, Kurtzke JF: Colles' fracture: A study of two thousand cases from the New York State Workmen's Compensation Board. J Bone Joint Surg 35A:643–658, 1953.
8. Bachdahl M: The caput ulnae in rheumatoid arthritis: A study of the morphology, abnormal anatomy, and clinical picture. Acta Rheumatol Scand 5:1–75, 1963.
9. Bednar MS, Arnoczky SP, Weiland AJ: The microvasculature of the triangular fibrocartilage complex: Its clinical significance. J Hand Surg 16A:1101–1105, 1991.
10. Bell MJ, Hill RJ, McMurtry RY: Ulnar impingement syndrome. J Bone Joint Surg 67B:126–129, 1985.
11. Blair FW, Berger RA, El-Khoury GY: Arthrotomography of the wrist: Experimental and preliminary clinical study. J Hand Surg 10A:350–359, 1985.
12. Bond JR, Berquist TH: Radiologic evaluation of hand and wrist motion. Hand Clin 7:113–123, 1991.
13. Bowers WH: Instability of the distal radioulnar articulation. Hand Clin 7:311–327, 1991.
14. Bowers WH: Problems of the distal radioulnar joint. In Advances in Orthopedic Surgery. Baltimore, Williams & Wilkins, 1984, pp 289–303.
15. Bowers WH: The distal radial ulnar joint. In Green DP (ed): Operative Hand Surgery, ed 2. New York, Churchill Livingstone, 1988, pp 939–989.
16. Bowers WH: The distal radial ulnar joint. In Green DP (ed): Operative Hand Surgery, ed 3. 1993, pp 973–1019.
17. Braunstein EM, Louis DS, Green TL, et al: Fluoroscopic and arthrographic evaluation of carpal instability. Am J Roentgenol 144:1259–1262, 1985.
18. Brown JA, Janzen DL, Adler BD, et al: Arthrography of the contralateral, asymptomatic wrist in patients with unilateral wrist pain. Can Assoc Radiol J 45:292–296, 1994.
19. Burgess RC, Watson HK: Hypertrophic ulnar styloid nonunions. Clin Orthop 228:215–217, 1988.
20. Burk DL Jr, Karasick D, Wechsler RJ: Imaging of the distal radial ulnar joint. Hand Clin 7:263–275, 1991.
21. Cabaud HE, Rodkey WG, Fitzwater JE: Medial meniscus repairs: An experimental and morphological study. Am J Sports Med 9:129–134, 1981.
22. Chan K, Huang P: Anatomic variations in radial and ulnar lengths in the wrists of Chinese. Clin Orthop 80:17–20, 1971.
23. Chidgey LK: Histologic anatomy of the triangular fibrocartilage. Hand Clin 7:249–262, 1991.
24. Chidgey LK, Dell PC, Bittar E, et al: Tear patterns and collagen arrangement in the triangular fibrocartilage. J Hand Surg 15A:826, 1990.
25. Chidgey LK, Dell PC, Bittar ES, Spanier SS: Histologic anatomy of the triangular fibrocartilage. J Hand Surg 16A:1084–1100, 1991.
26. Christensen JB, Adams JP, Cho KO, Miller L: A study of the interosseous distance between the radius and ulna during rotation of the forearm. Anat Rec 160:261, 1968.
27. Colles A: On the fractures of the carpal extremity of the radius. Med Surg J 10:181, 1814.
28. Cooney WP, Dobyns JH, Linscheid RL: Complications of Colles' fractures. J Bone Joint Surg 62A:613–619, 1980.
29. Dalinka MK, Myer S, Kricun ME, Vanel D: Magnetic resonance imaging of the wrist. Hand Clin 7:87–98, 1991.
30. Darrach W: Anterior dislocation of the head of the ulna. Ann Surg 56:801, 1912.
31. Darrach W: Colles' fractures. N Engl J Med 226:594–596, 1941.
32. Darrach W: Partial excision of the lower shaft of the ulna for deformity following Colles' fracture. Ann Surg 57:764, 1913.
33. Del PC: Distal radial ulnar joint dysfunction. Hand Clin 3:563–582, 1987.

34. Drewainy JJ, Palmer AK: Injuries to the distal radioulnar joint. Orthop Clin North Am 17:451–459, 1986.

35. Ekenstam FW, Hagert CG: Anatomical studies on the geometry and stability of the distal radial ulnar joint. J Plast Reconstr Surg 19:17–25, 1985.

36. Feldon P, Millender LH, Nalebuff EA: Rheumatoid arthritis in the hand and wrist. In Green DP (ed): Operative Hand Surgery, ed 3. New York, Churchill Livingstone, 1993, pp 1587–1690.

37. Feldon P, Terrono AL, Belsky MR: The "wafer" procedure, partial distal ulnar resection. Clin Orthop 275:124–129, 1992.

38. Frykman G: Fracture of the distal radius including sequelae—shoulder-hand-finger syndrome, disturbance in the distal radial ulnar joint and impairment of nerve function. ACTA Orthop Scand Suppl 108:1–153, 1967.

39. Galen: On the usefulness of the parts of the body (May MT, trans). Ithaca, NY, Cornell University Press, 1968.

40. Gelberman RH, Salamon P, Jurist J, Posch J: Ulnar variance in Kienböck's disease. J Bone Joint Surg 57A:674–676, 1975.

41. Gibson A: Uncomplicated dislocation of the inferior radioulnar joint. J Bone Joint Surg 7:180–189, 1925.

42. Gilula LA, Destouet JM, Weeks PM, et al: Roentgenographic diagnosis of the painful wrist. Clin Orthop 187:52–64, 1984.

43. Golumbu CN, Firooznia H, Melone CP Jr, et al: Tears of the triangular fibrocartilage of the wrist: MR imaging. Radiology 173:731–733, 1989.

44. Gundry CR, Kursunoglu-Brahme S, Schwaighofer B, et al: Is MR better than arthrography for evaluating the ligaments of the wrist? In vitro study. AJR 154:337–341, 1990.

45. Hagert CG: The distal radial ulnar joint in relation to the whole forearm. Clin Orthop 275:56–64, 1992.

46. Hamilin C: Traumatic disruption of the distal radioulnar joint. Am J Sports Med 5:93–97, 1977.

47. Hardy DC, Totty WG, Carnes KM, et al: Arthrographic surface anatomy of the carpal triangular fibrocartilage complex. J Hand Surg 13A:823–829, 1988.

48. Harrison MO, Freiberger RH, Ranawat CS: Arthrography of the rheumatoid wrist joint. AJR 112:480–486, 1971.

49. Hauck RM, Skahen J III, Palmer AK: Classification and treatment of ulnar styloid non-union. J Hand Surg 21A:418–422, 1996.

50. Heatley FW: The meniscus—can it be repaired? An experimental investigation in rabbits. J Bone Joint Surg 62B:397–402, 1980.

51. Heiple KG, Freehafer AA: Isolated traumatic dislocation of the distal end of the ulna or distal radioulnar joint. J Bone Joint Surg 44A:1387–1394, 1962.

52. Hinshaw WS, Andrew ER, Bottomley PA, et al: An in vivo study of the forearm and hand by thin section NMR imaging. Br J Radiol 52:36–43, 1979.

53. Hollingsworth R, Morris J: The importance of the ulnar side of the wrist in fractures of the distal end of the radius. Injury 7:263–266, 1976.

54. Hülten O: Über anatomische Variation der Hand Gelenkknochen. Acta Radiol 9:155–169, 1928.

55. Hyman G, Martin FR: Dislocation of the inferior radioulnar joint as a complication of fracture of the radius. Br J Surg 27:481–491, 1939.

56. Ishii S, Palmer AK, Werner FW, et al: Pressure distribution in the distal radioulnar joint. Presented at the 51st annual meeting of the American Society for Surgery of the Hand, Nashville, TN, 1996.

57. Jantea CL, Baltzer A, Ruther W: Arthroscopic repair of radial sided lesions of the triangular fibrocartilage complex. Hand Clin 11:31–36, 1995.

58. Kang HS, Kindynis P, Brahme SK, et al: Triangular fibrocartilage and intercarpal ligaments of the wrist: MR imaging—cadaveric study with gross pathologic and histologic correlation. Radiology 181:401–404, 1981.

59. Kessler I, Silberman Z: An experimental study of the radiocarpal joint by arthrography. Surg Gynecol Obstet 112:33–40, 1961.

60. Kihara H, Short W, Werner FW, et al: The stabilizing mechanism of the distal radioulnar joint during pronation and supination. J Hand Surg 20A:930–936, 1995.

61. King D: The function of semilunar cartilages. J Bone Joint Surg 18:1069–1076, 1936.

62. King GJ, McMurtry RY, Rubenstein JD, Gertzbein SD: Kinematics of the distal radioulnar joint. J Hand Surg 11A:798, 1986.

63. King GJ, McMurtry RY, Rubinstein JD, Ogston NG: Computerized tomography of the distal radioulnar joint: Correlation with ligamentous pathology in cadaveric model. J Hand Surg 11A:711–717, 1986.

64. Knirk JL, Jupiter JB: The interarticular fractures of the distal end of the radius in young adults. J Bone Joint Surg 68A:647–659, 1986.

65. Koman LA, Poehling GG, Toby EB, Kammire G: Chronic wrist pain: Indications for wrist arthroscopy. Arthroscopy 6:116–119, 1990.

66. Kulick MI, Chen C, Swearingen PS: Determining the diagnostic accuracy of wrist arthroscopy. Presented at 45th annual meeting of American Society for Surgery of the Hand, Toronto, 1990.

67. Levinsohn EM: Imaging of the wrist. Radiol Clin North Am 28:905–921, 1990.

68. Levinsohn EM, Palmer AK: Arthrography of the traumatized wrist. Radiology 146:647–651, 1983.

69. Levinsohn EM, Palmer AK, Coren AB, Zinberg EM: Wrist arthrography: The value of the three compartment injection technique. Skeletal Radiol 16:539–544, 1987.

70. Levinsohn EM, Rosen DI, Palmer AK: Value of the three compartment injection method. Radiology 179:231–239, 1991.

71. Linscheid RL: Biomechanism of the distal radioulnar joint. Clinical Orthop 275:46–55, 1992.

72. Linscheid RL, Dobbins JH: Rheumatoid arthritis of the wrist. Orthop Clin North Am 2:649–665, 1971.

73. Lippman RD: Laxity of the radioulnar joint following Colles' fracture. Arch Surg 35:772–786, 1937.

74. Mann FA, Wilson AJ, Gilula LA: Radiographic evaluation of the wrist: What does the hand surgeon want to know? Radiology 184:15–24, 1992.

75. Manaster BJ, Mann RJ, Rubinstein S: Wrist pain: Correlation of clinical and plain film findings with arthrographic results. J Hand Surg 14A:466–473, 1989.

76. Mayfield JKS, Johnson RP, Kilcoyne RF: Carpal dislocations: Pathomechanics and progressive perilunar instability. J Hand Surg 5:226, 1980.

77. Melone CP Jr: Articular fractures of the distal radius. Orthop Clin North Am 15:217–236, 1984.

78. Melone CP Jr: Open treatment for displaced articular fractures of the distal radius. Clin Orthop 202:103–111, 1986.

79. Melone CP, Nathan R: Traumatic disruption of the triangular fibrocartilage complex: Pathoanatomy. Clinical Orthop 275:65–73, 1992.

80. Metz VM, Mann FA, Gilula LA: Lack of correlation between site of wrist pain and location of non-communicating defect shown by three-compartment wrist arthroscopy. AJR 160:1239–1243, 1993.

81. Metz VM, Shratter M, Dock WI, et al: Age-associated changes of the triangular fibrocartilage of the wrist: Evaluation of the diagnostic performance of MR imaging. Radiology 184:217–220, 1992.

82. Mikic ZDJ: Age changes in the triangular fibrocartilage of the wrist. J Anat 126:367–384, 1978.

83. Milch H: So-called dislocation of the lower end of the ulna. Ann Surg 116:282–292, 1942.

84. Mino DE, Palmer AK, Levinsohn EM: The role of radiography and computerized tomography in the diagnosis of subluxation and dislocation of the distal radial ulnar joint. J Hand Surg 8:23–31, 1983.

85. Miura H, Uchida Y, Sugioka Y: Radial closing wedge osteotomy for Kienböck's disease. J Hand Surg 21A:1029–1034, 1996.

86. Morrissy RT, Nalebuff EA: Dislocation of the distal radioulnar joint: Anatomy and clues to prompt diagnosis. Clin Orthop 144:154–158, 1979.

87. Mourer AH: Nuclear medicine in evaluation of the hand and wrist. Hand Clin 7:183–200, 1991.

88. Mrose HE, Rosenthal DI: Arthrography of the hand and wrist: Imaging of the hand. Hand Clin 7:201–217, 1991.

89. Nagle DJ: Arthroscopic treatment of degenerative tears of the triangular fibrocartilage. Hand Clin 10:615–624, 1994.

90. Debate. 51st annual meeting of American Society for Surgery of the Hand, Nashville, TN, 1996.

91. Nathan R, Schneider LH: Classification of distal radial ulnar joint disorders. Hand Clin 7:239–247, 1991.

92. Nolan WB III, Eaton RG: The classic: Partial excision of the lower shaft of the ulna for deformity following Colles' fracture, William Darrach. Clinical Orthop 275:3–4, 1992.

93. O'Donovan TM, Ruby LK: The distal radial ulnar joint in rheumatoid arthritis. Hand Clin 5:249–256, 1989.

94. Osterman AL: Arthroscopic débridement of triangular fibrocartilage tears. Arthroscopy 6:120–124, 1990.

95. Osterman AL, Terrill RG: Arthroscopic treatment of TFCC lesions. Hand Clin 7:277–281, 1991.

96. Palmer AK: The distal radioulnar joint. In Lichtman DM (ed): The Wrist and Its Disorders. Philadelphia, WB Saunders, 1988, pp 220–231.

97. Palmer AK: The distal radioulnar joint. Hand Clin 3:31–40, 1987.

98. Palmer AK: Symposium on distal ulnar injuries. Contemp Orthop 7:81, 1983.

99. Palmer AK: Triangular fibrocartilage disorders: Injury patterns and treatment. Arthroscopy 6:125–132, 1990.

100. Palmer AK: Triangular fibrocartilage complex lesions: A classification. J Hand Surg 14A:594–606, 1989.

101. Palmer AK, Glisson RR, Werner FW: Ulnar variance determination. J Hand Surg 7:376–379, 1982.

102. Palmer AK, Glisson RR, Werner FW, Mech EM: Relationship between ulnar variance and triangular fibrocartilage complex thickness. J Hand Surg 9A:681–683, 1984.

103. Palmer AK, Levinsohn EM, Kuzma GR: Arthrography of the wrist. J Hand Surg 8:15–23, 1983.

104. Palmer AK, Loftus J: Wrist arthroscopy. In Cooney WP (ed): The wrist: Diagnosis and Operative Treatment. Chicago, Mosby Yearbook, tentative publication 1997.

105. Palmer AK, Werner FW: Biomechanics of the distal radial ulnar joint. Clin Orthop 187:26–34, 1984.

106. Palmer AK, Werner FW: The triangular fibrocartilage complex of the wrist—anatomy and function. J Hand Surg 6:153, 1981.

107. Palmer AK, Werner FW, Glisson RR, Murphy DJ: Partial excision of the triangular fibrocartilage complex. J Hand Surg 13A:403–406, 1988.

108. Pin PG, Semenkovich JW, Leroy Young V, et al: Role of radionucleotide imaging in the evaluation of wrist pain. J Hand Surg 13A:810–814, 1988.

109. Pirela-Cruz MA, Goll SR, Klug M, Windler D: Stress computed tomography analysis of the distal radial ulnar joint: A diagnostic tool for determining translational motion. J Hand Surg 16A:75–82, 1991.

110. Protas JM, Jackson WT: Evaluating carpal instabilities with fluoroscopy. AJR 135:137–140, 1980.

111. Reeves B: Excision of the ulnar styloid fragment after Colles' fracture. Int Surg 45:46–52, 1966.

112. Reinus WR, Hardy DC, Totty WG, Gilula LA: Arthrographic evaluation of the carpal triangular fibrocartilage complex. J Hand Surg 12A:495–503, 1987.

113. Rettig ME, Reskin KB, Melone CP Jr: Clinical applications of MR imaging in hand and wrist surgery—magnetic resonance imaging. Magn Reson Imaging Clin North Am 3:361–368, 1995.

114. Rhominger MB, Bernreuter WK, Kenney PJ, Lee DH: MR imaging of anatomy and tears of wrist ligaments. Radiographics 13:1233–1246, 1993.

115. Robbin ML, An KN, Linscheid RL, Ritman EL: Anatomic and kinematic analysis of the human forearm using high-speed computed tomography. Med Biol Eng Comput 24:164, 1986.

116. Rose-Innes AP: Anterior dislocation of the ulna at the inferior radio-ulnar joint: Case report with a discussion of the anatomy of rotation of the forearm. J Bone Joint Surg 42B:515–521, 1960.

117. Roth JH, Haddad RG: Radiocarpal arthroscopy and arthrography in the diagnosis of ulnar wrist pain. Arthroscopy 2:234–243, 1986.

118. Roth JH, Poehleng GG: Arthroscopic "ectomy" surgery of the wrist. Arthroscopy 6:141–147, 1990.

119. Sagerman SD, Zogby RG, Palmer AK, et al: Relative articular inclination of the distal radioulnar joint: A radiographic study. J Hand Surg 20A:597–601, 1995.

120. St Pierre RK, Sones PJ, Fleming LL: Arthroscopy and arthrography of the knee: A comparative study. South Med J 74:1322–1328, 1981.

121. Scalfani SJA: Dislocation of the distal radial ulnar joint. J Comput Assist Tomogr 5:450, 1981.

122. Schuind F, An KN, Berlund L, et al: The distal radioulnar ligaments: A biomechanical study. J Hand Surg 16A:1106–1114, 1991.

123. Schweitzer ME, Brahme SK, Hodler J, et al: Chronic wrist pain: Spin-echo and short tau inversion recovery MR imaging and conventional and MR arthrography. Radiology 182:205–211, 1992.

124. Skahen JR, Palmer AK, Levinsohn EM, et al: Magnetic resonance imaging of the triangular fibrocartilage complex. J Hand Surg 15A:552–557, 1990.

125. Smaill GB: Long-term follow-up of Colles' fracture. J Bone Joint Surg 47B:80–85, 1965.

126. Spinner M, Kaplan EB: Extensor carpi ulnaris: Its relationship to stability of the radioulnar joint. Clin Orthop 68:124–129, 1970.

127. Steinhauser J, Abele H, Schettler G: Anatomisch morphologische Studieen zer sogenannten Minusvariante der elle am Handgelenk. Z Orthop 3:36–40, 1973.

128. Straub LR, Ranawat CS: The wrist in rheumatoid arthritis—surgical treatment and results. J Bone Joint Surg 51A:1–20, 1969.

129. Sugimoto H, Shinozaki T, Ohsawa T: Triangular fibrocartilage in asymptomatic subjects: Investigation of abnormal MR signal intensity. Radiology 191:193–197, 1994.

130. Taleisnik J: The ligaments of the wrist. J Hand Surg 1:110–118, 1976.

131. Thiru-Pathi RG, Ferlic DC, Clayton ML, McClure DC: Arterial anatomy of the triangular fibrocartilage of the wrist and its surgical significance. J Hand Surg 11A:258–263, 1986.

132. Tolat AR, Sanderson PL, DeSmet L, Stanley JK: The gymnasts' wrist: Acquired positive ulnar variance following chronic epiphyseal injury. J Hand Surg 17B:678–681, 1992.

133. Totterman SMS, Miller RJ: Triangular fibrocartilage complex: Normal appearance on coronal three-dimensional gradient-recalled-echo MR images. Radiology 195:521–527, 1995.

134. Totterman SMS, Miller RJ, McCanc SE, Meyers SP: Lesions of the triangular fibrocartilage complex: MR findings with a three-dimensional gradient-recalled-echo sequence. Radiology 199:227–232, 1996.

135. Trentham DE, Hamm RL, Masi AT: Wrist arthrography: Review and comparison of normals, rheumatoid arthritis and gout patients. Semin Arthritis Rheum 5:105–120, 1975.

136. Vesely DG: The distal radioulnar joint. Clin Orthop 51:75–91, 1967.

137. Wechsler RJ, Wehbe MA, Rifkin, et al: Computed tomography diagnosis of distal radial ulnar joint subluxation. Skeletal Radiol 16:1–5, 1987.

138. Weiler PJ, Bogoch ER: Kinematics of the distal radial ulnar joint in rheumatoid arthritis: An in vivo study using centrode analysis. J Hand Surg 20A:937–943, 1995.

139. Werner FW, Palmer AK, Glisson RR: Forearm load transmission: The effect of ulnar lengthening and shortening. In Cracchiolo A (ed): Transactions of the 28th Annual Meeting of the Orthopedic Research Society. New Orleans, 1982, p 273.

140. Whipple TL: Arthroscopy of the distal radioulnar joint: Indications, portals, and anatomy. Hand Clin 10:589–592, 1994.

141. Whipple TL: Arthroscopic Surgery: The Wrist. Philadelphia, JB Lippincott, 1992.

142. Whipple TL, Cooney WP, Osterman AL, Viegas SF: Wrist arthroscopy. Instr Course Lect 44:139–145, 1995.

143. White SJ, Louis DS, Braunstein EM, et al: Capitate lunate

instability: Recognition by manipulation under fluoroscopy. AJR 143:361–364, 1984.

144. Wnorowski D, Palmer AK, Werner FW, Fortino MD: Anatomic and biomechanical analysis of the arthroscopic wafer procedure. Arthroscopy 8:204–212, 1992.

145. Zinberg EM, Palmer AK, Coren AB, Levinsohn EM: The triple injection wrist arthrogram. J Hand Surg 13A:803–809, 1988.

146. Zlatkin MB, Chao PC, Osterman AL, et al: Chronic wrist pain: Evaluation with high-resolution MR imaging. Radiology 173:723–729, 1989.

Treatment of Acute Injuries of the Triangular Fibrocartilage Complex

David S. Zelouf, MD, and William H. Bowers, MD

Acute injuries to the triangular fibrocartilage (TFC) are common and often difficult to manage. Interest in this subject continues to grow, as evidenced by the ever-increasing number of publications dealing with this structure. In this chapter, we discuss acute triangular fibrocartilage injuries and their management. Surgical approaches, both open and arthroscopic, are presented. Recommendations are based on our personal experience as well as published results. Anatomy, kinematics, and the treatment of chronic disorders of the distal radioulnar joint are covered elsewhere in this text.

SURGICAL APPROACHES

Surgical options for treatment of acute triangular fibrocartilage injuries generally involve either open or arthroscopic techniques. Because of the intimacy of contact between the radius, ulna, triangular fibrocartilage, and ulnar carpus, we frequently employ more than one approach to treat these difficult problems. We may, for example, perform arthroscopic inspection followed by open intervention either at the same sitting or in a delayed fashion. We now detail dorsal, volar, and arthroscopic approaches to the distal radioulnar joint.

Dorsal Approach

The dorsal approach is our most commonly employed technique for open exploration of the distal radioulnar joint. When properly performed, no significant alteration in kinematics or stability of the distal radioulnar joint should occur. This approach allows visualization of the dorsal 60 percent of the ulnar head and the carpal face of the triangular fibrocartilage, the lunotriquetral ligament, the triquetrum, the meniscus, the prestyloid recess, and the majority of the distal radioulnar joint synovial cavity.

PROCEDURE

Begin the procedure with the wrist in full pronation. Make a skin incision along the ulnar shaft that starts approximately three fingerbreadths proximal to the

ulnar styloid. Curve the incision gently around the distal side of the ulnar head so it ends dorsally at the midcarpus and can be extended distally in an ulnar fashion for more distal exposure. Lying just volar to the incision is the dorsal sensory branch of the ulnar nerve, which should be identified and protected during the procedure. Then, identify the extensor retinacular fibers and, beneath its proximal border, note the capsule overlying the ulnar head between the extensor digiti minimi and the extensor carpi ulnaris. Release the extensor digiti minimi from its sheath, and reflect the proximal and radial half of the extensor retinaculum ulnarward. Take care to leave the extensor carpi ulnaris undisturbed. Retract the extensor digiti minimi radialward, revealing the dorsal margin of the sigmoid notch of the radius and the triangular fibrocartilage. Next, sharply detach the distal radioulnar joint capsule from the radius, leaving a 1-mm cuff for later repair, and perform a transverse capsulotomy just proximal to the triangular fibrocartilage. The capsule can then be reflected ulnarward, allowing visualization of approximately 100 degrees of the total convexity of the ulnar head, the sigmoid notch, and the underside of the triangular fibrocartilage. We often employ a laminar spreader to improve visualization of the sigmoid notch.

Obtain exposure of the ulnar carpus and the distal articulating surface of the triangular fibrocartilage by incising the capsule in a hockey-stick fashion along the transverse-lying fibers of the dorsal radiotriquetral ligament. Should more distal exposure be required, the thick portion of the extensor retinaculum may be reflected as an ulnarly based flap with subperiosteal dissection of the unviolated sixth dorsal compartment. In general, we attempt to leave the thick portion of the retinaculum undisturbed, in order to avoid altering the stabilizing function of the extensor carpi ulnaris. Once completed, this dissection allows one to explore the distal radioulnar joint, the triangular fibrocartilage complex (TFCC), as well as the ulnar carpus, as shown diagramatically in Figure 22–1. At the conclusion of the procedure, repair all structures anatomically.

Volar Approach

The volar approach is indicated for release of soft tissue pronation contracture involving the volar cap-

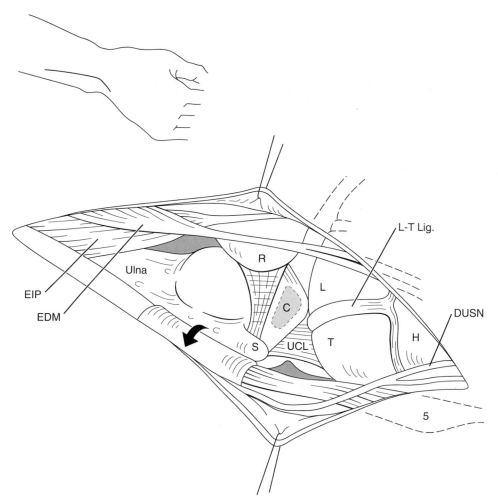

Figure 22–1. Dorsal approach to the DRUJ. *TFC* = triangular fibrocartilage complex; *C* = central portion of TFC; *H* = hamate; *L* = lunate; *R* = radius; *S* = styloid; *UCL* = ulnocarpal ligaments; *EDM* = extensor digiti minimi; *EIP* = extensor indicis proprius; *DUSN* = dorsoulnar sensory nerve; *T* = triquetrum; *L-T Lig.* = lunotriquetral ligament; *5* = fifth metacarpal. The *heavy double-dotted line* around the styloid that extends distally between the ulnolunate and ulnotriquetral ligaments represents the area in which a destabilizing tear of the ulnar wrist ligaments is most often found when the radiographic findings are negative. The same injury pattern may avulse the styloid.

sular structures, as well as occasionally to perform a Darrach procedure. The latter indication is especially useful for the anteriorly unstable distal ulna. This approach allows visualization of the volar sigmoid notch and the volar aspect of the ulnocarpal ligaments.

PROCEDURE

Use a volar ulnar incision, with the deep dissection proceeding between the flexor tendons and the ulnar neurovascular bundle. Retract the flexor carpi ulnaris ulnarward along with the ulnar neurovascular bundle. Visualize the pronator quadratus, and at its distal margin, identify and reflect the volar capsule of the distal radioulnar joint along with a portion of the pronator quadratus. We recommend a proximal-to-distal dissection to enable easier visualization of the volar limb of the triangular fibrocartilage, thus avoiding iatrogenic injury.

This soft tissue release alone may alleviate a pronation contracture in the post-traumatic setting. However, not all pronation contractures are relieved by a soft tissue release. In some cases, and especially in patients with distal radioulnar joint incongruity, a

resection of the distal radioulnar joint (DRUJ) may be required. The decision to perform DRUJ resection can be made following an adequate soft tissue release.

Arthroscopy

Arthroscopy as a technique continues to evolve rapidly. We now routinely employ the technique in the management of acute and chronic disorders of the distal radioulnar joint. It has added significantly to our diagnostic and therapeutic armamentarium and has become an indispensable tool in this regard. It offers unparalleled visualization of the ulnocarpal surface of the triangular fibrocartilage complex and is minimally invasive. The following synopsis offers several tips we have found to be helpful. See Chapters 10 and 11 for an in-depth discussion. We also recommend Whipple's text on arthroscopic surgery of the wrist[7] for additional information.

The procedure is performed using regional or general anesthesia with the patient in the supine position. The shoulder is abducted 90 degrees, and the forearm is allowed to rest in the neutral position. We use a hand table along with the Concept Traction

Tower Extremity Traction Device. We have found this device to offer several advantages; it is freestanding and completely self-contained, and is easy to use. It can be disassembled and autoclaved, thus reducing contamination. A universal joint allows for ease of adjustment, permitting radial/ulnar deviation, along with flexion/extension. This feature also enables easy positioning for use with intraoperative fluoroscopy. The traction tower is also equipped with a cassette holder, which allows one to obtain plain radiographs with the extremity in traction. Another notable feature is a built-in traction scale that can be easily adjusted from 0 to 15 lb.

Once the patient is positioned appropriately in the traction tower, the wrist joint is longitudinally distracted and distended with irrigation fluid. We have not found it necessary to exceed 15 lb of longitudinal distraction force. Entry into the radiocarpal articulation is facilitated by using a low-emission portable roentgen unit. This unit is very helpful in localizing the radiocarpal and midcarpal portals, thus reducing iatrogenic articular injury. We have also found the unit helpful in localizing entry into the distal radioulnar joint.

Standard instruments, including a 1.5-mm probe, a 2.9-mm suction basket, a basket forceps, a full-radius resector and a banana blade are most often employed for wrist arthroscopic surgery. A 2.7-mm diameter, 25-degree arthroscope is preferred. We continue to use gravity-feed irrigation and have not found it necessary to employ a mechanical pump.

PROCEDURE

Initial viewing is through the 3-4 radiocarpal portal, located between the extensor pollicis longus and extensor digitorum comminus tendons. After localizing the portal and distending the joint, longitudinally incise the skin with a no. 11 blade. Use a curved clamp to spread down to the capsule, and then use a cannula and blunt obturator to enter the radiocarpal joint. Take care to angle the trocar parallel to the distal radial articular surface. Establish inflow through the cannula, and perform a diagnostic survey. Next, localize a 4-5 radiocarpal portal with an 18-gauge needle under direct vision. Place a probe and continue the survey.

A 6R radiocarpal portal may also be established either for inflow or for further instrumentation. Other portals we routinely employ include the midcarpal radial portal, which is located 1 cm distal to the 3-4 radiocarpal portal, and the distal radioulnar joint portal, which is located 1 cm proximal to the 4-5 portal. Entry into both is facilitated by joint distension and radiographic visualization. We conclude our arthroscopic surgical procedures with copious irrigation of the joint, along with instillation of a combination of a water-soluble corticosteroid (Celestone) and a long-acting anesthetic (bupivacaine).

ACUTE INJURIES

Acute injuries to the triangular fibrocartilage complex may be isolated or may occur in conjunction with fractures of the distal radius and ulna. Their incidence is unknown, because many injuries heal uneventfully following a short period of disability. Others result in significant ulnar-sided wrist pain and distal radioulnar joint instability.

A classification of triangular fibrocartilage complex lesions reported by Palmer[5] has gained acceptance and serves as a useful starting point in this discussion (Table 22–1). This classification was based on TFCC lesions observed by Dr. Palmer over a period of years, and specifically, those that underwent surgical intervention. Most patients were initially treated conservatively, and thus, this classification of traumatic and degenerative lesions is applicable more in a global sense rather than in the acute setting. It is inferred, however, that acute tears, if untreated, may become chronic, and the treatment may be the same as in the acute setting. This scenario may not always be the case, and some injuries, if left untreated, may ultimately require a reconstructive approach.

We prefer to consider acute injuries to the triangular fibrocartilage complex in one of three categories: nondestabilizing, destabilizing, or associated with fractures of the distal radius and/or ulnar styloid.

Nondestabilizing TFC Injuries

Nondestabilizing triangular fibrocartilage injuries are those in which instability of the distal radioulnar joint is not obvious and the support structures (e.g.,

Table 22–1. CLASSIFICATION OF TFCC

CLASS I—Traumatic
  A. Central perforation
  B. Medial avulsion (ulnar attachment)
     with distal ulnar fracture
     without distal ulnar fracture
  C. Distal avulsion (carpal attachment)
  D. Lateral avulsion (radial attachment)
     with sigmoid notch fracture
     without sigmoid notch fracture

CLASS II—Degenerative (ulnocarpal impaction syndrome)
  Stage 1. TFCC wear
  Stage 2. TFCC wear
     + lunate and/or ulnar chondromalacia
  Stage 3. TFCC perforation
     + lunate and/or ulnar chondromalacia
  Stage 4. TFCC perforation
     + lunate and/or ulnar chndromalacia
     + L-T ligament perforation
  Stage 5. TFCC perforation
     + lunate and/or ulnar chondromalacia
     + L-T ligament perforation
     + ulnocarpal arthritis

From Palmer AK: Triangular fibrocartilage complex lesions: A classification. J Hand Surg 14A:594–606, 1989.

capsule, extensor carpi ulnaris sheath, and articular surface) are intact. Although clinically stable to the usual provocative testing, central or "core" lesions may allow abnormal joint displacement or dysfunction under conditions of physiologic loading. Hence, these lesions may be considered "potentially destabilizing." These tears typically occur following a fall on the outstretched pronated hand. In pronation, the distal radius is most proximal in relation to the ulna. It is postulated that this axial load results in a sudden proximal shift of the radius followed by a tear of the thin, central portion of the triangular fibrocartilage as it is draped over the ulnar head. The resultant linear tear is often found adjacent to the sigmoid notch and frequently includes an unstable flap of cartilage that may become impinged between the carpus and ulna. Clinically, this situation results in pain and a clicking sensation.

Following an adequate period of conservative management consisting of rest, splinting, nonsteroidal anti-inflammatory medications, and, occasionally, cortisone injections, surgical intervention is considered. We rarely consider operative intervention sooner than 3 months after injury and try to delay it for 6 months, because many injuries do improve in this time. We continue to employ arthrography in the diagnosis of triangular fibrocartilage tears.

Should the pain persist and surgery be indicated, the procedure chosen depends largely on grip-loaded ulnar variance. Positive ulnar variance, which increases loading through the ulnar column and through the triangular fibrocartilage, is thus a deterrent to successful treatment. The thin, central portion of the TFC, with its disorganized and random collagen arrangement, is poorly vascularized and has limited healing potential. Palmer and colleagues[6] and Adams[1] have convincingly demonstrated limited disk excisions have minimal effect on force transmission and on TFC deformation. We therefore treat nondestabilizing TFC injuries as follows: In the *negative* variant with a central tear, arthroscopic débridement alone is performed and is usually successful. We no longer perform open débridement of such a tear because of the greater morbidity and difficulty. In the setting of *neutral* variance, we perform arthroscopic débridement of the tear, which may be followed by arthroscopic débridement of the ulnar head through the hole made in the TFC during surgery. It should be emphasized that this approach is undertaken only in the setting of ulnar neutral variance.

For any *positive* variance (grip-loaded or static), a formal unloading procedure is performed. At this time, we favor the open method of Feldon and associates[3] for the minimally positive variant, and a formal ulnar-shortening osteotomy and plating at the diaphyseal level in patients with greater positive variance. We often perform the Feldon wafer procedure in addition to a TFC débridement. However, we have observed some difficulty in regaining supination following this combination of procedures, and we now recommend postoperative immobilization in supina-

tion for several weeks. The reason for this difficulty in regaining supination remains elusive, but we theorize that in the pronated position, the débrided TFC and distal ulna are not in direct contact with each other, whereas in supination, these structures do abut. Patients may naturally seek the more comfortable pronated position in the postoperative period, ultimately losing supination as a result.

It should be mentioned that a report by Cooney and associates[2] challenged the concept of the avascular nonrepair zone of the TFC and reported good functional results in a group of patients who underwent open repair of nondestabilizing TFC tears. Unfortunately, these researchers reported no confirmation of TFC healing following surgical repair.

Destabilizing TFC Injuries

Destabilizing triangular fibrocartilage tears in a symptomatic patient should be repaired when possible. Such a tear most often represents a peripheral detachment of the foveal insertion of the TFC.[4] This injury is analogous to an ulnar styloid avulsion at the base that destabilizes the distal radioulnar joint. Repair is usually straightforward, and we often perform a diagnostic arthroscopy prior to open surgical repair. Surgical repair may be performed at the same sitting or in a delayed fashion. We typically employ a dorsal approach and utilize suture anchors after appropriate preparation of the fovea. A portion of the styloid is often removed to facilitate exposure. We occasionally perform a "wafer" resection of the distal ulna in conjunction with a repair of the apically detached TFC, especially in the pathologically positive ulnar variant.

There continues to be interest in arthroscopic repair of peripheral ulnar-sided TFC tears that result in instability of the distal radioulnar joint. Zachee and coworkers[8] presented the technique of arthroscopic repair utilizing an outside-in suture method but offered no data to support its use. We have no experience with this technique, and we are concerned that this repair may not withstand the considerable forces about the distal radioulnar joint. An arthroscopic repair technique may be more applicable to TFC tears between the dorsal capsular ligament and the TFC. More research is required in this area prior to recommending arthroscopic suture techniques in the destabilizing TFC injuries.

TFC Injuries Associated with Distal Radius/Ulnar Styloid Fractures

The last area to be discussed concerns triangular fibrocartilage injuries associated with fractures of the distal radius and ulna. It should be stated that this injury pattern is most certainly underestimated, and distal radioulnar joint stability should always be assessed early on in the management of the distal radius fracture. This issue is further complicated by fractures that alter the normal anatomy of the sigmoid notch, thus affecting bony architecture and stability. In the isolated distal radius fracture without ulnar styloid involvement, we routinely assess stability of the distal radioulnar joint following reduction of the fracture. In unstable distal radius fractures that require operative intervention, radial length is reestablished and maintained by an external or internal fixation device. Following appropriate restoration of length, stability and rotation are checked. If the distal radioulnar joint remains unstable, it is explored and stability restored.

Instability following distal radius fractures more typically occurs in association with ulnar styloid fractures, including the typical Colles fracture and, similarly, Galeazzi fractures with associated ulnar styloid avulsion. The styloid may be avulsed at its base, compromising distal radioulnar joint stability. The same destabilizing injury may occur as a result of an isolated ulnar styloid avulsion-type fracture. Operative repair should be performed to restore distal radioulnar joint stability. Recommended techniques include a compression screw, interosseous wiring, and the tension band technique. Each can result in restoration of stability and union of the styloid fracture if attention is paid to detail.

The understanding of acute triangular fibrocartilage injuries associated with distal radius fractures will certainly continue to grow as more arthroscopically assisted reductions are performed.

Further discussion of this injury is found in Chapter 24.

CONCLUSION

The understanding of acute injuries to the triangular fibrocartilage complex continues to evolve. Arthroscopy has added substantially to the knowledge base. The management of these complex injuries requires a thorough understanding of the anatomy and injury patterns seen in this region. Our approach to the patient with a suspected acute tear is most often conservative, except when initial clinical testing reveals gross instability. In the latter case, early surgical intervention to restore distal radioulnar joint stability is our preferred management.

References

1. Adams BD: Partial excision of the triangular fibrocartilage complex articular disk: A biomechanical study. J Hand Surg 18A:334–340, 1993.
2. Cooney WP, Linscheid RL, Dobyns JH: Triangular fibrocartilage tears. J Hand Surg 19A:143–154, 1994.
3. Feldon P, Terrono AL, Belsky MR: The "wafer" procedure partial distal ulnar resection. Clin Orthop 275:124–129, 1992.
4. Hermansdorfer JD, Kleinman WB: Management of chronic peripheral tears of the triangular fibrocartilage complex. J Hand Surg 16A:340–346, 1991.
5. Palmer AK: Triangular fibrocartilage complex lesions: A classification. J Hand Surg 14A:594–606, 1989.
6. Palmer AK, Werner FW, Glisson RR, Murphy DJ: Partial excision of the triangular fibrocartilage complex. J Hand Surg 13A:391–394, 1988.
7. Whipple TL: Arthroscopic Surgery: The Wrist. Philadelphia, JB Lippincott, 1992.
8. Zachee B, DeSmet L, Fabry G: Arthroscopic suturing of TFCC lesions. Arthroscopy 9:242–243, 1993.

CHAPTER 23

Treatment of Acute Injuries of the Distal Radioulnar Joint

A. Herbert Alexander, MD, and David M. Lichtman, MD

Acute injuries of the distal radioulnar joint (DRUJ) frequently go undiagnosed or misdiagnosed, even by fully trained orthopedic surgeons. The physician's attention often is misdirected to an associated injury or the physician overlooks the findings on routine radiographs because they are subtle. Missing a DRUJ injury occurs commonly with isolated DRUJ injury, with distal radius fractures, and with forearm fractures.[2, 14, 17, 26, 46] In the isolated injury, the patient may have fallen on an outstretched hand or may have a hyperpronation or hypersupination injury of the forearm with no obvious radiographic findings. Wrist pain is regarded as a "sprain", and only when symptoms become chronic is the DRUJ injury retrospectively recognized. With severely displaced distal radius fractures, the surgeon frequently gives little thought to the consequences of an associated ulnar styloid fracture. Added to this tendency is the common misconception that a typical Colles fracture will do well and the ulnar styloid fracture need not be treated. With forearm fractures, and even with some elbow injuries, "tunnel vision" results in neglect of the DRUJ. Diagnosed and treated late, DRUJ injury is very likely to compromise the outcome.

To complicate matters, even when DRUJ injuries are successfully recognized, failure to distinguish between complex and simple dislocations can also compromise the long-term results.[13, 14] We discuss simple versus complex DRUJ dislocations in more detail later in the chapter.

DRUJ dislocation was first described by Desault[18] in 1777. Since that time, DRUJ dislocations have been reported as isolated injuries as well as with Essex-Lopresti injuries, both bone forearm fractures, Galeazzi fractures, distal radius fractures, and fracture-dislocation of the elbow, and in plastic deformation of the forearm.* The common theme in all these injuries is that the forearm is a two-boned structure linked securely at either end. Consequently, except for a "nightstick" fracture, it is difficult to compromise *just* the radius or *just* the ulna without compromising some other part of these two linked longitudinal struts. Therefore, with a radius fracture, we see either a disruption of the DRUJ, a fracture of the ulna,

or, in younger patients, plastic deformation of the ulna and/or Salter-Harris injuries to the distal ulnar epiphysis.

More severe injuries may also result in concomitant disruption of the radioulnar interosseous membrane—or radioulnar dissociation.[20, 21, 23, 56] Goldberg and associates[26] support this assertion. They conducted a prospective study of 119 consecutive forearm fractures and found a double injury to all but 5 (96 percent). Specifically, 96 percent of the "apparent" single bone forearm fractures had two or more sites of injury to either bone or ligament on closer scrutiny. Sixty percent of the patients also demonstrated an injury of the DRUJ. It is therefore correct to assume that there is a DRUJ injury in any patient with an isolated forearm fracture until proven otherwise. By observing the caveat "X-ray the joint above and the joint below" the injury, the physician can recognize most of these injuries.

The accepted nomenclature surrounding the DRUJ may be somewhat confusing.[2, 13] Anatomically, with forearm rotation, the ulna is stationary and the radius pronates and supinates about it. With hyperpronation or hypersupination, DRUJ restraints are torn, and the radius dislocates from the stationary ulna. However, by convention, when the DRUJ dislocates, we define the direction of the dislocation as if it were the ulna dislocating away from the radius. Therefore, in a dorsal dislocation of the DRUJ, the ulnar head is posterior to the radius; and in a volar dislocation of the DRUJ, the ulnar head is anterior to the radius.

DRUJ DISLOCATION—SIMPLE OR COMPLEX?

In 1991, we introduced the concept of simple versus complex dislocation of the DRUJ.[14] We defined a *simple* dislocation as one that reduces spontaneously or with minimal manipulation after internal fixation of the associated fracture. It may be stable or unstable; nonetheless, it is easily reducible. A *complex* dislocation is characterized by obvious irreducibility, incomplete reduction, or "mushy" reduction due to interposition of soft tissue or bone. This concept is important to understand, because the presence of either a sim-

---

*References 1–3, 5–11, 13–15, 17–21, 23–31, 34–42, 44–58.

ple or complex dislocation is pivotal in our decision-making for treatment. Therefore, we explain the rationale of this concept.

In looking at Galeazzi fracture dislocations reported in the literature up until about 1990, we found that no one had reported the incidence of irreducible DRUJ dislocation or recurrent subluxation in adults.[37, 44, 45, 49, 50] Mikic,[41] in 1975, however, noted a tendency toward redislocation of the DRUJ, in spite of rigid internal fixation of the radius. Persistent dislocation of the DRUJ was a common occurrence in nearly all of the series reporting nonoperative treatment.[32, 33, 41] In the later operative series prior to 1990, persistent or recurrent DRUJ dislocation received little attention.[37, 44, 45, 49, 50] Walsh and colleagues[57] in a series of 41 children with Galeazzi injuries, noted that 4 of 28 patients with adequate postreduction radiographs had persistent subluxation of the DRUJ. We had been acutely aware of the problem of irreducible DRUJ in Galeazzi fracture since we reported a case in 1981 in which the extensor carpi ulnaris (ECU) tendon had prevented reduction.[3] Our review of the literature demonstrated that there were others who had noted the same phenomenon then and since then.[9, 15, 30, 35, 47, 48] Because several of the standard texts paid little or no attention to the issue of the disrupted DRUJ, we decided to review our operative

experience with DRUJ dislocations over a 5-year period (1984–1989) to see whether we could determine how many DRUJ dislocations had a block to reduction.[14] During that period, we treated 11 patients with DRUJ dislocations, of which 4 (36 percent) were complex (not reducible by closed means). Two occurred in patients with severe fractures of both forearm bones, one in a Galeazzi fracture, and one in a patient with an unstable comminuted intra-articular distal radius fracture. All of the complex dislocations were associated with an ulnar styloid fracture (Fig. 23–1). We concluded that complex (unreducible) dislocation of the DRUJ most likely is underreported or not recognized.

ACUTE DRUJ DISLOCATIONS

Isolated dislocations of the DRUJ usually result from a supraphysiologic rotatory force applied to the forearm. The rotatory force is transmitted to the forearm when rotation occurs about a fixed hand, as in a fall, or when a twisting force is directly applied to the hand. Hyperpronation of the forearm causes a dorsal dislocation, and hypersupination, a volar dislocation. Volar dislocations are much less common than dorsal

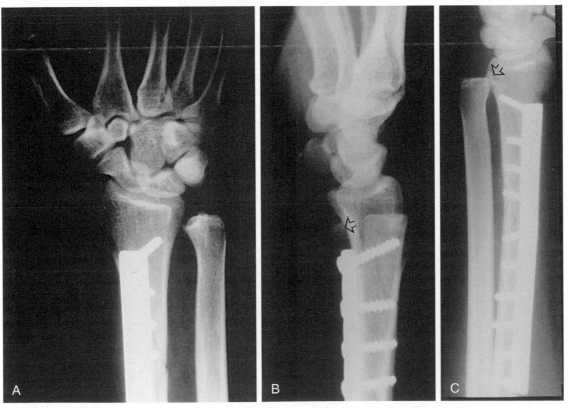

Figure 23–1. Anteroposterior (A), lateral (B), and oblique (C) radiographs of a patient referred to us after open reduction and internal fixation of a Galeazzi fracture. The distal radioulnar joint was reported as "reduced" by the treating surgeons. At 10 days, however, it was obvious that the ulna was dorsally dislocated. Note the displaced ulnar styloid fracture (arrow), which is volar to the distal ulna. A displaced ulnar styloid fracture is the hallmark of a "complex" distal radioulnar joint dislocation. At surgery, we found the extensor carpi ulnaris displaced into the distal radioulnar joint blocking reduction.

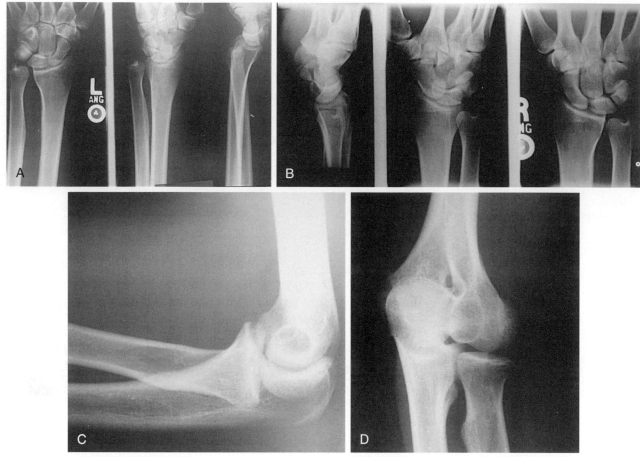

Figure 23–2. Essex-Lopresti injury. *A,* In the injured extremity, the ulna is displaced dorsally and distally. There is positive ulnar variance. Compare this to the normal contralateral wrist *(B).* Here, there is neutral ulnar variance. *C* and *D* show the fracture of the radial head. What cannot be seen on radiographs is the disruption of the interosseous membrane.

dislocations.[25, 51–53, 58] Rarely, an isolated dislocation of the DRUJ may be purely rotational.[29]

An Essex-Lopresti injury is a fracture or fracture-dislocation of the radial head associated with disruption of the interosseous membrane between the radius and ulna and dislocation of the DRUJ.[23] Commonly, the distal ulna is both longitudinally and dorsally displaced (Fig. 23–2). It may be associated with frank dislocation of the elbow as well.[10] The Essex-Lopresti injury, also known as radioulnar dissociation, usually occurs from a fall onto an outstretched hand.[56] Such a fall generates a longitudinal compression force that drives the radius proximally, disrupting the DRUJ and interosseous membrane and fracturing or dislocating the radial head. Needless to say, these are severe injuries with significant bone and soft tissue injury.

Both-bone forearm fractures may occur from a direct blow or from a fall. When a blow or fall is combined with a longitudinal load or with a hyperpronation or hypersupination force, disruption and dislocation of the DRUJ may accompany this injury. Attention may be drawn to the more significant forearm fracture and the DRUJ injury may be overlooked. Mikic[41] reported a 20 percent incidence of both-bone

forearm fractures in his 125 cases of Galeazzi fracture-dislocations. He theorized that this injury, both-bone forearm fracture, accompanied by DRUJ dislocation, is simply an extension of what happens when there is more energy to dissipate in the mechanism of injury than would ordinarily cause just a Galeazzi fracture. We agree with this concept on the basis of our experience[14] and that of Goldberg and associates.[26]

In our experience, most of the DRUJ dislocations have occurred in conjunction with Galeazzi fractures. Galeazzi fracture consists of a distal-third radius fracture accompanied by a dislocation of the DRUJ. The dislocation is usually dorsal but occasionally occurs volar, as demonstrated in Figure 23–3. The Galeazzi injury was originally described by Sir Astley Cooper[16] in 1822 but bears the name of Ricardo Galeazzi,[24] who reported 18 cases in 1934. It constitutes roughly 7 percent of forearm fractures.[45] Sometimes, high-energy trauma may also result in fracture of the ulna and/or segmental fracture of the radius and ulna as well as injury to the elbow and carpus.[14, 21] Galeazzi injuries can also occur in children but usually are treated successfully by closed means.[57] A Galeazzi variant in children consists of a fracture of the distal

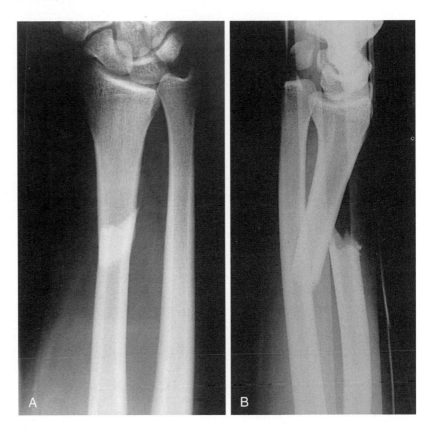

Figure 23–3. AP *(A)* and lateral *(B)* radiographs of a patient with a Galeazzi fracture and open volar dislocation of the distal radioulnar joint.

radial diaphysis and a Salter I fracture of the distal ulnar epiphysis;[27, 38] it, too, may be treated by closed means. Galeazzi fractures in adults have justly earned the reputation of being the "fracture of necessity"— implying that open reduction and internal fixation are necessary for successful treatment.[4]

DRUJ injuries also occur with distal radius fractures. The management of distal radius fractures is discussed in Chapter 19 but injury to the DRUJ, which often accompanies distal radius fractures, warrants additional mention. Surgeons commonly attribute poor results following treatment of distal radius fractures to symptoms at the distal radioulnar joint. Such results may occur, however, from chronic disruption of the TFCC, ulnar abutment due to radial shortening, post-traumatic arthritis of the distal radioulnar joint, and/or persistent instability or dislocation of the DRUJ. We believe that poor results due to ulnar-sided wrist pain following a distal radius fracture can best be prevented by recognizing and treating the injury immediately.

ASSESSMENT

The physical examination of a patient with a DRUJ dislocation is significantly affected by the presence of concomitant injuries (e.g., Galeazzi fracture, both-bone forearm fracture). The isolated dorsal DRUJ dislocation demonstrates a prominent ulna dorsally associated with tenderness and swelling. Invariably, the

forearm is locked in pronation, and the patient cannot supinate the forearm. In an isolated volar DRUJ dislocation, the wrist appears narrowed because the ulna is volar to the distal radius. There is swelling and tenderness and sometimes a dimple where the ulnar head belongs. This finding, however, may be obscured by swelling. Invariably, the forearm is locked in supination, and the patient is unable to pronate the forearm. One should check the neurovascular status in the hand, and should examine the elbow and wrist for additional injuries (see Fig. 23–2). In particular, the forearm should be checked for tenderness, which may be a clue to the presence of radioulnar dissociation (Essex-Lopresti injury).

Radiographs should be taken of the forearm, wrist, and elbow in at least two views to diagnose DRUJ dislocation. Though the posteroanterior (PA) view of the wrist may be helpful, the dislocation is usually best seen on the lateral view. On the PA view, in a dorsal dislocation, one should look for a slight diastasis between the distal radius and ulna along with a fracture of the ulnar styloid. Or, if the ulnar styloid is not fractured, it will appear closer to the radial border of the ulna than to the ulnar border, because the radius is pronated about the ulna and locked in this position. On the PA view, in a volar dislocation, the radius and ulna usually overlap distally. Naturally, on a lateral projection, the ulnar head is seen as prominent dorsally or volarly, depending on the direction of dislocation. Care must be taken, however, to position the wrist in a true lateral position for the radiograph, because a slight amount of obliqueness in the x-ray beam will cause the undisplaced distal ulna to appear prominent either dorsally or volarly. One method of ensuring the lateral view is "true," is to superimpose the four lesser metacarpals. Alternatively, one should ensure that the proximal pole of the scaphoid is superimposed over the lunate and the radial styloid appears in the center of the semilunar lunate when viewed on the lateral projection (Fig. 23–4). At some point prior to definitive treatment, radiographs of a patient's uninjured wrist should be taken for comparison, because they may help identify subtle degrees of subluxation.

Computed tomography (CT scanning) can accurately diagnose DRUJ dislocation or subluxation (Fig. 23–5.[43] It is important to obtain CT scans of both the injured and the uninjured wrist for comparison and to ensure that the CT scans are done with the forearms in the same degree of rotation (Fig. 23–6). Unfortunately, CT scanning cannot be used in the operating room; that is why it is important also to have an accurate lateral wrist radiograph.

The role of magnetic resonance (MR) imaging in diagnosing acute DRUJ injuries is still evolving. Like CT scans, axial MR images can show dorsal or volar subluxation or dislocation of the distal ulna, but they can also demonstrate injury to the ulnocarpal complex and the triangular fibrocartilage complex (TFCC). However, how to apply this information is subject to question.[19, 22] Currently, our decision to treat these injuries open rather than closed is based on reducibility and completeness of reduction, not on the presence or absence of clinically occult ligament or cartilage damage.

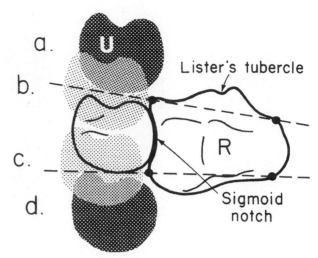

Figure 23–5. Schematic representation of a CT scan transverse section through the distal radioulnar joint. The distal ulna should fit snugly in the radius's *(R)* sigmoid notch. If in position *a*, the ulna is dorsally dislocated; in position *b*, the ulna is dorsally subluxed; in position *c*, the ulna is volarly subluxed; and, in position *d*, the ulna is volarly dislocated. (Redrawn from Mino DE, Palmer AK, Levinsohn EM: The role of radiography and computerized tomography in the diagnosis of subluxation and dislocation of the distal radioulnar joint. J Hand Surg 8:23–31, 1983.)

MANAGEMENT OF ACUTE DRUJ INJURIES

Simple Isolated Dislocation

Isolated dislocations of the DRUJ, when diagnosed in their acute stage, are generally easy to reduce, as follows: Using local anesthesia with or without parenteral sedatives or narcotics, reduce a dorsal dislocation by firm supination of the forearm with digital pressure over the ulnar head. Usually you will hear a clunk with reduction. Check forearm rotation, and determine whether the DRUJ is stable or unstable. If it is absolutely stable—usually the case—immobilize the forearm in slight to moderate supination for 3 to 4 weeks in a long-arm cast. If the DRUJ is stable but dislocatable, immobilize the forearm for 6 weeks.

If the DRUJ is grossly unstable, place a temporary 0.062-inch Kirschner (K) wire from the ulna into the radius. Insert the K wire with the forearm supinated and the DRUJ reduced to ensure maintenance of reduction. The optimal placement of the K wire is proximal to the radioulnar articulation in order to avoid any additional damage to the articular cartilage. Place the limb in a long-arm cast for 6 weeks to augment immobilization and prevent breakage of the wire. Remove the K wire at the time of cast removal.

Before embarking on 6 weeks of immobilization, obtain radiographs proving anatomic reduction. If radiographs are equivocal, you may obtain a CT scan in plaster to confirm reduction or to diagnose subtle degrees of subluxation (see Fig. 23–6).

An isolated volar dislocation may be somewhat

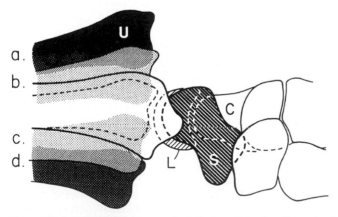

Figure 23–4. Schematic representation of a *true* lateral radiograph of the wrist in neutral position. In a *true* lateral view, the radial styloid is centered over the lunate *(L)*, and scaphoid *(S)*. If the x-ray beam is even slightly oblique to this position, one may incorrectly diagnose distal radioulnar joint dislocation. If in position *a*, the ulna is dorsally dislocated; if in position *b*, the ulna is dorsally subluxed; if in position *c*, the ulna is volarly subluxed; and if in position *d*, the ulna is volarly dislocated. (Redrawn from Mino DE, Palmer AK, Levinsohn EM: The role of radiography and computerized tomography in the diagnosis of subluxation and dislocation of the distal radioulnar joint. J Hand Surg 8:23–31, 1983.)

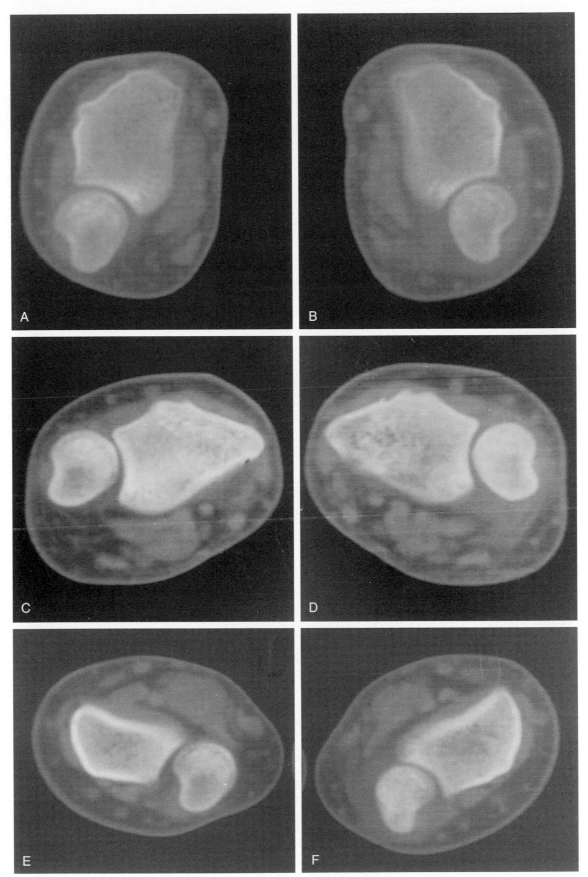

Figure 23–6. CT scans of a patient suspected of having distal radioulnar joint subluxation/dislocation following open reduction and internal fixation of a Galeazzi fracture. *A* and *B*, Left and right neutral forearm rotation. *C* and *D*, Left and right forearm pronation. *E* and *F*, Left and right forearm supination. It is important to obtain the CT scans with the patient leaning on flexed elbows so that the neutral, pronation, and supination rotation views obtained are actually rotation of the forearm and not of the shoulder. If this point is not clearly made to the CT technician and the elbow is extended during the CT study, the rotation views obtained may actually represent various degress of shoulder internal and external rotation. This DRUJ is normal, because the neutral, pronation, and supination views are comparable.

more difficult to reduce owing to the pull of the pronator quadratus muscle. As a consequence, regional or general anesthesia may be necessary along with muscle relaxation. With digital pressure over the volar surface of the ulnar head, reduce a volar dislocation by mobilizing the ulna ulnarward while pronating the forearm. Postreduction treatment and precautions are the same as described for dorsal dislocations, except that the forearm is immobilized in pronation.

Complex Isolated Dislocation

In our experience, isolated dislocations of the DRUJ are rarely complex. However, treatment for complex dislocations is the same whether for the isolated injury or following appropriate treatment of concomitant fracture of the forearm, distal intra-articular radius, distal radial diaphysis, or radial head. We thus discuss general principles of complex injuries here.

Complex dislocations (those that are irreducible or in which there is a "mushy" feel to the reduction) require exploration of the DRUJ, extrication of the material blocking reduction, suture repair of the damaged soft tissue (TFCC, sheath of the ECU, etc.), and internal fixation of the ulnar styloid fracture when present and if displaced more than 1 to 2 mm. We perform this exploration immediately after treating any associated bone injury as follows:

Approach the DRUJ dorsally through a straight longitudinal incision directly over the joint. After making the skin incision, we have found that additional dissection is rarely necessary, because the soft tissues, capsule, extensor retinaculum, and fibro-osseous canal of the extensor carpi ulnaris are disrupted. After removal of the offending material, reduction is easily accomplished. Reduce dorsal dislocations with forearm supination; reduce volar dislocations with forearm pronation. We prefer absorbable sutures for repair of the soft tissues and TFCC. Depending on the size of the ulnar styloid fragment, use small K wires, small bone screws, tension band technique, or suture anchors. Once the complex dislocation is converted to a simple one, proceed as you would for a simple dislocation, as outlined previously. In most instances, we utilize a temporary 0.062-inch K wire to transfix the ulna to the radius before placing the limb in a long-arm cast. Once again, obtaining radiographic documentation of anatomic reduction prior to leaving the operating room is paramount.

Galeazzi Fracture

Galeazzi fractures most commonly occur at the junction of the middle and distal thirds of the radius. We perform an open reduction and internal fixation of the radius through a volar approach utilizing an eight-hole, 3.5-mm dynamic compression plate (DCP). Important points for fracture fixation are as follows:

1. Contour the plate appropriately with a slight amount of pre-stress.
2. Use provisional fixation prior to plate application.
3. Engage at least eight cortices proximal and six cortices distal to the fracture.
4. Add autogenous bone graft for comminution.
5. Minimize periosteal stripping.
6. Utilize interfragmentary compression whenever possible.

Remember to prepare the iliac crest as a donor site for bone graft before starting the surgery if there is even the remotest chance that a bone graft will be required. There are new titanium, low-contact plates available, but as yet, they have not proved to be significantly better than the standard 3.5-mm DCP.

Only after stabilizing the radius fracture do we address the DRUJ. Usually, we find that the DRUJ spontaneously reduces with fracture fixation of the distal radius. We confirm the reduction with clinical examination and with the C-arm. Similarly, we determine stability of the DRUJ as outlined previously. If the reduction is "mushy" or uncertain, and definitely if it is still unreduced on C-arm image or on actual radiographs, we explore the DRUJ through a dorsal incision as previously described.

Both-Bone Forearm Fractures

We prefer to address the ulnar fracture first because it is usually easier to reduce and to approach. Our recommended incision is directly over its subcutaneous border. Applying fracture fixation principles as described previously, we internally fix the ulna with a 3-5 mm, eight-hole DCP. Following ulnar fixation, we proceed with open reduction and internal fixation of the radius, reduction of the DRUJ, assessment of stability of the DRUJ, and radiographs to ensure adequacy and completeness of reduction. Treatment of complex DRUJ dislocations proceeds as described previously.

Essex-Lopresti Injury (Radioulnar Dissociation)

Successful treatment of the Essex-Lopresti lesion is problematic, particularly if the radial head fracture is so comminuted that it is impossible to fix internally. When the interosseous membrane fails to heal, late proximal migration of the radius associated with symptoms at the DRUJ may occur. We recommend saving the radial head at nearly all costs. An immediate excision of the radial head is not necessary; Broberg and Morrey[12] have shown results of late excision of a radial head fracture to be satisfactory.

If the radial head fracture is severely comminuted and internal fixation is not possible, an appropriately sized Silastic radial head can be used as a temporary spacer. We counsel our patients that the Silastic radial head is *temporary* and that, because of fragmentation, it will require excision at 6 months.

Our recommended surgical approach to the radial head fracture is a Kocher incision carried down between the extensor carpi ulnaris and the anconeus. Avoid injury to the posterior interosseous nerve, which may occur with too distal dissection. By approaching the radial head with the forearm held in pronation, you are less likely to encounter the posterior interosseous nerve. Piece the fragments of the radial head together, and fix them provisionally with fine 0.045-inch K wires. Use Herbert screws and/or AO mini-screws for definitive fixation. In some cases, we have used a combination of Herbert or AO mini-screws with bioabsorbable pins. When the radial head is entirely detached from the metaphysis, we use an AO mini-plate, making sure that with forearm rotation there is no impingement of the plate on the ulna.

Whether replacing the radial head or internally fixing it, check the elbow for stability of reduction as well as valgus instability, because there may be concomitant medial collateral ligament disruption, which should be addressed if the elbow remains unstable. At this point, ensure that the DRUJ is reduced accurately, place the forearm in neutral rotation, and add a transfixing 0.062-inch K wire from the ulna to the radius just proximal to the distal radioulnar articular surface. We add the K wire in an Essex Lopresti injury, whether or not the DRUJ is unstable, to protect the interosseous membrane.[20] Immobilize the limb in a long-arm cast for 6 weeks, and remove the K wire when the cast is removed.

Distal Radius Fracture

Management of distal radius fractures is covered in detail in other chapters. As with other forearm fractures, we believe that most physicians give too little attention to the DRUJ when treating distal radius fractures. We recommend assessment and management of DRUJ reduction and stability just as described for Galeazzi fractures.

PITFALLS

Failure to diagnose and treat a complex dislocation may lead to ulnar wrist pain and chronic instability. Currently, there are no fail-safe treatments for chronic instability of the DRUJ. Though there are methods to address ulnar abutment syndrome and post-traumatic arthritis of the DRUJ (see Chapters 21, 22, 24), none is as good as avoiding the problem in the first place. In assessing reduction of the DRUJ following a Galeazzi fracture, for instance, it is possible to push so hard on the end of the ulna that the radiographs look normal even though there may be interposed tendon or soft tissue. When the pressure is removed, whether immediately or after a period of immobilization, the dislocation becomes apparent because the soft tissue is still interposed. Therefore, one should take care to ensure that reduction of the DRUJ is complete and is held without undue force; if not, the patient may have a complex rather than a simple dislocation.

Essex-Lopresti injuries may vary in severity; that is to say, the interosseous membrane may be partially torn or completely torn. With severe disruption of the interosseous membrane, diagnosis is obvious. In partial injuries, it may not be so apparent. In radial head fractures, it is extremely important to carefully examine the forearm for tenderness. Signs of DRUJ dislocation may be subtle. We recommend obtaining wrist radiographs as described previously as well as contralateral PA wrist radiographs in neutral rotation in order to compare ulnar variance. Asymmetric positive ulnar variance in the injured limb increases the likelihood of Essex-Lopresti injury.

Failure to immobilize a limb for sufficient time may allow the DRUJ to redislocate. Also, failure to immobilize a limb in which a transfixation K wire is placed as well as using a K wire that is too small may result in breakage of the wire.

Following immobilization, some patients may have difficulty regaining full range of motion. Therefore, in stable DRUJ dislocation that does not redislocate easily with provocative testing, we have shortened the period of immobilization to 3 weeks.

SUMMARY

Acute DRUJ dislocations occur as isolated injuries and along with Galeazzi fractures, both-bone forearm fractures, Essex-Lopresti injuries, and distal radius fractures. They may occur as simple or complex injuries. A simple DRUJ dislocation is easily reducible but may be stable or unstable. In complex dislocation, reduction is not possible or there is a "mushy" feel with a block to reduction because of interposed tendon, bone, or soft tissue. After the associated injury is dealt with, treatment for complex injuries requires exploration of the DRUJ, extrication of the interposed tissue, repair of the soft tissues, and open reduction with internal fixation of the ulnar styloid fracture, if present and displaced. Simple DRUJ dislocations require reduction and immobilization.

Dislocations, of the distal radioulnar joint, whether simple or complex, can be effectively treated immediately. Their early recognition is crucial, because chronic DRUJ conditions are much more difficult to manage.

References

1. Albert MJ, Engber WD: Dorsal dislocation of the distal radioulnar joint secondary to plastic deformation of the ulna. J Orthop Trauma 4:466–469, 1990.

2. Alexander AH: Bilateral traumatic dislocation of the distal radioulnar joint, ulna dorsal: Case report and review of the literature. Clin Orthop 129:238–244, 1977.
3. Alexander AH, Lichtman DM: Irreducible distal radioulnar joint occurring in a Galeazzi fracture. J Hand Surg 6:258–261, 1981.
4. Anderson LD, Meyer FN: Fracture of the shafts of the radius and ulna. In Rockwood CA, Green DP, Bucholz RW (eds): Fractures in Adults, ed 3, vol 1. Philadelphia, JB Lippincott, 1991, p 679.
5. Aulicino PL, Siegel JL: Acute injuries of the distal radioulnar joint. Hand Clin 7:283–293, 1991.
6. Beneyto FM, Renú JMA, Claramunt AF, Soler RR: Treatment of Galeazzi fracture-dislocations. J Trauma 36:352–355, 1994.
7. Bhan S, Rath S: Management of the Galeazzi fracture. Int Orthop 15:193–196, 1991.
8. Birch-Jensen A: Luxation of the distal radioulnar joint. Acta Chir Scand 101:312, 1951.
9. Biyani A, Bhan S: Dual extensor tendon entrapment in Galeazzi fracture dislocation: A case report. J Trauma 29:1295–1297, 1989.
10. Bock GW, Cohen MS, Resnick D: Fracture-dislocation of the elbow with inferior radioulnar dislocation: A variant of the Essex-Lopresti injury. Skeletal Radiol 21:315–317, 1992.
11. Braun RM: The distal joint of the radius and ulna. Clin Orthop 275:74–78, 1992.
12. Broberg MA, Morrey BF: Results of delayed excision of the radial head after fracture. J Bone Joint Surg 68A:669–674, 1986.
13. Bruckner JD, Alexander AH, Lichtman DM: Acute dislocations of the distal radioulnar joint. J Bone Joint Surg 77A:958–968, 1995.
14. Bruckner JD, Lichtman DM, Alexander AH: Complex dislocations of the distal radioulnar joint—recognition and management. Clin Orthop 275:90–103, 1992.
15. Cetti NE: An unusual cause of blocked reduction of the Galeazzi injury. Injury 9:59, 1977.
16. Cooper A: A Treatise on Dislocations and on Fractures of the Joints. London, J Churchill, 1822.
17. Dameron TB: Traumatic dislocation of the distal radioulnar joint. Clin Orthop 83:55–63, 1972.
18. Desault M: Extrait d'un mémoire de M. Desault sur la luxation de l'extrêmité inférieure du radius. J Chir (Paris) 1:78, 1791.
19. Dyer CR, Kuschner SH, Brien WW: The distal radioulnar joint following Galeazzi's fracture. Orthop Rev 23:587–592, 1994.
20. Edwards GS, Jupiter JB: Radial head fractures with acute distal radioulnar dislocation—Essex-Lopresti revisited. Clin Orthop 234:61–69, 1988.
21. Eglseder WA, Hay M: Combined Essex-Lopresti and radial shaft fractures: Case report. J Trauma 34:310–312, 1993.
22. Ekenstam FA, Jakobsson OP, Wadin K: Repair of the triangular ligament in Colles' fracture. No effect in a prospective randomized study. Acta Orthop Scand 60:393–396, 1989.
23. Essex-Lopresti P: Fractures of the radial head with distal radioulnar joint dislocation. J Bone Joint Surg 33B:244, 1951.
24. Galeazzi R: Über ein besonderes Syndrom bei Verletzungen im Bereich der Unterarmknochen. Arch Orthop Unfalchir 35:557–562, 1934.
25. Giangarra CE, Chandler RW: Complex volar distal radioulnar joint occurring in a Galeazzi fracture. J Orthop Trauma 3:76–79, 1989.
26. Goldberg HD, Young JW, Reiner BI, et al: Double injuries of the forearm: A common occurrence. Radiology 185:223–227, 1992.
27. Golz RJ, Grogan DP, Greene TL, et al: Distal ulnar physeal injury. J Pediatr Orthop 11:318–326, 1991.
28. Gordon L, Beaton W, Thomas T, Mulbry LW: Acute plastic deformation of the ulna in a skeletally mature individual. J Hand Surg 16A:451–453, 1991.
29. Graham HK, McCoy GF, Mollan RAB: A new injury of the distal radio-ulnar joint. J Bone Joint Surg 67B:302–304, 1985.
30. Hanel DP, Scheid DK: Irreducible fracture-dislocation of the distal radioulnar joint secondary to entrapment of the extensor carpi ulnaris tendon. Clin Orthop 234:56–60, 1988.
31. Heiple KG, Freehaher AA, Van't Hof A: Isolated traumatic dislocation of the distal end of the ulna or the distal radioulnar joint. J Bone Joint Surg 44A:1387, 1962.
32. Hughston JC: Fracture of the distal radial shaft: Mistakes in management. J Bone Joint Surg 39A:249–254, 1957.
33. Hughston JC: Fractures of the forearm. J Bone Joint Surg 44A:1664, 1962.
34. Itoh Y, Horiuchi Y, Takahashi M, et al: Extensor tendon involvement in Smith's and Galeazzi's fractures. J Hand Surg 12A:535–540, 1987.
35. Jenkins NH, Mintowt-Czyz WJ, Fairclough JA: Irreducible dislocation of the distal radioulnar joint. Injury 18:40–43, 1987.
36. Khurana JS, Kattapuram SV, Becker S, Mayo-Smith W: Galeazzi injury with an associated fracture of the radial head. Clin Orthop 234:70–71, 1988.
37. Kraus MB, Horne G: Galeazzi fractures. J Trauma 25:1093–1095, 1985.
38. Landfried MJ, Stenclik M, Susi JG: Variant of Galeazzi fracture-dislocation in children. J Pediatr Orthop 11:332–335, 1991.
39. Lichtman DM: Extensor tendon involvement in Smith's and Galeazzi's fractures [letter]. J Hand Surg 13A:313, 1988.
40. Merchan ECR, Corte H: Injuries of the distal radioulnar joint. Contemp Orthop 29:193–200, 1994.
41. Mikic ZD: Galeazzi fracture-dislocations. J Bone Joint Surg 57A:1071–1080, 1975.
42. Milch H: So-called dislocation of the lower end of the ulna. Ann Surg 116:282, 1942.
43. Mino DE, Palmer AK, Levinsohn EM: The role of radiography and computerized tomography in the diagnosis of subluxation and dislocation of the distal radioulnar joint. J Hand Surg 8:23–31, 1983.
44. Mohan K, Gupta AH, Sharma J, et al: Internal fixation in 50 cases of Galeazzi fractures. Acta Orthop Scand 59:314–320, 1988.
45. Moore TM, Klein JP, Patzakis MJ, Harvey JP: Results of compression-plating of closed Galeazzi fractures. J Bone Joint Surg 67A:1015–1021, 1985.
46. Morrissy RT, Nalebuff EA: Dislocation of the distal radioulnar joint: Anatomy and clues to prompt diagnosis. Clin Orthop 144:154–158, 1979.
47. Paley D, McMurtry RY, Murray JF: Dorsal dislocation of the ulnar styloid and extensor carpi ulnaris tendon into the distal radioulnar joint: The empty sulcus sign. J Hand Surg 12A:1029–1032, 1987.
48. Paley D, Rubenstein J, McMurtry RY: Irreducible dislocation of distal radioulnar joint. Orthop Rev 15:228–231, 1986.
49. Reckling FW: Unstable fracture-dislocation of the forearm (Monteggia and Galeazzi lesions). J Bone Joint Surg 64A:857–863, 1982.
50. Reckling FW, Cordell LD: Unstable fracture-dislocations of the forearm: The Monteggia and Galeazzi lesions. Arch Surg 96:999–1007, 1968.
51. Rose-Innes AP: Anterior dislocation of the ulna at the inferior radio-ulnar joint. J Bone Joint Surg 42B:515–521, 1960.
52. Schiller MG, Ekenstam F, Kirsch PT: Volar dislocation of the distal radio-ulnar joint. J Bone Joint Surg 73A:617–619, 1991.
53. Singletary EM: Volar dislocation of the distal radioulnar joint. Ann Emerg Med 23:881–883, 1993.
54. Strehle J, Gerber C: Distal radioulnar joint function after Galeazzi fracture-dislocations treated by open reduction and internal plate fixation. Clin Orthop 293:240–245, 1993.
55. Sumner JM, Khuri SM: Entrapment of the median nerve and flexor pollicis longus tendon in an epiphyseal fracture-dislocation of the distal radioulnar joint: A case report. J Hand Surg 9:711–714, 1984.
56. Trousdale RT, Amadio PC, Cooney WP, Morrey BF: Radioulnar dissociation: A review of twenty cases. J Bone Joint Surg 74A:1486–1497, 1992.
57. Walsh HPJ, McLaren CAN, Owen R: Galeazzi fractures in children. J Bone Joint Surg 69B:730–733, 1987.
58. Weseley MS, Barenfeld PA, Bruno J: Volar dislocation distal radioulnar joint. J Trauma 12:1083–1088, 1972.

Treatment of Chronic Disorders of the Distal Radioulnar Joint

William H. Bowers, MD, and David S. Zelouf, MD

This chapter presents a classification of chronic disorders of the distal radioulnar joint (DRUJ) and reviews surgical alternatives available for their management. We chose the listed procedures on the basis of published results, theoretical soundness, and our experience. We made no attempt to discuss or list many procedural variations that have appeared in the literature. Anatomy, methods of diagnosis, closed management, and the treatment of acute disorders of the DRUJ and of the triangular fibrocartilage complex (TFCC) are covered elsewhere in this book.

CLASSIFICATION

Table 24–1 lists conditions of the DRUJ and the procedures that may be applicable to their treatment. Acute problems, untreated, often become chronic problems, and commonly, the same surgical procedure that should have been applied in the acute interval is applicable in the chronic interval. In many cases, the development of arthritic and/or contracture problems dictates a reconstructive approach. This decision calls for surgical judgment. In general, if the bony structure is intact and the cartilage surfaces look good at the time of surgery, a restorative procedure as opposed to a salvage procedure should be attempted. The classification proposed in Table 24–1 is one we have found useful in thinking about the application of the current surgical armamentarium.[4, 8]

ARTHROSCOPIC DÉBRIDEMENT FOR CHRONIC LESIONS OF THE CENTRAL TFC

Tears, perforations or degenerative changes of the triangular fibrocartilage (TFC), when chronic, often become symptomatic through a painful premonition of instability even though the tear itself is nondestabilizing. These injuries are most often the result of wear produced by ulnocarpal loading. Undiagnosed traumatic tears may also become chronic. Treatment options include reducing the load and débriding the tear.

We recommend the arthroscopic procedures developed by the Poehling group.[15, 55] The traction tower developed by Whipple is useful. We prefer a 2.7-mm diameter, 25-degree arthroscope. The most useful tools are a suction punch and a full-radius resector and bur (Fig. 24–1). We have not found mechanically assisted joint distention necessary. The initial entry into the joint is greatly facilitated by the use of a low-emission portable roentgen unit, distention of the joint with irrigating fluid, and 15-lb longitudinal distraction of the joint. Using the 3-4 and 4-5 portals,

Table 24–1. CHRONIC DISTAL RADIOULNAR JOINT PROBLEMS AND THE PROCEDURES AVAILABLE FOR THEIR TREATMENT*

I. Chronic joint disruption (potential, intermittent, or continuous instability)
  A. Central TFC tears (potential instability—Herbert-Bowers stage I[4])
    1. Arthroscopic débridement
    2. Open repair and débridement
  B. Joint disruption due to chronic ligament or bony injury (Herbert-Bowers Stage II [dynamic] or III [static-reducible] instability)
    1. TFC peripheral tears
      a. Repair and/or reattachment
      b. Substitution
    2. TFC peripheral tears plus radial and/or ulnar angular shaft deformity
      a. Radial osteotomy
      b. Ulnar osteotomy
    3. Sigmoid notch and/or ulnar head deformity
      a. Corrective osteotomy
      b. Arthroplasty
II. Ulnocarpal impingement (impaction, abutment)
  A. Immature skeleton—growth arrest
  B. Adult skeleton
    1. Shortening intrinsic to joint ("wafer" procedure[20])
    2. Ulnar shaft shortening (Milch[44] type)
III. Procedures to address the arthritic joint
  A. Arthroplasty
    1. Partial resections (Bowers,[5–7] Watson[71, 72] procedures)
    2. Complete resections (Darrach procedure and its modifications)
    3. Joint replacement
  B. Arthrodesis
  C. Arthrodesis with surgical pseudarthrosis of ulna (Sauve-Kapandji[35] procedure)
IV. Other procedures
  A. Restoring the chronically unstable extensor carpi ulnaris
  B. Relieving rotational contracture

*Superscript numbers in table text refer to chapter references.

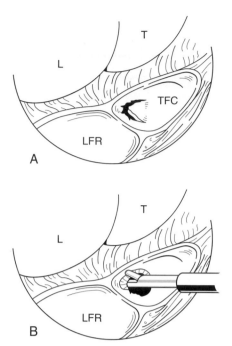

Figure 24–1. A and B, Arthroscopic débridement of chronic triangular fibrocartilage *(TFC)* tears. L = lunate; LFR = lunate facet of radius; T = triquetrum.

we switch the arthroscope and resectors as necessary to allow full débridement of the tear.

It is our practice to débride all observed wear to cartilage, ligament, and bone. We then decide what to do about the ulnocarpal loading. If the *grip-loaded* ulnar variance is negative or neutral, we débride the ulnar head through the hole made during the TFC débridement. We are not convinced that arthroscopic débridement of the ulnar dome can sufficiently unload any but the most minimal loading syndromes. Thus, for any positive variant ulna (grip-loaded or static), we do perform an open ulnar shortening (see later). The arthroscopic procedure should conclude with instillation of a few millileters of cortisone and bupivacaine into the joint to diminish postoperative discomfort.

OPEN DÉBRIDEMENT OF CHRONIC TFC TEARS

Open débridement has been utilized less commonly since the advent of wrist arthroscopy. Nevertheless, open débridement of chronic TFC tears, when coupled with correction of the ulnar loading, has paved the way for the technical success of arthroscopic débridement.[5, 33, 43, 50, 53, 70] Use of the arthroscope for visualization and débridement of the chronic tears of the triangular fibrocartilage complex currently has no peer in the surgical armamentarium.[52, 64]

Open débridement from the underside of the TFC can be done after an unloading procedure such as proposed by Feldon and associates[20] or Bowers.[6] These bone resections leave adequate room for both

visualization and resection. The open ulnocarpal approach remains difficult but can be accomplished by using distraction and small knives coupled with an angled suction punch.

OPEN REPAIR OF THE CHRONICALLY DISRUPTED TFC

The triangular ligament known as the TFC has two major attachments of concern to the distal radioulnar joint. The dorsal and volar marginal ligaments of the TFC attach to the radius at the two borders of the sigmoid notch and come together at their apical foveal insertion into the ulna.[8]

Repair of apical detachment is relatively straightforward. If detachment occurred via styloid fracture, a compression screw or interosseous wire technique of reattachment is recommended.[28, 30] Approach the distal ulna dorsally, and expose the area of detachment. In the case of the styloid fracture, insert a small compression screw from the styloid well into the medial cortex of the ulna. Take care not to overcompress, because the styloid fragment, although large enough to accept the screw, is not sufficiently strong to resist over-compression.

For an interosseous wire technique, it is advisable to retrograde the drill holes from the area of fracture. Using two Kirschner wires, drill holes from the styloid fracture site out to the axilla of the ulna beneath the ulnar head. Place appropriate wire suture through or around the ulnar styloid, pass it through the holes in the ulnar shaft, and twist it in the axilla to apply compression to the injury site (Fig. 24–2). Be careful to secure an anatomic reduction of the fracture.

If the TFC is avulsed from its foveal attachment without fracture,[30] a similar wiring technique can be employed. The advent of suture anchors has made

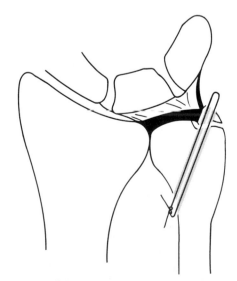

Figure 24–2. Internal fixation using the interosseous wire technique. The same method may be employed to repair a destabilizing tear of the TFCC when no fracture is present or when ulnar shortening is done in conjunction with the hemiresection arthroplasty.

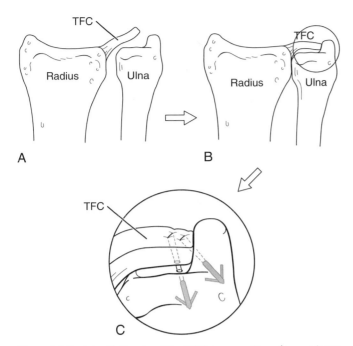

Figure 24–3. *A* to *C,* Repair of the TFC over positive ulnar variance. This procedure requires ulnar recession (shown as per Feldon and associates[20]). The use of suture anchors is shown.

standard suturing techniques more reliable. Insert the anchors into the foveal area. The styloid itself may be removed to secure adequate exposure. Note that an apically detached TFC cannot be successfully re-attached if it is stretched over a pathologically positive variant ulna. In these cases, we have found a sub-TFC "wafer" resection of the ulnar dome[20] to be useful in solving this dilemma if the positive variance is 2 mm or less (Fig. 24–3). More positive variance requires a formal ulnar shaft shortening.

Tears of the dorsal marginal ligament of the TFC may also occur. They are usually detachments from the radius. Direct suture repair, stabilized by Kirschner wires, is possible.[14] If the dorsal marginal ligament tear is chronic and associated with even mild instability, the repair should be augmented with local tendon grafts or transfers, as proposed by Leung and associates[40] and Scheker and colleagues.[60] Figure 24–4 demonstrates the way some local tissue may be utilized for these augmentations. Because of the torque placed on this structural relationship, all of these repairs should be tight and should be supported by cast immobilization for 6 to 8 weeks. We utilize an interosseous mold splint for 4 weeks after the cast immobilization.

TRIANGULAR FIBROCARTILAGE COMPLEX RECONSTRUCTION OR SUBSTITUTION FOR RECURRENT INSTABILITY OF THE DRUJ

The subject of recurrent DRUJ instability is complex. We have found the following points useful in under-standing this problem.[4]

Stability of the DRUJ is provided by:

1. Joint surface architecture and "fit" unique to each individual (ulnar head–sigmoid notch).
2. The alignment and length of the levers influencing the joint relationship (radius/ulna).
3. The major retaining ligaments of the joint (TFCC).

DRUJ stability may be lost if:

1. Joint architecture is disturbed (fracture of head or notch, surgery, etc). Containment of the ulnar head and the sigmoid notch may be lost in certain positions.
2. The attack angles or length relationships of the radius and/or ulna are altered. Alteration precipitates or magnifies the instability possible with either joint architecture disturbance or chronic ligament insufficiency.
3. Chronic ligament insufficiency exists.

Any procedure intended to restore DRUJ stability must:

1. Achieve a potentially satisfactory head-notch relationship. If this is not possible, a salvage measure (arthroplasty option) should be taken.
2. Restore TFCC integrity by repair or reconstruction.
3. Ensure the correctness of the radial-ulnar attack angles and length. If these parameters are not correct, attempts to achieve the goals in steps 1 and 2 will fail.

An understanding of these concepts is essential before one can proceed with surgical management of distal radioulnar joint instability.

Pain and limitation of function should dictate treatment for DRUJ instability, because some patients tolerate the instability itself with few complaints. Before proceeding with soft tissue reconstruction alone, the surgeon should ascertain that there is no evidence of arthritis and that the forearm bones are in normal alignment for the patient. The soft tissue procedures are contraindicated if rotational, angular, or translational malunions, length discrepancies, or arthritic changes are present and cannot be simultaneously corrected.

We believe, mainly on theoretic grounds, that for successful soft tissue reconstruction, the essential elements of the TFCC must be duplicated in an effective fashion. These essential elements are (1) a smooth carpal articulation, (2) a flexible rotational tether, radius to ulna, (3) suspension of the ulnar carpus to the radius, (4) an ulnocarpal cushion, and (5) ulnar shaft and ulnar carpal connection. The Bunnell-Boyes[9] reconstruction, as a working approach, is good but does not attempt to provide elements (1), (3), and (4) (Fig. 24–5). This technique is, however, innovative and carefully anatomic.

Reconstruction of the volar carpal ligaments, as diagrammed in Fig. 24–6*H,* was first conceptualized in a case reported by Hill.[31] Reports by Hui and Linscheid[32] (Fig. 24–7) and Tsai and Stillwell[68] (Fig.

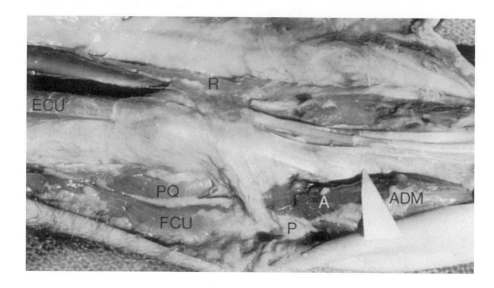

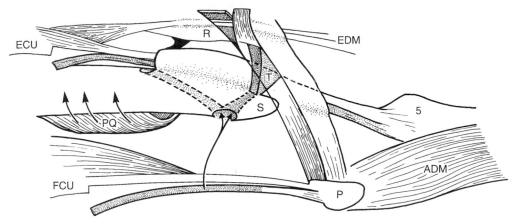

Figure 24–4. A strip of retinaculum, extensor carpi ulnaris *(ECU)*, or flexor carpi ulnaris *(FCU)* may be dissected distally to be utilized in augmentation or reconstruction of the TFCC. Suggested routes through the ulna allow relatively anatomic reconstruction. If the FCU or retinaculum is used, it should be woven through or sutured to firm capsular tissue proximal to the pisotriquetral joint in order to avoid abnormal stress on (and possibly pain from) this joint. The direction of pronator advancement is shown. *EDM* = extensor digiti minimi; *PQ* = pronator quadratus muscle; *ADM* = abductor digiti minimi; *P* = pisiform; *R* = radius; *T* = triangular fibrocartilage; *S* = styloid; *5* = fifth metacarpal.

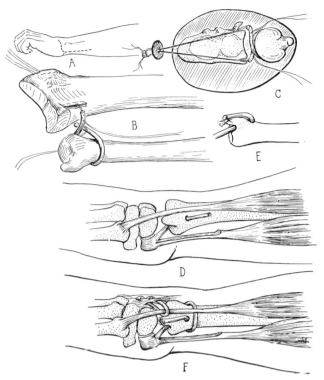

Figure 24–5. The Boyes-Bunnell reconstruction of the distal radioulnar joint.

24–8) use this feature of the Bunnell-Boyes reconstruction to advantage in operations for dorsal DRUJ instability. Both employ distally based portions of the flexor carpi ulnaris (FCU) harvested proximally and stripped distally to the pisiform attachment. This type of reconstruction has met with some success clinically. Untested but innovative procedures such as those proposed by Kuzma[37] may find some application, inasmuch as they more fully duplicate these normal TFCC elements (Fig. 24–9). Although making TFCC substitution in the manner suggested is difficult with the articular dome left intact, it is possible to selectively reconstruct the torn elements using locally available tissue (see Fig. 24–4).

Substitution for the normal triangular fibrocartilage complex has historically been by radioulnar tether procedures. These procedures attempt to supply one function of the triangular fibrocartilage complex; that of the radioulnar connection. As a group, they approach the problem at a level proximal to the radioulnar articulation and attempt, by weaving a tendon graft around or through the bones, to pull the bones together. Each series reports success in a limited number of patients; follow-up has been insufficient to allow meaningful statements to be made. Criticism generally reflects concerns that the procedures are ineffective in preventing instability or that rotation is restricted if anteroposterior stability is achieved. Some of these procedures are illustrated in Figure 24–6. We believe that achieving stability of the distal radioulnar joint connection should be directed to re-

pair or reconstruction of the TFC at its original anatomic site.

In dorsal instability of the distal ulna, some support can be given to the rationale of Johnson,[34] who has proposed advancing the pronator quadratus from its normal insertion on the ulna to a more lateral and dorsal insertion. This procedure could additionally be used to augment static repair of the triangular fibrocartilage, although Johnson[34] has not proposed its use for treating that disorder. This method may be conceptualized by review of Figures 24–4 and 24–10.

RADIAL OSTEOTOMY

Techniques of radial osteotomy are well described in the literature. This procedure should be utilized when correction of malunion or deformity of the radius is required to restore the proper relationship of the radius with the ulna at the distal radioulnar joint. The osteotomy may be midshaft, metaphyseal, or within the sigmoid notch. The desired result is to reestablish the radius's length, volar tilt, ulnar inclination, and translational relationships with the ulna. The technique usually requires a bone graft and the application of rigid internal fixation.

With regard to osteotomies about the metaphysis, some excellent results have been reported for the use of a wide radial approach and a strong volar plate with a trapezoidal bone graft.[21] Watson and Castle[74] described a technique using a limited dorsal approach to the radius and removing the trapezoidal graft from the radius to be corrected. This method converts a procedure requiring certain hospital stay into an outpatient-type procedure, and excellent results are reported.

If the original injury involved the sigmoid notch, one must presume that this surface is abnormal. An osteotomy done proximal to this level might not correct a sigmoid irregularity. An osteotomy done through the notch would be more direct but more difficult. If it cannot be done satisfactorily, arthroplasty options should be considered.

Malunions of the shaft of the radius associated with distal radioulnar joint instability are common. They are often the result of childhood fractures in which the instability is not recognized until the patient begins the provocative physical activities of adolescence or adulthood. Careful questioning often reveals the history of a childhood fracture. Comparison radiographs of both forearms in two planes (ensuring that the entire radius and ulna are shown on the films) reveal the deformity. Preoperative planning must be careful. A shaft osteotomy will provide relatively large movements of the distal radius in relation to the ulna with very small angular changes at the osteotomy site. A precise osteotomy is therefore required. Attempts to restore the radial bow and length of the radius relative to the ulna may require a small trapezoidal bone graft. Stable internal fixation is required.

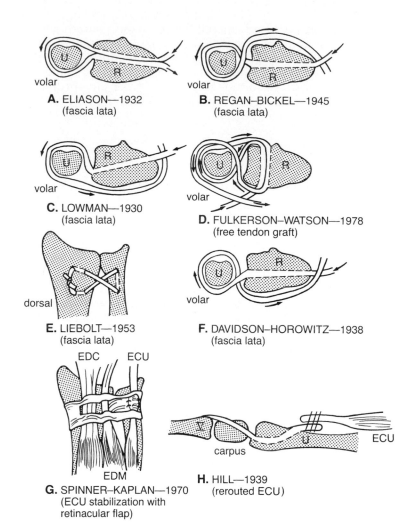

A. ELIASON—1932
(fascia lata)

B. REGAN–BICKEL—1945
(fascia lata)

C. LOWMAN—1930
(fascia lata)

D. FULKERSON–WATSON—1978
(free tendon graft)

E. LIEBOLT—1953
(fascia lata)

F. DAVIDSON–HOROWITZ—1938
(fascia lata)

G. SPINNER–KAPLAN—1970
(ECU stabilization with
retinacular flap)

H. HILL—1939
(rerouted ECU)

Figure 24–6. *A* to *H,* Radioulnar tenodesis procedures. *ECU* = extensor carpi ulnaris; *EDC* = extensor digitorum communis; *EDM* = extensor digiti minimi; *R* = radius; *U* = ulna.

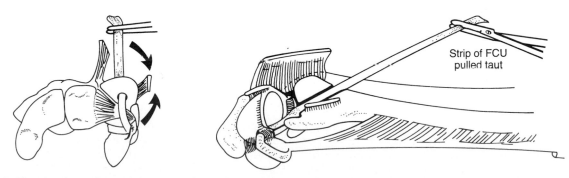

Figure 24–7. The ulnotriquetral augmentation tenodesis of Hui and Linscheid for dorsal instability. FCU = flexor carpi ulnaris. (From Hui FC, Linscheid RL: Ulnotriquetral augmentation tenodesis: A reconstructive procedure for dorsal subluxation of the distal radioulnar joint. J Hand Surg 7:230–236, 1982.)

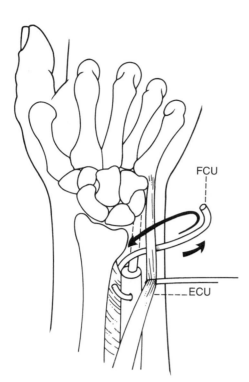

Figure 24–8. Stabilization of the ulnar stump using the flexor carpi ulnaris *(FCU)*—a modification of the Darrach procedure. *ECU* = extensor carpi ulnaris. (From Tsai T, Stillwell JH: Repair of chronic subluxation of the distal radioulnar joint [ulna dorsal] using flexor carpi ulnaris tendon. J Hand Surg 9B:289–293, 1984.)

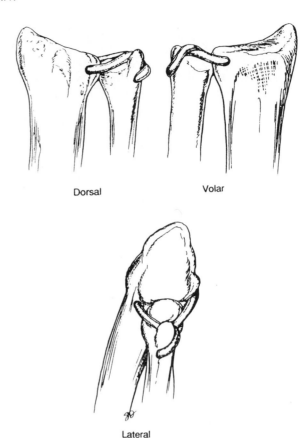

Figure 24–9. Stabilization of the distal radioulnar joint using Kuzma[37] reconstruction.

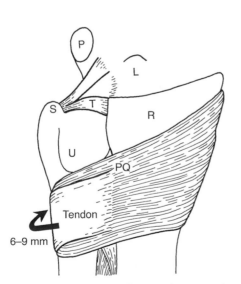

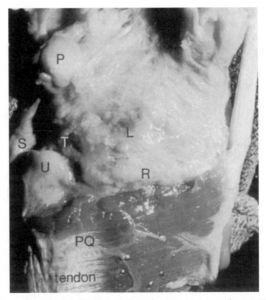

Figure 24–10. The drawing and photograph illustrate the approach to the volar distal radioulnar joint. The pronator quadratus *(PQ)* muscle-tendon unit as well as the direction and distance for advancement according to Johnson[34] are shown. (See also Fig. 24–4.) *L* = lunate; *P* = pisiform; *R* = radius; *S* = styloid; *T* = triangular fibrocartilage; *U* = ulna.

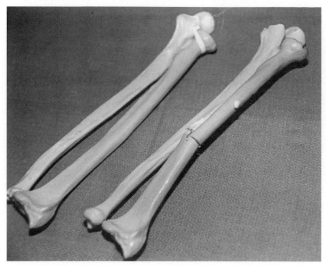

Figure 24–11. Supination dissociation following a midshaft radial fracture (normal left).

The result of such an osteotomy is often quite gratifying, with stability restored almost immediately postoperatively. Initially, we exposed the distal radioulnar joint to restore soft tissue relationships at the same time as the osteotomy, but in subsequent years, we have found that the osteotomy itself almost always suffices to restore stability. Figure 24–11 shows the normal radioulnar relationships in supination compared with an artificially created malunion at the midshaft level to indicate the type of deformity that will respond to corrective osteotomy.[67]

ULNAR OSTEOTOMY

Osteotomy of the ulna is used to correct rotational, angular, and length discrepancies of the ulna relative to the radius. Chevron, step-cut, transverse, and oblique osteotomies have been stabilized by wiring, compression screws, or plates (Fig. 24–12). The oper-

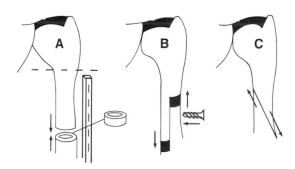

Figure 24–12. Techniques for ulnar osteotomy. The transverse osteotomy *(A)* may be used for shortening, lengthening (with bone graft), or rotational correction. The osteotomy should be planned so that the distal end of the plate does not impinge as the forearm rotates. Step-cut *(B)* and oblique *(C)* osteotomy techniques are applicable only for shortening. Compression screw or plate fixation can be used.

ation was popularized by Darrach,[16] who credits Dr. Kirby Dwight. Milch[44–47] developed the concept in the first half of this century and provided the best description of this procedure. Since then, precision techniques of osteotomy and internal fixation have achieved a more predictable outcome for this important procedure. A 1985 report by Darrow and colleagues[17] provided the first good evidence of its modern efficacy; a later report by Chun and Palmer[12] confirms this opinion.

We prefer the following surgical technique for ulnar shortening. Expose the distal ulna from the midshaft distally. Following exposure, perform all definitive maneuvers in zero rotation to ensure accurate measurements. We have been utilizing the arthroscopic traction tower as developed by Whipple for this procedure. The traction tower allows excellent exposure of the ulna and provides the zero rotation position during the osteotomy.

The planned site is several centimeters proximal to the proximal extent of the sigmoid notch. Place a four-hole or six-hole compression plate over the chosen site, and clamp it to the ulna. Carry the forearm to full supination. If impingement of the plate and radius occurs, adjust the site proximally. Then mark the site on the bone, and perform an osteotomy on the ulna transversely. Remove only bone proximal to the marked site, so that the distal margin of the plate does not change its relative position with the sigmoid notch. The amount to be removed should be predetermined by radiographic measurements. When the desired shortening is accomplished, stabilize the osteotomy by applying a plate with compression. Add bone graft from the removed bone or supplement it with bone graft from the radial metaphysis.

Use a long-arm cast with the forearm in zero rotation for 6 weeks, after which range of motion exercises can begin. Use an orthoplast forearm brace with the wrist and elbow free to protect the arm between exercise periods until the osteotomy is healed radiographically. Healing varies from 2 to 7 months, the usual time being less than 3 months. The hardware is often superficial and a source of patient complaints. Delayed union and non-union as well as re-fracture after plate removal can be problems. Linscheid[41] updated the original series reported by Darrow and co-workers[17] to include 150 patients with a 3 percent revision rate.

If rotational or angular correction is needed, the procedure is a little different. Angular changes are achieved with a wedge cut and a small bend in the plate. Rotational changes are best predetermined from a computed tomography (CT) scan and can be estimated at surgery using wires drilled into the shaft perpendicular to its long axis. We have noticed, however, that when ulnar rotational changes are needed, the distal ulnar fragment automatically derotates to assume the correct rotation relative to the radius upon completion of the osteotomy. This reaction is probably a result of the energy stored in an abnormally tensioned TFCC released by the osteotomy cut.

A precision technique of osteotomy has been developed by Rayhack and associates.[54] They employ a precision jig cut to the ulna. They use an oblique osteotomy coupled with a compression screw across the osteotomy site and three screws on either side of the osteotomy. The technique is technically demanding but straightforward, and with attention to detail, good results can be obtained. We have utilized this technique (as of this writing) in 12 cases, with one case of non-union and one of delayed union. Both of these problems could be attributed to technical errors. The technique holds promise and can be recommended.

PARTIAL ULNAR RESECTION: THE "WAFER" PROCEDURE

Feldon and colleagues[20] designed the "wafer" procedure to treat symptomatic TFC tears, ulnar impaction syndrome, or both by decompressing the ulnocarpal space. The distal 2 to 4 mm of the distal ulna (the "wafer") is resected, but the distal radioulnar joint articulation and the styloid process of the ulna as well as the triangular fibrocartilage are preserved (Fig. 24–13). The exposure is limited to the area of the inferior margin of the TFC. Small osteotomes are utilized to remove the "wafer." The procedure should be limited to no more than 4 mm of the distal ulna, with the goal to create approximately 2 mm of negative variance. The group's initial report detailed 12 patients ranging in age from 18 to 51 years, 69 percent of whom had excellent results, and 31 percent good results.

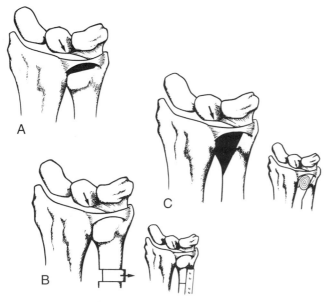

Figure 24–13. Procedures that may be useful in unloading the ulnocarpal axis. The Feldon wafer resection (A) is designed for this, as is the Milch osteotomy (B). C, The Bowers procedure is primarily a distal radioulnar joint resection and should be used only when arthritis of this joint is a primary feature of the loading syndrome.

We have used this procedure frequently over the past 5 years and found it to satisfy in all respects when utilized for the appropriate reasons. The results are similar to those of ulnar shortening by shaft osteotomy and compression plating. The "wafer" procedure obviates a secondary surgical procedure to remove the plates as well as the possibility of nonunion. Some surgeons have found the results not to be as satisfactory as Feldon and colleagues report.[20]

PARTIAL ULNAR RESECTION: THE HEMIRESECTION-INTERPOSITION TECHNIQUE OF ARTHROPLASTY[6]

The hemiresection-interposition (HIT) procedure is an outgrowth of what Dingman[18] described as the "best" Darrach procedures: those in which minimal resection was followed by regeneration of the ulnar shaft within the retained periosteal sleeve. The technique involves resection of only the ulnar articular head, leaving the shaft-styloid relationship intact.

There is a distinct difference between the HIT procedure and the previously discussed "wafer" procedure. The "wafer" procedure is designed specifically for unloading the ulnocarpal relationship, whereas the hemiresection-interposition arthroplasty is designed primarily for painful conditions of the radioulnar articulation (see Fig. 24–13). Such painful conditions are ulnocarpal impingement, contracture, arthritis, and/or instability. The HIT procedure, however, removes the entire articular surface of the distal ulna, thereby *creating* an unstable relationship between the radius and the ulna. By deleting the painful articulation, one substitutes less painful instability for the previously painful condition. The HIT procedure presupposes an intact or reconstructible triangular fibrocartilage complex. Otherwise, it has no advantage over the Darrach procedure. It should not be employed in situations in which the ulnar variance is markedly positive unless the ulna is shortened as part of the procedure.

Figure 24–14 illustrates the use of hemiresection-interposition arthroplasty and its modifications. The main advantage of this procedure over those in which completely the distal end of the ulna is completely resected (see later) is maintenance of some stability by the continued attachment of the ulnar shaft to the carpus to the radius. The stability is relative, however, as previously mentioned. We prefer it over the Darrach procedure in intra-articular ulnar head fractures, in arthritis, and in ulnocarpal impingement when shortening osteotomy or the "wafer" procedure alone cannot succeed because of arthritic or unstable joint surfaces.

The literature details the various techniques and problems of radioulnar joint hemiresection-interposition arthroplasty.[5–8, 71, 72] A similar procedure has been developed by Watson and colleagues[71, 72] and utilized for the same purpose.

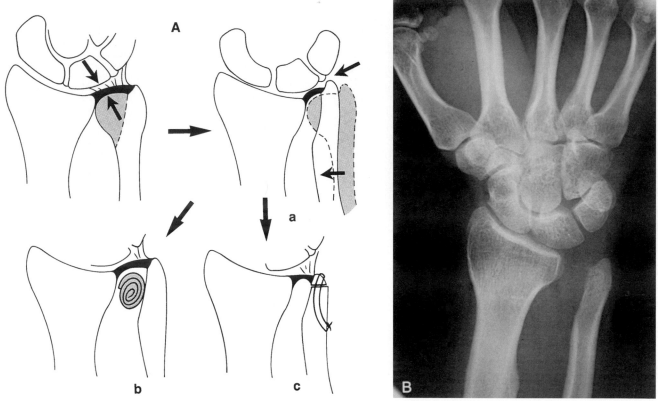

Figure 24–14. *A*, The hemiresection technique of arthroplasty employed in treatment of the ulnocarpal impingement syndrome. In view *a*, the still-too-long ulna produces stylocarpal impingement—a condition caused by the approximation of the radius and ulna that occurs when the articular dome is removed. To obviate this complication, interposition *(b)* or shortening *(c)* is necessary. In every instance in which the hemiresection technique is employed, intraoperative consideration of this possible complication is mandatory. *B*, Postoperative radiograph showing the usual case, i.e., no interposition or shortening is necessary.

COMPLETE ULNAR RESECTION: THE DARRACH PROCEDURE

The distal ulnar shaft and head are excised in the Darrach procedure. The general indication has been any condition that causes derangement of the joint, interfering with its action and resulting in limited or painful motion. The procedure has also been used in managing painful ulnar wrist instability in rheumatoid arthritis.

Complete ulnar resection has been used for many years and has been a worthy option for surgical treatment. It has become apparent that the best results are associated with minimal resection and brief immobilization. The procedure is not without its difficulties; however, two unsubstantiated criticisms are (1) increased ulnocarpal slide and (2) decreased grip strength. We know of no reports of ulnocarpal slide after the Darrach procedure in patients who have not also had their radiocarpal ligaments disrupted by trauma or rheumatoid arthritis. Thus, the "slide" is not a criticism of the procedure itself. There are no reports documenting grip strength. We have noted increased grip strength in patients in whom the procedure has been appropriately utilized.

The Darrach procedure does destroy the bone sup-

port of the triangular fibrocartilage complex. In addition to creating ulnocarpal instability, it results in "unstable" rotation of the radiocarpal unit around the ulnar axis. With muscular action, the ulnar stump may abut the radius or fray the overlaying tissues. This action may be evidenced by symptoms such as painful snapping or rupture of tendons, or both. Many papers have reported a significant number of dysfunctional results from Darrach procedures.* If such results occur, the temptation to remove more of the ulna must be resisted, because such a procedure may easily convert a poor result into a disaster.

There are no excellent salvage procedures for the painful instability of the "too short" Darrach procedure. We have found some success by instituting long-term use of the forearm brace (the elbow and wrist remain free with pronounced molding of the interosseous space), a concept borrowed from Sarmiento and associates.[58] For these reasons, the use of the Darrach procedure should be very selective. It may useful in the ulnocarpal loading syndrome when the distal radioulnar joint surfaces do not permit a successful shortening osteotomy or "wafer" procedure; in the patient with advanced rheumatoid arthri-

---

*References, 1, 2, 19, 22, 23, 26, 36, 49, 51, 56.

tis, it should be combined with a radiolunate fusion[11] or other radiocarpal stabilization procedures. Some options for stabilization of the distal ulnar stump following complete resection are described in the next section.

Technical Modifications to Improve Darrach's Procedure

In order to mitigate the instability created by Darrach's excision, a variety of modifications have been proposed. Swanson[65] has capped the distal ulna with a silicone implant, which has theoretic application in traumatic and attritional disorders. The greatest proven application of this modification is in the rheumatoid distal radioulnar joint. Disruption and dislocation of the implant are complicating problems.[42, 75]

Blatt and Ashworth[3] have sutured a flap of volar capsule to the ulnar stump to hold it down. Leslie and coworkers[39] have suggested tethering the distal ulnar stump with a distally based strip of extensor carpi ulnaris (ECU). The intact portion of the ECU is stabilized in a permanent dorsal position as Spinner and Kaplan[62] have suggested.

Kessler and Hecht[36] suggest a dynamic stabilization of the ulnar stump by looping a strip of tendon around the distal ulnar stump and the ECU and tying the two together. Goldner and Hayes[24] have formalized these recommendations by passing a strip of ECU (detached distally) through a drill hole in the ulnar stump with the forearm in supination. Tsai and coworkers have employed both flexor carpi ulnaris[65] (see Fig. 24–8) and ECU[69] tenodesis to stabilize the ulnar stump. We have successfully used their FCU procedure after failed Darrach procedures.

A further adjunct in the management of the unstable distal ulnar stump may be the pronator advancement proposed by Johnson.[34] Watson and Brown,[73] extending their success with their version of the hemiresection arthroplasty, have reported success after lengthening the short ulnar stump to approximate the appearance of a successfully done "matched" ulnar resection.

DISTAL RADIOULNAR FUSION WITH SURGICAL PSEUDARTHROSIS OF THE ULNA (THE SAUVE-KAPANDJI PROCEDURE)

In 1936, Sauve and Kapandji[59] proposed an operation consisting of a radioulnar joint fusion and creation of a pseudarthrosis proximal to the fusion (Fig. 24–15). This procedure was advanced as an alternative in the management of distal radioulnar joint disorders previously treated by excision of the ulnar head. Steindler[63] and Gonclaves[25] have apparently attributed this procedure erroneously to Lauenstein.

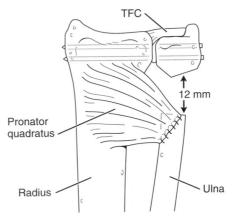

Figure 24–15. The Sauve-Kapandji procedure as modified by Taleisnik. (From Taleisnik J: Clin Orthop 275:110–123, 1992).

Elimination of pain, restoration of satisfactory forearm rotation, and few complications have led Taleisnik[66] to express general satisfaction with the procedure. He observed the theoretically predictable complication of an unstable ulnar stump in only 3 of 24 patients. Indications are similar to those for the Darrach procedure when dealing with a younger, more vigorous population. The indications are (1) osteoarthritis or severe chondromalacia of the distal radioulnar joint, (2) post-traumatic ulnocarpal impingement associated with distal radioulnar joint arthrosis, (3) in younger patients with rheumatoid arthritis who have ulnar translocation in addition to distal radioulnar joint disease, and (4) in patients with rheumatoid arthritis who may need a stable radioulnar surface for support of an arthroplasty or implant. Others have also expressed general satisfaction with the procedure, including Kapandji's son.[26, 35, 48]

The procedure is performed as follows: Expose the joint between the ECU and FCU tendons from 2 to 3 cm proximal to the prominence of the ulnar head to just distal to it. Expose the neck of the ulna subperiosteally. Completely excise the periosteum along the intended pseudarthrosis site for 12 to 15 mm. Grasp the ulnar head with a large towel clip, and perform an osteotomy transversely tangential to the proximal margin of the flair of the ulnar head no more than 1 to 2 mm proximal to the border of its articular cartilage.

If radial ulnar length discrepancy is present and needs correction—usually because the ulna is too long—recess the ulnar head proximally until it faces the sigmoid cavity of the radius. Then measure and cut a 12- to 15-mm section of ulna. Remove the articular surfaces to bare bone, and begin a fusion with compression screws or 0.0625-inch Kirshner wires. Bring the pronator quadratus into the pseudarthrosis gap and suture it to the sheath of the ECU.

Postoperative immobilization in a short-arm splint is required for 6 weeks with gradual resumption of function. The wires or screws are removed as necessary. We have had limited experience with this procedure, but in our patients for whom the procedure has been indicated, the results have been good.

ARTHRODESIS

If the need for a stable forearm is paramount and rotation can be sacrificed, the technique of Carroll and Imbriglia[10, 61] is trustworthy. The procedure may be a good choice in the paralytic instability of an otherwise unreconstructable brachial plexus injury or in spastic rotational contractures. The technique of arthrodesis is graphically demonstrated in Figure 24–16. The indication for this procedure is rare, and arthrodesis should be considered a salvage procedure.

STABILIZATION OF THE UNSTABLE EXTENSOR CARPI ULNARIS

The arrangement of the fibrous septa about the ECU creates an angular approach of the tendon to its insertion in the position of full supination. This angle results in an ulnar translocation stress on the tendon sheath during ECU contraction, particularly with the forearm in supination and the wrist ulnarly deviated. This is the position most often recalled by patients suffering traumatic dislocation of the tendon. The patient complains of a painful, soft snap.

For acute injuries, conservative management is immobilization with the forearm in pronation and the wrist dorsiflexed with slight radial deviation. Both acute and chronic injuries may be successfully repaired if the lesion within the sheath and its attachment to the ulna can be found. Rowland[57] has popularized this approach. Otherwise a surgical reconstruction of the tunnel as described by Spinner and Kaplan[62] and modified by the altered route for this flap suggested by Bowers[4] may be utilized (Fig. 24–17).

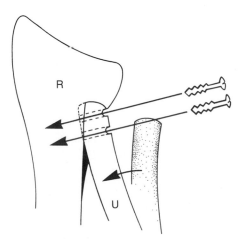

Figure 24–16. Distal radioulnar arthrodesis as described by Carroll and Imbriglia.[10] *R* = radius; *U* = ulna.

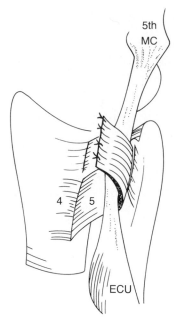

Figure 24–17. Modified retinacular sling stabilization of extensor carpi ulnaris *(ECU)* tendon. *4* and *5* = fourth and fifth metacarpals; *MC* = metacarpal.

Both stenosis of the extensor carpi ulnaris tendon[29] and a partial rupture[13] have been described. These conditions are treated surgically by exposure of the problem and limited débridement of the tendon and/or sheath without disrupting its integrity.

THE RELEASE OF CONTRACTURE ABOUT THE DISTAL RADIOULNAR JOINT

Contracture about the DRUJ should not be underestimated. Such a contracture may have had its genesis in a radioulnar dislocation or may have resulted from positions of immobilization after the fracture or ligamentous injuries of the wrist. The articular surfaces may be incompetent in the range of motion that has been lost, and the cartilage may be soft and poorly attached. Dystrophic changes may be present in soft and osseous tissue.

A full preoperative evaluation of DRUJ contracture should consist of: (1) comparison radiographic views of both forearms and wrists in several positions of rotation, (2) comparison CT scans of the distal radioulnar joint and carpal area in pronation, neutral, and supination, (3) arthrogram, and (4) bone scan. Preoperative hand therapy should include a baseline grip and motion evaluation. Two or more months of therapy are required to reach a preoperative plateau of improvement as well as to acquaint the patient and therapist with rehabilitation methods and techniques. The problem should not be approached surgically if therapy is missed or misunderstood.

The choice of operative approach should take into

consideration the information gained in the work-up. We use a dorsal and volar exposure with capsular contracture release as a primary goal before considering the hemiresection-interposition technique. If volar capsular release and limited interosseous division in the distal third of the foramen coupled with lysis of dorsal and volar ulnocarpal capsular adhesions is successful in achieving the rotation desired *and* the articulation is structurally competent, the forearm is immobilized in the desired range (usually 50 to 60 degrees of supination). Therapy is begun again 2 weeks after surgery. If the articulation is deficient (owing to chondromalacia, malformation, arthritis, instability, or markedly positive ulnar variance), we add the interposition technique with appropriate shortening. In some cases, the Darrach procedure may be required.

Therapy after surgery for DRUJ contracture may be prolonged. Pain control is essential. Initial patient-controlled analgesia is followed by oral medication. Transcutaneous nerve stimulation may also be helpful as therapy begins.

References

1. Bell MJ, Hill RJ, McMurtry RY. Ulnar impingement syndrome. J Bone Joint Surg 67B:126–129, 1985.
2. Bieber EJ, Linscheid RL, Dobyns JH, Beckenbaugh RD: Failed distal ulna resections. J Hand Surg 13A:193–200, 1988.
3. Blatt G, Ashworth CR: Volar capsule transfer for stabilization following resection of the distal end of the ulna. Orthop Trans 3:13–14, 1979.
4. Bowers WH: Instability of the distal radioulnar articulation. Hand Clin 7:311–327, 1991.
5. Bowers WH: Problems of the distal radioulnar joint. Adv Orthop Surg 7:289–303, 1984.
6. Bowers WH: Distal radioulnar joint arthroplasty: The hemiresection-interposition technique. J Hand Surg 10A:169–178, 1985.
7. Bowers WH: Distal radioulnar joint arthroplasty: Current concepts. Clin Orthop 275:104–109, 1992.
8. Bowers WH: The distal radioulnar joint. In Green DP (ed): Operative Hand Surgery, ed. 3. New York, Churchill Livingstone, 1993, pp 973–1019.
9. Boyes JH: Bunnell's Surgery of the Hand, ed 5. Philadelphia, JB Lippincott, 1970, pp 299–303.
10. Carroll RE, Imbriglia JE: Distal radioulnar arthrodesis. Orthop Trans 3:269, 1979.
11. Chamay A, Santa DD, Vilaseca A: Radiolunate arthrodesis: Factor of stability for the rheumatoid wrist. Ann Chir Main 2:5–17, 1983.
12. Chun S, Palmer AK: The ulnar impaction syndrome: Followup of ulnar shortening osteotomy. J Hand Surg 18A:46–53, 1993.
13. Chun S, Palmer AK: Chronic ulnar wrist pain secondary to partial rupture of the extensor carpi ulnaris tendon. J Hand Surg 12A:1032–1035, 1987.
14. Cooney WP, Linscheid RL, Dobyns JH: Triangular fibrocartilage tears. J Hand Surg 19A:143–154, 1994.
15. Cooper JL, Poehling GG, Chabon S, Koman LA: Wrist arthroscopy equipment, operating room set up and the surgical team. In McGinty JB, Caspari RB, Jackson RW, Poehling GG (eds): Operative Arthroscopy. New York, Raven Press, 1991, pp 607–612.
16. Darrach W: Partial excision of lower shaft of ulna for deformity following Colles fractures. Ann Surg 57:764–765, 1913.
17. Darrow JC, Linscheid RL, Dobyns JH, et al: Distal ulnar recession for disorders of the distal radioulnar joint. J Hand Surg 10A:482–491, 1985.
18. Dingman PVC: Resection of the distal end of the ulna (Darrach operation): An end result study of twenty-four cases. J Bone Joint Surg 34A:893–900, 1952.
19. Ekenstam F, Engvist O, Wadin K: Results from resection of the distal end of the ulna after fractures of the lower end of the radius. Scand J Plast Reconstr Surg 16:177–181, 1982.
20. Feldon P, Terrono AL, Belsky MR: The "wafer" procedure. Partial distal ulnar resection. Clin Orthop 275:124–129, 1992.
21. Fernandez DL: Radial osteotomy and Bowers arthroplasty for malunited fractures of the distal end of the radius. J Bone Joint Surg 70A:1538–1551, 1988.
22. Field J, Majkowski RJ, Leslie IJ: Poor results of Darrach's procedure after wrist injuries. J Bone Joint Surg 75B:53–57, 1993.
23. Friedman B, Yaffe B, Kamchin M, Engel J: Rupture of extensor digitorum communis after distal ulnar styloidecotmy. J Hand Surg 11A:818–822, 1986.
24. Goldner JL, Hayes MD: Stabilization of the remaining ulna using one-half of the extensor carpi ulnaris tendon after resection of the distal ulna. Orthop Trans 3:330–331, 1979.
25. Gonclaves D: Correction of disorders of the distal radioulnar joint by artificial pseudarthrosis of the ulna. J Bone Joint Surg 56B:462–463, 1974.
26. Gordon L, Levinsohn DG, Moore SV, et al: The Sauve-Kapandji procedure for the treatment of posttraumatic distal radioulnar joint problems. Hand Clin 7:397–403, 1991.
27. Hagert C-G: Functional aspects on the distal radioulnar joint [abstract]. J Hand Surg 4:585, 1979.
28. Hagert C-G: The distal radioulnar joint. Hand Clin 3:41–50, 1987.
29. Hajj AA, Wood MB: Stenosing tenosynovitis of the extensor carpi ulnaris. J Hand Surg 11A:519–520, 1986.
30. Hermansdorfer JD, Kleinman WB: Management of chronic peripheral tears of the triangular fibrocartilage complex. J Hand Surg 16A:340–346, 1991.
31. Hill RB: Habitual dislocation of the distal end of the ulna. J Bone Joint Surg 21:780, 1939.
32. Hui FC, Linscheid RL: Ulnotriquetral augmentation tenodesis: A reconstructive procedure for dorsal subluxation of the distal radioulnar joint. J Hand Surg 7:230–236, 1982.
33. Imbriglia JE, Boland DS: Tears of the articular disc of the triangular fibrocartilage complex: Results of excision of the articular disc [abstract]. J Hand Surg 8:620, 1983.
34. Johnson RK: Stabilization of the distal ulna by transfer of the pronator quadratus origin. Clin Orthop 275:124–129, 1992.
35. Kapandji IA: The Kapandji-Sauve operation: Its techniques and indications in non rheumatoid disease. Ann Chir Main 5:181–193, 1986.
36. Kessler I, Hecht O: Present application of the Darrach procedure. Clin Orthop 72:254–260, 1970.
37. Kuzma GK: Stabilization with a tendon graft. In Kasdan ML, Amadio PC, Bowers WH (eds): Technical Tips for Hand Surgery. Philadelphia, Hanley and Belfus, 1994, pp 307–308.
38. Lanz U, Kron W: Neue Technik zur Korrektur in Fehlstellung verheilter distaler Radiusfrakturen. Handchirurgie 8:203–206, 1976.
39. Leslie BM, Carlson G, Ruby LK: Results of extensor carpi ulnaris tenodesis in the rheumatoid wrist undergoing a distal ulnar excision. J Hand Surg 15A:547–551, 1990.
40. Leung PC, Hung LK: An effective method of reconstructing posttraumatic dorsal dislocated distal radioulnar joint. J Hand Surg 15A:925–928, 1990.
41. Linscheid RL: Ulnar lengthening and shortening. Hand Clin 3:69–79, 1987.
42. McMurtry RY, Paley D, Marks P, Axelrod T: A critical analysis of Swanson ulnar head replacement arthroplasty: Rheumatoid versus nonrheumatoid. J Hand Surg 15A:224–231, 1990.
43. Menon J, Wood VE, Shoene HR, et al: Isolated tears of the triangular fibrocartilage of the wrist: Results of partial excision. J Hand Surg 9A:527–530, 1984.
44. Milch H: Cuff resection of the ulna for malunited Colles fracture. J Bone Joint Surg 23:311–313, 1941.
45. Milch H: Dislocation of the end of the ulna—suggestion for a new operative procedure. Am J Surg 1:141–146, 1926.
46. Milch H: Cuff resection of the ulna for malunited Colles fracture. J Bone Joint Surg 23:311–313, 1941.

47. Milch H: So-called dislocation of the lower end of the ulna. Ann Surg 116:282–292, 1942.

48. Milroy P, Coleman S, Ivers R: The Sauve-Kapandji operation: Technique and results. J Hand Surg 17B:411–414, 1992.

49. Minami A, Ogino T, Minami M: Treatment of distal radioulnar disorders. J Hand Surg 12A:189–196, 1987.

50. Neviaser RJ, Palmer AK: Traumatic perforation of the articular disc of the triangular fibrocartilage complex of the wrist. Bull Hosp Joint Dis 44:376, 1984.

51. Newmeyer WC, Green DP: Rupture of extensor tendons following resection of the distal ulna. J Bone Joint Surg 64A:178–182, 1982.

52. Osterman AL: Arthroscopic debridement of triangular fibrocartilage tears. Arthroscopy 6:120–124, 1990.

53. Palmer AK, Werner FW, Glisson RR, Murphy DJ: Partial excision of the triangular fibrocartilage complex. J Hand Surg 13A:391–394, 1988.

54. Rayhack JM, Gasser SI, Latta LL, et al: Precision oblique osteotomy for shortening of the ulna. J Hand Surg 18A:907–918, 1993.

55. Roth JH, Poehling GG, Whipple TL: Arthroscopic surgery of the wrist. AAOS Instructional Course Lectures 37:183–194, 1988.

56. Rowland SA: Stabilization of the ulnar side of the rheumatoid wrist following radiocarpal arthroplasty and resection of the distal ulna following radiocarpal arthroplasty and resection of the distal ulna. Orthop Trans 6:474, 1982.

57. Rowland SA: Acute traumatic subluxation of the extensor carpi ulnaris tendon at the wrist. J Hand Surg 11A:809–811, 1986.

58. Sarmiento A, Kinman PB, Murphy RB: The treatment of ulnar fractures by functional brace. J Bone Joint Surg 58A:1104–1107, 1976.

59. Sauve, Kapandji: Nouvelle technique traitement chirurical des luxations récidivantes isolées de l'extrêmité inférieure du cubitus. J Chir (Paris) 47:589–594, 1936.

60. Scheker LR, Belliappa PP, Acosta R, German DS: Reconstruction of dorsal ligament of the triangular fibrocartilage complex. J Hand Surg 19B:310–318, 1994.

61. Schneider L, Imbriglia J: Radioulnar joint fusion for distal radioulnar instability. Hand Clin 7:391–396, 1991.

62. Spinner M, Kaplan EB: Extensor carpi ulnaris: Its relationship to stability of the distal radioulnar joint. Clin Orthop 68:124–129, 1970.

63. Steindler A: Orthopaedic Operations, Indications, Techniques and Results. Springfield, IL, Charles C Thomas, 1946.

64. Stokes HM, Poehling GG, Trainor BL, Crook ME: Results of arthroscopic debridement of isolated tears of the triangular fibrocartilage complex of the wrist. Presented at the American Society for Surgery of the Hand 45th Annual Meeting, Toronto, Sept 1990.

65. Swanson AB: Implant arthroplasty for disabilities of the distal radioulnar joint: Use of a silicone rubber capping implant following resection of the ulnar head. Orthop Clin North Am 4:373–382, 1973.

66. Taleisnik J: The Sauve-Kapandji procedure. Clin Orthop 275:110–123, 1992.

67. Thompson JS, Bowers WH, Schenck RC Jr: Supination dissociation of the distal radioulnar joint. Presented at the American Academy of Orthopaedic Surgery Annual Meeting, Atlanta, February, 1988.

68. Tsai T, Stillwell JH: Repair of chronic subluxation of the distal radioulnar joint (ulna dorsal) using flexor carpi ulnaris tendon. J Hand Surg 9B:289–293, 1984.

69. Tsai T-M, Shimizu H, Adkins P: A modified extensor carpi ulnaris tenodesis with the Darrach procedure. J Hand Surg 18A:697–702, 1993.

70. Van der Linden AJ: Disk lesion of the wrist joint. J Hand Surg 11A:490–497, 1986.

71. Watson HK, Ryu J, Burgess RC: Matched distal ulnar resection. J Hand Surg 11A:812–817, 1986.

72. Watson HK, Gabuzda GM: Matched distal ulna resection for posttraumatic disorders of the distal radioulnar joint. J Hand Surg 17A:724–739, 1992.

73. Watson HK, Brown RE: Ulnar impingement syndrome after Darrach procedure: Treatment by advancement lengthening osteotomy of the ulna. J Hand Surg 14A:302–306, 1989.

74. Watson HK, Castle TH Jr: Trapezoidal osteotomy of the distal radius for unacceptable articular angulation after Colles' fracture. J Hand Surg 13A:837–843, 1988.

75. White RE Jr: Resection of the distal ulna with and without implant arthroplasty in rheumatoid arthritis. J Hand Surg 11A:514–518, 1986.

PART V

Carpometacarpal Joints

CHAPTER 25

Carpometacarpal Joint of the Thumb

Stephen Flack Gunther, MD

The thumb is a fascinating structure. The fact that it is large and opposable sets humans and the other primates apart in the animal kingdom. The interphalangeal and metacarpophalangeal joints are relatively simple hinges, but the trapeziometacarpal joint at the base of the thumb is not. The full range of motion allowed by the joint and provided by the intrinsic and extrinsic muscles is best described by the term *circumduction* and is still being studied in laboratories with sophisticated equipment.[21] A detailed analysis of the kinematics and biomechanics of the thumb is not within the scope of this chapter. Rather, I present a simplified basis from which I can go on to address the pathologic conditions of the thumb, including ligament injuries, ligamentous attenuation over time, fractures, osteoarthritis, and rheumatoid arthritis.

FUNCTIONAL ANATOMY AND KINESIOLOGY

In order for the thumb to move into its many positions of function, the most important being opposition to the fingers, it has a very specialized anatomy at the trapeziometacarpal (carpometacarpal; CMC) joint. The matching articular surfaces of this saddle-shaped joint permit free motion in flexion-extension and in abduction-adduction. The very specialized interosseus ligaments and capsule provide enough stability to keep the metacarpal base stable during pinch but sufficiently lax to allow rotation of the metacarpal in the saddle, for which this joint would appear at first look not to have been designed. The intrinsic and extrinsic muscles that function across the joint coordinate to provide complex motions that have intrigued investigators for hundreds of years. I will consider these three aspects of functional anatomy and address the various traumatic and arthritic conditions that affect the thumb at this site.

Bones

In its resting position with fully innervated muscles, the thumb sits in a position of about 40° abduction (forward from the second metacarpal) and an equal amount of extension (radial to the second metacarpal) (Fig. 25–1). It has been likened to the boom of a sailboat, in that it is attached near the base of the rigid, main mast–like second metacarpal and is suspended by shrouds of ligament and muscle distally.[15] The resting position is determined by the direction of the articular facets of the trapezium and metacarpal base. The saddle-shaped surface of the trapezium is oriented so that a rider, the first metacarpal, seated comfortably in the saddle would look directly at the second metacarpal when the thumb is in its natural mid position (Fig. 25–2). The concave surface of the saddle allows the rider to rock back and forth into flexion and extension, toward and away from the second metacarpal. The saddle is convex in the sideways direction, and the metacarpal rider can rotate anteriorly away from the second metacarpal as if it were falling sideways from the saddle; this is abduction. Because the saddle is not terribly deep and because the metacarpal rider is usually not being compressed forcibly down into the saddle, it can also twist in its seat. This is what the metacarpal does when it rotates 15° to 20° into opposition.

Because of the alignment of the saddle, the truly congruent motions of the first metacarpal are not pure flexion-extension or abduction-adduction, but are roughly 45° from these motions.

Ligaments

The joint capsule is specialized in order (1) to keep the first metacarpal securely tethered to the trapezium during forceful pinch, an exercise that tends to subluxate the metacarpal base, and (2) to provide for rotation. The major strong ligament connects the beak of the metacarpal base to the anterior tubercle of the trapezium.[19, 22, 26, 31] This ligament has been referred to as the anterior oblique, the ulnar, the ulnar-volar, and the beak ligament (Fig. 25–3). There are two other discernible ligaments in the capsule. The lateral ligament is found under the abductor pollicis longus tendon insertion, and the posterior oblique ligament is under the extensor pollicis longus. These three ligaments are sufficiently taut in the normal state to

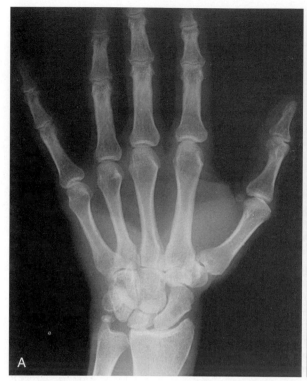

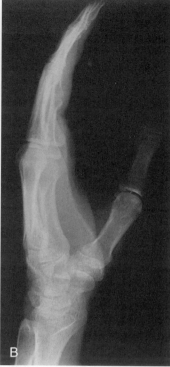

Figure 25–1. Anteroposterior *(A)* and lateral *(B)* radiographs of the normal thumb in resting position of approximately 40° abduction and 40° extension, both in relation to the second metacarpal.

secure the metacarpal base to the trapezium during function, but the whole capsule is sufficiently loose when the thumb is in the resting position that it can be distended with water.[26]

The ligaments have the dual functions of restraining the first metacarpal and limiting how far it can move and of guiding and determining the movements to a considerable extent. Haines[19] pointed out more than 50 years ago that the ligaments are arranged such that they determine the axial rotation of the metacarpal at the extremes of movement. Extension and adduction are accompanied by supination, whereas flexion and abduction are accompanied by pronation. Napier[31] pointed out in 1955 that there is passive mobility when the metacarpal is in its relaxed midposition. This is when the two saddle-shaped joint surfaces are least congruous and the restraining ligaments are relatively loose. However, the passive rotation is lost at the extremes of any motion, because the joint surfaces then become congruous, and the ligaments become taut.

Readers can demonstrate this concept on their own thumbs: Note the position of the thumbnail, and the passive rotation that is possible when the thumb is relaxed in tip-pinch position. Now note the involuntary pronation of the nail when the thumb is abducted away from the second metacarpal or flexed across the palm. Note as well the loss of passive rotation. Likewise, the nail rotates into supination when the thumb is adducted toward the second metacarpal or is extended. Cooney and associates[11] found that this rotation averaged 17° but that there was a great variation from one individual to another.

Muscles

The thumb is moved by a combination of extrinsic and intrinsic muscles. The extrinsics are the flexor pollicis longus (FPL), the extensor pollicis longus (EPL) and extensor pollicis brevis (EPB), and the abductor pollicis longus (APL). The intrinsics consist of two pairs of muscles whose actions on the metacarpal are fairly simple, the abductor pollicis brevis–opponens and the adductor pollicis–flexor brevis. These are relatively powerful, and they are arranged so that they can coordinate to put the thumb into any or all of its potential positions of function, exclusive of extension, assuming, of course, that the base is stabilized by normal ligaments.

TRAUMATIC DISLOCATIONS

Pure dislocation of the first metacarpal without fracture is quite rare (Fig. 25–4). There is only brief mention of it in most textbooks, and reported cases number less than 40. The dislocations are always dorsal, and the mechanism probably includes longitudinal compression of the flexed metacarpal against the trapezium,[12] with perhaps an adduction force distally, an abduction force proximally, or both. The causes of dislocation can range from simple falls to severe crush injuries. Strauch and colleagues[42] dissected 38 cadaver thumbs, and produced dorsal subluxations and dislocations mechanically after sectioning the ligaments in sequence. They concluded that the primary restraint to dorsal dislocation is the

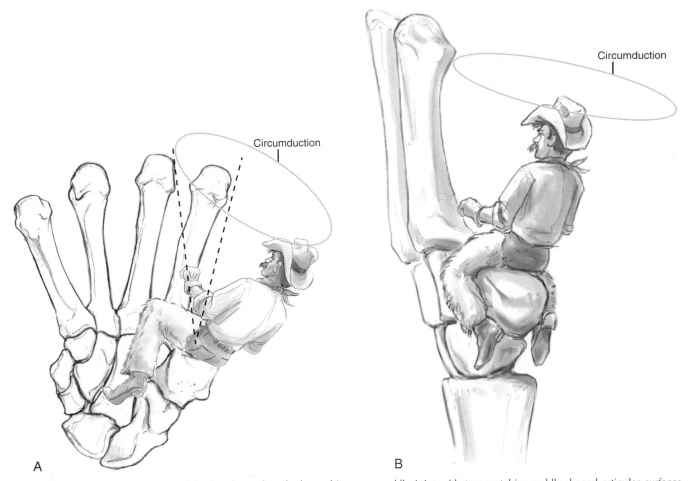

Figure 25–2. The trapeziometacarpal joint has been described as a biconcave saddle joint with two matching saddle-shaped articular surfaces. The terms flexion, extension, abduction, and adduction used in a proper anatomic sense do not describe the motions in which the joint surfaces are most congruous. In fact, if we envision the first metacarpal as a horseback rider seated in the saddle of the trapezium, we see that he looks at the second metacarpal at about a 40° angle. If he rocks to and fro or sideways in either direction, he is moving approximately midway between the motions. These are the natural positions of function. *A*, Here, the metacarpal rider has rocked back in his saddle. In this one dimension, all we see is extension of about 40°. His average flexion-extension arc is 53° in a plane in front of the second metacarpal. *B*, In his natural resting position, the rider sits in about 40° abduction as well. This is the direction at which the saddle points him. The average abduction arc is 48°.

The word *circumduction* describes all of the points at the extremes of metacarpal motion in all planes. Standard hinge joints such as the metacarpophalangeal and interphalangeal joints of the thumb do not allow this motion, a limitation explaining why the carpometacarpal joint is important, why it has a unique anatomy, and perhaps why it wears out. Opposition is the position in which the thumb is abducted, flexed, and pronated so that its pulp faces the pulps of the index and long fingers.

dorsoradial ligament. They found that the anterior oblique ligament strips subperiosteally up along the metacarpal. It is lax in the dislocated position, but it becomes tight again if the thumb is reduced, extended, and abducted.[42]

The best way to treat acute dorsal dislocation has not been determined. Cases of chronic instability have been reported,[23, 28] so it is obviously important that the metacarpal be reduced anatomically and held rigidly for 6 or 8 weeks. If reduction is accomplished with an audible clunk and the metacarpal seems fairly stable, it is reasonable to treat just in a thumb spica cast. This latter situation is usually not the case, however, so it is best to stabilize the reduction with a Kirschner wire. The wire can be passed either from the first metacarpal into the second[25] or from the metacarpal into the trapezium.[44] The former is more easily done and does not violate the joint surface. The metacarpal should be pinned in the comfortable position of about 45° extension and 45° abduction. The stripped anterior oblique ligament is taut again in this position and should heal. A word of caution: a smooth Kirschner wire should be used, because false passes across the palm with a threaded pin can damage important soft tissues. I have seen a woman in whom the motor branch of the ulnar nerve was destroyed in this way. The reduction and pinning can be carried out under local anesthesia, but the procedure should probably be done in an operating room after surgical preparation and under radiographic control.

Careful radiographic examination may demonstrate that tiny bits of bone have been avulsed from the metacarpal base by the anterior oblique ligament.

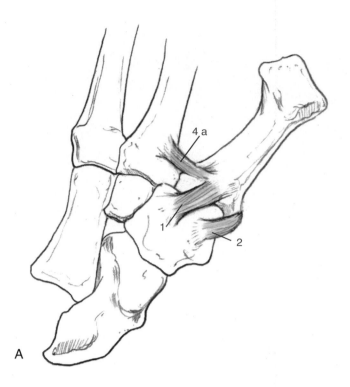

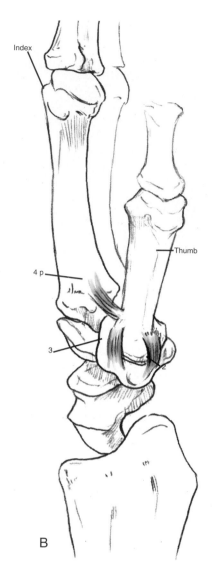

Figure 25–3. *A,* The ligaments as seen from the volar aspect and as described by Haines[19] in 1944: *1* = anterior oblique carpometacarpal ligament; *2* = radial carpometacarpal ligament; *3* = posterior oblique carpometacarpal ligament; *4* = intermetacarpal ligament, anterior *(a)* and posterior *(p)* divisions. *B,* The ligaments as seen from the posterolateral aspect. The posterior oblique ligament is responsible for pronation of the metacarpal in abduction and flexion, and this coupled motion is lost if the ligament is sectioned. Likewise, supination is determined by the intact anterior oblique ligaments when the thumb is abducted or extended.

This is a good sign, because bone-to-bone healing is possible and is always more reliable than ligament-to-bone healing.

If a good closed reduction cannot be accomplished or if time reveals the metacarpal to be unstable, open reduction and ligament reconstruction are indicated. Eaton[12] and Eaton and Littler[14] have described a procedure that entails passing a partial-thickness strip of distally based flexor carpi radialis (FCR) tendon through a hole drilled in the base of the metacarpal. The tendon enters the bone at the ulnovolar beak and emerges on the opposite radial surface, from which it is led back around the volar capsule under the first extensor compartment tendons to the remaining FCR. This transfer is designed to reconstruct an anterior oblique ligament and a radiodorsal ligament. The metacarpal is, of course, pinned for 6 weeks as previously described. In cases of chronic instability in which arthritis has already developed, it is better to perform arthrodesis (described later in this chapter).

BENNETT'S FRACTURE

Bennett's fracture is really a fracture-dislocation of the metacarpal base. It is more common than pure dislocation and most often occurs in falls or during fisticuffs.[10, 36] The mechanism of the two injuries is similar, and the difference between them is that in Bennett's fracture, an avulsed piece of metacarpal, including the ulnovolar beak and up to one third of the articular surface, remains in place with the ligament, but the remaining metacarpal dislocates radially (Fig. 25–5A).

Closed reduction of the metacarpal onto the trapezium can usually be accomplished with the help of local anesthesia if pressure is applied to the dorsum of the metacarpal base while axial traction is applied to the thumb phalanges. Unfortunately, reduction is difficult to maintain. The abductor pollicis longus and the other dorsoradial tendons exert a dislocating force proximally and radially at the base of the meta-

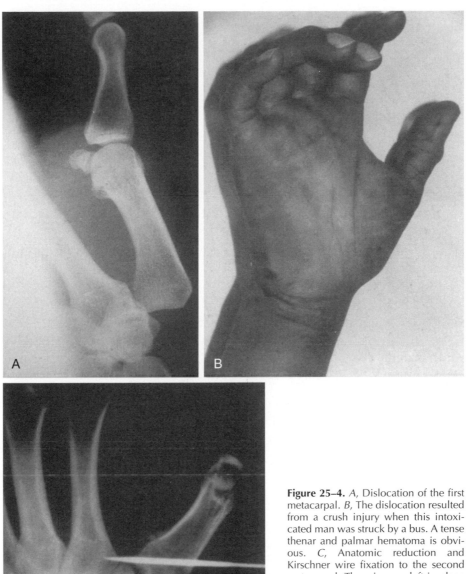

Figure 25–4. *A,* Dislocation of the first metacarpal. *B,* The dislocation resulted from a crush injury when this intoxicated man was struck by a bus. A tense thenar and palmar hematoma is obvious. *C,* Anatomic reduction and Kirschner wire fixation to the second metacarpal. The wire was left in place for six weeks. (*From* Gunther SF: The carpometacarpal joints. Orthop Clin North Am 15:259–277, 1984.)

carpal, and the adductor pollicis longus (APL) and flexor pollicis brevis (APB) tendons augment this tendency by their ulnar pull distally. The traditional position in plaster after closed reduction has been radial abduction of the thumb with careful molding of the cast over a felt pad at the base of the metacarpal.[4, 10] In the past, some surgeons have believed that dynamic traction should be added.[5] Others have judged that it is better to hold the metacarpal in a position of flexion and internal rotation (opposition), in line with the second metacarpal when the hand is viewed on its palmar aspect,[20] because this position more accurately matches the metacarpal to the avulsed piece. Whichever method is used, frequent radiographic checks must be made, because initial reduction is commonly lost over the ensuing

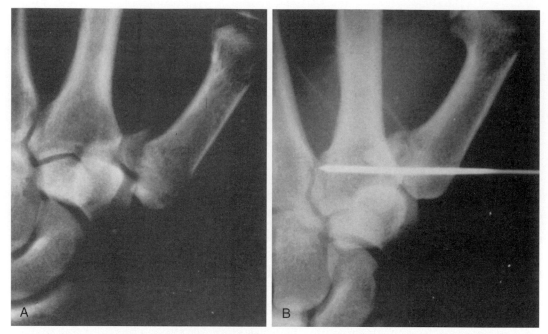

Figure 25–5. *A,* Bennett's fracture-dislocation. *B,* Percutaneous pin fixation after closed reduction. The metacarpal must be replaced in anatomic position on the trapezium. (*From* Gunther SF: The carpometacarpal joints. Orthop Clin North Am 15:259–277, 1984.)

weeks. In addition, the surgeon must be wary of causing pressure necrosis of the skin at the point of plaster molding at the base of the metacarpal.

A preferable alternative to uncertain closed reduc-

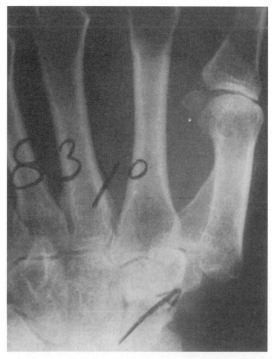

Figure 25–6. An untreated Bennett's fracture that occurred during the youth of an 83-year-old man. He was asymptomatic all his working life and continues to be so. The hand looks remarkably good. (*From* Gunther SF: The carpometacarpal joints. Orthop Clin North Am 15:259–277, 1984.)

tion is percutaneous pin fixation (Fig. 25–5*B*), as described in the previous section. It is not necessary that the pin traverse the avulsed piece, although this occurrence is helpful when the piece is large enough. The metacarpal should be anatomically positioned on the trapezium, but a 1-mm or 2-mm stepoff of the smaller fragment is not significant, provided that the piece is apposed to the metacarpal, where it can heal and provide stability. This is especially true when the piece is small and does not constitute a major portion of the articulation. Displacement is usually away from the joint surface and therefore should not cause arthritis.

Some authorities disagree, holding that any recognizable incongruity of the joint surface is reason to perform open reduction and pinning.[17, 32] The proponents of nonoperative treatment point out that there is no long-term study of Bennett's fracture results indicating that surgery is justified more than rarely, if ever.[10, 20, 36] Although they surely exist, I have never seen a patient who complained of arthritic pain years after Bennett's fracture, treated or untreated, and it is common to find old unreduced and asymptomatic Bennett's fractures in hand radiographs that are obtained for other reasons (Fig. 25–6).

If open reduction is required, it can be accomplished through a transverse incision around the base of the metacarpal from the dorsal to the volar aspect, extending approximately 1 cm onto the palmar skin over the thenar muscles. An alternative is the less cosmetic longitudinal incision along the subcutaneous border of the metacarpal, between the thenar muscles and the extensor pollicis brevis tendon. Through either incision, elevate the thenar muscles from bone and capsule volarly, allowing inspection of the fracture and reduction under direct vision. Pin both the fracture and the joint. Postoperative treatment is essentially the same as for the percutaneous procedure and for dislocation.

OTHER FRACTURES

Severely displaced and angulated fractures may occur in the proximal metaphysis of the metacarpal. Complete radiographic examination is important. Films should be ordered of the thumb specifically, and they should include three views, because major displacements can otherwise be overlooked (Fig. 25–7). When a fracture spares the joint, it can usually be handled nonsurgically. Closed reduction provides at least a general restoration of alignment, and the fracture heals despite a disquieting amount of displacement. The great range of motion at the CMC joint makes a moderate residual displacement and even angulation insignificant.

Rolando's T-condylar or other comminuted fractures into the joint commonly do require reduction and pinning (Fig. 25–8), particularly when the joint surface is broken into two or more pieces, none large enough to serve alone as a satisfactory articulation for the metacarpal. Although small plates and screws are available for this purpose, simple pinning with Kirschner wires is almost always preferable for its simplicity and for ease of hardware removal later on.

Plaster protection should be provided for approximately 6 weeks, but the pins can be left in place a few weeks longer if they do not penetrate the joint and if they are cut off beneath the skin.

Fractures of the trapezium are extremely rare. These are usually comminuted and are best left alone. Reconstruction can be accomplished later on by arthroplasty or arthrodesis, if necessary.

OSTEOARTHRITIS

Osteoarthritis of the thumb CMC joint is one of the most common conditions seen by the hand surgeon. The average patient is a woman in her fifties or sixties. She complains of pain and deformity at the base of the thumb. The duration has usually been from several months to years, and the pain has steadily increased up to the time of presentation. Pain with turning jar tops and keys can be relied upon as an indicator of this diagnosis. Commonly, the other thumb is symptomatic as well.

Physical examination reveals swelling and prominence at the joint. The base of the metacarpal is commonly luxated radially, and the thumb may be limited in abduction. Coincident with the adduction deformity of the metacarpal, there is compensatory hyperextension of the metacarpophalangeal (MP) joint in advanced cases. This joint is occasionally painful, but usually not. Although some authorities recommend longitudinal compression and grinding

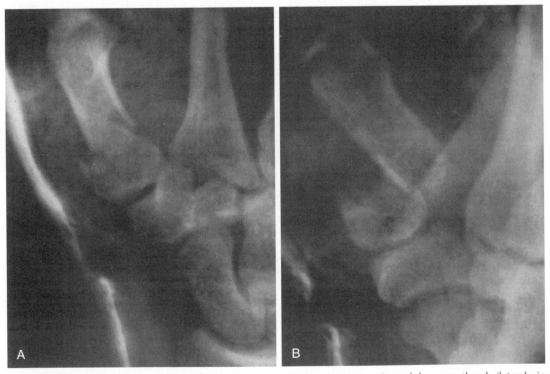

Figure 25–7. *A,* Proximal metaphyseal fracture of the thumb metacarpal. *B,* Anteroposterior view of the same thumb (lateral view of the hand) demonstrates the necessity for complete radiographic studies. This fracture is not uncommon. The position of the thumb can usually be improved by closed manipulation, and only rarely is open reduction or internal fixation necessary.

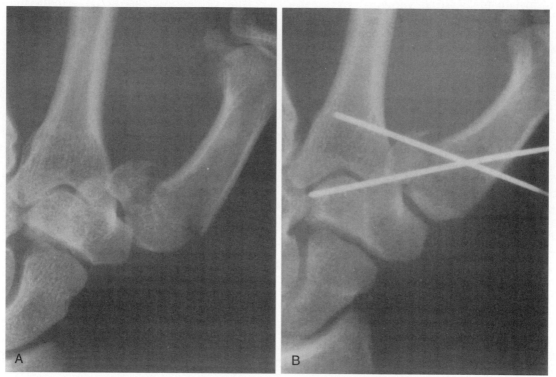

Figure 25–8. *A,* Rolando's fracture, a comminuted or T-condylar intra-articular fracture at the base of the first metacarpal. *B,* An excellent result was obtained by manipulation and percutaneous pin fixation. (*Radiographs courtesy of* Captain HJ Kimmich, MC, USNR, National Naval Medical Center, Bethesda, MD.)

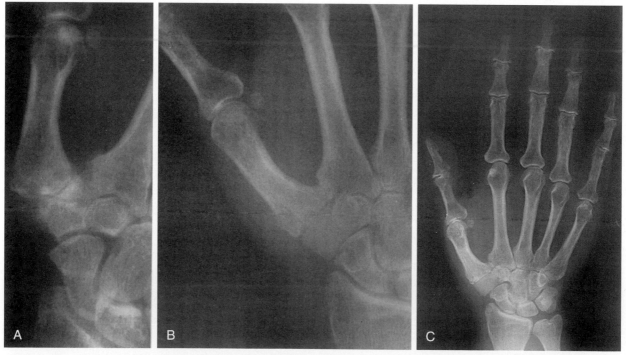

Figure 25–9. *A,* The patient, a 62-year-old woman, had experienced pain at the base of the first metacarpal for more than 2 years. An injection of triamcinolone brought relief for only a few months. Subluxation of the metacarpal base is obvious on this radiograph. *B,* Radiograph taken 11 weeks after Swanson Silastic trapezium arthroplasty was performed as described in the text. *C,* Minimal change in position and shape of the prosthesis is seen at 13 years. There is no sign of silicone synovitis, and the patient remains pain free and very happy with the result.

as a physical test to make the diagnosis, I find that the most reliable physical finding is point tenderness right on the joint. The surgeon can elicit this tenderness by holding the metacarpal in one hand and palpating the joint with the thumb tip of the other. By simply translating the base of the metacarpal, the surgeon can elicit crepitation and pain. This finding is helpful in the occasional case in which the patient describes a vague pain on the radial side of the hand and is having trouble localizing the problem. Radiographs reveal loss of joint space, subchondral sclerosis in both the metacarpal and the trapezium, and usually some subluxation (Fig. 25–9).

Although the thumb CMC ranks only seventh among hand joints in the incidence of arthritis, as determined by general radiographic screening of the population at large,[1] it easily ranks first in requiring treatment. The reason is obviously that the stresses on this joint are heavy during pinch and grasp, activities in which use of the thumb cannot really be avoided. It is interesting that some patients have severe symptoms with only moderate arthritic changes, whereas in others who are asymptomatic, advanced arthritic change is demonstrated on radiographs. Eaton and Littler[14] believe that primary laxity of the important ligaments of the CMC joint precedes and causes degenerative arthritis in many cases, and they have described a ligament reconstruction procedure to correct this laxity.

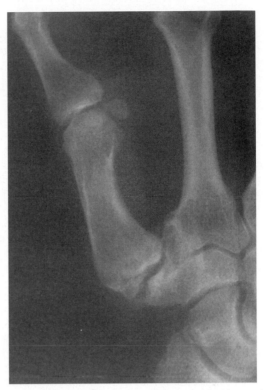

Figure 25–10. The patient, a 67-year-old man with advanced carpometacarpal arthritis, shown in the radiograph, has been asymptomatic for 4 years following injection of triamcinolone.

Conservative Management

When a patient presents with pain from arthritis in the CMC joint, the initial treatment should be nonsurgical. Some physicians use anti-inflammatory drugs and splinting with a special abduction orthosis, but I prefer an injection, which serves two purposes. The first purpose is diagnostic, because local anesthetic in the joint gives complete temporary relief if the pain truly is from the joint. The second purpose is therapeutic, because the pain is almost always relieved for some time by the corticosteroid. The pain generally returns in 2 to 6 months, but relief is occasionally accomplished for a much longer time (Fig. 25–10).

Accurate placement of the injection is easily accomplished by the experienced surgeon but may be difficult for the beginner. I prefer a 25-gauge needle and a small syringe with Xylocaine. I inject from the dorsoradial aspect of the joint while putting traction on the thumb with my opposite hand. The needle can be introduced to bone and walked a little distally or proximally until the joint is entered. A simple test for position can be accomplished by removing the syringe from the needle and watching to see whether Xylocaine flows back out. It will do so if the needle is in the joint but will not do so if the needle is in soft tissue. Approximately 0.4 mL of triamcinolone is injected through a second syringe after the needle position in the joint has been confirmed.

This treatment usually gives complete relief for some time, whereas the oral anti-inflammatory drugs give only partial relief and carry the risks of damage to the stomach wall and other body organs.

Selection of Surgical Procedure

If pain persists or recurs within a few months after injection and is severe enough to require medications and alter the patient's everyday activities, surgery is recommended. Deformity is a relative indication, but surgery is almost never performed for deformity alone. There are far more people in the population at large with asymptomatic deformities than there are patients with pain.

A number of different operations can be successful, and there is no consensus among hand surgeons today as to which is the best. As is true for treatment of arthritis in most joints, the general categories of operation are resection arthroplasty with or without interposition of autogenous material, resection with interposition of a prosthesis, and arthrodesis. Ten years ago, many hand surgeons were resecting the trapezium and replacing it with a silicone rubber prosthesis. This procedure has fallen out of favor even though the patients did well clinically. The problems are cold flow wear of the prosthesis and silicone particle–induced synovitis, which can cause bony changes within the wrist joint.[33, 34, 40] These are often evident on radiographs even in patients who feel well at 5 or 10 years.

Resection arthroplasty with interposition of autogenous tendon graft seems to be more popular than arthrodesis today,[45, 46] but I am not convinced that arthrodesis will not turn out to be better in the long run. After resection arthroplasty, patients take longer to become asymptomatic, and their thumbs are not as strong. The difference in motion between a resection and an arthrodesis is not really very significant once 2 years have passed, and of course, a successful arthrodesis ensures good thumb position permanently. I currently resect the distal half of the trapezium and form a biologic spacer in women who are not doing heavy work and who do not have severe deformity. I am much more likely to perform an arthrodesis in a man or in anyone with a severe adduction contracture of the metacarpal and compensatory hyperextension at the MP joint.

RESECTION ARTHROPLASTY WITHOUT PROSTHESIS

Resection includes procedures that entail removal of the base of the metacarpal,[27, 47] part of the trapezium,[3] or the whole trapezium.[18, 24, 30, 37, 48] The space that remains can be left empty or can be filled with a biologic spacer of tendon or fascia.[8, 13, 16, 47] The proponents of these operations argue that their procedures are simple, are sure to relieve most or all of the pain, and carry no risk of implant dislocation or wear in the future. There is also no risk of a non-union as there is when an arthrodesis is attempted.

Although resection arthroplasty has been done for many years, I believe that most hand surgeons do some version of the ligament reconstruction tendon interposition (LRTI) described by Burton and Pellegrini[8] in 1986. This is a modification of a procedure described by Eaton and colleagues[13] a year earlier. The principles are that resection arthroplasty is performed by removal of the trapezium, and a tendon graft is used to reconstruct as closely as possible the destroyed anterior oblique ligament. Although Burton and Pellegrini believe that the ligament reconstruction is the most important element in the procedure (after the bone resection, of course), they hold that the interposition of a wad of this tendon as a spacer is important as well. They use a Kirschner wire to secure position temporarily. If the thumb metacarpophalangeal joint hyperextends, they address that as well by tenodesis or arthrodesis.

There are a number of variations on this theme, and I do not know whether some are better than others. Good results can be obtained with resection of only the distal half of the trapezium, with using only a half-thickness of the flexor carpi radialis, with using one slip of the abductor pollicis longus APL instead of the FCR, or with resecting the trapezium without any interposition. The risk of the last is that the thumb will be unstable, and of course, it will shorten as the metacarpal base settles down on the scaphoid. Burton[7] believes strongly that a full thickness of FCR is better than any other tendon, because it gives adequate bulk and because the tendon attachment is already secure on the second metacarpal. He holds that the ligament reconstruction is the most important part of the operation but that the interposition of the remaining tendon rolled up into a ball is important as well. (RI Burton, MD, personal communication, 1995).

Ligament Reconstruction Tendon Interposition (LRTI) Procedures

LRTI with FCR Tendon. Stepwise, the surgical technique of Burton,[7] including current modifications on the original technique, is as follows:

1. Through a longitudinal skin incision, expose the trapezium between the APL and APB tendons. Remove the entire bone, taking care to preserve the capsule as much as possible (as seen in Fig. 13–13A to C).

2. Resect the articular surface of the thumb metacarpal with a saw or bur, and form a passage from the intramedullary space out through a hole in the radial cortex of the metacarpal near its base.

3. Through short transverse wrist and forearm incisions, transect the FCR tendon 8 to 10 cm above the wrist, free it of adhesions within its sheath, and pull it through the tunnel that runs under the transverse carpal ligament along the medial aspect of the trapezium. Deliver it into the cavity left by excision of the trapezium. It is still attached at its natural insertion on the second metacarpal base.

4. Place a suture through the capsule deep in the wound, and lead the two ends out through the wound; they will be passed through the bunched-up tendon graft later.

5. Draw the leading edge of the FCR tendon through the open base of the thumb metacarpal and out through the lateral hole, and suture it to the periosteum. Then, pass it back through the wound and suture it to itself (small needles are needed for work within this space). The tension should be such that the base of the thumb metacarpal cannot be moved more than 2 mm from the base of the second metacarpal. It should not be so tight as to cause abutment of the two bones, however.

6. Fold the remaining tendon on itself like a fire hose, and transfix it with two Keith needles, which are then used to draw the two suture ends mentioned in step 4 through the tendon interposition so that it can be tied snugly into the trapezium defect (Fig. 25–11).

7. Pass a Kirschner wire longitudinally from distal to proximal down the thumb metacarpal and into the scaphoid to fix the thumb metacarpal in a fist position, which is about 40° abduction and 45° extension from the second metacarpal.

8. Transfer the EPB tendon proximally to a bony insertion on the metacarpal shaft to augment metacar-

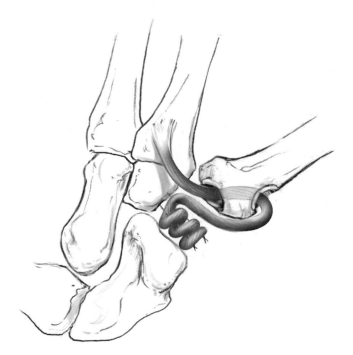

Figure 25–11. The ligament reconstruction tendon interposition (LRTI) as currently performed by Burton.[7] The full thickness of flexor carpi radialis tendon attached only to the second metacarpal base is led through a hole at the first metacarpal base and is sutured back on itself to reconstruct an anterior ulnar ligament. The remainder is sewn accordion-style to make an interposition wad that replaces the completely excised trapezium.

pal abduction and to remove a hyperextension force at the MP joint.

Apply a short-arm thumb spica cast for 4 weeks, after which time the cast and the Kirschner wire are removed, and an orthoplast thumb spica splint is fitted. Encourage isometric exercises of the thumb intrinsics now, as well as IP thumb exercises with the metacarpal stabilized. Have the patient begin pinch and full range-of-motion exercises 8 weeks after surgery and start weaning from the thumb spica splint. The exercise program is a long one and may extend for 6 to 12 months.

LRTI with APL Tendon. A variation on the LRTI involves use of the APL tendon instead of the FCR.[38, 39] I prefer a transverse incision in the skin lines over the CMC joint and a second transverse incision at the muscle-tendon junction of the APL on the dorsoradial aspect of the distal forearm. Cosmetically, these are far less noticeable than a longitudinal incision at the CMC and incisions in the volar aspect of the wrist and forearm when one takes the FCR.

Use the most radial slip of the APL if it is of adequate size. If there is only one tendon, use half. If the radial slip is small, use it and half of the main tendon. The tendon length is usually 6 or 7 cm, which is adequate. Various weaves have been described, but the simplest method is to lead the tendon through a hole in the radial base of the metacarpal, down around the FCR, and back. Then wrap the

tendon around or through the intact APL, and bunch the remainder up in the joint as described for the FCR tendon. This is actually fairly similar to the LRTI done with FCR, with the exception that the APL attachment deep in the wound is more proximal than in Burton's procedure. It should therefore not suspend the first metacarpal quite as well. Resect the trapezium and the base of the metacarpal in the same manner as described for the LRTI.

The procedure is simple, is quick, and I have been impressed that patients seem to have less discomfort postoperatively than with the FCR procedure. A Kirschner wire is very rarely necessary. I prefer a bulky dressing with the thumb in abduction for 10 days, followed by 5 weeks in a thumb spica cast.

Even with this procedure, patients have more discomfort in the early months than with a prosthesis, but I believe that both the patients undergoing the APL and those undergoing the FCR procedure are very close to asymptomatic by a year and generally completely asymptomatic by 2 years. Various researchers have stressed that it takes a year for patients to regain maximal strength and to recover from the procedure.

RESECTION ARTHROPLASTY WITH IMPLANT

Various implants have been used to fill the space when all or part of the trapezium has been resected.[6, 27, 43] In the first edition of this book, I wrote that I favored the Swanson trapezium arthroplasty. Although patients did well with it, and I have removed no more than two or three over the past 10 years, I have noticed worrisome changes on radiographs in many patients, and I tend to stay away from the procedure now. So-called silicone synovitis, a response to wear-induced free microparticles, can occasionally result in osteolysis and erosion of all the bones surrounding the implant, requiring implant removal and extensive débridement within the joint.[33] Pellegrini and Burton[35] reported a 25 percent failure rate in a series of 32 silicone implant arthroplasties followed for an average of only 3.9 years.

I will still use implant arthroplasty on the rare occasion in which an elderly person needs a procedure and the equally rare situation of bad rheumatoid disease. I do have patients who have done very well clinically and radiographically over many years after such a procedure (see Fig. 25–9). Because subluxation is the first stage of trouble, the surgeon should be careful with the surgical technique. It is relatively easy to obtain excellent, stable alignment when the alignment is good preoperatively. It is more difficult when the metacarpal is in a luxated position (Fig. 25–12). The joint angle at the base of the metacarpal varies considerably from patient to patient, so careful preoperative assessment is important.

A number of techniques have been described for reinforcing the CMC capsule around the prosthesis, but it is my contention that correct cutting of the base

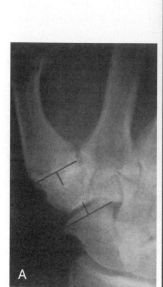

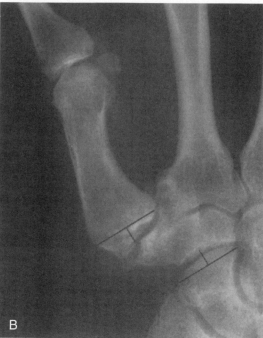

Figure 25–12. *A* and *B*, The T lines drawn on the radiographs of two patients with osteoarthritis demonstrate an obvious difference in the alignment of the metacarpal bases relative to the scaphoids. Stable silicone arthroplasty can be achieved more easily in the thumb shown in *A* than in that shown in *B*.

of the metacarpal is more important. The technique is illustrated in Figure 13. McGrath and Watson[29] published a series of 37 cases in which Swanson's trapezium replacement was performed without any capsule reinforcement and in which there were no dislocations. They stressed the importance of resecting the radial portion of the trapezoid in the depths of the wound. I do all of these procedures through a transverse skin incision, which is cosmetically very acceptable. Many surgeons prefer longitudinal incisions because they give a little better exposure.

Amadio and colleagues[2] reported an interesting study in which they compared 25 thumbs with silicone arthroplasty and 25 thumbs with resection arthroplasty. After 2 years, pain relief, motion, strength, and appearance were essentially the same in the two groups, although radiographs did show settling of the metacarpal base toward the scaphoid when there was no prosthesis.

ANCILLARY SURGICAL PROCEDURES

The procedures mentioned already may not be sufficient when there is severe postural deformity of the thumb. The combination of advanced subluxation of the metacarpal base, fixed adduction of the metacarpal, adduction contracture of the web fascia, and compensatory hyperextension of the MP joint carries a high risk of persistent postoperative deformity. Additional steps can be taken to prevent this sequela. In the rare case in which there is a true soft tissue contracture, the fascia of the thumb-index web can be released, and a formal resection of the adductor pollicis muscle can be carried out at either its origin or its insertion. The hyperextensible MP joint can be

pinned in slight flexion for 6 weeks, and in the most severe cases, a surgical tightening or free tendon graft substitution of the volar plate is indicated. I do not generally do either of these procedures. I believe that even a zigzag postural deformity of the thumb will be corrected by natural muscle tone if the metacarpal is held in proper position of abduction and extension. The best way to accomplish this position, of course, is through an arthrodesis.

ARTHRODESIS

A patient who would appear to require major correction of the position of the metacarpal and a procedure to correct MP joint hyperextension is probably better served by an arthrodesis at the CMC joint (Fig. 25–14). The incision is the same transverse one as described earlier, and a small amount of cancellous bone graft is taken through a transverse skin incision over the distal radius. The cartilage surfaces and subchondral bone plates are removed from the metacarpal base and the trapezium. Two or three Kirschner wires are placed across the joint, and they are cut off below the skin so that they can be left in place for 12 weeks. The proper position of the metacarpal is roughly the one that it naturally assumes in the making of the fist, 40° abduction and 45° extension. The only error that I have seen is in not obtaining enough extension, so the thumb metacarpal is in the way of the index finger when a full fist is made.

Secondary procedures are generally not necessary, because proper positioning of the metacarpal restores tendon balance, as has already been mentioned. In addition to patients with pronounced deformities, I recommend this operation to patients who will be

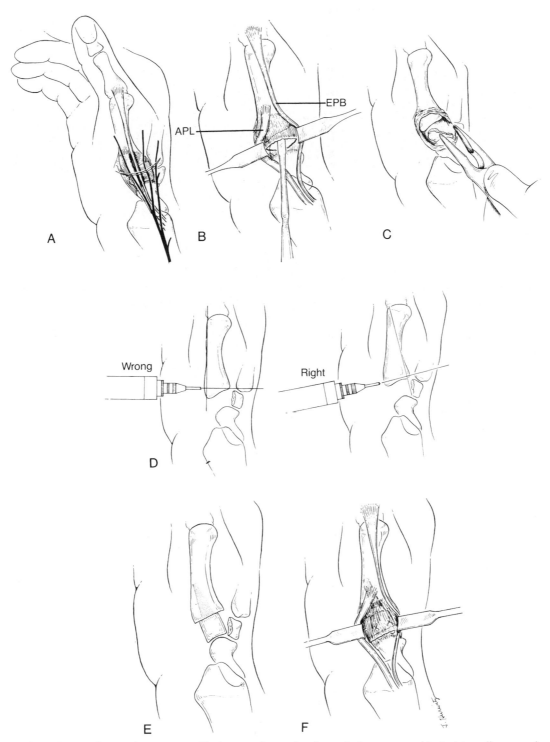

Figure 25–13. Outline of my technique for Swanson Silastic trapezium arthroplasty. *A,* A transverse skin incision allows good exposure and is cosmetically inconspicuous after healing. Identify and retract the sensory branches of the radial nerve in the subcutaneous tissue. *B,* Incise the joint capsule transversely between the retracted abductor pollicis longus *(APL)* and the extensor pollicis brevis *(EPB)* tendons. Elevate the capsule from the trapezium, and leave it attached to the scaphoid proximally and to the metacarpal distally. *C,* Remove the trapezium piecemeal. Small pieces of bone can be left rather than risk damage to the volar capsule. *D,* The wrong and right ways to cut the base of the metacarpal (see text). *E,* Close the capsule. *F,* The APL tendon can be incorporated in the closure if the capsule is deficient.

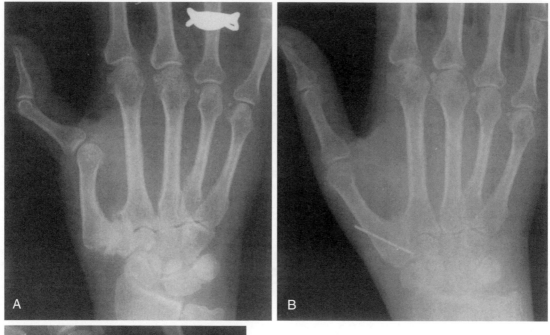

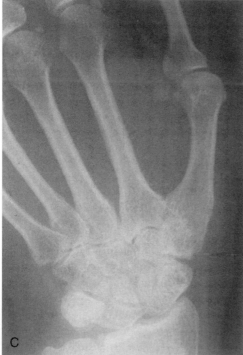

Figure 25–14. *A,* Severe deformity in a 57-year-old nurse who presented with pain, adduction contracture of the metacarpal, and compensatory hyperextension deformity of the metacarpophalangeal joint. *B,* Arthrodesis of the carpometacarpal joint has completely relieved pain and has restored normal thumb posture, without any further procedure being done, at 4 months. *C,* The other thumb is asymptomatic 16 years after arthrodesis. Note that there is some degenerative change at the scaphotrapezial joint. The patient remains pain free 14 years after surgery for the right thumb and 25 years after surgery for the left.

doing heavy work with their hands, whether on the job site or at home in the garden. I have been impressed by how little stiffness is evident when I examine patients 2 years after arthrodesis. Theoretically, fusion of the CMC joint increases stresses at the scaphotrapezial joint, but this is unlikely to pose a problem in patients who undergo this procedure after 50 years of age.

I am not aware of a study in which arthrodesis is compared with resection arthroplasty by the same surgeons and in the same series of patients. It is difficult, therefore, to say whether one is better than the other. Published series do show excellent functional results and patient satisfaction.[9, 41] I do know that I tend to do more arthrodeses as time goes on. They require the patient to be in plaster for a longer time, and Kirschner wires usually have to be removed eventually, but the patients feel better and stronger at 6 months than do those who undergo resection. Patients with arthrodeses are the only patients in my practice who are 100 percent asymptomatic at a year postoperatively.

RHEUMATOID ARTHRITIS

Rheumatoid arthritis presents special problems. The involvement of the basal joint of the thumb is rarely an isolated problem. Deformity, instability, and pain are commonly present at the metacarpophalangeal and interphalangeal joints, and arthrodesis is commonly necessary at one or both locations. This makes arthrodesis at the CMC joint unwise in most cases. In the rare instance in which any surgery is indicated, resection arthroplasty should be considered. If the bony architecture is good enough, a silicone prosthesis gives better results than it would in the higher demand osteoarthritic patient because silicone wear problems are unlikely. Wishing to preserve all bone stock possible, Pellegrini and Burton[35] prefer a condylar silicone implant, which does not require removal of the whole trapezium. My own experience with this is very limited, because patients with rheumatoid arthritis rarely require any surgery at all at this joint.

References

1. Acheson RM, Chan YK, Clemett AR: New Haven survey of joint diseases. XII: Distribution and symptoms of osteoarthritis in hands. Ann Rheum Dis 29:275–286, 1970.
2. Amadio PC, Millender LH, Smith RJ: Silicone spacer or tendon spacer for trapezium resection arthroplasty—comparison of results. J Hand Surg 7:237–244, 1982.
3. Ashworth CR, Blatt G, Chinard RG, et al: Silicone-rubber interposition arthroplasty of the carpometacarpal joint of the thumb. J Hand Surg 2:345–357, 1977.
4. Barton NJ: Fractures and joint injuries of the hands. In Wilson JN (ed): Watson-Jones, Fractures and Joint Injuries, ed 6. Edinburgh, Churchill Livingstone, 1982, pp 739–788.
5. Bradford CH, Dolphin JA: Fractures of the hand and wrist. In Flynn JE (ed): Hand Surgery. Baltimore, Williams & Wilkins, 1966, pp 142–143.
6. Braun RM: Total joint replacement at the base of the thumb—preliminary report. J Hand Surg 7:245–251, 1982.
7. Burton R: American Society for Surgery of the Hand Correspondence Newsletter, January 1995.
8. Burton RI, Pellegrini VD Jr: Surgical management of basal joint arthritis of the thumb. Part II: Ligament reconstruction with tendon interposition arthroplasty. J Hand Surg 11A:324–332, 1986.
9. Carroll RE, Hill NA: Arthrodesis of the carpometacarpal joint of the thumb. J Bone Joint Surg 55B:292–294, 1973.
10. Charnley J: The Closed Treatment of Common Fractures, ed 2. Edinburgh, ES Livingstone Ltd, 1957, pp 125–130.
11. Cooney WP, Lucca M, Chao E, Linscheid R: The kinesiology of the thumb trapeziometacarpal joint. J Bone Joint Surg 63A:1371–1381, 1981.
12. Eaton RG: Joint Injuries of the Hand. Springfield, Charles C Thomas, 1971, pp 66–69.
13. Eaton RG, Glickel SZ, Littler JW: Tendon interposition arthroplasty for degenerative arthritis of the trapeziometacarpal joint of the thumb. J Hand Surg 10A:645–654, 1985.
14. Eaton RG, Littler JW: Ligament reconstruction for the painful thumb carpometacarpal joint: A long-term assessment. J Bone Joint Surg 55A:1655–1666, 1973.
15. Flatt AE: The Care of Minor Hand Injuries, ed 3. St Louis, CV Mosby Co, 1972, pp 3–5.
16. Froimson AI: Tendon arthroplasty of the trapeziometacarpal joint. Clin Orthop 70:191–199, 1970.
17. Gedda KO, Mobert E: Open reduction and osteosynthesis of the so-called Bennett's fracture in the carpo-metacarpal joint of the thumb. Acta Orthop Scand 22:249–257, 1953.
18. Goldner JL, Clippinger FW: Excision of the greater multangular bone as an adjunct to mobilization of the thumb. J Bone Joint Surg 41A:609–625, 1959.
19. Haines RW: The mechanism of rotation at the first carpometacarpal joint. J Anat 78:44–46, 1944.
20. Harvey FJ, Bye WD: Bennett's fracture. Hand 8:48–53, 1976.
21. Imaeda T, Niebur G, Cooney W, et al: Kinematics of the normal trapeziometacarpal joint. J Orthop Res 12:197–204, 1944.
22. Imaeda T, Niebur G, An K, Cooney W: Kinematics of the trapeziometacarpal joint after sectioning of ligaments. J Orthop Res 12:205–210, 1944.
23. Jensen JS: Operative treatment of chronic subluxation of the first carpometacarpal joint. Hand 7:269–271, 1975.
24. Jervis WH: A review of excision of the trapezium for osteoarthritis of the trapeziometacarpal joint after 25 years. J Bone Joint Surg 55B:56–57, 1973.
25. Johnson ED: Fracture of the base of the thumb—a new method of fixation. JAMA 126:27–28, 1944.
26. Kaplan EB: Functional and Surgical Anatomy of the Hand, ed 2. Philadelphia, JB Lippincott, 1965, pp 88, 94–98.
27. Kessler I: Silicone arthroplasty of the trapeziometacarpal joint. J Bone Joint Surg 55B:285–291, 1973.
28. Kestler OC: Recurrent dislocation of the first carpometacarpal joint repaired by a functional tenodesis. J Bone Joint Surg 28:858–861, 1946.
29. McGrath MH, Watson HK: Arthroplasty of the carpometacarpal joint of the thumb in arthritis—emphasis on bone configuration. Orthop Rev 8:127–131, 1979.
30. Murley AHG: Excision of the trapezium in osteoarthritis of the first carpometacarpal joint. J Bone Joint Surg 42B:502–507, 1960.
31. Napier JR: The form and function of the carpo-metacarpal joint of the thumb. J Anat 89:362–369, 1955.
32. O'Brien ET: Fractures of the metacarpals and phalanges. In Green DP (ed): Operative Hand Surgery. New York, Churchill Livingstone, 1982, pp 583–635.
33. Peimer CA: Long-term complications of trapeziometacarpal silicone arthroplasty. Clin Orthop 220:86–98, 1987.
34. Peimer CA, Medige J, Eckert BS, et al: Reactive synovitis after silicone arthroplasty. J Hand Surg 11A:624–638, 1986.
35. Pellegrini VD Jr, Burton RI: Surgical management of basal joint arthritis of the thumb. Part I: Long-term results of silicone implant arthroplasty. J Hand Surg 11A:309–324, May 1986.

36. Pollen AG: The conservative treatment of Bennett's fracture-subluxation of the thumb metacarpal. J Bone Joint Surg 50B:91–101, 1968.

37. Poppen NK, Niebaurer JJ: "Tie-in" trapezium prosthesis: Long-term results. J Hand Surg 3:445–450, 1977.

38. Robinson D, Aghasi M, Halperin H: Abductor pollicis longus tendon arthroplasty of trapezio-metacarpal joint: Surgical technique and results. J Hand Surg 16A:504–509, 1991.

39. Sigfusson R, Lundborg G: Abductor pollicis longus tendon arthroplasty for treatment of arthrosis in the first carpometacarpal joint. Scand J Plast Reconstr Surg Hand Surg 25:73–77, 1991.

40. Smith RJ, Atkinson RE, Jupiter JB: Silicone synovitis of the wrist. J Hand Surg 10A:47–60, 1985.

41. Stark HH, Moore JF, Ashworth CR, et al: Fusion of the first metacarpotrapezial joint for degenerative arthritis. J Bone Joint Surg 59A:22–26, 1977.

42. Strauch RJ, Behrman MJ, Rosenwasser MP: Acute dislocation of the carpometacarpal joint of the thumb: An anatomic and cadaver study. J Hand Surg 19:93–98, 1994.

43. Swanson AB: Disabling arthritis of the base of the thumb: Treatment of resection of the trapezium and flexible silicone implant arthroplasty. J Bone Joint Surg 54A:456–471, 1972.

44. Wagner CJ: Method of treatment of Bennett's fracture-dislocation. Am J Surg 80:230, 1950.

45. Weilby A: Surgical treatment of osteoarthritis of the carpometacarpal joint of the thumb: Indications for arthrodesis, excision of the trapezium, and alloplasty. Scand J Plast Reconstr Surg 5:136–141, 1971.

46. Weinman DT, Lipscomb PR: Degenerative arthritis of the trapeziometacarpal joint: Arthrodesis or excision? Mayo Clin Proc 42:279–287, 1967.

47. Wilson JN: Arthroplasty of the trapeziometacarpal joint. Plast Reconstr Surg 49:143–148, 1972.

48. Wilson J, Bossley C: Osteotomy in the treatment of osteoarthritis of the first carpometacarpal joint. J Bone Joint Surg 65B: 179–181, 1983.

CHAPTER 26

Medial Four Carpometacarpal Joints

Stephen Flack Gunther, MD

The past few decades have seen a tremendous interest in the wrist. A copious literature on ligamentous and bony injuries has been followed by a large amount of basic research on normal kinematics and biomechanics as well as the abnormal states that follow ligamentous injuries. Nevertheless, extremely little has been written about the medial four carpometacarpal (CMC) joints. The obvious reason is that clinical problems there are less common than in the wrist, and their consequences are not usually as devastating. The result of this inattention is that many surgeons are not really familiar with the CMC joints. Architectural integrity and painless stability of the CMC joints and the bones that form them are essential to good hand and wrist function, especially in power grip.

This chapter addresses the anatomy and the results of both degenerative and traumatic disorders of the CMC joints. Infections and tumors are not covered here, because they are exceedingly rare and their treatment would not be specific to this anatomic area.

FUNCTIONAL ANATOMY

Eleven joints lie between the bones of the distal carpal row and the metacarpal bases. Each is invested with a heavy capsule and many well-defined capsular ligaments (Fig. 26–1). In general, the second and third metacarpal bones are rigidly fixed to the trapezoid and capitate bones, giving the hand a stable base around which the thumb, the phalanges, and the ulnar two metacarpals rotate during hand motion. With the help of the transverse carpal ligament, this central fixed unit maintains both the longitudinal and the transverse arches of the hand.[34] The second CMC joint is capable of only 1° or 2° of motion, and the third allows no more than 3°.[19] The normal motion is so slight that arthrodesis of either of these joints has no deleterious effect at all and is good treatment for traumatic disruption or for painful arthrosis. Different sources quote different figures, but my own observations during fresh cadaver dissection indicate that the fourth CMC joint allows some 8° to 10° of flexion-extension, and the fifth allows in excess of 15°. Flexion-rotation of the ulnar metacarpals, most obvious when the hand is cupped, is important for making a tight fist as well, although I am not aware of any studies showing that arthrodesis of these CMC joints reduces grip strength or leads to any clinical problem.

The joint surfaces are perpendicular to the axes of the metacarpal shafts and have neither a volar nor a dorsal tilt. The bases of the second and third metacarpals interlock with the distal surfaces of the trapezoid and capitate (Fig. 26–1B). In addition to these matched joint surfaces and the heavy ligamentous capsules, stabilizers of the second and third metacarpals include the radial wrist flexor and extensor tendons.

RADIOGRAPHIC EXAMINATION

The standard anteroposterior (AP) and lateral radiographic views of the hand may be enough to demonstrate traumatic and arthritic abnormalities to the practiced eye of an orthopedic radiologist or an experienced hand surgeon. Subtle findings in the overlapping articular surfaces and minor loss of symmetry may escape the average orthopedic surgeon, however, particularly if the radiographs have not been taken properly. Oblique views are very helpful, but unfortunately, they have been described in different terminology by different writers.[4, 12, 26, 33, 46] I will be very specific as to how these views can be accomplished. Because careful radiographic examination is essential to the conditions addressed in each of the following sections, I would like to go through the examination step by step:

1. Take a posteroanterior (PA) view with the hand flat and the wrist in neutral, neither flexed nor extended. At least the three medial CMC joint spaces should be demonstrated without bony overlap, and they should be parallel to one another (Fig. 26–2A).

2. Rotate (supinate) the hand up from the flat PA position 30°. This is the equivalent of 60° pronation down from a lateral position (thus the difficulties with terminology). X-ray technicians might call this an internal rotation view. This position shows the second and actually the first CMC joints nicely (Fig. 26–2B).

3. Rotate the hand further to a true lateral position with the wrist in neutral (Fig. 26–3C). Look for any angulation or asymmetry in the axes of the metacarpal shafts. Be aware that this view gives a lateral view of only the third CMC joint.

4. Continue the same rotation past the neutral po-

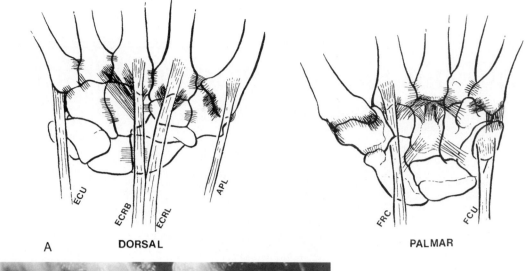

A DORSAL   PALMAR

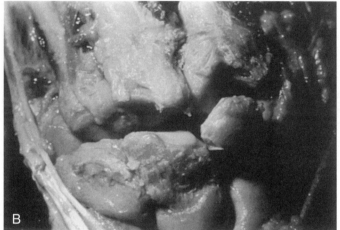

B

Figure 26–1. *A,* Sketch of the ligamentous investments of the carpometacarpal (CMC) joints, along with the tendons that insert in proximity to them. APL = Abductor pollicis longus; ECRB = extensor carpi radialis brevis; ECRL = extensor carpi radialis longus; ECU = extensor carpi ulnaris; FCU = flexor carpi ulnaris; FRC = flexor carpi radialis. *B,* Dorsal view of the radial CMC joints after division of the capsules and tendons. The interlocking architecture of the bones is obvious. (*From* Gunther SF: The carpometacarpal joints. Orthop Clin North Am 15:259–277, 1984.)

sition that was used for a lateral film and into 60° of supination, and then take the final film (Fig. 26–4). This beautifully demonstrates the fourth and fifth CMC joints en face. This is Bora's "30° pronated" view (Fig. 26–4)—pronated 30° from a flat AP position—and the technician's external rotation view.

For clear terminology, I find that it is easiest to think of these four positions as simple progressive rotations into supination from the palm-down-flat position. After studying the resultant radiographs shown in Figure 26–2, the reader is advised to look ahead to other figures in this chapter in which various pathologic conditions are demonstrated through one or more of these views.

DEGENERATIVE AND INFLAMMATORY DISORDERS

Arthritis

Although rarely mentioned, rheumatoid destruction of the medial four carpometacarpal joints is more common than many realize (see Fig. 26–3). Loss of

stability and shortening of the fixed CMC unit contribute to weakness and pain. Because this disorder occurs without great deformity and usually as a part of an overall wrist destruction that tends to capture the physician's attention, surgical stabilization is rarely performed. Nevertheless, it is worth consideration at the time of arthroplasty in the treatment of some wrist disorders.

Osteoarthritis without antecedent injury does not seem to be a problem in the CMC joints, but gout and other crystal deposition arthritides can manifest as acute inflammation. The principal differential is infection, and the treatment takes the form of anti-inflammatory medication and immobilization.

Fracture and fracture-dislocation can lead to degenerative arthritis in the CMC joints (see Fig. 26–4). The incidence and severity are undefined in the literature, but patients do gradually develop enlargement of these joints during the years following complete dislocation, and they can retain some symptoms with either prolonged or very heavy use.[20] I have rarely had to perform arthrodesis of the second and third metacarpals to their adjacent carpal bones for posttraumatic arthritis. I have even had to do so in a

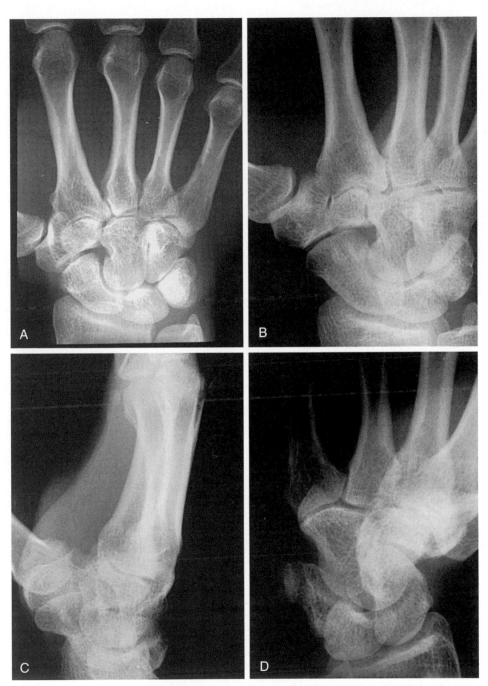

Figure 26–2. The four basic radiographic views that demonstrate the carpometacarpal joints. See text for full details. *A,* Posteroanterior (PA) view. *B,* Oblique 30° supinated from the PA view. *C,* Lateral (neutral) view. *D,* Oblique 60° supinated from the lateral view.

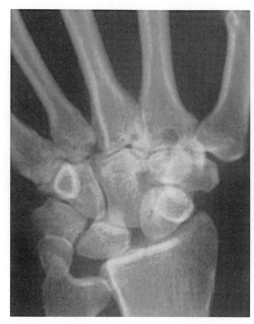

Figure 26–3. A 45-year-old patient with rheumatoid arthritis has the incidental finding of carpometacarpal arthritis in her wrist, which was being examined for radiocarpal pain.

golfer whose wrist had never undergone an acute traumatic event.

The architecture of the fifth CMC joint allows more motion than the other joints, while providing less intrinsic stability. The joint is gently slanted from the radial to the ulnar aspect. The extensor carpi ulnaris muscle is a deforming force, because it tends to pull the metacarpal base proximally and in an ulnar direction. Fracture-subluxation of the fifth metacarpal base is the ulnar counterpart of Bennett's fracture of the thumb (Fig. 26–5), and traumatic arthritis will surely follow if the need for anatomic reduction and pinning is overlooked[4, 42, 43, 47, 49] (Fig. 26–6). Nonoperative treatment of such arthritis with splinting and corticosteroid injection may control the symptoms, but the definitive treatment is either interposition arthroplasty or arthrodesis. Different Silastic prostheses have been modified for interposition in this joint, and good results have been reported.[17] There are no long-term studies, however. I believe that we know enough about the degradation of silicone prostheses over time that we can predict eventual trouble with them, and I advise against their use at this time. Interposition of rolled-up tendon or other biologic spacer is another option. As mentioned previously, there is little in the literature about arthrodesis of the mobile fourth and fifth CMC joints, but anecdotal experience indicates that patients maintain good strength and suffer no disability from loss of motion in those joints.[27, 28, 37, 42]

In the absence of data from comparative studies in the literature, treatment should be individualized to the patient, with the expectation that arthrodesis is a permanent remedy that will stand up to heavy use over time.

Carpal Boss

The term *carpal boss* describes a bony prominence of unknown etiology on the dorsal aspect of either the second or the third CMC joint (Fig. 26–7A). These prominences do not usually occur before early adulthood. Most are noticed as incidental findings on a hand being examined for some other reason,[2] because only a small percentage are painful. The bump is a buildup of new bone on both the metacarpal and the carpal bones (Fig. 26–7B).

Radiographically, the carpal boss suggests osteophyte formation as in osteoarthritis, and its gross appearance is similar to that of degenerative arthritis of these joints. However, there is no joint space narrowing and no subchondral bony sclerosis as one would expect in arthritis. It has been suggested that the bossing is sometimes an anomaly of an accessory ossification center in the styloid process of the third metacarpal base,[3, 10] and that it is the result of a periostitis initiated by some unknown form of microtrauma.[6, 30]

When patients do come for treatment of a carpal boss, it is generally because of the unsightly swelling. In about a third of cases that are severe enough to warrant surgery, the appearance is made worse by the presence of a sessile ganglion in addition to the bony prominence.[10] If the appearance is unsightly enough,

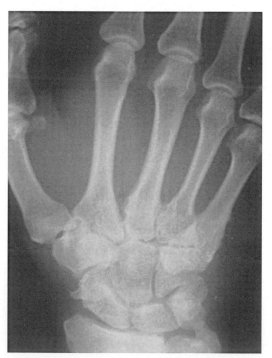

Figure 26–4. This radiograph was taken 7.5 years after this 37-year-old police officer dislocated all four carpometacarpal joints. He was treated initially by open reduction and pinning. He is back on full-time duty and has mild symptoms only in bad weather or after very heavy use of the hand. The joints are mildly prominent dorsally, both on observation and on palpation. They are not tender. (*From* Gunther SF, Bruno PD: Divergent dislocation of the carpometacarpal joints: A case report. J Hand Surg 10A:197–201, 1985.)

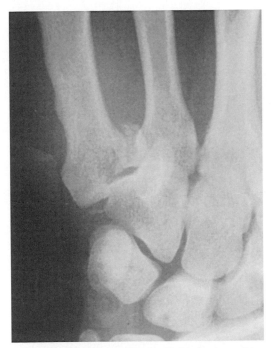

Figure 26–5. A 25-year-old man sustained this fracture-subluxation by punching another man's forehead.

or if the boss is chronically painful, surgery is the only effective treatment. As already mentioned, both the metacarpal base and the carpal bone contribute to the rounded prominence, so the protuberant portions of each bone must be removed by generous wedge resection that enters the joint well into its cartilaginous surface.

I prefer a transverse incision in the skin lines, as follows: Expose the boss, and identify the joint by inserting a small needle into it. Tease the insertion of the radial wrist extensor off the metacarpal base with a small scalpel blade, and then osteotomize matching wedges from both the metacarpal and the carpal bones at an angle of about 45° in order to truly enter the joint.

Early reports indicated a high rate of recurrence after surgical excision,[8] but a later study showed no recurrence in 16 patients treated as described here.[10] It has been my experience that some carpal bosses recur partially, even after a generous excision. As in other problems of the CMC joints, arthrodesis (see Fig. 26–11) is a good solution for persistent problems if simpler surgery fails.

Ganglions

Prominent dorsal ganglions sometimes arise over the second or third CMC joint, usually the second. They are clearly different from the far more common dorsal wrist ganglions that arise from the scapholunate ligament. They are commonly multilobulated, and they emerge from both sides of the adjacent radial wrist

extensor tendon. These ganglions are firmly anchored to the joint beneath, and they can become large enough to interfere with normal tracking of the index digital extensor tendons (Fig. 26–8). Sometimes they coexist with a carpal boss, as mentioned previously, and sometimes they occur alone. In either case, because they originate in the joint, they are very likely to recur unless a wedge resection of the dorsal portion of the CMC joint is carried out. Careful surgical technique is essential. You must remove an adequate amount of bone while preserving the important lateral ligaments. A case in point is that of a young woman with instability of the second CMC joint following ganglion excision (Fig. 26–9). Whether the instability existed prior to surgery is unknown, but the patient required arthrodesis for pain relief 2 years after the initial ganglionectomy.

TRAUMATIC DISORDERS

Sprains

Both acute and chronic sprains can be recognized by the sage physician. They seem to occur mostly in the second and third CMC joints, probably because these joints are loaded during almost any hand function. Acute sprains are evidenced by pain, diffuse swelling, and ecchymosis on both the dorsal and the palmar aspects of the hand (Fig. 26–10). There is local

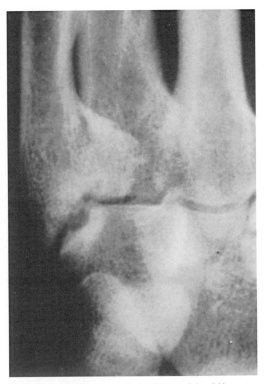

Figure 26–6. Advanced degenerative arthritis of the fifth carpometacarpal joint only 2 years after fracture-subluxation. (*From* Gunther SF: The carpometacarpal joints. Orthop Clin North Am 15:259–277, 1984.)

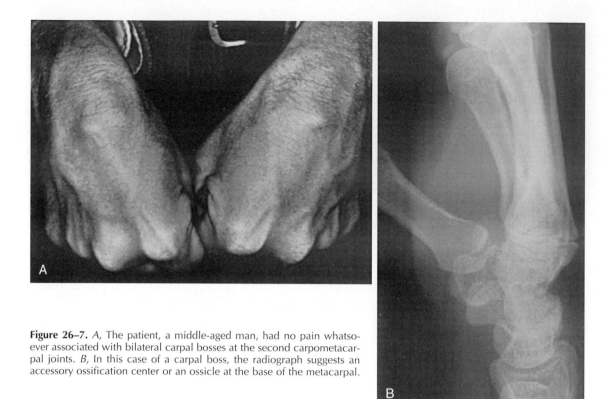

Figure 26–7. *A,* The patient, a middle-aged man, had no pain whatsoever associated with bilateral carpal bosses at the second carpometacarpal joints. *B,* In this case of a carpal boss, the radiograph suggests an accessory ossification center or an ossicle at the base of the metacarpal.

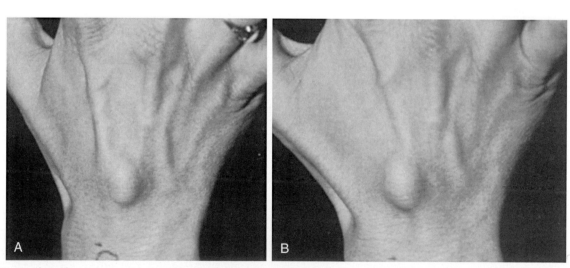

Figure 26–8. *A* and *B,* The patient, a 24-year-old woman, complained that the index extensor tendons snapped back and forth over the large ganglion shown here when she moved the finger in certain ways. The ganglion overlaid a small carpal boss. (*From* Gunther SF: The carpometacarpal joints. Orthop Clin North Am 15:259–277, 1984.)

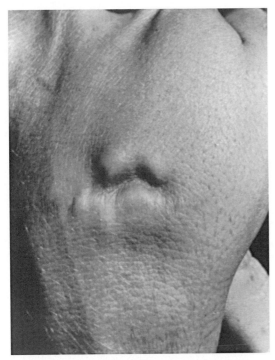

Figure 26–9. Instability of the second carpometacarpal joint was obvious when the examiner forced the metacarpal into flexion. This is the hand of an 18-year-old girl who had undergone ganglionectomy 2 years previously. At surgery, there were no dorsal ligaments and no evidence of the extensor carpi radialis longus tendon. Arthrodesis cured the pain that she had experienced with writing and any other prolonged activity.

tenderness on palpation, and pain when the examiner stresses the injured joints. The mechanisms of injury are similar to those that cause fracture-dislocations. After a thorough radiologic examination to rule out subluxation of the metacarpal bases, the acute sprain is treated with plaster immobilization until the pain subsides—generally for about 6 weeks.

Acute overuse in manual work or sports can cause

CMC joint pain severe enough to require treatment. I have seen this disorder at both the second and the fourth CMC joints in professional and low-handicap amateur golfers who were hitting practice balls for many hours a day. The same can happen in players of racquet sports. Immobilization and rest are the treatments for the acute phase of this disorder.

Chronic sprains of the second and third CMC joints are far more common than has been recognized. The diagnosis being used here applies to those patients with ongoing pain following significant injury as well as those more common patients with persistent or recurrent pain from overuse syndromes or even from seemingly trivial injuries. Chronic sprain as defined here is clearly different from carpal boss and arthritis. Patients have nagging pain deep in the hand during or after prolonged writing or during more strenous activities. The pain may be poorly localized by the patient, but the diagnosis is not difficult if the examiner looks specifically for this problem.

Diagnostic and therapeutic injection of local anesthetic and a corticosteroid into the joint or joints with chronic sprain is helpful in evaluation and treatment. It is performed as follows: Introduce a 25-gauge needle from straight dorsal. Use only local anesthetic at first, and walk the needle tip along the joint until it enters the joint space. Then remove the anesthetic syringe from the needle and replace it with a tuberculin syringe containing approximately 0.3 mL of a steroid compound.

I have cured chronic sprain by injection even when I was never confident that the needle had entered the joint completely.

Joseph and associates[27] reported a series of 28 chronic sprains that were treated successfully by arthrodesis. During the time in which these cases were collected, the authors recognized 20 other chronic sprains that were not severe enough to warrant surgery. Interestingly, they saw only 10 acute sprains. Arthrodesis is a reliable and apparently in-

Figure 26–10. Radiographs of the left hand of the patient were normal, but he had all the signs and symptoms of acute sprain of the second and third carpometacarpal joints in the involved left hand. The sprain did well with plaster immobilization.

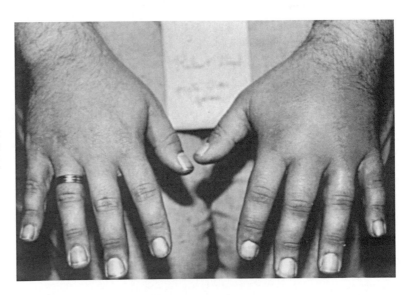

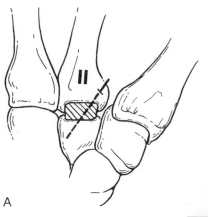

A   B

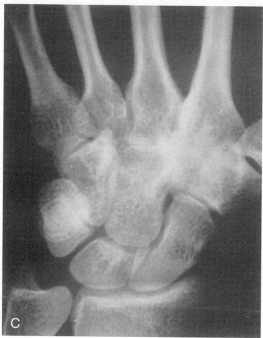

Figure 26–11. *A,* Arthrodesis of the second and third carpometacarpal joints. A tricortical iliac graft can be placed transversely in a slot prepared in the metacarpal and carpal bones. The subchondral bone plates are removed in this area. The normal distance between the metacarpal and carpal bones should be maintained. *B,* The graft can be replaced longitudinally. It should be supplemented with cancellous packing on either side. *C,* The 22-year-old policewoman whose radiograph is shown here presented with pain and an unsightly ganglion that had recurred after two separate surgical excisions. Preoperative grip strength in the involved hand was 57 percent that of the other, nondominant hand. She returned to full-time duty 6 months after surgery, and by 1 year, her grip strength had improved to 127 percent of that in the other hand. (*From* Gunther SF: The carpometacarpal joints. Orthop Clin North Am 15:259–277, 1984.)

nocuous remedy for chronic sprain. It can be accomplished through a dorsal approach with an inlay bone graft (Fig. 26–11). I have used tricortical iliac grafts oriented transversely, much like anterior interbody fusion in the cervical spine. Joseph and associates[27] used a longitudinally oriented graft. In either method, the graft is fashioned and inserted in such a way as to maintain the normal length of the ray. Kirschner wires are inserted across the fusion for fixation and left in place for about 12 weeks, which is long enough for the graft to incorporate. Care should be taken not to extend the wires into the scaphoid proximally or to disturb the wrist extensor tendon insertions. My results with arthrodesis have been excellent.

Fractures and Fracture-Dislocations

Although uncommon, fractures and fracture-dislocations do constitute the majority of clinical problems at the four medial CMC joints. Great and sudden force is required to disrupt the strong joint capsules. Multiple CMC dislocations are usually the result of a motorcycle accident during which the victim is gripping the handlebars at the moment of impact. Injuries limited to the ulnar side are more often from fist fights and falls. Early papers on the subject concentrated on simultaneous, dorsal dislocation of all four metacarpals,[44, 51, 52] but it now appears that the most common variant is dorsal or volar dislocation of the fifth metacarpal alone[4, 7, 9, 18, 19, 42] (Fig. 26–12). Next in frequency are the fourth and fifth together (Fig. 26–13), but just about every conceivable pattern of dorsal and volar dislocations of any or all metacarpals has been described.* For example, the fifth metacarpal may dislocate dorsally,[9, 22, 24, 25] volar-radially,[28, 35, 39] or volar-ulnarly.[40, 41, 47] There are even rotary injuries in which some metacarpals translate dorsally, and others volarly.[20, 21] Pure dislocation without fracture is rare. The heavy capsular ligaments usually avulse

---

*References 14, 19, 21–23, 26, 32, 38, 44, 50–52, 54–56.

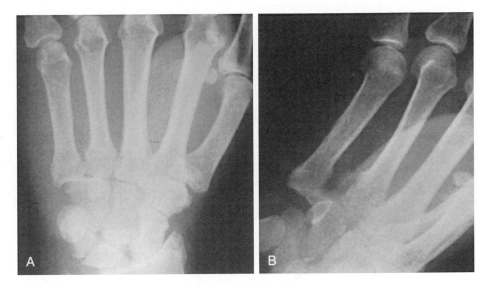

Figure 26–12. *A* and *B,* Dislocation of the fifth metacarpal. An 80-year-old man sustained this volar-ulnar dislocation of the fifth metacarpal base in a fall. Treatment was by open reduction and pinning for 8 weeks. The oblique view *(B)* demonstrates the severity and nature of the dislocation far better than the anteroposterior view *(A).* (*From* Gunther SF: The carpometacarpal joints. Orthop Clin North Am 15:259–277, 1984.)

pieces of bone from the carpus as the metacarpals dislocate, and sometimes the metacarpal bases themselves are fractured.

The importance of a complete radiographic workup cannot be overstated. Anteroposterior projection alone may be misleading, in that the dislocation may be poorly shown, whereas a good oblique or lateral film makes it very obvious (see Fig. 26–13). It is not uncommon for traumatic subluxations to be missed.

In my opinion, the best treatment for almost all major fracture-dislocations is open reduction and internal fixation with Kirshner wires (Fig. 26–14). Closed reduction of the metacarpals is usually accomplished easily, but in most cases it is immediately obvious that the reduction is unstable. Closed reduction is unlikely to bring avulsed pieces of the carpal bones back into position. Even when reduction can be maintained temporarily by careful cast molding, it is difficult to sustain for the full recovery period. Surgical visualization allows anatomic reduction of both the metacarpals and the avulsed carpal fragments. Because these fragments are attached to the capsular ligaments, bone healing should result in nearly normal ligament function. Some surgeons prefer closed reduction and percutaneous pinning,[18, 38, 40, 49] but this method runs the risk of less precise reduction and offers little advantage to the patient, because the hand and arm must be anesthetized anyway. I currently use this for dislocations and even fracture-dislocations of the fifth metacarpal, however.

Open reduction with Kirschner wire fixation is performed as follows. Approach the joint dorsally through a transverse skin incision. Mobilize and retract the extensor tendons to give ready access to the metacarpal bases. It is commonly not necessary to place a Kirschner wire in each dislocated metacarpal, because a pin across one joint stabilizes the adjacent joint if the interosseous ligaments at the metacarpal bases are intact (Fig. 26–14*C*). The appropriate number of pins is easily determined during surgery. Re-

attach major carpal fragments by pinning or by fixation with tiny screws. Remember to position the pins so as to avoid the extensor tendons, and cut them off well below the skin. I leave the pins in place for 12 weeks, although I usually discontinue plaster immobilization after 6 weeks.

Several years' follow-up has demonstrated that open reduction with Kirschner wire fixation results in excellent hand function. Grip strength returns to normal, and the only residual symptoms of the fracture-dislocation are usually mild aching during changes of weather or during extremely heavy work.

CMC subluxation and even frank dislocation may be overlooked in the patient with multiple injuries. Appropriate treatment of old injuries is arthrodesis, but of course, this is done only if there is enough pain to warrant an operation. An occasional patient has done sufficiently well with no treatment at all (Fig. 26–15).

Fractures of either the metacarpal bases or the carpal bones may predominate over dislocation as the most obvious injuries. Severely comminuted fractures may do best with simple splinting, but major displacement or angulations should be corrected with pins. There have been many case reports and short series of exceedingly rare fractures and dislocations in the distal carpal row[15, 29, 36, 48, 53] (Fig. 26–16). It is important to know that these fractures may be difficult to define on plain radiographs and that tomograms may be necessary to fully outline the injuries. For example, the hamate bone is rarely injured, but it can be dislocated either volarly or dorsally, and it can be fractured in a number of ways[1, 5, 11, 13, 16, 45] (Fig. 26–17). Aside from small dorsal avulsion fractures coincident with metacarpal dislocations, the hamate may be split in either the coronal or the sagittal plane, or the hamate hook may be avulsed. In particular, the coronal split is most difficult to recognize and very important to reduce and pin. Sometimes, these injuries are more obvious when radiographs are taken

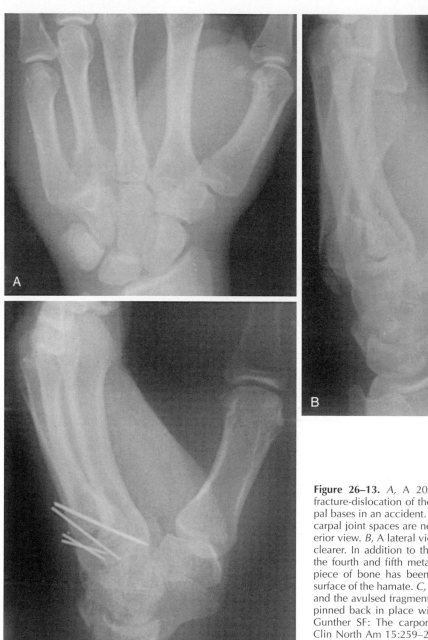

Figure 26–13. *A,* A 20-year-old man suffered a fracture-dislocation of the fourth and fifth metacarpal bases in an accident. The normal hamate-metacarpal joint spaces are not seen on this anteroposterior view. *B,* A lateral view makes the injury much clearer. In addition to the abnormal angulation of the fourth and fifth metacarpals, note that a large piece of bone has been avulsed from the dorsal surface of the hamate. *C,* Both the metacarpal bases and the avulsed fragment of the hamate have been pinned back in place with Kirschner wires. (*From* Gunther SF: The carpometacarpal joints. Orthop Clin North Am 15:259–277, 1984.)

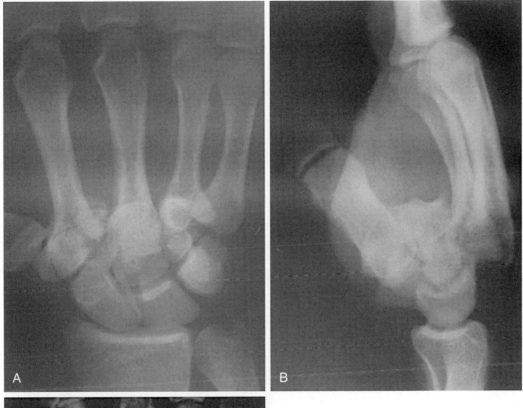

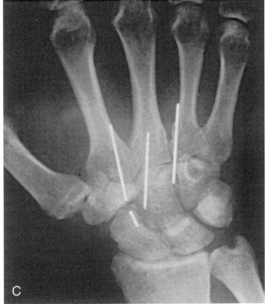

Figure 26–14. A 38-year-old man sustained dorsal dislocation of all four metacarpal bases in a motorcycle accident. *A,* Anteroposterior view. *B,* Lateral view. *C,* Open reduction was carried out, and the joints were pinned for 12 weeks. It was not necessary to pin the fifth metacarpal, because it was stable once the fourth metacarpal was pinned. One Kirschner wire broke where it crossed the scaphotrapezial joint. The result of the reduction was excellent. The patient was followed off and on for other reasons until he was killed in another motor vehicle accident 5 years later. (*From* Gunther SF: The carpometacarpal joints. Orthop Clin North Am 15:259–277, 1984.)

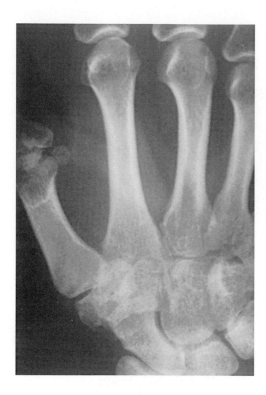

Figure 26–15. The patient, a 39-year-old multiple trauma victim from a motor vehicle accident, was too sick to complain at presentation of hand pain. When this dorsal dislocation of the trapezoid and trapezium was discovered 6 weeks later, it was irreducible by closed means. The patient did not seem to have pain sufficient to warrant open reduction. Nine months after injury, there was no residual pain whatsoever, but there was an obvious dorsal bump, and grip strength was reduced to 63 percent of that on the uninjured side.

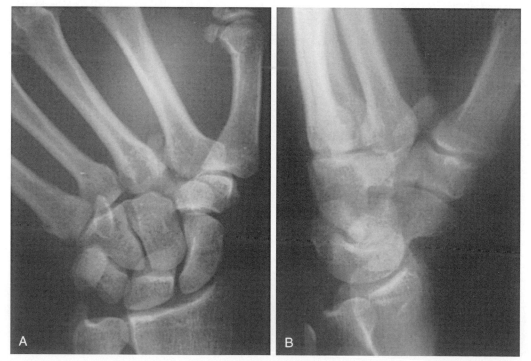

Figure 26–16. A 35-year-old bus driver sustained volar-radial subluxation of the second metacarpal base with anterior extrusion of a large portion of the articular surface when his steering wheel jolted in an accident and impacted forcibly against his hand. Because the articular surface was severely disrupted, primary arthrodesis was carried out with distal radius bone graft. The patient returned to bus driving 4 months after arthrodesis, and he continues to have an excellent result 39 months later. *A,* Anteroposterior view. *B,* Oblique view.

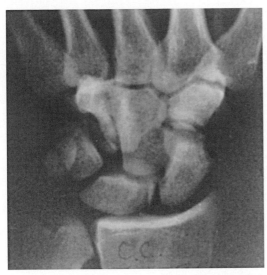

Figure 26–17. The hamate was fractured in the coronal plane and dislocated volarly when the patient, a 24-year-old lacrosse player, was struck with a stick. He returned to lacrosse 9 months after undergoing open reduction and pinning of both the hamate and the scapholunate injuries. He is asymptomatic at 16 years.

with traction or after closed reduction than they are on the initial films.

CONCLUSION

Architectural integrity and stability of the carpometacarpal joints are essential to normal hand and wrist function. With only a few exceptions, it can be said that fractures and dislocations should be accurately reduced and pinned, whereas arthritic conditions should be treated with arthrodesis. Fascial or Silastic arthroplasties seem to be effective at the fifth CMC joint, but long-term follow-up is not available yet. Surgical excision of a carpal boss or a symptomatic ganglion should include removal of some bone from both the metacarpal bone and the subjacent carpal bone. Carpometacarpal arthrodesis is a good salvage procedure after failure of treatment in any of these conditions.

References

1. Andress MR, Peckar VG: Fracture of the hook of the hamate. Br J Radiol 43:141–143, 1970.
2. Artz TD, Posch JL: The carpometacarpal boss. J Bone Joint Surg 55A:747–752, 1973.
3. Bassoe E, Bassoe H: The styloid bone and *carpe bossu* disease. AJR Am J Roentgenol 74:886–888, 1955.
4. Bora FW, Didizian NH: The treatment of injuries to the carpometacarpal joint of the little finger. J Bone Joint Surg 56A:1459–1463, 1974.
5. Bowen TL: Injuries of the hamate bone. Hand 5:235–238, 1973.
6. Boyes JH (ed): Bunnell's Surgery of the Hand. Philadelphia, JB Lippincott Co, 1964, pp 292–293.
7. Cain JE, Shepler TR, Wilson MR: Hamatometacarpal fracture-dislocation: Classification and treatment. J Hand Surg 12A(part 1):762–767, 1987.
8. Carter RM: Carpal boss: A commonly overlooked deformity of the carpus. J Bone Joint Surg 23:935–940, 1941.
9. Clement BL: Fracture-dislocation of the base of the fifth metacarpal. J Bone Joint Surg 27:498–499, 1945.
10. Cuomo CB, Watson HK: The carpal boss: Surgical treatment and etiological considerations. Plast Reconstr Surg 63:88–93, 1979.
11. Duke R: Dislocation of the hamate bone: Report of a case. J Bone Joint Surg 45B:744, 1963.
12. Fisher MR, Rogers LF, Hendrix RW: Systematic approach to identifying fourth and fifth carpometacarpal joint dislocations. AJR Am J Roentgenol 140:319–324, 1983.
13. Gainor BJ: Simultaneous dislocation of the hamate and pisiform: A case report. J Hand Surg 10A:88–90, 1985.
14. Garcia-Elias M, Bishop A, Dobyns J, et al: Transcarpal carpometacarpal dislocations, excluding the thumb. J Hand Surg 15A:531–540, 1990.
15. Garcia-Elias M, Dobyns J: Traumatic axial dislocations of the carpus. J Hand Surg 14A:446–457, 1989.
16. Geist DC: Dislocation of the hamate bone. J Bone Joint Surg 21:215–217, 1939.
17. Green WL, Kilgore ES Jr: Treatment of fifth digit carpometacarpal arthritis with Silastic prosthesis. J Hand Surg 6:510–514, 1981.
18. Greene TL, Strickland JW: Carpometacarpal dislocations. In Strickland JW, Steichen JB (eds): Difficult Problems in Hand Surgery. St Louis, CV Mosby Co, 1982, pp 189–195.
19. Gunther SF: The carpometacarpal joints. Orthop Clin North Am 15:259–277, 1984.
20. Gunther SF, Bruno PD: Divergent dislocation of the carpometacarpal joints: A case report. J Hand Surg 10A:197–201, 1985.
21. Hartwig RH, Louis DS: Multiple carpometacarpal dislocations: A review of four cases. J Bone Joint Surg 61A:906–908, 1979.
22. Harwin SF, Fox JM, Sedlin ED: Volar dislocation of the base of the second and third metacarpals. J Bone Joint Surg 57A:849–851, 1975.
23. Hazlet JW: Carpometacarpal dislocations other than the thumb: A report of 11 cases. Can J Surg 11:315–323, 1968.
24. Helal B, Kavanagh TG: Unstable dorsal fracture-dislocation of the fifth carpometacarpal joint. Injury 9:138–142, 1977.
25. Hsu JD, Cursti RN: Carpometacarpal dislocations on the ulnar side of the hand. J Bone Joint Surg 52A:927–930, 1970.
26. Jebson PJ, Engber WD, Lange RH: Dislocation and fracture-dislocation of the carpometacarpal joints. Orthopaedic Review: Aspects of Trauma, 19–28, February, 1994.
27. Joseph RB, Linscheid RL, Dobyns JH, et al: Chronic sprains of the carpometacarpal joints. J Hand Surg 6:172–180, 1981.
28. Ker HR: Dislocation of the fifth carpometacarpal joint. J Bone Joint Surg 37B:254–256, 1955.
29. Kopp JR: Isolated palmar dislocation of the trapezoid. J Hand Surg 10A:91–93, 1985.
30. Lamphier TA: Carpal bossing. Arch Surg 81:1013–1015, 1960.
31. Lawlis J, Gunther SF: Dislocation of the carpo-metacarpal joints: A long-term study. J Bone Joint Surg 73A:52–59, 1991.
32. Lewis HH: Dislocation of the second metacarpal: Report of a case. Clin Orthop 93:253–255, 1973.
33. Lewis RW: Oblique views in roentgenography of the wrist. Am J Roentgenol 50:119–121, 1943.
34. Littler JW: Hand structure and function. In Littler JW, Cramer LM, Smith JW (eds): Symposium on Reconstructive Hand Surgery. St Louis, CV Mosby Co, 1974, pp 3–12.
35. McWhorter GL: Isolated and complete dislocation of the fifth carpometacarpal joint: Open operation. Surg Clin Chicago 2:793–796, 1918.
36. Meyn MA, Roth AM: Isolated dislocation of the trapezoid bone. J Hand Surg 5:602–604, 1980.
37. Millender L: Joint injuries. In Lamb DW, Kuczynski K (eds): The Practice of Hand Surgery. St Louis, CV Mosby Co, 1981, pp 211–220.
38. Mueller J: Carpometacarpal dislocations: Report of five cases and review of the literature. J Hand Surg 11A:184–188, 1986.

39. Murless BC: Fracture-dislocation of the base of the fifth metacarpal bone. Br J Surg 31:402–404, 1943.

40. Nalebuff EA: Isolated anterior carpometacarpal dislocation of the fifth finger: Classification and case report. J Trauma 8:1119–1123, 1968.

41. North ER, Eaton RG: Volar dislocation of the fifth metacarpal. J Bone Joint Surg 62:657–659, 1980.

42. O'Brien ET: Fractures of the metacarpals and phalanges. In Green DR (ed): Operative Hand Surgery. New York, Churchill Livingstone, 1982, pp 583–635.

43. Petrie PWR, Lamb DW: Fracture-subluxation of base of fifth metacarpal. Hand 6:82–86, 1974.

44. Picchio A: Sulie lussazioni carpo-metacarpiale. Minerva Chir 9:43–50, 1954.

45. Polivy KD, Millender LH, Newburg A, et al: Fractures of the hook of the hamate—a failure of clinical diagnosis. J Hand Surg 10:101–104, 1985.

46. Rawles JG Jr: Dislocations and fracture-dislocations at the carpometacarpal joints of the fingers. Hand Clinics 4:103–112, 1988.

47. Roberts N, Holland CT: Isolate dislocation of the base of the fifth metacarpal. Br J Surg 23:567–571, 1936.

48. Russell TB: Carpal dislocations and fracture-dislocations: A review of fifty-nine cases. J Bone Joint Surg 31B:524–531, 1949.

49. Sandzen SC: Fracture of the fifth metacarpal (resembling Bennett's fracture). Hand 5:49–51, 1973.

50. Schrott E, Wessinghage D: Behandlungsverlauf einer Luxation in den Karpometakarpalgelenken IV and V unter Hamatumbeiteligung. Handchirurgie 15:25–28, 1983.

51. Shephard E, Solomon DJ: Carpometacarpal dislocation: Report of four cases. J Bone Joint Surg (Br) 42:771–777, 1960.

52. Shorbe HB: Carpometacarpal dislocations: Report of a case. J Bone Joint Surg 20:454–457, 1938.

53. Stein AH: Dorsal dislocation of the lesser multangular bone. J Bone Joint Surg 53A:377–379, 1971.

54. Waugh RL, Yancey AG: Carpometacarpal dislocations with particular reference to simultaneous dislocation of the bases of the fourth and fifth metacarpals. J Bone Joint Surg 30:397–404, 1948.

55. Weiland AJ, Lister GD, Villarreal-Rios A: Volar fracture dislocations of the second and third carpometacarpal joints associated with acute carpal tunnel syndrome. J Trauma 16:672–675, 1976.

56. Whiston RO: Carpometacarpal dislocation: A case report. Clin Orthop 6:189–195, 1955.

PART VI

Nerve, Sports, and Occupational Disorders

CHAPTER 27

Nerve Injuries Associated with Wrist Trauma and Entrapment

H. Relton McCarroll, Jr, MD

Orthopedic surgeons examine and treat many patients with wrist trauma or disease. Only a small percentage of these patients have involvement of a peripheral nerve.

The most common cause of nerve disorder at the wrist is open laceration produced by glass, a knife, or a saw. The structures disrupted are the soft tissues, and the focus of attention is on suture of the tendons and nerves. (For techniques of nerve suture, see reference 37.) This chapter focuses on peripheral nerve problems associated with closed wrist trauma.

ANATOMY

In the distal forearm, the median and ulnar nerves are surrounded by soft tissues and untethered by bone or dense ligamentous structures. Distal to the flexor digitorum superficialis muscle belly, the median nerve lies just deep to the fascia and is protected only by the palmaris longus tendon in those patients who have one. Within the carpal tunnel, the median nerve is in the most palmar layer of structures and is easily compressed by the transverse carpal ligament. The four unyielding walls of the carpal tunnel fix the volume of the tunnel and guarantee compression of the contained structures if edema or bone fragments occupy part of the available space.

The ulnar nerve enters the palm from the forearm through Guyon's canal. Although the radial, ulnar, and dorsal walls of the canal are firm and unyielding, the palmar ligament is less substantial. Compression within the ulnar canal is possible but less common than compression in the carpal tunnel. At the base of the palm, the ulnar nerve divides into two sensory branches and the deep motor branch. The sensory branches are minimally tethered by the palmar fascia and are uncommonly compressed. The deep motor branch is subject to compression over the distal carpal bones as it courses dorsally between the origins of the hypothenar muscles. In this area, the deep motor branch is tethered by unyielding structures.

The distal radius and ulna are separated from the median and ulnar nerves by several layers of soft tissue, including the pronator quadratus muscle belly. These structures provide considerable protection for the nerve when the bones are fractured. At the level of the carpal tunnel, only the wrist capsule separates the carpal bones from the tunnel. The proximity to the bony injury and the unyielding nature of the tunnel increase the incidence of nerve symptoms with injuries of the carpus. The radial nerve is subcutaneous at the level of the wrist. Although it is in close proximity to the distal radius, it is uncommonly injured except by lacerations.[14, 15]

DIAGNOSIS

Time of Onset

Nerve injuries that are associated with acute wrist trauma can occur at three different intervals during the clinical course. Immediate nerve injuries are contusions or lacerations related to the original trauma.

The second opportunity for injury is related to treatment. Postreduction nerve deficit usually occurs from a traumatic manipulation or a nerve caught between the fracture fragments. An avoidable cause of nerve compression is application of a cast that is too tight or that holds the wrist in extreme flexion. During the early postoperative period, a nerve deficit can also result from pressure secondary to swelling or hematoma.

A third period when the nerve is at risk occurs later after the original trauma has healed. At that time, nerve deficit can develop secondary to fracture callus and residual scarring. A tardy median nerve palsy is indistinguishable from an idiopathic carpal tunnel syndrome, except for the history of trauma.

When patients with Colles' fracture are carefully evaluated for signs of carpal tunnel syndrome, the incidence is as high as 12 percent at 6 months.[86] (See later discussion of carpal tunnel syndrome.)

Clinical Tests

It is important to include a brief examination of nerve function in the initial evaluation of any patient with trauma to the hand or wrist. Patients with laceration or contusion of a nerve have a deficit even if seen very soon after the injury. Most patients with compression of the nerve have intact motor function, at least clinically.[63] Nerve laceration results in loss of motor as well as sensory function. The loss of sweating that occurs after nerve division is an especially useful sign in children, in whom the other tests are impossible to perform or unreliable.

Reduction of a fracture or dislocation represents a second traumatic event for the nerve. A recheck of nerve function after the operative procedure detects those nerves with diminished sensibility because of entanglement at the fracture site.

In the presence of acute trauma with its associated pain and swelling, plus the often necessary plaster cast, diagnosis of nerve injury can be very difficult. Simple, practical tests are indicated.

One such test that requires no special equipment is to ask whether the patient can tell the *difference* between touch and scratch. The touch test is done with the pulp of the examiner's finger and the scratch test by light application of the examiner's fingernail. If the patient can tell the difference and the two activities feel normal to the patient, the nerve is probably intact.

If the patient reports an inability to tell the difference between fingernail scratch and simple touch, the fingernail test is abnormal. In most such cases, the involved nerve proves to be divided but it may be very severely compressed. If the patient has difficulty making the appropriate discrimination and the test produces paresthesias, there is a partial disruption of nerve function. The cause can be a contusion, excessive pressure, or a partial laceration.

As with all currently available tests of sensibility, this touch/scratch test is subjective; it requires the cooperation of the patient. Some patients are unable to provide useful answers to the test questions.

The number of patients categorized as having a sensory deficit depends on the tests used. Sensitive instruments such as the plastic ridge device detect diminished sensibility in the presence of swelling alone.[72] Less sensitive tests are more appropriate in the presence of acute trauma.

MEDIAN NERVE INJURIES

Fractures of the Distal Radius

Reports of large series of Colles' fractures suggest an incidence of median nerve involvement of approximately 0.2 to 12 percent.[4, 18, 86] The rate depends on what level of symptoms is defined as significant and on the duration of follow-up.

Median nerve injury occurring coincident with a Colles' fracture (laceration or contusion) is quite rare but should be considered when the fracture is compounded or with a Melone type III fracture pattern.[6, 55] However, most early median nerve problems are related to the progressive edema and hematoma that occur after injury and to reduction of the fracture. During the healing phase, exuberant fracture callus, especially in the presence of persistent bony deformity, can result in median nerve symptoms. The residual scarring and thickening that follow healing can eventually result in a carpal tunnel syndrome at a much later date (tardy median nerve palsy).[11, 81]

FRACTURE TREATMENT

Wrist Position

The relationship between median nerve symptoms and the position of immobilization used to maintain reduction of a fracture is of particular relevance to Colles' fractures. Numerous authorities have implicated the use of extreme pronation, ulnar deviation, and palmar flexion (the "Cotton-Loder position") as contributory causes of median nerve compression.[1, 60, 63] This is a major reason orthopedists now use more moderate wrist flexion in immobilizing Colles' fractures if a good reduction cannot be maintained in a neutral position.

Several experimental studies have demonstrated compression of the median nerve with the wrist flexed or extended.[1, 5] Bauman and associates[5] measured the pressure in the carpal tunnel of a patient with a comminuted Colles' fracture and found it to be elevated over the pressure in normal controls, even in neutral position. Indeed, in two of the four Colles' fractures these researchers reported with median nerve symptoms, the fracture was immobilized in neutral position using a pins-and-plaster technique.[5] Thus, the trend away from extreme positions of immobilization should decrease the incidence of early median nerve symptoms but is unlikely to eliminate the problem.

If significant nerve symptoms are present following closed reduction and plaster cast immobilization, the surgeon's first reaction should be to split all layers of the cast and ensure that the dressings are not too tight. If this maneuver does not improve the nerve symptoms, the wrist should be brought to a neutral position. It is unwise to maintain alignment at the risk of prolonged median nerve palsy.[84] Carpal tunnel release may be indicated for profound symptoms that do not respond to the preceding measures.

It is important to note that release of the transverse carpal ligament early in the course of treatment may dictate a change in treatment of the fracture. To circumvent bow-stringing of the flexor tendons from the carpal tunnel, it may be necessary to use an external fixator or "pins and plaster" even though cast immobilization would otherwise have been adequate for the fracture alone.[67]

Gelberman and colleagues[23] have recommended use of wick catheter pressure measurements to differentiate between median nerve symptoms secondary to compression and those caused by nerve contusion or laceration. In four cases of Colles' fracture complicated by median nerve symptoms, release of the transverse carpal ligament was accomplished in 36 to 96 hours after the trauma; only one of these patients had complete recovery. Gelberman[25] suggests that very early surgical release might improve the results in similar cases. I have managed several cases of acute carpal tunnel syndrome after wrist fusion in patients with a failed proximal row carpectomy. These patients did well if the transverse carpal ligament was released within 5 days of the wrist fusion. The contrast between the traumatic and iatrogenic cases suggests that in the cases associated with fracture, the median nerve injury is the result of both pressure and a direct contusion of the nerve. If such is the case, earlier surgery is not the solution to the problem of persistent paresthesias and sensory deficit (see Fig. 27–3).

Bone Fragments

Nerve symptoms can also result from displacement of the fracture fragments aided by surrounding hematoma and swelling.[54, 67] Displaced fractures of the volar lip of the radius (Melone type III fracture pattern) are especially likely to cause median nerve symptoms. These fragments are difficult or impossible to control by closed means. Open reduction is indicated.

Case Report

A 42-year-old, right-handed attorney fell forcefully on his outstretched left hand (Fig. 27–1A). He immediately felt paresthesias in the median nerve distribution. Sensation was impaired but not lost, and thenar muscle function remained intact. Radiographs of the affected wrist showed a very distal fracture of the radius with the palmar bone fragment displaced in the direction of the median nerve.

Open reduction, internal fixation, and release of the carpal tunnel were performed 4 days after the injury (Fig. 27–1B). The median nerve paresthesias resolved immediately following surgery. Although inserted through the palmar incision, the pins were left long on the dorsal surface and were removed 6 weeks after surgery through a dorsal incision. The patient's fracture healed, and he has normal median nerve function.

ASSOCIATED SUDECK'S ATROPHY

Although Sudeck's atrophy can occur after many different injuries, it is relatively common after Colles' fractures and accounts for some of the most troublesome management problems after that injury. Several authorities have commented on an apparent connection between pain, dysesthesia, prolonged disability, and a poor functional result with median nerve compression in the immediate postinjury period.[31, 50, 60, 63]

The clearest exposition of this thesis is Stein's[85] report of six patients (four with Colles' fractures) with signs of Sudeck's atrophy who demonstrated definite improvement after decompression of the median nerve at the carpal tunnel. Although this relationship is not universally accepted, it is certainly worth examining patients who have early complaints and findings suggestive of Sudeck's atrophy for signs of nerve compression at the carpal tunnel. The severe functional deficit that follows Sudeck's atrophy justifies removing the immobilization to measure the pressure in the carpal tunnel or to perform a nerve conduction study. Though median nerve decompression may not circumvent all cases of incipient Sudeck's atrophy, the procedure is worth considering.[20, 67]

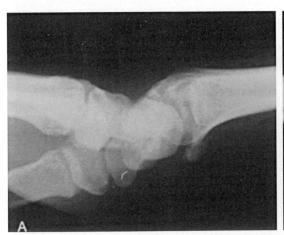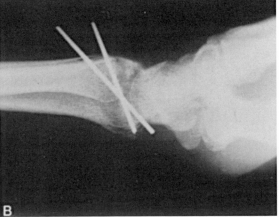

Figure 27–1. Median nerve compression by bone fragment. *A,* Displaced fracture of the volar lip of the radius. The displaced fragment and associated hematoma compressed the median nerve, producing paresthesias. *B,* Following open reduction and internal fixation of the fracture fragment and carpal tunnel release, the paresthesias resolved promptly. (Case courtesy of Dr. H. Edward Cabaud.)

Case Report

A 67-year-old woman fell on her outstretched left hand, sustaining a Colles' fracture of the wrist. A closed reduction was performed, and the fracture was immobilized in a plaster cast. The cast was split at 24 hours after reduction. At 9 days after injury, the fracture was well reduced, but the patient had stiffness of the fingers and numbness in the median nerve distribution. In spite of hand elevation and supervised exercises, the pain and numbness persisted.

One month after the fracture, the bivalved cast was removed for electromyography (EMG) and nerve conduction study. These tests documented severe prolongation of the median nerve sensory and motor latencies as well as partial denervation of the superficial thenar muscles.

Six weeks following the fracture, a carpal tunnel release was performed. After release of the transverse carpal ligament, the median nerve was observed to be slightly flattened and discolored. The skeletal structure of the carpal tunnel was normal to palpation. Although the operative wound and the Colles' fracture healed well, the patient's progress in regaining finger and wrist motion was poor. The severe pain and sensitivity did subside over 2 months following carpal tunnel release.

Three months after the carpal tunnel release, custom-made dynamic splints were fabricated, and joint-specific range-of-motion exercises were instituted (Fig. 27–2A and B). This concentrated program of hand therapy produced a gradual improvement in finger motion and in the subjective complaints of stiffness and pain. After 2½ months of therapy, the patient was able to start functional use of the involved hand (Fig. 27–2C and D).

The preceding case report emphasizes several important points. My clinical experience with Sudeck's atrophy suggests that there is a consistent natural history to this disease process. The patients generally have severe, increasing, or stable pain for a period of 3 to 4 months, followed by a longer period of decreasing pain and increasing motion. The total clinical course lasts about 1 year and then stabilizes, leaving a variable amount of permanent stiffness. The rapid improvement in the severe pain and hypersensitivity after the carpal tunnel release suggests that median nerve compression was causally related to the development of the Sudeck's atrophy. In this case, the carpal tunnel syndrome is well documented by the positive EMG and nerve conduction findings. It is important to exclude a specific, correctable cause before treatment is limited to the nonspecific treatment methods utilized for all types of reflex sympathetic dystrophy (see later).

A second important point is the difficulty in regaining joint motion once the fingers become stiff owing to Sudeck's atrophy. Hand therapists who have specialized training in hand and finger exercises and are capable of fabricating customized, dynamic splints are invaluable in rehabilitating these patients. Early release of the carpal tunnel helps avoid stiffness.

Median Nerve Injuries Associated with Carpal and Metacarpal Trauma

Acute compression of the median nerve has been very common in reported series of lunate dislocations

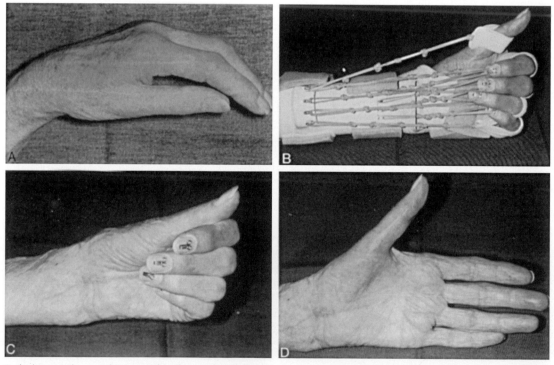

Figure 27–2. Sudeck's atrophy. *A,* Three months after a Colles' fracture, a 67-year-old homemaker had severe restriction of finger motion. The photograph demonstrates maximum active and passive finger flexion. *B,* A custom dynamic splint facilitated return of motion at all finger joint levels. After 2½ months of vigorous hand therapy, the active range of finger motion was markedly improved. *C,* Active flexion. *D,* Active extension.

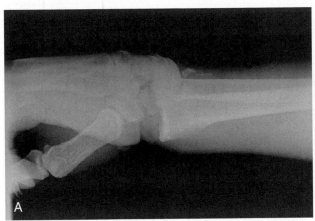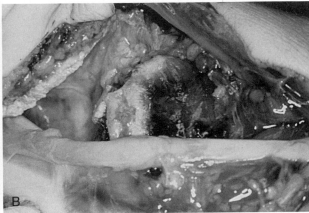

Figure 27–3. Median nerve contusion. *A,* A dorsal dislocation of the entire carpus in a 35-year-old man who fell from a roof. There was immediate numbness and tingling in the median nerve distribution. *B,* The palmar wrist capsule is avulsed from the radius, exposing its volar lip and the proximal carpus. The median nerve is drawn dorsally against the bare, prominent radius by the dorsal dislocation. The divided transverse carpal ligament and hand are to the left. There was a contusion of the median nerve but no visible disruption of fascicles or intraneural hematoma. At 10 months after injury, index finger sensibility recovered to 50 percent scratch—50 percent tingle with the fingernail test. The other digits demonstrated better recovery, and Tinel's sign was minimal.

(Fig. 27–3).[38, 73] Most of the cases have required treatment of the dislocation only, and the nerve has recovered without specific treatment. Rawlings,[73] however, did point out a relationship between the duration of nerve symptoms and persistent disability.

Carpal injuries are a common precursor of tardy median nerve palsy. Both the thickening and scarring that follow a carpal fracture or dislocation and the alteration of the volume of the carpal tunnel that results from imperfect realignment conspire over time to compress the median nerve. Even though Colles' fractures are more common than carpal injuries, Phalen[70] reported equal numbers of carpal tunnel syndromes resulting from the two types of injuries.

Carpal Tunnel Syndrome

Carpal tunnel syndrome (CTS) is the clinical symptom complex that results from compression of the median nerve at the carpal tunnel. It is characterized by numbness and tingling in the fingertips, by complaints of dropping things, and by being awakened at night from a sound sleep by pain in the hand. The hand is often described as feeling as if it were "asleep." Over time, the symptoms become more frequent and severe. In advanced carpal tunnel syndrome, the numbness becomes constant, and atrophy of the superficial thenar muscles develops. Any disorder that increases the pressure within the carpal tunnel can result in the syndrome.

ETIOLOGY

Measurement of pressure within the carpal tunnel by the wick catheter technique documents that patients with CTS have significantly higher carpal tunnel pressure than normal controls. In both patients with CTS and normal controls, the pressure is elevated at the extremes of wrist flexion and extension (Table 27–1).[22, 58, 75] Luchetti and coworkers[57, 58] found that the pressure is maximal in patients with CTS between 25 mm and 35 mm from the proximal border of the carpal tunnel.[57, 58]

Most cases of carpal tunnel syndrome are idiopathic, often occurring as normal aging processes. A number of specific causes of CTS must be excluded. The increased pressure on the median nerve can be the result of trauma, previous surgery, systemic arthritis, or medical problems such as amyloidosis and hypothyroidism. In some situations, there is an obvious mechanical cause for the increased pressure.

Table 27–1. PRESSURE IN THE CARPAL TUNNEL (mm Hg) IN PATIENTS WITH CARPAL TUNNEL SYNDROME (CTS) AND IN NORMAL CONTROLS

Study	Measurement Technique	Pressure in Normal Controls			Pressure in CTS Patients		
		Neutral	Extension	Flexion	Neutral	Extension	Flexion
Gelberman et al[22]	Wick catheter	2.5	30	31	32	110	94
Rojviroj et al[75]	Split catheter	3.48	12.68	9.32	11.87	32.76	26.60
Luchetti et al[57]	Continuous infusion	13	—	—	26	—	—

Both the displaced proximal half of a fractured capitate that rests within the carpal tunnel and the visible deposits of amyloid that complicate long-term dialysis provide easy explanations for the increased pressure. In many cases, however, the cause of the increased pressure is difficult to identify.

Experimental studies indicate that the increased pressure causes impairment of intraneural microcirculation and that the ischemia causes the symptoms. The thin afferent nerve fibers are affected most by the pressure and mediate the symptoms.[3, 59, 79]

CTS is often described as resulting from "tendinitis" of the flexor tendons at the wrist. Fuchs and colleagues[19] studied tenosynovial biopsy specimens from 177 wrists obtained at the time of surgical carpal tunnel release. Inflammation was present in only 10 percent of the specimens. Edema was present in 85 percent and did not correlate with inflammation. Vascular sclerosis was found in 98 percent and correlated with both patient age and the severity of edema. These researchers concluded that tenosynovitis is uncommon in patients undergoing surgery for idiopathic CTS.[19]

Schuind and associates[77] found that specimens from 21 patients with idiopathic CTS had histologic findings typical of "a connective tissue undergoing degeneration under repeated mechanical stresses." Similar synovial changes can be produced experimentally by decreasing the volume of the carpal tunnel.[56] These findings suggest that the synovial disease is not the cause of increased pressure but, rather, a secondary change.

REPETITIVE STRESS

In the last two decades, a growing number of cases of carpal tunnel syndrome have been diagnosed in patients engaged in repetitive activities such as typing and using grocery store scanners. The common connection among these various jobs appears to be flexion of the fingers while the wrist is palmar-flexed. This position causes the flexor tendons to displace palmarward and to force the median nerve against the transverse carpal ligament.[83]

Many such patients are involved in worker's compensation claims or some other legal process. Such cases usually entail third party payments that "pay the patient to stay sick." Although the entity of CTS is the same whether there is a third party payer or not, it is important to document the diagnosis with an electrodiagnostic test in such cases. Some patients have complaints that only sound like CTS, and some are very slow getting well after successful surgery. Studies of CTS treatment methods demonstrate that patients receiving worker's compensation take longer to go back to work than those who do not "suffer" from third party payer involvement.[2]

Discussions of arm symptoms in newspapers and magazines describe many patients for whom "carpal tunnel" or repetitive stress syndrome is a primary complaint. Their symptom complex commonly includes numbness and tingling in the fingers, but the precipitating events are not those usually reported by the patient with CTS. Such patients also have pains and tender areas in the forearm but not the typical pain that radiates up the forearm from the wrist. Their pains may also start more proximally and travel distally, a pattern very atypical of CTS. Some of these patients have a distinct, identifiable tendinitis like De Quervain's tenosynovitis, some have arthritis, and some actually have electrodiagnostically documentable CTS. Pronator syndrome and thoracic outlet syndromes are other uncommon disorders that must also be considered in these patients.

Many patients, however, have complaints of pain in the arm or hand without evidence of organic disease. They have already seen many physicians and arrive with reports indicating they have a positive Tinel's sign at the carpal tunnel. Many do indeed complain of tingling in the fingers when the examiner taps over the carpal tunnel; careful examination, however, reveals that they also complain of similar pain with tapping anywhere along the median nerve from the axilla distally, or at multiple separate spots along the nerve through the forearm. These clinical pictures do not document a positive Tinel's sign and are not indicative of CTS.

Some of these patients benefit from ergonomic changes in their workplace, including adjustable chairs, wrist supports, and adjustable monitors for their computers.[48] Those who are required to maintain a single position for long periods may benefit from variations in their work tasks, periods of relaxation, or stretching and strengthening exercises under the supervision of a therapist. Particular attention should be given to positive weight control and rehabilitation of tight, poorly conditioned cervicothoracic muscle groups. When these measures fail, I have found the insight of an experienced psychiatrist most informative. In many cases, the arm complaints originate from social problems; either anger at the employer or supervisor or difficulties at home. The pattern of using physical complaints to escape emotional conflicts has sometimes been learned from the patient's family of origin.

Hadler[32] regards this group of patients as having cases of *regional musculoskeletal symptoms* and views them as an epidemiologic problem. He points out that pain in the upper extremity in the absence of trauma is common but that choosing to be a patient because of such pain is an uncommon choice. He suggests that, rather than providing empirical treatment, "a far wiser approach, particularly in the setting of the illness of work incapacity, is to consider with patients the influences that caused them to process their predicaments so as to choose to become a patient rather than to cope on their own."[32]

DIAGNOSIS

A diagnosis of carpal tunnel syndrome is suggested by a history of numbness and tingling in the hand, especially the radial digits, that occurs with activities involving combined wrist and finger flexion or at night during sleep. The symptoms are commonly improved by dependency of the hand or shaking of the fingers. When the pain is moderately severe, it may radiate proximally up the arm toward the shoulder. A patient-administered hand symptom diagram is a useful time-saver in establishing the diagnosis.[41, 42, 52]

Clinical Tests

In early cases, physical examination is normal except for provocative tests for CTS. A Tinel's sign at the wrist flexion crease or carpal tunnel with radiation into the radial digits is suggestive of CTS. Phalen's test is a useful sign of CTS if symptoms occur promptly. With the wrist held in forced palmar flexion, the test is positive if symptoms occur in about 30 seconds. If the patient is asked to hold the forearms up and let gravity palmar-flex the wrists, as originally suggested by Phalen, the findings are significant if they begin in 60 seconds or less. Beyond these time limits, many patients with normal carpal tunnels develop symptoms.

All of the available clinical tests fall short of having ideal sensitivity and specificity.[26, 47] Koris and associates[45] found that measuring the Semmes-Weinstein monofilament threshold with the wrist in both neutral and flexed positions has a sensitivity of 82 percent and a specificity of 86 percent. Threshold tests such as the Semmes-Weinstein test are more sensitive for early CTS than are density tests such as static or moving two-point discrimination.

Electrodiagnostic Tests

The diagnosis of CTS is confirmed by electrodiagnostic testing. Most useful are two studies of the nerve conduction parameters of the median nerve, the distal sensory latency and the midpalmar latency. The distal sensory latency is measured between the tip of one finger and the forearm just proximal to the wrist flexion crease, and the result is expressed in milliseconds. The midpalmar latency is measured from the midpalm to the wrist. Because the distance involved in measuring midpalmar latency is short, the risk of error is relatively high. When CTS is quite advanced, the distal motor latency and the EMG of the thenar muscles are abnormal as well.

Electrodiagnostic testing requires skill to obtain accurate numbers and to interpret the results. The surgeon needs to ensure that the test is performed by a reliable electromyographer.

Several new tests may extend the sensitivity to detection of earlier cases of CTS. They include the Kimura inching technique and ring finger differential measurements.[13, 36, 43, 51]

CONSERVATIVE TREATMENT

Early CTS is commonly improved by simple protective measures, including application of a neutral-position wrist splint and avoiding use of the hand with the wrist in prolonged palmar flexion or extension.[48] If the patient is especially troubled by symptoms at night, use of a night splint can minimize symptoms. Daytime splinting can also be used for short periods to treat acute symptoms.

In conjunction with splints, steroid injections into the carpal canal can be effective. They are usually placed into the synovium surrounding the flexor tendons. The injections are most effective in mild, early cases.[21] Giannini and colleagues[28] have demonstrated electrophysiologic improvement as well as symptomatic improvement after steroid injection. Water-soluble steroid preparations are recommended because they are less likely to damage the median nerve if accidentally injected intraneurally.[17, 62]

Kaplan and coworkers[39] identified five factors that were useful in predicting a negative response to non-surgical management of CTS: age greater than 50 years, duration of symptoms greater than 10 months, a history of trigger finger, constant paresthesias, and a positive Phalen's test in less than 30 seconds. Medical management failed in 83 percent of patients with CTS who had two of these factors, and in 93 percent of those who had three factors.[39]

The natural history of CTS is one of gradual, slow progression. Unless a specific extrinsic or medical cause is identified and eliminated, conservative treatment is usually ineffective, and the syndrome recurs. When the patient presents with a history of increasing symptoms over several years, and the distal sensory latency of the median nerve is in excess of 8.0 milliseconds or "unobtainable," conservative treatment is generally ineffective.[21] In such cases it is reasonable to proceed directly to operative treatment.

OPERATIVE TREATMENT

When conservative treatment fails, surgical treatment of CTS is appropriate. After release of the transverse carpal ligament, most patients obtain good relief of symptoms and can return to their previous occupations. This statement assumes that the diagnosis is accurate and firmly established. In my experience, the most common cause of a failed carpal tunnel release is that the patient never had carpal tunnel syndrome.

Long-term studies of postoperative patients indicate success in 80 to 85 percent of cases. Kulick and associates[49] found three variables associated with persistent symptoms. Weakness or atrophy of the abductor pollicis brevis muscle is the most common cause, but the presence of a predisposing condition and failure to benefit from the initial steroid injection are also associated with unsuccessful surgery.[49]

Open Carpal Tunnel Release

The standard surgical technique for treatment of CTS is release of the transverse carpal ligament through an incision over the carpal tunnel. There are many

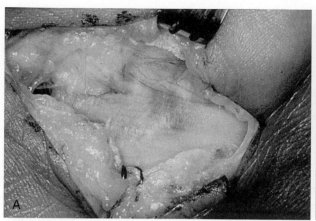
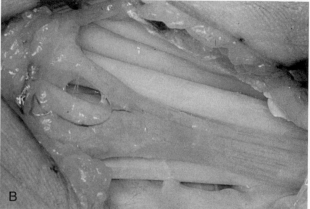

Figure 27–4. Open carpal tunnel release. *A*, A 40-year-old woman with bilateral carpal tunnel syndrome. Electrodiagnostic studies documented prolongation of the median nerve sensory and motor distal latencies. There are adherence of the surrounding synovium to the median nerve and its branches, and narrowing and injection of the nerve in the middle of the carpal tunnel. Histologic examination of the synovium showed "nonspecific fibrous thickening" but no inflammatory infiltrate. The hand is to the left, the thumb at the top. *B*, After epineurectomy, the narrowing is easily seen. The motor branch separates from the upper edge of the nerve. Two years postoperatively, a nerve conduction study was entirely normal.

variations in length and placement of the skin incision, but all approaches provide access to the ligament. The ligament is divided under direct vision, and the margins are allowed to retract.

The open approach allows inspection of the median nerve and its motor branch, neurolysis if indicated, and removal of excessive synovium if present (Fig. 27–4). The procedure has an excellent rate of success in relieving CTS and an acceptably low complication rate.

Endoscopic Carpal Tunnel Release

Use of the endoscope to facilitate carpal tunnel release is a relatively new technique. The method is designed to shorten the morbidity of carpal tunnel release surgery.[2, 10] Some patients, after an open carpal tunnel release, have persistent pain or soreness in the heel of the palm at the incision site. This complication is most likely to occur with the use of tools that place direct pressure on the operative scar. The single-incision endoscopic technique moves the incision to the wrist level and attempts to minimize the pain in the palm that occurs with direct pressure. Two-portal techniques also exist that use a small incision in the midpalm in addition to the wrist incision; one study shows that use of the second incision results in higher morbidity than the single-incision endoscopic technique.[68]

The single-incision endoscopic technique is performed as follows: Make an incision in the wrist flexion crease to gain access to the layer that is just deep to the deep fascia. After locating this layer, insert the endoscopic device into the carpal tunnel in line with the ring finger ray. Using the endoscope, visualize the undersurface of the transverse carpal ligament on a video monitor. Inspect the ligament to ensure there are no nerves or tendons trapped between the device and the ligament. Use the video picture and palpation to locate the distal edge of the transverse carpal ligament. There is a safety zone of several millimeters between the distal edge of the ligament and the superficial vascular arch.[76] When the distal edge of the transverse carpal ligament is clearly visualized and identified, elevate the blade and withdraw the device, cutting the ligament. Several passes may be needed to completely divide the ligament. Then visualize the cut ligament through the endoscope to confirm that a complete division has been accomplished.

Because it does not permit inspection of the structures in the carpal tunnel, neurolysis of the median nerve, or synovectomy of the flexor tendons, the endoscopic technique is not appropriate when any of these ancillary procedures is necessary (Fig. 27–5). Thus, the endoscopic approach is contraindicated in many patients with rheumatoid arthritis, amyloidosis, or bone fragments displaced into the carpal tunnel. Several studies show that the result of carpal tunnel release is not improved by neurolysis of the median nerve.[24, 61] Severely abnormal electrodiagnostic measurements and thenar atrophy are, therefore, not by themselves contraindications to the use of the endoscopic technique.

Initial studies show that the endoscopic approach is successful in relieving the symptoms of CTS and does allow patients to resume activities of daily living sooner and to return to work quicker than the standard open techniques.[2, 66] Reports of nerve damage associated with the endoscopic techniques indicate that training and experience are required before the devices can be used safely (Fig. 27–6).[10, 16] Considering the high cost of even very occasional inadvertent nerve injury, the overall costs of open versus endoscopic CTS surgery have not yet been fully analyzed. In the typical case, however, endoscopic tech-

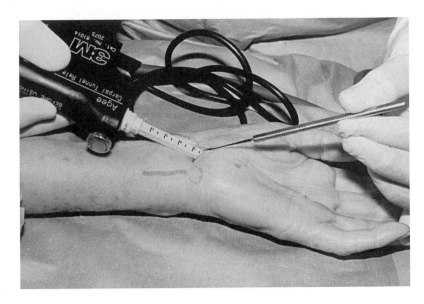

Figure 27–5. Endoscopic carpal tunnel release. The important anatomic landmarks are marked on the skin. A retrograde flap of deep fascia is elevated distally by a skin hook. The endoscopic release device is inserted into the carpal tunnel in line with the ring finger ray. Note that the device is not in line with the forearm. In this illustration, the photographic light obscures the light from the endoscope that can normally be seen through the skin.

nique does provide relief of carpal tunnel symptoms with about half the postoperative morbidity of the open method.[2] In skilled hands, the method can be effective, safe, and reliable.

ULNAR NERVE INJURIES

Injuries Associated with Wrist Trauma

Ulnar nerve injury is not commonly associated with fractures and dislocations about the wrist.[34, 46, 87, 90] Both laceration and compression of the ulnar nerve have been reported and are more common with carpal injuries than with distal forearm injuries. Considering the proximity of the nerve to the carpal bones, the rarity of compression problems must relate to the fact that the ulnar nerve is not as firmly tethered as

the median nerve in the carpal tunnel. Despite the fact that many of the cases of ulnar nerve injury initially have a complete ulnar nerve palsy, most of the cases described have recovered following treatment of the fracture only.

Isolated involvement of the deep motor branch of the ulnar nerve is associated with fracture-dislocation of the fifth metacarpal or ulnar carpal bone.[34] Exploration of the nerve shows that it is compressed against the fibrous hypothenar muscle origins by the displaced metacarpal.[29, 65] The nerve may recover equally well after reduction of the fracture alone.

Ulnar nerve palsy, especially involving the deep motor branch, has been described after numerous vocational and avocational activities. My own experience includes cases related to crutch-walking, kayaking, pressing large ledgers on a copy machine, and playing handball. In many instances, the symptoms

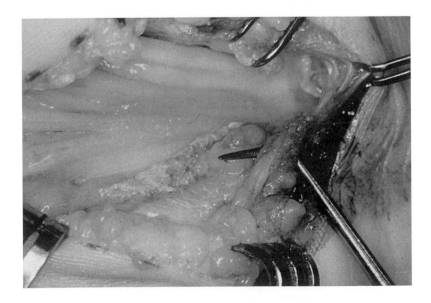

Figure 27–6. Anomalous nerve branch. The metal probe is under an anomalous branch of the median nerve that crosses the carpal tunnel structures from radial to ulnar at the wrist flexion crease. The branch separated from the radial margin of the median nerve 2 inches proximal to the carpal tunnel and entered the subcutaneous tissues over the hypothenar eminence at the proximal edge of the transverse carpal ligament. An anomalous branch like this one would be more at risk of division with endoscopic carpal tunnel release than the more common anomalies on the radial side of the tunnel. The ulnar edge of the divided transverse carpal ligament is at the point of the probe; the fingers are to the left; and the thumb is at the top.

are acute and the duration of the activity is limited. Affected patients usually do quite well and do not require surgery, only elimination of the external pressure. One patient who played handball had symptoms for a year and a half and continued to play the game regularly. At that advanced stage of repeated injury, neither neurolysis nor changing sports was helpful. At the time of surgery, this patient's ulnar nerve was noted to be severely scarred and abnormal over a 2-cm segment.

Compression by Ganglia

Although the ganglion cyst must be one of humankind's most common afflictions, it is an unusual cause of nerve compression. Several authorities have reported series in which ganglia compress the deep (motor) branch of the ulnar nerve as it courses from Guyon's canal to the level of the deep arch.[9, 78, 80] The sensory branches are usually not compressed, resulting in a pure motor lesion. Unlike most ganglia, these are too deep to palpate. Ultrasonography or magnetic resonance (MR) imaging may prove useful in identifying the mass preoperatively.[40] Because this is a curable lesion, patients with an unexplained deep motor branch paralysis should undergo exploration of the base of the palm and Guyon's canal. Successful removal of these ganglia requires reflection of part of the origin of the hypothenar muscles for adequate exposure.

Case Report

A 59-year-old contractor and carpenter sought medical attention because of symptoms in his left hand. He had noted muscle wasting in the left hand over 2 to 3 years with slow progression of the atrophy. He denied any alteration of sensibil-

ity. He finally sought medical attention because the atrophy had progressed to the point that, with firm pinch, the thumb was unstable and the proximal joint hyperextended. He gave a history of a number of minor injuries, but none that seemed likely to have produced a progressive problem. The patient did not admit to performing any repetitive activities that seemed likely to compress the motor branch of the ulnar nerve.

Examination was normal except for the muscles innervated by the deep motor branch of the ulnar nerve. The hypothenar muscles functioned normally, but there was complete paralysis of the adductor pollicis and deep head of the short flexor of the thumb. The patient had a markedly positive Froment's sign, and with firm pinch, the metacarpophalangeal (MP) joint of the thumb collapsed (Jeanne's sign), causing pain. He was unable to cross the index and long fingers. Key pinch strength was about a third that in the normal right hand.

An EMG and nerve conduction study showed a severe deficit in the deep motor branch of the ulnar nerve, with the other findings being normal. Exploration of the canal of Guyon and the base of the palm demonstrated a large ganglion originating from the distal ulnar carpus and compressing the deep motor branch between the heads of the hypothenar muscles (Fig. 27–7A). A large neuroma in continuity was visible proximal to the fascial band compressing the nerve (Fig. 27–7B). The ganglion was excised, and the nerve freed.

Evaluation 7 years after the operation documented return of excellent, stable pinch with a normal posture of the thumb. The adductor pollicis muscle had regenerated to good or normal strength, and the thumb MP joint no longer collapsed with firm pinch. The patient had regained good finger MP flexion power and independent abduction-adduction of the digits. The first dorsal interosseous muscle was slightly small but graded as good in power. The patient reported no problems with the hand.

Ulnar Artery Thrombosis

Trauma to the base of the palm, as when the hand is used as a mallet, can result in thrombosis of the ulnar artery as it passes over the carpal bones in the canal

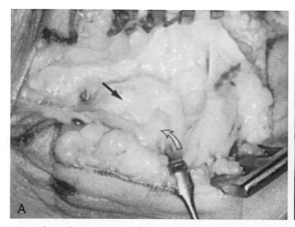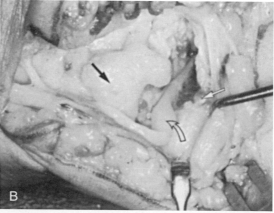

Figure 27–7. Motor branch compression by a ganglion. *A,* Ganglion from the triquetrohamate articulation protrudes through the hypothenar muscle origin. The deep motor branch of the ulnar nerve courses around the mass and is compressed as it penetrates the base of the muscle. *Black arrow* = ganglion; *white arrow* = neuroma. *B,* After release of the radial origin of the hypothenar muscles, a neuroma-in-continuity is visible proximal to the tendinous origin. *Black arrow* = ganglion; *open arrow* = neuroma; *white arrow* = tendinous muscle origin. (From McCarroll HR Jr: Nerve injuries associated with wrist trauma. Orthop Clin North Am 15:279–287, 1984.)

of Guyon. The resulting symptoms are often a combination of those produced by diminished blood supply and by compression of the adjacent ulnar nerve. The standard treatment for this condition is ligation and resection of the thrombosed segment of the artery. This procedure results in a temporary sympathectomy of the ulnar portion of the hand, reduces the vasospastic component of the problem, and decompresses the ulnar nerve. Reconstruction of the artery using a vein graft is appropriate when backflow from the radial side of the arch is insufficient. Otherwise, such reconstruction has not been shown to improve the result.

RADIAL SENSORY NERVE INJURIES

Most radial sensory nerve problems are related to open injuries, including a number that are iatrogenic.[55] The radial sensory nerve is at great risk when pins are inserted into the middle third of the radius during application of an external fixator. Percutaneous pin insertion is especially risky in this area. The branches of the nerve are also at risk of compression by the edge of a cast that is too tight.[86]

Several reports implicate either a tight wristwatch strap or the application of handcuffs as the cause of a transient radial neuropathy.[8, 74] Law enforcement officers are not the only persons who use handcuffs; we have seen several cases of nerve injury related to the friendly application of handcuffs by sexual partners. The patients complain of numbness and tingling in the distribution of the radial sensory nerve. All of our cases have resolved completely in about 3 months without specific treatment other than elimination of the external compression.

REFLEX SYMPATHETIC DYSTROPHY

Reflex sympathetic dystrophy (RSD) is an exaggerated, disordered response to trauma. The clinical picture includes four constant features: pain, vasomotor disturbances, diminished function, and trophic changes.[7, 12] Several labels are now encompassed by the term reflex sympathetic dystrophy, including causalgia, Sudeck's atrophy, traumatic dystrophy, post-traumatic pain syndrome, and shoulder-hand syndrome.[50]

The four cardinal features of RSD may vary in severity, but all must be present to establish the diagnosis. The pain associated with RSD is out of proportion to the traumatic event and more persistent than expected. It is commonly described as burning in character. The diminished function is in part due to increased pain with motion and is also out of proportion to the severity of the trauma.

The initial vasomotor changes include warm, flushed, and congested skin; later in the course, however, the skin becomes cool, pallid, and shiny. Edema is the earliest trophic change, with the late course characterized by soft tissue atrophy and osteopenia.

The diagnosis of RSD is based on the clinical picture, but several tests are useful in confirming the diagnosis. Radiographs suggest osteopenia in most cases, and in severe cases, a wormwood appearance is typical. Three-phase bone scans are positive in most cases. Isolated cold stress testing provides a quantitative assessment.[44] A good response to stellate ganglion block is a useful diagnostic test.[50] Regardless of the test results, the patient must have evidence of all four cardinal findings before being diagnosed as having RSD. The current trend to label all presentations of unexplained pain as cases of RSD will prove unproductive. In most cases of RSD, there is or has been a source of pain that triggered an exaggerated outflow by the sympathetic nervous system. Often, the sympathetic response is emotionally enhanced. Successful treatment targets one or more of these factors, and adjunctive measures emphasize the return to normal function.

A number of therapies have been recommended as means of breaking the circle of pain and swelling and allowing resumption of exercise and use of the hand and fingers. These varied approaches are well reviewed by Wilson.[89] No single treatment method is universally effective in relieving RSD. Early diagnosis is important, because treatment is most effective within the first 6 months of onset.[71]

Most therapies for RSD are directed toward interruption of the sympathetic nerve pathways that are thought to mediate much of the process. They include stellate ganglion blocks, intravenous guanethidine, oral phenoxybenzamine, and surgical sympathectomy.[27, 33] Other methods of pain reduction are injection of trigger points, desensitization procedures, and use of a transcutaneous nerve stimulator. Oral medications such as amitriptyline, fluoxetine, phenytoin, and nifedipine are also useful.[44]

Watson and Carlson[88] describe excellent results with an active "stress loading" program for RSD of the hand. The program consists of two activities designed to provide stressful stimuli without joint motion: scrub and carry. The scrub exercise has patients scrub the floor with a kitchen brush using as much force on the hand as they can tolerate. The carry part of the program has patients carry a weight throughout the day whenever they are standing or walking. Other therapy activities, including active range-of-motion exercise, are added after an initial response.[88]

It is important to recognize that the goal of these therapies is to allow resumption of exercise and functional use of the affected parts. The most successful treatment is a therapy program emphasizing active use and motion.[71] Regardless of the therapeutic approach chosen, a program of active use and exercise is indispensable in treatment of reflex sympathetic dystrophy.

INDICATIONS FOR SURGICAL EXPLORATION

The surgeon faces a difficult dilemma when trying to decide whether a particular patient would benefit from exploration of the median or ulnar nerves after wrist trauma. Statistically, most such nerve lesions resolve with treatment of the bony injury alone, suggesting caution in undertaking surgery. For a particular patient, however, if the nerve is too damaged or compressed to recover spontaneously, the potential for recovery is better with relatively early surgery. Unfortunately, none of the available tests clearly detects this situation.

Although surgical exploration and decompression of the median nerve at the carpal tunnel are not subject to many complications, their use can force a change in the preferred technique of fracture treatment. After the transverse carpal ligament is opened, the flexor tendons and median nerve must be prevented from bow-stringing, so the wrist cannot be immobilized in much flexion.[35] After decompression, an external fixator or pins and plaster are required for reduction and immobilization of some fractures for which, in the absence of the nerve decompression, a plaster cast would have been adequate.

The following guidelines are suggested for managing nerve problems associated with wrist trauma:

1. Treat an immediate, complete nerve lesion (detected by clinical examination) by closed reduction of the fracture or dislocation. If the nerve does not show prompt improvement, surgical exploration is justified.

2. If a nerve lesion develops after closed reduction or is significantly worse after reduction, explore the nerve.

3. If the fracture or dislocation requires open reduction and there is also a nerve lesion, strongly consider exploring the nerve at the same time even if the nerve lesion is incomplete.[64]

4. In the presence of disproportionate pain, swelling, and tingling suggesting Sudeck's atrophy, split the cast and padding; if symptoms do not promptly improve, change the wrist position to neutral. If symptoms still persist, consider carpal tunnel release, even if the clinical picture is not entirely typical of nerve compression.

5. Treat a partial nerve lesion that is part of a closed injury expectantly, unless there is a bone fragment in proximity to the nerve that is not reducible by closed means (Melone type III fracture). If improvement does not occur in the first week following reduction, consider surgical exploration of the nerve. Exploration is especially relevant if the deficit is in an important sensory or motor area.

Exploration of the ulnar nerve should comprise the canal of Guyon as well as the fracture site. Exploration of the median nerve should cover the fracture area as well as the carpal tunnel; compression by proximal hematoma has been described and could be missed if only the carpal tunnel is explored.[53]

CONCLUSION

Nerve injury is a rare accompaniment to orthopedic wrist problems. However, the nerve problem can have a profound influence on the end result and should, therefore, receive careful attention at all stages of treatment. This chapter presents guidelines for surgical release of the involved nerves. When a nerve injury is severe, the final result depends as much on careful management of the nerve injury as on treatment of the underlying orthopedic problem.

References

1. Abbott LC, Saunders JB, et al: Injuries of the median nerve in fractures of the lower end of the radius. Surg Gynecol Obstet 57:507, 1933.
2. Agee JM, McCarroll HR, Tortosa RD, et al: Endoscopic release of the carpal tunnel: A randomized prospective multicenter study. J Hand Surg 17:987, 1992.
3. Arendt-Nielson L, Gregersen H, Toft E, et al: Involvement of thin afferents in carpal tunnel syndrome: Evaluated quantitatively by argon laser stimulation. Muscle Nerve 14:508, 1991.
4. Bacorn RW, Kurtze JF: Colles fracture: A study of two thousand cases from the New York State Workman's Compensation Board. J Bone Joint Surg 35A:643, 1953.
5. Bauman TD, Gelberman RH, Mubarak SJ, et al: The acute carpal tunnel syndrome. Clin Orthop 156:151, 1981.
6. Bergfield TG, Aulicino PL, DePuy TE: The carpal tunnel syndrome. Orthop Rev 12:39, 1983.
7. Betcher AM, Casten DF: Reflex sympathetic dystrophy: Criteria for diagnosis and treatment. Anesthesiology 16:994, 1955.
8. Braidwood AS: Superficial radial neuropathy. J Bone Joint Surg 57B:380, 1975.
9. Brooks DM: Nerve compression by simple ganglia: A review of thirteen collected cases. J Bone Joint Surg 34B:391, 1952.
10. Brown RA, Gelberman RH, Seiler JG, et al: Carpal tunnel release: A prospective, randomized assessment of open and endoscopic methods. J Bone Joint Surg 75A:1265, 1993.
11. Cannon BW, Love JG: Tardy median palsy; median neuritis; median thenar neuritis amenable to surgery. Surgery 20:210, 1946.
12. Casten DF, Betcher AM: Reflex sympathetic dystrophy. Surg Gynecol Obstet 100:97, 1955.
13. Charles N, Vial C, Chauplannaz G, et al: Clinical validation of antidromic stimulation of the ring finger in early electrodiagnosis of mild carpal tunnel syndrome. Electroencephalogr Clin Neurophysiol 76:142, 1990.
14. Cooney WP, Dobyns JH, Linscheid RL: Complications of Colles fractures. J Bone Joint Surg 62A:613, 1980.
15. Cotton FJ: Wrist fractures: Disabilities following restorative operations. Trans Am Surg Assoc 40:289, 1922.
16. Feinstein PA: Endoscopic carpal tunnel release in a community-based series. J Hand Surg 18A:451, 1993.
17. Frederick HA, Carter PR, Littler JW: Injection injuries to the median and ulnar nerves at the wrist. J Hand Surg 17A:645, 1992.
18. Frykman G: Fractures of the distal radius including sequelae—shoulder-hand-finger syndrome, disturbance in the distal radio-ulnar joint and impairment of nerve function: A clinical and experimental study. Acta Orthop Scand Suppl 108:1, 1967.
19. Fuchs PC, Nathan PA, Myers LD: Synovial histology in carpal tunnel syndrome. J Hand Surg 16A:753, 1991.
20. Gaul JS: Letter to the editor. Orthopaedics 1:252, 1978.
21. Gelberman RH, Aronson D, Weisman MH: Carpal-tunnel syndrome: Results of a prospective trial of steroid injection and splinting. J Bone Joint Surg 62A:1181, 1980.
22. Gelberman RH, Hergenroeder PT, Hargens AR, et al: The carpal tunnel syndrome: A study of carpal canal pressures. J Bone Joint Surg 63A:380, 1981.
23. Gelberman RH, Szabo RM, Mortensen WW: Carpal tunnel pressures and wrist position in patients with Colles fractures. J Trauma 24:747, 1984.
24. Gelberman RH, Pfeffer GB, Galbraith RT, et al: Results of

treatment of severe carpal-tunnel syndrome without internal neurolysis of the median nerve. J Bone Joint Surg 69A:896, 1987.

25. Gelberman RH: Acute carpal tunnel syndrome. In Gelberman RH (ed): Operative Nerve Repair and Reconstruction. Philadelphia, JB Lippincott, 1991, p 939.

26. Gellman H, Gelberman RH, Tan AM, et al: Carpal tunnel syndrome: An evaluation of the provocative diagnostic tests. J Bone Joint Surg 68A:735, 1986.

27. Ghostline SY, Comair YG, Turner DM, et al: Phenoxybenzamine in the treatment of causalgia. J Neurosurg 60:1263, 1984.

28. Giannini F, Passero S, Cioni R, et al: Electrophysiologic evaluation of local steroid injection in carpal tunnel syndrome. Arch Phys Med Rehabil 72:738, 1991.

29. Gore DR: Carpometacarpal dislocation producing compression of the deep branch of the ulnar nerve. J Bone Joint Surg 53A:1387, 1971.

30. Green DP: Diagnostic and therapeutic value of carpal tunnel injection. J Hand Surg 9A:850, 1984.

31. Grundberg AB, Reagan DS: Compression syndromes in reflex sympathetic dystrophy. J Hand Surg 16A:731, 1991.

32. Hadler NM: Cumulative trauma: Carpal tunnel syndrome in the workplace—epidemiological and legal aspects. In Gelberman RH (ed): Operative Nerve Repair and Reconstruction. Philadelphia, JB Lippincott, 1991, p 949.

33. Hannington-Kiff JG: Relief of Sudeck's atrophy by regional intravenous guanethidine. Lancet 1:1019, 1974.

34. Howard FM: Ulnar-nerve palsy in wrist fractures. J Bone Joint Surg 43A:1197, 1961.

35. Inglis AE: Two unusual operative complications in the carpal-tunnel syndrome. J Bone Joint Surg 62A:1208, 1980.

36. Jetzer TC: Use of vibration testing in the early evaluation of workers with carpal tunnel syndrome. J Occup Med 33:117, 1991.

37. Jewitt DL, McCarroll HR (eds): Nerve Repair and Regeneration: Its Clinical and Experimental Basis. St Louis, CV Mosby, 1980.

38. Jones RW: Primary nerve lesions in injuries of the elbow and wrist. J Bone Joint Surg 12:121, 1930.

39. Kaplan SJ, Glickel SZ, Eaton RG: Predictive factors in the nonsurgical treatment of carpal tunnel syndrome. J Hand Surg 15B:106, 1990.

40. Kato H, Ogino T, Nanbu T, et al: Compression neuropathy of the motor branch of the median nerve caused by palmar ganglion. J Hand Surg 16A:751, 1991.

41. Katz JN, Larson MG, Sabra A, et al: The carpal tunnel syndrome: Diagnostic utility of the history and physical examination findings. Ann Intern Med 112:321, 1990.

42. Katz JN, Stirrat CR, Larson MG, et al: A self-administered hand symptom diagram for the diagnosis and epidemiologic study of carpal tunnel syndrome. J Rheumatol 17:1495, 1990.

43. Kimura J: The carpal tunnel syndrome: Localization of conduction abnormalities within the distal segment of the median nerve. Brain 102:619, 1979.

44. Koman LA, Poehling GG: Reflex sympathetic dystrophy. In Gelberman RH (ed): Operative Nerve Repair and Reconstruction. Philadelphia, JB Lippincott, 1991, p 1497.

45. Koris M, Gelberman RH, Duncan K, et al: Carpal tunnel syndrome: Evaluation of a quantitative provocational diagnostic test. Clin Orthop 251:157, 1990.

46. Kornberg M, Aulicino PL, DuPuy TE: Laceration of the ulnar nerve with a closed fracture of the distal radius and ulna. Orthopaedics 6:729, 1983.

47. de Krom MC, Knipschild PG, Kester ADM, et al: Efficacy of provocative tests for diagnosis of carpal tunnel syndrome. Lancet 335:393, 1990.

48. Kruger VL, Kraft GH, Deitz JC, et al: Carpal tunnel syndrome: Objective measures and splint use. Arch Phys Med Rehabil 72:517, 1991.

49. Kulick MI, Gordillo G, Javidi T, et al: Long-term analysis of patients having surgical treatment for carpal tunnel syndrome. J Hand Surg 11A:59, 1986.

50. Lankford LL, Thompson JE: Reflex sympathetic dystrophy, upper and lower extremity: Diagnosis and management. American Academy of Orthopaedic Surgeons Instructional Course Lectures 26:163, 1977.

51. Lauritzen M, Liguori R, Trojaborg W: Orthodromic sensory conduction along the ring finger in normal subjects and in patients with a carpal tunnel syndrome. Electroencephalogr Clin Neurophysiol 81:18, 1991.

52. Levine DW, Simmons BP, Koris MJ, et al: A self-administered questionnaire for the assessment of severity of symptoms and functional status in carpal tunnel syndrome. J Bone Joint Surg 75A: 1585, 1993.

53. Lewis MH: Median nerve decompression after Colles fracture. J Bone Joint Surg 60B:195, 1978.

54. Lin E, Ezra E, Nerubay J, et al: Acute carpal tunnel syndrome following Colles' fracture. Orthop Rev 13:524, 1984.

55. Linscheid RL: Injuries to radial nerve at wrist. Arch Surg 91:942, 1965.

56. Lluch AL: Thickening of the synovium of the digital flexor tendons: Cause or consequence of the carpal tunnel syndrome? J Hand Surg 17B:209, 1992.

57. Luchetti R, Schoenhuber R, De Cicco G, et al: Carpal-tunnel pressure. Acta Orthop Scand 60:397, 1989.

58. Luchetti R, Schoenhuber R, Alfarano M, et al: Carpal tunnel syndrome: Correlations between pressure measurement and intraoperative electrophysiological nerve study. Muscle Nerve 13:1164, 1990.

59. Lundborg G, Gelberman RH, Minteer-Convery M, et al: Median nerve compression in the carpal tunnel—functional response to experimentally induced controlled pressure. J Hand Surg 7:252, 1982.

60. Lynch AC, Lipscomb PR: The carpal-tunnel syndrome and Colles fractures. JAMA 185:363, 1963.

61. MacKinnon SE, McCabe S, Murray JF, et al: Internal neurolysis fails to improve the results of primary carpal tunnel decompression. J Hand Surg 16A:211, 1991.

62. McConnell JR, Bush DC: Intraneural steroid injection as a complication in the management of carpal tunnel syndrome. Clin Orthop 250:181, 1990.

63. Meadoff N: Median nerve injuries in fractures in the region of the wrist. Calif Med 70:252, 1949.

64. Mullen GB, Lloyd GJ: Complete carpal disruption of the hand. Hand 12:39, 1980.

65. Murphy TP, Parkhill WS: Fracture-dislocation of the base of the fifth metacarpal with an ulnar motor nerve lesion. J Trauma 30:1585, 1990.

66. Nagle D, Harris G, Foley M: Prospective review of 278 endoscopic carpal tunnel releases using the modified Chow technique. Arthroscopy 10:259, 1994.

67. Paley D, McMurtry RY: Median nerve compression by volarly displaced fragments of the distal radius. Clin Orthop 215:139, 1987.

68. Palmer DH, Paulson JC, Lane-Larsen CL, et al: Endoscopic carpal tunnel release: A comparison of two techniques with open release. Arthroscopy 9:498, 1993.

69. Peterson P, Sacks S: Fracture-dislocation of the base of the fifth metacarpal associated with injury to the deep motor branch of the ulnar nerve. J Hand Surg 11A:525, 1986.

70. Phalen GS: The carpal-tunnel syndrome: Seventeen years' experience in diagnosis and treatment of six hundred fifty-four hands. J Bone Joint Surg 48A:211, 1966.

71. Poplawski ZJ, Wiley AM, Murray JF: Post-traumatic dystrophy of the extremities: A clinical review and trial of treatment. J Bone Joint Surg 65A:642, 1983.

72. Poppen NK, McCarroll HR, Doyle JR, Neibauer JJ: Recovery of sensibility after suture of digital nerves. J Hand Surg 4:212, 1979.

73. Rawlings ID: The management of dislocations of the carpal lunate. Injury 12:319, 1981.

74. Rayan GM, Foster DE: Handcuff compression neuropathy. Orthop Rev 13:527, 1984.

75. Rojviroj S, Sirichativapee W, Kowsuwon W, et al: Pressures in the carpal tunnel: A comparison between patients with carpal tunnel syndrome and normal subjects. J Bone Joint Surg 72B:516, 1990.

76. Rotman MB, Manske PR: Anatomic relationships of an endoscopic carpal tunnel device to surrounding structures. J Hand Surg 18A:442, 1993.

77. Schuind F, Ventura M, Pasteels JL: Idiopathic carpal tunnel syndrome: Histologic study of flexor tendon synovium. J Hand Surg 15A:497, 1990.
78. Seddon HJ: Carpal ganglion as a cause of paralysis of the deep branch of the ulnar nerve. J Bone Joint Surg 34B:386, 1952.
79. Seiler JG, Milek MA, Carpenter GK, et al: Intraoperative assessment of median nerve blood flow during carpal tunnel release with laser Doppler flowmetry. J Hand Surg 6:986, 1989.
80. Shea JD, McClain EJ: Ulnar-nerve compression syndromes at and below the wrist. J Bone Joint Surg 51A:1095, 1969.
81. Short DW: Tardy median nerve palsy following injury. Glasgow Med J 32:315, 1951.
82. Siegel RS, Weiden I: Combined median and ulnar nerve lesions complicating fractures of the distal radius and ulna. J Trauma 8:1114, 1968.
83. Skie M, Zeiss J, Ebraheim NA, et al: Carpal tunnel changes and median nerve compression during wrist flexion and extension seen by magnetic resonance imaging. J Hand Surg 15A:934, 1990.
84. Sponsel KH, Palm ET: Carpal tunnel syndrome following Colles fracture. Surg Gynecol Obstet 121:1252, 1965.
85. Stein AH: The relation of median nerve compression to Sudeck's syndrome. Surg Gynecol Obstet 115:713, 1962.
86. Stewart HD, Innes AR, Burke FD: The hand complications of Colles' fractures. J Hand Surg 10B:103, 1985.
87. Vance RM, Gelberman RH: Acute ulnar neuropathy with fractures at the wrist. J Bone Joint Surg 60A:962, 1978.
88. Watson HK, Carlson L: Treatment of reflex sympathetic dystrophy of the hand with an active "stress loading" program. J Hand Surg 12A:779, 1987.
89. Wilson RL: Management of pain following peripheral nerve injuries. Orthop Clin North Am 12:343, 1981.
90. Zoega H: Fracture of the lower end of the radius with ulnar nerve palsy. J Bone Joint Surg 48B:514, 1966.

CHAPTER 28

Occupational and Sports Injuries of the Wrist

Steven R. Novotny, MD, David M. Lichtman, MD, and
Ellison H. Wittels, MD

The disciplines of sports medicine and occupational health share two primary objectives: to prevent injury and to return the injured participant to full activities as soon as possible. The goal of this chapter is to raise the consciousness of upper extremity physicians about degenerative and pathologic conditions commonly associated with occupational or athletic activity. We do not cover major traumatic events that are nonspecific to a particular activity; these problems are covered elsewhere in the text. Instead, we concentrate on repetitive stress or chronic injuries that can be closely linked to a particular occupation or sport. In addition to the strictly medical aspects of these injuries, the treatment of these conditions is often complicated by psychosocial factors that affect the patient's compliance with various therapeutic regimens. We stress the epidemiologic aspects of the disorders along with the special problems encountered in returning the injured worker or athlete to full productivity.

OCCUPATIONAL INJURIES

Impact of Work-Related Injury and Illness

On January 11, 1994, Dr. David Satcher, Director of the Centers for Disease Control and Prevention, stated that with more people now employed than ever before, work "will continue to be a primary influence on the health of this nation for many years to come."[1] With the larger workforce size, there has also been an accompanying increase in reported work-related injuries and illnesses.

The physician should not only understand the reasons to diagnose and treat an injured worker, but also appreciate the legal need to report the injury and the importance of preventing recurrence in the injured worker and similar injury in others at the same worksite. A compensable work injury or illness is generally defined as arising out of and in the course and scope of employment.[2] For practical purposes, this means that the work itself has been the cause of the injury or illness or has made worse a pre-existing condition.

The health and economic impacts of occupational injury and illness are enormous. Nationwide, it has been estimated that 10,000 workers are killed and 100,000 die from occupational diseases each year.[3] The cost to employers of providing workers' compensation was estimated to be $62 billion in 1991.[4]

Over the last few years, there has also been a shift in the type of work-related injuries reported. Previously, acute illness or injuries reported constituted the majority of on-the-job injuries. In 1981, cumulative trauma disorders (CTDs) accounted for 18 percent of all occupational illness; by 1991, CTDs accounted for 61 percent of all occupational illness, and for 3.5 percent of all occupational injuries and illness. An analysis of Liberty Mutual Insurance Companies' 1989 workers' compensation claims found that CTDs of the upper extremity accounted for 0.83 percent of all claims and 1.64 percent of all claim costs, approximately $563 million; the mean cost per case was $8,070, and the median cost was $1,824.[5] In addition, the average CTD claim costs more than an average traumatic injury claim and causes more time lost from work than other musculoskeletal problems.[6]

Workplace illness and injury produce direct medical care costs, indirect medical costs from lost production, foregone opportunities, and diminished investment and noneconomic costs, including pain and suffering, disrupted careers, and devastated families.[7] Employer costs consist of repeat medical treatment, lost worker productivity, higher insurance premiums, reduced work force efficiency, and higher temporary employee costs. Clearly, identification of the work-relatedness of an injury or illness is necessary, especially in a CTD.

Identifying Work-Related Illness or Injury

Occupational disease can be difficult to diagnose. It has been estimated that 60 to 95 percent of occupational diseases are undiagnosed. In one study, a relevant occupational exposure was considered only 17 percent of the time among patients who were hospitalized with illnesses that could have had an occupational basis.[8]

An epidemiologic study attempts to link an illness or injury by establishing the presence of certain relationships, as follows:

1. Symptoms consistent with the diagnosis.
2. Signs consistent with the diagnosis.
3. Temporal relationship between exposure and disease.
4. Fellow workers with similar problems.
5. Workplace monitoring data.
6. Biologically plausible explanation.
7. Lack of nonoccupational exposure.
8. Evidence that supports the causal association.

An occupational *sentinel health event (SHE)* "is a disease, disability, or untimely death that is occupationally related and whose occurrence may provide the impetus for epidemiological industrial hygiene surveys or serve as a warning signal that material substitution, engineering control, personal protection, or medical care may be required."[9] Most sentinel health events are not only expensive but also preventable. A sentinel health event identifies the need to develop occupational health care surveillance and to initiate preventive and therapeutic medical care. Requesting an industrial hygienist or ergonomist to perform an ergonomic evaluation of a person's work site may be very helpful in identifying common risk factors for other employees and in providing the opportunity to prevent continued injury to the worker.

In 1700, Bernardino Ramazzini, the father of occupational medicine, wrote of the medical history, "I may venture to ask one more question: What occupation does he follow?" For the physician, an occupational history is an essential first step in establishing the work-relatedness of a work-related problem. The occupational history, as part of the medical history, may be abbreviated, expanded, or specifically focused, but it should never be omitted.[10]

Inquiry into the current work, including type of industry, place of work, general and specific job duties, need for personal protective equipment, previous occasions of missed work because of health problems, and similar illness in coworkers can give the physician important information. A person's job title may not reveal what that person actually does. The most important piece of information is an accurate job description that includes having the patient describe and demonstrate the activity required at work. This may also include a job description provided by the employer, or even a job-site inspection or videotape of the actual job duties. A description of the worker's past work history and years worked in each position is especially important in a CTD.

It is useful to obtain a description of the relationship of symptoms to work periods. Especially important is the time needed for the symptoms to abate after work ends. Whether the symptoms abate after 10 minutes of rest or persist between work days makes a statement as to the severity of the condition. A report of any change in work routine, work activity, or production quotas in relation to the development of symptoms provides valuable clues to etiology and a rationale for immediate work restrictions. Finally, careful evaluation of home activities and avocational interests may provide information as to work-relatedness of an injury, especially in patients for whom conservative care has failed.

Identifying Those at Risk

Employers are concerned about the rising rate of work-related musculoskeletal injuries and their direct and indirect costs. Screening prospective employees to identify those more likely to develop musculoskeletal injuries has been attempted. With a marked increase in the workplace of carpal tunnel syndrome, several tests have been developed to screen workers.[11–13] At this time, no screening test has the necessary sensitivity and specificity to predict whether an asymptomatic individual will develop a CTD in the future. Neither current perception threshold testing (CPT) nor vibrotactile thresholds (VTs) have proved useful in diagnosing carpal tunnel syndrome or possible cases of carpal tunnel syndrome in workers.[14]

The Americans with Disabilities Act (ADA) prohibits an employer from asking specific medical questions at a job interview. Moreover, the ADA requires that before a candidate can be disqualified from a job, the tests must clearly demonstrate that performing the essential job functions poses a direct threat to the employee's health and safety or to the health and safety of those around the employee. The physician must make recommendations for "reasonable accommodations" for the employee. The focus has shifted from "screening out" prospective employees to providing engineering changes, administrative controls, and personal protective equipment.

Formal Definition of Work-Related Injury and Illness

Work-related injury or illness causes the same problems (e.g., tendinitis, myositis, nerve compression), symptoms, and signs, and requires the same treatment as a non–work-related injury or illness. It is the nonspecificity of work versus nonwork medical injury or illness that requires extra diligence from the physician in establishing a work-related medical problem. The ability to provide long-term preventive care, decrease the risk of recurrence, and protect others who could also be at risk depends on correctly identifying the work-relatedness of an injury or illness. The objective of occupational medicine is the management and prevention of medical problems associated with hazards in the workplace.[15]

The 1990 Ergonomic Program Management Guidelines for Meatpacking Plants issued by the Occupational Safety and Health Administration (OSHA),[16] commonly referred to as the "Red Meat Guidelines," is a model for ergonomic safety. To have an OSHA-recordable injury requires a combination of a physical finding, and either a subjective symptom or a contributing action. *Physical findings* may consist of erythema, edema, deformity, restricted motion, tenderness, or a positive Tinel's, Phalen's, or Finkelstein's test. *Subjective symptoms* may include, but are not limited to, pain, tingling, aching, and stiffness, but they must occur in conjunction with the worker's acting upon the symptoms. A *contributing action* would be seeking medical care, including self-administered treatment when made available through employee health benefits, lost work days or restricted work activity, or transfer to another job.

The reader is referred to Hansen's[17] review of these guidelines and their implications as well as insightful commentary on their pitfalls.

CTD Overview

OSHA's "Red Meat Guidelines"[16] define *cumulative trauma* as a "class of musculoskeletal disorders involving damage to the tendons, tendon sheaths, synovial lubrication of tendon sheaths, and the related bones, muscles, and nerves of the hands, wrists, elbows, shoulders, and back."

Cumulative trauma disorders include both clearly identifiable and nonspecific diagnoses. Although arthritis, tendinitis, and local entrapment neuropathies are more easily diagnosed and treated, a large number of injured workers have nonspecific upper extremity pain. Pain often involves the whole or most of the extremity, paresthesia, or numbness that does not always follow dermatomal or clearly defined nerve distributions. Cramping and aching of muscles in the shoulder, forearm, and hand are reported.

Mackinnon and Novak[18] proposed that prolonged maintenance of abnormal postures produces three major adverse effects on the soft tissues. First, certain positions place direct pressure around nerves at various entrapment points and subsequently cause chronic nerve compression. Examples would be cubital tunnel compression with elbow flexion, carpal tunnel compression with wrist flexion, and radial sensory nerve entrapment between the brachioradialis and the extensor carpi radialis longus muscles with prolonged forearm pronation. At these entrapment points, edema and fibrosis tether nerves, eliminating normal nerve excursion with movement. Nerves thought of as purely motor, such as the anterior interosseous nerve, carry sensory afferent fibers that can produce dull aching in the innervated muscles when the nerves are compressed. The double-crush phenomenon also helps explain the large cumulative effect produced by multiple minor compressions as well as the usually normal nerve conduction studies obtained in affected patients.

Mackinnon and Novak's[18] second point is that prolonged maintenance of abnormal posture allows muscle groups to tighten in a shortened position. Tightened muscles can cause nerve compression directly, such as of the pronator teres with prolonged keyboard activity. The tightened muscle can compress the median nerve and can also cause pain when it is subsequently stretched. Mackinnon and Novak[18] also believe that shortened muscles operate ineffectively, resulting in a secondary overuse by another group of compensatory muscles. Muscle imbalance develops that may be self perpetuating. A general strengthening program may maintain the imbalance. The initial goal is to identify the tight structures and direct early therapy toward stretching. Once a pain-free range of motion is achieved, strengthening is directed toward the deficient muscles.

There is also concern about the role that psychosocial factors play in the development of a CTD. Himmelstein and colleagues[6] reported that individuals with upper extremity injury and disability had more anger with their employer, and a greater reactivity to pain, than employees with upper extremity disorders who had returned to full work. Although it is difficult to separate cause and effect, such a finding does indicate the need to deal with psychosocial issues with this patient population. The World Health Organization[31] also concluded that psychosocial factors are "at least as important as physical characteristics of the workplace in influencing health and well-being."

Australian Experience

In the early 1980s, Australia experienced an epidemic of repetition strain injury (RSI) diagnosed in workers suffering from occupational disease. This occupational phenomenon affected the upper extremities of Australian workers. The phenomenon was not exclusively associated with repetitive tasks. Interestingly, a dramatic rise in complaints was noted in occupations in which the manual tasks and work practices had not substantially changed for a decade before the epidemic.

Hocking's[19] 1987 study of Telecom Australia employees revealed that the lowest rates of RSI complaints (3 percent) were in keyboard workers performing approximately 12,000 keystrokes per hour. The highest complaints of RSI were in telephonists (34 percent), who performed the lowest number of keystrokes, a few hundred per hour, during their work. Graham[20] and Ryan and Pimble[21] have found inconsistent relationships between RSI symptoms and the ergonomics of the workstation, but a stronger relationship with job satisfaction. Hocking[19] also demonstrated that part-time employees have a significantly higher rate of complaints compared with full-time employees. The group he studied had a disproportionate and statistically significant higher rate of complaints by women compared with men at the same work position.

Ireland[22, 23] critically reviews the history of RSI in Australia, comparing it with historical outbreaks of workers' musculoskeletal complaints that eventually disappeared when the complaints were determined to be nonphysiologic in nature. He clearly states that all patients need a thorough evaluation to separate commonly accepted overuse conditions—impingement syndrome, tennis elbow, cubital tunnel, De Quervain's stenosing tenosynovitis, flexor tenosynovitis causing median nerve compression—from complaints of pain not conforming to any known neurologic pathways, anatomic structures, or physiologic pattern. This latter group of cases called RSI in Australia are now generally accepted to represent a psychosomatic symptom complex[24] and not a physical disorder. Ireland[23] believes that because the RSI complaint is now clearly defined and accepted as a nonphysical condition, medical practitioners are less willing to certify patients as unable to work. This development eliminated the secondary gain from the equation and resulted in a precipitous drop in RSI complaints. Ireland[23] attributes the acceptance of this view by medical practitioners and the lay public to three main events. First, in 1986, the *Australian Medical Journal* changed its editorial perspective to allow publication of articles emphasizing the nonphysical origin of RSI. This included a strong statement issued by the Australian Hand Club[25] in 1985 stating that RSI was a costly national epidemic and that in only a small number of patients does a pathologic basis for continuing symptoms exist. The statement went on that the condition is reversible and that the majority of cases stem from nervous causes and can be categorized as occupational neuroses. Second, a well-coordinated educational campaign by the hand specialists working with the College of General Practitioners and the media was employed. Third, several court cases, most significantly *Cooper v. the Commonwealth* (1987), decided by the Australian Supreme Court, found that the employer was not guilty of negligence and that the plaintiff had not suffered an injury, and awarded all costs against the plaintiff. Since the court has taken this action, virtually all pending RSI cases have been withdrawn.

Ergonomics

Ergonomics is the application of human biology and engineering science to achieve the optimum benefits of human efficiency and well-being. Ergonomics adapts the workplace and the tools to the worker, rather than the worker to them. The main emphasis is three-fold. First, biomechanical evaluation of the physical demands of the required task is performed. Second, workplace design relates the physical characteristics and capabilities of the worker to the design of equipment and work space layout. Anthropomorphic data are used to integrate the required functional body movements and special accommodations of the work space into the optimum performance of the task. Thirdly, the ergonomist must consider the behavioral demands of the job when making recommendations. The industrial hygienist is trained to recognize environmental stressors that adversely affect the worker, to evaluate the magnitude of these stressors, and to implement measures to correct or control the problem.[26]

VIDEO DISPLAY TERMINALS

The vast majority of clerical workers are now video display terminal (VDT) users. More than 12 million VDTs were in use in 1987,[27] with a ten-fold increase anticipated in the next decade. The shear number of VDT users makes any problem associated with their use potentially monumental. Clerical workers provide a prime example of the multiple potential anatomic sites affected by CTDs. Higher rates of eye strain, headaches, neck and shoulder pain, cubital and carpal tunnel syndromes, wrist tendinitis, and low back pain have been reported.

The maximum work capacity of the musculoskeletal system is not obtained in VDT work, even in the most extreme positions. These jobs involve prolonged periods of static loading of muscles. The immediate effect may be reduced muscular blood flow, metabolic changes, and fatigue. If this effect represents a significant daily occurrence, chronic problems may result. Arndt[28] pointed out that workstation design must minimize muscular load but also must allow relief in the form of movement or variations in posture to avoid the long-term effects of static loading.

Rossignol[27] demonstrated that 0.5 to 3 hours per day of VDT use was not associated with increased musculoskeletal complaints. Persons working 7 hours or more at a VDT had a higher incidence of musculoskeletal complaints. It is likely that there were fewer interruptions among this group. This group would benefit from taking more breaks or scheduling alternative work to decrease prolonged VDT use.

The general guideline for positioning VDT users starts with a comfortable rolling chair with lumbar support (Fig. 28–1). An adjustable foot rest is used as needed to allow the knees to rest at 90° of flexion. The primary work surface should be at or slightly below elbow height to allow the shoulders to rest. The elbow should work in the 45° to 60° flexion range. Minor adjustments may be needed to ensure that the wrist works in a neutral position. The top of the video display should be at eye level and at a comfortable reading distance. Data entry personnel should work from a document holder to minimize head, neck, and shoulder movement. Accessory work items should be nearby to prevent excessive reach. The shoulders should not be moved more than 20° from the resting position for long periods, to minimize shoulder impingement trauma.

During break periods, stretching exercises for the whole body should be performed to prevent muscle contracture and improve circulation.[29] The World Health Organization[30] and others[5] have clearly shown

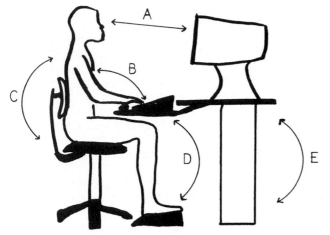

Figure 28–1. The illustration demonstrates several ergonomic principles. *A,* The line top of the monitor is at eye level, and the screen is slightly angled upwards diminishing glare. The viewing distance varies from 18 to 30 inches. Special eyewear for computer use may be necessary to allow for two depths of near vision (screen and keyboard distances) along with far vision. *B,* The shoulder is at 0 to 20° of flexion diminishing fatigue, the elbow is flexed to less than 90° to minimize cubital tunnel symptoms, and the wrists are in neutral. Though a wrist support pad is shown here, some question positioning that encourages the worker to apply pressure directly on the median nerve by resting the wrists on any surface. *C,* The back should be supported and the chair should be moveable if possible. *D,* Demonstrates the foot support with the ankle in neutral or slight dorsiflexion and the knees bent to 90°. *E,* Denotes that table height should be adjustable to accommodate persons of differing body habitus.

that psychologic factors may be as important as ergonomic designs. Job design should include some user discretion in task organization. Short, frequently taken breaks are more satisfactory than infrequent, longer breaks. These breaks should be taken away from the VDT. Rest periods are more effective for work requiring continuous attention than for jobs that leave employees discretionary time.

HAND TOOLS

The hand and upper extremity become susceptible to injury from improper tool design. The force applied to the hand and arm is both external from the weight of the tool and internal from muscle contraction. Heavier tools have the benefit of dampening vibratory stresses and can be counterbalanced by overhead springs to reduce the external load.

Contact stresses are localized applications of intrinsic and extrinsic forces where edges of the tool contact the skin. Neurovascular bundles and tendon sheaths are very susceptible to these stresses. The stresses can be minimized by enlarging grip areas to distribute the forces over a larger area or by using more than one finger to activate a trigger mechanism. The intrinsic hand muscles and wrist extensors are very susceptible to static overloading. The work environment should be designed for the lowest possible isometric effort required to complete the task. The lower muscle tension impairs blood flow the least,

resulting in prolonged work periods before peak muscle fatigue occurs.

Hand tools that deviate the wrist from a neutral position ultimately decrease grip strength. Redesigning handle shapes and tool offset and angle can overcome the problem. Grips should allow the control area to be as large as possible. The handle should distribute the force over the thenar and hypothenar eminences and the lesser digits. Torque bars on power tools reduce rotational force transmission, and antivibration gloves reduce vibration transmission. Handles and hand grips should be designed for power grip, as opposed to precision grip or three-point chuck. Power grip generates more force and it is less fatiguing, because less overall force is needed to control the tool.

VIBRATION INJURY

Vibration-induced Raynaud's phenomenon often has been called "vibration white finger." By international agreement, it is now called *hand-arm vibration syndrome* (HAVS). The syndrome is defined as a disease with the following peripheral components: circulatory disturbances (vasospasm with local finger blanching), sensory and motor disturbances (numbness, loss of dexterity), and musculoskeletal disturbances (muscle, joint, bone disorders). Though a large number of tools and situations can lead to this disorder, hand-held compressed air tools and gasoline and electric-drive tools such as polishers, grinders, and chain saws are easily recognized as vibration-producing agents.

After a variable latent exposure period (the time between starting exposure and developing symptoms), and depending on the subject's susceptibility, blanching of the fingertips occurs after cold exposure. The finger is blanched and numb during the attack, and there may be persistent sensory changes or reduced sensitivity between attacks. The attacks are precipitated by exposure to cold, damp conditions. They occur more often in the morning and with handling wet or cold objects. With continued exposure, the attacks become more frequent.

A sequence of pathologic and physiologic changes occurs in the tissues to produce the clinical syndrome.[31] The first response to vibration is a dilation of the small vessels, increased permeability, extravasation of fluid, and a thickening of local tissue. Hypertrophy of the vessel's smooth muscle layer occurs. As its lumen size decreases, the vessel may become susceptible to thrombosis secondary to sluggish blood flow.

Workers with HAVS have been shown to have decreased sensory nerve conduction velocity from the finger to the wrist[32] and increased motor and sensory latency with reduced conduction velocity in the medial and ulnar nerves of the forearm.[33, 34] Such study findings suggest a direct injury pattern of the peripheral nerve unrelated to the vascular spasm.

A grading scale that separates the vascular and

Table 28–1. VASCULAR STAGES IN HAND-ARM VIBRATION SYNDROME

Stage	Grade	Symptoms
0		No clinical symptoms
1	Mild	Occasional attacks
2	Moderate	Occasional attacks involving finger up to the middle phalanx
3	Severe	Frequent attacks affecting potentially all phalanxes
4	Very severe	Frequent attacks with trophic changes on the fingertip

From Gemne G, Pyyko I, Taylor W, Pelmear PL: Scand J Work Environ Health 13:275, 1987, and Brammer AJ, Taylor W, Lundborg G: Scand J Work Environ Health 13:279, 1987.

sensorineural symptoms into separate categories has been proposed (Tables 28–1 and 28–2). The vascular stages are rated from 0 to 4 and the sensorineuronal (SN) stages are from 0 SN to 3 SN. The higher the stage, the more severe or persistent the symptoms. Recovery from neuropathy after elimination of exposure is less likely than reversal of the vascular effects. Workers under age 40 with early disease usually recover after elimination of exposure.[37]

Prevention of the problem is as important as treatment. Treatment starts with the identification of hazards and the elimination of vibration transmission through tool design and the use of antivibration gloves and antivibration pads. Work rotation or alternative work methods reduce exposure. Educating workers to avoid smoking and to wear appropriate warm and dry clothes to maintain core temperature during inclement weather is important. For severe cases, electrically heated mittens are recommended during winter.

New therapies are directed to reduce vasospasm. Nifedipine in a slow-release preparation can be effective along with peripheral vasodilators such as isosorbide dinitrate and nitroglycerine ointment. Pentoxifylline may enhance red blood cell flexibility and promote platelet deaggregation, improving circulation. Surgical sympathectomy is of little help in this disease process.

Table 28–2. SENSORINEURAL (SN) STAGES IN HAND-ARM VIBRATION SYNDROME

Stage	Symptoms
0 SN	Exposed without symptoms
1 SN	Intermittent numbness with or without tingling
2 SN	Intermittent or persistent numbness reducing sensory perceptions
3 SN	Intermittent or persistent numbness reducing tactile discrimination or manual dexterity

From Gemne G, Pyyko I, Taylor W, Pelmear PL: Scand J Work Environ Health 13:275, 1987, and Brammer AJ, Taylor W, Lundborg G: Scand J Work Environ Health 13:279, 1987.

SPORTS INJURIES

The upper extremity, specifically the wrist and hand, is often the initial point of contact in sports, as in catching a pass or tackling in football, blocking a shot in basketball, and swinging a racquet in tennis. The same could be said for everyday life: holding the steering wheel in an automobile accident, falling off a bicycle, or slipping and falling on an icy sidewalk. Fractures, ligament sprain, and contusions can all occur, although fractures are surely the most dramatic injury.

In a review of their 11-year experience of treating intercollegiate athletes, Whiteside and colleagues[38] noted that the hand, fingers, and wrist were the most common locations of fractures, regardless of sport or gender. Hand and wrist fractures represented more than one third of all fractures. The contact sports football and basketball led the men's teams in number of injuries, whereas in women's sports, gymnastics and lacrosse led the list. Phalangeal and metacarpal fractures were the most common sites of injury. Canale and associates[39] reviewed their collegiate football team over a 4-year period and reported that 3 percent of injuries were to the hand and wrist; 90 percent of these were listed as mild injuries, resulting in less than a 1-week loss of sports participation.

A change in the level of competition can alter the profile of hand injuries. Ellsasser and Stein,[40] while taking care of a professional football team, reported 46 major hand injuries over 15 years. Of five scaphoid fractures, one required bone grafting to treat a delayed union. These investigators recommend aggressive treatment of intra-articular fractures and protection with appropriate splints and casts. No wound problems or fracture complications occurred, and the players returned to competition sooner as a result of the aggressive approach. Raab and colleagues[41] identified ten lunate and perilunate injuries in professional football players over a 10-year period. The majority of the players returned to competition after appropriate treatment. In a survey of a variety of sports, most hand injuries involved the phalanges and metacarpals, a pattern that corresponded to ball-handling and tackling activities.[42–44] Injury more proximal than the hand was documented in a series of 2,774 consecutive, prospectively evaluated fractures of the distal radius in Great Britain.[45] Two hundred and twenty-five (8 percent) were the result of sports injuries. Soccer produced 50 percent of the injuries, influenced largely by cultural and geographic factors. Skiing, skating, and equestrian events produced more complex injuries according to the Arbeitgemeineschaft fur Osteosynthesesfragen (AO) classification. High-energy sports and rising participant age resulted in more severe and increasingly complex injuries.

Strickland[46] reminds treating physicians that it is their "responsibility" to athlete patients to provide a thorough explanation of an injury and the implications of compromising treatment by returning to play sooner than recommended. With an increasing level of play, there can be untoward pressure to return the athlete to competition prematurely. For professional athletes, financial implications can be tremendous. Strickland states, "Nonetheless, the need for the treating physicians to completely advise the athlete of the potential short and long term consequences of such premature participation cannot be understated."[46] The care of these common wrist and hand fractures can be found in selected readings and recommended texts on the subjects.[47-49] The following discussion represents only a partial list of conditions affecting the wrist and related structures.

Hamate Fractures

In 1972, Torisu[50] described an acute hook of the hamate fracture in a golfer. It failed to unite and subsequently caused an ulnar nerve palsy. In 1977, Stark and colleagues[51] reported on 20 athletes with hamate hook fractures: 7 golfers, 9 baseball players, and 4 tennis players. The etiology of the injury is believed to be striking of the hamate hook by the butt end of the club, bat, or racquet. It more often occurs with a checked swing in baseball or a duffed shot in golf. These investigators treated 17 of the patients using excision of the hamate hook fragments, all of whom had complete recovery. Carter and associates[52] reported on 9 hamate fractures with similarly good results. Stark and colleagues[53] in 1989 reported an expanded series of 62 patients. In 47, hamate hook fractures had occurred at the base or proximal one third of the hook. Of the 10 acute fractures seen, 3 were treated early with immobilization and subsequent failure of conservative care. These investigators advise surgical removal of the hook fragment as the treatment of choice.

Radiologically, the fracture can be seen on a carpal tunnel view in most people.[54, 55] If the patient is too symptomatic to dorsiflex the wrist for the radiograph, a supinated oblique view will profile the hamate hook (Fig. 28–2).[56] If the lesion is suspected but not confirmed on plain radiographs, a computed tomography (CT) scan of the region will most likely demonstrate the lesion.[57] A technetium Tc 99m bone scan may confirm an injury in the region but cannot specifically diagnose a hamate fracture.

Complications from this injury have been noted. Howard[58] and Shea and McClain[59] have described ulnar nerve palsies secondary to hamate hook fractures. Two of the patients reported by Stark and colleagues[53] and Torisu's[50] patient complained of ulnar nerve–related symptoms. Favorable response was noted with surgical intervention. Clayton[60] reported on two patients with a flexor tendon rupture in the carpal canal and associated hamate hook fracture. No history or treatment was reported for either patient. Crosby and Linscheid[61] reported on two patients with flexor digitorum profundus tendon rupture and hamate hook fracture, one of whom was treated with cortisone injections. Stark and colleagues[51] also noted

the association between tendon rupture and steroid injection in their series. Milek and Boulas[62] reported on four patients with a hamate hook fracture and associated tendon rupture. All of their cases responded well to excision of the bone fragment and an end-to-side repair of the tendon.

Not all authorities agree that hamate excision is the preferred treatment. Whalen and coworkers[63] reported on eight hamate fractures treated by a short-arm cast with inclusion of the ring and little finger metacarpal phalangeal joints. Six patients with acute fractures were seen within 7 days of injury. The other two fractures were subacute when seen. Immobilization averaged 11 weeks. Seven of the eight patients had documented union on trispiral tomography and were asymptomatic at 8 months' follow-up. Thus, immediately recognized fractures may respond to conservative care.

Our preferred method of treatment for hamate fracture is a trial of immobilization for up to 3 months, especially if the fracture is diagnosed early. Once sclerosis of the fracture fragment occurs, we excise the fragment through an incision made directly over Guyon's canal.

Soft Tissue Injury

Soft tissue injury can be broken down into four stages: inflammation, proliferation, maturation, and fibrosis.[64] A more effective treatment plan can be devised if the correct stage at initial presentation can be identified.

Inflammation begins early after injury. The initial inflammatory cells release bioactive factors to increase vascular permeability, promote vascular ingrowth, and attract other inflammatory cells.[65, 66] Pain, swelling, and edema are the identifiers of this stage. Rest, ice, compression, and elevation are the important treatment modalities. Avoiding provocative maneuvers, possibly with the use of immobilization in the early stages, reduces further injury. Nonsteroidal anti-inflammatory drugs (NSAIDs) can reduce symptoms.

The proliferative stage lasts 1 to 2 weeks. Early collagen production is of disorganized bundles. The alignment of these bundles is not oriented to accept maximal stress. Controlled early motion allows proper maturation of the new tissue.

The maturation stage, when the collagen matures through cross-linking and organizing along lines of stress, takes 6 to 12 weeks to complete. Muscle atrophy associated with prolonged rest and improved tendon healing with controlled stress can be influenced during this time.[65-67] Isometric exercises, flexibility drills, and a gradual return to resistive exercises are instituted during this phase. Modalities such as ultrasound, electrical stimulation, and iontophoresis are often helpful adjunctive therapy during this phase.

Fibrosis occurs when the inflammatory cycle is

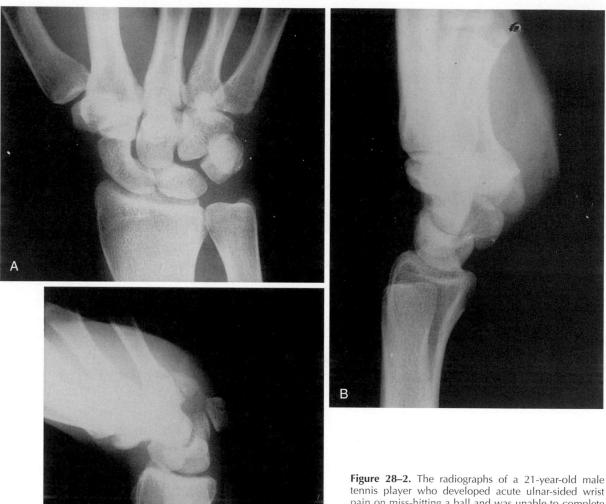

Figure 28–2. The radiographs of a 21-year-old male tennis player who developed acute ulnar-sided wrist pain on miss-hitting a ball and was unable to complete the game. *A,* Standard posteroanterior view. *B,* Standard lateral view. *C,* A hamate fracture is demonstrated on a supinated oblique view. (Courtesy of David H. Hildreth, MD.)

continuous or recurs frequently. This results in thickened tendon sheaths and restricted tendon excursion.[68, 69] Surgical release is often necessary once this point is reached.

De Quervain's Tenosynovitis

De Quervain's stenosing tenosynovitis is a common cause of radial-sided wrist pain. Whether the disorder starts in the tenosynovium or in the tendon sheath is unclear. What is clear is the increased rate of occurrence with repetitive gripping, ulnar and radial deviation of the wrist, and thumb adduction.[64, 70] Commonly a disorder of middle aged women, De Quervain's tenosynovitis can develop in any person of either sex and any age given the right provocation. Clerical work, racquet sports, and golf are very commonly identified as precipitating events.

The patients have various complaints ranging from inability to abduct the thumb to swelling, crepitance, and localized pain on the radial side of the wrist. Finkelsteins's test is diagnostic. We have the patient clasp the thumb in the palm and ulnarly deviate the wrist. If this recreates the symptoms, the diagnosis is confirmed. Localized tenderness or swelling over the first dorsal compartment is a complementary finding. Basal joint arthritis, Wartenberg's syndrome, intersection syndrome, and flexor carpi radialis tendinitis are included in the differential diagnosis, and possibly could be concomitant disease processes.

Management consists of immobilization in a forearm-based thumb spica splint, oral NSAIDs, and strong consideration of a local cortisone injection. Adjuvant therapy may consist of heat and ice alone or combined with modalities such as ultrasound, galvanic stimulation, and iontophoresis. With failure of conservative care, surgical release of the first dorsal compartment is undertaken.[71]

SURGICAL PROCEDURE

Make a curvilinear or chevron incision over the radial border of the distal radius through the dermis. While the assistant retracts the skin edges, gently spread the subcutaneous tissue. This allows easy identification of the radial sensory nerve branches. Protect them with a blunt retractor such as Ragnell's retractors. Identify the fibro-osseous tunnel over the abductor pollicis longus (APL) tendon and extensor pollicis brevis (EPB) tendon from the tip of the radial styloid to its most proximal extent. Now make an incision on the dorsal-most attachment of the sheath at its periosteal attachment. Retract both the APL and the EPB tendons, ensuring their complete release. Look for any additional subcompartments at this time. Close the skin and apply a protective splint for 2 to 3 weeks before starting the patient on a strengthening program.

The dorsal tenovaginotomy allows the sheath to retract volarly and act as a buttress to volar tendon subluxation. After 2 weeks, therapy is begun for scar management and range of motion, followed by a strengthening program. Racquet and club sports can be started in 6 to 8 weeks as determined by symptoms.

To prevent complications, carefully avoid the radial sensory branches and diligently search for "hidden" subcompartments. Recurrence of symptoms may require re-exploration of the sheath. Postoperative palmar dislocation of the tendon can occur. Prevent this by proper dorsal, longitudinal division of the sheath.

If dislocation does occur, loose reconstruction of the sheath or, preferably, excision of the longitudinal bony ridge, which acts as the palmar insertion of the first compartment, eliminates the symptoms.

Intersection Syndrome

Intersection syndrome is a cause of swelling, pain, and crepitance 5 cm proximal to Lister's tubercle on the radial side of the forearm.[72–74] This area overlies the junction where the first extensor compartment tendons cross over the radial wrist extensor tendons. Though common in players of racquet sports, the syndrome is more common in weight lifters and rowers.[70] Wood and Linscheid[75] reported the cause as an adventitial bursitis at the crossing of the tendons, whereas Grundberg and Reagan[73] reported a stenosing tenosynovitis of the radial wrist extensors' sheath.

Conservative care is highly successful. Wrist immo-

bilization in 20° of dorsiflexion combined with NSAIDs and judicious rest is recommended. Occasionally, a cortisone injection directly into the area of tenderness is required. Six weeks of conservative care is recommended before operative intervention is considered.

SURGICAL PROCEDURE

Because opinion is varied as to the exact etiology of the intersection syndrome,[72, 73, 75] we agree with Kiefhuber and Stern's[64] algorithm for order and choice of steps in surgery for intersection syndrome. Surgical treatment is performed as follows:

Start with a 3-cm to 4-cm oblique incision, following the course of the APL and EPB muscle bellies on the radial half of the dorsal forearm 5 cm proximal to Lister's tubercle. Spread the subcutaneous tissue in line with the muscle bellies. Now, inspect the intersection area and débride any inflamed tissue with a rongeur. Divide the APL and EPB fascial sheaths longitudinally from their musculotendinous junction as far proximally as can be seen. Once the muscle bellies are decompressed, inspect the extensor carpi radialis longus (ECRL) and extensor carpi radialis brevis (ECRB) tendons, following them distally to the extensor retinaculum. Any evidence of tenosynovitis or constriction of the second dorsal compartment is an indication for synovectomy and release. Extend the incision longitudinally 1 to 2 cm distally to visualize the wrist extensor tendons. Open the second compartment longitudinally, and débride the synovium from the tendons and fibro-osseous tunnel. Replace the tendon in the tunnel, but do not close the retinaculum. If the second compartment was opened, apply a plaster splint with the wrist in neutral.

Once the sutures are removed, a cock-up wrist splint is used until little pain is experienced with activity. Otherwise, a soft dressing is applied, and the patient is encouraged to start using the hand a few days postoperatively.

Extensor Carpi Ulnaris Tendinitis

Wood and Dobyns[70] state that the sixth dorsal compartment is the second most common site of stenosing tenosynovitis in the upper extremity. Extensor carpi ulnaris (ECU) tendinitis is commonly encountered in players of sports requiring repetitive wrist motion. ECU tendinitis and subluxation are included in the differential diagnosis of ulnar-sided wrist pain. In the supinated position, the ECU tendon is located in a dorsal position, whereas when the forearm is pronated, the ECU tendon is found ulnarly. The extensor retinaculum lies over the sixth compartment. A septum anchors the fibro-osseous tunnel to the radius dorsally, and the retinaculum attaches volarly to the pisiform and triquetrum.[76] The ECU tendon is bound to the ulna by a distinct subsheath that merges with the capsule of the distal radioulnar joint (DRUJ) proximally and the triangular fibrocartilage complex (TFCC) distally.

ECU tendinitis produces pain and swelling dorsally over the ulna. Occasionally, crepitance is noted. A diagnostic and therapeutic injection of lidocaine and cortisone is often required to confirm and treat the process. Treatment starts with splinting and NSAIDs. Rest, ice, compression, and elevation are the mainstays of conservative care. If the disorder is treated in the inflammatory stage, cortisone is usually curative. Progressive fibrosis of the sixth compartment may require surgical release.[77]

Traumatic rupture of the ECU subsheath can cause a painful subluxation syndrome. If the extensor retinaculum is also disrupted, chronic dislocation can occur. This extensive an injury occurs after forced supination, palmar flexion, and ulnar deviation of the wrist. An acute injury is treated with a long-arm cast in full supination and neutral wrist position for 4 to 6 weeks. A chronic or recalcitrant condition requires open reconstruction of the retinaculum.[78–82]

SURGICAL PROCEDURE

Surgical treatment of these conditions is uncommon, but is performed as follows: Use a dorsal longitudinal incision over the sixth compartment and ulnar head. Spare branches of the dorsal sensory ulnar nerve with gentle dissection. In stenosing tenosynovitis, open the extensor retinaculum sharply longitudinally over the top of the tendon. Open the subsheath on the radial border, and release the radial septum of the sixth compartment. Repair the extensor retinaculum securely. For an unstable ECU tendon, the extensor retinaculum can be repaired. If a direct repair is not possible, or for a chronic dislocation, develop a strip of extensor retinaculum for the repair as an ulnarly based flap from the fourth and fifth compartments. Suture the retinacular flap over the ECU tendon, attaching it firmly to the remnant of the sixth dorsal compartment septa both ulnar and radial to the ECU tendon.

After a release procedure, the arm is immobilized in 20° of wrist extension for 3 weeks. Then a gradual rehabilitation program is initiated. The postoperative regimen for a reconstructive procedure is a long-arm cast at 90° of elbow flexion and 20° to 30° of wrist extension in neutral forearm rotation and deviation. After 6 weeks of immobilization, a rehabilitation protocol is initiated. Activity is restricted for 6 weeks more before the patient is allowed to resume full activity. It may take 6 to 9 months before a return to normal function is achieved.

Flexor Carpi Radialis Tendinitis

Volar wrist pain is a common complaint in both athletic and occupational settings. Flexor carpi radialis (FCR) tendinitis is not an often-diagnosed condition,[83] possibly owing to a lack of awareness, failure of diagnosis, and high prevalence of other conditions on the volar radial side of the wrist. Carpal tunnel syndrome, volar ganglions, scaphoid fractures and non-unions, basal joint instability, and arthritis are common entities that produce volar radial wrist pain. Linburg syndrome—anomalous tendon slips between the flexor pollicis longus and flexor digitorum profundus—is an often-quoted cause of radial volar wrist pain.[84, 85]

Repetitive wrist motions using a racquet, club, or bat can cause synovitis, tendinitis, and subsequent stenosis. The patient complains of pain with wrist flexion, which often radiates along the course of the FCR tendon. Swelling is rarely noted. Pain with resisted wrist flexion and palpation of the FCR tendon is highly suggestive of the disorder, especially if it recreates the patient's symptoms. Lister[86] has reported a Finkelstein-type test for FCR disease that entails suddenly dorsiflexing the relaxed wrist. Confirmation can be obtained by an anesthetic injection into the FCR sheath, and cortisone, if added, often is curative in the early stages.

Fitton and colleagues[87] in 1968 demonstrated that FCR tendinitis is predominantly a problem of the "over-fifty" population. With more aggressive leisure activity and prolongation of sports careers, the disease is being identified more commonly in recreational athletes. The FCR tendon passes through a separate sheath in the wrist that runs over the scaphoid tubercle before taking a 30° dorsal turn. It next courses over the trapezial ridge before inserting on the second and third metacarpals. A small slip of FCR does insert into the trapezium. Ninety percent of the tunnel is occupied by the FCR tendon,[32] making it a snug fit. The close association of the tendon with the scaphoid and trapezium may make this syndrome a concomitant disease in the older patient with a basal joint disorder.

Initial treatment comprises rest, NSAIDs, restricted activity, splinting, and a cortisone injection if necessary. Surgical treatment for this problem has been described.[87, 88]

SURGICAL PROCEDURE

Center the incision over the FCR tendon sheath, beginning proximal to the wrist crease volarly and extending distally over the proximal thenar eminence. Protect the palmar cutaneous branch of the medial nerve, superficial radial sensory branches, and lateral antebrachial cutaneous nerves. Elevate the origin of the thenar muscles from the transverse carpal ligament, thereby exposing the sheath of the FCR tendon. Incise the sheath from the distal aspect of the forearm to the trapezial crest. The tendon now can be seen entering the FCR tunnel. Incise the tunnel along the ulnar margin of the trapezial crest (about 3 cm). Verify that the tendon has been completely released by pulling it out of the trapezial groove. Inspect the floor of the sheath and tunnel, and excise any bony spicules or osteophytes that may be rubbing on the tendon.

Suture flaps of local soft tissue over exposed bone to prevent adhesions. Débride thickened synovium from the tendon, and repair partial ruptures and attritional areas with nylon core sutures and an epitenon running stitch if possible.

Splint the wrist in slight dorsiflexion until the sutures are removed, and then start an active range-of-motion program. Resistance exercises are not started for 6 weeks if the tendon was repaired.

Flexor Carpi Ulnaris/Pisotriquetral Disorders

Flexor carpi ulnaris (FCU) tendinitis and disorders of the pisiform are relatively common entities in racquet sports players and golf enthusiasts. Active flexion and extension of the wrist, while firmly gripping and ulnarly deviating, increase direct pressure on the sesamoid and FCU tendon insertion. Instability of the pisotriquetral joint and ulnar nerve symptoms can occur. Helal[89] treated patients with hyperligamentous laxity as well as local trauma, and believed that the laxity could contribute to pisotriquetral instability and arthritis.

Resisted flexion of the wrist and palpation of the FCU tendon can produce pain in patients with a tendinitis or pisiform disorder. The diseased pisiform causes symptoms if a direct load is placed on it, grinding it into the triquetrum, or if attempts are made to sublux the pisiform. Radiographs in a 20° supinated oblique projection[90] show the pisotriquetral joint, possibly demonstrating degenerative changes. The radiographs may also show evidence of calcific tendinitis.

The initial treatment is the same for both conditions. Resting the wrist in 20° of extension, NSAIDs, and limited activity are instituted. FCU tendinitis usually responds to conservative care, but often, a peritendinous injection of cortisone at the tendon pisiform junction is required. For pisotriquetral disorders, the injection is made into the pisotriquetral joint. Palmieri[91] reports a 35 to 40 percent success rate of conservative care for these disorders. If conservative measures fail, surgical removal of the pisiform is recommended.[89–91]

SURGICAL PROCEDURE

The surgical approach is centered over the pisiform: Make a zigzag incision in the hypothenar eminence centered over the pisiform. Extend the incision proximally in a longitudinal fashion along the FCU tendon if greater exposure is required. For patients with ulnar nerve symptoms, open Guyon's canal completely and inspect the ulnar nerve. Subperiosteally, shell out the pisiform from the FCU tendon. Inspect the triquetral articulation of the pisiform, and remove any spurs.[92] Repair the cleft in the FCU tendon with a nonabsorbable suture, preferably burying the knots.

Immobilize the wrist in 20° of dorsiflexion until the sutures are removed.

A removable orthosis is used to rest the tissues. A range-of-motion exercise program, scar management, and desensitization techniques form the cornerstone of postoperative management. Resistive exercises are started at 6 weeks.

Triangular Fibrocartilage Complex Disorders

Another cause of ulnar sided wrist pain in the athlete is triangular fibrocartilage complex (TFCC) disorders. They can be secondary to acute trauma or degeneration. Palpation along the ulnar head and the dorsal and palmar TFCC attachments can localize the problem. Flexion and extension of the wrist in ulnar deviation reproduce symptoms. An unstable tear produces a click with motion.

Gymnast's Wrist

Gymnastics provides a perfect example of injuries that can occur to the musculoskeletal systems from constant overuse. Any high-energy sport can cause acute fractures and injuries. Scaphoid fractures, scapholunate ligament tears, radius and ulna fractures, and finger dislocations and fractures all can result from a miscalculated or unforeseen event during practice or competition.

To the chronic injuries and overuse phenomenon associated with gymnastics must be added a different dimension to the problem: injury to a developing musculoskeletal system. Entry into gymnastics starts at an early age, often as early as 7 years old. The career may be short, usually ending competition by age 20. Training for an elite athlete may involve 30 hours per week. This practice allows ample time to overuse the upper extremities, especially in a weight-bearing mode for which they were not designed. The injury rate for female gymnasts ranges from 0.7/100 per year in noncompetitive participants to 5/100 per year in those competing at the Olympic level.[93] Overall, the upper extremity accounts for 25 to 31 percent of these injuries.[94]

Many authorities can attest to the dramatically increased popularity of gymnastics over the past 20 years.[93–96] The sheer number of people becoming involved increases the likelihood that the average orthopedic or hand surgeon will treat gymnasts with these problems or, for that matter, athletes in other sports with similar injuries.

Markoff and associates[97] instrumented a standard pommel horse with specially designed load cells to study the wrist-loading patterns of male gymnasts. They showed that the wrist impact forces and loading rates for a gymnast aggressively performing an exercise routine are comparable to those recorded at heel strike in a runner. A force magnitude up to two times body weight and a loading rate up to 219 body weights per second were recorded. These are exceptionally high for a joint not regularly under such a compressive load. The shear stresses involved in pivoting on the loaded wrist adds further insult to the distal radius.

Gymnast's wrist is not a single pathologic entity but represents one or a combination of related clinical entities. The common disorders that affect the wrist in this group of athletes are discussed individually in the following sections.

DISTAL RADIAL PHYSIS STRESS REACTION

Read[98] in 1981 reported on three gymnasts and Aubergé[99] in 1984 reported on 84 of 105 young gymnasts with radiographic changes in the distal radius growth plate. Roy and associates[100] found that 42 percent (11 of 26) of the gymnasts they studied had similar stress reactions on radiographic examination. Carter and Aldridge[101] provided more detail about the radiographic changes, describing widening of the distal radius growth plate, particularly on its volar aspect, with narrowing of the adjacent epiphysis (Fig. 28–3). The physis had a radiographically hazy quality owing to irregularity of the border between the cartilage and the metaphyseal zone of ossification. The distal ulnar epiphysis was also narrowed. Other reports of ulnar growth plate changes have emerged.[102] Szot and Galaj,[103] in reviewing elite gymnasts, have shown a strong correlation between the duration of training, radiographic changes, and wrist symptoms. Carter and Aldridge[101] have demonstrated a retardation of bone age of the distal radius in their group of gymnasts.

Mendelbaum and colleagues,[95] and DeSmet and co-workers,[104] have shown a statistically significant increase in positive ulnar variance in female gymnasts. Albanese and colleagues[105] reported on three cases of premature distal radial physeal closure in skeletally immature competitive gymnasts. Their patients were symptomatic from ulnar abutment syndrome. They propose that ulnar shortening can be used to treat the condition definitively but recommend limitation of activity at the first sign of symptoms to prevent physeal closure. Vender and Watson[106] report a case of acquired bilateral Madelung-like deformity in a gymnast. Asymmetric closure of the distal radial physis occurred, resulting in an increased radial-ulnar slope. The more symptomatic side eventually required a matched hemiresection arthroplasty for distal radioulnar joint arthrosis.[107]

To treat the symptomatic physeal stress reaction, Roy and colleagues[100] and Carter and Aldridge[101] propose similar recommendations. For patients with symptoms but without radiographic changes, 4 weeks of rest usually allows the condition to resolve. The patient should be precluded from weight-bearing activity on the wrist until all symptoms have abated.

Splints or casts can be used for the more symptomatic patient. If radiographic changes are seen, the prognosis is not as good, and it often takes 3 to 4 months for the symptoms to resolve. During the healing phase, the gymnast can continue other workout activities, such as stretching, strengthening of unaffected limbs, and floor moves without tumbling. No weight bearing on the affected wrist is allowed until the physical examination is benign and all the patient's complaints have resolved. A gradual progressive workout is initiated, and a taping program to prevent maximal wrist dorsiflexion is instituted. Most importantly, coaches and family members need to be educated about the causes and potential problems of the disease process. This step enables the coaching staff to ensure that proper technique is enforced in training and to recognize an injury so appropriate treatment can be started earlier.

Gymnasts use a variety of grip and wrist supports as standard equipment (Figs. 28–4 and 28–5) and as prophylactic and therapeutic devices (Figs. 28–6 and 28–7) to reduce stress across the wrist or to prevent the extremes of wrist positioning in the loaded position.

CARPAL STRESS REACTION

Carpal stress injuries, though uncommon or underdiagnosed, have been reported. To date, five cases of stress fractures of the scaphoid have been reported, four of which occurred in gymnasts.[108, 109] Stress fractures occurred through the waist region. It was believed that repeated loads in compression and dorsiflexion resulted in the stress reaction. In all four patients who had bone scans, there was increased bony uptake in the scaphoid. Plain radiographs are not always diagnostic, but for a suspicious history, anatomic snuffbox tenderness, and any subtle changes on conventional radiographs, empiric treatment should be given or a confirmatory bone scan obtained.[110] If this reaction is recognized and treated early, the duration of symptoms can be shortened, and the risk of a complete fracture with displacement or of a non-union leading to surgery can be reduced. Magnetic resonance (MR) imaging of the wrist can confirm the diagnosis.

Two collegiate gymnasts have been reported to have developed avascular necrosis of the capitate.[111] The two cases had similar presentations, consisting of chronic progressive wrist pain of more than a year's duration without an identifiable inciting event. Radiographs revealed resorption of the proximal capitate. Physical examination demonstrated hand and wrist swelling, focal tenderness over the capitolunate interval, and significantly restricted range of motion. The capitate receives nutrient vessels at the neck-body junction. It is proposed that trauma by repeated capitate dorsiflexion with impingement on the dorsal lunate ridge interrupts the capitate blood supply. Both patients were successfully treated by resection of the affected bone and drilling of the capitate sur-

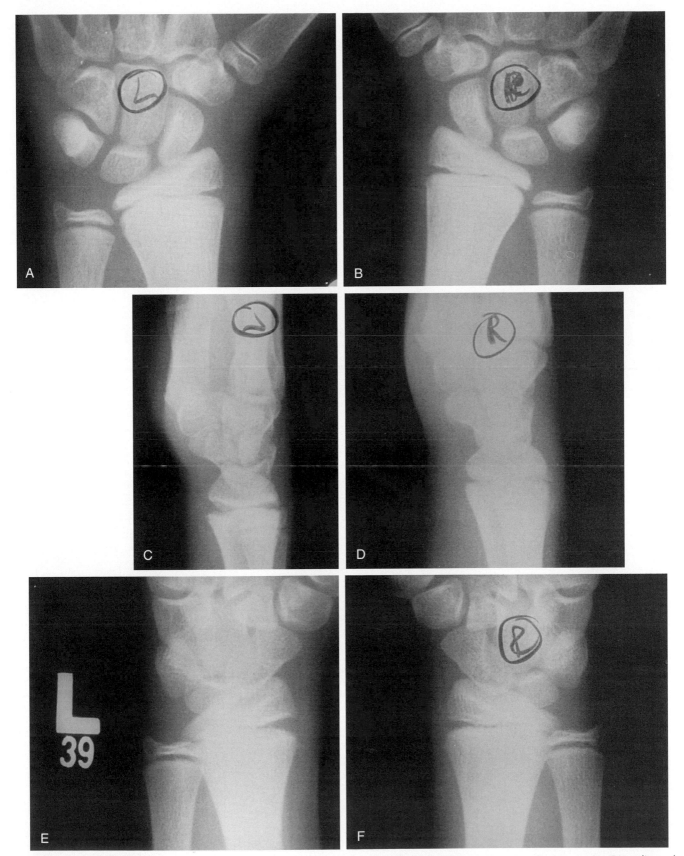

Figure 28–3. Radiographs show evidence of a left distal radius physis injury in an 11-year-old competitive gymnast. Posteroanterior (PA) radiographs of the symptomatic left (A) and right (B) wrists are normal. C and D, The lateral radiographs demonstrate slight physeal widening volarly on the left wrist. PA radiographs taken with the wrist in midpronation clearly demonstrate widening of the volar radial physis in the left wrist (E), compared with the right (F). (Courtesy of Gerard T. Gabel, MD.)

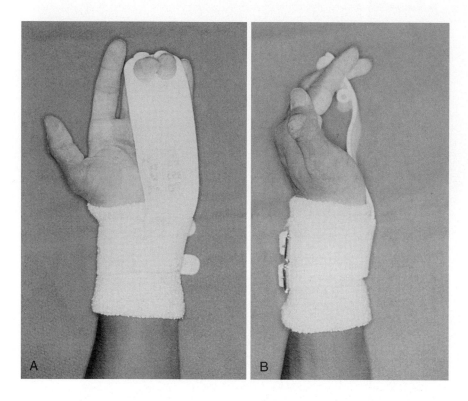

Figure 28–4. *A* and *B*, A gymnast wearing a dowel grip. (Courtesy of US Glove, Inc., Albuquerque, NM.) The device transfers the load across the wrist, and decreases friction on the skin when the hands are gripping a bar apparatus. The dowel increases the ability to grasp the bar without requiring supramaximal grip strength.

Figure 28–5. *A* and *B*, A gymnast wearing a wrist support that provides a less restricted range of motion.

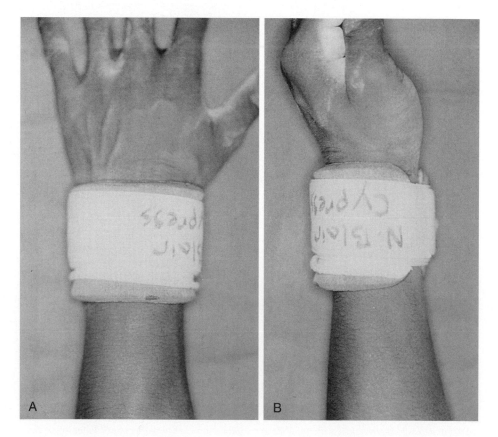

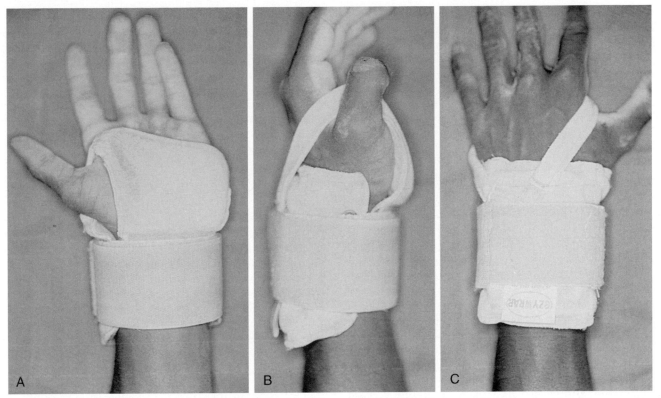

Figure 28–6. *A* to *C,* A brace that provides more support to the wrist, prevents maximum dorsiflexion, and includes a cushion palmar support pad. (Courtesy of eZYWRAP, Gibson, Englewood, CO.)

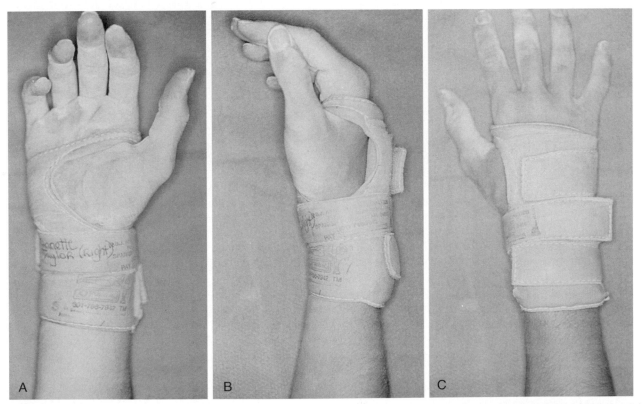

Figure 28–7. *A* to *C,* The lion's paw brace restricts dorsiflexion and is used by gymnasts and platform divers. (Courtesy of RBJ Athletic Specialties, Spanish Fork, UT.)

face. It is possible that late reconstruction will be necessary after such a procedure, and a limited intercarpal fusion required.

IMPINGEMENT

Several common entities that cause dorsal wrist pain have not yet been discussed. Scaphoid and lunate impingement syndrome, occult dorsal ganglion, and "wrist capsulitis" in a gymnast fit in this category. The wrist ganglion, triangular fibrocartilage complex tear, ulnar impaction syndrome, carpal instability, and intercarpal ligament tear may be more common; their description and treatment are well covered in other chapters of this text.

Scaphoid and lunate impingement syndromes result from repetitive maximum dorsiflexion in which the carpal bones abut against the dorsal lip of the distal radius.[96, 112] The symptoms are pain, decreased grip strength, and focal tenderness aggravated by wrist dorsiflexion. Radiographs may be negative or may show sclerosis of the bones, but they often reveal a small ossicle in the soft tissue contiguous with the dorsal rim of the radius. Hypertrophic ridging or osteophytes on the dorsal scaphoid, lunate, or radius can also be identified. Lateral radiographs and occasionally tomograms are necessary to define the pathology. Rest, NSAIDs, avoidance of dorsiflexion enforced by a splint or cast, and perhaps a steroid injection along the dorsal rim are the mainstays of care. Once symptoms are controlled, a gradual return to activity is allowed. Special splints or taping can prevent maximum dorsiflexion with activity and a subsequent recurrence of the symptoms. If symptoms return, excision of ossicles or a cheilectomy is indicated. If the impingement is between the scaphoid and radial styloid, a styloidectomy can be considered. A synovectomy is occasionally helpful for chronically thickened dorsal synovium.

OCCULT GANGLIA

When the active athlete has dorsal wrist pain without a palpable mass, the diagnosis of occult ganglia is often overlooked. Gunther[113] reports that a traumatic event is not usually part of the history in patients with occult ganglia. In his series of ten patients, eight were skilled musicians or avid atheletes, and the remaining two did significant work with their hands. Sanders[114] reported on nine patients treated for occult ganglia. None had a palpable ganglion, though one had a 2-mm to 3-mm intracapsular ganglion at the time of surgery, and two had obvious mucinous degeneration at the attachment of the dorsal capsule to the scapholunate ligament. In the remaining six patients, the diagnosis was confirmed with microscopic examination. In all nine patients pathologic areas of mucinous degeneration consistent with incipient ganglion formation were observed on the permanent pathology sections.[114]

Of the 19 patients studied in Sander's[114] and

Gunther's[113] reports, only 1 reported no improvement in symptoms following ganglion excision. Nine patients had complete relief of symptoms and return of full range of motion. Six patients had an "odd" feeling or tightening after significant activity, 2 patients had improvement but did not return to unlimited activity, and 1 patient was lost to follow-up. Gunther[113] reported that his patients who had reported a deep continuous ache preoperatively obtained almost complete symptomatic relief immediately after surgery. Those initially affected only after strenuous activity or musical performances noted significant pain relief at 2 months, though it usually took 5 months for a full return of motion. Gunther[113] also reported that of the 5 patients with follow-up radiographs, none demonstrated scapholunate instability or widening.

With a negative plain radiograph, MR imaging would be the advanced imaging study of choice. Hollister and associates[115] reported a case in which MRI imaging showed a nonpalpable dorsal ganglion in a patient with wrist pain. The high water content of the ganglion enhances on a T_2-weighted image. Vo and colleagues[116] reported a series of 14 patients with chronic dorsal wrist pain of unknown etiology who underwent MR imaging formatted to show the scapholunate region. Ten of the patients had evidence of occult ganglia on the MR images. In 7 patients, the diagnosis was confirmed at surgery, 1 patient's ganglion subsequently became palpable, and the other 2 declined operative intervention. The dimension of the ganglia ranged from 2 to 7 mm with an average of 4.7 mm.

Of the four patients reported by Vo and colleagues[116] in whom MR imaging was negative, one patient underwent surgical exploration, and pathologic examination showed an occult ganglion. The other three patients did not have a final diagnosis. For patients with dorsal wrist pain in whom conservative care fails, MR imaging is warranted. Surgical intervention can be planned on the basis of the MR findings.

Surgical Procedure

Our operative technique is as follows: Make a 4-cm transverse incision centered over the area of maximal tenderness. After incision of the skin, bluntly dissect the subcutaneous tissue to avoid injury to superficial nerve branches. Open the interval between the third and fourth compartments by longitudinally incising the distal fourth of the extensor retinaculum. By this time, a small ganglion or area of degeneration is usually evident. Remove the small ganglion in standard fashion by excising a small margin of surrounding capsule that includes the stalk. If an area of degeneration is encountered, curette or sharply remove the material without disturbing normal scapholunate ligament. If the dorsal capsule appears normal, make a 1-cm transverse incision in the dorsal capsule proximal to the scapholunate ligament. Inspect the undersurface of the dorsal capsule and intra-articular scapholunate ligament. Remove the ganglion or area of degeneration sharply, and repair the dorsal capsule. If the posterior interosseous is compressed, or if a neuroma is present, excise up to 1 cm of the nerve. Close the distal retinaculum and skin. Apply a splint for 5 to 10 days before starting the patient on a rehabilitation program.

CAPSULITIS

Wrist capsulitis and synovitis probably are an early stage of the dorsal impingement syndrome. Dorsiflexion causes impingement of the soft tissue between the carpus and distal radius. Most patients have a diffuse pain with warmth, swelling, and limited use of the hand. When the physical examination localizes the pain to one area, a more specific diagnosis is offered. Capsulitis is a diagnosis of exclusion. If plain radiographs or an MR image has localized findings, a more specific diagnosis is made.[117] Aronsen[118] believes that inflammation is the most common cause of dorsal wrist pain in athletes and that treatment should be directed to decreasing the symptoms, allowing the athlete to continue competing. We believe that the diagnoses of stress fractures and ligament injuries need to be excluded before symptomatic treatment is instituted. Treatment includes judicious rest, NSAIDs, strengthening of the wrist flexors, and taping or splinting of the wrist to prevent maximum dorsiflexion. Cortisone can reduce the local synovitis.

Cyclist's Palsy

Cycling is not a new sport, but its increasing popularity in the United States over the past 20 years has exposed the medical community to a variety of musculoskeletal disorders related to cycling. Most hand and wrist conditions in cyclists are the result of repetitive motion and compressive injuries, which are not unfamiliar in an occupational medicine setting.

Destot[119] is credited with describing the first report of cyclist's palsy in 1896, and Hunt[120] described a neuritis of the ulnar nerve in the hand of occupational origin. Harris[121] added to Hunt's work, reporting his cases of occupational pressure neuritis of the ulnar nerve. Treatment and follow-up were not reported. Since Destot's[119] first description, numerous reports have surfaced in the literature of cycling-related ulnar nerve compressive neuropathy.[122–126] Hoyt[127] reported the largest series of cyclist's neuropathy; 117 cases were seen over 4 years. All of his patients returned to cycling without recurrence of the neuropathy by making the proper adjustments to their bicycles or their cycling techniques.

The symptoms reported in cyclists include pain in the hypothenar region, and paresthesia, dysesthesia, or anesthesia in the ulnar border of the hand along with the ring and little fingers. Weakness of grip strength, atrophy of the intrinsic muscles, and claw-ing of the ring and little fingers can be found, depending on the duration and severity of the symptoms. Tenderness is often elicited over Guyon's canal, the pisiform, and the hook of the hamate. The dominant hand is more often affected.[126]

Eckman and colleagues[122] reported prolonged bilateral distal motor latency in the deep branch of the ulnar nerve in a cyclist. Noth and associates[126] demonstrated both motor and sensory latency prolongation in their two patients who underwent nerve conduction studies. Jackson[128] performed nerve conduction studies on 20 members of a cycling club chosen at random. Nine had complaints of hand or finger numbness during cycling that resolved after completion of the ride. The results of nerve conduction studies were normal for all 20 cyclists. The cyclists reported diminished symptoms after adjusting their bicycles and modifying their cycling techniques.

Shea and McClain[59] provided a classification system for ulnar neuropathy in the hand. They described three clinical syndromes corresponding to the anatomic site of compression (Table 28–3).

Type I syndrome is combined motor and sensory loss. All ulnar innervated hand muscles are weak. Also, there is sensory loss over the hypothenar eminence and the volar aspect of the ring and little fingers. The compressive lesion is just proximal to or in Guyon's canal before the bifurcation of the ulnar nerve. Normal sensation over the dorsal ulnar area of the hand indicates that the dorsal sensory branch of the ulnar nerve is intact; thus, the lesion is not proximal to the wrist. The type II syndrome is solely motor loss. The deep branch of the ulnar nerve is involved, sparing the superficial sensory branch. This involvement occurs as the nerve exits Guyon's canal or more distally. It is also possible to produce the lesion by traction of the nerve against the hook of the hamate, which occurs with prolonged hyperextension of the wrist. Type III syndrome has only sensory changes,

Table 28–3. CLASSIFICATION OF ULNAR NEUROPATHY IN THE HAND

Type		Symptoms
I	Sensory:	Hypothenar eminence and volar ring and little finger
	Motor:	Ulnar intrinsic muscle weakness
	Location:	Distal to dorsal ulnar sensory nerve branch takeoff, proximal to superficial sensory branch takeoff in Guyon's canal
II	Sensory:	None
	Motor:	Ulnar intrinsic muscle weakness
	Location:	Distal to superficial sensory branch takeoff in Guyon's canal or distal to it
III	Sensory:	Hypothenar eminence and volar ring and little finger
	Motor:	None
	Location:	Superficial sensory ulnar nerve involvement only

From Shea JD, McClain EJ: Ulnar-nerve compression syndrome at and below the wrist. J Bone Joint Surg 51A:1095–1103, 1969.

manifested as hypesthesia over the hypothenar eminence and the volar ring and little fingers.

Cyclists with ulnar neuropathy were reported by Haloua and coworkers.[189] Their series included 55 hands with disorders classified according to Shea and McClain[59] system. Of these hands, 67 percent had type I, 12.5 percent had type II, and 8 percent had type III syndromes. The remaining hands had more proximal lesions.

Median nerve symptoms are reported with less frequency than ulnar nerve dysfunction. Maimaris and Zadeh[130] reported their survey results of 89 coast-to-coast bicycle tour participants, of whom 23 complained of some hand numbness. Though the group manifested mostly ulnar-sided symptoms, 10 cyclists experienced median nerve symptoms as well. Braithwaite[131] described acute bilateral carpal tunnel symptoms in a novice cyclist after a prolonged bicycle ride. The symptoms responded to conservative care.

Evaluation of the cyclist's complaint of hand numbness or weakness includes a careful history of the symptoms and of the individual's occupational and recreational activities. Specific questions elicit information about the type of bicycle and handlebar, protective equipment, including gloves and handlebar padding, preferred riding posture, and frequency of hand position changes. A detailed physical examination including a sensory and motor neurological evaluation should be performed.

Because most cases respond to conservative care alone, it should be used before one proceeds to diagnostic testing.[127] A progressive treatment regimen consists of restricted activity, NSAIDs, and splinting. Once the patient shows a response, prevention of recurrence should be addressed. Hoyt[132] advises changing hand position frequently while riding. The use of gloves, a padded handlebar, and a properly fitted bicycle distributes the body weight evenly on the hands and reduces nerve compression. Burke[133, 134] states that the gloves should have adequate palmar padding but should not restrict flexibility. He believes that gel padding may offer better protection than the standard foam pads, which may compress with time and lose their energy-absorbing capacity. Proper bicycle fit requires that the distance from the "toe" of the seat to the handlebar be the same as the distance from the elbow to the fingertips, measured with the seat and handlebar at the same level. This fit prevents excessive reaching and the resultant increasing pressure on the palm.

Handlebar adjustments can also improve a rider's posture. Drop handlebars come in a variety of sizes and curves to accommodate the rider. If a satisfactory drop handlebar can not be fitted, consideration should be given to an upright handlebar. The upright handlebar keeps the wrist in less ulnar deviation with less weight bearing on the hypothenar region.

If adequate response is not obtained with these adjustments, electrodiagnostic studies to confirm the location of the compression neuropathy are indicated. MR imaging of Guyon's canal will help evaluate for mass lesions such as a ganglion[59, 135] before surgical exploration is considered. If electrodiagnostic studies demonstrate a conduction block across Guyon's canal, exploration and surgical release are indicated. If median nerve symptoms predominate, a carpal tunnel release alone will most likely be effective.[136]

Vasculitis/Thrombosis

Baseball,[137–140] among other sports,[140–143] has been associated with vascular compromise of the hand and fingers. Lowrey and colleagues[137] studied the effect of repeated trauma in baseball catchers. Twenty professional, one collegiate, and one retired catchers were evaluated using a modified Allen's test and Doppler flow studies. Ten volunteers from the group had a perfusion scan with radioactive technetium Tc 99m. Only 5 had evidence of normal circulation to the index finger of the catching hand. These investigators concluded that repetitive impact could result in vascular changes and that extra padding in the mitt may be protective.

Sugawara and associates[138] reported on eight baseball players who developed digital ischemia as a result of repetitive impact. Their symptoms were coolness, numbness, cyanosis, and a positive digital Allen test. No treatment was described. By surveying baseball players at various ages, these researchers found no digital ischemia in junior high school players and a 40 percent incidence in college age players. They showed that accumulated play time correlated with the probability of developing digital ischemia.

Nuber and coworkers[140] reported that 2 of their 13 athletes with ischemic symptoms required hospitalization because of severe hand ischemia. Evaluation by arteriogram showed nonfilling of the ulnar artery in one patient and superficial arch occlusion in the other. Both cases responded to intravenous papaverine followed by intravenous dextran and heparin. Itoh and colleagues[139] reported on three baseball pitchers with fingertip necrosis due to ischemia. They all required surgical release of the entrapped vascular bundles. One required release of Cleland's ligament, and the other two showed response to decompression of the vessels in the lumbrical canal. All returned to pitching without a decrease in performance.

Microvascular repair of sports-related vascular trauma has been reported. Ho and associates[14] reported successful repair of an ulnar artery aneurysm and a digital artery aneurysm in symptomatic athletes that resulted from blunt trauma. Follow-up showed no recurrence and a resumption of full activity. In one report, Porubsky and colleagues[142] reported on a 22-year-old hockey player who was struck in the hypothenar area by a hockey stick. Immediate pain was noted, and grip strength weakness resolved after 2 months. The symptoms on presentation included coolness of the ulnar digits and decreased sensation of the ulnar half of the hand with awakening at night.

Arteriograms demonstrated complete ulnar artery occlusion. Symptoms resolved after a 15-cm section of the ulnar artery was replaced from the mid-forearm to the superficial arch with reversed saphenous vein graft (Fig. 28–8).

Koman and Urbaniak[144] proposed a patient-oriented treatment algorithm for patients with symptomatic ulnar artery insufficiency. No single treatment is suitable for every patient, especially considering a high incidence of some persistent symptoms. Surgery is indicated in patients who have local disease or persistent symptoms, or for whom digital survival is in question. The affected segment is resected. If adequate backflow is observed, ligation is all that is necessary; otherwise, end-to-end anastamosis or vein grafting is required.

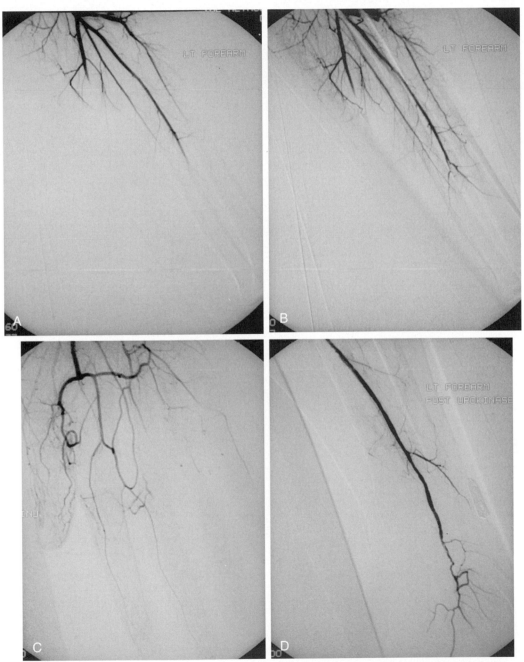

Figure 28–8. Angiograms of a 21-year-old university football defensive lineman who frequently used his forearm to slap opposing players' helmets. He acutely developed pain, pallor, and paresthesia in the ulnar half of his left hand. *A* and *B*, Sequential angiogram pictures demonstrate nonfilling of the ulnar artery proximally. *C*, Shows poor filling of half of the long, ring, and little fingers through the arch connections to the radial artery. The patient was treated with priscoline and selective catheterization of the ulnar artery, followed by urokinase infusion. *D*, Demonstrates patency of the ulnar artery, though distally, evidence of thrombus remains. The patient continues to have minor symptoms of a cool sensation with almost complete resolution of the paresthesias. He has not returned to playing football, nor has he had surgical revascularization. (Courtesy of David H. Hildreth, MD.)

CONCLUSION

There is a large overlap of disorders and illnesses that can be categorized either as occupational disease or as sports injury. The common ground affords a natural grouping of these topics into a single discussion as we have done here. Many practicing physicians have had little exposure to the realm of occupational medicine—the ergonomics involved, the unique injuries, and the legal foundation. Moreover, the field of sports medicine is dominated by knee and shoulder injuries, which are often the only exposure the resident physician receives. Our intent is to provide the clinician with a solid core of material upon which the clinician can build through experience and future study.

References

1. 23 OSH Rep (BNA) 23 (1994).
2. The Texas Workers' Compensation Act, Texas Labor Code Title 5 Subtitle A 9/1/93.
3. Keller B: U.S. health aide urges logging of job injury data. NY Times, June 21, 1984.
4. Medical Cost Containment in Workers' Compensation: A National Inventory, 1991–1992. Cambridge, MA: Workers' Compensation Research Institute, 1994.
5. Webster BS, Snook SH: The cost of compensable upper extremity cumulative trauma disorders. J Occup Environ Med 36:713–717, 1994.
6. Himmelstein JS, Feuerstein M, Stanek EJ, et al: Work related upper extremity disorders and work disability: Clinical and psychosocial presentation. J Occup Environ Med 37:1278–1285, 1995.
7. Fahs MC, Markowitz SB, Fischer E, et al: Health costs of occupational disease in New York State. Am J Ind Med 16:437–449, 1989.
8. Brancati FL, Hodgson MJ, Karpf M: Occupational exposures and diseases among medical inpatients. J Occup Environ Med 35:161–165, 1993.
9. McCunney RJ (ed): A Practical Approach to Occupational and Environmental Medicine, ed 2. Boston, Little, Brown, 1994, p 205.
10. The Occupational and Environmental Health Committee of the American Lung Association. Taking the occupational history. Ann Intern Med 88:641–651, 1983.
11. Franzblau A, Werner RA, Johnston E, Torrey S: Evaluation of current perception threshold testing as a screening procedure for carpal tunnel syndrome among industrial workers. J Occup Environ Med 35:1015–1021, 1994.
12. Checkosky CM, Bolanowski SJ, Cohen JC: Assessment of vibrotactile sensitivity in patients with carpal tunnel syndrome. J Occup Environ Med 38:593–601, 1996.
13. Gerr F, Letz R, Harris-Abbott D, Hopkins LC: Sensitivity and specificity of vibrometry for detection of carpal tunnel. J Occup Environ Med 37:1108–1115, 1995.
14. Occupational Injury and Illness in Texas: Report to the Texas Legislature. University of Houston, 1993.
15. DeHart RL: Guidelines for Establishing an Occupational Medical Program. The American Occupational Medicine Association, Washington D.C., 1987.
16. Ergonomic Program Management Guides for Meatpacking Plants, OSHA 3123. Washington, DC, Occupational Safety and Health Administration, 1990.
17. Hansen JA: OSHA Regulation and Ergonomic Health. J Occup Environ Med 35:42–46, 1993.
18. Mackinnon SE, Novak CB: Clinical commentary: Pathogenesis of cumulative trauma disorder. J Hand Surg 19A:873–883, 1994.
19. Hocking B: Epidemiological aspects of "repetition strain injury" in Telecom Australia. Med J Aust 147:218–222, 1987.
20. Graham G: Job satisfaction and repetition strain injury [dissertation]. Adelaids, Elton-Mayo School of Management, SA Institute of Technology, Australia, 1985, p 32.
21. Ryan A, Pimble J: Repetition strain injury and the influence of the work environment. Presented to the Australia-New Zealand Association for the Advancement of Sciences 55th Congress, Melbourne, Aug 26–30, 1985.
22. Ireland DCR: Psychological and physical aspects of occupational arm pain. J Hand Surg 13B:5–10, 1988.
23. Ireland DCR: Repetition strain injury: The Australian Experience—1992 update. J Hand Surg 20A:553–556, 1995.
24. Lucire Y: Neurosis in the workplace. Med J Aust 145:323–327, 1986.
25. Morgan RG: RSI. Med J Aust 1244:56, 1986.
26. Plog BA: Fundamentals of Industrial Hygiene, ed 3. Chicago, National Safety Council, 1988, pp 3–28.
27. Rossignol AM, Morse EP, Summers VM, Paynotto LD: Video display terminal use and reported health symptoms among Massachusetts clerical workers. J Occup Environ Med 29:112–118, 1987.
28. Arndt R: Working posture and musculoskeletal problems of video display terminal operators—review and reappraisal. Am Industrial Hygiene Association Journal 44:437–446, 1983.
29. Ergonomics User Manual, Brea, CA, IAC Industries, 1994.
30. World Health Organization: Work with visual display terminals: Psychosocial aspects and health. J Occup Environ Med 31:957–968, 1989.
31. Pelmear PL, Taylor W: Hand-arm vibration syndrome: Clinical evaluation and prevention. J Occup Environ Med 33:1144–1149, 1991.
32. Sakaurai T, Matoba T: Peripheral nerve responses to hand-arm vibrations. Scand J Work Environ Health 12:432–434, 1986.
33. Seppalainen AM: Nerve conduction in the vibration syndrome. Scan J Work Environ Health 1:82–84, 1970.
34. Seppalainen AM: Peripheral neuropathy in forestry workers: A field study. Scan J Work Environ Health 3:106–111, 1972.
35. Gemne G, Pyyko I, Taylor W, Pelmear PL: The Stockholm workshop scale for the classification of cold-induced Raynaud's phenomenon in the hand-arm vibration syndrome (revision of the Taylor-Pelmear scale). Scand J Work Environ Health 13:275–278, 1987.
36. Brammer AJ, Taylor W, Lundborg G: Sensorineural stages of the hand-arm vibration syndrome. Scand J Work Environ Health 13:279–282, 1987.
37. Pelmear P, Taylor W: Hand-arm vibration syndrome. J Fam Pract 38:180–184, 1994.
38. Whiteside JA, Fleagle SB, Kalenak A: Fractures and refractures in intercollegiate athletes. Am J Sports Med 9:369–377, 1981.
39. Canale ST, Cantler ED, Sisk TD, Freeman BL: A chronicle of injuries of an American intercollegiate football team. Am J Sports Med 9:384–389, 1981.
40. Ellsasser JC, Stein AH: Management of hand injuries in a professional football team: Review of 15 years of experience with one team. Am J Sports Med 7:178–182, 1979.
41. Raab DJ, Fischer DA, Quick DC: Lunate and perilunate dislocations in the professional football player. Am J Sports Med 22:841–845, 1994.
42. Henry JH, Lareau B, Neigut D: The injury rate in professional basketball. Am J Sports Med 10:16–18, 1982.
43. Shewring DJ, Matthewson MH: Injuries to the hand in Rugby Union Football. J Hand Surg 18B:122–124, 1993.
44. Degroot H, Mass DP: Hand injury patterns in softball players using a 16 inch ball. Am J Sports Med 16:260–265, 1988.
45. Lawson GM, Hajducka C, McQueen MM: Sports fractures of the distal radius—epidemiology and outcome. Injury 26:33–36, 1995.
46. Strickland JW: Philosophy of the treatment of athletes. Clin Sports Med 14:285–288, 1995.
47. Culver JE, Anderson TE: Fractures of the hand and wrist in the athlete. Clin Sports Med 11:101–128, 1992.

48. Markiewitz AD, Andrish JT: Hand and wrist injuries in the preadolescent and adolescent athlete. Clin Sports Med 11:203–225, 1992.

49. Green DP: Operative Hand Surgery. Ed 3, Vol 1 and 2. Churchill Livingstone, 1993.

50. Torisu T: Fracture of the hook of the hamate by a golf swing. Clin Orthop 83:91–94, 1972.

51. Stark HH, Jobe FW, Boyes JH, Ashworth CR: Fracture of the hook of the hamate in athletes. J Bone Joint Surg 59A:575–582, 1972.

52. Carter PR, Eaton RG, Little JW: Ununited fracture of the hook of the hamate. J Bone Joint Surg 59A:583–588, 1977.

53. Stark HH, Chao E-K, Zemel NP, et al: Fracture of the hook of the hamate. J Bone Joint Surg 71A:1202–1207, 1989.

54. Hart VL, Gaynor V: Roentgenographic study of the carpal canal. J Bone Joint Surg 23A:382–383, 1941.

55. Wilson JN: Profiles of the carpal canal. J Bone Joint Surg 36A:127–132, 1954.

56. Andress MR, Peckar VG: Fracture of the hook of the hamate. Br J Radiol 43:141–143, 1970.

57. Egawa M, Asai T: Fracture of the hook of the hamate: Report of six cases and the suitability of computerized tomography. J Hand Surg 8A:393–398, 1983.

58. Howard FM: Ulnar-nerve palsy in wrist fractures. J Bone Joint Surg 43A:1197–1201, 1961.

59. Shea JD, McClain EJ: Ulnar-nerve compression syndrome at and below the wrist. J Bone Joint Surg 51A:1095–1103, 1969.

60. Clayton ML: Rupture of the flexor tendons in carpal tunnel with specific reference to fracture of the hook of the hamate. (Proceedings of the American Society for Surgery of the Hand.) J Bone Joint Surg 51A:798–799, 1969.

61. Crosby EB, Linscheid RL: Rupture of the flexor profundus tendon of the ring finger secondary to ancient fracture of the hook of the hamate. J Bone Joint Surg 56A:1076–1078, 1974.

62. Milek MA, Boulas HJ: Flexor tendon ruptures secondary to hamate hook fractures. J Hand Surg 15A:740–744, 1990.

63. Whalen JL, Bishop AT, Linscheid RL: Nonoperative treatment of acute hamate hook fractures. J Hand Surg 17A:507–511, 1992.

64. Kiefhuber TR, Stern PJ: Upper extremity tendinitis and overuse syndrome in the athlete. Clin Sports Med 11:39–55, 1992.

65. Curwin S, Stanish WD: Tendinitis: Its Etiology and Treatment, Lexington, MA, The Collamore Press, 1984, pp 1–43.

66. Pitner MA: Pathophysiology of overuse injuries in the hand and wrist. Hand Clin 6:355–364, 1990.

67. Renstrom P, Johnson RJ: Overuse injuries in sports: A review. Sports Med 2:316–333, 1985.

68. Morgan ML, Arnold WJ: Mechanically induced synovitis. In Leadbetter WB, Buckwalter JA, Gordon SL (eds): Sports-Induced Inflammation. Park Ridge, IL, American Academy of Orthopaedic Surgeons, 1990, pp 331–335.

69. Wahl S, Renstrom P: Fibrosis in soft-tissue injuries. In Leadbetter WB, Buckwalter JA, Gordon SL (eds): Sports-Induced Inflammation. Park Ridge, IL, American Academy of Orthopaedic Surgeons, 1990, pp 637–647.

70. Wood MD, Dobyns JH: Sports related extraarticular wrist syndrome. Clin Orthop 202:93–102, 1986.

71. Froimson A: Tenosynovitis and tennis elbow. In Green DP (ed): Operative Hand Surgery, ed 3. New York, Churchill Livingstone, 1992, pp 1989–2006.

72. Howard NJ: Peritendinitis crepitans: A muscle-effort syndrome. J Bone Joint Surg 19A:447–459, 1937.

73. Grundberg AB, Reagan DS: Pathologic anatomy of the forearm: Intersection syndrome. J Hand Surg 10A:299–302, 1985.

74. Dobyns JH, Sim FH, Linscheid RL: Sports stress syndromes of the hand and wrist. Am J Sports Med 6:236–253, 1978.

75. Wood MB, Linscheid RL: Abductor pollicis bursitis. Clin Orthop 93:293–296, 1973.

76. Spinner M, Kaplan EB: Extensor carpi ulnaris: Its relationship to the stability of the distal radio-ulnar joint. Clin Orthop 68:124–129, 1970.

77. Hajj AA, Wood MB: Stenosing tenosynovitis of the extensor carpi ulnaris. J Hand Surg 11A:519–520, 1986.

78. Osterman AL, Moskow L, Low DW: Soft tissue injuries of the hand and wrist in racquet sports. Clin Sports Med 7:329–348, 1988.

79. Eckhardt WA, Palmer AK: Recurrent dislocation of the extensor carpi ulnaris tendon. J Hand Surg 61:629–631, 1981.

80. Burkhart SS, Wood MB, Linscheid RL: Post traumatic recurrent subluxation of the extensor carpi ulnaris tendon. J Hand Surg 7A:1–3, 1982.

81. Rayan GM: Recurrent dislocation of the extensor carpi ulnaris in athletes. Am J Sports Med 11:183–184, 1983.

82. Rowland SA: Acute traumatic subluxation of the extensor carpi ulnaris tendon at the wrist. J Hand Surg 11A:809–811, 1986.

83. Bishop AT, Gabel GT, Carmichael SW: Flexor carpi radialis tendonitis. Part I: Operative anatomy. J Bone Joint Surg 76A:1009–1013, 1994.

84. Linburg RM, Comstock BE: Anomalous tendon slips from the flexor pollicis longus to the flexor digitorum profundis. J Hand Surg 4:79–83, 1979.

85. Stern PJ: Tendonitis, overuse syndrome, and tendon injuries. Hand Clin 6:467–476, 1990.

86. Lister G: The Hand, ed 2. Edinburgh, Churchill Livingstone, 1984, p 244.

87. Fitton JM, Shea FW, Goldie W: Lesions of the flexor carpi radialis tendon and sheath causing pain at the wrist. J Bone Joint Surg 50B:359–363, 1968.

88. Gabel GT, Bishop AT, Wood MB: Flexor carpi radialis tendonitis. Part II: Results of operative treatment. J Bone Joint Surg 76A:1014–1018, 1994.

89. Helal B: Racquet players pisiform. Hand 10:87–91, 1978.

90. Carroll RE, Coyle MP: Dysfunction of the pisotriquetral joint: Treatment by excision of the pisiform. J Hand Surg 10A:703–707, 1985.

91. Palmieri TJ: Pisiform area pain treatment by pisiform excision. J Hand Surg 7:477–480, 1982.

92. Takami H, Takahashi S, Ando M, Kabata K: Rupture of the flexor tendon secondary to osteoarthritis of the pisotriquetral joint: Case report. J Trauma 31:1703–1706, 1991.

93. Pettrone FA, Ricciandelli E: Gymnastic injuries: The Virginia experience, 1982–1983. Am J Sports Med 15:59–62, 1987.

94. McAuley F, Hudash G, Shields K, et al: Injuries in women's gymnastics: The state of the art. Am J Sports Med 15:558–565, 1987.

95. Mendelbaum BR, Bartolozzi AR, Craig AD, et al: Wrist pain syndrome in the gymnast: Pathogenic, diagnostic, and therapeutic considerations. Am J Sports Med 17:305–317, 1989.

96. Dobyns JH, Gabel GT: Gymnast's wrist. Hand Clin 6:493–505, 1990.

97. Markolf KL, Shapiro MS, Mendelbaum BR, Teurlings L: Wrist loading patterns during pommel horse exercises. J Biomechanics 23:1001–1011, 1990.

98. Read MTF: Stress fractures of the distal radius in adolescent gymnasts. Br J Sports Med 15:272–276, 1981.

99. Aubergé T, Zenny JC, Duvallet A, et al: Etude de la maturation osséuse et des lésions ostéoarticulare des sportifs de haut niveau. J Radiol 65:555–561, 1984.

100. Roy S, Carne D, Singer K: Stress changes of the distal radial epiphysis in young gymnasts. Am J Sports Med 13:301–308, 1985.

101. Carter SR, Aldridge MJ: Stress injury of the distal radial growth plate. J Bone Joint Surg 70B:834–836, 1988.

102. Yong-Hing K, Wedge JH, Bowen CV: Chronic injury to the distal ulnar and radial growth plates in an adolescent gymnast. J Bone Joint Surg 70A:1087–1089, 1988.

103. Szot ZB, Galaj Z: Overloading changes in the motor system occurring in elite gymnasts. Int J Sports Med 6:36–40, 1985.

104. DeSmet L, Claessens A, Lafevre J, Beunen G: Gymnast's wrist: An epidemiologic survey of ulnar variance and stress changes of the radial physis in elite female gymnasts. Am J Sports Med 22:846–850, 1994.

105. Albanese SA, Palmer AK, Kerr DR, et al: Wrist pain and distal growth plate closure at the radius in gymnasts. J Pediatr Orthop 9:23–38, 1989.

106. Vender MI, Watson HK: Acquired Madelung-like deformity in a gymnast. J Hand Surg 13A:19–21, 1988.

107. Watson HK, Ryu J, Burgess RC: Matched distal ulnar resection. J Hand Surg 11A:812–817, 1986.
108. Manzione M, Pizzutillo PD: Stress fracture of the scaphoid waist: A case report. Am J Sports Med 9:268–269, 1981.
109. Hanks GA, Kalenak A, Bowman LS, Sebastianelli WJ: Stress fractures of the carpal scaphoid. J Bone Joint Surg 71A:938–941, 1989.
110. Patel N, Collier BD, Carrera GF, et al: High-resolution bone scintigraphy of the adult wrist. Clin Nucl Med 17:449–453, 1992.
111. Murakami S, Nakajima H: Aseptic necrosis of the capitate bone in two gymnasts. Am J Sports Med 12:170–173, 1984.
112. Linscheid RL, Dobyns JH: Athletic injuries of the wrist. Clin Orthop 198:141–151, 1985.
113. Gunther SF: Dorsal wrist pain and the occult scapholunate ganglion. J Hand Surg 10A:697–703, 1985.
114. Sanders WE: The occult dorsal carpal ganglion. J Hand Surg 10B:257–260, 1985.
115. Hollister AM, Sanders RA, McCann S: The use of MRI in the diagnosis of an occult ganglion cyst. Orthop Rev 28:1210–1212, 1989.
116. Vo P, Wright T, Hayden F, et al: Evaluating dorsal wrist pain: MRI diagnosis of occult dorsal wrist ganglion. J Hand Surg 20A:667–670, 1995.
117. Teitz CC: Sports medicine concerns in dance and gymnastics. Clin Sports Med 2:571–593, 1983.
118. Aronsen JG: Problems of the upper extremity in gymnasts. Clin Sports Med 4:67–71, 1985.
119. Destot J: Paralysié cubital par l'usage de la cyclette. Gazette des Hôpital 68:1176–1177, 1896.
120. Hunt JR: Occupational neuritis of the deep palmar branch of the ulnar nerve: A well defined clinical type of professional palsy of the hand. J Nerv Ment Dis 35:673–689, 1908.
121. Harris W: Occupational pressure neuritis of the deep palmar branch of the ulnar nerve. Br Med J 1:98, 1929.
122. Eckman PB, Perlstein G, Altrocchi PH: Ulnar neuropathy in bicycle riders. Arch Neurol 32:130–131, 1975.
123. Converse T: Cyclist's palsy. N Engl J Med 301:1397–1398, 1979.
124. Finelli PF: Handlebar palsy. N Engl J Med 292:702, 1975.
125. Gardiner KM: More on bicycle neuropathies. N Engl J Med 292:1245, 1975.
126. Noth J, Dietz V, Mauritz KH: Cyclist's palsy. J Neurol Sci 47:111–116, 1980.
127. Hoyt CS: Ulnar neuropathy in bicycle riders. Arch Neurol 33:372, 1976.
128. Jackson DL: Electrodiagnostic studies of median and ulnar nerves in cyclists. Phys Sportsmed 17:137–148, 1989.
129. Haloua JP, Collin JP, Coudeyre L: Paralysis of the ulnar nerve in cyclists. Ann Chir Main 6:282–287, 1987.
130. Maimaris C, Zadeh HG: Ulnar nerve compression in the cyclist's hand: Two case reports and review of the literature. Br J Sports Med 24:245–246, 1990.
131. Braithwaite MA: Bilateral median nerve palsy in a cyclist. Br J Sports Med 26:27–28, 1992.
132. Hoyt CS: Numb hands: A sequel. Bike World 2:30–31, 1973.
133. Burke E: Hands—get a grip on several common problems. Bicycling May:161–167, 1990.
134. Burke E: Ulnar neuropathy in bicyclists. Phys Sportsmed 9:53–56, 1981.
135. Seddon HJ: Carpal ganglion as a cause of paralysis of the deep branch of the ulnar nerve. J Bone Joint Surg 34B:386–390, 1952.
136. Silver MA, Gelberman RH, Gellman H, Rhoades CE: Carpal tunnel syndrome: Associated abnormalities in ulnar nerve function and the effect of carpal tunnel release on these abnormalities. J Hand Surg 10:710–713, 1985.
137. Lowrey CW, Chadwick RU, Waltman EN: Digital vessel trauma from repetitive impact in baseball catchers. J Hand Surg 1:236–278, 1976.
138. Sugawara M, Ogino T, Minami A, Ishii S: Digital ischemia in baseball players. Am J Sports Med 14:329–334, 1986.
139. Itoh Y, Wakano K, Takeda T, Murakami T: Circulatory disturbances in the throwing hand of baseball pitchers. Am J Sports Med 15:264–269, 1987.
140. Nuber GW, McCarthy WJ, Yao JS, et al: Arterial abnormalities of the hand in athletes. Am J Sports Med 18:520–523, 1990.
141. Ho PK, Dellon AL, Wilgis EF: True aneurysms of the hand resulting from athletic injury. Report of two cases. Am J Sports Med 13:136–138, 1985.
142. Porubsky GL, Brown SI, Urbaniak JR: Ulnar artery thrombosis: A sports-related injury. Am J Sports Med 14:170–175, 1986.
143. Kostianen S, Orava S: Blunt injury of the radial and ulnar arteries in volleyball players: A report of three cases of the antebrachial-palmar hammer syndrome. Br J Sports Med 17:172–176, 1983.
144. Koman LA, Urbaniak JR: Ulnar artery insufficiency: A guide to treatment. J Hand Surg 6:16–24, 1981.

PART VII

Developmental and Degenerative Disorders

CHAPTER 29

Congenital and Developmental Wrist Disorders in Children

Sudhir B. Rao, MD, Paul W. Esposito, MD, and
Alvin H. Crawford, MD

Congenital and developmental abnormalities of the wrist are quite rare in comparison with traumatic and acquired disorders. The incidence of congenital anomalies affecting the upper limb is estimated to be 11.4 per 10,000 live births.[98] In 17 to 21 percent of cases, there is an associated skeletal or visceral anomaly.[105, 136] Five to seven percent of all patients may be classified as having some syndrome complex.[98, 105] Congenital skeletal defects have been created experimentally by a variety of physical and chemical agents.[49, 163] They are also known to be associated with certain genetic abnormalities and drugs such as thalidomide.[190] From a clinical standpoint, however, the underlying cause remains unknown in 85 to 90 percent of cases.[158] The classification adopted by the International Federation of Societies for Surgery of the Hand[180] is widely used (Table 29–1). There is no significant geographic variation in the types of anomalies, except that transverse deficiencies appear to be less common, and ring constrictions more common, among Asians, than among Caucasians.[98, 105, 136]

Congenital and developmental disorders rarely affect the wrist in isolation. In radial hemimelia, for example, thumb hypoplasia is extremely common, requiring reconstruction in addition to correction of the clubhand. In generalized afflictions such as arthrogryposis, the status of the shoulder and elbow often dictates what useful function the hand may have. It is clear, therefore, that the whole upper extremity must be evaluated and treated. Such an all-inclusive approach is beyond the scope of this chapter; nevertheless, to facilitate understanding of the basic principles of management, we have briefly discussed the treatment of associated deformities where appropriate.

DEVELOPMENTAL ANATOMY

At the end of the fourth week of intrauterine life, the upper limb bud arises from the lateral ridge of Wolff at the level of the caudal cervical segments. This limb bud consists of a core of proliferating mesenchyme covered by ectoderm. The apical ectodermal ridge (AER) is a specialized region of ectoderm at the tip of the limb bud that develops in response to a stimulus from the underlying mesoderm.[45] The AER regulates subsequent development and differentiation of the mesoderm and influences polarity of the limb bud. Experiments have shown that transverse limb deficiencies result from removal of the AER.[163] There appears to be a complex set of reciprocal interactions between the AER and underlying mesoderm that influences morphogenesis, cellular differentiation, pattern formation, and growth in the developing limb bud.[194]

A small group of cells located on the postaxial border of the tip of the limb bud (polarizing region) controls cellular differentiation across the radioulnar axis. The pattern of digit formation is probably reflective of the concentration gradient of a diffusable morphogen from the polarizing region. Anomalous occurrence of an additional polarizing region on the preaxial border may account for duplication anomalies such as ulnar dimelia.[193, 214] Occurring concur-

Table 29–1. CLASSIFICATION OF CONGENITAL LIMB ANOMALIES

I	Failure of formation of parts	V	Undergrowth (hypoplasia)
II	Failure of differentiation (separation) of parts	VI	Congenital constriction band syndrome
III	Duplication	VII	Generalized skeletal abnormalities
IV	Overgrowth (gigantism)		

Adapted from Swanson AB: A classification of congenital limb malformations. J Hand Surg 1:8–22, 1976.

rently is a sequence of programmed cell death in select regions of the limb bud, which leads to separation of digits and joint formation.

By the sixth week, the distal part of the limb bud has broadened into the hand plate. By the seventh week, individual digits have formed and separated. Axial mesenchymal cells condense into primitive cartilaginous precursors of the skeleton, and by the seventh week, primary ossification centers appear in the long bones. The interzonal mesenchyme condenses into a trilaminar structure. Cavitations develop within the central layer, leading ultimately to the formation of a joint space with a synovial lining. The surrounding mesenchyme differentiates into capsuloligamentous structures. Myogenic cells migrating from the somites differentiate into muscle groups that later become innervated by ingrowing nerves.[194]

A secondary ossification center arises in the distal radius at the end of the first year and fuses in the 17th and 19th years in females and males, respectively. The distal ulna epiphysis ossifies in the 5th and 6th years and fuses in the 17th and 18th years in females and males, respectively. Carpal bones develop by endochondral ossification. The capitate ossifies in the second month, the hamate by the end of the third month, and the triquetrum and lunate in the third and fourth years, respectively. The scaphoid, trapezium, and trapezoid follow in the fourth year in females and the fifth year in males. The pisiform is the last carpal bone to ossify at 9.5 years in females and 11 years in males.

An accessory carpal ossicle is seen in 1 percent of the population. More than 25 different ossicles have been described, the most common being the os centrale.[132] This normally appears in the second month of intrauterine life and fuses with the scaphoid, forming its tubercle. Occasionally, it may persist as a separate ossicle, lying between the scaphoid, capitate, and trapezoid. Although the pattern of secondary ossification shows some variation, it forms the basis for estimation of skeletal age.

TRANSVERSE DEFICIENCY

Transverse failure of formation affects any level and is almost always sporadic in occurrence.[158] Transverse deficiency at the wrist is seen in acheiropodia of the Brazil type and Robert's syndrome, both of which show autosomal recessive inheritance, and occasionally in Poland's syndrome.[59, 174] In the upper extremity, deficiency occurs most commonly through the upper third of the forearm. The incidence of transverse deficiency at the wrist (acheiria) is 0.6 per 10,000 live births.[101, 158] The actual level may be radiocarpal, transcarpal, or carpometacarpal. Unossified carpal bones are not apparent on a radiograph, but the child may show some active motion at the radiocarpal joint (Fig. 29–1). The stump, which may be tapered or bulbous, is usually well padded, and vestigial digits and dimpling may be present. Transverse deficiency at the wrist may represent an ex-

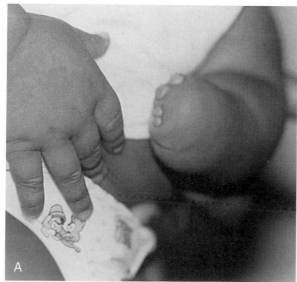
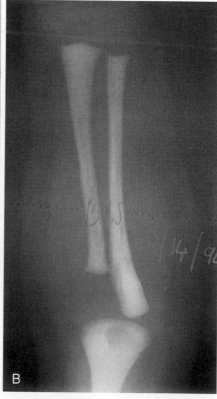

Figure 29–1. *A,* An 8-month-old infant with transverse absence at the wrist. There is a well-padded stump with vestigial digits. *B,* Although the radiograph does not demonstrate any carpal elements, the child could actively flex and extend the stump, indicating a functional radiocarpal articulation.

treme form of symbrachydactyly.[128] Associated anomalies are rare[219]; they include radial head dislocation, radioulnar synostosis, and transverse defects of the lower limb.[191]

Many patients with acheiria whose opposite limb is normal function satisfactorily without a prosthesis. If some radiocarpal motion exists, a "volar plate" may be used to assist in prehension. This device is cheap and simple, and it preserves sensory input. Alternatively, a prosthetic hand with pinch powered by wrist motion may be prescribed.[217] In transverse deficiency through the forearm, a passive prosthesis is fitted at 4 to 5 months of age to aid in crawling. An active prothesis with a terminal hook is fitted at 12 to 16 months. Most children accept and adapt very well to their prostheses.[181, 217] Myoelectric prostheses offer an expensive alternative, but not all children continue using them for active prehension.[96]

Children with bilateral congenital amputations at the wrist or distal forearm are best served with a Krukenburg procedure on one limb and a prosthesis on the other. Swanson[183] recommends performing the procedure as early as is feasible. Although the result is not cosmetically pleasing, the operation creates a strong, sensate, prehensile pincer, much like chopsticks, that no prosthesis can match.[31, 62, 183] If present, the distal radial and ulnar epiphyses should be preserved to maintain length.

PHOCOMELIA

Phocomelia is an extreme form of longitudinal deficiency, representing failure of formation of an entire segment of the limb. Although rare, in the 1950s it affected over 50 percent of children born to mothers taking thalidomide in the fourth to eighth week after conception.[190] There are three types: (1) complete, in which the hand is attached directly to the trunk, (2) proximal, in which the arm is missing and the forearm attaches to the trunk, and (3) distal, in which the forearm is absent and the hand attaches directly to the arm. The ipsilateral hand is usually hypoplastic, and additional skeletal and visceral anomalies may coexist. Although limb lengthening by distraction or bone grafting is theoretically possible, affected patients obtain maximum benefit from prosthetic fitting.

RADIAL CLUBHAND

Radial clubhand refers to the deformity associated with congenital radial dysplasia. It may be characterized by a stiff, extended elbow and a radially deviated hand. It is a form of preaxial longitudinal deficiency and principally involves the radius and the radial aspect of the hand. The incidence of radial clubhand is estimated to be 0.8 per 10,000 births.[88, 158] Bilateral involvement occurs more commonly, and in unilateral cases, the right side is involved more often than

the left.[9, 17, 74, 90, 100] Petit,[144] in 1733, is credited with the first description of radial clubhand.

Etiology

Most cases of radial clubhand occur sporadically. In Europe, the disorder was seen in the 1950s in children born to mothers taking thalidomide during the early weeks of gestation.[98, 100, 190, 219] Rare instances of familial clubhand have been documented.[74, 90] Geneticists have described several syndromes with autosomal dominant or recessive inheritance, in which radial dysplasia is but one component (Table 29–2). The coexistence of several musculoskeletal and visceral anomalies with radial dysplasia points to an embryonic insult occurring around the fifth week of intrauterine life.

Associated Anomalies

Between 25 and 81 percent of patients with radial clubhand, especially with bilateral cases, have at least one associated congenital anomaly.[28, 38, 64, 100] About half of all cases can be classified as a recognizable syndrome complex.[38] Some of the accompanying musculoskeletal defects are rib hypoplasia and fusion, Sprengel's deformity, congenital scoliosis and kyphosis, torticollis, sacral agenesis, short or absent humerus, syndactyly, clinodactyly, hip dysplasia, genu varum, foot deformities such as pes planus, clubfoot, and pes cavus, constriction bands, and congenital pseudarthrosis of the contralateral radius.[10, 17, 28, 38, 74, 90, 140] Visceral abnormalities include a wide spectrum of cardiac, pulmonary, gastrointestinal, genitourinary, hematologic, and neurologic aberrations.

Thrombocytopenia–absent radius (TAR) syndrome is an autosomal recessive disorder characterized by hypomegakaryocytic thrombocytopenia and bilateral radial dysplasia. The thumbs are always present, and associated anomalies include cardiac defects and facial hemangioma. Low platelet count and spontaneous hemorrhages require treatment during infancy, but the platelet condition shows spontaneous resolution with time, and affected patients who survive the first 2 years have an excellent prognosis. Surgery should be postponed until platelet counts have stabilized to 100,000/mm³ or more. Up to 86 percent of patients with TAR syndrome have associated bilateral knee dysplasia, necessitating multiple surgical procedures during childhood.[165] Knee dysplasia may include varus, flexion and rotational deformity, instability, stiffness, and patellar abnormalities.

In contrast, patients with *Fanconi's syndrome*, which is also an autosomal recessive disorder, have radial dysplasia with an absent thumb. In addition, these patients may have pigmentary skin changes as well as cardiac and renal anomalies. The platelet count is normal at birth, but pancytopenia secondary

Table 29–2. CONDITIONS ASSOCIATED WITH RADIAL DYSPLASIA (ADAPTED FROM[55, 64, 174])

Condition	Inheritance*
Syndromes with blood dyscrasias	
TAR syndrome	AR
Fanconi's pancytopenia syndrome	AR
Aase syndrome (hypoplastic anemia–triphalangeal thumb)	?
IVIC syndrome (thrombocytopenia, hearing loss, and atresia)	AD
Syndromes with congenital heart disease	
Holt-Oram syndrome	AD
Syndromes with craniofacial abnormalities	
Nager syndrome (acrofacial dysostosis)	SP/AD
Juberg-Hayward (orocraniodigital) syndrome	AR
Baller-Gerold syndrome (craniosynostosis-oligodactyly)	AR
Rothmund-Thomson syndrome (short stature, poikiloderma, brachydactyly, brachymetacarpal)	AR
Levy-Hollister syndrome (lacrimoauriculodentodigital [LADD])	AD
Duane's syndrome (eye, radial dysplasia)	AD
Goldblatt-Viljoen syndrome (choanal atresia–radial deficiency)	AD
Radial deficiency–hemifacial microsomia	AD?
Syndromes with vertebral abnormalities	
VACTERS†	
Klippel-Feil syndrome	AD
Goldenhar's syndrome (occuloauriculovertebral dysplasia)	SP; AD
Keutel's syndrome (costovertebral dysplasia; radiohumeral synostosis)	AR
Syndromes with chromosomal abnormalities	
Trisomy 13	
Trisomy 18	
Trisomy 21	
Chromosome 4	
Deletion and ring chromosomes	
Triploidy	
Syndromes with mental retardation	
Seckel's syndrome (bird-headed dwarfism)	AR
Hutteroth syndrome (short stature, cardiac defects)	?
Cornelia de Lange's syndrome (microcephaly, cardiac and genital anomalies)	SP
Syndromes with genitourinary anomalies	
Siegler's syndrome (renal ectopia, hydronephrosis)	AR
Sofer's syndrome (short stature, renal and ear anomalies)	AD
Schmitt's syndrome (radial hypoplasia–triphalangeal thumb–hypospadias)	AD
Teratogenic syndromes	
Thalidomide embryopathy	
Aminopterin-induced syndrome	
Varicella embryopathy	

*AD, autosomal dominant; AR, autosomal recessive; SP, sporadic; ?, unknown.
†V, vertebral anomalies; A, anal atresia; C, cardiac; TE, tracheoesophageal fistula; R, renal defects; S, single umbilical artery.

to marrow aplasia develops between 5 and 10 years of age, leading to a fatal outcome within 2 to 3 years.

Holt-Oram syndrome is an autosomal dominant disorder characterized by atrial septal and other cardiac defects, as well as radial dysplasia with absence or hypoplasia of the thumb. Other upper limb anomalies may occur, but the absence of lower limb involvement, visceral abnormalities, and mental retardation differentiates this disorder from other syndromes.[64]

The *VATER association*[149] occurs sporadically. It consists of three or more nonrandom associations of the following anomalies, the first letters of which confer the acronym: *v*ertebral abnormalities, *a*nal atresia, *t*racheoesophageal fistula, *e*sophageal atresia, *r*adial clubhand. Associated anomalies include cardiac and renal defects, lower limb anomalies, and a single umbilical artery.

The distinguishing feature in children with *thalidomide* embryopathy is the occurrence of bilateral longitudinal upper limb deficiencies, often in association with lower limb defects.[100, 219]

Pathoanatomy

The dysplasia in radial clubhand involves, to a lesser or greater extent, the entire upper extremity.[113, 140, 157] The abnormal anatomy of radial clubhand has been examined in some depth in several autopsy and clinical studies.[74, 90, 133, 157, 175]

BONES

The scapula and clavicle often show varying degrees of hypoplasia. The humerus is usually short with considerable abnormality of its distal end. The radius may be completely absent, partially absent (usually the distal two thirds), or present in its entirety but short.[74] A fibrous anlage may replace the missing portion and contribute to deformity.[24, 55, 140, 204] The ulna is always short, being half to two thirds of its usual length[9, 17, 55, 74, 100] (Fig. 29–2). There is delay in appearance and early closure of the distal ulnar epiphysis.[74] At birth, the ulna shows some thickening and posteromedial bowing. This usually progresses with growth and persistent muscular imbalance.[9, 100] Especially following centralization, the distal end of the ulna becomes wide and cupped, resembling the radius. The scaphoid and trapezium are absent in approximately 82 to 98 percent and 67 to 100 percent of wrists, respectively.[55, 100, 134] The capitate, hamate, and triquetrum are usually normal, although in a patient nearing skeletal maturity, carpal coalitions may be evident,[100] the most common being triquetrolunate. Thumb ray abnormality ranges from total absence to mild hypoplasia, and the incidence of each type may vary with the reported series (Table 29–3). In general, but not always, the extent of thenar dysplasia correlates with the severity of radial dysplasia.[74]

MUSCLES

Muscles may be absent, hypoplastic, or fused with other muscles, or they may have abnormal attachments. In general, preaxial muscles are more pro-

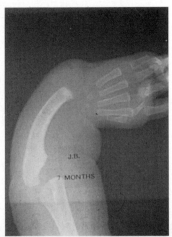

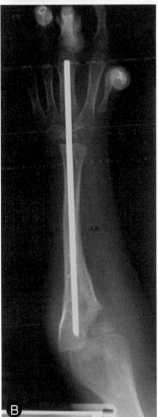

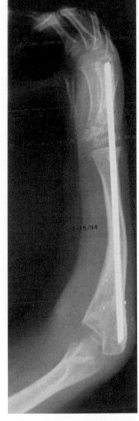

Figure 29–2. A child with unilateral complete absence of the radius who was treated by centralization using an indwelling intramedullary rod. *A,* Radiograph at 7 months of age. Other forearm shown for comparison. Note that the affected ulna, which is thickened and bowed, is about two thirds the length of the normal ulna. The carpus is angulated and displaced radially. *B,* Anteroposterior and lateral radiographs taken 8 years following surgery. Despite having undergone three rod exchanges, the ulna appears to be growing satisfactorily. There is no significant bowing and its distal end has broadened to resemble the radius.

Table 29–3. TYPES AND INCIDENCE OF THUMB DYSPLASIA IN RADIAL CLUBHAND*

Series	Type and Incidence (%)			
	Absent	Floating	Hypoplastic	Normal
Lamb[100] (117)	86 (101)	9 (11)	4 (5)	0
Bayne[9] (101)	Types not specified			15
Heikel[74] (82)	36.6 (30)	8.5 (7)	34.1 (28)	20.7 (17)
Pardini[140] (39)	49 (19)	0	21 (8)	31 (12)†
Manske[116] (21)	66.6 (14)		33.3 (7)	0

*Figures in parentheses indicate numbers of cases.
†Described as "present."

foundly affected than their postaxial counterparts. The latissimus dorsi, triceps, flexor carpi ulnaris, extensor carpi ulnaris, extensor digiti minimi, ulnar lumbricals (third and fourth) and interossei are usually normal. The long head of the biceps is usually absent. The short head of the biceps muscle is usually present and may be fused with the coracobrachial muscle or the antebrachial flexors; it may insert abnormally into the elbow joint capsule, forearm fascia, or radial anlage. The brachialis, brachioradialis, supinator, anconeus, flexor carpi radialis, extensor carpi radialis longus, extensor carpi radialis brevis, pronator quadratus, and extrinsic and intrinsic thenar muscles are either absent or grossly abnormal. The flexor digitorum sublimis and flexor digitorum profundus muscles, especially the former, may be partially fused or hypoplastic and may have abnormal carpal and metacarpal insertions. The extensor digitorum communis may be fused with adjacent extensor muscles. The long flexor tendons to the index finger and the extensor indicis proprius may be absent. Accessory muscles may arise from the humerus, ulna, or antebrachial soft tissue and may insert abnormally into the carpus or metacarpals.

JOINTS

The carpus is displaced radially and volarly, forming a thick fibrous articulation with the radial aspect of the distal ulna. Some elbow stiffness is usual at birth, with motion averaging 85° of flexion.[9, 74, 170] Fingers show decreased range of flexion at the metacarpophalangeal and interphalangeal joints. The metacarpophalangeal joints are generally hyperextended, whereas the proximal interphalangeal joints show a fixed flexion contracture. The loss of finger mobility is secondary to both intra- and extra-articular causes, and the severity of involvement decreases from the index to little finger.[7, 74, 100, 116]

VASCULATURE

The brachial artery may divide high in the arm. The ulnar artery is usually normal, and the radial artery is usually absent. The superficial palmar arch may be incomplete, and rarely, the radial digital artery to the index finger may be absent.[23] In some instances, the median artery may substitute in the formation of the superficial palmar arch.[82] In the absence of a radial artery, the interosseous arteries are large and dominant.[90, 140, 55]

NERVES

The brachial plexus may derive some contribution from higher cervical segments. The ulnar and axillary nerves are usually normal. Very rarely, the ulnar nerve may be absent.[90] The musculocutaneous nerve is usually absent and its motor and sensory distribution is taken over by the median nerve. The radial nerve ends at the elbow after innervating the triceps. The median nerve supplies the anterior brachial muscles and usually divides into two main branches in the forearm, the more radial of which innervates the territory of the superficial radial nerve. Less commonly, the median nerve divides into several terminal branches in the forearm. The median nerve runs an aberrant course in the forearm. It may manifest as a tight fibrous band immediately deep to the deep fascia and must be protected during surgery.

The Deformity

The hand is radially deviated to 90° or more with the digits pointing toward the elbow and arm (Fig. 29–3A). The average arc of flexion-extension at the ulnocarpal articulation has ranged between 45° and 83°.[74, 170] With weakness or absence of extensors, an unstable ulnocarpal articulation, and radial deviation deformity, the long finger flexors are at a mechanical disadvantage and dissipate their amplitude and moment at the wrist. This perpetuates the wrist deformity and contributes to decreased active finger flexion and strength.[17, 100, 113, 116, 157] Emphasizing that the carpus is not only angulated, but also displaced radially in relation to the distal ulna, Manske and colleagues[113] have described certain quantifying parameters. The longitudinal axes of the distal and proximal ulna are defined by a line perpendicular to the distal and proximal physes, respectively. The hand forearm angle is the angle between the longitudinal axis of the long metacarpal and the longitudinal axis of the distal ulna. The hand-forearm position is the perpendicular distance from the base of the small finger metacarpal to the longitudinal axis of the distal ulna. Ulnar bowing is the angle between the longitu-

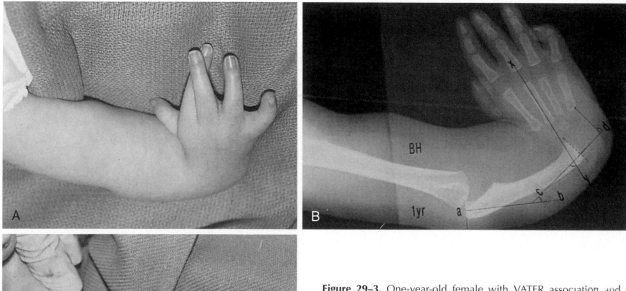

Figure 29–3. One-year-old female with VATER association and a unilateral radial clubhand who underwent centralization of the hand. *A,* Note the typical radial deviation of the hand, short forearm, and hypoplastic thumb. *B,* Radiograph showing hand-forearm angulation, hand-forearm displacement, and ulnar bowing. Lines *ab* and *cd* represent longitudinal axes of the proximal and distal ulna, respectively, and line *xy* represents the longitudinal axis of the long finger metacarpal (see text for details). *C,* Surgical correction was performed using a longitudinal volar and transverse ulnar approach. The hand was centralized over the index metacarpal ("radialization"[24]).

dinal axes of the distal ulna and proximal ulna (Fig. 29–3*B*).

CLASSIFICATION

The current classification proposed by Bayne and associates[9, 46] is a modification of previous descriptions by Heikel[74] and Krichler.[95] It is as follows:

Type I *Short distal radius:* The distal radial physis has inhibited growth, but the proximal physis is normal. The radius is short and present in its entirety. Radial deviation of the hand is minimal.

Type II *Hypoplastic radius:* Both the proximal and distal physes are abnormal. The radius is complete but very short, essentially a miniature. Radial deviation can vary from mild to severe.

Type III *Partial aplasia:* Most often, the distal two thirds or more is absent. Exceptionally, the proximal portion is missing, in which instance there is minimal hand deformity, but instability and valgus deformity occur at the elbow.[74]

Type IV *Total aplasia:* This is the most common variety. In both types III and IV, the missing radius may be replaced by a fibrocartilaginous anlage.

Owing to delay in ossification, the differentiation between partial and total aplasia cannot be made with certainty until a patient is 2.5 years of age.[74] Hand deformity and ulnar bowing are generally proportional to the extent of radial dysplasia.[157] Absence of the radius without a clubhand deformity is seen in extreme radioulnar synostosis and ulna dimelia,[74] whereas radial deviation of the hand can occur with a normal radius and hypoplastic radial carpal bones.[116] The incidences of various types of radial dysplasia in several large series are shown in Table 29–4.

FUNCTIONAL DEFICIT*

The major factors restricting function in radial clubhand are a short forearm, an unstable and deformed wrist, absence of a functioning thumb, and weakness and limitation of finger motion. In unilateral involvement, the affected limb is always used as a helper limb. Patients with bilateral involvement have more difficulty with feeding, toilet care, and reaching for their head or feet. The ulnar border of the hand be-

---

*References 9, 17, 18, 24, 44, 55, 74, 106, 113, 116, 140.

Table 29–4. TYPES AND INCIDENCE OF RADIAL DYSPLASIA*

Series	Type and Incidence (%)		
	Hypoplasia (I, II)	*Partial Aplasia (III)*	*Total Aplasia (IV)*
Bayne and Klug[9] (101)	25 (25)	9 (9)	67 (67)
Heikel[74] (82)	39 (32)	14.6 (12)	46.3 (38)
Kato[90] (253)		14.6 (37)	85.4 (216)
Lamb[100] (117)	19 (22)	3 (4)	78 (91)
Manske[116] (21)	10 (2)	0	90 (19)
Pardini[140] (39)†	2.6 (1)	23 (9)	61.5 (24)

*Figures in parentheses indicate numbers of cases.
†Five cases (12.8%) were undetermined.

comes prehensile, and large objects are held between the fingers and the arm, forearm, or trunk. Absence of an opposable digit places serious restrictions on grasping large objects, power grip, cylindrical grip, and fine dexterous work. Small objects are held with a lateral pinch between the index and long or long and ring fingers. Larger objects may be held in a spherical type of grip, with the index finger pronating (autopollicization) and the small finger supinating. Finally, the limb is not aesthetically pleasing. Thus, although patients with radial clubhand may cope with their daily activities, they are at a disadvantage from a functional and cosmetic point of view.

Treatment

Previous methods of treatment have been reviewed extensively[17, 74, 90, 100] and are not discussed in detail here. Some techniques were designed to provide skeletal support to the carpus by tibial or proximal fibular grafts or radial xenograft, by splitting the ulna longitudinally, or by creating a periosteal tube from the distal ulna. Realignment procedures included ulnar osteotomy, trapezoidal ulna resections, and implantation of the sharpened distal ulna into the split carpus. Kangaroo tendon, silkworm gut, silver or gold wire, and ivory pegs were used for internal fixation and stabilization. These techniques were used singularly or in combination with tenotomies and soft tissue release.

Surgical treatment of radial clubhand has come a long way since Kato[90] concluded in 1924 that "cases of complete absence offer a gloomy outlook" and "the consensus of opinion seems to be that of pessimism." Centralization of the carpus on the distal ulna is now the accepted method of treatment. Initially described by Sayre[164] in 1893, the procedure has evolved slowly into its present form.* There are two fundamental variations to the procedure. One, which is also termed *implantation,*[17, 44, 100, 106, 113, 123] aims to create a

---

*References 17, 24, 44, 100, 106, 113, 155, 204.

stable and mobile ulnocarpal pseudarthrosis by implanting the distal ulna into a carpal slot. The other variation involves accurately realigning the intact carpus over the distal ulna.[9, 24, 46, 204] This latter approach has the theoretic advantage of preserving more motion. Both variations emphasize careful soft tissue repair and balancing. Ulnocarpal arthrodesis should be reserved as a salvage procedure in recurrent deformity.[100, 152]

GOALS OF SURGERY

The goals of surgical treatment of radial clubhand are as follows:[17, 18, 44, 74, 113, 116, 204]

1. To provide a stable, balanced, mobile well-aligned one-bone forearm-hand unit. Some loss of wrist mobility is inevitable. However, this is compensated by a gain in limb length, increase in grip strength, and improvement in finger motion.
2. To retain the maximum growth potential of the distal ulna.
3. To reconstruct the thumb.

CONTRAINDICATIONS

Surgery is contraindicated in the following situations:

1. A child with severe congenital anomalies and a short life expectancy.
2. An adult with well-established patterns of use.
3. Uncorrected clubhand with severe elbow and wrist contractures. Correction of such a deformity may risk the neurovascular structures.

PREREQUISITES FOR SURGERY

Before surgery can be contemplated, the following requirements must be met:

1. A complete work-up must be undertaken to rule out thrombocytopenia and other potentially life-threatening conditions.
2. The child should be 6 months of age or older.[9, 204]
3. There should be active elbow flexion of 90° or more.[17, 55]

The incidence of elbow stiffness in radial clubhand has ranged from 4 to 23 percent. In most instances, improvement occurs with time and manipulation.[9, 100] Splinting the wrist in a corrected position will encourage active elbow motion.[100] Centralizing is contraindicated in the absence of elbow flexion, because such a maneuver would make it impossible to place the hand near the body or face. If active elbow flexion is lacking, centralization is likely to be followed by a recurrence of deformity.[113] In the small number of patients who do not gain sufficient elbow flexion with treatment, a posterior soft tissue release and capsulotomy with triceps transfer to the coronoid process may be indicated.[100, 123]

Serial manipulation and casting is begun soon after birth. The aims are to obtain maximum elbow flexion and to realign the hand over the distal ulna as much as possible. Once a plateau is reached, the correction is maintained in a custom-made splint. Nonoperative treatment may be successful in type I and some type II deformities. However, recurrence of deformity necessitates a soft tissue release and muscle balancing.[55] In addition, lengthening of the radius should be considered to provide radial support of the carpus.[116]

SURGICAL TECHNIQUE

Centralization of the carpus is the procedure of choice for type III and IV and most type II deformities.[46] Surgery is generally undertaken when the patient is around 6 to 12 months of age.[9, 17, 24, 113]

Surgical Approach

Approach the deformity through either a single dorsoradial sinuous incision[17, 24, 44, 55] or separate radial and ulnar incisions.[9, 46, 204] If two incisions are used, make the radial incision in the form of a Z-plasty. The ulnar incision, which is taken as a horizontal ellipse, gives ample access to the ulnocarpal articulation (Fig. 29–3C). On completion of centralization, excise redundant soft tissue within the elliptical incision to leave a more pleasing contour.[46, 113] If preoperative manipulation has achieved sufficient correction, the entire surgical procedure may be carried out through a single ulnar approach.[113]

Soft Tissue Release

Through the radial incision, release the deep fascia widely. Identify the median nerve immediately deep to the fascia.[55, 100, 204] The nerve, which divides into two terminal branches, may appear thick and fibrous and must be protected from inadvertent division. Release all tight musculotendinous units on the radial side. Identify the long finger flexors and test their excursion. Release any abnormal carpal or metacarpal insertions. If a fibrous anlage of the radius is found, excise it completely.[24, 55, 204] If an ulnar incision is used, reflect the extensor retinaculum. Identify the extensor carpi ulnaris, flexor carpi ulnaris, and extensor digiti minimi muscles, the ulnar neurovascular bundle, and the dorsal cutaneous branch of the ulnar nerve. Expose the distal ulna by reflecting a distally based capsular flap. Avoid extensive soft tissue stripping to prevent devascularization of the physis.

Centralization

Sufficient soft tissue release must be obtained to avoid tension on the realigned carpus. If implantation is to be performed, create a carpal slot.[17, 44, 100, 113] To provide stability, the slot should be at least as deep as the width of the distal ulna.[100] Satisfying this requirement usually entails excising the lunate and capitate.[17] Gently pare hypertrophic cartilage off the distal ulna, taking care not to damage the physis. For unilateral cases, implant the hand in midpronation[55] or neutral[17] position. In bilateral cases, one hand should be in 45° of pronation and the other in 45° of supination.[17] Some surgeons do not create a carpal slot, but prefer to accurately align the carpus over the distal ulna, in line with the long finger metacarpal.[9, 204]

Internal Fixation

Drill a 0.054-inch or 0.062-inch smooth Kirschner (K) wire distally into the long metacarpal. Position the hand with the long metacarpal perpendicular to the distal ulnar physis,[9, 17] and advance the K wire proximally into the ulna. The wire usually exits along its subcutaneous border; at this point, attach the drill to the wire and withdraw the wire until its distal tip is beneath the metacarpal head. If ulnar bowing exceeds 30°, an osteotomy may be performed simultaneously.[9] Obtain a radiograph to confirm correct positioning.

Soft Tissue Repair

Draw the capsular flap proximally and repair it over the distal ulna.[24, 100, 113] Careful balancing of musculotendinous units is crucial to the success of centralization. Some commonly used techniques are proximal advancement of the hypothenar muscle origin, imbrication or distal advancement of the extensor carpi ulnaris,[9, 17, 24, 106, 113] dorsoulnar advancement of the flexor carpi ulnaris,[9] dorsal transfer of the flexor carpi radialis,[24] and transfer of the long and ring finger sublimis tendons around the ulnar border of the forearm to the index and long metacarpals.[17]

Postoperative Care

The limb is immobilized in an above the elbow cast. The K wire is usually removed at 6 to 12 weeks. We agree with Bayne and colleagues[9, 46] that bracing should be used until the patient reaches skeletal maturity to prevent recurrence of the deformity.

ALTERNATIVE SURGICAL TECHNIQUES

Buck-Gramcko[24] introduced the concept of radialization, wherein the distal ulna is aligned with the index finger metacarpal. K-wire fixation is performed with the hand held in some ulnar deviation. The radially located wrist flexors and extensors, which are often fused and difficult to distinguish, are detached from their abnormal insertion. These are transferred to the imbricated extensor carpi ulnaris tendon. Radialization aims to improve balance by increasing the mechanical advantage of ulnar located muscles.

Kessler[93] has described external fixation and gradual distraction for correction of severe untreated radial clubhand deformity, thereby avoiding the need for extensive soft tissue surgery. Once alignment has been attained, the hand is stabilized by a Kirschner wire inserted across the metacarpals into the ulna.

In response to concerns about growth arrest with the use of current techniques of centralization, Tsuge and Watari[198] have described a one-stage wrist stabilization and pollicization. The index ray is pronated, abducted, and transposed proximally in its entirety so that the base of its metacarpal rests against the ulna. No formal attempt is made to realign the carpus, and the transposed ray is expected to act as an osseous strut with growth potential. In their two cases, these surgeons describe satisfactory cosmetic and functional results.[198]

Delorme[44] centralized the wrist using the largest possible intramedullay rod. The rod was left in place indefinitely to act as an internal splint (see Fig. 29–2). In his five cases, frequent rod changes were needed. Complications of this method included premature growth arrest in the distal ulna and metacarpal, as well as breakage and migration of the rod. This is the preferred technique of the author (AHC).

Despite successful centralization, the short forearm will limit reach. Catagni and associates[30, 203] have reported lengthening of the forearm in a small group of patients.[30, 203] Although up to 13 cm in length was gained, virtually all patients had notable complications; they included nerve dysfunction, neuroma formation, permanent finger stiffness, delayed union, flexion deformity, and wound breakdown. However, these researchers concluded that despite the morbidity, all patients had functional, cosmetic, and psychological improvement.

Nonvascularized fibular grafting was abandoned by its proponents because the physis promptly closed and the graft often resorbed, leading to recurrence of deformity.[29, 156, 177] Free vascularized fibular transfer has been performed in a few cases,[140, 197, 206] but long-term follow-up is unavailable. Growth from the transplanted physis is unpredictable, and a composite osteocutaneous flap may be required for coverage and monitoring of perfusion. We believe that this procedure fails to confer any significant benefit over centralization.

COMPLICATIONS

Recurrence of radial deviation has occurred in 5 to 28 percent of cases.[9, 17, 18, 100, 113] Up to 30° of angulation is functionally acceptable. Recurrence has been attributed to technical errors[17, 100, 113, 116, 177, 204] (failure to release tight structures and balance muscles, failure to align the long metacarpal perpendicular to the distal ulnar physis, failure to anchor the ulna in an adequate carpal slot, failure to stabilize with a K wire), centralization in the absence of active elbow flexion,[113] poor postoperative brace compliance,[46] and recurrence of deformity at the intercarpal and carpometacarpal joints.[9, 55]

Distal ulnar growth arrest may result from the use of a large intramedullary rod,[44] from inadequate soft tissue release,[9] and from centralization performed in a child more than 8 years of age.[100]

Other complications reported are (1) delayed healing, skin necrosis, and superficial infection[24, 46, 198]; (2) K-wire migration and breakage[24, 44, 100]; (3) accidental division of a superficially located median nerve[100]; (4) spontaneous ulnocarpal and intercarpal fusion from iatrogenic injury; and (5) vascular compromise following correction of severe deformity.[9] We have seen a compartment syndrome that followed corrective osteotomy for ulna bowing, which was performed several years after the centralization.

THUMB RECONSTRUCTION

Thumb reconstruction should be considered in every case of radial clubhand. For milder forms of thumb hypoplasia (Blauth grade II and some grade III), soft tissue reconstruction is appropriate. This procedure entails web release, metacarpophalangeal joint stabilization, opponensplasty, and attention to extrinsic tendon abnormalities.[108, 112, 114]

In more severe forms of hypoplasia and aplasia (Blauth grades III, IV, and V), pollicization of the index finger is the method of choice.[23, 100, 114, 185] although absence of its long flexors may dictate the choice of another digit. A third to half of patients with pollicized digits need an additional procedure such as opponensplasty, scar revision, excision of bony spikes, extensor tendon shortening, and arthrodesis of interphalangeal joints.[114, 185] Transfer of the abductor digiti minimi is perhaps ideally suited to restore opposition, because this muscle is virtually unaffected in radial dysplasia. It is synergistic with the abductor pollicis brevis muscle, has suitable amplitude, and does not require construction of a pulley.[114] It is generally recommended that pollicization be performed before the first birthday.[23, 24, 108] Because the index finger is cortically represented as the radialmost digit, function after repositioning does not appear to require special sensory reeducation. Hence, the timing for pollicization may not be as critical as previously believed.[114]

In the case of an untreated, inoperable bilateral radial clubhand in a patient with stiff elbows, pollicization of the small finger has been performed.[216] In such instances, the ulnar digits are prehensile. Repositioning the small finger ray on the ulnar aspect of the hand, in much the same manner as a conventional index finger pollicization, may restore useful pinch and grasp function.

RESULTS

It is generally believed that the best results are obtained when treatment of radial clubhand is begun in the first year of life.[9, 24, 18] Although criteria for assessing results may vary, several authorities[9, 17, 18, 24, 113, 100, 204] have reported successful outcome in the majority of cases following centralization. Manske and associates,[113] at an average of 34 months of fol-

low-up, reported satisfactory results in 20 of 21 patients with radial clubhand who underwent centralization of the ulna into a carpal slot. Bayne and Klug,[9] at average of 8.6 years of follow-up, reported only two unsatisfactory results in 39 limbs undergoing centralization without carpal implantation. Wrist motion following centralization has ranged from 0 to 40° of flexion.[9, 24, 204] Some radial deviation tends to recur, but generally no more than 30°.

Bora and colleagues[18] reviewed 10 patients at an average of 14 years after initial presentation. Eight had undergone centralization, and two were untreated. There was no significant change in ulnar bowing, percentage of shortening of the ulna, handforearm angle, or wrist and elbow motion in either group of patients for the duration of follow-up. However, active finger motion in patients with centralization averaged 54 percent of normal, compared with 27 percent for the untreated group.

Long-term review of results of pollicization has confirmed continued use and function of the transposed digit, especially for grasping large objects.[114, 185] Small objects are preferentially held with a side-to-side pinch between fingers. Functional improvement following pollicization for radial clubhand is less spectacular than that for isolated thenar dysplasia because of the presence of associated musculoskeletal abnormalities.

ULNAR HEMIMELIA

Longitudinal deficiency of the ulna is among the least common congenital anomalies affecting the upper limb, with an incidence of 0.2 per 10,000 births.[88, 158] Fewer than 200 cases have been reported in the literature.[84] Between 10 and 35 percent of patients have bilateral involvement.[126, 135, 179]

Ulnar deficiency differs from its preaxial counterpart, the radial clubhand, in several respects. Virtually all cases of ulnar deficiency are sporadic in occurrence.[84, 126, 135, 176, 179] Associated malformations are common, but they are almost always musculoskeletal. Hand anomalies occur commonly and are not confined to the postaxial rays. Ulnar deviation at the wrist is rarely severe enough to warrant surgical treatment. Radiohumeral instability or radiohumeral synostosis may, however, warrant operative attention.

Associated Anomalies

Almost half the patients with ulnar hemimelia have at least one associated anomaly[58, 84, 126, 179] (Table 29–5). These generally are musculoskeletal, although cardiac and genital malformations occur in some syndromes (Table 29–6). Hematologic, pulmonary, and gastrointestinal anomalies have not been associated with ulnar deficiency. Between 23 and 52 percent of patients with unilateral ulnar hemimelia have some abnormality of the opposite extremity; the abnormali-

**Table 29–5. ASSOCIATED ANOMALIES IN
ULNAR HEMIMELIA**

Upper limb	Glenohumeral instability
	Hand anomalies (see text)
	Radial head dislocation
	Short humerus
	Shoulder girdle hypoplasia
	Transverse deficiency
Lower limb	Absence of patellae
	Clubfeet
	Congenital coxa vara
	Congenital hip dislocation
	Fibular and tibial hemimelia
	Proximal focal femoral deficiency, short femur
	Transverse deficiency
Other	Bicornuate uterus
	Branchial cyst
	Diaphragmatic hernia
	Hypospadias
	Microcephaly
	Orofacial abnormalities
	Scoliosis, torticollis

Data from references 20, 26, 55, 84, 126, 179.

ties include oligodactyly, polydactyly, transverse deficiency, radial ray deficiency, phocomelia, and radial head dislocation.[20, 55, 126, 135, 179]

The Deformity

The ulna may be hypoplastic or partially or completely aplastic (Table 29–7). The missing portion is usually replaced by a fibrocartilaginous anlage. The radius is short and bowed to a varying extent; its distal articular surface may be inclined steeply. The

**Table 29–6. CONDITIONS ASSOCIATED WITH
ULNAR HEMIMELIA**

Syndrome	Inheritance*
Al-Awadi limb deficiency	AR
CHILD (congenital *h*emidysplasia, *i*chthyosiform erythroderma, *l*imb *d*efects)	XLD
Cornelia de Lange's (growth retardation, microcephaly, hirsutism, cardiac and genital abnormalities)	SP
di Bella's: ulnar agenesis (cardiac defects)	?
Pallister's clefting (facial abnormalities, mental retardation)	XLD
Pallister's ulnar-mammary (hypogenitalism, hypoplasia of apocrine glands)	AD
Pfeiffer's: absent fibulae–oligodactyly (cleft lip/palate, brain malformation)	AR
Pillay's: ophthalmomandibulomelic	AD
Richieri-Costa's limb deficiency	AD
Robert's limb deficiency (cleft lip/palate, blond hair, enlarged phallus)	AR

*AD, autosomal dominant; AR, autosomal recessive; SP, sporadic; XLD, X-linked dominant; ?, unknown.
Adapted from Stevenson RE, Meyer LC: The Limbs. In Stevenson RE, Hall JG, Goodman RM (eds): New York, Oxford University Press, 1993, pp 699–720.

**Table 29–7. INCIDENCE AND TYPES OF ULNAR
HEMIMELIA***

Series	Types and Incidence (%)		
	Hypoplasia	*Partial Aplasia*	*Complete Aplasia*
Broudy and Smith[20] (26)	15 (4)	54 (14)	31 (8)
Carroll and Bowers[26] (23)	13 (3)	74 (17)	13 (3)
Ogden et al[135] (12)	25 (3)	67 (8)	8 (1)
Swanson et al[179] (88)	25 (22)		75 (66)

*Figures in parentheses indicate number of cases.

pisiform, triquetrum, hamate, and capitate are usually missing.[55, 135] Ulnar deviation of the wrist occurs in 30 to 40 percent of cases and is related to the loss of ulnar carpal support, tethering from a fibrocartilaginous anlage, and an increased slope of the distal radius (Fig. 29–4).

It is believed that the wrist deformity is nonprogressive in the majority of cases.[20, 84, 117, 126] The elbow may be nearly normal or may show varying degrees of abnormality. There is no strong correlation between the extent of ulnar dysplasia and the state of the elbow.[20, 55, 120] The radial head may be subluxed or dislocated. However, 17 to 53 percent of limbs may show a radiohumeral synostosis.[20, 26, 135, 179] In these cases, the radiohumeral angulation varies from 15° to 100°. In some instances, extreme pronation and anterior bowing of the entire limb cause the palm to face posteriorly ("hand on flank" deformity).[126]

Associated hand abnormalities are extremely common.[20, 26, 126, 176, 179] Only 5 to 12 percent of hands in patients with ulnar hemimelia show a full complement of digits.[20, 126, 179] A two- or three-digit hand is usual (Fig. 29–5). Absence of ulnar rays occurs most commonly, but central and radial rays may be deficient as well. Two thirds of hands may show camptodactyly,[126] and syndactyly is seen in 13 to 54 percent of cases.[20, 26, 126, 179] Thumb ray anomalies, consisting of absence, floating, hypoplasia, supination, or duplication of thumbs, have been noted in 35 to 100 percent of cases.[20, 26, 126, 55, 179] Other abnormalities are hypoplastic digits, delta phalanx, symphalangism, absence of carpal bones, carpal coalition, and metacarpal synostosis.[26]

CLASSIFICATION

Because the severity of ulnar dysplasia bears little correlation with the type of the elbow or hand abnormality, anatomic classifications have little functional significance. The Bayne classification[46] is widely used but is by no means comprehensive, and any therapeutic plan should take the overall status of the limb into consideration. This classification is as follows:

Type I   *Hypoplasia of the ulna:* Proximal and distal physes are present and show decreased growth. The is no

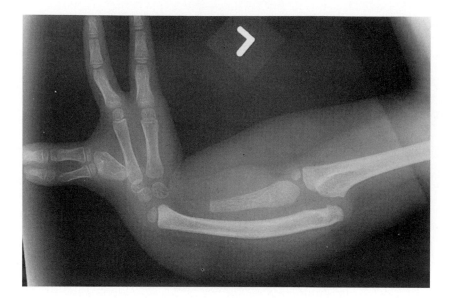

Figure 29–4. Radiographs showing partial aplasia of the ulna (type II) with radiohumeral dislocation. The ulnar carpus and the ring and small finger rays are absent. The hand shows a marked ulnar deviation deformity, and the thumb is duplicated.

anlage, and wrist deformity is usually minimal and static.

Type II *Partial aplasia:* The distal portion is absent and is replaced by a fibrocartilaginous anlage. The proximal portion, which may not ossify until the patient is 3 years of age,[135] articulates with the humerus. The proximal radius may articulate with the capitellum, although more commonly, the radiohumeral joint is dislocated. Radial bowing is present and is less severe if the radial head is dislocated.

Type III *Total aplasia:* The radiohumeral joint is usually dislocated and unstable. An anlage may be present.[135] The elbow may show a

pterigium and severe flexion deformity. Radial bowing is minimal.

Type IV Radiohumeral synostosis is present along with any grade of ulnar dysplasia. The radiohumeral angle is variable, and often, the entire limb is pronated and anteriorly bowed, causing the hand to face posteriorly. An anlage is usually present, and radial bowing can be severe.

Treatment

There is controversy in the literature regarding the indications for surgical treatment of ulnar hemimelia.

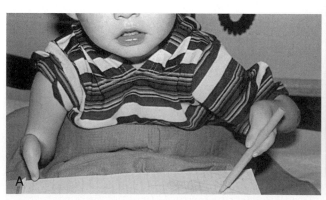
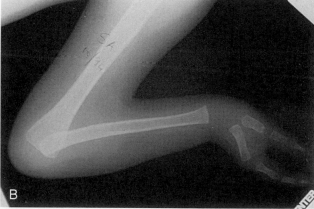

Figure 29–5. A 3-year-old child with bilateral type III (complete aplasia) ulnar hemimelia. *A,* Both elbows show a fixed flexion contracture. Prehension is achieved with the thumb and index finger of the left hand. The monodactylous hand is used for support. *B,* Radiograph of the left upper limb showing complete absence of the ulna and a two-ray hand.

On the assumption that the anlage causes progressive ulnar deviation of the hand, radial bowing, and radiohumeral dislocation, some surgeons have advocated its early excision.[26, 55, 135, 154] Others have recommended creating a one-bone forearm in patients with radiohumeral dislocation.[26, 154, 173, 176]

Blair and colleagues[16] performed a functional assessment of eight patients with ulnar hemimelia who had undergone no surgical treatment for their elbows, wrists, or forearms. The group's average total range of motion was 43 percent of normal, and average grip strength was 27 percent of that on the other side. Most patients completed tests of function and dexterity, and none reported any difficulty with activities of daily living. Many surgeons share the view that in general, patients with ulnar deficiency cope well with their deformity.[20, 55, 84, 117, 126] The indications for surgical treatment have therefore become more selective. The status of the hand and elbow are more important functional determinants than the severity of ulnar dysplasia. A small number of patients with severe flexion contractures of the elbow and skin webbing may be better served by early prosthetic fitting.[58]

Indications for and summaries of the surgical options follow.

EXCISION OF THE ANLAGE

Periodic stretching and casting are commenced after birth.[84, 117] Once a satisfactory alignment has been achieved, correction is maintained by long-term bracing. Some surgeons have advocated routine early excision of the anlage, at 6 to 12 months of age,[26, 135, 159] whereas others have discounted its prophylactic value.[20, 126] A compromise approach appears more reasonable. Failure of manipulation to improve ulnar deviation beyond 30° or the presence of severe fixed ulnar deviation[55, 84, 117, 126] is a reasonable indication for excision of the anlage along with soft tissue release.

ONE-BONE FOREARM

Patients with radiohumeral dislocation may show some elbow instability but may still retain a useful range of elbow motion and forearm rotation. In the patient with partial ulnar aplasia, functionally disabling elbow instability and painful radial head dislocation can be addressed by creating a one-bone forearm. The procedure, which may be carried out in one or two stages,[46, 55] involves excision of the anlage and proximal radius followed by osteosynthesis of the proximal ulna and distal radius. Care should be taken to maintain maximal forearm length.

ROTATIONAL OSTEOTOMY

In patients with radiohumeral synostosis showing the "hand on flank" deformity, the forearm can be derotated and flexed with an appropriately placed wedge osteotomy, thereby placing the hand in a more suitable position.

CORRECTION OF HAND ANOMALIES

No effort should be spared in providing timely correction of thumb ray abnormality, syndactyly, and other surgically treatable anomalies.

CARPAL COALITION

Approximately 0.1 percent of Caucasians have a carpal coalition. The condition is far more common among persons of West African ancestry; it is seen in 9.5 percent of Hausa females in Nigeria.[34] A coalition may be seen between any two adjacent carpal bones, and coalitions occur bilaterally in over half the cases.[34, 43, 70, 132] Carpal coalition may be classified into four types, as follows[127]:

Type I   Synchondrosis.

Type II   (Incomplete) synostosis with a notch

Type III Complete synostosis.

Type IV   Complete synostosis associated with other carpal anomalies.

A carpal coalition represents failure of separation during embryologic development. Triquetrolunate coalition is by far the most common (Fig. 29–6), followed by capitohamate and pisohamate. Because the pisiform is a sesamoid bone, a pisohamate coalition probably arises from metaplasia of the pisohamate ligament.[34] Carpal coalitions occur in conditions such as arthrogryposis, Ellis–van Creveld syndrome, hand-foot-uterus syndrome, hereditary symphalangism, diastrophic dwarfism, dyschondrosteosis, Holt-Oram syndrome, and otopalatodigital syndrome.[147]

Virtually all carpal coalitions are asymptomatic and discovered incidentally on a radiograph.[34, 35, 43, 127] The involved wrist shows a full range of motion with no functional limitation. A type I coalition may, on rare occasions, become symptomatic. Pain may follow acute or repetitive trauma or may arise insidiously. Most such case reports involve adults,[61, 70] in whom surgical exploration has revealed degenerative changes necessitating a limited intercarpal arthrodesis. Simmons and McKenzie[169] reported a 15-year-old girl with painful triquetrolunate synchondrosis following a fall, which was treated successfully with a triquetrolunate arthrodesis. Rarely, a bony coalition may fracture after a fall,[61, 145] but such injuries have not been described in children. Ulnar nerve entrapment within Guyon's canal has been described in two teenagers with type I pisohamate coalition.[14] In both instances, the nerve was compressed between an enlarged pisiform, the hamate hook, and cartilaginous coalition. Complete recovery followed decompression and excision of the coalition.

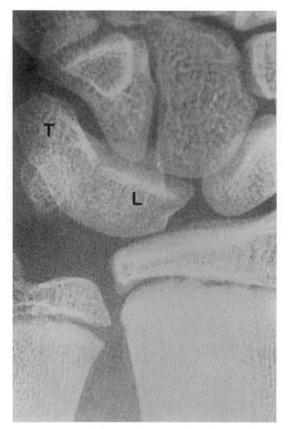

Figure 29–6. Triquetrolunate coalition incidentally noted on a wrist radiograph of an asymptomatic 13 year old male. *L* = lunate; *T* = triquetrum. (*From* Oestreich AE, Crawford AH: Atlas of Pediatric Orthopedic Radiology, New York, Thieme Inc., 1985.)

CONGENITAL RADIOULNAR SYNOSTOSIS

Congenital radioulnar synostosis represents a failure of segmentation. In virtually all cases, the synostosis occurs proximally and extends a variable distance along the shafts of both bones. Distal radioulnar synostosis is exceedingly rare,[92] and we have not encountered a case so far. Rotational osteotomy would be indicated to improve disabling pronation or supination deformity.

ULNAR DIMELIA

Ulnar dimelia, or mirror hand, is characterized by duplication of the ulna, the ulnar carpus, and its attending complement of digits. There is absence of normal preaxial structures, namely the radius, scaphoid, trapezium, and thumb ray. There are usually seven digits, although six or eight may exist.[73, 199] The medialmost digit is the small finger, followed by the ring and middle fingers. The lateralmost digit also resembles the small finger, followed by a ring and middle finger. The central digit probably represents the index finger. This is an extremely rare condition

that occurs sporadically. Except for one reported case of bilateral ulnar and fibular duplication,[103] ulnar dimelia is not accompanied by other abnormalities.

Pathoanatomy[7, 8, 73, 199]

The carpus shows symmetric duplication of the triquetrum, hamate, capitate, and pisiform. The lunates are fused into one wide bone. Each of the two capitates has a triangular facet distally to accommodate a single trapezoid. The distal end of both ulnae are broad and articulate with the carpus. Their proximal ends are rotated such that the trochlear surfaces face each other. The distal end of the humerus, especially the lateral condyle, is abnormal. This, along with a misshapen lateral olecranon, constitutes a bony block to flexion. Muscles may be absent or hypoplastic or may have abnormal attachments. The biceps, brachialis, and triceps muscles are usually abnormal. The extensor digitorum may be attenuated or absent. The pronators, supinator, and wrist extensors are usually absent. The flexor carpi ulnaris is duplicated but otherwise normal. The flexor digitorum sublimis and flexor digitorum profundus may be fused. The nerve supply may be symmetric, with two sets of "ulnar" and "median" nerves. In contrast, the vascular supply is not symmetric, and abnormal digital vessels may be encountered during surgery.

Clinical Features

The wrist and elbow appear broad. A flexion and ulnar or radial deviation deformity exists at the wrist, and the elbow is usually stiff in extension with very little forearm rotation.[7, 8, 46, 69, 199] The fingers are usually flexed, and active extension is weak or absent. The fingers may be rotated toward the central digit. Syndactyly may coexist. The entire upper limb has some dysplasia,[8, 73] and in general, the postaxial structures show less involvement.

Treatment

Surgery is indicated to improve appearance and function. The goals include correction of wrist deformity, excision of extra digits, and pollicization, performed preferably in one stage. A volar soft tissue release including wrist capsulotomy is always necessary, and proximal row carpectomy[199] may also be required to position the wrist in neutral. The flexor carpi ulnaris or flexor digitorum sublimis from an excised digit is transferred to a wrist extensor tendon to provide muscle balance. The most functional digit is pollicized, and the adjacent two digits are filleted and excised. The resulting skin is used to construct a web space. Intrinsic muscles and tendons from the digits to be excised may be judiciously used to augment the intrinsic and extrinsic muscles of the pollicized digit.[7, 69, 199]

Loss of elbow flexion is disabling. Reshaping of the articular surfaces, excision of the proximal lateral ulna, and anterior transfer of the abnormal biceps insertion have been described, but lasting improvement is unlikely.[7, 46, 69, 199] A rotational osteotomy may be necessary to improve forearm position in patients with extreme pronation or supination deformity.

CONGENITAL PSEUDARTHROSIS OF THE RADIUS AND ULNA

Congenital pseudarthrosis of the radius and ulna is rare; only 53 cases have been reported in the literature.* Both bones have been involved simultaneously in 13 cases, and in the remainder, one or the other has been affected with equal frequency. At least two thirds of affected patients are known to have neurofibromatosis when the pseudarthrosis is first diagnosed. It is conceivable that the true incidence is much higher, because cutaneous stigmata of neurofibromatosis may not be apparent in the very young. Histologic evidence of neurofibromatosis at the fracture site has been found in only a few instances.[2, 33, 213] Rarely, pseudarthrosis follows a fracture through

---

*References 4, 12, 32, 50, 86, 89, 110, 119, 121, 166, 189, 213, 221.

a cystic lesion, suggestive of fibrous dysplasia.[21, 33] Multiple limb involvement is extremely rare, and there is only one reported case of fibular pseudarthrosis occurring concurrently with forearm pseudarthrosis.[221]

True congenital bowing or pseudarthrosis accounts for approximately one fourth of reported cases. In the remainder, one or both bones fracture following an injury and progress to frank non-union (Fig. 29–7). Although no site is immune, pseudarthrosis typically occurs in the distal third of the forearm, leading to progressive shortening and angular deformity. In most cases, some preexisting osseous dysplastic changes predispose to fracture, but pseudarthrosis has followed fracture through apparently normal bone.[12, 86] Once fracture occurs, the radiographic appearance steadily evolves to one of frank pseudarthrosis, with narrowing and sclerosis of bone ends, obliteration of the medullary canal, and even disappearance of a segment of bone. Ulnar pseudarthrosis can lead to radial head dislocation.[1, 12, 32, 119]

Such fractures do not heal with simple cast immobilization,[10, 12, 138, 153] and surgical treatment is indicated when non-union is impending or established. The union rate following internal fixation and conventional bone grafting is around 50 percent. Vascularized fibular grafting, however, offers several advantages. It carries a 100 percent union rate,[2, 12, 32, 119, 166, 213] although refracture has been reported.[121] The procedure is particularly suitable in cases with a

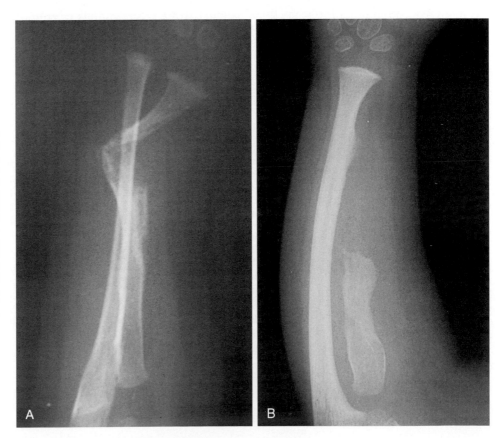

Figure 29–7. This 3-year-old child with neurofibromatosis sustained a fracture through the distal third of the radius, which failed to heal following cast immobilization. Despite an attempt at bone grafting, the fracture progressed to a frank non-union. Because of pain and increasing deformity, the distal radius was excised, and the hand was centralized over the distal ulna. This procedure resulted in correction of deformity and a stable wrist. *A,* Radiograph showing a non-union through the distal third of the radius with marked angulation. *B,* Radiograph taken 3 years after surgery shows a well-aligned carpus over a hypertrophied distal ulna.

short distal fragment. Because graft length is not an issue, wide excision of diseased tissue, preliminary lengthening, and correction of angular deformity with a distraction device can be carried out.

In those instances in which repeated attempts at bone grafting have failed or severe deformity or radial head dislocation exists, a one-bone forearm procedure offers a suitable alternative. It may be performed using conventional techniques[10, 32, 138] or with a vascularized fibular graft.[121] The Ilizarov fixator has been used to simultaneously correct deformity and obtain healing.[4, 50] Although this method may have its place in selected cases, its potential morbidity and duration of treatment makes it less attractive to us than vascularized fibular grafting.

CONGENITAL CONSTRICTION RING SYNDROME

Congenital constriction ring syndrome accounts for less than 5 percent of congenital upper limb anomalies,[55, 98, 105, 136] and its estimated incidence is 1 in 15,000 births.[141] It occurs sporadically[3, 94, 98, 129, 141, 188] and is more common among Asians.[98, 105, 136] There is a higher incidence of prematurity and low birth weight in affected patients.[3, 57]

The etiology of this condition remains controversial.[141] One theory proposes a primary germ cell dysplasia. Others believe that intrauterine constriction from amniotic bands is responsible. In a set of elegant experiments involving amniocentesis, Kino[94] reproduced defects in mice similar to those seen in humans. This led him to conclude that excessive uterine contractions caused soft tissue hemorrhage and cell necrosis, leading to the formation of constriction rings.

Involvement of the upper extremity alone or in combination with the lower extremity occurs in up to 75 percent of cases.[3, 94] In the upper limb, some 85 percent of constriction rings are located distally, in the hand and digits. Wrist and distal forearm rings account for 2 to 7 percent of cases.[3, 129, 188] The constriction ring may vary in depth from being very superficial to being adherent to the periosteum. There is one reported case of a midforearm fracture associated with a deep constriction ring that healed following immobilization.[226]

In the extreme form of constriction ring syndrome, an intrauterine amputation may result; this occurrence may be difficult to differentiate from transverse deficiency at the wrist. In constriction ring syndrome, the proximal parts are usually well developed, whereas in transverse deficiency, some proximal hypoplasia exists. Constriction rings usually run at right angles to the long axis of the limb, but those at the wrist may run obliquely on to the hand.[141]

Occasionally at birth, granulation tissue and constricting "amniotic bands" may be present in the trough of the ring. Depending on its depth, underlying structures may be constricted. Distal edema and cyanosis are indicative of lymphatic and venous obstruction. In severe cases, the whole hand is ballooned, with unrecognizable digits. Nerve involvement, ranging from mild sensory loss to complete paralysis of the median and ulnar nerves, may be associated with a forearm or wrist constriction ring.[3, 129, 188, 200] A temperature gradient is present across the ring, especially in proximal rings associated with a neurologic deficit.[129]

Patterson[141] has classified ring constrictions into four groups: (1) simple ring constrictions, (2) ring constriction accompanied by deformity of the distal part with or without lymphedema, (3) ring constrictions accompanied by fusion of distal parts (acrosyndactyly), and (4) intrauterine amputations.

Up to 87 percent of patients have associated hand anomalies, including additional ring constrictions, amputations, syndactyly, acrosyndactyly, hypoplastic phalanges, nail abnormalities, short digits, and symphalangism.[3, 57, 94, 141, 129, 188] Central digits are affected more often, and the thumb is rarely involved. Acrosyndactyly may vary in its extent and generally involves soft tissues, although bony fusion may occur rarely.[3, 94] Additional anomalies such as clubfoot, cleft lip, and cleft palate occur in a third to half of patients.[3, 57, 129, 141]

Constriction can increase with growth and development.[129, 201] Surgical treatment is indicated to improve appearance and distal edema. Single-stage correction is appropriate in most cases; deep rings with marked distal edema are preferably excised in two stages. Upton and Tan[201] have refined earlier techniques of ring excision and Z-plasty, resulting in a more aesthetic appearance of the digit and limb. They emphasize careful dissection using magnification to preserve veins. An appropriately sized flap of subcutaneous fat is raised after skin edges have been mobilized. This fatty apron is then advanced across the defect to augment contour. Skin repair is accomplished using Z-plasty along the midlateral axes and a straight line closure dorsally.

Following healing, there is a gradual and steady improvement in distal swelling. In patients with paralysis or circulatory embarrassment, ring excision should be carried out with some urgency. Although circulatory improvement invariably occurs, nerve recovery may be unpredictable. Uchida and Sugioka[200] reported three cases of proximal constriction rings that were associated with severe flattening and degeneration of the median and ulnar nerves. Nerve recovery did not follow excision of the rings.

MADELUNG'S DEFORMITY

Madelung's deformity is a developmental growth disturbance of the distal radial physis that manifests clinically during adolescence. In 1878, Madelung[111] reported on a "spontaneous forward subluxation of the hand" in a 20-year-old woman. The condition that now bears his name was probably first described by Malgaigne in 1855.[131] Madelung's deformity is rare in occurrence[99] but is more common in the West Indies.[75] It predominantly affects females and is usually bilateral, although one side may be symptomatic. Clinically, the carpus and hand appear to be displaced anterior to the forearm and the distal ulna is dorsally subluxed, forming a prominence that is most marked in pronation (Fig. 29–8). Dorsiflexion, radial deviation, and supination may show varying degrees of restriction.

Radiographic findings are characteristic.[39, 102, 150] The radius is short with a dorsolateral curvature. Its distal articular surface shows excessive volar and ulnar inclination. The distal radial epiphysis is triangular and medially beaked. A lucent area is seen in the ulnar aspect of the distal radius, and osteophytes may be noted here in later stages. The anteromedial quadrant of the distal radial physis consistently undergoes premature closure. The distal ulna is relatively long and subluxed dorsally. Its head is enlarged and deformed, and the distal physis is radially inclined. The carpus assumes a triangular shape as it translates proximally, volarly, and ulnarwards. The lunate becomes wedged in the widened distal radioulnar interosseous space. In the lateral view, the carpus shows a dorsal curvature in continuation with radial bowing. Reverse Madelung's deformity is very rare, fewer than 10 cases having been reported.[51] The radius displays an anterior convexity, and its distal articular surface is inclined dorsally, carrying the carpus with it.

Etiology

The distal radius deformity arises from a focal dysplasia of the growth plate, the exact nature of which is unknown. Biopsy specimens of the physis have shown normal chondrocytes with abnormally arranged cell columns.[202]

Madelung's deformity is considered a manifestation of dyschondrosteosis, a form of mesomelic dwarfism, which was first described by Leri and Weill[104] in 1929. Inheritance of this disorder is autosomal dominant with 50 percent penetrance,[42] and males show lesser expression.[102] Characteristically,

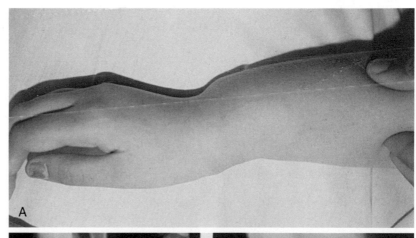
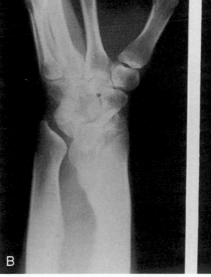
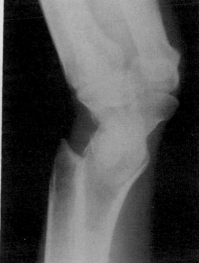

Figure 29–8. Madelung's deformity in an asymptomatic 15-year-old female. *A,* Note the dorsally prominent ulnar head and volar displacement of the hand. *B,* Anteroposterior *(left)* and lateral *(right)* radiographs showing triangularization of the carpus, increased inclination of the radial articular surface with proximal migration of the lunate, and dorsal subluxation of the ulna (or volar displacement of the radius and carpus).

patients have near normal to moderate short stature, normal facies, and normal intelligence.[42, 52] The radius-to-humerus ratio is 0.65:1 (normal 0.72 to 0.75:1), and the tibia-to-femur ratio is 0.7:1 (normal 0.83 to 0.85:1), indicating short middle segments of limbs. Although most patients will show a "Madelung's deformity," some with equal shortening of both forearm bones show minimal deformity.[42] Associated skeletal changes in dyschondrosteosis include thickening of the proximal radius, flattening and tilting of the radial head, cubitus valgus, restricted elbow motion, genu varum, ankle varus, coxa valga, abnormalities of the proximal humerus, exostosis of the proximal medial tibia, and brachydactyly.[39, 42, 102]

There appears to be another variety of Madelung's deformity (primary or idiopathic) that is nonheritable, occurs bilaterally, affects only females, and is not associated with dyschondrosteosis.[65] Other rare causes of a similar deformity are trauma, infection, sickle cell disease, tumor, Turner's syndrome, nail-patella syndrome, and multiple epiphyseal dysplasia.[42, 46, 65, 102, 131]

Clinical Presentation

Madelung's deformity may occasionally be evident in infancy,[102] but most patients present in adolescence with pain, deformity, loss of motion, and weakness. Pain in the younger patient is usually the result of ligamentous stretching accompanying carpal translocation.[52] This generally improves with skeletal maturity.[131] Later on, pain is due to mechanical derangement of the distal radioulnar joint[52] or radiocarpal osteoarthrosis. There appears to be little correlation between symptoms and radiographic appearance.[52, 99] Attrition rupture of extensor tendons over a deformed ulnar head has been described in adults but not in children.[48] An acute median neuropathy following a fall has been described in an adult and a 9-year-old.[51, 46] Both patients had reverse Madelung's deformity with marked obliquity of the carpal tunnel.

Treatment

The natural history of Madelung's deformity is one of progressive radiographic deterioration. In most cases, symptoms can be controlled by bracing.[52, 99, 131] Surgical treatment should be considered for persistent pain, loss of motion, weakness of grip, and severe deformity.[46, 99, 120, 131, 150, 202]

Several operations have been described in the literature: resection of the distal ulna (Darrach procedure), the Sauve-Kapandji procedure, distal ulnar recession, open or closed wedge radial osteotomy, correction with external fixators, epiphysiodesis of the distal ulna and radius, and radiocarpal and total wrist fusion.[46, 52, 75, 120, 131, 209] Procedures confined to the distal ulna are indicated when radial deformity

is not severe. Nielsen[131] reported subjective improvement in 9 of 13 patients following surgery; 4 were unchanged, and only 1 patient had improved motion. Ranawat and colleagues[150] reported improvement in pain, strength, and forearm rotation in 12 of 13 patients at an average 8-year follow-up. They recommended a closed-wedge radial osteotomy with distal ulna resection for severe deformity. A distal ulna resection was performed in patients with mild deformity. In these patients, the researchers noted continued carpal translocation, although this was asymptomatic.[150]

Instead of such salvage procedures, Vickers and Nielsen[202] have advocated prophylactic excision of the physeal bar in symptomatic adolescents. In the 15 cases they reviewed, all patients showed significant improvement in pain and motion. Progression was arrested in every instance, and 10 cases showed an improvement of deformity. An anomalous pronator quadratus muscle[107] or thickened ligament[202] has been found by some to tether the carpus to the distal radius. Release of these abnormal structures may prevent progressive carpal shift.

ARTHROGRYPOSIS MULTIPLEX CONGENITA

Arthrogryposis (from the Greek for "curved joint") multiplex congenita is a congenital disorder characterized by multiple rigid joint contractures, marked limitation of active and passive motion, muscle weakness, and hypotonia. The condition, first described by Otto[139] in 1841, has an incidence of 1 to 2 per 10,000 births.[218] Quadrimelic involvement is most typical (Fig. 29–9), and isolated upper extremity involvement occurs infrequently.[60, 220] The deformities are usually bilaterally symmetric, and distal joints are more severely involved.[63, 220] The affected limb appears tubular and featureless with smooth waxy skin and absent joint creases. Skin dimpling and webbing may be seen. The extent of muscle weakness varies; in some patients, it may be profound and global.[109, 205] Facial muscle involvement results in a "wooden doll" appearance.[87] Superficial and deep sensation is normal, and reflexes are diminished or absent.[63] Although muscle weakness is non-progressive, joint deformities may progress if left untreated.[63, 218] Some increase in flexibility occurs with time and stretching,[60] and functional improvement is noted as the affected child adapts to the deformities.[212]

Etiology

Arthrogryposis is broadly classified into two types, neurogenic and myogenic.[5, 47, 87] Myogenic arthrogryposis, which may be an autosomal recessive disorder, accounts for less than 10 percent of cases. Pathologic changes in muscles are similar to those seen in

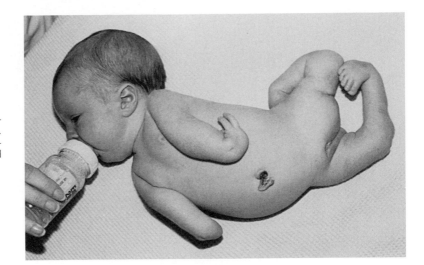

Figure 29–9. A newborn with arthrogryposis multiplex congenita showing typical deformities affecting all four limbs. At 6 months of age, this child underwent bilateral midcarpal wedge resection to improve wrist/hand position and bilateral talectomy for clubfoot deformities.

congenital myopathies.[5, 6, 47] Conventionally, neurogenic arthrogryposis excludes syndromes with congenital joint contracture or obvious neurologic lesions such as myelodysplasia (Table 29–8). It is sporadic in occurrence and shows no familial association with clubfoot, hip dislocation, or neuromuscular disease.[22, 41, 218] Neurogenic arthrogryposis is associated with a high incidence of congenital anomalies such as scoliosis, rib cage abnormalities, Klippel-Feil syndrome, orofacial anomalies, inguinal hernia, genitourinary abnormalities, pulmonary hypoplasia, and congenital heart disease.[6, 60, 63, 218]

Evidence from animal, autopsy, electrodiagnostic, and muscle biopsy studies suggests that neurogenic arthrogryposis is associated with a decrease in or absence of anterior horn cells in the cervical and lumbar cord enlargements.[15, 40, 87, 97, 211] Brown and coworkers[22] have shown a correlation between the pattern of deformity and the length of anterior horn cell columns, as is seen in poliomyelitis. Muscles with a long cell column, such as the pectoralis major, showed minimal involvement. The almost constant occurrence of foot and ankle deformity in arthrogryposis, however, seemed to correlate well with the fact that extrinsic foot muscles have short cell columns. An apparent sharp increase in the incidence of arthrogryposis in the 1950s and 1960s in contrast to scanty prior reports, coupled with a high incidence of prenatal maternal complications, has led some investigators to implicate an environmental factor, possibly a virus, in the genesis of arthrogryposis.[41, 218]

On the basis of examination of 74 cases, including 53 at autopsy, Banker[6] has subclassified neurogenic and myogenic arthrogryposis into 17 subgroups. It appears that a variety of factors—chromosomal defects, mutagenic agents, chemicals, and viruses—may adversely influence the early embryonic development of the motor neuron, peripheral nerve, motor end plate, or muscle fiber. The result is muscle hypoplasia, a compensatory connective tissue response, periarticular and muscle fibrosis, and consequent failure of normal joint development.[6, 184] Hall and associates[72] have described a group of patients with distal arthrogryposis predominantly affecting the hands and feet. Inheritance in some cases is autosomal dominant. Abnormalities of stature, spine, jaw, face, and oral cavity may coexist; the joint deformities in these patients respond well to treatment, suggesting that they may be a special subset of patients with arthrogryposis.

Clinical Features

Upper limb involvement (Fig. 29–10) is seen in 55 to 87 percent of cases.[13, 22, 60, 109, 220] The shoulders are fixed in adduction and internal rotation. The elbows show a fixed extension contracture or, less commonly, a flexion contracture. Significant wrist deformity occurs in 40 to 50 percent of cases.[37, 60, 63, 109, 220]

Table 29–8. DISORDERS ASSOCIATED WITH MULTIPLE CONGENITAL JOINT CONTRACTURES*

Cerebral palsy
Congenital muscular dystrophy
Diastrophic and metatropic dwarfism
Fetal alcohol syndrome
Fetal hydantoin syndrome
Freeman-Sheldon syndrome
Intrauterine postural malformations
Laxity syndromes
Mietens' syndrome
Möebius's syndrome
Osteogenesis imperfecta
Potter's syndrome
Sacral agenesis
Schwartz's syndrome
Spinal dysraphism
Trisomy 18
Turner's syndrome
Zellweger's syndrome

Data from references 6, 22, 109, 218.

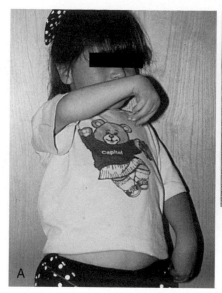

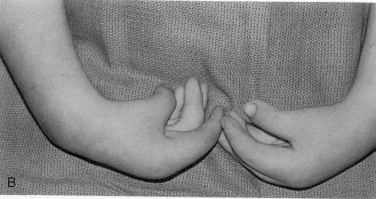

Figure 29–10. Five-year-old child with arthrogryposis multiplex congenita. *A,* There is a fixed adduction and internal rotation contracture at both shoulders. The elbows cannot be flexed actively, and the forearm shows a fixed pronation contracture. With this combination of deformities, the child is unable to place her hand in her mouth. *B,* Both wrists show a fixed flexion contracture. Digits appear tubular with absence of joint creases. The thumb is adducted with a narrow web space.

Typically, the wrist shows a flexion or flexed and ulnar-deviated deformity. An extension deformity is uncommon.[60, 109] The thumb may be flexed and adducted across the palm. Fingers may show an intrinsic-plus or intrinsic-minus deformity or any intermediate pattern.[63, 109, 220] Occasionally, marked ulnar deviation at the wrist and metacarpophalangeal joints gives rise to a "windblown" hand. The severity of hand involvement is variable. At one extreme, the patient may have stiff, spiderlike fingers with a rigid, flexed wrist, and at the other, the patient may retain some active finger motion that improves with treatment.

Weeks[205] has classified patients with upper extremity involvement in arthrogryposis into three groups: In group I, there is single localized deformity, such as fixed forearm pronation or a wrist flexion contracture. Group II patients have contractures affecting the entire upper extremity. Group III patients have generalized involvement with no functional muscles.

Treatment

Patients with arthrogryposis are usually intelligent and highly motivated, with a good life expectancy if they survive the first few years.[13, 22, 63] Stretching, splinting, and judicious corrective casting should be commenced soon after birth. This treatment, combined with active exercises in the form of play and swimming, may result in some improvement of deformity and stiffness. Lower limb surgery takes precedence to provide stable, aligned limbs by the time the child is ready to ambulate.[109, 212] The goal of upper extremity surgery is to achieve a functional limb so that the patient is capable of independent feeding and toilet activity and of performing adequately in

other activities of daily living.[13, 212] This goal may be achieved by correcting the fixed deformity, increasing the range of motion, and providing an active motor where feasible. Certain points of treatment need to be emphasized, as follows:

1. Despite severe involvement, children learn "trick" movements utilizing unusual patterns of prehension and may be functionally independent.[13, 63, 220] Every effort should be made to provide modified implements for feeding, toileting, dressing, and other basic functions.[212]

2. Several authorities have noted better results with early reconstruction.[13, 60, 63, 124, 220] Although some believe that good results are obtained by correcting elbow and wrist contractures between 3 and 6 months of age,[124] we agree with others that upper extremity reconstruction should be performed after 2 years. Elbow release should be deferred until ambulation has been achieved. If the child requires the use of crutches or a wheelchair, the triceps must be retained as an elbow extensor.

3. It is imperative that the whole limb be considered in reconstruction planning. Surgery at one joint level should not compromise the function of another. One extremity should be operated on at a time.

4. When possible, especially at the wrist, tendon transfers should be used to achieve muscle balance. Soft tissue procedures take preference over bony realignment because of a potential for recurrence.

5. Children who have global weakness (Weeks group III) or severe contractures are not candidates for reconstruction.[109, 205]

Using these principles, several authorities have described satisfactory results for upper extremity surgery in children with arthrogryposis.[13, 60, 63, 109, 124, 205] At the *shoulder,* a severe internal rotation contracture in combination with fixed forearm pronation causes the palm to face posteriorly. The child cannot hold crutches or a walker and is unable to place the palm against the mouth or perineum.[109, 212] An external rotation osteotomy of the humerus repositions the extremity and improves reach. Some patients with internal rotation contracture at the shoulder and wrist flexion deformity hold objects between the backs of their hands. Those having active shoulder abduction develop a "crossover grip" between the palms of the hands. In such cases, humeral derotation should be accompanied by correction of the wrist deformity to allow effective grasp.[212] Forearm pronation deformity may be addressed by release or rerouting of the pronator teres in cases in which some motion is preserved. A rotational osteotomy of both bones is indicated if no motion exists.

One *elbow,* preferably in the dominant arm, should be capable of active flexion to allow feeding. An extension contracture is corrected by a posterior capsulotomy and triceps lengthening.[13, 109] Because the elbow flexors are usually nonfunctional, active flexion is restored by transfer of the pectoralis major,[109] latissimus dorsi,[222] or triceps.[13, 27, 109] The Steindler flexorplasty has not proved reliable.[37, 109, 212] The nondominant elbow should be capable of extension for toileting needs; a triceps transfer is contraindicated here.[109, 212]

Correction of *wrist* deformity is especially rewarding when the child has active elbow and finger motion. If severe finger stiffness exists, the wrist is better off flexed, because the radial borders of the hands are prehensile.[109] Depending on its severity, correction of flexion and ulnar deviation deformity is accomplished by a combination of soft tissue and bony procedures. These involve release of contracted deep fascia, musculotendinous units, and wrist capsule,[13, 60, 109, 124] supplemented with a partial or total carpectomy[13, 60, 124, 220] or shortening osteotomy of the radius and ulna.[205] Transfer of the flexor carpi ulnaris or other flexors to the extensor carpi radialis brevis[13, 63, 124] achieves some muscle balance. Prolonged postoperative bracing is essential in preventing recurrence.[13, 46, 60, 125] Following correction of wrist deformity, some active digital extension may return. Extension osteotomy of the distal radius and ulna for correction of wrist flexion is not recommended in children, owing to risk of recurrence.[109, 124] In a patient nearing skeletal maturity, wrist arthrodesis can be performed for recurrent deformity.[63, 109, 208]

A *thumb-in-palm* deformity should be approached with a web release, stabilization of the metacarpophalangeal joint, and transfers to augment extension and abduction.[13, 205, 220] Surgical attempts to improve finger motion at the proximal interphalangeal joints are unrewarding,[13, 212] although some surgeons have reported a successful outcome following soft tissue release and skin grafting[220] or release of abnormal lumbrical and sublimis insertions.[46] Phalangeal osteotomy or proximal interphalangeal joint arthrodesis is more dependable for correction of deformity.

DYSPLASIA EPIPHYSEALIS HEMIMELICA

A rare disorder of unknown etiology and also known as Trevor's disease, dysplasia epiphysealis hemimelica is characterized by an asymmetric enlargement of a long bone epiphysis or a tarsal or carpal bone owing to multiple abnormal ossification centers, which eventually coalesce with the main epiphysis.[53] Radiographically and histologically, the lesion appears identical to an osteochondroma. In essence, therefore, this is an intra-articular osteochondroma. On rare occasions, dysplasia epiphysealis hemimelica may coexist with a typical metaphyseal osteochondroma,[54, 151, 172] suggesting a common etiology. There is no known hereditary transmission or risk of malignant degeneration.

The condition usually affects one side of a lower limb, although generalized involvement may rarely occur. Fewer than 25 cases of upper extremity involvement have been reported.[151] The carpus is involved in about half these cases, the scaphoid being most commonly affected (Fig. 29–11). In the remaining cases, virtually every epiphysis in the upper

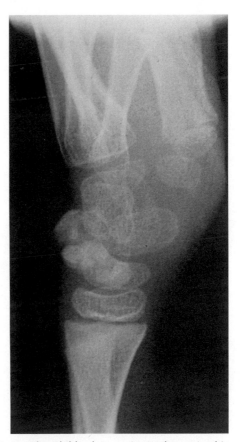

Figure 29–11. The child whose wrist is shown in this radiograph presented with a hard, painless swelling on the dorsoradial aspect of the wrist. The lesion arising from the dorsal aspect of the scaphoid shows multiple ossification centers typical of dysplasia epiphysealis hemimelia. In essence, this condition represents an intra-articular osteochondroma. (Courtesy of Dr. Christopher Hull.)

extremity has been involved. Clinically, the patient presents with a hard, painless mass that may cause articular deformity and restrict motion. Symptomatic lesions should be excised.

MULTIPLE HEREDITARY EXOSTOSIS

Multiple hereditary exostosis, also known as multiple hereditary osteochondromas or diaphyseal aclasis, is the most common generalized developmental skeletal anomaly.[83] It is a disorder of endochondral growth characterized by osteocartilaginous tumors, failure of metaphyseal remodeling, and retardation of longitudinal growth. Transmission is autosomal dominant with reduced expression in females.[172, 215] Osteochondroma is the most common benign bone tumor.[143] Bone ends with the greatest growth potential show the most common involvement, and accordingly, osteochondromas occur around the knee in 95 percent of cases.[167, 171, 172]

The forearm bones are involved in some 85 percent of patients, and at least half of these show significant deformity.[167, 171, 172] Osteochondromas occur in the distal radius and ulna at least twice as frequently as they do proximally.[25, 167, 171, 172] The earliest radiographic sign is an asymmetric beaking of the metaphyseal cortex adjacent to the physis.[172] Later on, typical sessile or pedunculated metaphyseal outgrowths become apparent. These have a radiolucent cartilaginous cap, which may reach a considerable size in children. Osteochondromas usually arise near the interosseous surface of the bones. On rare occasions, opposing tumors ("kissing lesions") may interlock and restrict forearm rotation. Tumors of the proximal radius or ulna can cause radial head dislocation. Metacarpal and phalangeal involvement results in brachydactyly and angular deformity. Carpal bones are rarely affected.[171, 172] Forearm deformity is usually detected in the first decade[172] and may consist of one or more of the following features (Fig. 29–12):

1. Shortening and bowing of both bones. The ulna shows disproportionately greater shortening. Its distal end is tapered and radially tilted, giving it a carrot-shaped or licked-candystick appearance.[56, 172]

2. Steeper inclination of the distal radial articular surface.

3. Ulnar translation of the carpus.

4. Dislocation of the radial head. In such circumstances, the radius shows less bowing.[118, 167]

Clinically, the forearm appears short, with the hand in ulnar deviation. Forearm rotation and radial wrist deviation are reduced. A large osteochondroma or dislocated radial head may be easily apparent. The wrist in multiple hereditary exostosis differs from that in Madelung's deformity. The latter shows a dorsally prominent ulnar head with positive ulnar variance and an anteriorly subluxed wrist.

Two radiographic parameters[56] are useful in assessing forearm deformity (see Fig. 29–12). The radial articular angle is the angle between two lines, one

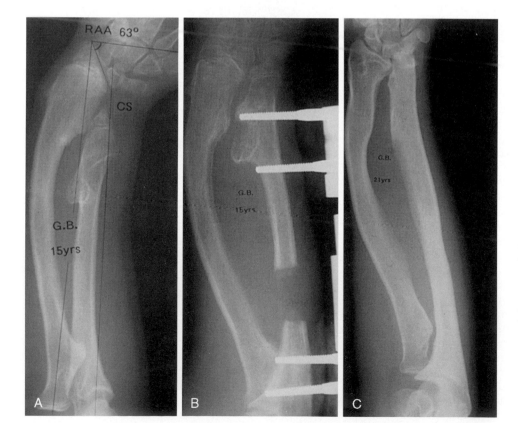

Figure 29–12. Anteroposterior radiographs of a patient with multiple hereditary exostosis who underwent surgery for progressive forearm deformity. *A,* At age 15 years, there is bowing of the radius, a negative ulnar variance, and increased inclination of distal radial articular surface. Distal radial and ulnar osteochondromas can be appreciated. *RAA* = radial articular angle; *CS* = carpal slip. (See text for details.) *B,* Patient underwent lengthening of the ulna followed by lateral radial physeal stapling and excision of osteochondromas. *C,* Six years after surgery, radial bowing has not progressed and the distal radial articular inclination has improved. The distal radioulnar relationship has remained unchanged since surgery.

along the distal articular surface of the radius and the other perpendicular to a line drawn from the center of the radial head to the radial edge of the distal radial epiphysis (normally less than 30°). In carpal slip, a line drawn from the center of the olecranon to the ulnar edge of the distal radial epiphysis intersects the lunate. (Normally, at least 50 percent of the lunate articulates with the distal radius).

Masada and colleagues[118] have classified forearm deformities seen in multiple hereditary exostosis into three types, as follows:

Type I Relative ulnar shortening. The radius is bowed with increased inclination of its distal articular surface.

Type II Associated radial head dislocation secondary to a proximal radial osteochondroma (type IIa) or due to ulnar shortening (Type IIb).

Type III Distal radial osteochondroma with radial shortening.

In their series of 39 forearms, the frequency of these deformities was 61 percent for type I, 20 percent for type II, and 19 percent for type III.

The cause of deformity is subject to conjecture. Osteochondromas are thought to affect longitudinal growth and metaphyseal remodeling by "squandering growth potential"[83] or by tethering the physis.[171, 172, 215] Disproportionate ulnar shortening may be related to two factors. First, its distal physis has a smaller cross-sectional area and contributes proportionately more to overall bone length as compared to the distal radial epiphyseal plate; hence, the potential for defective growth is greater.[171, 172] Second, the short ulna acts as a tether and results in progressive radial bowing, ulnar tilt of the distal radial articular surface, and dislocation of the radial head.[171, 172, 215] A 1993 report, however, failed to substantiate any correlation between the ulnar tether theory and wrist deformity.[25]

The natural history of forearm osteochondromas is one of progressive enlargement during growth that causes deformity and functional impairment.[142, 143] An isolated distal radius osteochondroma, however, may cause little deformity. Small tumors may be incorporated by appositional growth and may spontaneously "disappear."[171] Sarcomatous change is exceedingly rare in children.[143]

Treatment

The goal of treatment in multiple hereditary exostosis is to prevent progressive deformity and loss of motion. Early detection and excision is especially indicated for distal ulnar and proximal radial osteochondromas, which have a high deforming potential. The ideal age for surgery is not known, but results appear to be better in younger patients.[118]

Excision of osteochondromas as a prophylactic procedure is of value in young patients with minimal deformity. Although there is a risk of recurrence, which would necessitate a repeat excision, one may expect improvement of the deformity with growth.[56, 143] In older patients, excision of tumors can arrest progression of the deformity. Improvement in forearm rotation occurs only if the tumors were mechanically restrictive. Peterson[142] has cautioned against simultaneous excision of lesions from both bones through a single incision because of the risk of synostosis, although this is contrary to our experience. We have seen growth arrest following excision of a distal ulnar osteochondroma (Fig. 29–13).

Progressive deformity as indicated by a radial articular angle greater than 30°, a carpal slip exceeding 60 percent, an ulnar shortening of more than 1.5 cm, and a radial head instability requires more extensive procedures.[56, 148, 215] Excision of osteochondromas combined with ulnar lengthening and hemiepiphyseal stapling of the distal radius has been shown to decrease progression of deformity, improve radial articular inclination and carpal slip, correct ulnar deviation of the hand, and occasionally improve forearm rotation.[56] Ideally, radial hemiepiphyseal stapling should be performed between 10 years of age and skeletal maturity. Once the physis has closed, a corrective osteotomy of the distal radius may be performed.[118, 142, 215] Ulnar lengthening of up to 2.5 cm can be attained in a single stage, whereas greater lengths require a distraction device. Some overcorrection is desirable to compensate for the inherent loss of growth potential in the distal ulna.[142, 146] Lengthening of the ulna may prevent radial head dislocation. For established radial head subluxation or dislocation, ulnar lengthening can reposition the radial head alongside the capitellum. The annular ligament must then be reconstructed to retain the radial head. Forearm rotation does not improve,[142] and there is a risk of posterior interosseus nerve palsy or radioulnar synostosis.[118] We prefer not to operate for a dislocated radial head. In those rare patients who have severe pain, a one-bone forearm is a satisfactory option.

CEREBRAL PALSY

Cerebral palsy is the result of a nonprogressive encephalopathy resulting from a wide variety of prenatal, intranatal, and postnatal causes. Although involvement of the motor system is the hallmark of this condition, a varying proportion of affected children may show sensory, visual, auditory, speech, cognitive, behavioral, and emotional disturbances as well as epilepsy. The upper motor neuron lesion results in weakness, paralysis, incoordination, alteration of tone, involuntary movements, and impairment or loss of selective voluntary control of muscles. Predominant involvement of the pyramidal system causes spasticity, whereas extrapyramidal involvement may result in athetosis, rigidity, ataxia, or tremor.[162, 225] Spastic cerebral palsy accounts for 70 to

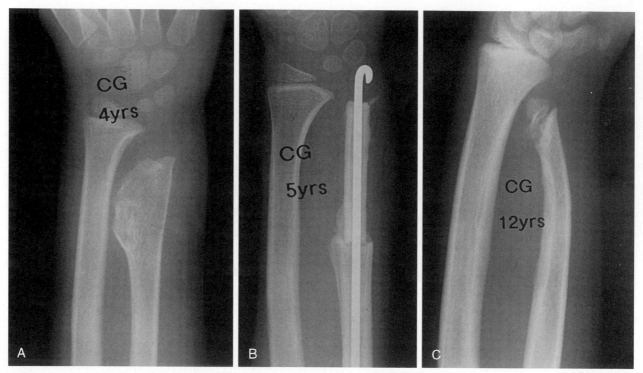

Figure 29–13. A 4-year-old boy presented with a swelling and restricted forearm rotation due to a large distal ulnar osteochondroma. The tumor was excised, and a nonvascularized fibular graft was used to bridge the defect. *A*, Radiograph showing a large expansile osteochondroma in the distal ulna. *B*, Postoperative radiograph showing healing of the fibular graft. *C*, Seven years after surgery, there is obvious growth arrest of the distal ulna, indicated by shortening and bowing.

75 percent of cases.[115, 168] The distribution of motor involvement may be classified as a monoplegia, hemiplegia, diplegia, double hemiplegia, or quadriplegia.

Spastic cerebral palsy is characterized by hypertonia and an exaggerated stretch reflex. Normal muscles are electrically silent at rest. Spastic muscles, on the other hand, show continuous electrical activity at rest and during contraction of antagonistic muscles; this is termed synchronous activity or co-contraction.[162] The typical upper limb deformity consists of adduction and internal rotation at the shoulder, elbow flexion, forearm pronation, flexion and ulnar deviation at the wrist, an adducted thumb, and fingers with flexion or swan-neck deformity (Fig. 29–14). Much less often, one encounters a wrist dorsiflexion and thumb-in-palm deformity or fixed supination of the forearm. In a minimally affected patient, this abnormal posturing may not be apparent at rest but is readily accentuated when the child performs any physical activity or is emotionally upset. Although the underlying neurologic lesion remains static, joint deformity and muscle contracture may show progression owing to the influence of growth and development.

"Cortical" epicritic sensation involving discrimination and spatial relationship is affected in half to two thirds of patients.[186, 223] Protopathic sensations such as pain, touch, and temperature are generally intact. A study involving 64 patients with spastic hemiplegia revealed astereognosis in 47 percent, loss of two-point discrimination in 34 percent, and loss of position sense in 16 percent. Patients with profound loss of cortical sensation effectively ignore the limb, and any attempts to improve function prove futile. There appears to be an increased incidence of Kienböck's disease in patients with severe wrist flexion contractures, suggesting that this posture may interfere with the blood supply.[85, 159]

Examination

Examination of the upper extremity should include assessment of active and passive range of motion, dynamic and fixed deformity, power, and overall function. Dynamic deformity at the wrist results from spasticity of the flexor-pronator group of muscles in combination with weakness of the extensor and supinator muscles. This can be corrected by sustained stretching to overcome the stretch reflex. Fixed deformity results from musculotendinous and joint contracture, which commonly coexist.[79]

Selective proximal nerve blocks can abolish spasticity and are useful in assessing the extent of dynamic versus fixed deformity. The child should be observed during play and when performing simple tasks. Coordination, dexterity, reach, and prehension are assessed. Two-handed activity indicates some volitional control of the affected limb. Grasp and release patterns may vary according to the severity of muscle involvement. Continuous activity of the flexor carpi ulnaris may result in incomplete digital flexion and weak grasp. Complete finger extension (release) may be achieved only in full wrist flexion using tenodesis effect.[115, 162, 224]

Grading the power in spastic muscles with poor voluntary control is difficult, and one may obtain a rough estimate by palpating contraction during active motion. Depending on the child's age, sensory assessment is made by texture discrimination, object identification, graphesthesia, or two-point discrimination.[79]

Classification

Zancolli[225] has classified wrist deformity into three groups on the basis of the severity of flexor spasticity and extensor weakness, as follows:

Group I   Complete finger extension is achieved with the wrist flexed 20° or less. Spasticity is minimal and mainly involves the flexor carpi ulnaris.

Group II   Complete finger extension is possible only with the wrist flexed more than 20°. This indicates spasticity in the wrist and digital flexors. This group may be further divided as follows:
IIa: The wrist can be actively extended if the fingers are flexed, indicating functioning wrist extensors. The predominant spasticity lies in the finger flexors.
IIb: The wrist cannot be extended even with the fingers flexed, indicating nonfunctioning wrist extensors.

Group III   Fingers or wrist extension is not possible in any position, indicating severe spasticity and contracture in the flexor group and marked weakness of the extensors.

Treatment

GOALS OF SURGICAL TREATMENT

Reconstructive surgery in cerebral palsy aims to improve reach, grasp, release, pinch, and range of motion. The improvement in appearance that occurs consequently is no less important than the functional gains.[81, 91, 115, 224, 225] In severely affected individuals, correction of fixed deformity may be indicated for hygiene purposes or to prevent development of painful arthroses. It is important for the patient and family to appreciate that normal function can never be

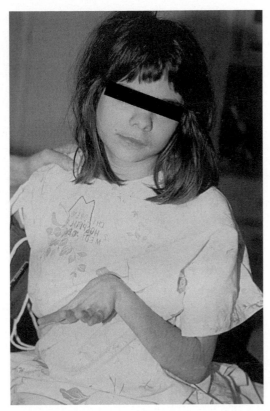

Figure 29–14. Typical posturing of the upper extremity in a girl with spastic hemiplegia. Note the adducted arm, flexed elbow, and flexed and ulnarly deviated wrist. She is able to extend her fingers only by completely flexing her wrist.

achieved and that the patient will continue to use the unaffected limb as the dominant one.

PREREQUISITES FOR SURGERY

Depending on selection criteria, surgical objectives, and specialty interest of the surgeon, between 5 and 20 percent of patients with cerebral palsy may be suitable candidates for upper limb reconstructive surgery.[67, 80, 91, 115, 210] The remainder are either functional or too severely affected. If the child voluntarily uses the affected limb in some capacity during play or other activity, there is some cortical representation. This is perhaps the best predictor of a successful outcome following surgery.* A strong drive and motivation on the part of the patient and family ensure cooperation with postoperative rehabilitation.[68, 91, 162, 210]

Surgery is usually recommended after 5 years of age, when the child's functional pattern has been established and an accurate assessment of the limb can be made.[161, 210, 224, 225] We do not use an upper age limit, because some of our patients are teenagers who become acutely aware of their deformity and request surgery for cosmesis. Although the presence of stereognosis is beneficial, its absence is not a contraindica-

---

*References 11, 68, 80, 81, 115, 178, 223–225.

tion for surgery,[68, 162, 178, 195, 207] because some compensation can occur through eye-hand coordination.[66, 115] In general, however, hands with poor epicritic sensation have the most deformity and are least likely to improve functionally.[11, 67, 68, 186, 223–225] Surgery is beneficial for spastic muscles or patients with a mixed pattern in which spasticity predominates. For athetosis, rigidity, and other extrapyramidal motion disorders, surgery is contraindicated, because an opposite deformity is likely to occur following muscle release or transfer.[91, 210, 223–225] Patients with emotional instability, behavioral problems, low intelligence, marked spasticity, or severe weakness are not suitable for reconstructive surgery. The ideal patient is a mildly affected hemiplegic with good stereognosis and strong motivation.

ELECTROMYOGRAPHY

Dynamic electromyography has been used to determine which muscles are active during grasp and release. It is believed that spastic muscles rarely change phase postoperatively and that the best results are obtained by transferring muscles that contract in phase with the recipient muscle.[77] Although this belief is generally true, phasic conversion has been known to occur, and even continuously active muscles may become phasic postoperatively.[130, 162]

GUIDELINES FOR TREATMENT

Upper extremity orthoses are neither functional nor well tolerated by spastic children, but night-time bracing may be useful in preventing fixed deformity. Surgery aims to improve balance in the hand by weakening spastic muscles, augmenting weak antagonists, and stabilizing joints.[66, 67, 91, 115, 223–225] In general, the various procedures employed are: (1) proximal muscle release, (2) recession at musculotendinous junction, (3) tendon lengthening, (4) release of tendon insertion, (5) tendon transfer, and (6) joint stabilization by tenodesis, capsulodesis or arthrodesis.

Zancolli's classification, shown here, offers conceptually sound guidelines for treatment,[195, 223–225] and we follow it without significant modification:

Group I Patients have effectual grasp and release. Distal tenotomy of the flexor carpi ulnaris can balance the hand and optimize function.

Group II Patients have spastic wrist and digital flexors. A flexor carpi ulnaris tenotomy along with myoaponeurotic release of the flexor-pronator origin is indicated. In the latter procedure, a 3-cm segment of aponeurosis and all deep septae are excised at a level 6 cm distal to the medial epicondyle.[225] Any residual muscle contracture is released as well.

Fractional lengthening of the flexors at their musculotendinous junction is an equally effective alternative.[11, 187] Patients in groups I and IIa with weak wrist extension and all patients with absence of wrist extension (group IIb) require a tendon transfer of flexor carpi ulnaris to the extensor carpi radialis brevis.

Group III Patients have fixed muscle and joint contracture and functional goals are limited. Flexor-pronator muscle slide,[76, 81] Z-lengthening of tendons,[66, 224, 225] superficialis-to-profundus transfer,[19, 76] or a proximal row carpectomy[137] can correct wrist flexion deformity. A tendon transfer of flexor carpi ulnaris to extensor carpi radialis brevis may be added to improve balance.

Zancolli[225] believes that the extensor digitorum communis recovers sufficient power postoperatively and does not advocate routine transfers to augment digital extension. He has cautioned against excessive weakening of digital flexors for fear of creating an intrinsic-plus deformity. Using these guidelines, Tonkin and Gschwind[195] reported satisfactory results in 27 of 34 patients without the need to augment finger extension in any case.

AUGMENTATION OF WRIST EXTENSION

Green transfer, which involves transfer of the flexor carpi ulnaris to the extensor carpi radialis longus or brevis, changes a spastic deforming force into a force that provides active wrist extension.[68] The flexor carpi ulnaris contracts in phase with digital flexion and hence improves grasp following transfer.[11, 76, 79, 115, 225] As a prerequisite, active finger extension should be possible with the wrist passively positioned at neutral, and the flexor carpi radialis should be intact to avoid an extension deformity of the wrist.[195] Although the range of dorsiflexion increases, the total arc of motion does not change appreciably.[11, 207] Some increase in supination occurs in addition. If a myoaponeurotic release is to be performed simultaneously, the flexor carpi ulnaris must be left intact. We prefer to anchor the tendon into the extensor carpi radialis brevis. The transfer should be tensioned to maintain the wrist at neutral[11] rather than in dorsiflexion.[76, 192] This avoids a fixed extension deformity that would interfere with release. When performed on carefully selected patients, the Green transfer reliably improves function and appearance.[11, 68, 162, 192, 207]

Using similar indications, others have advocated transferring the pronator teres[36] or flexor carpi radialis[79] or brachioradialis[80, 122] to the extensor carpi radialis longus or brevis to improve wrist extension. If the wrist shows marked ulnar deviation, the extensor carpi ulnaris may be transferred to the extensor carpi radialis brevis.[67, 195]

IMPROVING FINGER EXTENSION

On the basis of electromyographic data, Hoffer and associates[76, 77] believe that most patients with cerebral palsy have weak release (finger extension) rather than weak grasp. Clinically, such a patient is unable to extend the fingers with the wrist passively held in neutral. The flexor carpi ulnaris is active in phase with the extensor digitorum communis. A Green transfer in such cases will improve wrist extension, but release is difficult. Accordingly, Hoffer and associates[76, 77] recommend transferring the flexor carpi ulnaris to extensor digitorum communis and have reported successful long-term results.[76] The flexor digitorum sublimis, brachioradialis, or extensor carpi ulnaris may be transferred to the extensor digitorum communis, if indicated by electromyography.[76, 77, 79, 122]

WRIST ARTHRODESIS

Wrist motion is important for grasp and release by tenodesis effect.[182, 223] In a severely deformed wrist with no potential for useful function, wrist arthrodesis may be indicated to facilitate hygiene and improve appearance in the young. In the older individual, it may relieve pain of arthritis or dislocation. A soft tissue release may be required in addition for release of severely flexed digits.[78] Arthrodesis may rarely be indicated for wrist instability in dystonia or athetosis.[66, 223]

CORRECTION OF PRONATION DEFORMITY

Although most prehensile activity occurs in pronation,[223] fixed pronation deformity and loss of active supination can be disabling. Procedures used to correct wrist flexion deformity in patients with cerebral palsy, such as the Green transfer, myoaponeurotic release, and flexor-pronator slide, result in some incidental improvement in supination.[11, 68, 81, 192, 225] A pronator teres tenotomy[178, 182, 223] or pronator quadratus release[162, 71, 229] gives additional correction. Pronator teres rerouting converts a spastic muscle into an active supinator and results in an average increase of 45° in supination.[161, 178] The procedure is performed by releasing the tendon at its insertion and redirecting it around the interosseous border to be implanted into the radius laterally.[115, 168] We prefer to divide the tendon in a Z-fashion, reroute the distal end, and repair it to its proximal member, keeping the forearm in 45° of supination. This maneuver is easier to perform and avoids the risk of a postoperative fracture.

TREATMENT OF THUMB DEFORMITY

Adduction contracture of the carpometacarpal joint in cerebral palsy may be accompanied by hyperextension and instability at the metacarpophalangeal joint or flexion deformity at the metacarpophalangeal and interphalangeal joints (thumb-in-palm deformity).[80] These deformities interfere with grasp and pinch. Stepwise release of the adductor pollicis, first dorsal interosseous, and flexor pollicis brevis, Z-lengthening of the flexor pollicis longus, and Z-plasty of the thumb web space are essential to correct the deformity.[66, 80, 91, 115] The palmaris longus, brachioradialis, flexor carpi radialis, or flexor digitorum sublimis should be transferred either to the abductor pollicis longus and extensor pollicis brevis, or to the rerouted extensor pollicis longus to help maintain correction.[66, 67, 80, 91, 122, 162, 182] Other alternatives for stabilization are an abductor pollicis longus tenodesis to the distal radius[225] and rerouting the extensor pollicis longus through the first dorsal interosseous compartment.[115] An unstable metacarpophalangeal joint can be stabilized by sesamoid-metacarpal synostosis[196, 224, 225] or a formal metacarpophalangeal arthrodesis.[182]

SUMMARY

In this chapter, we have discussed a spectrum of congenital and developmental wrist disorders. Given that they occur infrequently, not many surgeons would be fortunate enough to acquire a large clinical experience dealing with these conditions. Although treatment priorities and goals may differ among the various disorders, the surgeon's primary concern should be directed toward restoration and improvement of function. Some children with these disorders may have involvement of other musculoskeletal and visceral structures. In the management of these patients, upper limb surgery is but one part of a well-coordinated, multispecialty team approach.

References

1. Ali MS, Hooper G: Congenital pseudarthrosis of the ulna due to neurofibromatosis. J Bone Joint Surg 64B:600–602, 1982.
2. Allieu Y, Gomis R, Yoshimura M, et al: Congenital pseudarthrosis of the forearm: Two cases treated by free vascularized fibular grafting. J Hand Surg 5A:475–481, 1981.
3. Askins G, Ger E: Congenital constriction band syndrome. J Pediatr Orthop 8:461–466, 1988.
4. Atar D, Lehman WB, Posner M, et al: Ilizarov technique in treatment of congenital hand anomalies. Clin Orthop 273:268–274, 1991.
5. Banker BQ, Victor M, Adams RD: Arthrogryposis multiplex due to congenital muscular dystrophy. Brain 80:319–334, 1957.
6. Banker BQ: Neuropathological aspects of arthrogryposis multiplex congenita. Clin Orthop 194:30–43, 1985.
7. Barton NJ, Buck-Gramcko D, Evans DM, et al: Mirror hand treated by true pollicization. J Hand Surg 11B:320–336, 1986.
8. Barton NJ, Buck-Gramcko D, Evans DM: Soft-tissue anatomy of mirror hand. J Hand Surg 11B:307–319, 1986.

9. Bayne LG, Klug MS: Long-term review of the surgical treatment of radial deficiencies. J Hand Surg 12A:169–179, 1987.

10. Bayne LG: Congenital pseudarthrosis of the forearm. Hand Clinics 1:457–465, 1985.

11. Beach WR, Strecker WB, Coe J, et al: Use of the Green transfer in treatment of patients with spastic cerebral palsy: 17-year experience. J Pediatr Orthop 11:731–736, 1991.

12. Bell DF: Congenital forearm pseudarthrosis: Report of six cases and review of the literature. J Pediatr Orthop 9:438–443, 1989.

13. Bennett JB, Hansen PE, Granberry WM, Cain TE: Surgical management of arthrogryposis in the upper extremity. J Pediatr Orthop 5:281–286, 1985.

14. Berkowitz AR, Melone CP, Belsky MR: Pisiform-hamate coalition with ulnar neuropathy. J Hand Surg 17A:657–662, 1992.

15. Bharucha EP, Pandya SS, Dastur DK: Arthrogryposis multiplex congenita. Part 1: Clinical and electromyographic aspects. J Neurol Neurosurg Psychiatr 35:425–434, 1972.

16. Blair WF, Shurr DG, Buckwalter JA: Functional status in ulnar deficiency. J Pediatr Orthop 3:37–40, 1983.

17. Bora FW Jr, Nicholson JT, Cheema HM: Radial meromelia: The deformity and its treatment. J Bone Joint Surg 52A:966–979, 1970.

18. Bora FW Jr, Osterman AL, Kaneda RR, Esterhai J: Radial club-hand deformity: Long-term follow-up. J Bone Joint Surg 63A:741–745, 1981.

19. Braun RM, Vise GT, Roper B: Superficialis-to-profundus transfer. J Bone Joint Surg 56A:466–472, 1974.

20. Broudy AS, Smith RJ: Deformities of the hand and wrist with ulnar deficiency. J Hand Surg 4A:304–315, 1979.

21. Brown GA, Osebold WR, Ponseti IV: Congenital pseudarthrosis of long bones: A clinical, radiographic, histological and ultrastructural study. Clin Orthop 128:228–242, 1977.

22. Brown LM, Robson MJ, Sharrard WJW: The pathophysiology of arthrogryposis multiplex congenita neurologica. J Bone Joint Surg 62B:291–296, 1980.

23. Buck-Gramcko D: Pollicization of the index finger: Methods and results in aplasia and hypoplasia of the thumb. J Bone Joint Surg 53A:1605–1617, 1971.

24. Buck-Gramcko D: Radialization as a new treatment for radial club hand. J Hand Surg 10A:964–968, 1985.

25. Burgess RC, Cates H: Deformities of the forearm in patients who have multiple hereditary osteochondromas. J Bone Joint Surg 75A:13–18, 1993.

26. Carroll RE, Bowers WH: Congenital deficiency of the ulna. J Hand Surg 2A:169–174, 1977.

27. Carroll RE, Hill NA: Triceps transfer to restore elbow flexion: The study of fifteen patients with paralytic lesions and arthrogryposis. J Bone Joint Surg 52A:239–244, 1970.

28. Carroll RE, Louis DS: Anomalies associated with radial dysplasia. J Pediatr 84:409–411, 1974.

29. Carroll RE: Use of the fibula for reconstruction in congenital absence of the radius. J Bone Joint Surg 48A:1012, 1966.

30. Catagni MA, Szabo RM, Cattaneo R: Preliminary experience with the Ilizarov method in late reconstruction of radial hemimelia. J Hand Surg 18A:316–321, 1993.

31. Chan KM, Ma GFY, Cheng JCY, Leung PC: The Krukenberg procedure: A method of treatment for unilateral anomalies of the upper limb in Chinese children. J Hand Surg 9A:548–551, 1984.

32. Cheng JCY, Hung LK, Bundoc RC: Congenital pseudarthrosis of the ulna. J Hand Surg 19B:238–243, 1994.

33. Cleveland RH, Gilsanz V, Wilkinson RH: Congenital pseudarthrosis of the radius. Am J Roentgenol 130:955–957, 1978.

34. Cockshott WP: Carpal fusions. Am J Roentgenol 89:1260–1271, 1963.

35. Cockshott WP: Pisiform hamate fusion. J Bone Joint Surg 51B:778–780, 1969.

36. Colton CL, Ransford AO, Lloyd-Roberts GC: Transposition of the tendon of pronator teres in cerebral palsy. J Bone Joint Surg 58B:220–223, 1976.

37. Cooney WP, Schutt AH: Arthrogryposis multiplex congenita. In Bora FW Jr (ed): The Pediatric Upper Extremity: Diagnosis and Management. Philadelphia, WB Saunders, 1986, pp 339–348.

38. Cox H, Viljoen D, Beighton P: Radial ray defects and associated anomalies. Clin Genet 35:322–330, 1989.

39. Dannenberg M, Anton JI, Spiegel MB: Madelung's deformity: Considerations of its roentgenological diagnostic criteria. Am J Roentgenol 42:671–676, 1939.

40. Dastur DK, Razzak ZA, Bharucha EP: Arthrogryposis multiplex congenita. Part 2: Muscle pathology and pathogenesis. J Neurol Neurosurg Psychiatry 35:435–450, 1972.

41. Davidson J, Beighton P: Whence the arthrogrypotics? J Bone Joint Surg 58B:492–495, 1976.

42. Dawe C, Wynne-Davies R, Fulford GE: Clinical variation in dyschondrosteosis. J Bone Joint Surg 64B:377–381, 1982.

43. Delaney TJ, Eswar S: Carpal coalitions. J Hand Surg 17A:28–31, 1992.

44. Delorme TL: Treatment of congenital absence of the radius by transepiphyseal fixation. J Bone Joint Surg 51A:117–129, 1969.

45. Dhouailly D, Kieny M: The capacity of the flank somatic mesoderm of early bird embryos to participate in limb development. Dev Biol 28:162–175, 1972.

46. Dobyns JH, Wood VE, Bayne LG: Congenital hand deformities. In Green DP (ed): Operative Hand Surgery, ed 3. New York, Churchill Livingstone, 1993, pp 251–548.

47. Drachman DB, Banker BQ: Arthrogryposis multiplex congenita. Arch Neurol 5:77–93, 1961.

48. Ducloyer P, Leclercq C, Lisfranc R, Saffar P: Spontaneous ruptures of extensor tendons of the fingers in Madelung's deformity. J Hand Surg 16B:329–333, 1991.

49. Duraiswami PK: Experimental causation of congenital skeletal defects and its significance in orthopaedic surgery. J Bone Joint Surg 54B:646–698, 1952.

50. Fabry G, Lammens J, Van Melkebeek J, Stuyck J: Treatment of congenital pseudarthrosis with the Ilizarov technique. J Pediatr Orthop 8:67–70, 1988.

51. Fagg PS: Reverse Madelung's deformity with nerve compression. J Hand Surg 13B:23–27, 1988.

52. Fagg PS: Wrist pain in the Madelung's deformity of dyschondrosteosis. J Hand Surg 13B:11–15, 1988.

53. Fairbank TJ: Dysplasia epiphysealis hemimelica (tarso-epiphyseal aclasis). J Bone Joint Surg 38B:237–257, 1956.

54. Fasting OJ, Bjerkreim I: Dysplasia epiphysealis hemimelica. Acta Orthop Scand 47:217–225, 1976.

55. Flatt AE: The Care of Congenital Hand Anomalies, ed 2. St Louis, Quality Medical Publishing, 1994.

56. Fogel GR, McElfresh EC, Peterson HA, Wicklund PT: Management of deformities of the forearm in multiple hereditary osteochondromas. J Bone Joint Surg 66A:670–680, 1984.

57. Foulkes GD, Reinker K: Congenital constriction band syndrome: A seventy-year experience. J Pediatr Orthop 14:242–248, 1994.

58. Frantz DH, O'Rahilly R: Ulnar hemimelia. Artif Limbs 15:25–35, 1971.

59. Freire-Maia A: Genetics of acheiropodia (the handless and footless families of Brazil). Clin Genet 7:98–102, 1975.

60. Friedlander HL, Westin GW, Wood WL Jr: Arthrogryposis multiplex congenita. J Bone Joint Surg 50A:89–112, 1968.

61. Ganos DL, Imbriglia JE: Symptomatic carpal coalition of the pisiform and hamate. J Hand Surg 16A:646–650, 1991.

62. Garst RJ: The Krukenberg hand. J Bone Joint Surg 72B:385–388, 1991.

63. Gibson DA, Urs NDK: Arthrogryposis multiplex congenita. J Bone Joint Surg 52B:483–493, 1970.

64. Goldberg MJ, Bartoshesky LE: Congenital hand anomaly: Etiology and associated malformations. Hand Clin 1:405–415, 1985.

65. Golding JSR, Blackburne JS: Madelung's disease of the wrist and dyschondrosteosis. J Bone Joint Surg 58B:350–352, 1976.

66. Goldner JL: Surgical reconstruction of the upper extremity in cerebral palsy. Hand Clin 4:223–265, 1988.

67. Goldner JL: Upper extremity reconstructive surgery in cerebral palsy or similar conditions. In Reynolds FC (ed): AAOS Instructional Course Lectures, vol 18. St Louis, CV Mosby, 1961, pp 169–177.

68. Green WT, Banks HH: Flexor carpi ulnaris transplant and its use in cerebral palsy. J Bone Joint Surg 44A:1343–1352, 1962.

69. Gropper PT: Ulnar dimelia. J Hand Surg 8A:487–491, 1983.
70. Gross SC, Watson HK, Strickland JW, et al: Triquetral-lunate arthritis secondary to synostosis. J Hand Surg 14A:95–102, 1989.
71. Gschwind C, Tonkin M: Surgery for cerebral palsy. Part 1: Classification and operative procedures for pronation deformity. J Hand Surg 17B:391–395, 1992.
72. Hall JG, Reed SD, Greene G: The distal arthrogryposes: Delineation of new entities—review and nosologic discussion. Am J Med Genet 11:185–239, 1982.
73. Harrison RG, Pearson MA, Roaf R: Ulnar dimelia. J Bone Joint Surg 42B:549–555, 1960.
74. Heikel HVA: Aplasia and hypoplasia of the radius. Acta Orthop Scand Suppl 39:9–155, 1959.
75. Henry A, Thorburn MJ: Madelung's deformity: A clinical and cytogenetic study. J Bone Joint Surg 49B:66–73, 1967.
76. Hoffer MM, Lehman M, Mitani M: Long-term follow-up on tendon transfers to the extensors of the wrist and fingers in patients with cerebral palsy. J Hand Surg 11A:836–840, 1986.
77. Hoffer MM, Perry J, Melkonian GJ: Dynamic electromyography and decision-making for surgery in the upper extremity of patients with cerebral palsy. J Hand Surg 4A:424–431, 1979.
78. Hoffer MM, Zeitzew S: Wrist fusion in cerebral palsy. J Hand Surg 13A:667–670, 1988.
79. Hoffer MM: Cerebral Palsy. In Green DP (ed): Operative Hand Surgery, ed 3. New York, Churchill Livingstone, 1993, pp 215–223.
80. House JH, Gwathmey FW, Fidler MO: A dynamic approach to the thumb-in-palm deformity in cerebral palsy. J Bone Joint Surg 63A:216–225, 1981.
81. Inglis AE, Cooper W: Release of the flexor-pronator origin for flexion deformities of the hand and wrist in spastic paralysis: A study of eighteen cases. J Bone Joint Surg 48A:847–857, 1966.
82. Inoue G, Miura T: Arteriographic findings in radial and ulnar deficiencies. J Hand Surg 16B:409–412, 1981.
83. Jaffe HL: Hereditary multiple exostosis. Arch Pathol 36:335–357, 1943.
84. Johnson J, Omer GE Jr: Congenital ulnar deficiency: Natural history and therapeutic implications. Hand Clin 1:499–510, 1985.
85. Joji S, Mizuseki T, Katayama S, et al: Aetiology of Kienböck's disease based on a study of the condition among patients with cerebral palsy. J Hand Surg 18B:294–298, 1993.
86. Kaempffe FA, Gillespie R: Pseudarthrosis of the radius after fracture through normal bone in a child who had neurofibromatosis. J Bone Joint Surg 71A:1419–1421, 1989.
87. Kakulas BA, Adams RD: Diseases of Muscle: Pathological Foundations of Clinical Myology, ed 4. Philadelphia, Harper and Row, 1985, pp 321–328.
88. Kallen B, Rahmani T M-Z, Winberg J. Infants with congenital limb reduction registered in the Swedish register of congenital malformations. Teratology 29:73, 1984.
89. Kameyama O, Ogawa R: Pseudarthrosis of the radius associated with neurofibromatosis: Report of a case and review of the literature. J Pediatr Orthop 10:128–131, 1990.
90. Kato K: Congenital absence of the radius. With review of literature and report of three cases. J Bone Joint Surg 22:589–625, 1924.
91. Keats S: Surgical treatment of the hand in cerebral palsy: Correction of thumb-in-palm and other deformities. J Bone Joint Surg 47A:274–284, 1965.
92. Kelikian H: Congenital Deformities of the Hand and Forearm. Philadelphia, WB Saunders, 1974, pp 939–967.
93. Kessler I: Centralisation of the radial club hand by gradual distraction. J Hand Surg 14B:37–42, 1989.
94. Kino Y: Clinical and experimental studies of the congenital constriction band syndrome, with an emphasis on its etiology. J Bone Joint Surg 57A:636–643, 1975.
95. Krichler U: Uber die Variationsbreite der kongenitalen Fibula- und Radiusaplasien. Z menschl Vererb-u Konstit-Lehre 24:480, 1940.
96. Kruger LM, Fishman S: Myoelectric and body-powered prosthesis. J Pediatr Orthop 13:68–75, 1993.
97. Krugliak L, Gadoth N, Behar AJ: Neuropathic form of arthrogryposis multiplex congenita. J Neurol Sci 37:179–185, 1978.
98. Lamb DW, Wynne-Davies R, Soto L: An estimate of the population frequency of congenital malformations of the upper limb. J Hand Surg 7A:557–562, 1982.
99. Lamb DW: Madelung deformity. J Hand Surg 13B:3–4, 1988.
100. Lamb DW: Radial club hand: A continuing study of sixty-eight patients with one hundred and seventeen club hands. J Bone Joint Surg 59A:1–13, 1977.
101. Lamb DW: Upper limb dysplasia: Form and function. J R Coll Surg Edinb 28:203–213, 1983.
102. Langer LO Jr: Dyschondrosteosis, a heritable bone dysplasia with characteristic roentgenographic features. Am J Roentgenol 95:178–188, 1965.
103. Laurin CA, Fevreau JC, Labelle P: Bilateral absence of the radius and tibia with bilateral duplication of the ulna and fibula: A case report. J Bone Joint Surg 46A:137–142, 1964.
104. Leri A, Weill J: Une affection congénitale et symétrique du developpement osseux: La dyschondrostéose. Bull Mém Soc Med Hop Paris 53:1491–1494, 1929.
105. Leung PC, Chan KM, Cheng JCY: Congenital anomalies of the upper limb among the Chinese population in Hong Kong. J Hand Surg 7:563–565, 1982.
106. Lidge RT: Congenital radial deficient club hand. J Bone Joint Surg 51A:1041–1042, 1969.
107. Linscheid RL: Madelung's deformity. American Society for Surgery of the Hand. 1979 Correspondence letter, no 24. Correspondence Club, 1979.
108. Lister G: Reconstruction of the hypoplastic thumb. Clin Orthop 195:52–65, 1985.
109. Lloyd-Roberts GC, Lettin AWF: Arthrogryposis multiplex congenita. J Bone Joint Surg 52B:494–508, 1970.
110. Lloyd-Roberts GC: Treatment of defects of the ulna in children by establishing cross-union with the radius. J Bone Joint Surg 55B:327–330, 1973.
111. Madelung O: Die Spontane Subluxation der Hand nach vorne. Arch Klin Chir 23:395–412, 1878.
112. Manske PR, McCarroll HR Jr, James M: Type III-A hypoplastic thumb. J Hand Surg 20A:246–253, 1995.
113. Manske PR, McCarroll HR, Swanson K: Centralization of the radial club hand: An ulnar surgical approach. J Hand Surg 6A:423–433, 1981.
114. Manske PR, Rotman MB, Dailey LA: Long-term functional results after pollicization for the congenitally deficient thumb. J Hand Surg 17A:1064–1072, 1992.
115. Manske PR: Cerebral palsy of the upper extremity. Hand Clin 6:697–709, 1990.
116. Manske PR: Radial deficiency. In Barr JS Jr (ed): AAOS Instructional Course Lectures, vol XXXVIII. Chicago, American Academy of Orthopaedic Surgeons, 1989, pp 43–57.
117. Marcus NA, Omer GE Jr: Carpal deviation in congenital ulnar deficiency. J Bone Joint Surg 66A:1003–1007, 1984.
118. Masada K, Tsuyuguchi Y, Kawai H, et al: Operations for forearm deformity caused by multiple osteochondromas. J Bone Joint Surg 71B:24–29, 1989.
119. Masterson E, Earley MJ, Stephens MM: Congenital pseudarthrosis of the ulna treated by free vascularized fibular graft: A case report and review of methods of treatment. J Hand Surg 18B:285–288, 1993.
120. Matev I, Karagancheva S: The Madelung deformity. Hand 7:152–158, 1975.
121. Mathoulin C, Gilbert A, Azze RG: Congenital pseudarthrosis of the forearm: Treatment of six cases with vascularized fibular graft and a review of literature. Microsurgery 14:252–259, 1993.
122. McCue FC, Honner R, Chapman WC: Transfer of the brachioradialis for hands deformed by cerebral palsy. J Bone Joint Surg 52A:1171–1180, 1970.
123. Menelaus MB: Radial club hand with absence of the biceps muscle treated by centralization of the ulna and triceps transfer: Report of two cases. J Bone Joint Surg 58B:488–491, 1976.
124. Mennen U: Early corrective surgery of the wrist and elbow in arthrogryposis multiplex congenita. J Hand Surg 18B:304–307, 1993.

125. Meyn M, Ruby L: Arthrogryposis of the upper extremity. Orthop Clin North Am 7:501–509, 1976.

126. Miller JK, Wenner SM, Kruger LM: Ulnar deficiency. J Hand Surg 11A:822–829, 1986.

127. Minnaar AB DeV: Congenital fusion of the lunate and triquetral bones in the South African Bantu. J Bone Joint Surg 34B:45–48, 1952.

128. Miura T, Nakamura R, Horii E: The position of symbrachydactyly in the classification of congenital hand anomalies. J Hand Surg 19B:350–354, 1994.

129. Moses JM, Flatt AE, Cooper RR: Annular constricting bands. J Bone Joint Surg 61A:562–565, 1979.

130. Mowery CA, Gelberman RH, Rhoades CE: Upper extremity tendon transfers in cerebral palsy: Electromyographic and functional analysis. J Pediatr Orthop 5:69–72, 1985.

131. Nielsen JB: Madelung's deformity: A follow-up study of 26 cases and a review of the literature. Acta Orthop Scand 48:379–384, 1977.

132. O'Rahilly R: Developmental deviations in the carpus and in the tarsus. Clin Orthop 10:9–18, 1957.

133. O'Rahilly R: Morphological patterns in limb deficiencies and duplications. Am J Anat 89:135–193, 1951.

134. O'Rahilly R: Radial hemimelia and the functional anatomy of the carpus. J Anat 80:179–183, 1946.

135. Ogden JA, Watson HK, Bohne W: Ulnar dysmelia. J Bone Joint Surg 58A:467–475, 1976.

136. Ogino T, Minami A, Fukuda K, Kato H: Congenital anomalies of the upper limb among the Japanese in Sapporo. J Hand Surg 11B:364–371, 1986.

137. Omer GE, Capen DA: Proximal row carpectomy with muscle transfers for spastic paralysis. J Hand Surg 1:197–204, 1976.

138. Ostrowski DM, Eilert RE, Waldstein G: Congenital pseudarthrosis of the ulna: A report of two cases and a review of the literature. J Pediatr Orthop 5:463–467, 1985.

139. Otto AW: Monstrum humanum extremitatibus incurvatus: Monstrorum Sexcentorum descriptio Anatomica in Vratislaviae Museum. Anatomico-Pathologieum Breslau, 1841, p 322.

140. Pardini AG Jr: Radial dysplasia. Clin Orthop 57:153–177, 1968.

141. Patterson TJS: Congenital ring-constrictions. Br J Plast Surg 14:1–31, 1961.

142. Peterson HA: Forearm deformities in children with multiple hereditary osteochondromata. J Pediatr Orthop 14:92–100, 1994.

143. Peterson HA: Multiple hereditary osteochondromas. Clin Orthop 239:222–230, 1989.

144. Petit JL: Rémarques sur un enfant nouveau-né, dont les bras étaint difformes. Med Acad R Soc 1733, p 17.

145. Peyton RS, Moore JR: Fracture through a congenital carpal coalition. J Hand Surg 19A:369–371, 1994.

146. Pho RWH, Patterson MH, Kour AK, Kumar VP: Free vascularised epiphyseal transplantation in upper extremity reconstruction. J Hand Surg 13B:440–447, 1988.

147. Poznanski AK, Holt JF: The carpals in congenital malformation syndromes. Am J Roentgenol 112:443–459, 1971.

148. Pritchett JW: Lengthening the ulna in patients with hereditary multiple exostosis. J Bone Joint Surg 68B:561–565, 1986.

149. Quan L, Smith DW: The VATER association: Vertebral defects, anal atresia, tracheoesophageal fistula with esophageal atresia, radial dysplasia. Birth Defects 8:75–78, 1972.

150. Ranawat CS, DeFiore J, Straub LR: Madelung's deformity: An end result study of surgical treatment. J Bone Joint Surg 57A:772–775, 1975.

151. Rao SB, Roy DR: Dysplasia epiphysealis hemimelica: Upper limb involvement with associated osteochondroma. Clin Orthop 307:103–109, 1994.

152. Rayan GM: Ulnocarpal arthrodesis for recurrent radial clubhand deformity in adolescents. J Hand Surg 17A:24–27, 1992.

153. Richin PF, Kranik A, Van Herpe L: Congenital pseudarthrosis of both bones of the forearm. J Bone Joint Surg 58A:1032–1033, 1976.

154. Riordan DC, Mills EH, Alldredge RH: Congenital absence of the ulna. J Bone Joint Surg 43A:614, 1961.

155. Riordan DC: Congenital absence of the radius or ulna. J Bone Joint Surg 54B:381, 1972.

156. Riordan DC: Congenital absence of the radius: A fifteen-year follow-up study. J Bone Joint Surg 45A:1783, 1963.

157. Riordan DC: Congenital absence of the radius. J Bone Joint Surg 37A:1129–1140, 1955.

158. Rogala EJ, Wynne-Davies R, Littlejohn A, Gormley J: Congenital limb anomalies: Frequency and aetiological factors. J Med Genet 11:221–233, 1974.

159. Rooker GD, Goodfellow JW: Kienböck's disease in cerebral palsy. J Bone Joint Surg 59B:363–365, 1977.

160. Roth JH, O'Grady SE, Richards RS, Porte AM: Functional outcome of upper limb tendon transfers performed in children with spastic hemiplegia. J Hand Surg 18B:299–303, 1993.

161. Sakellarides HT, Mital MA, Lenzi WD: Treatment of pronation contractures of the forearm in cerebral palsy by changing the insertion of the pronator radii teres. J Bone Joint Surg 63A:645–652, 1981.

162. Samilson RL, Morris JM: Surgical improvement of the cerebral-palsied upper limb. J Bone Joint Surg 46A:1203–1216, 1964.

163. Saunders JW Jr: The proximo-distal sequence of origin of the parts of the chick wing and the role of the ectoderm. J Exp Zool 108:363–403, 1948.

164. Sayre RH: A contribution to the study of clubhand. Trans Am Orthop 6:208–216, 1893.

165. Schoenecker PL, Cohn AK, Sedgwick WG, et al: Dysplasia of the knee associated with the syndrome of thrombocytopenia and absent radius. J Bone Joint Surg 66A:421–427, 1984.

166. Sellers DS, Sowa DT, Moore JR, Weiland AJ: Congenital pseudarthrosis of the forearm. J Hand Surg 13A:89–93, 1988.

167. Shapiro F, Simon S, Glimcher MJ: Hereditary multiple exostosis. J Bone Joint Surg 61A:815–824, 1979.

168. Sharrard WJW: Paediatric Orthopaedics and Fractures, ed 3. Oxford, Blackwell Scientific Publications, 1994, p 923.

169. Simmons BP, McKenzie WD: Symptomatic carpal coalition. J Hand Surg 10A:190–193, 1985.

170. Skerik SK, Flatt AE: The anatomy of congenital radial dysplasia: Its surgical and functional implications. Clin Orthop 66:125–155, 1969.

171. Solomon L: Bone growth in diaphyseal aclasis. J Bone Joint Surg 43B:700–716, 1961.

172. Solomon L: Hereditary multiple exostosis. J Bone Joint Surg 45B:292–304, 1963.

173. Spinner M, Freundlich BD, Abeles ED: Management of moderate longitudinal arrest of development of the ulna. Clin Orthop 69:199–202, 1970.

174. Stevenson RE, Meyer LC: The limbs. In Stevenson RE, Hall JG, Goodman RM (eds): Human Malformations and Related Anomalies, vol 2. New York, Oxford University Press, 1993, pp 699–720.

175. Stoffel A, Stempel E: Anatomische studien über die klumphand. Z Orthop Chir 23:1–15, 1909.

176. Straub LR: Congenital absence of the ulna. Am J Surg 109:300–305, 1965.

177. Straub LR: Congenital absence of the radius and of the ulna. J Bone Joint Surg 54A:907, 1972.

178. Strecker WB, Emanuel JP, Dailey L, Manske PR: Comparison of pronator tenotomy and pronator rerouting in children with spastic cerebral palsy. J Hand Surg 13A:540–543, 1988.

179. Swanson AB, Tada K, Yonenobu K: Ulnar ray deficiency: Its various manifestations. J Hand Surg 9A:658–664, 1984.

180. Swanson AB: A classification of congenital limb malformations. J Hand Surg 1:8–22, 1976.

181. Swanson AB: Phocomelia and congenital limb malformations: Reconstruction and prosthetic replacement. Am J Surg 109:294–299, 1965.

182. Swanson AB: Surgery of the hand in cerebral palsy and the swan-neck deformity. J Bone Joint Surg 42A:951–964, 1960.

183. Swanson AB: The Krukenburg procedure in the juvenile amputee. J Bone Joint Surg 46A:1540–1548, 1964.

184. Swinyard CA, Bleck EE: The etiology of arthrogryposis (multiple congenital contractures). Clin Orthop 194:15–29, 1985.

185. Sykes PJ, Chandraprakasam T, Percival NJ: Pollicisation of the index finger in congenital anomalies. J Hand Surg 16B:144–147, 1991.

186. Tachdjian MO, Minear WL: Sensory disturbances in the hands of children with cerebral palsy. J Bone Joint Surg 40A:85–90, 1958.

187. Tachdjian MO: Paediatric Orthopaedics, ed 2. Philadelphia, WB Saunders, 1990, p 1738.

188. Tada K, Yonenobu K, Swanson AB: Congenital constriction band syndrome. J Pediatr Orthop 4:726–730, 1984.

189. Talab YA: Congenital pseudarthrosis of the ulna. Clin Orthop 291:246–250, 1993.

190. Taussig HB: A study of the German outbreak of phocomelia: The thalidomide syndrome. JAMA 180:1106–1114, 1962.

191. Temtamy SA, McKusick VA: In Bergsma D (ed): The Genetics of Hand Malformations. Birth Defects 14:36–71, 1978.

192. Thometz JG, Tachdjian M: Long-term follow-up of the flexor carpi ulnaris transfer in spastic hemiplegic children. J Pediatr Orthop 8:407–412, 1988.

193. Tickle C, Summerbell D, Wolpert L: Postaxial signaling and specification of digits in chick embryo morphogenesis. Nature 254:199–202, 1975.

194. Tickle C: Experimental embryology as applied to the upper limb. J Hand Surg 12B:294–300, 1987.

195. Tonkin M, Gschwind C: Surgery for cerebral palsy. Part 2: Flexion deformity of the wrist and fingers. J Hand Surg 17B:396–400, 1992.

196. Tonkin MA, Beard AJ, Kemp SJ, Eakins DF: Sesamoid arthrodesis for hyperextension of the thumb metacarpophalangeal joint. J Hand Surg 20A:334–338, 1995.

197. Tsai T, Ludwig L, Tonkin M: Vascularized fibular epiphyseal transfer: A clinical study. Clin Orthop 210:228–234, 1986.

198. Tsuge K, Watari S: New surgical procedure for correction of club hand. J Hand Surg 10B:90–94, 1985.

199. Tsuyuguchi Y, Tada K, Yonenobu K: Mirror hand anomaly: Reconstruction of the thumb, wrist, forearm and elbow. Plast Reconstr Surg 70:384–388, 1982.

200. Uchida Y, Sugioka Y: Peripheral nerve palsy associated with congenital constriction band syndrome. J Hand Surg 16B:109–112, 1991.

201. Upton J, Tan C: Correction of constriction rings. J Hand Surg 16A:947–953, 1991.

202. Vickers D, Nielsen G: Madelung deformity: Surgical prophylaxis (physiolysis) during the late growth period by resection of the dyschondrosteosis lesion. J Hand Surg 17B:401–407, 1992.

203. Villa A, Paley D, Catagni MA, et al: Lengthening of the forearm by the Ilizarov technique. Clin Orthop 250:125–137, 1990.

204. Watson HK, Beebe RD, Cruz NI: A centralization procedure for radial clubhand. J Hand Surg 9A:541–547, 1984.

205. Weeks PM: Surgical correction of upper extremity deformities in arthrogryposis. Plast Reconstr Surg 36:459–465, 1965.

206. Weiland AJ, Kleinert HE, Kutz J, Daniels RK: Free vascularized bone grafts in surgery of the upper extremity. J Hand Surg 4A:129–144, 1979.

207. Wenner SM, Johnson KA: Transfer of the flexor carpi ulnaris to the radial wrist extensors in cerebral palsy. J Hand Surg 13A:231–233, 1988.

208. Wenner SM, Saperia BS: Proximal row carpectomy in arthrogrypotic wrist deformity. J Hand Surg 12A:523–525, 1987.

209. White GM, Weiland AJ: Madelung's deformity: Treatment by osteotomy of the radius and Lauenstein procedure. J Hand Surg 12A:202–204, 1987.

210. White WF: Flexor muscle slide in the spastic hand: The Max Page operation. J Bone Joint Surg 54B:453–456, 1972.

211. Whittem JH: Congenital abnormalities in calves: Arthrogryposis and hydranencephaly. J Pathol 73:375–387, 1957.

212. Williams PF: Management of upper limb problems in arthrogryposis. Clin Orthop 194:60–67, 1985.

213. Williamson DM, Copeland SA, Landi A: Pseudarthrosis of the radius treated by free vascularized bone graft. J Hand Surg 14B:221–225, 1989.

214. Wolpert L: Pattern formation in limb morphogenesis. Fortschr Zool 26:142–152, 1981.

215. Wood VE, Sauser D, Mudge D: The treatment of hereditary multiple exostosis of the upper extremity. J Hand Surg 10A:505–513, 1985.

216. Wood VE: Small finger pollicization in the radial club hand. J Hand Surg 13A:96–99, 1988.

217. Wynne-Davies R, Kuczynski K, Lamb DW, Smith RJ: Congenital abnormalities of the hand. In Lamb DW, Hooper G, Kuczynski K (eds): The Practice of Hand Surgery. Oxford, Blackwell Scientific Publications, 1989, pp 475–526.

218. Wynne-Davies R, Williams PF, O'Connor JCB: The 1960's epidemic of arthrogryposis multiplex congenita. J Bone Joint Surg 63B:76–82, 1981.

219. Wynne-Davies R, Lamb DW: Congenital upper limb anomalies: An etiologic grouping of clinical, genetic, and epidemiological data from 387 patients with "absence" defects, constriction bands, polydactylies, and syndactylies. J Hand Surg 10A:958–964, 1985.

220. Yonenobu K, Tada K, Swanson AB: Arthrogryposis of the hand. J Pediatr Orthop 4:599–603, 1984.

221. Younge D, Arford C: Congenital pseudarthrosis of the forearm and fibula. Clin Orthop 265:277–279, 1991.

222. Zancolli E, Mitre H: Latissimus dorsi transfer to restore elbow flexion: An appraisal of eight cases. J Bone Joint Surg 55A:1265–1275, 1973.

223. Zancolli EA, Goldner LJ, Swanson AB: Surgery of the spastic hand in cerebral palsy: Report of the Committee on Spastic Hand Evaluation. J Hand Surg 8:766–772, 1983.

224. Zancolli EA, Zancolli EA Jr: Surgical management of the hemiplegic spastic hand in cerebral palsy. Surg Clin North Am 61:395–406, 1981.

225. Zancolli EA: Structural and Dynamic Bases of Hand Surgery, ed 2. Philadelphia, JB Lippincott, 1979, pp 263–283.

226. Zionts LE, Osterkamp JA, Crawford TO, Harvey JP Jr: Congenital annular bands in identical twins. J Bone Joint Surg 66A:450–453, 1984.

CHAPTER 30

Traumatic and Acquired Wrist Disorders in Children

Sudhir B. Rao, MD, and Alvin H. Crawford, MD

In contrast to congenital and developmental disorders of the wrist, traumatic and acquired disorders of the distal forearm and wrist are among the most common conditions encountered in a pediatric orthopedic practice. The natural playfulness of children results in frequent accidental injury, and fractures of the upper extremity, especially those of the distal forearm and hand, are seen more commonly than any other. The tremendous increase in organized sports participation at school and club levels has resulted in a greater awareness of chronic overuse injuries to the wrist. The presence of a physeal plate is unique to growing children, and the attendant potential for growth and remodeling allows us a certain leeway in treating fractures of the distal forearm that is not applicable in adults. Damage to the physis from trauma or infection, however, may lead to premature growth arrest, which can have serious implications. This chapter emphasizes some of the more common traumatic and acquired conditions affecting the distal forearm and wrist.

FRACTURES OF THE DISTAL FOREARM

In the growing child, injuries to the upper extremity outnumber those to the lower extremity.[110] Fractures of the distal radius and ulna account for 35 to 47 percent of all fractures and are more common in boys. Seventy-five to eighty-six percent of all forearm fractures occur in the distal third.[27, 49, 81, 97, 107, 153] Metaphyseal fractures are more common before 10 years of age, whereas physeal injuries peak at 12 to 14 years for boys and 11 to 13 years for girls.[97] Despite their frequency, the majority of these injuries can be treated successfully. Most of these injuries occur following a fall on the outstretched hand (FOOSH injury).

The incidence of serious complications is low if one pays careful attention to detail. Clinical examination is the key to diagnosis. Whereas displaced fractures may be plainly visible as a "dinner-fork" deformity, tenderness, swelling, and a painful range of motion are important clues to a subtle fracture that may otherwise be missed on the initial radiograph.

The entire extremity should be examined because, not uncommonly, fractures of the distal humerus, clavicle, or, rarely, carpal bones[24, 64, 141] may coexist. An assessment of the neurovascular status concludes the examination.

Anteroposterior and lateral radiographs show the extent of displacement and angulation and offer a guide to management. We currently use intravenous sedation when manipulating fractures in the emergency room. Intravenous regional or hematoma blocks may also be used. If we do not obtain satisfactory alignment, or if the fracture subsequently becomes displaced, we recommend re-manipulation using general anesthesia.

Types

DISTAL RADIAL AND ULNAR METAPHYSIS

Buckle and greenstick fractures are most common, constituting between 52 and 88 percent of all forearm fractures.[31, 49, 153] A buckle or torus fracture represents one end of the spectrum (Fig. 30–1), whereas more severe injuries may show considerable volar angulation and dorsal displacement. The reverse pattern with dorsal angulation is much less common. Fractures of the distal radius may occur in isolation or may be accompanied by an epiphyseal, physeal, or metaphyseal ulnar fracture.

Buckle fractures need to be immobilized for the duration of pain. Most greenstick fractures can be reduced without completing the fracture,[27] although on occasion, such a maneuver may be necessary to achieve a satisfactory stable reduction.[107] Displaced fractures should be reduced by applying traction and increasing the deformity, followed by manipulation to achieve apposition and alignment of the fragments. Although pronation of the distal fragment is usually recommended, one should judge the position of immobilization from the best alignment achieved.

The reduction is maintained with a well-molded sugar-tong splint employing three-point fixation, although an above-elbow cast is an acceptable alternative. A below-elbow cast may be substituted 3 weeks later, and healing usually occurs within 4 to 6 weeks.

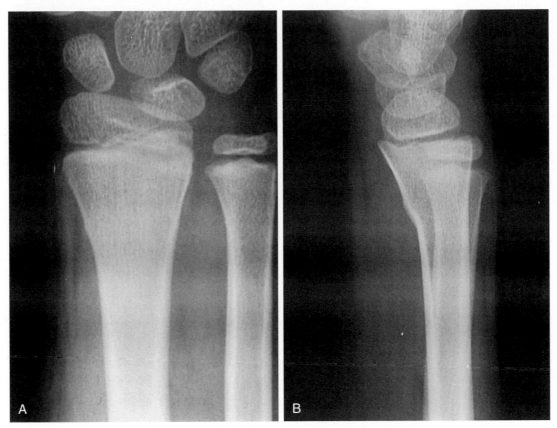

Figure 30–1. *A* and *B,* Torus fracture of the distal radius.

PHYSEAL FRACTURES

Physeal injuries of the distal radius and ulna are less common than metaphyseal fractures.[97, 107] They occur more commonly in children 11 to 14 years of age, with a significantly higher incidence in boys. Physeal injuries in the distal radius account for 17.9 to 50 percent of all physeal injuries (Fig. 30–2) and are second in incidence only to physeal fractures in the fingers.[97, 107, 110]

In a series of 100 cases, Mizuta and colleagues[97] found seven Salter-Harris type I, 90 type II, one type III, and two type IV injuries. Peterson[111] has described a new type of physeal injury (Peterson type I), characterized by a transverse metaphyseal fracture with an extension to the physis. There is minimal disruption of the growth plate and an extremely low incidence of growth arrest. In his series, this type accounted for 32.9 percent of distal radial physeal fractures. There is controversy regarding the existence of a true Salter-Harris type V injury, although chronic repetitive stress such as occurs in young gymnasts has been shown to result in premature growth arrest.

Distal radial physeal fractures are usually accompanied by a fracture of the ulna. Often, the unossified ulnar styloid is avulsed, and the avulsion becomes evident at a later date as an apparently non-united ossicle, which, rarely, in itself gives rise to symptoms.[108] These injuries should be treated by closed reduction in the same fashion as metaphyseal fractures.

In contrast, distal ulnar physeal injuries are much less common and have an incidence of less than 4.5 percent.[2, 39, 97, 110] These are usually Salter-Harris type I, II, or III injuries and may show considerable displacement. The incidence of growth arrest following this fracture is high.[59] Every attempt should be made to reduce these fractures by closed means, failing which, open reduction is indicated. We recommend closed reduction of the displaced epiphysis followed by fixation using percutaneous smooth Kirschner (K) wires.

COMPLETE FRACTURE OF THE RADIUS WITH INTACT ULNA

Complete fracture of the radius with an intact ulna is an infrequent injury.[53, 120] Closed reduction may be difficult, and subsequent loss of alignment is common. Roy[120] has shown that up to 16° of radial deviation, 20° of dorsal angulation, and shortening will remodel satisfactorily in a patient less than 12 years of age. Fractures that are unstable or difficult to reduce should be percutaneously pinned.[120] We prefer threaded K wires, which may be used as a "joystick" to obtain acceptable alignment.

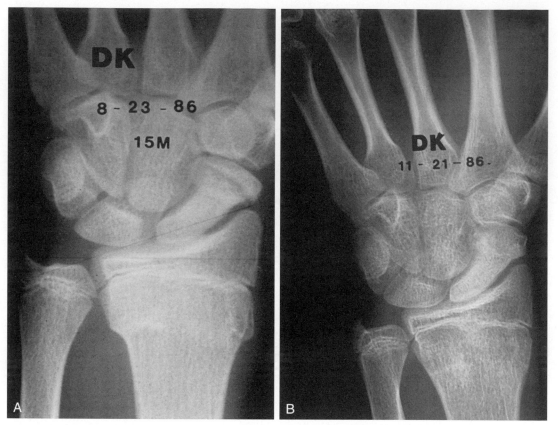

Figure 30–2. *A,* An acute fracture of the distal radius in a 13-year-old male, including an incidentally noted non-union in the distal third of the scaphoid. The scaphoid fracture was presumably sustained in a fall 9 months prior to diagnosis. *B,* Radiograph taken after 12 weeks of thumb spica cast immobilization, demonstrating complete union of the radial and scaphoid fractures.

ISOLATED DISLOCATION OF THE DISTAL ULNA

Forced pronation or supination may result in a dorsal or volar dislocation of the distal ulna. The injury results in disruption of the radioulnar joint capsule and the triangular fibrocartilaginous cartilage complex (TFCC). Actually, however, it is the radius along with the carpus that displaces in relation to the ulna. This injury is rare in the skeletally immature.[29] Closed reduction is accomplished by rotating the forearm in the opposite direction. For dorsal dislocation of the ulna, the forearm should be immobilized in full supination. For volar dislocation of the ulna, some manual pressure may be necessary to dislodge the ulna prior to immobilization in full pronation. Failure to attain a congruent reduction may necessitate open reduction of the distal radioulnar joint (see Chapter 23).

GALEAZZI FRACTURE

Fracture of the distal radius accompanied by dislocation of the distal radioulnar joint is an uncommon injury in children, accounting for less than 3 percent of all forearm fractures.[145] The radial fracture may occur at the junction of the middle and distal thirds (Fig. 30–3) or distally as a metaphyseal or physeal fracture. In the former instance, the radius is usually displaced anteriorly, and in the latter, posteriorly. In a Galeazzi-equivalent injury,[78, 82] the distal radioulnar joint remains intact, but instead, there is an ulnar physeal fracture. A true lateral radiograph shows abnormal dorsal or volar displacement of the ulna. Closed reduction is usually successful provided that the forearm is immobilized in supination with an above-elbow cast.

Walsh and colleagues[145] reviewed 41 cases of Galeazzi fractures in children. In 41 percent of cases, the injury to the distal radioulnar joint was not recognized. Overall, 88 percent of patients had excellent or fair results. A satisfactory outcome correlated with immobilization of the forearm in supination in an above-elbow cast. In this reduced position of the distal radioulnar joint, adequate healing of the TFCC seems more likely to occur in children. Mikic[96] similarly reported excellent results in 10 of 12 children with Galeazzi fracture-dislocation, of whom only 2 required internal fixation of the radius.[96]

ESSEX-LOPRESTI INJURY

Essex-Lopresti injury consists of distal radioulnar joint dislocation accompanied by a fracture or dislo-

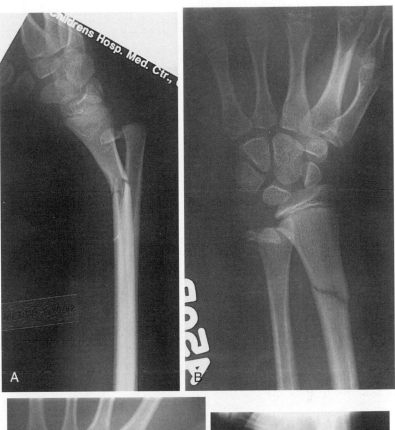

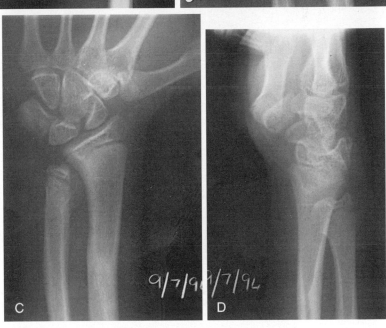

Figure 30–3. *A* and *B*, Galeazzi fracture-dislocation of the distal radius with a completely displaced Salter II fracture of the distal ulna in a 12-year-old male. *C* and *D*, One year following closed reduction and immobilization, there is premature growth arrest of the distal ulna, resulting in shortening. Note the Park-Harris line in the *distal* radius parallel to the physis, indicating normal growth.

cation of the humeroradial joint. The latter may be a fracture of the proximal radius or capitellum, or a radial head dislocation as in a Monteggia injury.[138] There is substantial disruption of the interosseous membrane and triangular fibrocartilaginous ligament complex, leading to proximal migration of the radius. This radioulnar dissociation may not always be evident initially, and it is critical to examine the wrist clinically and radiologically to assess the status of

the distal radioulnar joint. The best results are obtained by early treatment.[37, 138]

Radial length should be restored by internal fixation of the radial head or capitellar fracture. The distal radioulnar joint may be stabilized by transfixing the radius to the ulna with Kirschner wires or by immobilizing the forearm in full supination. The TFCC and interosseous membrane may be amenable to repair in the acute situation, although we are unaware of a published series describing results. Radial head excision should be avoided at all costs in children.

Complications

FAILURE OF REDUCTION

Entrapment of flexor or extensor tendons, or neurovascular structures within the fracture site, may necessitate open reduction.[42, 73, 93, 131] Rarely, excessive swelling may dictate a period of elevation prior to attempting closed reduction. In general, we accept bayonet apposition of the fracture in patients less

than 10 years of age provided that alignment is acceptable (Fig. 30–4).

LOSS OF REDUCTION AND MALUNION

Failure to apply a well-molded cast may result in loss of alignment once swelling has decreased. Up to 9 percent[53, 144] of forearm fractures may require re-manipulation. If the loss of reduction is significant, we prefer to re-manipulate the fracture under general anesthesia. Although osteoclasis may be performed in distal-third fractures up to 3 weeks after injury, caution should be exercised in re-manipulating physeal injuries over a week old. In one series, recurrent angulation was seen in 10 percent of greenstick frac-

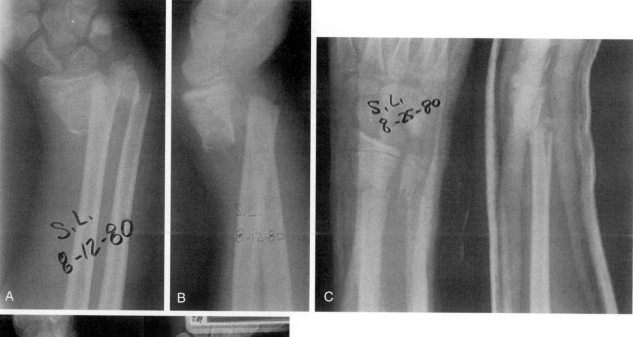

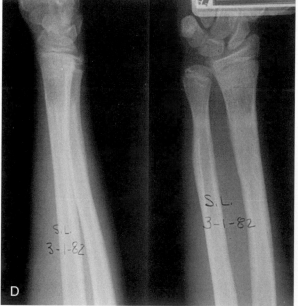

Figure 30–4. An 11-year-old child with a completely displaced fracture of the distal radius and ulna, which was reduced and immobilized in bayonet apposition. The fracture remodeled completely, restoring normal anatomic alignment. *A* and *B,* Anteroposterior and lateral radiographs showing a completely displaced fracture of the distal radius and ulna. *C,* Post-reduction radiographs showing satisfactory alignment and bayonet apposition. *D,* Anteroposterior and lateral radiographs taken 1½ years following injury. There has been complete remodeling of both bones. The Park-Harris growth arrest line in the distal radius has progressed symmetrically away from the physis, indicating normal growth. The child regained a full range of motion. (From Crawford AH: Pitfalls and complications of fractures of the distal radius and ulna in childhood. Hand Clinics 4:403–413, 1988.)

tures and 25 percent of complete fractures of the distal radius and ulna.[31]

More often than not, this angular malalignment is a manifestation of rotatory deformity, which can be easily corrected by pronation of the distal fragment.[44] In Daruwalla's[30] series of 53 patients with forearm fractures, angular or rotational malunion occurred in 49 percent of cases. Of the 30 patients with distal radius fractures, significant angular and rotational malalignment was seen in 9 and 4 patients, respectively. Overall, limitation of forearm rotation, chiefly pronation, occurred in 28 patients, 15 of whom had distal-third fractures. An angular deformity of one or both bones was responsible in 20 cases, rotational malalignment in 6, and inferior radioulnar joint disruption in 2. Although none of the patients in the study had functional disability, Daruwalla[30] noted that 10° or more of angulation always resulted in loss of rotation, and that any angular deformity of 10° or more in a child older than 10 years was unlikely to correct, as was any rotational malalignment. Gandhi and associates[49] have noted an almost complete correction of angular deformity 5 years following distal forearm fractures, thus reaffirming the excellent remodeling capacity in children less than 10 years of age. When malunion results in significant loss of motion, corrective osteotomy is indicated (Fig. 30–5).

PREMATURE GROWTH ARREST

Despite the frequency of distal radial physeal fractures, growth arrest following this injury is uncommon,[31, 81, 97, 110] although the exact incidence is not known. Mizuta and colleagues[97] found no case of distal radial growth arrest among 100 fractures, whereas Lee and associates[81] found a 7 percent incidence in a select group of 100 patients. In our experience, growth arrest has been rare and has followed severe open fractures. Factors predisposing to growth arrest include severity of injury, repeated manipulations, vascular compromise of the growth plate following open reduction or compartment syndrome, and transgression of the physis with threaded Kirschner wires.[18, 81, 97] There is no convincing evidence that the use of smooth wires for a short time causes growth arrest.[116]

Complete growth arrest of the distal radial physis results in shortening, loss of radial tilt, and relative ulnar lengthening, whereas a Madelung-like deformity may occur with a partial growth arrest of the ulnar, volar physis of the radius. If growth arrest is recognized early, excision of the bar may be worthwhile.[18] However, in complete growth arrest, ulnar epiphyseodesis or shortening may be indicated, in addition to radial osteotomy with bone grafting to restore normal anatomy.[18, 67, 81, 155]

Growth arrest following distal ulnar physeal injury is much more common (see Fig. 30–3). Golz and coworkers[59] described premature growth arrest in 55 percent of their 18 patients. Although radial bowing, carpal translocation, and radioulnar impingement

have been known to occur, functional disability is rare.[104]

RADIOULNAR SYNOSTOSIS

Cross-union is a rare complication resulting in complete loss of forearm rotation. Vince and Miller[143] classified these complications into three types. Type 1 involves the distal intra-articular radius and ulna; type 2, the distal and middle thirds; and type 3, the proximal third. Predisposing factors include severe trauma, open reduction, and repeated manipulation. The results of surgical excision in children have been complicated by recurrence, perhaps owing to the increased osteogenic potential. If indicated, excision may be performed at 6 to 12 months, when the synostosis has matured.[46, 143] Despite the use of various interposition materials, results have been rather unsatisfactory. The use of postoperative low-dose radiation appears promising,[28] but we would not recommend its use in children.

ACUTE NEUROPATHY

Stretching, impingement at the fracture site, and compression by hematoma may result in an acute neuropathy of the median nerve. Prompt reduction and percutaneous K-wire fixation in unstable fractures should result in resolution in the majority of cases.[146] An acute volar compartment syndrome following distal fractures of the radius and ulna is rare and is related primarily to the severity of injury. In the presence of severe swelling, a hematoma block may precipitate a compartment syndrome by acutely increasing pressure in an already compromised situation.[67, 154]

FRACTURES OF THE THUMB METACARPAL

O'Brien[106] has classified fractures through the base of the thumb metacarpal in children into four types. Type A is a laterally angulated metaphyseal fracture (Fig. 30–6); types B and C are Salter-Harris type II injuries that are angulated medially or laterally (Fig. 30–7); and type D is a Salter-Harris type III injury, which is the equivalent of a Bennett's fracture in adults. Types A, B, and C should be reduced by closed manipulation. Up to 30 percent of angulation may remodel. Type C fractures have a reputation for frequently being irreducible because of soft tissue buttonholing, and one should not hesitate to proceed to open reduction, as for all displaced type D fractures.

CARPOMETACARPAL INJURIES

Pure dislocation or fracture-dislocation of one or more carpometacarpal joints is a rare injury in chil-

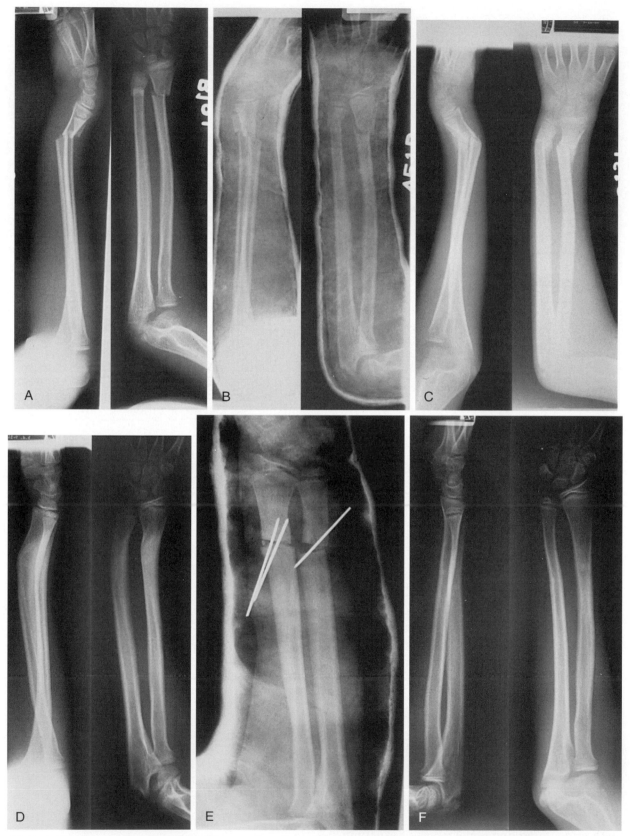

Figure 30–5. *A,* This 10-year-old boy sustained a fracture through the distal radius and ulna that was treated by closed reduction and casting. *B,* Check radiographs at 1 week showed satisfactory alignment. The patient subsequently removed his cast and when seen 5 weeks later *(C)* was noted to have recurrence of angulation. This was treated expectantly for a year. *D,* At 1 year, there was failure of complete remodeling along with loss of forearm rotation. *E,* The patient underwent corrective osteotomy of the distal radius and ulna. *F,* Following uneventful healing, the patient regained full wrist pronation and supination. (From Crawford AH: Pitfalls and complications of fractures of the distal radius and ulna in childhood. Hand Clinics 4:403–413, 1988.)

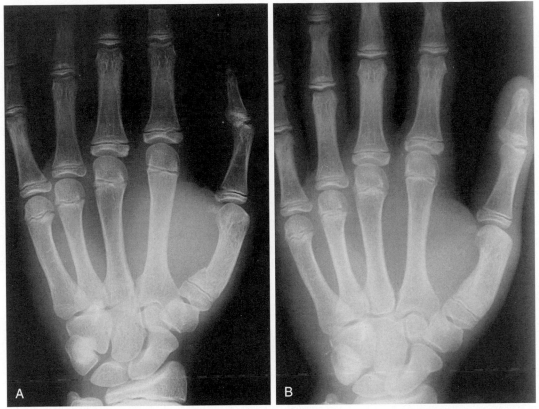

Figure 30–6. *A,* Laterally angulated fracture through the base of the thumb metacarpal in an 11-year-old boy. *B,* Radiograph taken 4 weeks later shows healing.

dren and often follows a severe crushing injury. Skeletal stabilization is essential for soft tissue healing. The displacement is easily reducible and maintained by K-wire fixation (Fig. 30–8). Dislocation of the basal thumb joint is also rare, because the adjacent physis or metaphysis fractures preferentially.

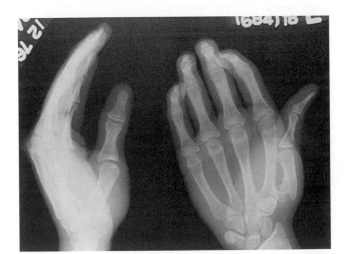

Figure 30–7. A displaced Salter-Harris II fracture of the thumb metacarpal in an 8-year-old boy. This is the pediatric equivalent of a Bennett fracture.

CARPAL INJURIES

Given the frequency of FOOSH injuries in children, carpal injuries are surprisingly uncommon. The thick cartilaginous shell of carpal bones may have a cushioning effect.[65] Subtle fractures through largely unossified elements may be missed on plain radiographs, although magnetic resonance (MR) imaging can detect these fractures with greater sensitivity. Eccentric ossification of the scaphoid makes evaluation of scapholunate diastasis difficult. Nevertheless, we cannot overemphasize the importance of a careful and diligent clinical examination. A child with a tender, swollen wrist and normal radiograph should be treated with cast immobilization until subsequent clinical examination and radiographs establish a definite diagnosis or conclusively rule out a fracture.

Fracture of the Scaphoid

The scaphoid is the most commonly fractured carpal bone in children, accounting for 0.39 percent of all childhood fractures and between 0.45 and 1.7 percent of all upper limb fractures.[23, 141] The peak age of occurrence in children is between 10 and 14 years, when the ossified scaphoid has assumed an adult shape. A fall on the outstretched hand is the most

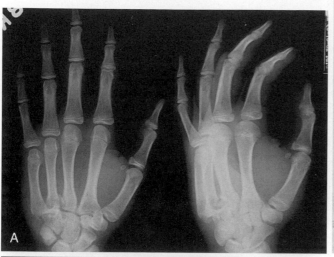

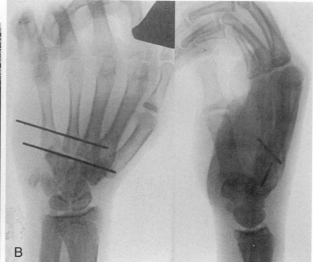

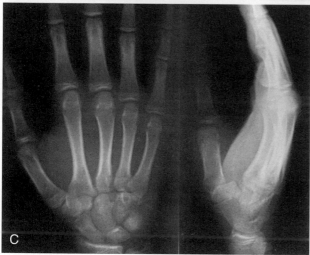

Figure 30–8. *A,* Fracture-dislocation of the fourth and fifth carpo-metacarpal joints. This injury is easy to reduce but usually unstable, requiring internal fixation. *B,* Closed reduction and percutaneous Kirschner-wire fixation. *C,* Radiograph taken 6 months later shows healing in anatomic alignment.

common mode of injury, but direct trauma, especially in younger children, may result in multiple carpal bone fractures.[17, 79] A careful clinical examination is important, because up to 12 percent of fractures may be missed on the initial radiograph.[23, 141]

Scaphoid fractures in children differ from those in adults in several respects. In children, between 59 and 87 percent of scaphoid fractures occur in the distal third, and half to two thirds of these are avulsions of the tubercle or dorsoradial surface[23, 101, 141] (Fig. 30–9). The remainder occur mostly at the waist (Fig. 30–10). In young children, a fracture through the proximal chondro-osseous junction may not be evident radiologically; this situation can result later in a bipartite scaphoid.[79] Eccentric ossification of the scaphoid may account for the erroneous labeling of some injuries as proximal pole fractures.[79, 112] In contrast to scaphoid fractures in adults, up to 23% of scaphoid fractures in children may be incomplete, and less than 8 percent show significant displacement.[23, 141]

In children, virtually all scaphoid fractures heal

uneventfully if recognized and treated promptly. There is ample evidence that use of a below-elbow thumb spica cast for 4 to 10 weeks suffices in children.[23, 65, 141] Non-united fractures are rare; fewer than 20 have been reported in the literature (Fig. 30–11). Virtually all have occurred at the waist. Non-union may follow a missed diagnosis, inadequate immobilization, or severe displacement. The infrequency of non-union in children may be a consequence of the preponderance of distal pole fractures combined with good healing potential. Established non-unions respond successfully to anterior bone grafting,[127] but there may be a place for prolonged cast immobilization in delayed unions.[141, 151] Owing to lack of adequate data on the long-term outcome of scaphoid non-union in children,[122] some authorities treat asymptomatic non-unions expectantly. Although it is said that the vascular supply of the scaphoid does not change appreciably with growth,[135] we are not aware of any reported case of avascular necrosis in children. Larson and associates[79] described one case of non-union with increased radiodensity of the prox-

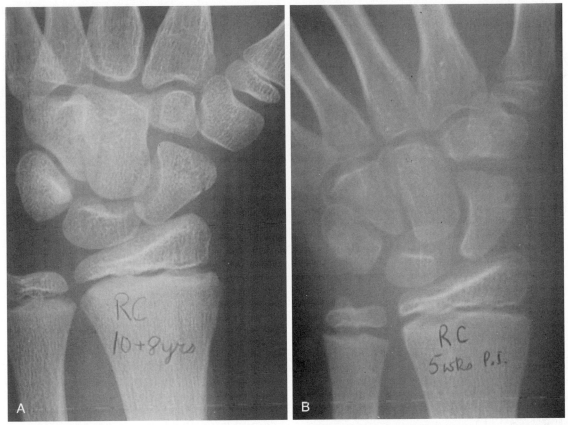

Figure 30–9. *A*, Fracture through the distal tuberosity of the scaphoid in a 9-year-old child. *B*, Healing following 5 weeks of immobilization.

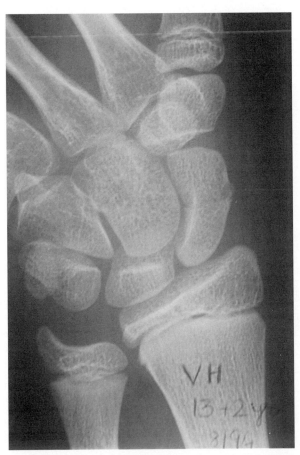

Figure 30–10. Fracture through the scaphoid waist in a 13-year-old boy.

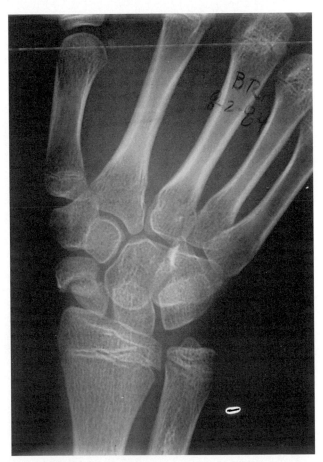

Figure 30–11. Asymptomatic non-union of the scaphoid in a 12-year-old girl 1 year following a fall.

imal pole, but this finding in itself may not constitute evidence of avascularity.

Fracture of Other Carpal Bones

Injuries to other carpal bones are rare enough to merit case reports. The capitate is the next most commonly fractured bone.[106] A fall on the outstretched hand causes impingement of the dorsal radial cortex against the neck of the capitate, resulting in a fracture. Indeed, the same mechanism may also cause an associated scaphoid fracture.[5, 60] These injuries heal uneventfully with a period of immobilization. Any displacement of the fracture may suggest a more significant injury. Although fragment rotation is not reported in children, the proximal fragment may rotate through 180 degrees, the so-called naviculocapitate syndrome, necessitating open reduction. Severe direct trauma has been reported to cause fracture of the hamate (Fig. 30–12), trapezium, and capitate,[4, 17] and other rare injuries, such as fracture of the triquetrum and posterior dislocation of the trapezium and trapezoid, have also been reported.[48]

CARPAL INSTABILITY

Perilunar dislocations of the carpus and its variants are rare in children. There are two case reports of trans-scaphoid–perilunar dislocation in the literature.[23, 114] Published series in the adult literature have also included cases of carpal dislocations in the skel-

etally immature.[25, 68] We recommend that these injuries be treated with the same degree of urgency and aggressiveness as in the adult.

Both dissociative and nondissociative carpal instability patterns have been reported in the skeletally immature. Zimmerman and Weiland[156] reported on a 13-year-old boy with scapholunate dissociation and a dorsal intercalated segment instability (DISI), which was treated with soft tissue reconstruction. Gerard[51] described a 7-year-old girl with a long-standing palmar intercalated segment instability and carpal collapse, which was treated with preliminary traction and ligament reconstruction. Suzuki and Herbert[133] reported on two children with symptomatic DISI deformity secondary to malunited fracture of the scaphoid. Over a 4-year period, there was complete remodeling of the deformity and resolution of symptoms. Midcarpal instability, a form of nondissociative carpal instability, has been described in adolescents and adults.[72, 83, 148] It may be secondary to trauma, malunited distal radius fracture, or developmental ligament laxity. The instability may be volarly or dorsally directed and is best detected by cineradiography. We recommend that symptomatic carpal instability in the skeletally immature be treated nonoperatively or with soft tissue reconstruction. Limited wrist arthrodesis should be avoided.

SPORTS INJURIES

Acute bony and soft tissue injuries are the result of a single unpredictable event. Diagnosis and manage-

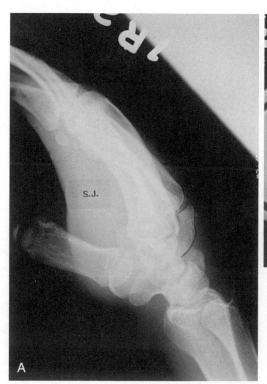

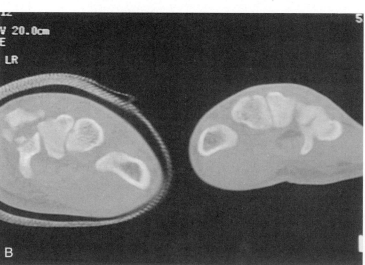

Figure 30–12. Lateral radiograph (A) and CT scan (B) showing a coronal split fracture of the hamate in a 15-year-old male.

ment of these injuries is usually straightforward. Chronic oft-repeated stress, however, results in the so-called "overuse injury." The incidence of injury varies with the sport and the level of competitiveness. Goldberg and colleagues[57] reported that hand and wrist injuries accounted for 27.6 percent of all injuries in youth football. Lorish and associates[87] reported wrist injuries in 6 of 73 injuries in wrestling. Ferkel and colleagues[47] reported a wrist injury rate of 47 percent in roller skating injuries, the majority of which were distal radius fractures.

The wrist is particularly vulnerable in gymnastics because of the repeated weight-bearing loads and stresses entailed. The incidence of chronic wrist pain in competitive gymnasts is reported to be as high as 87.5 percent.[91] The uniqueness of this situation is appreciated when one considers the training profile of an elite gymnast. Entry usually occurs at 6 or 7 years of age, with peak performance in middle to late teens and retirement soon thereafter.[31, 92] Class I athletes may train 3 to 4 hours a day during these years of skeletal growth and development. Up to 2 million people participate in organized gymnastics at school, college, or club level. Injury rate in gymnastics is higher among elite and competitive athletes.[95] Floor exercises are responsible for the highest number of injuries in general,[50] whereas the pommel horse is responsible for the very high incidence of wrist pain in men.[20, 91] Accidental failure of the dowel grip to disengage has resulted in serious fracture-dislocations of the wrist.[147]

This section deals with chronic wrist problems seen in athletes. A large proportion of those injuries occur in gymnasts. Chronic wrist pain may have multiple causes, and a thorough clinical and radiographic examination, with arthrography, arthroscopy, or MR imaging if indicated, is essential to establish an accurate diagnosis.

Stress Injury to the Distal Radius and Ulna

Continued stressful use of the wrist in gymnastics has been shown to result in widening and irregularity of the distal radial growth plate and volar spurring of the metaphysis along with cystic and sclerotic changes and flattening and beaking of the epiphysis.[19, 20, 121] Similar changes can occur in the distal ulna.[19, 52] More than 80 percent of elite gymnasts may have such changes,[10] which are evident on the radiograph and represent an adverse reaction of the growth plate to excessive compressive loading and may ultimately lead to premature growth arrest of the distal radial physis.[3, 137] The predominant involvement of the ulnar and volar part of the physis attests to major load transmission through the capitolunate axis and may result in a Madelung-like deformity.[3, 20, 142] Positive ulnar variance has been shown to be more common in gymnasts than in a control population and to be correlated with the intensity and duration of training.[91]

The usual presentation is one of diffuse activity-related dorsal wrist pain aggravated by dorsiflexion. Clinical and radiographic improvement can occur with cessation of stressful activity.[19, 20] In more advanced cases, the acquired positive ulnar variance may result in painful abutment against the lunate and triquetrum in addition to TFCC and lunotriquetral ligament tears. Distal ulnar shortening may be indicated in recalcitrant cases.[84, 137]

Impaction Syndromes

Acute or repetitive hyperextension and compression forces in gymnasts, weight lifters, and roller skaters can cause impingement lesions consisting of chondromalacia, reactive sclerosis, and resultant synovitis. A lateral radiograph may show sclerosis or spurring in the distal radius and carpal bones or the presence of a small ossicle.[84, 147] Rest, anti-inflammatory medication, and physical modalities should be tried initially. For cases that fail to respond to such treatment, an arthroscopic or open débridement and cheilectomy may be indicated.

Soft Tissue Lesions

Soft tissue lesions in athletes include de Quervain's tenovaginitis, intersection syndrome (inflammation of the bursa between the radial wrist extensor and abductor pollicis longus tendons), and dorsal wrist ganglia.[147] *Wrist splints* refers to ulnar-sided forearm pain of unknown etiology that usually responds to nonoperative measures. *Dorsal capsulitis* and *dorsiflexion jam syndrome* are nonspecific terms used to describe a gymnast's wrist with diffuse dorsal pain, swelling, and tenderness, which may represent synovitis secondary to carpal chondromalacia.

Miscellaneous Sports Injuries

Repetitive submaximal compressive loading can result in stress fractures of the distal radius, scaphoid, and capitate.[66, 94, 100, 118] Diagnosis is established by bone scanning and MR imaging. Immobilization in a cast should result in healing. Nakamura and associates[102] have described sports-related Keinböck's disease in teenagers. Repetitive tensile loading of volar wrist ligaments may result in a spectrum of carpal instabilities.[35]

INFECTIONS

Bacterial Infections

ACUTE HEMATOGENOUS OSTEOMYELITIS

Acute hematogenous osteomyelitis in children affects the radius and ulna in 5 to 9 percent of cases. Carpal bone osteomyelitis is extremely rare.[45, 69, 80, 124, 134, 140] Males are affected more commonly, and a history of trauma or recent infection is often obtained. *Staphylococcus aureus* is the primary offender in 60 to 80 percent of cases,[32, 69, 80, 134] followed by group A *Streptococcus* and gram-negative rods. *Haemophilus influenzae* is an uncommon pathogen confined to children less than 3 years of age.[32, 45, 103]

Hematogenous bacterial seeding occurs initially in the metaphysis. Infection spreads due to pressure of exudate, pus, and secondary vascular thrombosis. In children more than 12 months of age, the growth plate acts as a barrier. Because the distal radial and ulnar metaphysis is extra-articular, secondary joint involvement does not occur as a rule.

Clinically, there is severe pain and refusal to move the limb. Exquisite tenderness is elicited over the metaphysis, and in late cases, fluctuation or brawny induration suggests pus in the subperiosteal or intermuscular plane. A sympathetic joint effusion may coexist. Radiographs are nonspecific in the early stages, showing soft tissue changes. After 10 days or so, diffuse or spotty osteopenia, periosteal elevation, and new bone formation are seen.

A bacteriologic diagnosis can be established in 55 to 85 percent of cases by multiple-site cultures.[32, 45] Positive blood cultures are obtained in less than 60 percent of cases, whereas direct bone and soft tissue aspiration has a 69 percent positive yield. Technetium Tc 99m bone scanning has an 80 to 90 percent accuracy.[123, 140] A "cold" scan indicates an avascular segment of bone and has a 100 percent positive predictive value.[140]

Initial treatment consists of broad-spectrum penicillinase-resistant antibiotic coverage. If the child presents within 24 hours of the onset of symptoms, successful resolution of infection may be obtained. Later presentation, failure to improve with antibiotics, and the presence of pus or exudate on aspiration are absolute indications for surgical decompression (Fig. 30–13). There is ample evidence to show that 4 to 6 weeks of appropriate antibiotics result in a significantly reduced incidence of recurrence and chronic osteomyelitis.[16, 32, 103]

NEONATAL OSTEOMYELITIS

Staphylococcus aureus, group B *Streptococcus,* and gram-negative rod infections predominate in neonates. Sixty-five percent of patients have predisposing factors, such as prematurity, umbilical sepsis, and jaundice.[75, 150] The hip is most commonly affected, but half the patients have multiple bone involvement. These children may have overwhelming septicemia, and often, the absence of physical findings leads to a late diagnosis.[75] Tc 99m bone scanning is known to be unreliable in these patients.[9] Prior to the development of a secondary ossification center, metaphyseal vessels are not restricted by the growth plate and hence extend to the cartilaginous epiphysis.[139] This fact accounts for the very high incidence of associ-

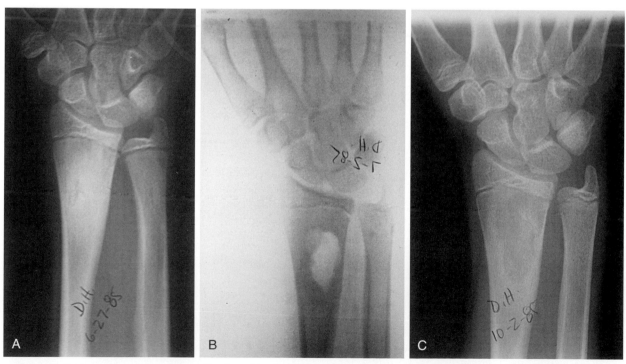

Figure 30–13. *A,* Osteomyelitis of the distal radius in a 14-year-old female presenting with a 6-week history of wrist pain. *B,* Intraoperative radiograph at the time of débridement and saucerization. *C,* Radiograph 4 months following surgery. Early surgical drainage and appropriate antibiotic treatment are vital to prevent sequestrum formation and growth arrest. Patients such as this one must be followed over a period of several years to detect the onset of late deformity.

ated septic arthritis and irreparable damage to the growth plate in these cases.[75, 139, 150]

INFECTIONS IN SICKLE CELL DISEASE

Salmonella osteomyelitis is a hundred times more common in patients with sickle cell disease (hemoglobin SS, SC, AS, and other variants) than in the general population.[33, 40] Positive bacterial cultures may be obtained in up to 74 percent of cases.[40, 56] Epps and colleagues[41] reported isolating S. aureus in 8 of 15 patients with sickle cell disease. Multiple and often symmetric bone involvement, subacute onset, chronicity, and recurrences may be seen.[40, 41] Osteomyelitis may be difficult to differentiate from aseptic bone infarction. The hand-foot syndrome is a painful aseptic bony infarction affecting hands and feet that typically presents between 6 and 24 months of age (Fig. 30–14). Bone infarction at any site may be complicated by secondary infection.[41] A child with sickle cell disease who presents with a painful extremity should be regarded as having osteomyelitis, and every attempt should be made to establish a diagnosis by repeated blood and bone aspirate cultures.

SEPTIC ARTHRITIS

The incidence of acute bacterial arthritis of the wrist is 4 percent.[69, 134] The infection is usually hematogenous in origin but may occur secondary to an open injury or spread of metaphyseal osteomyelitis prior to development of the growth plate.[139] A bacteriologic diagnosis is established in only two thirds of cases.[99, 103] The offending pathogens are similar to those seen in acute hematogenous osteomyelitis, with S. aureus being isolated in approximately 50 percent of cases.[26, 103] A notable difference is seen in children between 1 month and 2 years of age, in whom influenza B accounts for the majority of infections.[103, 134] In the newborn and the sexually active teenager, Neisseria gonorrhoeae may account for up to 7 percent of infections and is the most common cause of infective polyarthritis.[69] Gonococcal infection should be suspected in the sexually abused child.

Clinically, the wrist shows a warm effusion with extreme pain on attempted movement. Maximum tenderness is elicited at the joint level. The most efficacious method of diagnosis is joint aspiration, which may have a positive yield in up to 83 percent of cases[32] and also accomplishes some decompression. Broad-spectrum antibiotic coverage effective against S. aureus and H. influenzae should be commenced immediately. Failure of response within 24 hours or frank pus on aspiration of the wrist is an indication for open or arthroscopy-assisted drainage.

COMPLICATIONS

Timely aggressive medical and surgical management of bacterial infection should result in a low rate of complications. Chronic osteomyelitis or recurrent infection may occur if the duration of antibiotic coverage is less than 3 weeks or if a sequestrum has developed. Damage to the growth plate may occur, especially in neonatal infections, leading to shortening and deformity (Fig. 30–15). Radial lengthening has been described for such complications.[115] Marked cortical osteopenia and destruction may result in a pathologic fracture. Joint stiffness may occur secondary to extra-articular or intra-articular adhesions.

Atypical Infections

The wrist is the most commonly affected site in atypical mycobacterial infections. Children are affected less frequently than adults. The usual presentation is as a chronic extensor or flexor tenosynovitis, with joint involvement in some cases. There is a firm or boggy swelling with minimal tenderness and inflammation. Diagnosis may be delayed for several months.[34, 76] Infection with Mycobacterium fortuitum can occur following penetrating wounds and steroid injections,[68] whereas infection with Mycobacterium marinum or Mycobacterium terrae may follow exposure to a marine or farm environment, respectively.[76] Mycobacterium kansasii and Mycobacterium avium-intracellulare appear to be the most commonly isolated pathogens in deep mycobacterial infections.[76, 132] Mycobacterium tuberculosis infection occurs less commonly at the wrist, however, than at other sites, such as the spine and hip, although the clinical pre-

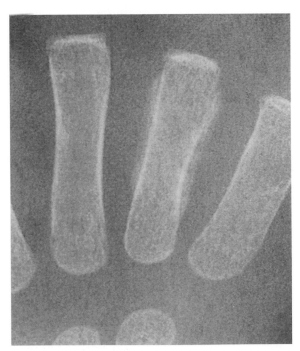

Figure 30–14. A 9-month-old male infant presented with wrist swelling. This radiograph showed periosteal reaction around the fourth metacarpal. This was the first indication that the child had sickle cell anemia. (From Oestreich AE, Crawford AH: Atlas of Pediatric Orthopedic Radiology. New York, Thieme, Inc, 1985.)

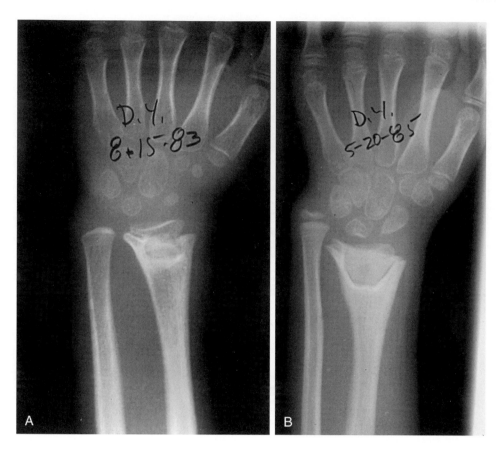

Figure 30–15. *A,* Growth arrest of the distal radial physis following medical and surgical management of acute hematogenous osteomyelitis. *B,* Two years following excision of physeal bar and Silastic interposition. There is failure of growth and resultant severe shortening of the radius.

sentation is similar. In addition, dactylitis involving the metacarpals may present as a swollen wrist (Fig. 30–16). Successful treatment of mycobacterial infection consists of surgical débridement along with long-term antibiotic therapy.

Cutaneous, tendon sheath, and joint infection may be caused by *Sporothrix schenckii.*[12] A variety of unusual bacterial, mycobacterial, and fungal infections may occur in the immunocompromized patient and are difficult to eradicate.[126] *Bacteroides* infection may follow a human bite wound.[117]

Chronic recurrent multifocal osteomyelitis is an inflammatory disorder of unknown origin often affecting the skeletally immature. It is characterized by repeated episodes of fever, local pain, and swelling over the metaphyseal region of tubular bones and clavicle. The radiographic appearance is similar to that of osteomyelitis. Antibiotics produce no response, although the condition shows eventual spontaneous remission.[15]

JUVENILE RHEUMATOID ARTHRITIS

Wrist and hand involvement occurs in over 50 percent of patients with juvenile rheumatoid arthritis (JRA),[22, 61] and its frequency is second to only that of knee involvement. Twenty percent of cases are seropositive, and these tend to have more severe involvement. Early clinical findings include synovitis and a

loss of complete wrist extension. With time, an ulnar deviation of the wrist and radial deviation of the digits appear. There is often limitation of flexion at the metacarpophalangeal and interphalangeal joints.[61] The wrist deformity is in contrast to the usual pattern of radial deviation seen in adults. It may be related in part to shortening of the ulna secondary to premature physeal arrest. This, in conjunction with attenuation of the volar wrist ligaments, results in ulnar and volar translocation of the carpus, leading to a bayonet deformity.[22] Secondary changes occur in the distal radial epiphysis consisting of wedging and fragmentation of its ulnar half. Swan neck and boutonnière deformities of the fingers are uncommon,[61] and spontaneous tendon ruptures and carpal tunnel syndrome are rare.[7] Involvement of the basal joint of the thumb may lead to dorsal subluxation and adduction contracture of the first web space.[125] Early radiographic changes include premature appearance of the carpal bones, soft tissue swelling, and periarticular osteopenia (Fig. 30–17). Later on, there is a decrease in the intercarpal and radiocarpal joint spaces with premature cessation of growth. Spontaneous intercarpal or radiocarpal fusion occurs more commonly in children with JRA than in adults.

Pharmacotherapeutic treatment is the mainstay in JRA, and surgical intervention is necessary in a small proportion of patients.[61] From an orthopedic standpoint, it is important to assess the hand closely and to institute splinting of the wrist and metacarpophalangeal joints in a functional position. Established deformity may respond to serial corrective splints or plaster casts. Intra-articular steroid injections have been shown to decrease pain and swelling and improve range of motion.[43]

The role of synovectomy is controversial.[43, 61, 62, 71] Improvement in pain and swelling may be expected if synovectomy is performed for medically unresponsive synovitis in the absence of degenerative changes. Evans and associates[43] have described lengthening of the ulna as a means to arrest progressive wrist deformity. Soft tissue release for contracture at the wrist or metacarpophalangeal joints may rarely be indicated.[43, 61]

REFLEX SYMPATHETIC DYSTROPHY

It has been suggested that reflex sympathetic dystrophy or sympathetically maintained pain syndrome is more common in children than previously thought.[14] Upper extremity involvement occurs far less commonly than lower limb involvement, and in one series, the wrist was involved in 7 percent of cases.[149]

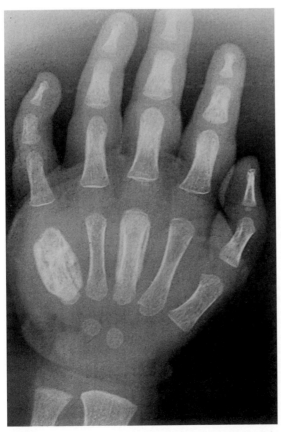

Figure 30–16. A 2-year-old child presented with swelling in the wrist and dorsum of the hand. The periosteal reaction about the small and long finger metacarpals is fairly typical of that seen in tuberculous dactylitis. A similar reaction may occur in the phalanges. (From Oestreich AE, Crawford AH: Atlas of Pediatric Orthopedic Radiology. New York, Thieme, Inc, 1985.)

The condition generally occurs in the teen years and has a predilection for girls. A high proportion of patients are involved in an organized sport. A history of significant trauma is obtained in less than half the patients,[14, 149] and in some, the disorder may follow operative intervention.

Diagnosis of reflex sympathetic dystrophy should be based on the presence of pain disproportionate to the injury, neuropathic pain pattern such as allodynia, hyperalgesia, and dysesthesia, and signs of autonomic imbalance such as cyanosis, mottling, hyperhidrosis, and coldness of the limb. Radiologic signs such as periarticular osteopenia are usually absent, and radionuclide bone scanning commonly shows decreased uptake in most children.[58] Intravenous phentolamine has been used as a diagnostic and prognostic indicator quite effectively.[8] Treatment should employ a multidisciplinary approach consisting of aggressive physical therapy, transcutaneous nerve stimulation, and pharmacologic measures such as nonsteroidal anti-inflammatory medication, opiates, and tricyclic antidepressants. Sympathetic blocks can be effective in resistant cases. Underlying emotional conflicts if detected should be resolved with psychological counseling.

CHILD ABUSE

Unexplained injury, especially in the very young child, should lead one to suspect child abuse. Metaphyseal "corner" or bucket-handle fractures have a high specificity for child abuse,[21] whereas physeal fractures and spiral fractures of the radius and ulna do not commonly result from nonaccidental trauma. Other highly suggestive fractures are those of the ribs, scapula, vertebrae, skull, and femur, especially if these are in different stages of healing. The injury pattern in conjunction with an inappropriate or changing history should lead one to suspect child abuse. Social services should be notified immediately so that such a child is removed from the harmful environment. Patients with osteogenesis imperfecta and Menkes's kinky-hair syndrome may present with multiple fractures and should be differentiated from possible victims of child abuse.

CARPAL AND TARSAL OSTEOLYSIS

A rare condition of unknown etiology, carpal and tarsal osteomyelitis is characterized by painful swelling of the wrist and feet accompanied by destruction of the carpal and tarsal bones.[13, 105] It is first recognized in early childhood and may be mistaken for juvenile rheumatoid arthritis. Except for nonspecific elevation of sedimentation rate and blood alkaline phosphatase level, laboratory studies are normal. There is progressive involvement of wrists, feet, and often elbows, resulting in stiffness and fixed deformity. Associated findings include scoliosis, abnormal

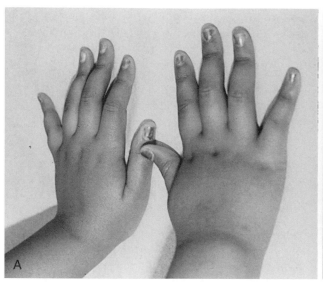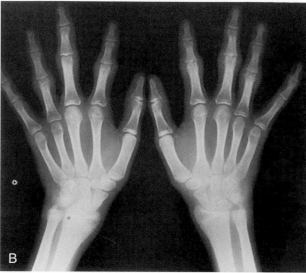

Figure 30–17. A 13-year-old female with pauciarticular juvenile rheumatoid arthritis. *A,* There is generalized swelling of both hands, which is most notable around the proximal interphalangeal joints. *B,* Anteroposterior radiograph of both hands. There is soft tissue swelling around the wrist and proximal interphalangeal joints along with diffuse carpal osteopenia and some loss of radiocarpal joint space.

skull shape, early degenerative changes in the hip, knee, and sacroiliac joints, joint laxity, and generalized muscle weakness. Radiologically, there is failure of appearance of carpal bones, progressive destruction of carpal and tarsal bones, and shortening and tapering of metacarpals, metatarsals, and proximal and distal forearm bones (Fig. 30–18). The condition may be associated with nephropathy, and in some cases appears to be inherited by autosomal dominant or recessive transmission. There are other causes of carpal osteolysis; Beals and Bird[13] have reviewed the subject in depth.

GANGLION

Ganglia, perhaps the most common soft tissue tumors in children, have a predilection for the wrist.[90] There is evidence to suggest that a significant proportion of ganglia in children resolve spontaneously with time. Rosson and Walker[119] found that 22 of 29 ganglia disappeared spontaneously at an average of 10.5 months. MacCollum[89] reported that 9 of 14 untreated wrist ganglia resolved spontaneously between 4 months and 5 years, whereas there were two recurrences among the 7 ganglia that were excised.

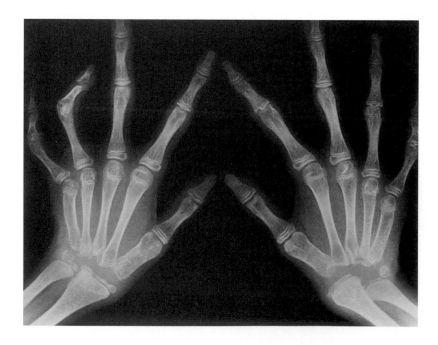

Figure 30–18. Severe carpal destruction, flattening of the distal radius and ulna epiphyses, expansion of the thumb and small metacarpals, and diffuse osteopenia characterize the hands of this boy with carpal osteolysis. Similar changes were noted in his father. (From Oestreich AE, Crawford AH: Atlas of Pediatric Orthopedic Radiology. New York, Thieme, Inc, 1985.)

A wrist ganglion arises in association with the joint capsule or tendon sheath and manifests as a tense, cystic, transilluminant, and often multiloculated swelling. Pain is generally not a presenting feature, although persistent wrist pain may be the only finding in an occult dorsal ganglion. Dorsal ganglia are more common and usually overlie the scapholunate joint.[6] A volar ganglion usually occurs in the interval between the flexor carpi radialis and abductor pollicis longus tendons.

Given the natural history of ganglia, we recommend that they simply be observed unless symptomatic. Lesions that cause pain should be excised with meticulous care. A volar ganglion may be adherent to the radial artery, which should be protected during dissection. Often, the ganglion's pedicle takes a sinuous path to the scaphotrapezial or scapholunate joint. This pedicle must be carefully dissected and excised along with a portion of the joint capsule.

Jacobs and Govaers[70] reviewed the results in 71 patients in all age groups who underwent excision of a volar wrist ganglion. Twenty-eight percent of patients each had either a recurrence, injury to the palmar cutaneous branch of median nerve, or an unsatisfactory scar. MacKinnon and Azmy[90] reported on the treatment of wrist ganglia by various methods in 74 children. The overall recurrence rate was 30.5 percent, but only 12.5 percent of ganglia that were surgically excised recurred.

Intraosseous ganglia are rare and may be seen in any carpal bone.[6, 85] They may occur in isolation or along with extraosseous cysts. Curettage and bone grafting are the treatment of choice in symptomatic cases.

HEMOPHILIA

The clinical manifestations of hemophilia A and hemophilia B are indistinguishable. Hemorrhage may occur spontaneously or following minor trauma in patients whose clotting factor level is less than 3 percent.[1] Immediate replacement of the deficient factor is the single most important and effective measure in acute bleeds. The wrist is involved much less often than the knee, ankle, and elbow,[1, 55] and in one series, an acute wrist hemarthrosis was seen in only 3 percent of patients.[77] Although the issue is controversial, we believe that a tense hemarthrosis should be aspirated once a satisfactory plasma level of the deficient factor has been achieved.

Chronic arthropathy is the consequence of repeated intra-articular bleeds and is not common in children.[1] Enzymatic degradation of articular cartilage in addition to mechanical and chemical factors[130] results in synovial thickening, deformity, and ankylosis. In rare cases, synovectomy may be indicated for persistent hypertrophic synovitis.

Intramuscular hemorrhage into the forearm can result in a compartment syndrome, necessitating decompression. Untreated patients present with Volkmann's ischemic contracture.[1, 77, 129] Median and ulnar neuropathy occur next in frequency to femoral nerve involvement[36, 38] and may follow compression from a soft tissue or joint hemorrhage, distal radial pseudotumor, or, rarely, an intraneural bleed. In the absence of compartment syndrome, acute neuropathy usually responds to nonoperative treatment. Failure of resolution may necessitate operative decompression.[98]

Bone cysts or pseudotumors involve the peripheral parts of the skeleton in children. They result from subperiosteal or intraosseous bleeding and manifest as painful, enlarging swellings of the wrist or hand.[54, 129] Immobilization and replacement therapy usually result in resolution.

METABOLIC DISORDERS

Rickets

Children occasionally present with wrist or forearm pain, or both, in whom radiographic studies reveal metabolic defects. Rickets is a condition that may manifest as isolated wrist discomfort or swelling. The swelling is a result of disorganized endochondral growth at the distal radial physis (Fig. 30–19). The swelling is occasionally painful and is noted at the ends of all long bones.

Bachrach and coworkers[11] reported on vitamin D deficiency secondary to nutritional, racial, cultural,

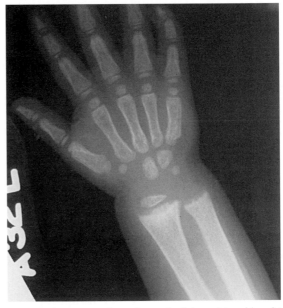

Figure 30–19. Anteroposterior radiograph of the wrist and hand in a 3-year-old child with nutritional rickets. The child had been put on a strict low-fat diet without meat or dairy products. Note the widening, cupping, and fraying of the distal radius and ulna metaphyses with an associated increase in the thickness of the physis. These changes are the consequence of disordered endochondral growth. In addition, there is delay in ossification along with osteopenia.

and environmental factors.[11] Their patients presented with swollen wrists and other musculoskeletal symptoms, including refusal to use the extremity and developmental regression. In their 24 cases, all the infants were breast-fed and all were African-American. Meat and dairy products were not part of the diets of 21 of the 24 patients, and none were being given vitamin D supplementation.

The importance of making the diagnosis early is demonstrated by the fact that although patients with rickets show early response to vitamin D supplementation, few catch up on lost growth.[11, 109, 113] Rickets has been noted on radiographs taken for dysmorphology evaluation and also as a diagnostic finding in neonates being given prolonged parenteral nutrition with chronic lung disease. The presence of rickets can also be indicated by wrist pain and swelling in patients with unrecognized renal disease, in those on prolonged anticonvulsant medications, in cases of delayed developmental milestones, and in patients with chronic liver disease.[88] Rickets may also simulate child abuse.[109]

Copper Deficiency in Total Parenteral Nutrition

Long-term total parenteral nutrition (TPN), especially in neonates, can lead to changes in the wrist as a result of copper deficiency. The peak incidence occurs at 7 to 9 months of age, when the large hepatic reserves of copper have been used up. The earliest changes are generalized demineralization with retardation or failure of epiphyseal ossification centers to appear. Late changes include metaphyseal widening and irregularity, extensive subperiosteal new bone formation, and ring-like or bucket-handle deformities. There is a striking similarity between this disorder and scurvy, both of which are caused by defects in collagen formation.[74, 152]

Hypervitaminosis A

Hypervitaminosis A may occur in the young child secondary to excessive ingestion of this substance. Our experience with this condition has been in adolescents who, after being prescribed vitamin A for their acne, believed that the more vitamin tablets they took, the more quickly their pimples would go away. These patients present with hyperostosis of the ulna. This condition promptly resolves with cessation of vitamin A intake.[86]

Caffey's disease—idiopathic cortical hyperostosis occurring in the young child—frequently manifests as forearm and wrist pain and swelling because of involvement of the radius and ulna. The clinical and radiographic features of this condition are similar to those of hypervitaminosis A. A low-vitamin diet does not result in improvement, and corticosteroid therapy may be indicated for treatment.

References

1. Ahlberg A: Haemophilia in Sweden. VII. Incidence, treatment and prophylaxis of arthropathy and other musculo-skeletal manifestations of haemophilia A and B. Acta Orthop Scand Suppl 77:1–132, 1965.
2. Aitken AP: End results of the fractured distal radial epiphysis. J Bone Joint Surg 17:302–302, 1935.
3. Albanese SA, Palmer AK, Kerr DR, et al: Wrist pain and distal growth plate closure of the radius in gymnasts. J Pediatr Orthop 9:23–28, 1989.
4. Ali MS: Fracture of the body of the hamate bone associated with compartment syndrome and dorsal decompression of the carpal tunnel. J Hand Surg 11B:207–210, 1986.
5. Anderson WJ: Simultaneous fracture of the scaphoid and capitate in a child. J Hand Surg 12A:271–273, 1987.
6. Angelides AC: Ganglions of the hand and wrist. In Green DP (ed): Operative Hand Surgery, ed 3. New York, Churchill Livingstone, 1993, pp 2157–2171.
7. Ansell BM: Juvenile arthritis. Clin Rheum Dis 10:657–672, 1984.
8. Arner S: Intravenous phentolamine: Diagnostic and prognostic use in reflex sympathetic dystrophy. Pain 46:17–22, 1991.
9. Ash JM, Gilday DL: The futility of bone scanning in neonatal osteomyelitis: Concise communication. J Nucl Med 21:417–420, 1980.
10. Auberge T, Zenny JC, Duvallet A, et al: Etude de la maturation osseuse et des lesions ostéoarticulaires des sportifs de haut niveau. J Radiol 65:555–561, 1984.
11. Bachrach S, Fisher J, Parks JS: An outbreak of vitamin D deficiency rickets in a susceptible population. Pediatrics 64:871–877, 1979.
12. Bayer AS, Scott VJ, Guze LB: Fungal arthritis III: Sporotrichal arthritis. Semin Arthritis Rheum 9:66–74, 1979.
13. Beals RK, Bird CB: Carpal and tarsal osteolysis: A case report and review of the literature. J Bone Joint Surg 57A:681–686, 1975.
14. Bernstein BH, Singsen BH, Kent JT, et al: Reflex neurovascular dystrophy in children. J Pediatr 93:211–215, 1978.
15. Bjorksten B, Boquist L: Histopathological aspect of chronic recurrent multifocal osteomyelitis. J Bone Joint Surg 62B:376–380, 1980.
16. Blockley NJ, Watson JT: Acute osteomyelitis in children. J Bone Joint Surg 52B:77–88, 1970.
17. Bloem JJA: Fracture of the carpal scaphoid in a child aged 4. Arch Chir Nederl 23:91–94, 1971.
18. Boyden EM, Peterson HA: Partial premature closure of the distal radial physis associated with Kirschner wire fixation. Orthopaedics 14:585–587, 1991.
19. Carter SR, Aldridge MJ, Fitzgerald R, Davies AM: Stress changes of the wrist in adolescent gymnasts. Br J Radiol 61:109–112, 1988.
20. Carter SR, Aldridge MJ: Stress injury of the distal radial growth plate. J Bone Joint Surg 70B:834–836, 1988.
21. Carty HML: Fractures caused by child abuse. J Bone Joint Surg 75B:849–857, 1993.
22. Chaplin D, Pulkki T, Saarimaa A, Vainio K: Wrist and finger deformities in juvenile rheumatoid arthritis. Acta Rheumatol Scand 15:206–223, 1969.
23. Christodoulou AG, Colton CL: Scaphoid fractures in children. J Pediatr Orthop 6:37–39, 1986.
24. Compson JP: Trans-carpal injuries associated with distal radial fractures in children: A series of three cases. J Hand Surg 17B:311–314, 1992.
25. Cooney WP, Bussey R, Dobyns JH, Linscheid RL: Difficult wrist fractures: Perilunate fracture-dislocations of the wrist. Clin Orthop 214:136–147, 1987.
26. Cooper C, Cawley MID: Bacterial arthritis in an English health district: A 10 year review. Ann Rheum Dis 45:458–463, 1986.
27. Crawford AH: Pitfalls and complications of fractures of the distal radius and ulna in childhood. Hand Clin 4:403–413, 1988.
28. Cullen JP, Pellegrini VD, Miller RJ, Jones JA: Treatment of

traumatic radioulnar synostosis by excision and postoperative low-dose irradiation. J Hand Surg 19A:394–401, 1994.

29. Dameron TB: Traumatic dislocation of the distal radio-ulnar joint. Clin Orthop 83:55–63, 1972.

30. Daruwalla JS: A study of radioulnar movements following fractures of the forearm in children. Clin Orthop 139:114–120, 1979.

31. Davis DR, Green DP: Forearm fractures in children: Pitfalls and complications. Clin Orthop 120:172–184, 1976.

32. Dich VQ, Nelson JD, Haltalin KC: Osteomyelitis in infants and children. Am J Dis Child 129:1273–1278, 1975.

33. Diggs LW: Bone and joint lesions in sickle-cell disease. Clin Orthop 52:19–143, 1967.

34. Dixon JH: Non-tuberculous mycobacterial infection of the tendon sheaths in the hand. J Bone Joint Surg 63B:542–544, 1981.

35. Dobyns JH, Gabel GT: Gymnast's wrist. Hand Clin 6:493–505, 1990.

36. Duthie RB, Matthews JM, Rizza CR, Steel WM: Peripheral nerve lesions. In The Management of Musculoskeletal Problems in Haemophiliacs. Oxford, Blackwell Scientific, 1972.

37. Edwards GS Jr, Jupiter JB: Radial head fractures with acute distal radioulnar dislocation: Essex-Lopresti revised. Clin Orthop 234:61–69, 1988.

38. Ehrmann L, Lechner K, Mamoli B, et al: Peripheral nerve lesions in haemophilia. J Neurol 225:175–182, 1981.

39. Eliason EL, Ferguson KL: Epiphyseal separation of the long bones. Surg Gynecol Obstet 58:85–99, 1934.

40. Engh CA, Hughes JL, Abrams RC, Bowerman JW: Osteomyelitis in the patient with sickle-cell disease. J Bone Joint Surg 53A:1–15, 1971.

41. Epps CH Jr, Bryant D'OD, Coles M, Castro O: Osteomyelitis in patients who have sickle-cell disease. J Bone Joint Surg 73A:1281–1294, 1991.

42. Evans DL, Stanber M, Frykman GK: Irreducible epiphyseal plate fracture of the distal ulna due to interposition of the extensor carpi ulnaris tendon: A case report. Clin Orthop 251:162–165, 1990.

43. Evans DM, Ansell BM, Hall MA: The wrist in juvenile arthritis. J Hand Surg 16B:293–304, 1991.

44. Evans EM: Fractures of the radius and ulna. J Bone Joint Surg 33B:548–561, 1951.

45. Faden H, Grossi M: Acute osteomyelitis in children: Reassessment of etiologic agents and their clinical characteristics. Am J Dis Child 145:65–69, 1991.

46. Failla JM, Amadio PC, Morrey BF: Post-traumatic proximal radio-ulnar synostosis. J Bone Joint Surg 71A:1208–1213, 1989.

47. Ferkel RD, Mai LL, Ullis KC, Finerman GAM: An analysis of roller skating injuries. Am J Sports Med 10:24–30, 1981.

48. Fischer L, Moulin R, Deidier CH, et al: Luxation postérieure du trapéze et du trapézoide chez une enfant en fin de croissance, avec fracture de l'apophyse antérieure du trapéze, traitée orthopédiquement. Lyon Med 12:556–559, 1969.

49. Gandhi RK, Wilson P, Mason Brown JJ, Macleod W: Spontaneous correction of deformity following fractures of the forearm in children. Br J Surg 50:5–10, 1963.

50. Garrick JG, Requa RK: Epidemiology of women's gymnastic injuries. Am J Sports Med 8:261–264, 1980.

51. Gerard FM: Post-traumatic carpal instability in a young child. J Bone Joint Surg 62A:131–133, 1980.

52. Gerber SD, Griffin SD, Simmons BP: Break dancer's wrist. J Pediatr Orthop 6:98–99, 1986.

53. Gibbons CLMH, Woods DA, Pailthorpe C, et al: The management of isolated distal radius fractures in children. J Pediatr Orthop 14:207–210, 1994.

54. Gilbert MS, Kreel I, Hermann G: The hemophilic pseudotumor. In Hilgartner M, Pochedly C (eds): Hemophilia in the Child and Adult. New York, Raven Press, 1989, pp 149–160.

55. Gill JC, Thometz J, Scott JP, Montgomery RR. Musculoskeletal problems in hemophilia. In Hilgartner M, Pochedly C (eds): Hemophilia in the Child and Adult. New York, Raven Press, 1989, pp 27–43.

56. Givner LB, Luddy RE, Schwartz AD: Etiology of osteomyelitis in patients with major sickle hemoglobinopathies. J Pediatr 99:411–413, 1981.

57. Goldberg B, Rosenthal PP, Robertson LS, Nicholas JA: Injuries in youth football. Pediatrics 81:255–261, 1988.

58. Goldsmith DP, Vivino FB, Eichenfield AH, et al: Nuclear imaging and clinical features of childhood reflex sympathetic dystrophy: Comparison with adults. Arthritis Rheum 32:480–485, 1989.

59. Golz RJ, Grogan DP, Greene TL, et al: Distal ulnar physeal injury. J Pediatr Orthop 11:318–326, 1991.

60. Gouldesbrough C: A case of fractured scaphoid and os magnum in a boy ten years old. Lancet 2:792, 1916.

61. Granberry MW, Mangum GL: The hand in the child with juvenile rheumatoid arthritis. J Hand Surg 5:105–113, 1980.

62. Granberry WM, Brewer EJ Jr: Results of synovectomy in children with rheumatoid arthritis. Clin Orthop 101:120–126, 1974.

63. Green DP, O'Brien ET: Open reduction of carpal dislocations: Indications and operative techniques. J Hand Surg 3:250–265, 1978.

64. Greene WB, Anderson WJ: Simultaneous fracture of the scaphoid and radius in a child. J Pediatr Orthop 2:191–194, 1982.

65. Grundy M: Fractures of the carpal scaphoid in children. Br J Surg 56:523–524, 1969.

66. Hanks G, Kalenak A, Bowman L, et al: Stress fracture of the carpal scaphoid: A report of four cases. J Bone Joint Surg 71A:938–941, 1989.

67. Hernandez J, Peterson HA: Fracture of the distal radial physis complicated by compartment syndrome and premature physeal closure. J Pediatr Orthop 6:627–630, 1986.

68. Ip FK, Chow SP: Mycobacterium fortuitum infections of the hand. J Bone Joint Surg 17B:675–677, 1992.

69. Jackson MA, Nelson JD: Etiology and medical management of acute suppurative bone and joint infections in pediatric patients. J Pediatr Orthop 2:313–323, 1982.

70. Jacobs LGH, Govaers KJM: The volar wrist ganglion: Just a simple cyst? J Hand Surg 15B:342–346, 1990.

71. Jacobsen ST, Levinson JE, Crawford AH: Late results of synovectomy in juvenile rheumatoid arthritis. J Bone Joint Surg 67A:8–15, 1985.

72. Johnson RP, Carrera G: Chronic capitolunate instability. J Bone Joint Surg 68A:1164–1176, 1986.

73. Karlsson J, Appelqvist R. Irreducible fracture of the wrist in a child. Acta Orthop Scand 58:280–281, 1987.

74. Karpel JT, Peden VH: Copper deficiency in long-term parenteral nutrition. J Pediatr 80:32–36, 1972.

75. Knudsen CJM, Hoffman EB: Neonatal osteomyelitis. J Bone Joint Surg 72B:846–851, 1990.

76. Kozin SH, Bishop AT: Atypical Mycobacterium infections of the upper extremity. J Hand Surg 19A:480–487, 1994.

77. Lancourt JE, Gilbert MS, Posner MA: Management of bleeding and associated complications of hemophilia in the hand and forearm. J Bone Joint Surg 59A:451–460, 1977.

78. Landfried MJ, Stenclik M, Susi JG: Variant of Galeazzi fracture-dislocation in children. J Pediatr Orthop 11:332–335, 1991.

79. Larson B, Light T, Ogden JA: Fracture and ischemic necrosis of the immature scaphoid. J Hand Surg 12A:122–127, 1987.

80. Lauschke FHM, Frey CT: Hematogenous osteomyelitis in infants and children in the northwestern region of Namibia. J Bone Joint Surg 76A:502–510, 1994.

81. Lee BS, Esterhai JL, Das M: Fracture of the distal radial epiphysis. Clin Orthop 185:90–96, 1984.

82. Letts M, Rowhani N: Galeazzi-equivalent injuries of the wrist in children. J Pediatr Orthop 13:561–566, 1993.

83. Lichtman DM, Bruckner JD, Culp RW, Alexander CE: Palmar midcarpal instability: Results of surgical reconstruction. J Hand Surg 17A:307–315, 1992.

84. Linscheid RL, Dobyns JH: Athletic injuries of the wrist. Clin Orthop 198:141–151, 1985.

85. Logan SE, Gilula LA, Kyriakos M: Bilateral scaphoid ganglion cysts in an adolescent. J Hand Surg 17A:490–495, 1992.

86. Lonon WD, Jost LA, Perlman AW, et al: Chronic hypervitaminosis A. Orthop Rev 10:93–97, 1981.

87. Lorish TR, Rizzo TD, Ilstrup DM, Scott SG: Injuries in adolescent and preadolescent boys at two large wrestling tournaments. Am J Sports Med 20:199–202, 1992.

88. Lumpkins L, Oestreich AE: Rickets as an unexpected x-ray finding. J Natl Med Assoc 75:255–258, 1983.

89. MacCollum MS: Dorsal wrist ganglia in children. J Hand Surg 2:325, 1977.

90. MacKinnon AE, Azmy A: Active treatment of ganglia in children. Postgrad Med J 53:378–381, 1977.

91. Mandelbaum BR, Bartolozzi AR, Davis CA, et al: Wrist pain syndrome in the gymnast: Pathogenetic, diagnostic, and therapeutic considerations. Am J Sports Med 17:305–317, 1989.

92. Mandelbaum BR: Gymnastics. In Reider B (ed): Sports Medicine: The School-Age Athlete. Philadelphia, WB Saunders, 1991, pp 415–428.

93. Manoli A: Irreducible fracture separation of the distal radius epiphysis. J Bone Joint Surg 64A:1095–1096, 1982.

94. Manzione M, Pitzzutillo P: Stress fracture of the scaphoid waist: A case report. Am J Sports Med 9:268–269, 1981.

95. McAuley E, Hudash G, Shields K, et al: Injuries in women's gymnastics: The state of the art. Am J Sports Med 15:558–565, 1987.

96. Mikić Z Dj: Galeazzi fracture-dislocations. J Bone Joint Surg 57A:1071–1080, 1975.

97. Mizuta T, Benson WM, Foster BK, et al: Statistical analysis of the incidence of physeal injuries. J Pediatr Orthop 7:518–523, 1987.

98. Moneim MS, Gribble TJ: Carpal tunnel syndrome in hemophilia. J Hand Surg 9A:580–583, 1984.

99. Morrey BF, Bianco AJ Jr, Rhodes KH: Septic arthritis in children. Orthop Clin North Am 6:923–951, 1975.

100. Murakami S, Nakajima H: Aseptic necrosis of the capitate bone in two gymnasts. Am J Sports Med 12:170–173, 1984.

101. Mussbichler H: Injuries of the carpal scaphoid in children. Acta Radiol 56:361–368, 1961.

102. Nakamura R, Imaeda T, Suzuki, Miura T: Sports-related Kienböck's disease. Am J Sports Med 19:88–91, 1991.

103. Nelson JD: The bacterial etiology and antibiotic management of septic arthritis in infants and children. Pediatrics 50:437–440, 1972.

104. Nelson OA, Buchanan JR, Harrison CS: Distal ulnar growth arrest. J Hand Surg 9A:164–171, 1984.

105. Normand ICS, Dent CE, Smellie JM: Disappearing carpal bones. Proc Roy Soc Med 55:978–979, 1962.

106. O'Brien ET: Fractures and dislocation of the wrist region. In Rockwood CA, Wilkins KE, King RE (eds): Fractures in Children. Philadelphia, JB Lippincott, 1991, pp 372–413.

107. Ogden JA: Skeletal injury in the child. Philadelphia, WB Saunders, 1990. pp 451–526.

108. Onne L, Sandblom PH: Late results in fractures of the forearm in children. Acta Chir Scand 98:549–567, 1949.

109. Paterson CR: Vitamin D deficiency rickets simulating child abuse. J Pediatr Orthop 1:423–425, 1981.

110. Peterson HA, Madhok R, Benson JT, et al: Physeal fractures. Part 1: Epidemiology in Olmstead County, Minnesota, 1979–1988. J Pediatr Orthop 14:423–430, 1994.

111. Peterson HA: Physeal Fractures. Part 3: Classification. J Pediatr Orthop 14:439–448, 1994.

112. Pick RY, Segal D: Carpal scaphoid fracture and non-union in an eight year old child. J Bone Joint Surg 65A:1188–1189, 1983.

113. Pierce DS, Wallace WM, Herndon CH: Long-term treatment of vitamin D–resistant rickets. J Bone Joint Surg 46A:978–995, 1964.

114. Piero A, Mertos F, Mat T, et al: Transcaphoid perilunate dislocation in a child. Acta Orthop Scand 52:31–34, 1981.

115. Price CT, Mills WL: Radial lengthening for septic growth arrest. J Pediatr Orthop 3:88–91, 1983.

116. Pritchett JW: Does pinning cause distal radial growth plate arrest? Orthopedics 17:550–552, 1994.

117. Raff MJ, Melo JC: Anaerobic osteomyelitis. Medicine 57:83–103, 1978.

118. Read M: Stress fractures of the distal radius in adolescent gymnasts. Br J Sports Med 15:272–276, 1981.

119. Rosson JW, Walker G: The natural history of ganglia in children. J Bone Joint Surg 71B:707–708, 1989.

120. Roy DR: Completely displaced distal radius fractures with intact ulnas in children. Orthopedics 12:1089–1092, 1989.

121. Roy S, Caine D, Singer KM: Stress changes of the distal radial epiphysis in young gymnasts: A report of twenty-one cases and a review of the literature. Am J Sports Med 13:301–308, 1985.

122. Ruby LK, Stinson J, Belsky MR: The natural history of scaphoid non-union. J Bone Joint Surg 67A:428–432, 1985.

123. Scoles PV, Hilty MD, Sfakianakis GN: Bone scan patterns in acute osteomyelitis. Clin Orthop 153:210–217, 1980.

124. Seimon LP, Stram RA: Staphylococcal osteomyelitis of the carpal scaphoid. J Pediatr Orthop 4:123–125, 1984.

125. Simmons BP, Nutting JT: Juvenile rheumatoid arthritis. Hand Clin 5:157–168, 1989.

126. Snook GA: Injuries in women's gymnastics. Am J Sports Med 7:242–244, 1979.

127. Southcott R, Rosman MA: Non-union of the carpal scaphoid in children. J Bone Joint Surg 59B:20–23, 1977.

128. Sponseller PD, Malech HL, McCarthy EF, et al: Skeletal involvement in children who have chronic granulomatous disease. J Bone Joint Surg 73A:37–51, 1991.

129. Steel WM, Duthie RB, O'Connor BT: Haemophilic cysts: Report of five cases. J Bone Joint Surg 51B:614–626, 1969.

130. Stein H, Duthie RB: The pathogenesis of chronic haemophilic arthropathy. J Bone Joint Surg 63B:601–609, 1981.

131. Sumner JM, Khuri SM: Entrapment of the median nerve and flexor pollicis longus tendon in an epiphyseal fracture dislocation of the distal radioulnar joint: A case report. J Hand Surg 9A:711–713, 1984.

132. Sutker WL, Lankford LL, Tompsett R: Granulomatous synovitis: The role of atypical mycobacteria. Rev Infect Dis 1:729–735, 1979.

133. Suzuki K, Herbert TJ: Spontaneous correction of dorsal intercalated segment instability deformity with scaphoid malunion in the skeletally immature. J Hand Surg 18A:1012–1015, 1993.

134. Syriopoulou V Ph, Smith AL: In Feigin RD, Cherry JD (eds): Textbook of Pediatric Infectious Diseases, ed 3. Philadelphia, WB Saunders, 1992, pp 727–746.

135. Taleisnik J, Kelly P: The extraosseous and intraosseous blood supply of the scaphoid bone. J Bone Joint Surg 48A:1125–1137, 1966.

136. Taleisnik J, Watson HK: Midcarpal instability caused by malunited fractures of the distal radius. J Hand Surg 9A:350–357, 1984.

137. Tolat AR, Sanderson PL, De Smet L, Stanley JK: The gymnast's wrist: Acquired positive ulnar variance following chronic epiphyseal injury. J Hand Surg 17B:678–681, 1992.

138. Trousdale RT, Amadio PC, Cooney WP, Morrey BF: Radioulnar dissociation: A review of twenty cases. J Bone Joint Surg 74A:1486–1497, 1992.

139. Trueta J: The three types of acute haematogenous osteomyelitis: A clinical and vascular study. J Bone Joint Surg 41B:671–680, 1959.

140. Tuson CE, Hoffman EB, Mann MD: Isotope bone scanning for acute osteomyelitis and septic arthritis in children. J Bone Joint Surg 76B:306–310, 1994.

141. Vahvanen V, Westerlund M: Fracture of the carpal scaphoid in children. Acta Orthop Scand 51:909–913, 1980.

142. Vender MI, Watson HK: Acquired Madelung-like deformity in a gymnast. J Hand Surg 13A:19–21, 1988.

143. Vince KG, Miller JE: Cross-union complicating fractures of the forearm. J Bone Joint Surg 69A:654–661, 1987.

144. Voto SJ, Weiner DS, Leighley B: Redisplacement after closed reduction of forearm fractures in children. J Pediatr Orthop 10:79–84, 1990.

145. Walsh HPJ, McLaren CAN, Owen R: Galeazzi fracture in children. J Bone Joint Surg 69B:730–733, 1987.

146. Waters PM, Kolettis GJ, Schwend R: Acute median neuropathy following physeal fractures of the distal radius. J Pediatr Orthop 14:173–177, 1994.

147. Weiker GC: Hand and wrist problems in the gymnast. Clin Sports Med 11:189–202, 1992.

148. White SJ, Louis DS, Braunstein EM, et al: Capito-lunate instability: Recognition by manipulation under fluoroscopy. AJR 143:361–364, 1984.

149. Wilder RT, Berde CB, Wolohan M, et al: Reflex sympathetic dystrophy in children. J Bone Joint Surg 74A:910–919, 1992.

150. Williamson JB, Galasko CSB, Robinson MJ: Outcome after acute osteomyelitis in preterm infants. Arch Dis Child 65:1060–1062, 1990.

151. Wilson-MacDonald J: Delayed union of the distal scaphoid in a child. J Hand Surg 12A:520–522, 1987.

152. Wiss DA, Peden VH: Copper deficiency in long-term parenteral nutrition. Orthopedics 3:969–973, 1980.

153. Worlock P, Stower M: Fracture patterns in Nottingham children. J Pediatr Orthop 6:656–660, 1986.

154. Younge D: Hematoma block for fractures of the wrist: A cause for compartment syndrome. J Hand Surg 14B:194–195, 1989.

155. Zehntner MK, Jakob RP, McGanity PLJ: Growth disturbance of the distal radial physis after trauma: Operative treatment by corrective radial osteotomy. J Pediatr Orthop 10:411–415, 1990.

156. Zimmerman NB, Weiland AJ: Scapholunate dissociation in the skeletally immature carpus. J Hand Surg 15A:701–705, 1990.

CHAPTER 31

Tumors of the Wrist

George P. Bogumill, PhD, MD

With the exception of the ubiquitous ganglion, tumors and tumorous conditions of the wrist are distinctly uncommon.[8] The true incidence of such lesions is almost impossible to ascertain, because most reports include them with lesions of the hand in general, and do not restrict their description to lesions of the wrist alone. As is true of the hand, most tumors that occur in or about the wrist are benign, although malignancies do appear sporadically. Lesions may occur at any age, and size alone gives no specific clues as to whether they are benign or malignant. The majority of lesions arise in local tissues, although they may be associated with a generalized metabolic disorder, such as gout or xanthomatosis, or may develop following trauma (e.g., a foreign body granuloma).

Some of the smaller, more superficial lesions may be readily treated in outpatient surgery units; however, this statement presupposes that there is an adequate operating room with good lighting and good instruments as well as trained staff. Preoperative evaluation of the lesion includes a carefully taken history, in which are recorded symptoms such as pain and numbness, duration of the lesion, history of trauma, and any other related factors. A careful general physical examination should evaluate the epitrochlear and axillary nodes. Laboratory studies and radiographic evaluations should be done prior to biopsy; these may occasionally consist of computed tonography (CT) scans, magnetic resonance (MR) images, tomograms, arteriograms, or bone scans. A chest radiograph should be obtained if there is any suspicion that the lesion may be malignant.

Adequate anesthesia at the time of surgery is necessary. It may occasionally be local anesthesia, but the patient frequently requires axillary block or even general anesthesia. Some authorities have questioned use of the pneumatic tourniquet because of the fear that aggregates of tumor cells may be trapped at the level of the tourniquet and freed as an embolus at the time of tourniquet release. Others argue that with the tourniquet inflated and no blood flowing, the likelihood that individual cells or clusters of cells would be washed the full length of the extremity to the tourniquet is unlikely, and that the benefits to be gained by operating in a bloodless field outweigh the theoretic risks of tumor aggregates.

A nerve stimulator is occasionally useful. One must remember that nerves stop conducting after the tourniquet has been inflated for 15 or 20 minutes.

Standard extensile skin incisions and closures are used when possible but may need to be modified, depending on the location of the tumor or of a previous biopsy.

A full catalog of the lesions that might possibly appear in the wrist would be impractical and would serve no useful purpose. Therefore, the discussion here is limited to some of the more common entities.

BENIGN SOFT TISSUE LESIONS

Lesions of Synovial Tissues

GANGLIA

The dorsal wrist ganglion arising from the capsule over the scapholunate joint is the most common tumor in the hand in all reported series[1, 2, 4, 8, 12, 21, 24] (Fig. 31–1A). It can appear in patients of almost any age but tends to predominate during the third to fifth decades. It is rare in old age and infancy. Two thirds to three fourths of dorsal wrist ganglia occur in women. Although such a lesion may disappear spontaneously, particularly in children, it usually persists for a prolonged period. The main symptom or presenting complaint is a painless mass. There is a history of trauma in approximately one third of affected patients. Weakness of grip, occasional pain when the ganglion first appears, and, rarely, paresthesias or paralysis from nerve compression or irritation may bring the patient to see the doctor.

Most volar wrist ganglia also originate from the wrist joint capsule (Fig. 31–1B and C). Some originate from the trapezioscaphoid joint. They usually appear near the radial artery and may cause compression of the artery or distortion of its pathway. They may also be found in the carpal tunnel or in Guyon's canal, with compression of the deep branch of the ulnar nerve (Fig. 31–2A). A ganglion may dissect medially or laterally for a distance to reach the subcutaneous regions. The cavity, which is filled with a mucinous material, may appear to be loculated but seldom has true compartmentation (see Fig. 31–1B). Early in its course, the wall of the ganglion is quite thin and easily ruptured; however, with the passage of time, the wall becomes thicker and more resilient. Even then, the wall is easily transilluminated with a penlight, the classic diagnostic test (Fig. 31–1D).

The etiology of ganglia is still being debated. The

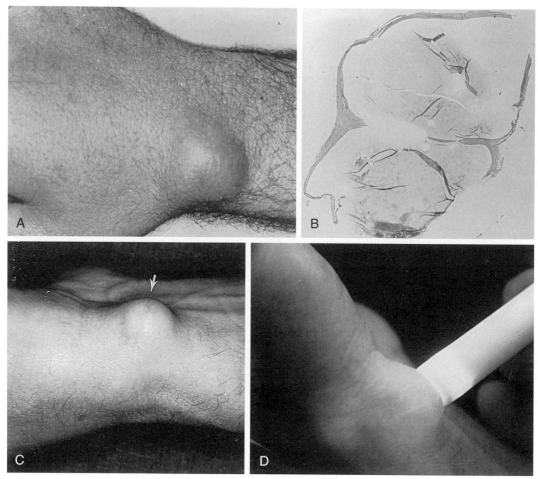

Figure 31–1. Ganglion. *A*, Typical dorsal wrist ganglion in the classic location. *B*, Microscopic section of the ganglion. The apparent trabeculation and multiloculation are deceiving; ganglia almost always have a single cavity. *C*, Volar wrist ganglion in the typical position. *Arrow* indicates a previous attempt at surgical excision. *D*, Transillumination of the ganglion confirms the diagnosis.

commonly accepted theory involves remodeling of the fibrous capsular tissue of the joint.[2, 21, 26] Collagen fiber breakdown products and intercellular mucin collect in microscopic pools; as these collections of mucin coalesce, expand, and dissect their way toward the subcutaneous tissues, fibrous tissue around them is compacted, creating a pseudocapsule. Initially, the thin pseudocapsule is easily ruptured, but it thickens with time, making aspiration or rupture less likely to prevent recurrence. Even resection of the ganglion may not be curative if the capsule adjacent to the attachment of the stalk is not also removed. This joint capsular tissue, which is also remodeling, could be the source of a new, not a truly recurrent, ganglion.

Many attempts have been made to inject ganglia with radiopaque or colored dyes in an effort to see whether the dye will pass from the ganglion into the adjacent joint. These efforts have been quite uniformly unsuccessful. However, Andren and Eiken[1] injected the wrist in their patients on the aspect opposite the ganglion until the joint space became distended. A significant percentage of the ganglia filled with dye from the joint, suggesting a one-way valve effect.[1]

Treatment of a ganglion is also controversial.[2, 4, 10, 12, 26] Aspiration or rupture by striking with a heavy book, the so-called Bible treatment, is followed by recurrence in more than 50 percent of cases. Injection of sclerosing agents or steroids is followed by recurrence in 40 to 50 percent of patients. Surgical excision under adequate anesthesia and tourniquet control, with removal of a portion of the joint capsule surrounding the stalk at the site of origin, may require extensive dissection but has reduced the recurrence rate to 15 percent or lower. When removing a volar ganglion, the surgeon must be aware of danger to the radial artery and should be prepared to repair or replace a segment of artery that is firmly adherent to the ganglion. For the surgeon's protection, the results of Allen's test should have been recorded in the preoperative record.

Surgical Treatment

Many surgeons (and patients) question the need for treatment of a ganglion at all, because the risks associ-

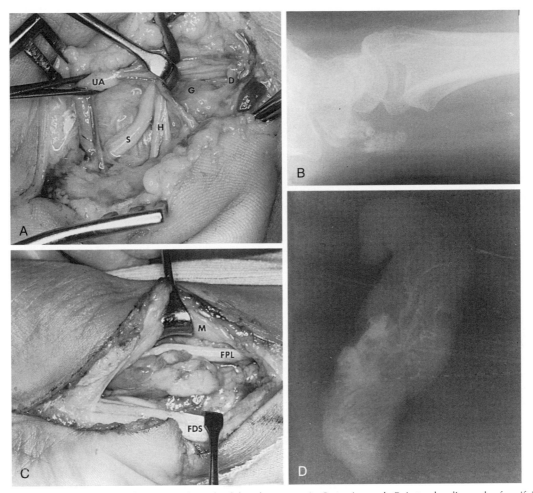

Figure 31–2. *A,* Ganglion compressing the deep motor branch of the ulnar nerve in Guyon's canal. *B,* Lateral radiograph of ossifying myxolipoma illustrates its tenuous connection to the volar surface of the capitate. *C,* Myxolipoma presenting between flexor pollicis longus and flexor digitorum-superficialis, after division of the flexor retinaculum. *D,* Lacy mineralization throughout the lesion proved to be bone on H & E preparation. *D* = deep motor branch of ulnar nerve; *FDS* = flexor digitorum superficialis; *FPL* = flexor pollicis longus; *G* = ganglion arising from hamate-metacarpal joint; *H* = branch of ulnar nerve to hypothenar eminence; *M* = median nerve; *S* = sensory branch of ulnar nerve; *UA* = Ulnar artery.

ated with surgery may indeed be more undesirable than the mild cosmetic deformity and minimal symptoms associated with the presence of the lesion. When surgical excision is chosen by the patient, I usually operate under local or intravenous regional anesthesia in same-day surgery, as follows:

For dorsal ganglia, I prefer a transverse incision placed in one of the dorsal wrist creases. Identify and retract branches of the superficial sensory radial nerve. Use scissors dissection on the capsule of the ganglion to outline the bulk of the lesion. Attempt to identify the stalk, or at least the origination of the ganglion from the dorsal wrist capsule, and remove a portion of it with the ganglion. Minimal to no attempt should be made to exise the ganglion without rupture; rather, deliberately drain the ganglion to facilitate dissection.

For volar wrist ganglia, I utilize a longitudinal or zigzag incision so it can be readily extended along the course of the radial artery to protect, and if necessary, to repair any damage to the vessel. Again, take a portion of the wrist joint capsule.

Postoperative Care

After the usual wound closure, a bulky compression dressing with incorporated plaster splints is applied for the initial 3 or 4 postoperative days; this dressing is then changed to a short-arm cast for 2 weeks to promote benign early wound healing and allow for some capsular repair. Restriction of range of motion usually is present for a number of months, or even permanently in some cases, but I believe that this regimen results in a recurrence rate of less than 5 percent.

SYNOVIAL OSTEOCHONDROMATOSIS

The term *synovial osteochondromatosis* is used for metaplastic foci of cartilage that develop in the synovial lining of bursae, tendons, or joints. When pedunculated, they may break loose from their synovial attachments. The bony centers become avascular, but the cartilage can continue to grow because of nourishment by synovial fluid. The foci can become so numerous and large that they completely fill the joint space and hinder movement. Small, loose "joint mice" may get caught between the bone ends during joint motion, causing pain and joint locking. The disorder usually affects young adult males and is uncommon before puberty.

Clinically, the patients experience low-grade pain for prolonged periods, but it is the restriction of motion, especially episodic, that brings the patient in for treatment. Open or arthroscopic removal of all the loose bodies and as much of the affected synovium as possible is the only effective treatment, although complete excision is seldom possible, and recurrences are common.[7]

Lesions of Fat

Lipomas are common about the hand, appearing in areas where fat normally is found in relatively large quantities, such as the thenar and hypothenar eminences and the midpalm.[8, 18] Ordinarily, there is not much fat around the wrist, but occasionally a lipoma may arise there or may extend there from the hand or forearm. A lipoma may be a surprise finding during carpal tunnel release, and there are numerous reports of large lipomas in the median nerve.[11, 20]

Lipomas are usually soft, lobulated, and slow growing. Radiographically, they have the typical density of fat and are shaped by the surrounding tissues, such as the thenar space. They have a thin capsule and are quite clearly defined from the surrounding tissues. Deeper masses tend to follow the tissue planes and may extend far proximally or distally into the palm or hand. When lipomas are widely spread or arborized, excision may be difficult and may require great patience. On rare occasions, the basic fatty tissue undergoes metaplastic change and appears as a mixture of fat and myxoid material and, if traumatized, may actually undergo osseous metaplasia (Fig. 31–2B through 2D). Of course, when that happens, the change may be visible on radiograph.

GIANT CELL TUMORS

Giant cell tumors of tendon sheath, known by a variety of names (histiocytoma, benign synovioma, etc.) are much more common in the fingers than about the wrist, but they may arise in association with synovial tissue of the joints or tendon sheaths on either the flexor or the extensor side. These lesions are benign growths containing numerous histiocytes and foreign body giant cells adjacent to hemosiderin deposits from minor bleeding episodes secondary to trauma (Fig. 31–3). When tendon sheath tumors do appear about the wrist, like those appearing around the fingers, they often have a long history by the time they are brought to the attention of a doctor, because they are slow-growing, painless masses. They may be large enough or have enough active circulation to cause hyperemic removal of adjacent bones, but this sce-

nario is uncommon. Simple excision is the treatment of choice.

Lesions of Vessels

HEMANGIOMA

Cavernous and capillary hemangiomas are very common around the hand and are frequently seen about the wrist. They can vary considerably in size and in symptoms. In relation to the complex development of the vascular tree, angiomas can be predominantly cavernous (Fig. 31–4A to C) or capillary. Marginal excision of small, well-defined lesions is usually simple, and there is seldom a recurrence. Larger lesions may extend widely into surrounding tissues, such as muscle and bone, and may be very difficult to eradicate without significant functional loss. Serious consideration and extensive experience are advised if one is contemplating surgical treatment of cavernous angiomas.

ARTERIOVENOUS SHUNT

Arteriovenous shunts are common and are characterized by large dilated vessels resulting from the direct shunting of the blood from artery to vein through abnormal vascular channels. These anomalous shunts can be either congenital or acquired. When the shunt is congenital, the vessels have histologic characteristics of both artery and vein in the same vessel.[5]

The true nature of the vascular lesion is often best demonstrated by an arteriogram. The concern of major importance in arteriovenous fistulas is to recognize them as such and to avoid ligating the feeder vessels. The arterial head of pressure may be essential for perfusion of distal tissues; ligation of the feeder vessel often results in tissue infarction. If surgical treatment is required for unremitting pain or avascular necrosis of distal parts, amputation may be the only solution. Lesser procedures are seldom helpful. Partial rather than thorough limb exsanguination prior to inflation of the tourniquet facilitates dissection and ligation of associated feeder and drainage vessels.

THROMBOSIS

Thromboses of vessels are frequently of concern to the patient; they manifest as firm, often tender masses. They are most common after intravenous infusions but may occur spontaneously following trauma.

ANEURYSM

Aneurysms also tend to appear following trauma; the most common site is the hypothenar area, owing to repeated use of this region as a hammer (e.g., installing a hubcap) (Fig. 31–4D). These aneurysms can also

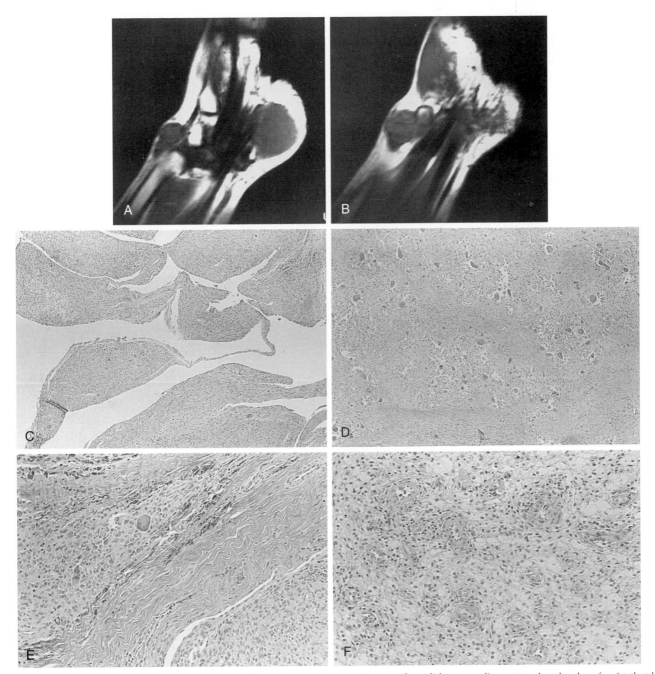

Figure 31–3. Giant cell tumor of tendon sheath. *A* and *B*, Magnetic resonance images of a solid tumor adjacent to ulnar border of wrist that had grown rapidly over less than 6 months. *C*, Photomicrograph illustrating the combined nodular and villous nature typical of many of these lesions. *D*, Numerous giant cells in field of histiocytes. *E*, Fibrosis is common, as are hemosiderin deposits from microtrauma. Tendon or tendon sheath elements are often found in excised specimens. *F*, Xanthoma cells intermingle with numerous vessels; this hypervascularity rather than pressure may be the source of erosions into adjacent bones.

thrombose, causing changes in the digits if collateral circulation is inadequate.

GLOMUS TUMOR

Glomus tumors have been described in the carpal area.[15] As in the fingers, diagnosis is difficult and delayed, because the lesion is small and rarely palpable. Also, it is seldom considered in the differential diagnosis of wrist and hand pain. Simple excision is curative, although multiple lesions do occur.

Lesions of Nerves

NEUROMA

The most common lesion at the wrist, as elsewhere, is a traumatic neuroma following section of the nerve,

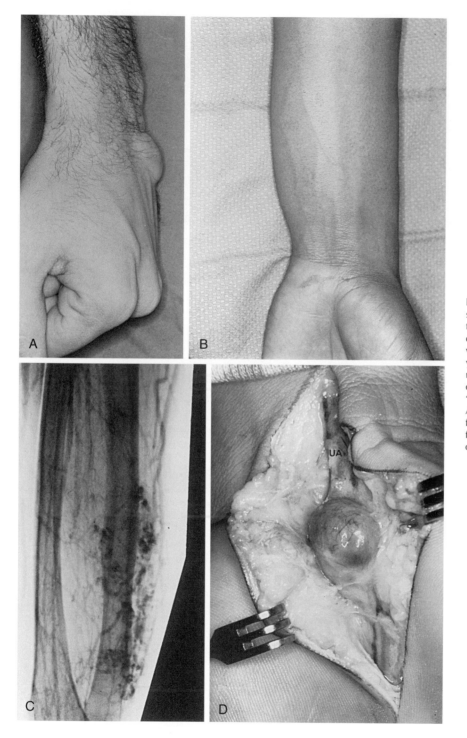

Figure 31–4. *A,* Cavernous hemangioma. This lesion consisted primarily of a large sacular dilatation that filled with blood when the hand was dependent and emptied readily when the hand was elevated. *B,* Clinical view of forearm of 25-year-old man who had intermittent pain and fullness over a period of years. *C,* Venous phase of arteriogram in this patient demonstrating "puddling" of the dye in abnormal vessels. D, Aneurysm in the ulnar artery (*UA*) that appeared following repeated trauma to the heel of the hand from playing pinball machines for prolonged periods.

with or without repair. It can present as a moderate-sized tender mass, but usually neuromas are diagnosed by means of history and a positive percussion test. Lesions of the superficial radial and palmar cutaneous branch of the median are particularly troublesome.

NEURILEMOMA

Any of the nerves crossing the wrist can give rise to either a neurofibroma or a neurilemoma[13, 22, 29, 30] (Fig. 31–5). A neurilemoma is often associated with pain, tenderness, and paresthesias. It is peeled away from the nerve fibers with minor difficulty and without significant damage to function if the surgeon uses magnification loupes or a microscope. A neurilemoma arises from Schwann's cells and usually is composed of two distinct types of tissue (Fig. 31–5*B*). The Antoni A cells compose the more cellular portions of the tumor; they appear as well-defined, orderly groups of cells and fibers. The Antoni B cells are in

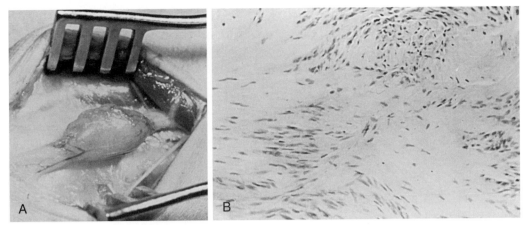

Figure 31–5. A, Neurilemoma in median nerve. This mass on the nerve was a surprise finding at carpal tunnel release for median nerve compression. It was readily dissected from the nerve with no loss of nerve function. B, Photomicrograph of typical field in a neurilemoma showing clusters of cells closely grouped (Antoni A) and other areas of fewer cells with abundant intercellular myxoid matrix that may further modify to form cystic spaces.

areas of myxomatous degeneration, leading to looser texture and haphazard fiber and cell arrangement, with sparse cellularity. These areas may actually break down and form cystic areas, which may coalesce into one large cyst and lead to loss of the typical structure of the neurilemoma. This may be the origin of case reports of intraneural ganglia.

NEUROFIBROMA

The neurofibroma originates from the fibrous tissue of the epineurium or endoneurium and tends to infiltrate more thoroughly between the nerve bundles. It is less clearly defined and, therefore, impossible to remove without causing significant damage to the nerve in which it arises.

LIPOFIBROMA

Lipofibroma of nerve, of which Déjèrine-Sottas disease may be a manifestation, is a hamartomatous enlargement of the median nerve, often accompanied by macrodactyly of the fingers or overgrowth of portions of the hand.[19, 23] It is fortunately a very rare condition but causes great problems in management. Attempts have been made to excise the involved portion of the nerve and to use a nerve graft to bridge the resulting defect. The recommended treatment at present, however, is merely carpal tunnel release, possibly combined with an epineurotomy of the median nerve. Excising the lesion without removing the nerve is impossible.

Fibrous Lesions

Fibrous lesions comprise a gamut of lesions, both benign and malignant. Stout[28] in 1954 and Soule[27] in 1956 tried to classify these lesions to bring order out of chaos, but there is still a great deal of difficulty in defining the borderline between the well-differenti-

ated fibrosarcoma and the benign, but aggressive, fibrous lesion.

Fibrous lesions can occur in the skin or the immediate subdermal tissues (Fig. 31–6A and B); these lesions are relatively common, may be single or multiple, and are most often self-limited and benign. Most fibrous lesions are poorly circumscribed because of the very nature of the tissue of which they are composed. They tend to infiltrate the adjacent fibrous planes, and it is almost impossible to identify this spread with the naked eye. Many fibrous lesions tend to be quite cellular and locally invasive; they may or may not have fine stippled calcifications, but this feature is seldom enough to be evident radiographically. Fibrous lesions may be fixed to deeper structures and, unlike most of the other soft tissue lesions, seldom have a pseudocapsule.

Lesions of the Skin

To my knowledge, there are no specific lesions that are more apt to occur in the region of the wrist than anywhere else. The whole range of benign to malignant lesions can be seen on either dorsal or palmar aspects of the wrist. The malignant lesions tend to create problems for the surgeon, because the wrist area is not considered well compartmented; all of the nerves, vessels, and tendons pass through the wrist area on their way from the forearm to the hand, making a localized resection of a malignancy very difficult to accomplish. Malignancy that invades the deeper tissues usually requires amputation through the forearm rather than localized resection (see Fig. 31–16B).

Lesions of Muscle

The most commonly seen mass of muscle tissue is normal muscle in an abnormal location (Fig. 31–7); for example, the extension of a flexor digitorum su-

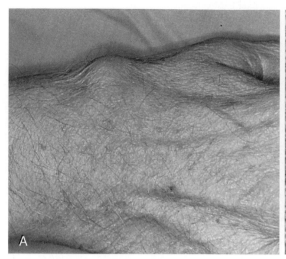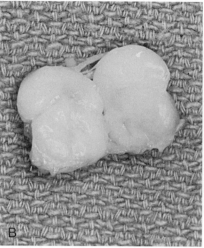

Figure 31–6. Fibroma. *A,* This mass appeared and grew rapidly over a period of 3 or 4 months in a 76-year-old man who had severe involvement with Dupuytren's disease in both hands. *B,* Cut section of the mass showed a glistening, white, shiny surface; it appeared to be well contained within a pseudocapsule.

perficialis muscle belly into the carpal tunnel may present diagnostic problems or may cause carpal tunnel syndrome (Fig. 31–7*B*). Likewise, a muscle originating in the palm and extending proximally into the carpal tunnel can cause symptoms of median nerve compression (Fig. 31–7*A*). With the exception of myositis ossificans, tumors of muscle are decidedly rare.

BENIGN LESIONS OF THE WRIST SKELETON

Lesions of the Distal Radius and Ulna

A variety of lesions appear in the radius and ulna.

BENIGN GIANT CELL TUMOR

The distal radius is one of the more common locations for benign giant cell tumor of bone, the distal ulna somewhat less common. Because neither is a weight-bearing bone, there is often a delay before the patient presents to a physician. The delayed diagnosis results in extensive osteoclastic resorption and

remodeling, leaving an irregular, thin shell of expanded bone and periosteum that does not lend itself well to curettage (Fig. 31–8). Resection of the involved bone end is the preferred treatment for cure (Fig. 31–8*B*). In the case of the ulna, replacement is seldom necessary for function.

The distal radius, however, presents more of a treatment problem. Often, the reparative bone shell in the more aggressive lesions is incomplete, and the tumor is contained merely by periosteum (Fig. 31–8*C*), making the risk of leaving tumor cells in crevices uncomfortably high. For this reason, ancillary treatment of the cavity resulting from curettage is desirable. Attempts to reduce the high rate of recurrence in benign giant cell tumor with liquid nitrogen have been made by some surgeons, but I believe that this complicated technique is destructive to tissues outside the desired bone and places vessels and nerves at risk. For this reason, my preferred technique for treatment of small lesions that are seen early is thorough curettage, followed by treatment of the cavity with 89 percent sterile phenol and then absolute alcohol to absorb remaining phenol.[6] It is a good idea to surround the cortical window with petroleum jelly–impregnated

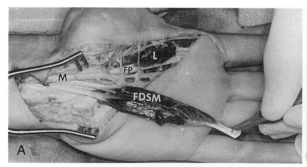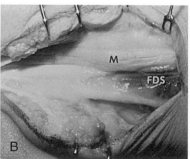

Figure 31–7. *A,* Anomalous muscle belly presented in the hand of an 18-year-old man who had had symptoms consistent with carpal tunnel syndrome for 3 months. *B,* Prolongation of the flexor digitorum superficialis muscle into the carpal tunnel is not an unusual cause of carpal tunnel syndrome. *FDS* = flexor digitorum superficialis; *FDSM* = flexor digitorum superficialis manus; *FP* = flexor digitorum profundus; *L* = first lumbrical; *M* = median nerve.

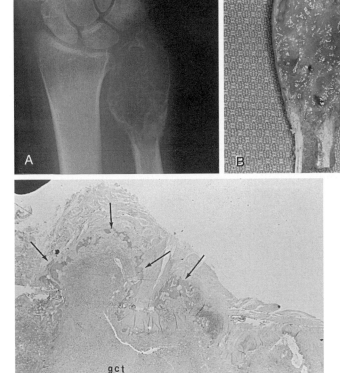

Figure 31–8. Benign giant cell tumor of distal ulna in 23-year-old man with symptoms for less than 1 year. *A,* Radiograph illustrates expansion of bone with very thin periosteal shell surrounding central tumor. *B,* Resection specimen reveals solid nature of the lesion with several small cystic areas. *C,* Photomicrograph at low power. Solid cellular areas are poorly contained by periosteal bony shell *(arrows)* with many areas entirely deficient in bone but still covered with fibrous periosteum. *gct* = giant cell tumor.

gauze to protect the soft tissues, particularly the skin, from spill of the phenol. The phenol is left in the cavity for approximately 1 minute, followed by aspiration and a repeat application. After the alcohol is instilled into the cavity for 1 or 2 minutes, the entire wound is thoroughly irrigated with saline solution.

If the lesion is small enough that adequate remaining bone may be left for functional support during the early postoperative months, many cases of giant cell tumors (and other benign lesions) of the upper limb can be managed without filling of the cavity with bone or methacrylate. This is seldom the case in the distal radius, however, and even small lesions may require bone grafting or cementation to provide support for the articular surface.[14] Filling with autograft may be possible if the lesion is small enough, but larger lesions may require allograft (Fig. 31–9*B* and *C*).

Most authorities advise resection of the involved bone completely if destruction is extensive or if the lesion recurs after curettage. The surgeon is then faced with a problem of replacement, and many techniques have been developed to solve it. Generally, bone grafting of some sort is preferred over prosthetic replacement. The choice of graft source varies considerably among different surgeons.

My personal experience with 11 cases includes 9 in which iliac bone was used to create a bone bridge between the remaining proximal radial shaft and the proximal carpal row. Including the distal ulna in the fusion created a one-bone forearm in effect, but abutment of the tumor against the distal ulna required removal of a portion of the ulna in two cases. In the subsequent 7 cases, the distal ulna was not included in the fusion. Although forearm rotation was retained, second operations were required in several cases for fracture of the graft or failure of the graft to unite to the radius. A long corticocancellous graft from the ilium is necessary, with a plate and screws holding the graft to the radius and Kirschner wires joining the graft to a groove cut into the scaphoid and lunate.

Occasionally, a patient refuses fusion of the wrist. In such cases, I prefer replacement with an allograft radius, which in one case has been dramatically successful, with normal range of motion adequate stability, and freedom from pain for 9 years (Fig. 31–10). Several points of technique are important. A fresh-frozen allograft from the contralateral upper limb of a cadaveric donor similar in size to the patient allows the normal volar tilt of the articular surface to be reversed, placing the normal dorsal overhang volar to the proximal row and providing support to the carpus in resisting the tendency of the wrist and hand to displace palmarward.

When a patient prefers to retain as much wrist motion as possible but does not want to use banked bone for fear of disease transmission, autogenous

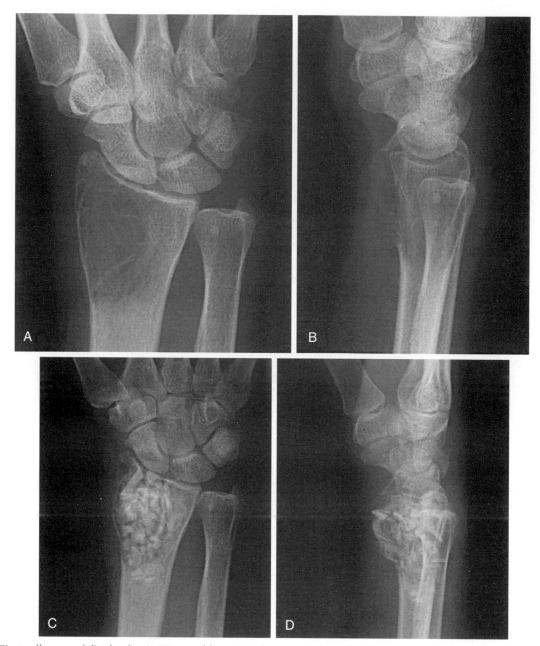

Figure 31–9. Giant cell tumor of distal radius in 51-year-old woman who presented with less than 3 months of symptoms because of worry about recurrence of a previously treated lymphoma. *A* and *B*, Preoperative radiographs show typical eccentric location at end of long bone. *C* and *D*, Radiographs taken after curettage, treatment of cavity with 89 percent phenol and absolute alcohol, and grafting with corticocancellous chips of allograft.

fibula with or without vascularization (Fig. 31–11) has been utilized with some success in retaining a stable wrist with some mobility.

The recurrence rate after curettage with or without bone graft or other ancillary treatment for giant cell tumors of the distal radius approaches 100 percent in larger lesions in the distal radius, whereas the recurrence rate after resection is approximately 7 percent.[14] Curettage of giant cell tumors, even with phenol cautery, does not have the same high rate of cure in the metacarpals, although I have seen only one recurrence in five cases.

OTHER BENIGN LESIONS OF BONE

Bone cysts, nonossifying fibromata, and a wide variety of other benign lesions also can be found in any of the bones about the wrist and are treated with conventional measures, usually curettage with or without bone grafting. It has been my experience that bone grafting to fill the cavity is seldom necessary in the upper limb, because the cavities fill with new, reactive bone quite quickly, and bone strength has reached preoperative levels within 6 to 8 weeks for functional purposes.

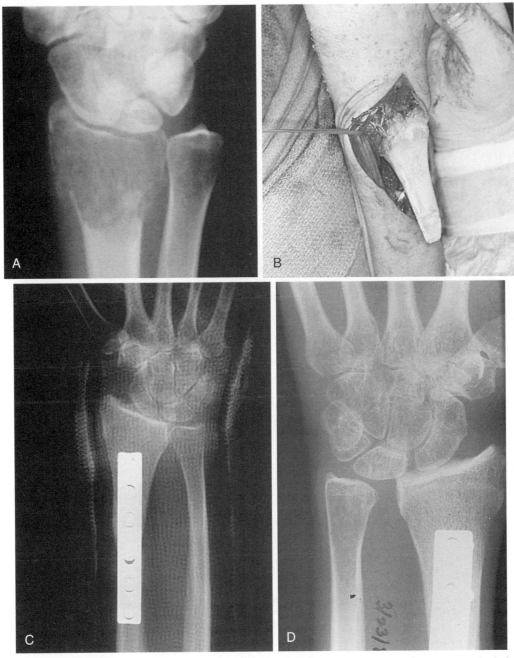

Figure 31–10. Giant cell tumor of radius in 37-year-old female. She had symptoms of pain and swelling for 6 months before presentation. *A,* Radiograph illustrates almost total removal of bone with poor periosteal recovery. Note pathologic fracture. *B,* Allograft replacement of distal radius. Ligaments of graft are sutured to remnants of joint capsule, and a plate fastens the proximal end of the graft to the distal radius. *C,* Anteroposterior (AP) radiograph taken 3 months after surgery. The radius and ulna remain in close approximation, but the carpus is sliding ulnarward off the articular surface of the allograft. *D,* AP radiograph taken at 3 years shows no further drift of the carpus on the allograft, but the radius and ulna show significant separation.

Illustration continued on following page

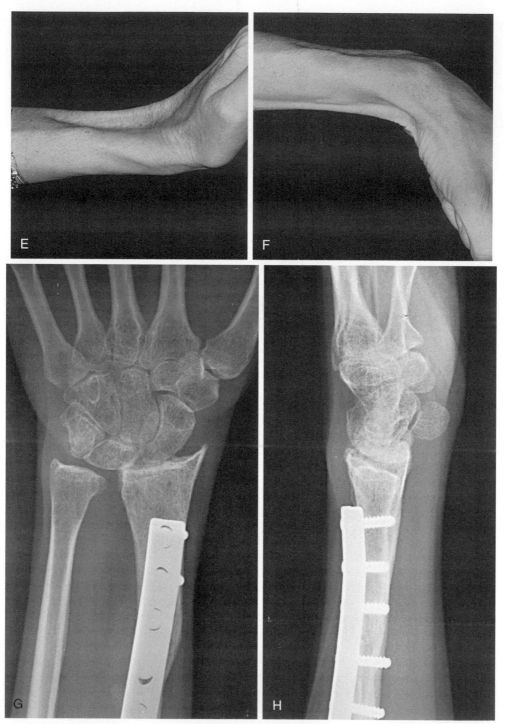

Figure 31–10 *(Continued).* *E* and *F,* Patient has maintained excellent range of motion with full pronation and supination, and good flexion and extension in spite of tendon bow-stringing of both flexors and extensors. *G* and *H,* There has been no further shift of the carpus, separation of the radius from the ulna, or loss of motion after 5 more years. Progressive degenerative changes are evident.

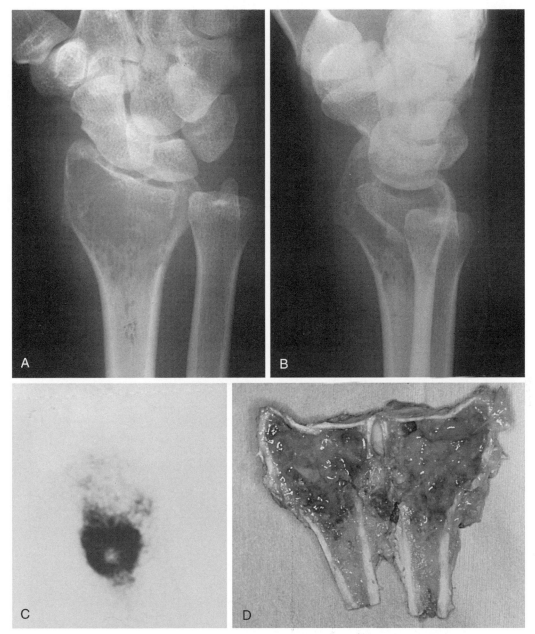

Figure 31–11. Giant cell tumor of distal radius in 37-year-old man who had had symptoms for only 3 months. *A* and *B*, Extensive resorption of bone with periosteal expansion is evident on preoperative radiographs. *C*, Bone scan illustrates the typical picture of the "hot" periphery, where bone repair is attempted, and "cool" center, where lesion has overcome all attempts at repair. *D*, Resection specimen shows solid tumor mass and lack of penetration through articular cartilage into joint.

Illustration continued on following page

RECURRENCE

With the previously described techniques, tumor has not recurred after resection in cases of giant cell tumor in the upper limb that I have treated. Resection for other benign lesions in the wrist bones has not been necessary.

Lesions of the Carpal Bones

A wide variety of accessory bones occurs in the carpal area; some of them are common enough to be named, such as the os epilunatum (Fig. 31–12*A*). Some can actually become large enough to be palpated as excrescences, the most common being the metacarpal boss at the base of the third or, occasionally, the second metacarpal.

CARTILAGINOUS LESIONS

Cartilaginous lesions, such as benign enchodromas, are relatively common and are commonly seen in conjunction with other enchondromas in the hand skeleton. Osteochondromas are quite unusual but can

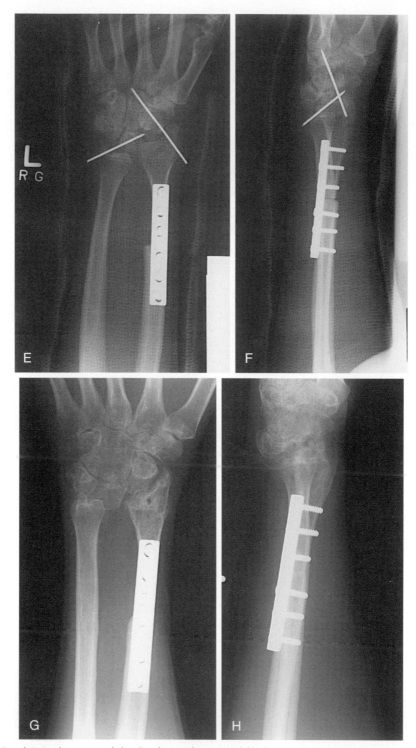

Figure 31–11 *(Continued). E* and *F,* Replacement of distal radius with proximal fibula to attempt to retain some wrist motion. Even though the fit is poor, stability and 60° of total motion were obtained. *G* and *H,* At 9 months, the carpus has shifted dorsally and ulnarward, but the construct is pain free and has enough motion to satisfy the patient and allow him to do light work.

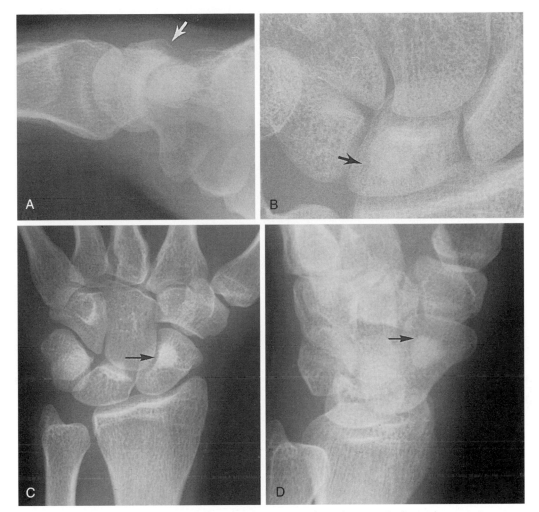

Figure 31–12. *A,* Os epilunatum. An example of an accessory ossicle occurring about the wrist. Such ossicles are quite common and many have been given names. The *arrow* indicates the ossicle overlying the lunate bone dorsally. This patient also had a ganglion adjacent to this accessory bone. *B,* Osteoma, lunate bone *(arrow).* Histologic examination showed that this lesion consisted of portions of very dense reactive bone, without significant medullary space. Portions of this reactive bone showed avascular necrosis. *C* and *D,* Bone island *(arrow).* This lesion was present in a 16-year-old girl who had had symptoms in her wrist for 3 years. The lesion was "warm" on bone scan but did not change in appearance over a 3-year period.

occur in the wrist as they do in the foot, including intra-articular varieties. Seldom is treatment required.

OSTEOBLASTIC LESIONS

Osteoblastic lesions vary from the benign inactive bone island (Fig. 31–12*C* and *D*) or osteoma (Fig. 31–12*B*) to aggressive, fortunately rare, osteosarcoma. Bone islands are common, can occur in any carpal bone, are usually asymptomatic, and are picked up as incidental findings. Occasionally, one may be "hot" on bone scan, but more commonly, increased radionuclide uptake represents a more active process, such as an osteoid osteoma (Fig. 31–13).

For some reason, osteoid osteoma is not an infrequent finding in the wrist area. It usually manifests as pain that is relieved more or less completely by salicylates. A tomogram, CT scan, or MR image may

be necessary to delineate the nidus. It is not unusual for symptoms to be present for a year or more before a diagnosis is made. Curettage of the nidus is curative.

LYTIC LESIONS

Lytic (cystic) lesions are very common in the carpal bones. Radiographically, they usually appear as rounded lucencies that are sharply demarcated by an endosteally reinforced trabecular margin (Fig. 31–14). They usually contain mucinous material and probably represent degenerative cysts. Occasionally, they are called "intraosseous ganglia,"[16] and because they originate in the same location as the routine ganglia (Fig. 31–14*C* and *D*), they may indeed be similar to such entities, in that they represent remodeling of the bone and capsular tissues.

It is often difficult to determine the relationship of a carpal bone lucency to symptoms of wrist pain or

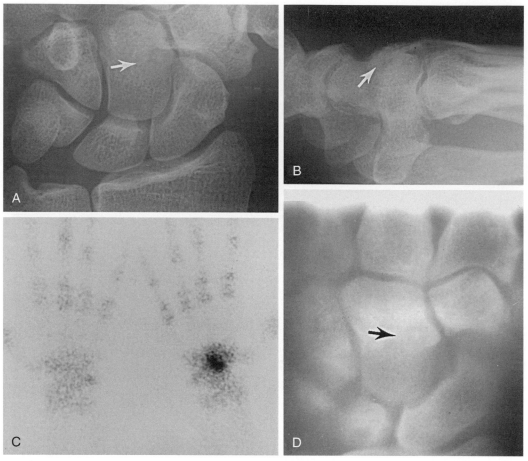

Figure 31–13. Osteoid osteoma of the capitate. *A* and *B*, Anteroposterior and lateral radiographs of a relatively dense island of bone surrounded by a lucent zone and increased reactive sclerosis in the spongiosa of the capitate. *C*, Bone scan showed significant radionuclide uptake in the center of the wrist. *D*, Tomograms delineate the osteoid osteoma nidus clearly *(arrow)*.

limitation of motion. Commonly, the lucencies are surrounded by an endosteal rim of bone, indicating a long-standing process, which may not be consistent with symptoms of short duration. If no other cause for the symptoms is apparent, and the pain is unresponsive to conservative measures such as nonsteroidal anti-inflammatory drugs (NSAIDs) and splinting, curettage with postoperative splinting may solve the problem. Bone grafting may be advisable to fill a defect that is large enough to compromise the involved bone and to lead the surgeon to anticipate possible collapse with the normal compressive forces involved in normal use of the hand.

Lesions of the Metacarpals

The short, tubular metacarpal bones are prey to any of the lesions that one can find in the long tubular bones. Enchondromas are particularly common, but osteochondromas are not rare.

Giant cell tumors are also quite common in the metacarpals, appearing more often in the distal metaphysis than near the proximal end. Simple curet-

tage has been condemned as leading to a recurrence rate higher than 90 percent[3]; however, that has not been my personal experience. A trial of thorough curettage—opening the cortex widely enough to see the entire endosteal cavity for excision of the full extent of the lesion, and cauterizing the remaining cavity with 89 percent phenol—has resulted in prolonged freedom from the disease for periods ranging from 4 to 7 years in three of my patients. Most recurrences happen within the first year, so I am encouraged that these results may last. Curettage with phenol cautery is less disabling than attempts at resection and allografting or other replacement, particularly of centrally placed metacarpals. Bone grafting of these lesions after curettage has not been shown to be helpful, because the metacarpals are not weight-bearing bones. There is usually enough structural stability remaining after curettage to preserve length and shape until the body can refill the canal with normal bone; the refilling is sufficient to provide strength for most activities within a few months, and restoration of the bone is usually quite complete within a year. On the basis of studies in rabbits, I find the phenol treatment with its death

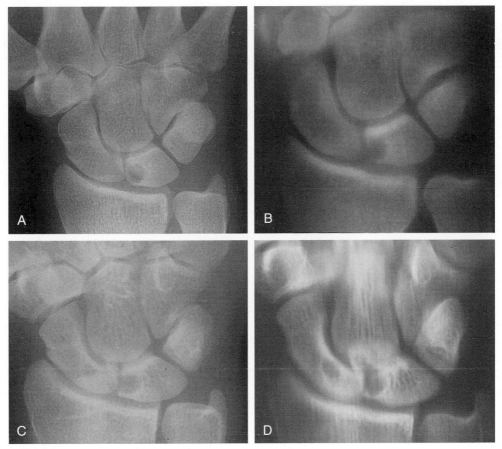

Figure 31–14. Examples of cystic lesions in bone. *A* and *C*, Plain films of two patients with well-defined cystic lesions. *B* and *D*, Tomograms through these areas. Note the rim of endosteal bone outlining the cysts.

of bone to be a strong stimulant to endosteal bone production, and I see no reason to use autogenous bone graft, with its increased morbidity, nor allograft, with its risk, admittedly small, of disease transmission.

MALIGNANT TUMORS OF THE WRIST

Malignant wrist tumors are rare enough to cause problems in treatment for the surgeon who sees only an occasional malignant tumor of the extremities. Primary malignant tumors of the wrist are rare enough to deserve a case report. Affected patients often present to the physician early because of the superficial nature of the tissues and the fact that the tumors cause a mass or pain; because they are found early, there is a good chance of cure. The question of incisional biopsy versus excisional biopsy continues to be debated.[24, 25] Certainly, if the lesion is large or is situated in an area in which wide resection would create considerable disability in the hand, an incisional biopsy would be appropriate. This is true for most aggressive malignant tumors but may actually

be true for many benign ones as well, particularly the fibrous types of lesions. By its nature, excisional biopsy in a malignant lesion usually results in a marginal resection that goes through the pseudocapsule of the tumor, leaving tumor cells behind. In many cases, this result would make attempts at a limb-sparing procedure impossible. If the lesion is small and readily accessible, in an area that can be easily removed such as in a finger, excisional biopsy may be acceptable; however, such characteristics of size and accessibility are rare in lesions about the wrist.

Metastatic Tumors

Although reports of metastatic tumors of the bones of the hand are quite uncommon,[9] a large number of malignant tumors of the wrist are metastatic.[17] There is no specific predilection for any given primary tumor to metastasize to the bones of the wrist. The incidence of any type tends to match that of the tumors that metastasize to bone (breast, lung, kidney, and so forth). When tumors do metastasize to the carpus, they tend to cause destruction in several bones simultaneously (Fig. 31–15), which is often a

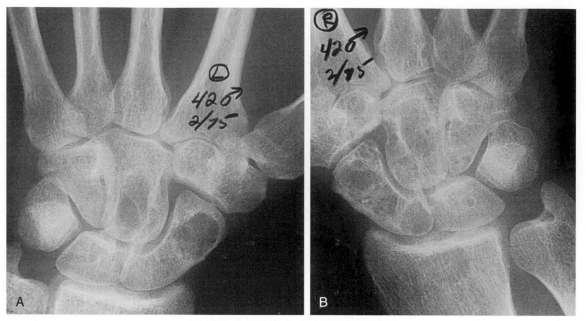

Figure 31–15. *A* and *B*, Amyloid deposits from widespread multiple myeloma. The erosions seen in the carpal bones were detected during work-up for carpal tunnel syndrome. Numerous amyloid deposits were also found in and around the flexor tendons passing through the carpal tunnel.

clue to the aggressive nature of the process. Generally, the tumor is treated systemically, although occasionally, a local approach may be necessary for diagnostic reasons and for stabilization or pain relief.

Primary Malignant Tumors of the Wrist

Primary skeletal malignancies of the carpus are decidedly rare. Because of the central location of the wrist, in terms of structures passing through it from forearm to hand and in the reverse direction (Fig. 31–16*A*), a localized limb-sparing resection is seldom feasible. As in malignancies elsewhere, control of the primary tumor is usually surgical. Staging is essential to determine whether the tumor is indeed retained within a compartment, and the tumor must also be sampled for biopsy to determine the grade. As mentioned previously, through-forearm amputation is usually required for malignancies in the region of the wrist, whether skeletal or soft tissue in origin.

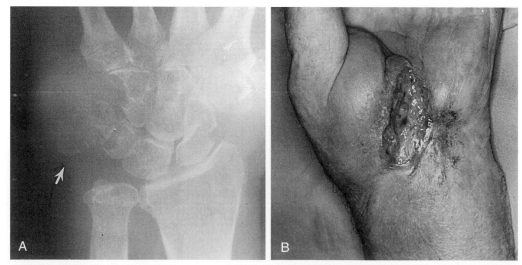

Figure 31–16. *A*, Malignant skeletal tumor with admixture of cartilage and fibrous elements. Note the aggressive nature of the lesion with erosion of multiple bones and a soft tissue mass that shows very little mineralization. Multiple bone destruction is characteristic of the more aggressive lesions, whether primary or metastatic. *B*, Squamous cell carcinoma. The central location of this lesion precludes attempts at limb-sparing procedures, because compromise in the form of resection in an effort to retain function leads to a high incidence of recurrence.

References

1. Andren L, Eiken O: Arthrographic studies of wrist ganglion. J Bone Joint Surg 53A:299–302, 1971.
2. Angelides AC, Wallace PF: The dorsal ganglion of the wrist: Its pathogenesis, gross and microscopic anatomy, and surgical treatment. J Hand Surg 1:228–235, 1976.
3. Averill RM, Smith RJ, Campbell CC: Giant cells tumors of the bones of the hand. J Hand Surg 5:39–50, 1980.
4. Barnes WE, Larsen RD, Posch JL: Review of ganglia of the hand and wrist with analysis of surgical treatment. Plast Reconstr Surg 34:570–578, 1964.
5. Bogumill GP: Clinicopathological correlation in a case of congenital arterio-venous fistulae. Hand 9:60–64, 1977.
6. Bogumill GP: Tumors of the Hand. In Evarts CMcC (ed): Surgery of the Musculoskeletal System, ed 2, vol II. New York, Churchill Livingstone, 1990, p 1197.
7. Bogumill GP, Nelson MC, Lack EE: Lesions of cartilage. In Bogumill GP, Fleegler EF (eds): Tumors of the Hand and Upper Limb. Edinburgh, Churchill Livingstone, 1993.
8. Bogumill GP, Sullivan DJ, Baker GI: Tumors of the hand. Clin Orthop 108:214–222, 1975.
9. Chung TS: Metastatic malignancy to the bones of the hand. J Surg Oncol 24:99–102, 1983.
10. Crawford GP, Taleisnik J: Rotatory subluxation of the scaphoid after excision of dorsal carpal ganglion and wrist manipulation. J Hand Surg 8:921–925, 1983.
11. Friedlander HL, Rosenberg NJ, Graubard DJ: Intraneural lipoma of the median nerve. J Bone Joint Surg 51A:352–362, 1969.
12. Holm PCA, Pandey SD: Treatment of ganglia of the hand and wrist with aspiration and injection of hydrocortisone. Hand 5:63–68, 1973.
13. Jenkins SA: Solitary tumors of peripheral nerve trunks. J Bone Joint Surg 34B:401–411, 1952.
14. Johnston JO: Differential diagnosis and treatment of giant cell lesions. In Bogumill GP, Fleegler EF (eds): Tumors of the Hand and Upper Limb. Edinburgh, Churchill Livingstone, 1993.
15. Joseph FR, Posner MA: Glomus tumors of the wrist. J Hand Surg 8:918–920, 1983.
16. Kambolis C, Bullough PG, Jaffe HL: Ganglionic cystic defects of bone. J Bone Joint Surg 55A:496–505, 1973.
17. Kerin R: Metastatic tumors of the hand: A review of the literature. J Bone Joint Surg 65A:1331–1335, 1983.
18. Leffert RD: Lipomas of the upper extremity. J Bone Joint Surg 54A:1262–1266, 1972.
19. Louis DS, Dick HM: Ossifying lipofibroma of the median nerve. J Bone Joint Surg 55A:1082–1084, 1973.
20. Mikhail IK: Median nerve lipoma in the hand. J Bone Joint Surg 46B:726–730, 1964.
21. Nelson CL, Sawmiller C, Phalen GS: Ganglions of the wrist and hand. J Bone Joint Surg 54A:1459–1464, 1972.
22. Rinaldi E: Neurilemomas and neurofibromas of the upper limb. J Hand Surg 8:590–593, 1983.
23. Rowland SA: Case Report: Ten year followup of lipofibroma of the median nerve in the palm. J Hand Surg 2:316–317, 1977.
24. Schultz RJ, Kearns RJ: Tumors in the hand. J Hand Surg 8:803–806, 1983.
25. Smith RJ: Tumors of the hand: Who is best qualified to treat tumors of the hand? J Hand Surg 2:251–252, 1977.
26. Soren A: Pathogenesis and treatment of ganglion. Clin Orthop 48:173–179, 1966.
27. Soule EH: Tumors of fibrous tissues: A classification and problems in diagnosis and treatment. Instr Course Lect 13:265–274, 1956.
28. Stout AP: Juvenile fibromatoses. Cancer 7:953–978, 1954.
29. Strickland JW, Steichen JB: Nerve tumors of the hand and forearm. J Hand Surg 2:285–291, 1976.
30. White NB: Neurilemomas of the extremities. J Bone Joint Surg 49A:1605–1610, 1967.

CHAPTER 32

Degenerative Disorders of the Carpus

H. Kirk Watson, MD, and Samuel D. Kao, MD

Degenerative arthritis of the wrist follows specific patterns. On examination of more than 4,000 radiographs of the wrist, 210 demonstrated some form of degenerative arthritis.[27] The joints were evaluated for joint space narrowing, extent of cartilage loss, cyst formation, sclerosis, and progression of degeneration. After categorization of the patterns of degeneration in the human wrist, 95 percent of observed changes were found to involve the scaphoid. These occurred in three distinct patterns.

The most common pattern observed was the scapholunate advanced collapse pattern (SLAC wrist). Changes observed in this pattern manifest initially as degeneration of the proximal scaphoradial articulation, with subsequent development of capitolunate articular destruction. In its most advanced form, there is complete destruction of the scaphoradial, capitolunate, and scaphocapitate joints with capitate impingement on the radius and secondary hamate-lunate joint narrowing. The radiolunate joint usually is surprisingly intact (Fig. 32–1). As the name implies, these changes develop as result of ligamentous disruption and laxness, resulting in malpositioning of the scaphoid and lunate. SLAC wrist accounts for 55 percent of cases of unselected degenerative arthritis occurring in the human wrist.

The second most common form of degenerative arthritis is "triscaphe" arthritis which occurs in 20 percent of cases of wrist degenerative arthritis. This disease pattern involves disease of the articulation of the scaphoid, the trapezium, and the trapezoid. In a random cadaveric study of the triscaphe joint, 15 percent of the specimens taken from cadavers with an average age of 74.9 years showed degenerative changes.[14] The scaphotrapezial involvement alone (19 percent) was more than twice as common as scaphotrapezoidal involvement alone (9 percent). In only one instance was the trapezotrapezoidal joint involved, and this involvement was considered to be mild.

The third most common form of degenerative arthritis occurs as a combination of the SLAC wrist and triscaphe arthritis and is found in approximately 10 percent of degenerative wrist disorders. The remaining 5 percent of degenerative disorders noted are ulnolunate, triquetrolunate and radiolunate joint disease. The first two are often noted to be secondary to ulnar impingement type problems. The radiolunate joint is very rarely involved, for reasons discussed later.

The triquetrolunate joint is also the most common location of the rare occurrence of incomplete separation of carpal bones, a process that results in a symptomatic arthrosis that resembles degenerative arthritis. This manifestation of partial congenital coalition has the pathognomonic radiologic finding of a "fluted champagne glass" appearance to the joint as it narrows down to the point of abnormal joint separation (Fig. 32–2).

Isolated intracarpal arthroses that do not correspond to the common degenerative patterns, in an otherwise stable wrist, are usually best treated by a simple fusion of the involved joint. Ulnar impingement may also need to be addressed by ulnar shortening or a matched ulnar arthroplasty (see Chapter 24 and reference 30).

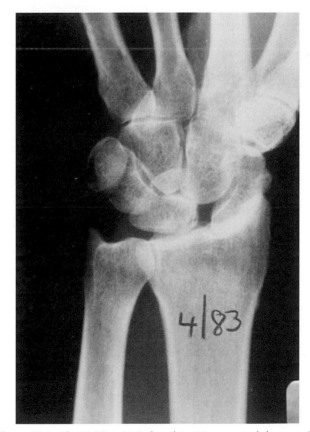

Figure 32–1. The SLAC wrist is found in 55 percent of degenerative arthritis of the wrist. Degenerative changes are found in the radioscaphoid and capitolunate joints. The radiolunate joint is spared, even in advanced disease.

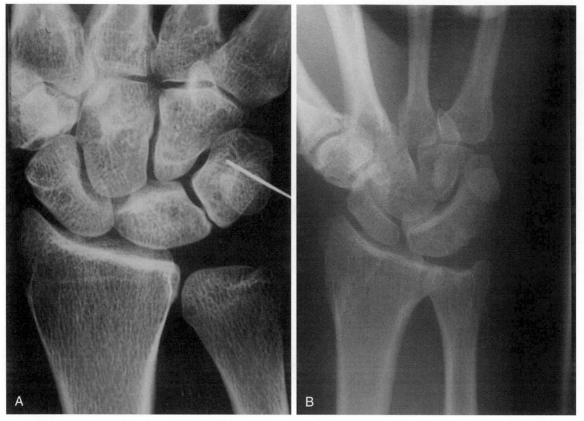

Figure 32–2. *A,* incomplete separation of the triquetrolunate joint may be diagnosed by the "fluted champagne glass" appearance of the joint. *B,* treatment is by fusion of the lunate and triquetrum.

PATHOPHYSIOLOGY

The normal wrist does not usually develop arthritis. Arthritis develops as a consequence of abnormally high shear stresses over small contact surfaces. When they occur over articular surfaces, permanent damage of the joint results. However, when high shear stress develops as a consequence of perimeter impingement, osteophytes may develop instead. This distinction is critical in situations such as radiolunate impingement from significant dorsal intercalary segment instability (DISI) disorders. With this condition, osteophytes develop on the lip of the radius and on the dorsal ridge of the lunate. These osteophytes do not progress to destroy the radiolunate joint and are easily excised during reconstructive surgery. The joint itself is spared.

SLAC Wrist

The most common etiology of SLAC wrist is rotary subluxation of the scaphoid (RSS) due to scapholunate or periscaphoid dissociation. Clinically, the disorder manifests in a progression of disease. In its mildest form, there is no abnormal radiographic finding on either static or dynamic views; this form may be termed predynamic RSS. The next stage of disease is dynamic RSS, in which static radiographic views are normal and abnormalities such as increased scapholunate gap, scaphoid ring sign, and lunate instabilities are manifested only at extremes of range of motion and loading. In more advanced cases, static RSS is observed, and radiographic signs may be seen on static, unloaded views (Fig. 32–3). This stage ultimately progresses to radioscaphoid or triscaphe arthrosis and SLAC wrist.

In addition to RSS, SLAC wrist may be caused by other conditions that result in ligamentous instability of the wrist and/or abnormal articular loading patterns between the carpal bones. These conditions include Kienböck's disease, scaphoid fracture nonunion or malunion, radioscaphoid and capitolunate intra-articular fractures, Preiser's disease, and other idiopathic causes.

SLAC degeneration may initially involve the radioscaphoid joint or triscaphoid joint. As the scaphoid cartilage degenerates, further shift and collapse of the scaphoid occur, resulting in an increasing load on the capitolunate joint. The loaded capitate is driven off the radial side of the lunate between the lunate and scaphoid, with shear loading of the capitolunate cartilage. Rapid degeneration of the capitolunate joint follows, allowing the capitate to migrate proximally between the scaphoid and lunate, with complete scapholunate dissociation.

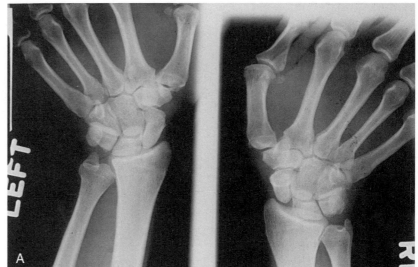

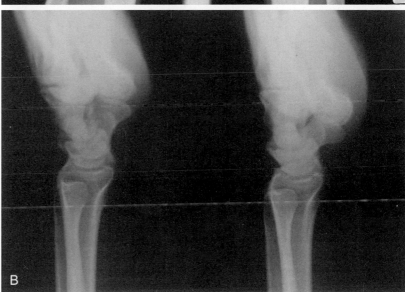

Figure 32–3. Static rotary subluxation of the scaphoid (RSS) is diagnosed by radiographs. *A,* Comparison AP view exhibits foreshortening of the scaphoid, scapholunate gap and scaphoid ring sign on the right. *B,* Lateral view shows the DISI instability of the lunate and abnormal (>70°) scapholunate angle.

The radiolunate and radioscaphoid joints are the load-bearing surfaces between the carpus and the distal radius. The radioscaphoid joint, however, is particularly susceptible to changes in articulation and load patterns because of its ovoid ("jai alai basket") anatomy. If one pictures the joint as two stacked spoons with their handles aligned and their bowls nestled one within the other, one can see that within certain limitations, excellent joint contact may be maintained. However, with any change in the rotational alignment of the two spoons—that is, if one handle were to rotate away from the other—normal articular contact would be dramatically disrupted. The upper spoon bowl would rise out of the lower bowl, and the subsequent contact between the two bowls would be concentrated around the rim of the lower bowl as it contacts the undersurface of the upper bowl (Fig. 32–4). These are exactly the sort of

concentrated high shear loads on small contact surfaces that result in rapid cartilaginous destruction.

The radiolunate joint, however, is a spherical surface that thus accommodates dramatic changes in rotation and alignment while maintaining adequately smooth articular contact to avoid abnormal shear loading.

These mechanics may be illustrated by the degenerative changes that occur with scaphoid non-union. In these situations, the distal fragment rotates in the radioscaphoid fossa, and the proximal, more spherical fragment lies in the rounder region toward the ulnar side of the radioscaphoid fossa. As a result, rapid degenerative changes occur along the scaphoid only along the distal fragment up to the fracture site. The proximal fragment sits within the more spherical portion of the articular surface and is usually spared (Fig. 32–5). This process supports the theory of

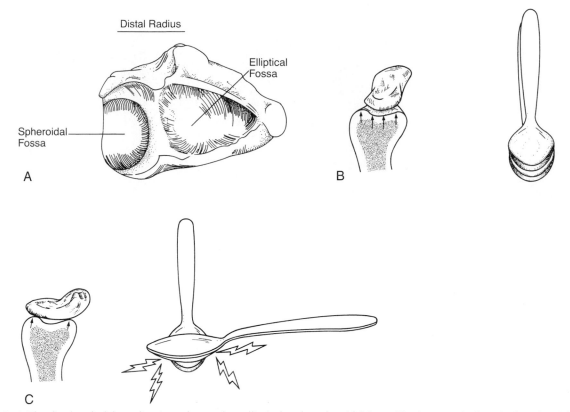

Figure 32–4. *A*, The distal end of the radius is made up of an elliptical and a spheroidal fossa. The lunate articulates in the spheroidal fossa, and the scaphoid in the elliptical fossa. *B* and *C*, The articular shape of the radioscaphoid joint is not unlike that of two stacked spoons. With even the slightest amount of rotational instability, as in rotary subluxation of the scaphoid, the congruous joint surface contact is lost, with all the load now transferred along the edges of the radius and the center of the scaphoid, as demonstrated by the perpendicular spoons. This results in rapid degeneration of the joint.

scaphoid rotation as the basis of SLAC degeneration and emphasizes the importance of grafting of scaphoid non-unions, even in less symptomatic cases.

Triscaphe Arthritis

Triscaphe arthritis occurs as a result of load changes and articular abnormalities analogous to those in the SLAC wrist. The destruction of the trapezioscaphoid and trapezoidoscaphoid joints results from disruptions in the ligamentous support of the scaphoid distally. The radial column collapse allows the trapezium and trapezoid to migrate proximally and come to rest on the nonarticular dorsum of the distal scaphoid, immediately proximal to the distal articular cartilage. This, along with any rotational changes and lateral displacement of the distal scaphoid, leads to abnormal shear stresses that result in the degeneration observed.

TREATMENT

Conservative Treatment

The conservative treatment for osteoarthritis of the wrist is fairly well established. The two primary

approaches consist of immobilization and anti-inflammatory treatment. In the latter category are oral nonsteroidal anti-inflammatory drugs as well as intra-articular steroid injections. These treatments are ideal for acute exacerbations of chronic arthritic disorders. Steroid injections in particular may be effective for up to 2.5 months. One may, thus, obtain dramatic relief of acute synovitis. However, it should be emphasized that these regimens do not change the permanent damage sustained across the articular surface. More significantly, these regimens do not improve the abnormal kinematics and articulations that resulted in the arthritis. As a result, these approaches are often temporizing for young and active patients. For sedentary individuals, regardless of age, such conservative measures often suffice.

Operative Techniques

GENERAL PRINCIPLES

Approach the wrist through a dorsal exposure. Place the transverse incision immediately distal to the radiostyloid. Spare the dorsal veins and superficial nerves using a tissue-spreading dissection technique. Incise the distal extensor retinaculum along the ex-

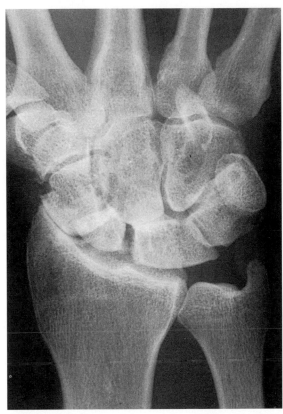

Figure 32–5. Degenerative changes occurring with non-union of the scaphoid tend to support the hypothesis of RSS as a primary etiology of SLAC wrist. Degenerative changes occur between the radius and distal scaphoid segment but progress only as far as the non-union site. The proximal pole, having been detached from the elongated scaphoid, acts within the wrist as if it were a second lunate. It is spheroidal, and degenerative arthritis does not occur between the proximal pole and the radius, just as it does not occur between the lunate and the radius. Destruction does occur, however, between the capitate and proximal scaphoid fragments as well as the capitate and lunate.

tensor pollicis longus tendon. Then enter the capsule over the appropriate joint. Longitudinal traction on the index and middle finger contribute to wide exposure.

The following points regarding small bone fusion in the wrist are worth emphasizing. Remove the appropriate cartilaginous surfaces down through the subcortical bone until raw cancellous bone is exposed. Avoid high-speed burs, because thermal necrosis can interfere with healing. Rather, use dental rongeurs and angled curettes. Ultimately, obtain broad surface areas to allow for fusion. Inadequate bone stock across the fusion site, even with successful fusion, is often inadequate to bear the large loads that are demanded upon the wrist. As a result, postoperative pain will continue to be a problem. Also, be sure to maintain the external dimensions of the fused bones so as not to disrupt the balance between these bones and the remaining wrist bones.

Excellent cancellous bone for grafting can usually be obtained from the radius. Make the dorsoradial transverse incision approximately 2.5 cm proximal to the radial styloid. Use spread dissection here also to expose the flat periosteal region between the first and second dorsal compartments. A small periosteal artery can usually be identified; incise the periosteum directly along this vessel. Then dissect the periosteum off the bone dorsally and volarly with retraction of the first and second dorsal compartments. Use a 4-mm osteotome to elevate a tear-shaped cortical window measuring 2.5 by 1.5 cm. Bevel the window cuts inward. Remove the cancellous bone using an 8-mm curette, taking care along the volar side of the radius, which is particularly thin. Replace the window that is held in place once the tendons are released.

Immobilize the bones using percutaneous Kirschner wire pins. These pins allow a minimal but important amount of compaction across the fusion site. Cut the pins off at the skin level and bury them beneath the subcutaneous fat. The pins may be removed at the appropriate time in the office via small incisions over the pin sites with the aid of small amounts of lidocaine for anesthesia.

Immobilization after limited wrist fusion consists of an initial bulky hand dressing and long-arm splint applied immediately postoperatively. One week postoperatively, the dressing is removed and the arm is then immobilized in a "Groucho Marx" long-arm cast. With this cast, the thumb is held in opposition and the index and middle fingers in the intrinsic-plus position up to the proximal interphalangeal (PIP) joint. At 4 weeks postoperatively, the long-arm cast is changed to a short-arm thumb spica cast after the skin closure wire sutures are removed. This cast is removed at 6 weeks postoperatively, and a radiograph is obtained to verify adequate bone healing. Smokers and diabetics in particular may require an additional week or two of immobilization. The pins are then removed as described previously, and physical therapy for full range of motion is initiated.

Previously described techniques utilizing Silastic implants of various designs are emphatically contraindicated. The silicone not only offers very poor load-bearing properties, but also at times results in catastrophic particulate synovitis and subsequent permanent bone loss from large degenerative cysts.

SLAC WRIST RECONSTRUCTION

Technique

Approach the wrist dorsally as previously described. Then enter the capsule between the tendons of the extensor carpi radialis longus and extensor carpi radialis brevis. Remove the diseased scaphoid in its entirety. Take care to protect the radial and palmar ligaments. No prosthetic filler is needed, and a radial styloidectomy is unnecessary.

Next, retract the extensor pollicis longus and extensor carpi radialis longus and extensor carpi radialis brevis radialward and the extensor digitorum communis and extensor digitorum indicis proprius ulnarward. Make a transverse incision in the capsule over the capitate-lunate joint. Remove the cartilage entirely from the adjacent surfaces of the lunate, capitate, hamate, and triquetral articulations. Preset (0.045-inch) pins to run from capitate to lunate, from triquetrum to lunate, from hamate to lunate, and from triquetrum to hamate. Place cancellous bone graft between capitate and lunate. Ulnar and volar shift the capitate and hamate on the lunate and triquetrum. Drive the pins across the assigned joints, but never into the radius or ulna. Pack the remaining cancellous bone graft into place with a dental tamp.

The single most important surgical point is that the lunate must be reduced into a slight volar intercalary segment instability (VISI) position to correct the nearly universal tendency for DISI deformity of the lunate. This goal can usually be achieved by volarly displacing the capitate on the lunate to rotate the lunate volarly. Dorsiflexing the hand often helps in accomplishing this maneuver. Occasionally, the lunate must be held in the VISI position by a buttress pin placed percutaneously across the distal dorsal edge of the radius into the lunate to maintain the lunate position. If the abnormal DISI alignment of the lunate is not corrected, the subsequent wrist dorsiflexion will be limited and painful.

Although we emphasize that in limited wrist arthrodesis, it is usually critical to maintain the external dimensions of the fused bones, some collapse of the capitate and hamate onto the lunate and triquetrum may be allowed in SLAC reconstruction, because no other wrist joints are affected by the fusion. In addition, less bone graft is required.

Mechanics and Indications

This technique of reconstruction of SLAC wrist is based on the fact that the radiolunate joint is highly resistant to degenerative changes. Fusion of the capitolunate joint transfers the entire wrist load across this preserved joint (Fig. 32–6). Adding the hamate and triquetrum to the capitolunate fusion increases significantly the surface area available for healing of the arthrodesis but does not change the subsequent range of motion. A proximal row carpectomy for non-union fractures of the scaphoid and rotary subluxation of the scaphoid not only needlessly discards the intact proximal lunate articular surface, but also replaces it with a less congruous and often diseased and eburnated surface of the proximal capitate.

SLAC reconstruction is indicated for the symptomatic diseased wrist with the SLAC pattern that has not responded to a program of conservative management. SLAC reconstruction is not designed for treatment of systemic inflammatory arthritis conditions (see Chapter 33).

Results

Evaluation of 100 such procedures over an average follow-up of 44 months has verified an excellent long-lasting functional result with a high rate of pa-

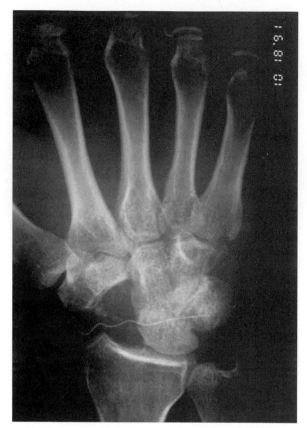

Figure 32–6. The wrist following SLAC reconstruction exhibits proper alignment of the capitate on the lunate and return of the lunate to a slight VISI configuration. No Silastic implant is used.

tient satisfaction.[2] More than 50 percent of patients had no pain and another 34 percent had pain only with heavy labor. The average flexion-extension range of motion was 72° (53 percent of that in the other, normal wrist) and radioulnar deviation averaged 37° (59 percent of that in the other, normal wrist)), and a grip strength 91 percent of that on the other side. Radiographs revealed only two instances of radiolunate destruction, both in conjunction with ulnar translation of the carpus. Significant ulnar translation is now an absolute contraindication to SLAC wrist reconstruction.

The other most significant postoperative complications were as follows. Three cases of non-union were successfully treated by secondary bone grafting. Seven of the 80 patients who underwent reconstruction with silicone implants developed significant particulate synovitis requiring removal of the implant. The most common late postoperative complication was dorsal radiocarpal impingement in 13 wrists, requiring limited resection of both the dorsal radial articular margin and the abutting ridge of the dorsal capitate. This problem should not occur if the lunate is reduced properly as described.

Overall, 80 percent of these 100 patients returned to their original jobs, 79 percent resumed their previous wrist-related recreational activities, and 92 percent indicated that they would readily choose the same surgical solution if faced with the same problem.

TRISCAPHE ARTHRODESIS

Technique

Approach the triscaphe joint by entering the wrist capsule between the tendons of the extensor carpi radialis longus and extensor carpi radialis brevis. Inspect the radioscaphoid joint to ensure that good cartilaginous surfaces are available for load bearing after fusion. We have seen cases in which the central portion of the scaphoid was noted to be eburnated, leaving a rim of intact cartilage. These wrists have done remarkably well following fusion, because, it appears, the load was adequately borne by the remaining cartilage. If significant irreversible radioscaphoid disease is found, a SLAC wrist procedure is indicated instead.

First, excise the radial styloid (5 mm). Then identify the triscaphe joint and remove the adjacent articular surfaces of the trapezium, trapezoid, and scaphoid. Include the proximal vertical, non–load-bearing portion of the trapezoid and trapezium. Next, take the bone graft through a separate transverse incision over the distal radius (see earlier). Preset two Kirschner wire pins (both 0.045-inch for females; one 0.062-inch and one 0.045-inch for males) in the trapezoid directed toward the scaphoid. Place a 5-mm spacer, such as the handle of a small rake, between the trapezoid and scaphoid. Reduce the scaphoid by dorsiflexing the wrist 45° with maximal radial deviation. Then apply thumb pressure on the distal volar prominence of the scaphoid to maintain scaphoid dorsiflexion within these constraints. Drive the pins into place to the proximal subcortical bone of the scaphoid. The pins should not enter the radioscaphoid joint or cross into the radius. Pack cancellous bone graft into place between the raw surfaces of the three bones. The fused scaphoid should lie approximately 50° to 65° to the long axis of the radius when viewed from a lateral position (Fig. 32–7). Check the range of motion of the wrist prior to closure.

Mechanics and Indications

Some surgeons have made the mistake of attempting to over-reduce the scaphoid in a position aligned with the axis of the radius and capitate. After triscaphe fusion, the wrist has different mechanics. With flexion and extension, the scaphoid moves as a unit with the trapezium and trapezoid, transferring the entire range of motion across the capitolunate and radiocarpal joints. With radial deviation, the scaphoid no longer flexes but rather must translocate across its fossa ulnarly. The radial styloid must, there-

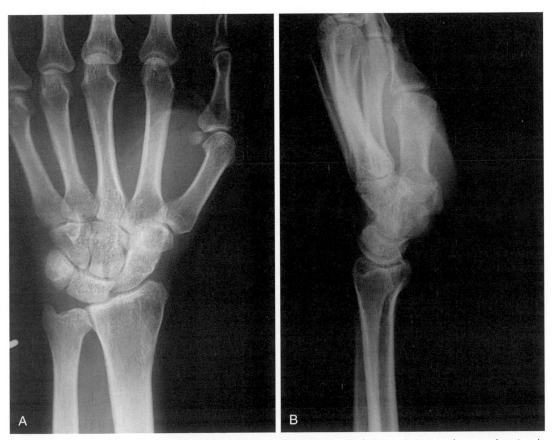

Figure 32–7. A and B, Triscaphe arthritis as treated by triscaphe arthrodesis. Residual VISI or DISI is no longer a functional concern.

fore, be removed to prevent impingement of the distal scaphoid against the radius. Most importantly, this wrist fusion allows for ulnar deviation and extension for maximal power grip.

Others have recommended scaphoid-capitate arthrodesis as an alternative to triscaphe fusion.[16a] These procedures are, in principle, two very different operations. Whereas the scaphoid-capitate fusion transmits the wrist's load directly across the fusion site from capitate to scaphoid and then on to the radius (i.e., analogous to mechanics in a fused knee) the triscaphe arthrodesis transfers the load across normal cartilage between the capitate, scaphoid, and radius. The triscaphe arthrodesis merely maintains the scaphoid in position to carry the load; the fusion does not carry the load. In addition, the normally small amount of motion between the capitate and scaphoid gradually increases as the ligaments accommodate the fusion. The result is greater range of motion and grip strength.

Results

Our follow-up of 200 triscaphe arthrodeses, more than 4 years after surgery, showed that wrist extension, flexion, and ulnar deviation averaged 75 percent of those in the other, normal wrist. Grip strength averaged 84 percent and key pinch and tip pinch were greater than 90 percent of those on the other side. Eighty-eight percent of patients returned to their original jobs, and 8 percent to modified duties. Furthermore, 85 percent of patients resumed wrist-related recreational activities. Overall, 86 percent of patients described their wrist function as better or much better than preoperatively. Perhaps most interesting, those patients who underwent triscaphe arthrodesis for triscaphe arthritis all returned to their original employment and had the best results as determined objectively and subjectively.

Surgery for a Combination of SLAC Wrist and Triscaphe Degenerative Arthritis

In the 10 percent of patients who present with a combination of SLAC wrist and triscaphe degenerative arthritis, the treatment is usually SLAC wrist reconstruction. The decision is made intraoperatively, upon direct inspection of the radioscaphoid and capitolunate joints. Although preoperative radiographs often suggest significant articular damage with narrowing of the joint space, surgical exposure allows the surgeon to determine the extent and location of preserved cartilage as well as the severity of permanent sclerotic changes along the articular surfaces. Narrowed cartilage without sclerosis usually responds to improved mechanics and proper loading. Therefore, in cases in which the triscaphe disease is severe but the changes on the radioscaphoid and capitolunate joints are milder, one should consider triscaphe fusion. The salvage procedure for an unsuc-

cessful triscaphe fusion (i.e., continued pain and weakness) would be SLAC wrist reconstruction.

CONCLUSION

Degenerative arthritis of the wrist manifests in very specific patterns of progression. Almost 95 percent of cases occur as a result of problems involving the scaphoid. The scaphoid plays a critical role in both wrist motion and wrist function. The most common arthritis pattern is the SLAC wrist, which is most commonly the result of disruptions of the ligamentous support of the proximal scaphoid. Because the elliptic articulation between the scaphoid and the radius does not tolerate rotational changes well, degeneration develops between the radius and scaphoid, subsequently progressing to capitolunate joint destruction and finally to hamatolunate destruction. Similarly, triscaphe arthritis is often the result of rotational changes of the distal scaphoid following significant ligamentous disruptions.

The goal in treating patients who present with these problems is to restore to the patient a painless, full-power grip that allows the patient to return to both occupational and recreational activities. The limited wrist arthrodeses described here are the surgeon's tools to achieve that goal.

References

1. Allende BT: Osteoarthritis of the wrist secondary to non-union of the scaphoid. Int Orthop 12:201–211, 1988.
2. Ashmead D, Watson HK, Damon C, et al: Scapholunate advanced collapse wrist salvage. J Hand Surg 19[Am]:741–750, 1994.
3. Bonnevialle P, Mansat M, Railhac JJ, et al: Radiocarpal and inter-carpal degenerative arthritis in sequela of scaphoid injuries. Ann Chir Main 6:89–97, 1987.
4. Brenner LH, Watson HK, Strickland JW, et al: Triquetral-lunate arthritis secondary to congenitally incomplete carpal separation. J Hand Surg 14[Am]:95–102, 1989.
5. Campbell CJ, Koekarn T: Total and subtotal arthrodesis of the wrist. J Bone Joint Surg [Am] 46:1520–1533, 1964.
6. Carstam N, Eiken O, Andren L: Osteoarthritis of the trapezio-scaphoid joint. Acta Orthop Scand 39:354–358, 1968.
7. Chernin MM, Pitt MJ: Radiographic disease patterns at the carpus. Clin Orthop 187:72–80, 1984.
8. Cockshott WP: Pisiform hamate fusion. J Bone Joint Surg [Am] 51:778–780, 1969.
9. Crosby EB, Linscheid RL, Dobyns JH: Scapho-trapezial trapezoid arthrosis. J Hand Surg 3:223–234, 1978.
10. Inglis AE, Jones EC: Proximal-row carpectomy for diseases of the proximal row. J Bone Joint Surg [Am] 59:460–463, 1977.
11. Kempf L, Copin B, Forster JP: Wrist arthrodesis, critical study, à propos of 28 cases. Ann Chir 23:81–88, 1969.
12. Kleinman WB, Steichen JB, Strickland JW: Management of chronic rotary subluxation of the scaphoid by scaphotrapezio-trapezoid arthrodesis. J Hand Surg 7:125–136, 1982.
13. Mack GR, Bosse MJ, Gelberman RH, et al: The natural history of scaphoid non-union. J Bone Joint Surg [Am] 66:504–509, 1984.
14. North ER, Eaton RG: Degenerative joint disease of the trapezium: A comparative radiographic and anatomic study. J Hand Surgery 8:160–166, 1983.

15. Patterson AC: Osteoarthritis of the trapezioscaphoid joint. Arthritis Rheum 18:375–379, 1975.
16. Peterson HA, Lipscomb PR: Intercarpal arthrodesis. Arch Surg 95:127–134, 1967.
16a. Pisano SM, Peimer CA, Wheeler DR, et al: Scaphocapitate intercarpal arthrodesis. J Hand Surg 16:328–333, 1981.
17. Rechnasel K: Arthrodesis of wrist. Acta Orthop Scand 42:441, 1971.
18. Resnik CS, Miller BW, Gelberman RH, et al: Hand and wrist involvement in calcium pyrophosphate deposition disease. J Hand Surg 8:856–863, 1983.
19. Ricklin P: L'arthrodèse radiocarpienne partialle. Ann Chir 30:909–911, 1976.
20. Rotman MB, Manske PR, Pruitt DL, Szerzinski J: Scaphocapitolunate arthrodesis. J Hand Surg 18A:26–33, 1993.
21. Schwartz S: Localized fusion at the wrist joint. J Bone Joint Surg [Am] 49:1591–1596, 1967.
22. Simmons BP, McKenzie WD: Symptomatic carpal coalition. J Hand Surg 10:190–193, 1985.
23. Smith RJ, Atkinson RE, Jupiter JB: Silicone synovitis of the wrist. J Hand Surg 1:47–60, 1985.
24. Watson HK, Hempton RF: Limited wrist arthrodesis. Part I: The triscaphoid joint. J Hand Surg 5:320–327, 1980.
25. Watson HK, Goodman ML, Johnson TR: Limited wrist arthrodesis. Part II: Intercarpal and radial carpal combinations. J Hand Surg 6:223–233, 1981.
26. Watson HK, DiBella A: Triscaphe Arthrodesis—Operative Technique. (Sound Slide Program #791.) Anaheim, CA, American Academy of Orthopaedic Surgeons, 1983.
27. Watson HK, Ballet FL: The SLAC wrist: Scapholunate advanced collapse pattern of degenerative arthritis. J Hand Surg 9A:358–365, 1984.
28. Watson HK, Ryu J, Akelman E: Limited triscaphoid intercarpal arthrodesis for rotary subluxation of the scaphoid. J Bone Joint Surg 68A:345–349, 1986.
29. Watson HK, Ryu J, DiBella A: An approach to Kienböck's disease: Triscaphe arthrodesis. J Hand Surg 10:179–187, 1985.
30. Watson HK, Gabuzda GM: Matched distal ulna resection for posttraumatic disorders of the distal radioulnar joint. J Hand Surg 17:724–730, 1992.
31. Zielinski CJ, Gunther SF: Congenital fusion of the scaphoid and trapezium—case report. J Hand Surg 6:220–222, 1981.

CHAPTER 33

Inflammatory and Rheumatoid Arthritis

Donald C. Ferlic, MD

The wrist is commonly involved in the patient with inflammatory arthritis, and occasionally, the first presenting symptom is wrist pain or deformity. Hand surgeons need to be familiar with the diagnosis, treatment, and pathomechanics of the various conditions that can involve and destroy the wrist. In the early stages, inflammation and synovitis may be controlled with rest and a short course of anti-inflammatory medications, but the wrist with destroyed cartilage, pain, and deformity may need tendon reconstruction, bone resection, arthroplasty, or fusion.

DIFFERENTIAL DIAGNOSIS

There are more than 100 types of arthritis and rheumatic disorders, but rheumatoid arthritis is second only to degenerative joint disease in occurrence. Patterns of joint involvement are helpful in the diagnosis of arthritis. Clinically, the disease is polyarticular and symmetric. Typically, the small joints of the hands and feet swell initially, but wrist disease is almost invariably noted.[67] Active synovitis can be observed on the dorsum of the wrist as a boggy soft tissue swelling. Median nerve compression may develop owing to volar tenosynovitis. Later in the diseased wrist, immobility results from fibrous or bony ankylosis. Commonly, forearm rotation is painful or limited because of distal radioulnar joint involvement.

Systemic lupus erythematosus (SLE) can manifest as wrist and hand deformities similar to those seen in rheumatoid arthritis. Joint involvement is the most common manifestation of SLE.[68] Joint pain or swelling may precede the onset of this multisystem disease by many years. Arthritis, with objective evidence of painful motion, tenderness, or effusion, is present in 75 percent of patients with SLE at the time of diagnosis. The joints most commonly involved are the proximal interphalangeal (PIP) joints, knees, wrists, and metacarpophalangeal joints. Joint involvement is remarkably symmetric.[67] Generally, the deformities are passively correctible, but over time, they can also become fixed.[40] The articular cartilage is usually well preserved until late in the disease, with joint spaces radiographically normal. Because of the severe deformities in patients with normal radiographs, planning of reconstructive surgery may be puzzling. Of-

ten, soft tissue reconstruction of the wrist with painful carpal collapse and volar subluxation is inadequate. In these cases, wrist arthroplasty should be considered.[20]

Progressive systemic sclerosis incorporates scleroderma as one of its components. Hand involvement is almost universal with this condition, in that 98 percent of the patients have Raynaud's phenomenon.[67] Polyarthralgias and joint stiffness affecting both small and large peripheral joints are common. Many patients develop severe deformities of the fingers and wrists owing to intense fibrosis of the synovium. Skin breakdown may occur over the small joints (Fig. 33–1). Radiographs reveal subcutaneous calcinosis (Fig. 33–2) as well as absorption of the tufts of the terminal phalanges. Other areas of bone absorption are the distal portions of the radius and ulna as well as the ribs and mandible.[67]

Psoriatic arthritis classically affects the distal interphalangeal joints but can affect any of the joints, including the wrists. It has a pattern of symmetric polyarthritis clinically indistinguishable from that in rheumatoid arthritis. Arthritis mutilans may be a component, and except for this condition, psoriatic arthritis tends to cause less pain and disability than rheumatoid arthritis.

Arthritis mutilans is an extremely debilitating condition that sometimes is present with psoriatic or rheumatoid arthritis[94] (Fig. 33–3). Nalebuff and Garrett[62] performed six wrist arthrodeses for marked instability with resorption of the radiocarpal joint in patients with arthritis mutilans. In four wrists, the carpal bones had been totally resorbed. The thumb, index, and middle finger metacarpals were articulating with the distal radius.

Belsky and colleagues[7] found patterns of psoriatic hand and wrist involvement to differ from those typically seen in rheumatoid disease. Their patients had multiple joint involvement in the hands with joint destruction and stiffness as characteristic findings, rather than the typical instability seen in rheumatoid arthritis. Palmar subluxation of the carpus, common in the rheumatoid patient, was not found, but spontaneous wrist fusion was common in their patients.

Osteoarthritis is the most common joint disease. This condition can be either primary or secondary, depending on the presence of some preexisting con-

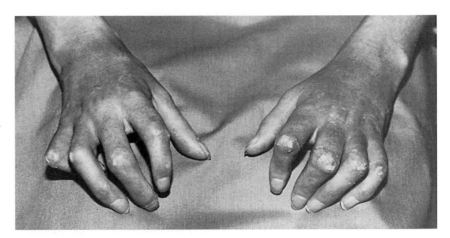

Figure 33–1. Hands of a patient with scleroderma. Note the finger contractures and the ulcerations over the proximal interphalangeal joints.

dition. Although primary osteoarthritis commonly involves the thumb basal joints and the digits with Heberden's nodes in the distal and proximal interphalangeal joints, wrist involvement is uncommon. Secondary degenerative arthritis of the wrist due to old trauma is very common.

Gouty arthritis is caused by sodium urate crystals present in the synovium as a result of chronic hyperuremia. In the majority of patients, recurrent bouts of acute joint inflammation constitute the first manifestation of the disease, but in 10 to 15 percent of pa-

tients, it is preceded by nephrolithiasis.[67] A family history is common. Gouty arthritis is a disease of middle-aged and older men, but women can also be affected. The initial attacks are typically monarticular and most often affect the great toe or other foot joints, ankles, and knees. The acute episode can be confused with sepsis because of the swelling, redness, and localized heat. The patient may also have a low-grade fever and leukocytosis. Initially, the attacks are separated by long periods, but as the disease progresses, they become more frequent and affect fingers, wrists, and elbows. Primarily, the joints return to normal during the remissions, but later, permanent, chronic arthritis persists. Before effective control of hyperuricemia was available, up to 60 percent of gout patients developed tophi (Fig. 33–4). Medical treatment with uricosuric agents is usually all that is necessary to control or shrink gouty tophi, but it may be necessary to débride and decompress tendons and nerves involved by gouty tenosynovitis in the wrist[59, 79] or to remove gouty tophi that may be painful.

Pseudogout, caused by a deposition of calcium pyrophosphate crystals, is marked by inflammation in one or more joints lasting for several days or longer. It is usually self-limited and is less painful than gout.[67] This disease can be similar to rheumatoid arthritis, with multiple, symmetric joint involvement lasting for weeks or months. The wrists are the second most commonly affected joints after the knees, followed by the metacarpophalangeal joints, hips, shoulders, elbows, and ankles. Flexion deformities develop. Radiographs demonstrate crystal deposition in articular cartilage in the menisci of the knees, the intervertebral disks, the symphysis pubis, and the articular fibrocartilage of the wrist (Fig. 33–5). As in rheumatoid arthritis, intra-articular wrist ligaments can be weakened, causing perilunate instabilities and, eventually, generalized carpal arthritis. Surgical reconstruction of wrists with these other disorders is similar to that of the wrist with rheumatoid arthritis.

Some of the other conditions that result in wrist deformities similar to those seen in rheumatoid arthritis are juvenile rheumatoid arthritis, mixed con-

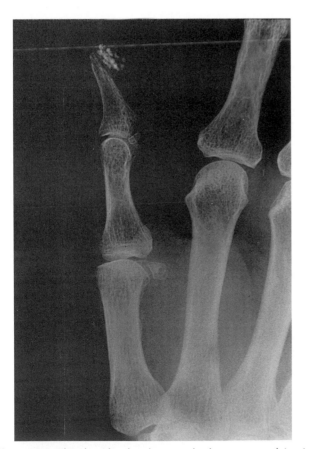

Figure 33–2. Thumb with scleroderma and subcutaneous calcinosis.

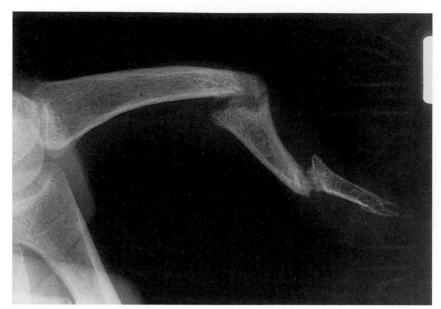

Figure 33–3. Psoriatic arthritis with arthritic mutilans.

nective tissue disease, ankylosing spondylitis, Reiter's syndrome, rheumatic fever with Jacoud's syndrome, infectious arthritis, sarcoidosis, and hemochromatosis. All of these conditions must be consideredand ruled out through history, physical examination, and appropriate laboratory studies in a patient presenting with wrist pain and deformity.

MEDICAL CONSIDERATIONS AND MANAGEMENT

Rheumatoid arthritis is a generalized systemic disease, and surgeons are called upon to treat it only when the disease process cannot be controlled medically. At this time, there is no cure for rheumatoid arthritis, although there are many claims of cures. The Arthritis Foundation states that frauds and rackets have robbed arthritis victims of hundreds of millions of dollars and that, for every dollar spent by responsible organizations in legitimate research into the cause and cure of arthritis, many more are spent on useless quack cures and remedies.

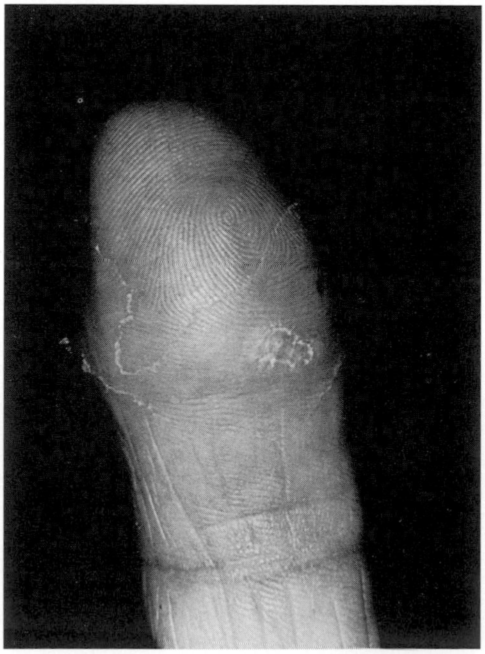

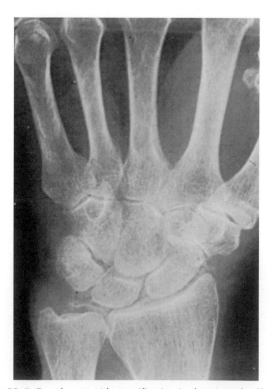

Figure 33–4. A finger with gout. Note the erythema, swelling, and tophus.

Figure 33–5. Pseudogout with opacification in the triangular fibrocartilage of the wrist.

One reason charlatans can claim a cure for rheumatoid arthritis is the unpredictable behavior of this disease. Rheumatoid arthritis can follow any of three hypothetic courses: monocyclic, polycyclic, or progressive.[23, 75] (Fig. 33–6). According to the best available estimates,[75] rheumatoid arthritis might be expected to follow a monocyclic course with complete spontaneous recovery in 35 percent of patients, a polycyclic course with periods of unpredictable swings in disease activity in 50 percent, and a progressive, unremitting course in 15 percent. Because of the variable potential courses that this illness may follow without any therapy, it is exceedingly difficult to judge the response to any of the modes of therapy, either drug, physical, or surgical. One must, therefore, be constantly aware that what appears to be a favorable change may be due to a natural remission rather than a beneficial response to therapy and, conversely, that an unfavorable change may reflect a spontaneous relapse rather than the ill effect of an agent or procedure being used. It is for this reason that surgical treatment is avoided in the early stages of this disease.

A Stepwise Approach

It is useful to consider a stepwise approach to the treatment of rheumatoid arthritis.[27, 76] The therapeutic pyramid shown in Figure 33–7 offers a realistic approach to the treatment of patients in various stages of the disease, as discussed here.

LEVEL I

The basic program is the foundation of the pyramid; it consists of patient and family education, rest, pain relief with salicylates, measures to combat anemia, controlled exercise, and a well-balanced diet. Psychologic support is extremely important, because patients in whom the diagnosis of rheumatoid arthritis is made may present with relatively few symptoms and no joint destruction, but they will see other patients in the waiting rooms who have severe destruction and disability.

For many patients with low-grade disease and little disability, this basic program (level I) may provide adequate control for long periods, and no additional measures are necessary.

LEVEL II

For patients with moderately severe rheumatoid arthritis with multiple joint involvement and considerable constitutional disturbance and disability, if the basic medical treatment proves inadequate after several weeks of trial, additional measures are needed. These level II treatments include the use of nonsteroidal anti-inflammatory drugs (NSAIDs), antimalarials, and anthranilic acid derivatives. Also included in this second level of therapy are intra-articular injections of corticosteroids.

LEVEL III

The drugs that make up the third level of the treatment pyramid are gold, D-penicillamine, and corticosteroids.

Gold. Of all the anti-inflammatory agents commonly used in treatment of rheumatoid arthritis, only gold salts may alter the clinical course or stop the progression of the disease.

Toxic reactions to gold are of the utmost importance and may even be fatal. The most common toxic manifestation is dermatitis, and gold should be stopped when itching appears.

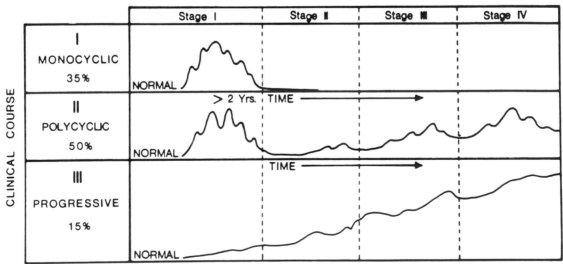

Figure 33–6. Various clinical courses of rheumatoid arthritis. (From Ferlic DC: Extensor indicis proprius transfer for extensor pollicis longus rupture. In Blair W, Steyers C (eds): Techniques in Hand Surgery. Baltimore, Williams & Wilkins Co., 1996, 649–653, and Ranawat CS: Orthop Nurs J 6:61, 1979.)

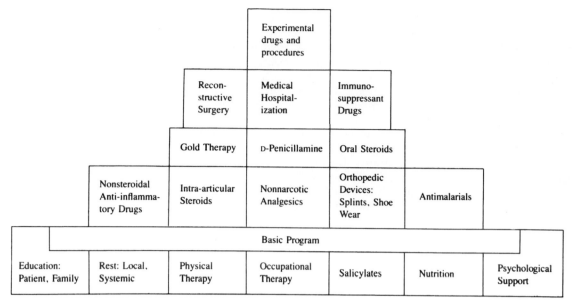

Figure 33–7. Pyramidal approach to the treatment of rheumatoid arthritis. (From Ferlic DC: Extensor indicis proprius transfer for extensor pollicis longus rupture. In Blair W, Steyers C (eds): Techniques in Hand Surgery. Baltimore, Williams & Wilkins Co., 1996, 649–653, and Rasmussen KB, Sneppen O: Nord Med 77:433, 1967.)

D-Penicillamine. D-Penicillamine (3-mercaptova-line) is used in the treatment of patients with rheumatoid arthritis that has not responded to NSAIDs. Its use is limited by side effects that are similar to those encountered with gold and that may be equally hazardous. Nausea, vomiting, and diminution of the sense of taste can be annoying, whereas thrombocytopenia and proteinuria are more hazardous.

Oral Corticosteroids. The corticosteroids are the most powerful anti-inflammatory compounds available. There is no convincing evidence to show that corticosteroids can stop or significantly alter the natural course of the underlying disease. They are used for their palliative effect in supressing symptoms and alleviating general fatigue. Candidates for oral corticosteroid therapy are patients who have severe unremitting disease with fever, anemia, weight loss, effusion, neuropathy, vasculitis, and deformities in spite of an adequate trial of conservative treatment. Few people can take therapeutic amounts of corticosteroids without some unwanted side effects.

LEVEL IV

The patient with severe rheumatoid athritis may require level IV treatment, consisting of hospitalization either for reconstructive surgery or for lack of response to the measures already mentioned.

There is growing recognition of the effectiveness of a team approach for management of the patient with severe rheumatoid arthritis. The cooperative efforts of professional personnel trained in rheumatology, orthopedic surgery, hand surgery, and rehabilitation medicine have proved to be of great value in providing a truly comprehensive and maximally effective approach to the care of the patient with rheumatoid arthritis.

Immunosuppressive drugs are indicated in level IV. These are used only in patients who have progressive rheumatoid arthritis unresponsive to all other of the usual forms of therapy or who require large doses of steroids for adequate control of synovitis. The side effects—bone marrow suppression, loss of hair, hematuria, sterility, and liver inflammation—are not to be taken lightly. A major unanswered question is the risk of induction of malignant changes with the use of immunosuppressive drugs.

LEVEL V

Treatment at level V is investigational in nature. It includes orthopedic procedures and devices as well as drugs and such modalities as radiation of lymphoid tissue, "cryopheresis," and, in the future, immunization against the very agent that causes rheumatoid arthritis.

Conservative Treatment

The wrist is the most commonly involved upper extremity joint in the patient with rheumatoid arthritis. It is the one part of the hand that can be splinted for long periods with some success. Resting the wrist with a simple splint may provide relief of pain and some subsidence of inflammation. A complex, burdensome device is likely to be abandoned.[13] A single steroid injection may be useful, but local steroid injections have been implicated in tendon rupture, so they are used sparingly for dorsal tenosynovitis. My colleagues and I also use joint positioning and joint education techniques and call upon hand therapists to instruct patients in these areas.

Indications for Surgery

Indications for surgery in rheumatoid arthritis are progressive pain and deformity in the joints and progression of the synovial disease in tendon sheaths despite adequate medical treatment. In general, any patient with rheumatoid arthritis who is selected for surgery should be properly motivated and willing to cooperate in the preoperative and postoperative regimens. Surgery of the wrist, however, may be indicated even in the lackadaisical patient because of the known disastrous natural course of tendon rupture, which occurs if surgery is withheld, and because a good result may be obtained without a formal postoperative exercise program.

Conservative surgery for inflammatory joint disease has received less attention than the dramatic surgery of salvage and replacement. This conservative surgery also leads to the question, Does early synovectomy improve long-term function of the patient? Surgeons have for years advocated early synovectomy and tenosynovectomy, but Stanley[77] has stated that although he believes conservative surgery is indicated, there are no long-term studies with sufficient control to provide clear evidence of significant long-term benefits from synovectomy and that well-designed trials of soft tissue surgery need to be undertaken.

In an earlier study, Hindley and Stanley[42] studied the radiographic patterns of disease progression in the rheumatoid wrist and found a relative sparing of the midcarpal joint with a significant correlation between a high incidence of triquetrolunate disease and changes in the ulnar styloid. Wrist disease was found to "protect" the hand for the first 5 years but not after this time. On the basis of these results, they proposed earlier surgical intervention with the intention of shifting the emphasis of surgery from salvage to prophylactic or reconstructive procedures.[42]

PATHOGENESIS AND SURGICAL TREATMENT

Radiocarpal-Intercarpal Joints

Radiocarpal involvement by proliferative synovitis begins beneath the radioscaphocapitate or sling ligament in the region of the deep volar radiocarpal ligament.[24, 85–87] Destruction of these ligaments eventually results in rotary instability of the scaphoid, which assumes a volar-flexed position. There is secondary loss of carpal height and radial rotation of the carpus. The midcarpal joint may not be involved early in the disease process, leaving alternatives such as radial carpal fusion open. Fixed palmar flexion of the lunate may be seen, resulting in palmar displacement of the capitate. This is similar to a volar intercalary segment instability (VISI) deformity, and progression may be a cause of palmar dislocation of the carpus.[50]

Triangular Fibrocartilage Complex (TFCC)

Involvement of the TFCC and instability of the distal radioulnar joint are often present, producing the so-called caput ulna syndrome.[5] The clinical manifestations of this syndrome are as follows:

1. Increasing weakness of the wrist, crepitation on movement, especially on rotation, and pain, which may be sudden, sharp, and severe and may momentarily prevent use of the hand.
2. Loss of rotation and dorsiflexion of the wrist.
3. Dorsal prominence and instability of the head of the ulna.
4. Soft tissue swelling over the ulnar dorsal surface of the wrist caused by synovial proliferation.
5. Descent of the ulnar wrist column, including the fourth and fifth metacarpals.
6. Occasional rupture of the extensor tendons to the digits.
7. Loss of normal action of the extensor carpi ulnaris, which produces some of the deformities seen in the rheumatoid hand, including radial rotation of the wrist.[83, 84]

Dorsal Tenosynovitis

Rheumatoid tenosynovitis on the dorsum of the wrist begins beneath the dorsal carpal retinaculum and extends distally, causing swelling below this rigid ligament. Occasionally, this swelling is misdiagnosed as a ganglion.

If dorsal tenosynovitis persists despite splinting, rest, and adequate medication, surgical treatment is indicated to prevent tendon damage.

Rupture of the extensor tendons at the wrist level has been blamed solely on the erosive effect of the distal end of the ulna, but tendon rupture has occurred after distal ulnar resection in patients in whom no other wrist surgery has been performed. Clayton[14] has indicated that extensor tendon rupture results from a combination of three factors: (1) erosion caused by bone irregularity; (2) compressive effect of the dorsal carpal retinaculum; and (3) direct rheumatoid invasion of the tendons. Other causes, demonstrated at least in flexor tendons, are local steroid injections and occlusion by hypertrophic rheumatoid tissue around vincular vessels, which causes localized infarcts in the tendon.[51]

The diagnosis of rupture of the extensor tendons at the wrist usually poses no problem (Fig. 33–8), but three other conditions must be considered in the differential diagnosis of this occurrence in the rheumatoid patient. The first is metacarpophalangeal synovitis, in which the extensor tendons have slipped off the metacarpal heads into the intermetacarpal areas so that the extensor tendons are below the axis of rotation, impeding their mechanical advantage. The second is posterior interosseous nerve palsy second-

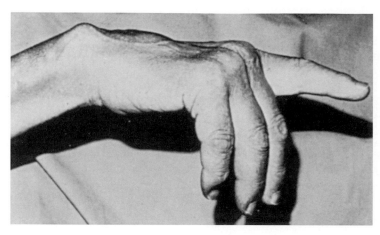

Figure 33–8. Rupture of the extensor tendons of the ulnar three digits.

ary to rheumatoid involvement at the elbow, usually a ganglion[55] (Fig. 33–9). The third possibility is rupture of the extensor tendons over the metacarpal heads.[17]

Tendon rupture of the extensor tendons at the wrist in rheumatoid arthritis is not just an academic issue. Beginning with Vaughan-Jackson,[90] who reported two cases in 1948, there have been many articles in the literature dealing with spontaneous tendon rupture in the arthritic wrist.[14, 46, 56, 58, 64, 66, 78, 84]

DORSAL WRIST RECONSTRUCTION

Early dorsal wrist surgery, consisting of tenosynovectomy, synovectomy, resection or hemiresection of the distal end of the ulna (or the Sauve-Kapandji fusion-osteotomy), and transposition of the dorsal carpal ligament beneath the extensor tendons, will indeed prevent tendon rupture. Abernathy and Bennyson[1] do not believe that tenosynovectomy is even necessary, finding that dorsal tenosynovitis resolved in 81.5 percent of their 54 cases after simple transposition of the dorsal carpal ligament.

What of wrist synovectomy itself? Allieu and associates[4] reported on the long-term results of synovectomy with ulnar head resection in 60 wrists with an average follow-up of 5 years. More than two thirds of the patients were free of constant pain, and synovitis, which had been present in 95 percent of patients initially, was absent in 80 percent after surgery. A useful range of motion was preserved, although reduced, as was grip strength. Synovectomy did not prevent a decrease in carpal height nor a shift of the carpus.[4]

TREATMENT OF THE DISTAL END OF THE ULNA

In most cases, the distal 1 to 2 cm of ulna is resected along with dorsal wrist surgery in rheumatoid arthritis. A hemiresection arthroplasty is another alternative, but it has not worked as well in our rheumatoid patients doing to impingement of the ulnar styloid, continued pain, and failure to obtain the postoperative rotation that was expected.

The Sauve-Kapandji procedure is being used more often now, especially when the carpus is ulnarly translocated. Vincent and associates,[92] reporting on 21 rheumatoid wrists, concluded that significant ulnarward and palmarward translocation of the carpus was prevented and that this procedure provides a stable ulnar-side support in the rheumatoid wrist with distal radioulnar degeneration. We also believe that this operation may prevent or minimize further ulnar sliding of the carpus, and we use it when the carpus is already ulnarly translocated instead of a simple ulnar resection (Fig. 33–10).

SURGICAL TECHNIQUE

Make a straight-line, longitudinal, dorsal incision. It may be diagonal or may be placed more to the radial or ulnar side, depending on where the tenosynovitis is most prominent. Make the incision long enough so that retraction is gentle. Do not undermine the skin, but leave the subcutaneous fat attached in order to minimize the chance of skin necrosis. Preserve dorsal

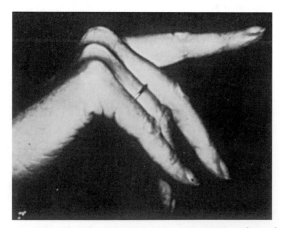

Figure 33–9. Hand with posterior interosseous nerve palsy, which is similar to a hand with tendon rupture or a hand unable to extend the fingers because of metacarpophalangeal destruction.

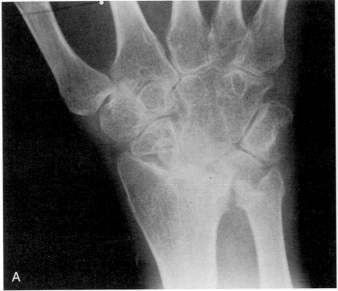
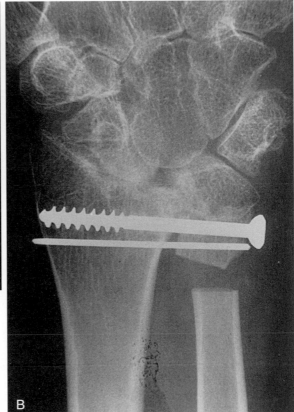

Figure 33–10. *A,* Radiograph of wrist in a patient with juvenile rheumatoid arthritis with marked ulnar translocation of the lunate. *B,* Radiograph taken after Sauve-Kapandji procedure.

veins as much as possible. Protect the dorsal sensory nerves. Reflect the dorsal carpal ligament from the ulnar side, leaving it attached radially (Fig. 33–11).

Open the second through sixth extensor compartments, and isolate each extensor tendon. Excise the diseased tenosynovium with sharp dissection or with a rongeur. Remove bony spicules from the carpus and the distal radius. Incise the capsule of the distal ulna longitudinally, and resect the distal 1 to 2 cm of the

ulna if the carpus is not ulnarly translocated; if it is, I perform the Sauve-Kapandji operation, whereby the distal ulna is fused to the distal radius along with a resection osteotomy of 1 to 2 cm of the ulna proximal to the fusion site. The radioulnar disk usually is destroyed. Distract the wrist using a rongeur, and perform a synovectomy of the radiocarpal joint.

Reconstruct the wrist. Pass the ulnar retinaculum beneath the extensor carpi ulnaris, suturing the reti-

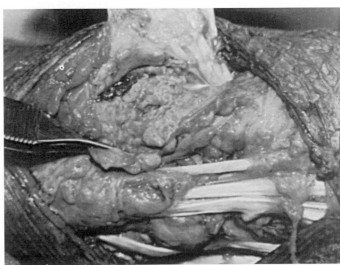

Figure 33–11. Marked dorsal tenosynovitis. The dorsal retinaculum is reflected, exposing each extensor compartment.

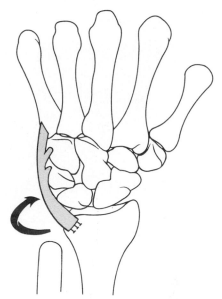

Figure 33–12. Reconstruction of the ulnar side of the wrist. (From Thirupathi RG, Ferlic DC, Clayton ML: Dorsal wrist synovectomy in rheumatoid arthritis. A long-term study. J Hand Surg 8:848, 1983.)

naculum and ulnar carpal capsule to the dorsum of the distal radius. This maneuver reconstructs the radioulnocarpal complex and helps prevent later ulnar sliding and supination deformities; it is the key to the reconstruction (Fig. 33–12). Pass the dorsal carpal ligament beneath the extensor tendons, and suture it to its cut edge on the ulnar side, leaving a small strip to be passed around the extensor carpi ulnaris to keep it dorsalized and help stabilize the distal ulna (Fig. 33–13). I do not use a silicone cap on the distal ulna.

Lower the tourniquet before wound closure, and insert suction drains. Splint the arm from above the elbow to the metacarpal heads until the sutures are removed at 10 to 14 days. Then shorten the splint to below the elbow. After 2 to 4 weeks, actively and passive motion of the wrist is started with a removable splint for comfort.

DISCUSSION

Using this operative technique before tendons rupture usually prevents this complication in the rheumatoid wrist.[16, 88]

Wound breakdown is a complication encountered with dorsal wrist surgery. We have seen it in about 5 percent of our cases. Most often, wound breakdown involves a very small area and heals without any problem. It rarely will involve a more significant area, necessitating débridement or even grafting. This complication can be minimized by (1) making an almost straight, longitudinal, ample incision, (2) not undermining the skin, (3) leaving all the fat on the skin flaps, (4) preserving all possible dorsal veins, avoiding strong retraction, (5) lowering the tourniquet and obtaining hemostasis, (6) ensuring wound drainage, (7) dressing to the fingertips with much padding, and (8) using only light compression and splinting.

One complication of moving the entire retinaculum may be bow-stringing of the extensor tendons (Fig. 33–14). This problem may be avoided by leaving intact the dorsal fascia in the forearm proximal to the dorsal carpal ligament. If this fascia is released, it may be necessary to make a check-rein ligament with a thin strip of dorsal carpal ligament. To prevent the carpus from sliding off the radius, the key suture is made to join the ulnar volar wrist capsule and retinaculum to the dorsal radius.

Instability of the distal ulna may result after distal ulnar resection, especially in the patient with the loose type of rheumatoid arthritis who already has some dorsal bowing of the ulna. This complication

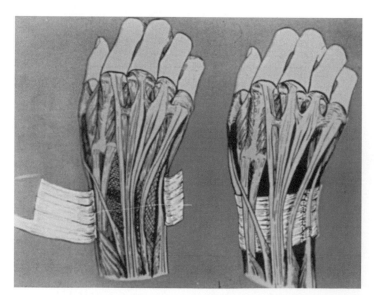

Figure 33–13. The dorsal carpal ligament is passed beneath the extensor tendons, and a flap is used to dorsalize the extensor carpi ulnaris.

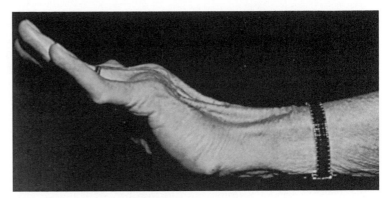

Figure 33–14. Bow-stringing of extensor tendons after dorsal tenosynovectomy.

has been treated with various stabilization techniques using the extensor carpi ulnaris, flexor carpi ulnaris, or volar capsule. Leslie and coworkers[49] used a distally based slip of extensor carpi ulnaris in 26 rheumatoid wrists. Ninety-six percent of the wrists in their series were stabilized using this technique. These additional procedures usually are not necessary but are useful in selected cases.

The use of the silicone ulnar cap also remains controversial. According to Swanson,[83] the advantages of the implant over simple resection are as follows:

1. Less bone needs to be removed.
2. The physiologic length of the ulna is maintained, thus helping to prevent ulnar carpal shift and to provide greater wrist stability.
3. A smooth articular surface in contact with the radius and carpus provides freer movements of the distal radioulnar and carpoulnar joints.
4. There is a smooth surface on which the overlying extensor tendons can glide.
5. The incidence of bone overgrowth is decreased.
6. Ligament reconstruction is possible.
7. The important extensor carpi ulnaris tendon may be rerouted over the dorsum of the ulna.
8. The cosmetic appearance is improved.

We believe that the use of a silicone ulnar cap does not prevent the complications it is supposed to avoid, and that stabilizing the ulnar side of the wrist and the distal ulna by soft tissue reconstruction is the preventive measure one should take.

The last point of emphasis about the surgical technique is the reconstruction of a flap of retinaculum around the extensor carpi ulnaris, which keeps this tendon on the dorsum of the wrist. This measure helps stabilize the distal ulna and keeps the ulnar wrist column and the bases of the fourth and fifth metacarpals from descending and adding to the supination deformity of the hand.

RESULTS

We are confident that synovectomy, tenosynovectomy, dorsal retinaculum transfer, capsular reconstruction, and selected treatment of the distal ulna will minimize extensor tendon rupture, but what happens to the wrist joint itself after synovectomy? Does the reconstruction on the dorsal side prevent further destruction of the wrist with collapse of the carpus and ulnar translocation? In order to answer these questions, my colleagues and I[88] reviewed our patients after a minimum 5-year follow-up and found that 95 percent had excellent relief of pain. Motion increased somewhat. Seventy percent of the patients maintained good carpal height. In those who had carpal collapse of more than 5 mm the collapse occurred linearly over 2 years, not just suddenly. Ulnar translocation of more than 5 mm also occurred in a linear fashion. Progressive carpal collapse was associated with an increase in ulnar deviation of the fingers. An attempt was made to predict which wrists would deteriorate with time; this long-term study showed that once collapse and ulnar translocation progressed beyond 5 mms, the wrist was likely to continue to change further. Synovectomy does not cure the disease, but it is an effective procedure to minimize the destructive effects of the arthritis in the wrist.

Our long-term follow-up of wrist synovectomy and tenosynovectomy can be compared with others' results. Kulik and associates[44] had similar satisfactory results, but synovitis recurred in 20 percent of their patients. In a study with follow-up of 3 to 20 years in 102 wrist procedures, Brumfield and colleagues[10] found pain diminished in all but 17 wrists. Synovitis recurred in 16 wrists, and radiographic evidence of progressive intra-articular destruction was seen in 45. Revision surgery was necessary in 28.

Ishikawa and associates[43] reported on 43 wrists followed for an average of 11 years and compared with opposite, untreated wrists. They found that pain was reduced, forearm rotation was increased with wrist extension, and flexion had changed little. Radiographically, carpal collapse and palmar carpal subluxation progressed nearly parallel to the process in the other wrist, but ulnar carpal shift was much greater in the surgically treated wrist.

We continue to recommend dorsal wrist reconstruction in the patient with chronic tenosynovitis and to see favorable long-term results with tenosynovectomy, synovectomy, dorsal retinaculum transposition, and distal ulnar resection or Sauve-Kapandji fusion.

Extensor Tendon Rupture

Many patients with dorsal tenosynovitis experience rupture of the extensor tendons, and repair of these structures needs to be considered at the time of wrist reconstruction. Rarely, if ever, can a ruptured extensor tendon in the rheumatoid wrist be repaired primarily. In order to reconstruct these tendons, it is necessary to resect a considerable amount of frayed tendon, leaving it too short for end-to-end suture. The wrist with an acute rupture should, however, be treated with some urgency,[56, 57] because a single rupture is often followed by a second rupture, which may be prevented by prompt surgery. The result of surgery for ruptured tendons is directly proportional to the number of tendons ruptured. Surgery in a hand with a triple rupture (extensor tendons to the little, ring, and long fingers) cannot be expected to turn out as well as that in a hand in which only the tendons to the little finger are separated.

Extensor pollicis longus. Extensor pollicis longus rupture is common. It is often overlooked because it results in minimal functional deficit owing to the action of the intrinsic thumb muscles. In the isolated case, a number of alternatives are available. Arthrodesis of the interphalangeal joint of the thumb may be all that is warranted if the joint is already destroyed or does not have satisfactory passive motion. In cases in which thumb motion needs to be preserved, our preferred treatment for this rupture is to transfer the extensor indicis proprius.[25] Others have also reported satisfactory results using this transfer.[56, 69] We have also successfully used a free graft in thumbs in which the tissue bed is relatively unaffected. The brachioradialis, or extensor carpi radialis longus may also be used as a motor.[34, 70]

Finger Extensor Tendons. For treatment of ruptured finger extensors, individual transfers work better than mass transfer of one tendon into all that are ruptured. If the extensor tendons to the little finger are gone, transfer of the extensor digitorum communis into the adjacent intact ring finger extensor works well. The same principle applies if any single finger extensor tendon is ruptured. If the extensors to the little and ring fingers have ruptured, the ring finger extensor is sutured into the long finger tendon, and the extensor indicis proprius is used to motor the little finger. The proximal muscles of the ruptured tendon are sutured into the transfer tendon motor. If the adjacent tendon is frayed, it may not be suitable for transfer and should be bypassed for the next tendon. In such a case, a tendon graft is used to reinforce the weakened area.

In the case of triple rupture, several options are available, but goals will be limited. The extensor carpi radialis longus can be transferred into all three ruptured tendons. This is often the best method, con-

sidering the extensive pathology involved. Normal finger motion cannot be expected because of the limited excursion of this muscle. If the wrist is supple, a tenodesis effect helps with the motion, but usually, the wrist has limited motion in such a case. Another alternative is to transfer the ruptured long finger tendon into the intact index extensor, transfer the extensor indicis proprius to the little finger, and use a flexor superficialis into the ring finger. One may consider the possibility of using the extensor pollicis longus for transfer if the metacarpophalangeal or interphalangeal joints of the thumb are to undergo arthrodesis at the same time.

Many other possibilities of tendon transfer have been advocated,[32, 38, 56, 70, 89, 91] and alternatives often need to be considered because of the local conditions found at the time of surgery. In cases in which the wrist as well as the finger extensors are ruptured, reconstruction is not possible unless the wrist is fused. The wrist tendons can then be used for transfers. Surgery in such hands certainly has limited goals, and the patient must be made aware of the limitations before reconstructive attempts are made.

Postoperatively, an outrigger rubber-band splint is fitted after 3 to 5 days, and active flexion is started, but no active extension is permitted for 4 weeks after surgery.

The hand with ruptured finger extensors and fixed volar subluxed metacarpophalangeal joints presents a special problem in reconstruction. The metacarpophalangeal joints must be mobilized, and the tendon transfers need to be immobilized; thus, performing both these procedures together is not advisable. In these cases, the metacarpophalangeal joints should be replaced first and held in extension with dynamic rubber-band traction. Motion is started as usual. Wrist surgery and tendon transfers are then performed at a second operation.

ARTHROSCOPIC SYNOVECTOMY

The specific role of arthroscopy of the wrist in rheumatoid arthritis and other inflammatory conditions of the wrist involves two specific areas.

The primary experience has been the use of arthroscopy for the diagnosis of inflammatory conditions of the wrist. Specifically, arthroscopy can assist rheumatologists, physiatrists, and infectious disease specialists to obtain appropriate biopsy specimens of the wrist synovium to confirm the diagnosis of rheumatoid arthritis, psoriatic arthritis, crystalline arthritis, and infectious monarticular arthritis at a variety of stages of presentation. In several circumstances, patients have been referred to our office specifically for arthroscopic examination because an accurate diagnosis of multisystem disease was not present. By using selected portals for wrist arthroscopy (see Chapter 10), one can separately sample the preradial styloid recess, the volar capsule beneath the radioscapholunate ligament, and the ulnar prestyloid recess and sacculus recessiformis. The articular cartilage can be inspected and probed for loss of substance, intra-articular cyst formation, and integrity of interosseous ligaments. Loose calcium or urate crystal deposits can be retrieved and then removed through a second arthroscopic portal. In addition, midcarpal biopsy can be performed through a separate portal, and with the combination of radiocarpal and midcarpal arthroscopy, the condition of the articular cartilage can be carefully determined and correlated with the radiographic appearance of the wrist.

A second potential, but currently limited application of arthroscopy of the wrist is in the definitive treatment of noninfectious inflammatory synovitis. With the advent of high-speed, constant suction-irrigation arthroscopic shavers, synovectomy of the radiocarpal joint and, to a limited extent, the midcarpal joint can be performed arthroscopically. As a result of the arthroscopic exposure of the entire joint surface and internal capsule and synovial lining, one could argue the point that wrist arthroscopy may be the preferred procedure for radiographic stage I and stage II rheumatoid arthritis. Morbidity associated with such a procedure is low; postoperative wrist mobilization could be initiated early; and the injury to soft tissue required for exposure of the radiocarpal joint is significantly reduced. Both the midcarpal and radiocarpal joints are amenable to arthroscopic synovectomy.[26] Adolfsson and Nylander,[2] reporting on 18 wrists in 16 patients with rheumatoid arthritis treated using arthroscopic synovectomy, found good pain relief, increased grip strength, and no postoperative stiffness. Ferlic and Cooney[26] reported on ten wrist arthroscopies for rheumatologic disease. These were diagnostic in only five cases which were subsequently treated medically. Two cases were treated with arthroscopic synovectomy, and in the remaining three, after the arthroscopic examination, an open synovectomy was performed.

SURGICAL TECHNIQUE FOR TREATMENT OF EXTENSOR (TENDON RUPTURES)

Carry out tenosynovectomy, synovectomy, and surgery of the distal ulna as described previously. Choose the tendons for transfer. If the extensor indicis proprius is chosen, harvest it with a narrow strip of hood expansion by detaching it from the ulnar side of the extensor mechanism just proximal to the metacarpophalangeal (MP) joints. A deficit is created in the extensor mechanism, which must be closed with sutures to prevent an extensor lag at the PIP joint. Carry out transfers by interweaving the distal end of the ruptured tendon into the intact tendon. Suture with 3-0 nonabsorbable undyed suture.

This technique will provide adequate fixation so that early motion is possible using dynamic extension splints. If sufficient length to obtain this type of suture is not possible, then longer immobilization may be necessary but it is to be avoided. In setting tension, err on the side of increased tension. Suture the tendon with the MP joints in slight flexion, the wrist in slight extension, and maximal passive excursion of the transferred tendon.[60] Lower the tourniquet, obtain hematosis, insert a suction drain, and close the wound.

Apply a bulky dressing with the wrist splinted in neutral and the affected digits extended to neutral. Change the postoperative dressings in 3 to 5 days, when motion is started. Have dynamic extension splints made by the hand therapist. A static splint may be used for sleeping. The transferred tendons are protected for 4 weeks, but longer if an extensor lag develops.[25]

RESULTS

The outcome is variable. If a single rupture is present and the hand is otherwise minimally involved, near-normal function may be anticipated. If there are multiple ruptures and if the wrist and finger joints are involved, the goals and expectations are limited.

Ulnar Drift

The hypothesis that radial rotation and deviation of the carpals and metacarpals initiates ulnar drift of the fingers has been presented elsewhere.[12, 31, 48, 63, 68, 72] Ulnar drift with a proliferative synovitis of the metacarpophalangeal joints causes loss of dorsal, radial, and volar support. Thus, the fingers may progressively drift toward the ulnar side because of dynamic influences within the hand,[13, 21, 80, 95] the normal anatomy of the hand,[21, 32, 36] and external forces acting upon the hand.[6, 30, 31]

Although radial rotation of the metacarpals may not be the sole initiating factor, it is an important one (Fig. 33–15). If radial rotation of the wrist is not corrected, ulnar drift is more prone to recur after ulnar deviation has been corrected. In addition to tenosynovectomy, synovectomy of the wrist, resection of the distal ulna, and transposition of the dorsal carpal ligament, it has been our practice to transfer the extensor carpi radialis longus (ECRL) to the extensor carpi ulnaris (ECU) in patients who do not have the ability to actively ulnar-deviate the wrist or in whom the extensor carpi ulnaris is attentuated or ruptured[15] (Fig. 33–16). This transfer may also help prevent "metacarpal descent," which Zancolli[95] believes to be an important factor in producing ulnar deviation of the long extensor tendons.

The extensor carpi radialis longus inserts on the radial side of the second metacarpal, making this tendon a strong radial deviator. Therefore, using this muscle for a transfer not only provides active ulnar deviation of the metacarpals but also removes a strong deforming force.

SURGICAL TECHNIQUE

After the dorsal wrist surgery and after the dorsal retinaculum has been sutured beneath the extensor

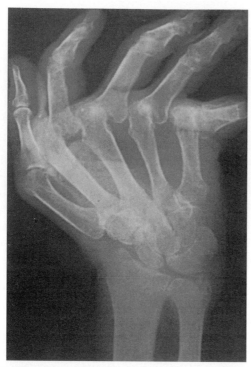

Figure 33–15. Rheumatoid hand with ulnar deviation of the fingers and radial rotation of the wrist. (From Clayton ML, Ferlic DC: Tendon transfer for radial rotation of the wrist in rheumatoid arthritis: Clin Orthop 100:176–185, 1974.)

tendons, detach the ECRL from its insertion on the radial side of the base of the second metacarpal. With the wrist in neutral, pass the ECRL across the top through the ECU three times. Put maximum tension on the transferred ECRL, and suture in place. Postoperatively, splint the wrist in ulnar deviation and neutral flexion for 4 weeks. Then start active and passive motion with a removable splint for 2 to 4 weeks longer.

RESULTS

Others have contradicted the concept that radial rotation of the wrist effects ulnar deviation of the fingers.[8, 39] In spite of these conflicting reports, we continue to perform the transfer, and we believe we have shown that it favorably affects ulnar deviation of the fingers.

Flexor Tenosynovitis

In many patients, hand pain may be interpreted as arthritic pain but is, in fact, pain from carpal tunnel syndrome due to rheumatoid arthritis.[41] Carpal tunnel syndrome may also be the initial symptom of rheumatoid arthritis.[11, 61] There may actually be locking or triggering of tendons at the level of the transverse carpal ligament[14] (Fig. 33–17). Initial treatment consists of splinting and perhaps a local injection of

steroid into the carpal canal. Failure of response to this treatment after a single injection is an indication for surgery.

As well as incising the volar carpal ligament to decompress the nerve, a flexor tenosynovectomy is carried out when hypertrophic synovium is found. It is also necessary to inspect the floor of the carpal canal, because we have seen bony spicules from the carpus as well as synovium ruptured through the volar capsule.[51]

The ulnar nerve may also be entrapped at the wrist when it passes through Guyon's canal. Surgical decompression of the nerve in Guyon's canal is the preferred treatment for ulnar nerve compression at the wrist. More common than with the median nerve, the so-called "double crush"[61] phenomenon may compress the ulnar nerve in more than one place, and in the patient with rheumatoid arthritis, involvement at the elbow or cervical radiculopathy may also be present.

Rupture of the flexor tendons is not nearly as common as rupture of the extensor tendons in rheumatoid arthritis, but the flexor tendons are more difficult to reconstruct satisfactorily. The most common flexor tendon to rupture is the flexor pollicis longus, followed by the flexor digitorum profundus to the index finger (Fig. 33–18). Flexor tendons rupture from infiltrative flexor tenosynovitis or from attrition caused by bony prominence. Ertel and associates[22, 23] found that all 24 ruptures in the palm and digits, as well as 30 of 91 ruptures in the wrist, were attributed to invasion of the tendons by rheumatoid synovium. The other ruptures in the wrist were caused by attrition of the flexor tendons by spurs within the carpal canal. Walker[93] reported a flexor pollicis longus rup-

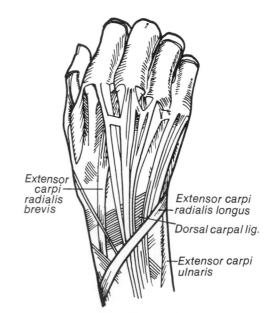

Figure 33–16. Transfer of the extensor carpi radialis longus to the extensor carpi ulnaris. (From Clayton ML, Ferlic DC: Tendon transfer for radial rotation of the wrist in rheumatoid arthritis: Clin Orthop 100:176–185, 1974.)

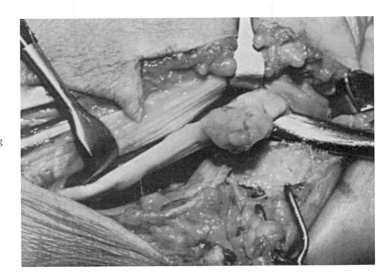

Figure 33–17. Rheumatoid granuloma of a flexor tendon causing triggering beneath the volar carpal ligament.

ture in a rheumatoid thumb secondary to attrition on a sesamoid. Mannerfelt and Norman[51] reported on 25 flexor tendon ruptures, 11 from bony attrition in the carpal canal and 14 from synovial invasion. The bone spurs arose from the scaphoid or trapezium and pierced the floor of the carpal tunnel in relation to the tendon of the flexor pollicis longus. These researchers described the combination of rupture of the flexor pollicis longus and the two flexor tendons to the index finger due to bony attrition in the carpal canal; this combination has become known as the Mannerfelt lesion.

With regard to reconstruction of the ruptured flexor tendons, one must keep in mind that it is necessary to start motion early after volar tenosynovectomy, or motion may be lost forever. It may be more advisable to perform arthrodesis or tenodesis of the distal joint of a finger if only the flexor digitorum profundus is ruptured. Tendon transfers, free tendon grafts, direct repair, and arthrodesis have been described as giving satisfactory results.[22, 23, 51, 93] If only a flexor digitorum superficialis is ruptured, no reconstruction is indicated. To reconstruct a ruptured flexor pollicis longus, the ring flexor digitorum superficialis may be

transferred, but a free tendon graft can be used if there is minimal tenosynovitis. Arthrodesis of the interphalangeal joint of the thumb is the treatment of choice if the thumb is destroyed or if there is little chance of mobilizing it. Reconstruction of the finger in which both flexor tendons are ruptured at the wrist can usually be carried out by transferring one of the intact flexor digitorum superficialis tendons to the distal stump of the ruptured distal flexor digitorum profundus. The anastomosis site must be secure enough to allow motion to be started immediately.

Probably the most important treatment for flexor tendon rupture at the wrist is to prevent additional tendons from rupturing by performing a flexor tenosynovectomy, decompressing the volar carpal ligaments, exploring the carpal canal, and removing bony spicules that could cause further tendon damage.

Role of Wrist Arthroplasty

A stable, balanced, and painless wrist is necessary for optimal hand function. A wrist arthrodesis in the neutral position with preserved forearm pronation and supination is compatible with useful hand function, but elimination of wrist motion may be unnecessary or even objectionable in the patient with progressive disease in adjacent joints. To be acceptable, an arthroplasty must relieve pain, be stable, correct deformity, provide motion, and leave a reasonable alternative for salvage in case of failure.

Arthroplasties without implants have been used. Proximal row carpectomy has been useful in the traumatic wrist. We have performed this procedure in eight patients with rheumatoid arthritis in whom the articular surface of the capitate and the lunate fossa of the radius have been preserved, but long-term results were unsatisfactory because of progressive deterioration.[28]

The second type of arthroplasty for the rheumatoid wrist without an implant is palmar shelf arthro-

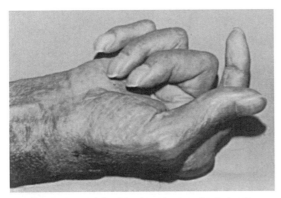

Figure 33–18. Rupture of the flexor tendons to the index finger and the flexor pollicis longus.

plasty.[3, 33, 73] Instead of removal of bone from the carpus, the distal end of the radius is shaped, and a volar lip of bone is preserved, giving the wrist stability.

Our experience with this procedure is limited. We encountered one case of persistent lateral deviation that could possibly have been prevented by a longer period of splinting. We do not use this procedure today.

Role of Implant Arthroplasty

Joint replacement at the wrist level has significantly influenced the treatment of the rheumatoid wrist. Our experience with the silicone wrist was quite favorable initially, but with time, there was a high rate of failure due to particulate synovitis and breakage.[45] We rarely recommend this procedure today.

Our experiences with the total wrist replacement is more promising, but results with its use also have deteriorated with time. Loosening and imbalance problems are the most significant reasons for failure.[19, 29, 47] Both of these procedures are discussed in Part V of this book.

Role of Arthrodesis

There is still a place for arthrodesis of the wrist in selected patients with rheumatoid arthritis. Wrist fusion is sometimes desirable. Occasionally, bilateral wrist fusion may be necessary, and patients sometimes retain better function in the distal joints after wrist arthrodesis.[74] Indications for wrist fusion are (1) ankylosis in marked flexion, (2) marked instability as the result of carpal destruction, (3) rupture of the extensor carpi radialis longus and extensor carpiradialis brevis, and (4) moderate changes in the wrist but marked pain with the use of crutches.

The general recommendation has been fusion in 10° of dorsiflexion[35]; Boyes[9] has recommended 20° to 30°. For bilateral wrist fusions, it has sometimes been recommended that one wrist be fused in dorsiflexion and the other in palmar flexion. We recommend fusion in the neutral position for unilateral or bilateral cases.[18] With the wrist placed at neutral, the arc of motion of pronation and supination substitutes for palmar flexion and dorsiflexion without shoulder or elbow substitution.

Our technique for wrist arthrodesis[18, 54] is a modification of that described by Mannerfelt and Malmsten[52] in 1971. Bone graft other than local bone has usually not been found to be necessary. The largest intramedullary rod that will fit into the third metacarpal is inserted into the radius and then driven into the third metacarpal. Two Kirschner wires are crossed from the carpus to the radius for additional support. Wrist fusion is discussed in detail in Chapter 38.

SUMMARY

The wrist destroyed by inflammatory arthritis has characteristic deformities. The patterned or cookbook approach to solving these problems is not always indicated, because each patient must be evaluated for multiple joint involvement. Hand surgeons need to be familiar with the diagnosis and treatment of various inflammatory arthritides that affect the wrist because they may be the first physicians to see patients in whom a disease is still in its monarticular form.

Early surgery for persistent dorsal tenosynovitis is likely to prevent tendon rupture. It has not been proven that wrist synovectomy prevents continued destruction of the wrist joint. Reconstruction of ruptured extensor tendons is usually very satisfactory, but the results are not as good as in wrists in which the tendons have not ruptured. Flexor tenosynovitis of the wrist may manifest as carpal tunnel syndrome, wrist pain, swelling, or ruptured flexor tendons. Surgery is necessary to decompress the nerve and to remove the diseased tenosynovium. Repair of ruptured flexor tendons is rewarding, but the results are not as satisfactory as those of surgery on the extensor side. Wrist arthroplasty and arthrodesis both have a place in treatment of the wrist with marked destruction.

References

1. Abernathy PJ, Bennyson WG: Decompression of the extensor tendons at the wrist in rheumatoid arthritis. J Bone Joint Surg 61B:64, 1979.
2. Albright JA, Chase RA: Palmar-shelf arthroplasty of the wrist in rheumatoid arthritis. J Bone Joint Surg 52A:896, 1970.
3. Adolfsson L, Nylander G: Arthroscopic synovectomy of the rheumatoid wrist. J Hand Surg 18B:92–96, 1993.
4. Allieu Y, Lussiez B, Asencio G: The long-term results of synovectomy in the wrist: A report of 60 cases. French J Orthop Surg 3:188–194, 1989.
5. Backdahl M: The caput ulna syndrome in rheumatoid arthritis. Acta Rheum Scand (Suppl) 5:1, 1963.
6. Backhouse KM: The mechanics of normal digital control in the hand and an analysis of the ulnar drift of rheumatoid arthritis. Ann R Coll Surg 43:154, 1968.
7. Belsky MR, Feldon P, Millender LH, et al: Hand involvement in psoriatic arthritis. J Hand Surg 7:203, 1982.
8. Boyce T, Youm Y, Sprague BL, Flatt AE: Clinical and experimental studies on the effect of extensor carpi radialis longus transfer in the rheumatoid hand. J Hand Surg 3:390, 1978.
9. Boyes JH: Bunnell's Surgery of the Hand, 5th ed. Philadelphia, JB Lippincott, 1970, p 296.
10. Brumfield R Jr, Kuschner SH, Gellman H, et al: Results of dorsal wrist synovectomy in the rheumatoid hand. J Hand Surg 15A:733–735, 1990.
11. Chamberlain MA, Corbett M: Carpal tunnel syndrome in early rheumatoid arthritis. Ann Rheum Dis 29:149, 1970.
12. Chaplin D, Pulkki T, Saarimaa A, Vainio K: Wrist and finger deformities in juvenile rheumatoid arthritis. Acta Rheum Scand 15:206, 1969.
13. Clayton ML: Surgery of the rheumatoid hand. Clin Ortho 36:47, 1964.
14. Clayton ML: Surgical treatment at the wrist in rheumatoid arthritis. J Bone Joint Surg 47A:741, 1965.
15. Clayton ML, Ferlic DC: Tendon transfer for radial rotation of the wrist in rheumatoid arthritis. Clin Orthop 100:176, 1974.

16. Clayton ML, Ferlic DC: The wrist in rheumatoid arthritis. Clin Orthop 106:182, 1975.
17. Clayton ML, Thirupathi R, Ferlic DC, Goldberg B: Extensor tendon rupture over the metacarpal heads. Hand 15:149, 1983.
18. Clayton ML, Ferlic DC: Arthrodesis of the arthritic wrist. Clin Orthop 187:89, 1984.
19. Dennis DA, Ferlic DC, Clayton ML: Long-term results of Volz total wrist arthroplasty. J Hand Surg 11A:790–797, 1986.
20. Dray GJ, Millender LH, Nalebuff EA, Phillips C: The surgical treatment of hand deformities in systemic lupus erythematosis. J Hand Surg 6:339, 1981.
21. Ellison M, Flatt AE, Kelly KJ: Ulnar drift of the fingers in rheumatoid disease. J Bone Joint Surg 53A:1061, 1971.
22. Ertel AN, Millender LH: Flexor tendon involvement in rheumatoid arthritis. In Hunter JM, Schneider LH, Makin EJ (eds): Tendon Surgery in the Hand. St Louis, CV Mosby, 1987, pp 370–384.
23. Ertel AN, Millender LH, Nalebuff E, et al: Flexor tendon ruptures in patients with rheumatoid arthritis. J Hand Surg 13A:860–866, 1988.
24. Feldon P, Millender LH, Nalebuff EA: Rheumatoid arthritis in the hand and wrist. In David Green (ed): Operative Hand Surgery. New York, Churchill Livingstone, 1993, pp 1623–1624.
25. Ferlic DC: Extensor indicis proprius transfer for extensor pollicis longus rupture. In Blair W, Steyers C (eds): Techniques in Hand Surgery. Baltimore, Williams & Wilkins Co., 1996, pp 649–653.
26. Ferlic DC, Cooney WP: The wrist in inflammatory arthritis. Metcalf PG (ed): Operative Arthroscopy. New York, Raven Press, 1991, pp 641–646.
27. Ferlic DC, Smyth CJ, Clayton ML: Medical considerations and management of rheumatoid arthritis. J Hand Surg 8 Supplement:662–666, 1983.
28. Ferlic DC, Clayton ML, Mills MF: Proximal row carpectomy—a review of rheumatoid and nonrheumatoid patients. J Hand Surg 16A:420–424, 1991.
29. Ferlic DC, Clayton ML: Results of CFV total wrist arthroplasty: Review and early report. Orthopaedics 18:1167–1171, 1995
30. Flatt AE: Some pathomechanics of ulnar drift. Plast Reconstr Surg 37:295, 1966.
31. Flatt AE: Ulnar Drift. The Care of the Arthritic Hand, 5th ed. St. Louis, Quality Medical Publishing, 1995, pp 343–383.
32. Flatt AE: The Care of the Arthritic hand, ed 4. St Louis, CV Mosby, 1983.
33. Gellman H, Rankin G, Brumfield R, et al: Palmar shelf arthroplasty in the rheumatoid wrist. J Bone Joint Surg 71A:223–227, 1989.
34. Goldner JL: Tendon transfers in rheumatoid arthritis. Orthop Clin North Am 5:425, 1974.
35. Haddad RJ Jr, Riordan DC: Arthrodesis of the wrist. J Bone Joint Surg 49A:950, 1967.
36. Hakstian RW, Buriana R: Ulnar deviation of the fingers. J Bone Joint Surg 48A:608, 1966.
37. Hamas RS: A quantitative approach to total wrist arthroplasty—development of a precentered total wrist prosthesis. Orthopedics 2:245, 1979.
38. Harrison S, Swannell AJ, Ansell BM: Repair of extensor pollicis longus using extensor pollicis brevis in rheumatoid arthritis. Ann Rheum Dis 31:490, 1972.
39. Hastings DE, Evans JA: Rheumatoid wrist deformities and their relation to ulnar drift. J Bone Joint Surg 57A:930, 1975.
40. Hastings DE, Evans JA: The lupus hand—a new surgical approach. J Hand Surg 3:1979, 1978.
41. Henderson ED, Lipscomb P: Surgical treatment of the rheumatoid hand. JAMA 175:431, 1961.
42. Hindley CJ, Stanley JK: The rheumatoid wrist—patterns of disease progression. J Hand Surg 16B:275–279, 1991.
43. Ishikawa H, Hanyu T, Tajima T: Rheumatoid wrist treated with synovectomy of the extensor tendons and the wrist joint combined with a Darrach procedure. J Hand Surg 17A:1109–1117, 1992.
44. Kulick RG, DeFiore JC, Straub LR, Ranawat CS: Long-term results of dorsal stabilization in the rheumatoid wrist. J Hand Surg 6:272, 1981.
45. Jolly SL, Ferlic DC, Clayton ML, et al: Swanson silicone arthroplasty of the wrist in rheumatoid arthritis—a long-term follow-up. J Hand Surg 17A:142–149, 1992.
46. Laine VAI, Vainio KJ. Spontaneous rupture of tendons in rheumatoid arthritis. Acta Orthop Scand 24:250, 1955.
47. Lamberta FJ, Ferlic DC, Clayton ML: Volz total wrist arthroplasty in rheumatoid arthritis: A preliminary report. J Hand Surg 5:245, 1980.
48. Landsmeer JMF: Studies in the anatomy of articulation. II: Patterns of movement of bimuscular biarticular systems. Acta Morph Neerl Scand 3:304, 1960.
49. Leslie BM, Carlson G, Ruby LK: Results of extensor carpi ulnaris tenodesis in the rheumatoid wrist undergoing a distal ulnar excision.
50. Linscheid RL, Dobyns JH: J Hand Surg 15A:547–551, 1990. Rheumatoid arthritis of the wrist. Orthop Clin North Am 2:649, 1971.
51. Mannerfelt L, Norman O: Attrition ruptures of flexor tendons in rheumatoid arthritis caused by bony spurs in the carpal tunnel. J Bone Joint Surg 51B:270, 1969.
52. Mannerfelt L, Malmsten M: Arthrodesis of the wrist in rheumatoid arthritis. A technique without external fixation. Scand J Plast Reconstr Surg 5:124, 1971.
53. Marmor L, Lawrence JF, Duboid EL: Posterior interosseous nerve palsy due to rheumatoid arthritis. J Bone Joint Surg 49A:381, 1967.
54. Millender LH, Nalebuff EA: Arthrodesis of the rheumatoid wrist. J Bone Joint Surg 55A:1026, 1973.
55. Millender LH, Nalebuff EA, Holdsworth DE: Posterior interosseous nerve syndrome secondary to rheumatoid arthritis. J Bone Joint Surg 55A:753, 1973.
56. Millender LH, Nalebuff EA, Albin R, et al: Dorsal tenosynovitis and tendon ruptures in the rheumatoid hand. J Bone Joint Surg 56A:601, 1974.
57. Millender LH, Nalebuff EA: Preventative surgery: Tenosynovectomy and synovectomy. Orthop Clin North Am 6:765, 1975.
58. Moberg E: Tendon grafting and tendon suture in rheumatoid arthritis. Am J Surg 109:375, 1965.
59. Moore JR, Weiland AJ: Gouty tenosynovitis in the hand. J Hand Surg 10A:291, 1985.
60. Moore JR, Weiland AJ, Valdata L: Tendon ruptures in the rheumatoid hand—analysis of treatment and functional results in 60 patients. J Hand Surg 12A:9–14, 1987.
61. Nakaro KK: The entrapment neuropathy of rheumatoid arthritis. Orthop Clin North Am 6:837, 1975.
62. Nalebuff EA, Garrett J: Opera glass hand in rheumatoid arthritis. J Hand Surg 1:210–220, 1976.
63. Pahle I, Raunio P: The influence of wrist position in finger deviation in the rheumatoid hand. J Bone Joint Surg 51B:664, 1969.
64. Rana NA, Taylor AR: Excision of the distal end of the ulna in rheumatoid arthritis. J Bone Joint Surg 55B:96, 1973.
65. Ranawat CS: Anatomical considerations and design features of total wrist joint. Orthop Nurs J 6:61, 1979.
66. Rasmussen KB, Sneppen O: Operativ behandlung of polyarthritis. Nord Med 77:433, 1967.
67. Rodman GP, Schumacher R (eds): Primer on the Rheumatic Diseases, ed 8. Atlanta, Arthritis Foundation, 1983.
68. Rothfield NT: Systemic lupus erythematosis: Clinical and laboratory aspects. In McCarty DJ (ed): Arthritis and Allied Conditions, ed 9. Philadelphia, Lea & Febiger, 1979.
69. Schneider LH, Rosenstein RG: Restoration of extensor pollicis longus function by tendon transfer. Plast Reconstr Surg 71:533–537, 1983.
70. Shannon FT, Barton NJ: Surgery for rupture of extensor tendons in rheumatoid arthritis. Hand 8:279, 1976.
71. Shapiro JS: The etiology of ulnar drift. J Bone Joint Surg 48:634, 1968.
72. Shapiro JS: A new factor in the etiology of ulnar drift. Clin Orthop 68:32, 1970.
73. Skoff HD: Palmar shelf arthroplasty: A follow-up note. J Bone Joint Surg 70A:1377–1388, 1988.
74. Smith-Peterson MM, Aufranc OE, Larson CB: Useful surgical procedures for rheumatoid arthritis involving joints of the upper extremity. Arch Surg 36:764, 1943.

75. Smyth CJ: Optimum therapeutic program in seropositive nodular rheumatoid arthritis. Med Clin North Am, 52:687, 1968.

76. Smyth CJ: Therapy of rheumatoid arthritis. A pyramidal plan. Postgrad Med J 51:31, 1972.

77. Stanley JK: Conservative surgery in the management of rheumatoid disease of the hand and wrist. J Hand Surg 17B:339–342, 1992.

78. Straub LR, Wilson EH: Spontaneous rupture of extensor tendons in the hand associated with rheumatoid arthritis. J Bone Joint Surg 38A:1208, 1956.

79. Straub LR, Smith JW, Carpenter GK Jr, Dietz GH: The surgery of gout in the upper extremity. J Bone Joint Surg 43A:731, 1961.

80. Straub LR: Surgical rehabilitation of the hand and upper extremity in rheumatoid arthritis. Bull Rheum Dis 12:265, 1962.

81. Straub LR, Ranawat CS: The wrist in rheumatoid arthritis. J Bone Joint Surg 51A:1, 1969.

82. Summers B, Hubbard MJS: Wrist joint arthroplasty in rheumatoid arthritis: Comparison between the Mueli and Swanson prostheses. J Hand Surg 9B:171, 1984.

83. Swanson AB: The ulnar head syndrome and its treatment by implant resection arthroplasty J Bone Joint Surg 54A:906, 1972.

84. Swanson AB, Swanson G de G: Pathogenesis and pathomechanics of rheumatoid deformities in the hand and wrist. Orthop Clin North Am 4:1039, 1973.

85. Taleisnik J: The ligaments of the wrist. J Hand Surg 1:110–118, 1976.

86. Taleisnik J: Rheumatoid synovitis of the volar compartment of the wrist joint: Its radiographical signs and its contribution to wrist and hand deformities. J Hand Surg 4:526–535, 1979.

87. Taleisnik J: Rheumatoid arthritis of the wrist. Hand Clin 5:257–278, 1989.

88. Thirupathi R, Ferlic DC, Clayton ML: Dorsal wrist synovectomy in rheumatoid arthritis: A long-term study. J Hand Surg 8:848, 1983.

89. Vainio KJ: Hand. In Milch RA (ed): Surgery of Arthritis. Baltimore, Williams & Wilkins, 1964, p 130.

90. Vaughan-Jackson OJ: Rupture of extensor tendons by attrition at the inferior radio-ulnar joint. J Bone Joint Surg 30B:528, 1948.

91. Vaughan-Jackson OJ: Tendon ruptures in the hand. Hand 1:122, 1969.

92. Vincent KA, Szabo RM, Agee JM: The Sauve-Kapandji procedure for reconstruction of the rheumatoid distal radioulnar joint. J Hand Surg 18A:978–983, 1993.

93. Walker LG: Flexor pollicis longus rupture in rheumatoid arthritis: Secondary to attrition on a sesamoid. J Hand Surg 18A:990–991, 1993.

94. Walton RL, Brown RE, Giansiracusa DF: Psoriatic arthritis mutilans: Digital distraction lengthening: Pathophysiological and current therapeutic review. J Hand Surg 13A:510–515, 1988.

95. Zancolli E: Structural and Dynamic Basis of Hand Surgery. Philadelphia, JB Lippincott, 1972.

PART VIII

Surgical Options for Common Wrist Disorders

CHAPTER 34

Soft Tissue Arthroplasty About the Wrist

Gregory G. Degnan, MD, and David M. Lichtman, MD

The goals of treatment for destructive radiocarpal and intercarpal arthrosis are pain relief, stability, strength, and mobility. However, it is rarely possible to achieve all of these desired goals. Historically, the most popular and predictable procedure has been complete wrist arthrodesis. In conditions, however, which are limited to only one or several of the articulations that make up the wrist joint, the complete loss of motion associated with total wrist arthrodesis may be unnecessary as well as unacceptable to the patient. This situation has led to the continued search for alternative salvage procedures.

Implant arthroplasty and total wrist arthroplasty have been used extensively in the rheumatoid population with favorable results. They have not, however, met with similar success in post-traumatic arthritis and degenerative arthritis related to the carpal instabilities. Interest in the use of limited intercarpal arthrodesis in the treatment of these disorders has therefore increased.[18] The limited procedure offers the advantages of pain relief and stability while maintaining some motion.

Early results using limited fusions for carpal instabilities, scapholunate advanced collapse deformity (SLAC wrist), and Kienböck's disease have been encouraging. These procedures are not, however, without potential problems.[19] Clinically, the range of motion achieved has not consistently matched that produced in cadaver studies. Nelson and colleagues[13a] reported a non-union rate of 28 percent with lunotriquetral fusions; and McAuliffe and associates[12] reported non-unions in 45 percent of fusions involving the proximal row. Another disadvantage of these procedures is the prolonged immobilization required.

Perhaps the greatest controversy surrounding limited intercarpal fusion concerns the long-term effects on adjacent joints. Few authorities have reported on long-term follow-up in such cases, and these few reports have demonstrated a number of patients with radiographic evidence of progressive degenerative disease at adjacent joints. Thus, the question arises as to whether limited intercarpal fusion can be considered a definitive procedure or whether a significant number of patients undergoing the procedure will require further surgery. A more complete discussion of the advantages and disadvantages of these fusions is presented in Chapter 37.

Fascial implant arthroplasty has been used with success for replacement of small avascular proximal pole scaphoid fragments and also for reconstruction of the degenerative thumb carpometacarpal (CMC) joint[4]; these procedures are also covered elsewhere in this text, and so are not discussed. Fascial interpositional arthropasties have been used with success in the treatment of degenerative joint disease of the wrist in patients with rheumatoid arthritis.[18] Tillman and Thabe[18] described the use of the palmar capsule or dorsal retinaculum as an interpositional material with or without partial resection of the proximal row (see section on techniques).

In 1944, T. T. Stamm[17] first reported on the use of proximal row carpectomy as a salvage procedure in the wrist. He credits Lambrinudi, however, with conceiving the notion that excising the proximal row for scaphoid non-union would convert an unstable link joint system into a simple hinge joint. Stack[16] first reported on proximal row excision in this country for treatment of transcaphoid perilunate dislocations in 1948.

Since its initial description in 1944, proximal row carpectomy has developed an undeservedly poor reputation. Almost every report in the literature makes mention of this poor reputation, and yet there is no large series to substantiate this perception. Every published series of proximal row carpectomy has shown favorable long-term results when the procedure was used to treat post-traumatic disorders limited to the proximal row.[1, 2, 5, 8–10, 13] As a result, proximal row carpectomy has been gaining popularity as a salvage for these difficult problems.

609

INDICATIONS AND CONTRAINDICATIONS

Commonly, in long-standing post-traumatic disorders of the scaphoid or lunate, collapse and degeneration of both bones will occur with the potential for subsequent radiocarpal arthritis (Fig. 34–1). Proximal row carpectomy is often well suited for this situation. These disorders include long-standing scaphoid nonunions, rotary subluxation of the scaphoid with radioscaphoid arthritis, stage IV osteonecrosis of the lunate, and severe perilunate dislocations and fracture-dislocations.[1, 8, 10, 14, 18] Less common indications are severe flexion deformities related to arthrogryposis, septic arthritis, and Volkmann's ischemic contracture.[20] Omer and Capen[15] also describe its use in spastic paralysis.

In our experience, calcium pyrophosphate deposition disease (CPPD) has also been an occasional indication for this procedure. Late in the disease, the wrist ligaments are stiffened by crystal deposition. The stiffness predisposes them to rupture and leads to scapholunate dissociation with eventual radioscaphoid degenerative changes.[3] Crystal deposition in articular cartilage also hastens joint degeneration. These changes respond well to proximal row carpectomy.

The one absolute contraindication to proximal row carpectomy performed in the classic manner is significant degeneration of the proximal articular surface of the capitate or lunate fossa of the radius.[1, 5, 8, 10] Mild to moderate changes can be tolerated, and the procedure can be performed with expectation of good results.[2] A relative contraindication is in a patient who cannot be trusted to perform an aggressive postoperative regimen.[5] The procedure is also contraindicated in patients who demand a totally stable and pain-free wrist rather than one that retains partial mobility. For these patients, we would recommend limited intercarpal or total wrist arthrodesis. Rheumatoid arthritis also represents a relative contraindication to proximal row carpectomy. The surfaces of the capitate and radius are often severely involved in this disease. If not severely involved at the time of surgery, such surfaces are likely to become involved later, because the articular surfaces of the capitate and radius must be left intact and are therefore susceptible to subsequent destruction by persistent synovitis. In such cases, consideration should be given to arthrodesis as well as total wrist arthroplasty or silicone interposition arthroplasty as described by Swanson.[17a] The details of these procedures and their specific indications are discussed elsewhere in this text.

PROXIMAL ROW CARPECTOMY: SURGICAL TECHNIQUE

Proximal row carpectomy can be carried out under regional anesthesia. Because bone graft is not necessary and operative times are routinely less than 2 hours, axillary block or interscalene block anesthesia is adequate. More commonly, however, we use a general anesthetic so that an iliac crest bone graft may be harvested if intraoperative conditions (severe degeneration of the capitate or lunate fossa) dictate a

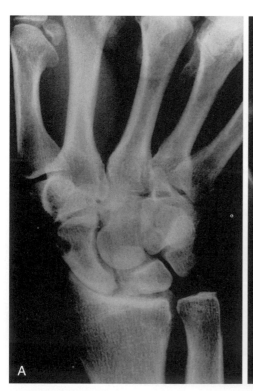
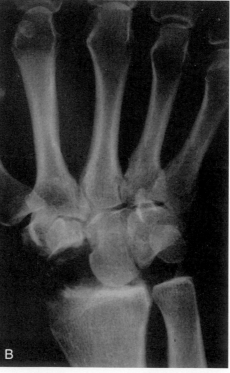

Figure 34–1. A, Degenerative arthritis limited to the radioscaphoid and radiolunate joints. The patient is a 62-year-old man with a history of repeated "wrist sprains" sustained in college football. In recent years, wrist stiffness and pain interfered with his avocational activities. B, Postoperative radiograph depicting proximal row carpectomy with radial styloidectomy.

change from proximal row carpectomy to intercarpal arthrodesis or wrist arthrodesis. The technique is performed as follows:

After the extremity is surgically prepared and draped, identify the external landmarks of the wrist, and outline them on the skin with a marking pen. Outline the radial styloid, proximal pole of the scaphoid, base of the third metacarpal, and Lister's tubercle (Fig. 34–2). Make a straight dorsal longitudinal incision extending from the base of the third metacarpal to a point 2 to 3 cm proximal and just ulnar to Lister's tubercle. Carry the dissection down to extensor retinaculum in line with the skin incision. After defining the level of the retinaculum, develop radial and ulnar flaps in this plane to ensure thick subcutaneous flaps containing the superficial nerves and vessels. Develop these flaps in one of two ways. While maintaining straight dorsal retraction with heavy skin hooks, develop the plane either using a spread and snip technique with the scissors or using an inverted no. 15 blade to feather or paint the subcutaneous

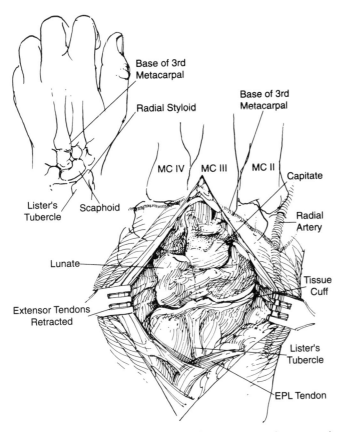

Figure 34–2. *Top,* The landmarks used to map out the approach. *Bottom,* The exposure of the radiocarpal and midcarpal joints after the subperiosteal capsular dissection. Note the position of the radial artery and its branches in the radial flap. These vessels must be dissected and protected during excision of the distal pole of the scaphoid and styloidectomy. This dissection depicts a central longitudinal capsular incision. As described in the text, we usually perform a transverse capsular incision. This incision can be converted to a flap arthroplasty, if needed, at the time of capsular closure. EPL = extensor pollicis longus; MC = metacarpal, with Roman numerals.

tissues off the retinaculum. As the radial flap is developed, take care to identify and protect the superficial sensory branch of the radial nerve. Similarly, identify and protect the dorsal sensory branch of the ulnar nerve in the ulnar flap.

Divide the distal half to third of the extensor retinaculum between the third and fourth compartments. Mobilize the tendons of the second, third, and fourth compartments, and remove the extensor pollicis longus out of the groove at Lister's tubercle. Retract the tendons of the second and third compartments radially, and the tendons of the fourth compartment ulnarly, to expose the dorsal wrist capsule. At this point, we identify the posterior interosseous nerve in the floor of the fourth compartment and excise a 0.5 to 1 cm segment.

Identify the level of the radiocarpal joint while flexing and extending the wrist. Incise the wrist capsule transversely over the proximal row, taking care to ensure that a large enough cuff of tissue remains proximally along the dorsal rim of the radius to allow subsequent repair. Elevate the dorsal capsule from the bones of the proximal row using sharp dissection with a knife blade. When approaching the distal pole of the scaphoid, take great caution not to injure the radial artery, which overlies the scaphotrapeziotrapezoid joint. Identify the vascular bundle with blunt dissection, and then retract it gently to the radial side with a small Meyerding retractor (see Fig. 34–1). After inspecting the head of the capitate, "T" the incision centrally and distally to the level of the midthird of the capitate (see Fig. 34–1).

As an alternative approach, incise the retinaculum and dorsal capsule longitudinally between the second and fourth compartments after freeing the extensor pollicis longus from the third compartment. Then perform a subperiosteal dissection of the medial and lateral flaps, exposing all the bones of the proximal row as well as their joint surfaces. This exposure is excellent but will not permit a dorsal capsular flap arthroplasty closure, which will be required if the head of the capitate is severely degenerated (see discussion of pitfalls and technical alternatives).

Prior to excising the proximal row, inspect the articular surfaces of the capitolunate and radiolunate joints. The inspection is facilitated by manual distraction of the wrist combined with forced flexion (Fig. 34–3). If either of these surfaces shows significant wear or degenerative changes, perform an alternative procedure. Mild wear is not considered a contraindication to proximal row excision, because studies have shown that mild wear does not adversely affect the clinical outcome and that significant progression of the degenerative arthritis does not occur.[2, 14] The order of excision is usually from ulnar to radial (see Fig. 34–3), although some surgeons prefer to excise the lunate first. It should be noted that the pisiform, a sesamoid bone palmar to the wrist, should not be excised with the remainder of the proximal row. Excision of the proximal row is challenging, and it is easier to remove the individual bones in a piecemeal

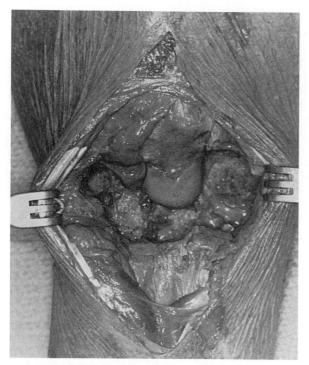

Figure 34–3. In this cadaver specimen, the wrist is flexed to visualize the articular surface of the capitate. The lunate fossa will be similarly inspected. Significant degenerative change would result in selection of an alternative procedure.

fashion. Use an osteotome to split the bone and then to strip the soft tissues while stabilizing the fragments with rongeurs (Fig. 34–4). Use rongeurs to reduce the size of the fragments, facilitating removal. The distal pole of the scaphoid is by far the most difficult portion to remove, so using a 0.062-inch Kirschner (K)

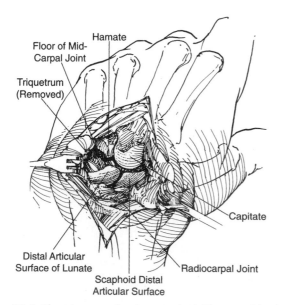

Figure 34–4. The triquetrum has been excised. The carpal bones are removed from ulnar to radial without disturbing the pisiform.

wire as a joystick to manipulate the bone can be extremely helpful (Figs. 34–5 and 34–6).

During excision of the proximal row, there are two key points to remember. First, it is essential to avoid damage to the articular surfaces of the lunate fossa and the capitate. Second, it is crucial to preserve the volar capsule and ligaments. In particular, as previously noted by Green,[8] preservation of the radioscaphocapitate ligament is critical. This ligament is the major stabilizing force keeping the capitate in the lunate fossa.

After removing the proximal row, position the capitate in the lunate fossa, and move the wrist from neutral to radial deviation to check for impingement of the radial styloid on the trapezium. If impingement is present, perform a radial styloidectomy. An index finger placed on the styloid tip can detect impingement when the wrist is radially deviated.

To perform styloidectomy, "T" the proximal capsule and dorsal periosteum centrally and proximally, then develop the radial flap subperiosteally using a no. 15 blade and periosteal elevator. Carry this dissection around the styloid to the volar aspect of the radius. During this subperiosteal dissection, entry into the first dorsal compartment is almost inevitable, so take care not to damage the abductor tendons. Excise no more than 1 to 1.5 cm of articular surface using a sharp osteotome or sagittal saw (see Fig. 34–1B). Be sure not to disturb the origin of the stout volar radiocarpal ligaments.

At this point, release the tourniquet and obtain hemostasis. Pay special attention to the area of the deep branch of the radial artery in the region of the proximal trapezium. After 10 minutes, re-inflate the tourniquet prior to closure. Next, perform copious irrigation with antibiotic solution, then seat the capitate in the lunate fossa, place the wrist in neutral, and close the dorsal capsule with interrupted sutures. The capsule is usually redundant, so advance the distal flaps proximally to aid in stabilizing the capitate. After capsular closure, assess the stability of the capitate. If translation does not seem excessive, continue closure. If, however, translation does seem excessive, place crossed K wires across the radiocarpal joint into the capitate, avoiding the articular portions of the capitate and the lunate fossa (Fig. 34–7). Place the K wires in such a fashion that the capitate is distracted slightly away from the radius to avoid pressure across these articular surfaces.

Re-approximate the extensor retinaculum with 5-0 nylon, specifically taking care to avoid making the repair too tight. Use a Z-plasty closure of the retinaculum if the closure is tight. Stenosing tenosynovitis can be a troublesome complication if this step is overlooked. The extensor pollicis longus tendon may be left free above the retinaculum if necessary. Approximate the skin with 4-0 nylon using horizontal mattress sutures, and apply a bulky sterile dressing to the fingertips. Keep the wrist in neutral position by applying a palmar or dorsal splint.

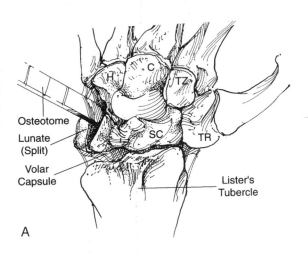

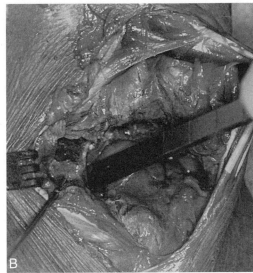

Figure 34–5. *A,* The osteotome is being used to split the lunate after previous triquetral excision. *B,* The osteotome will then be used to lever the fragments and dissect soft tissue free from the bone, as demonstrated here in a cadaver specimen. Note that the K wire has been placed in the bone to be used as a joystick. This technique significantly facilitates removal of these bones. C = capitate; H = hamate; SC = scaphoid; TZ = trapezium; TR = trapezoid.

PITFALLS AND TECHNICAL ALTERNATIVES

Proximal row carpectomy is occasionally performed through a transverse dorsal incision along the line from the ulnar styloid to the radial styloid.[5, 8, 11] Although this is certainly an acceptable technique, we believe that the straight dorsal longitudinal incision is more versatile. If the articular surface of either the capitate or lunate fossa is degenerative, the longitudinal incision provides excellent exposure for limited intercarpal fusion or wrist arthrodesis.

Some surgeons expose the proximal row through two capsular incisions, one on either side of the fourth compartment. We believe, however, that this exposure makes it more difficult to visualize the posi-

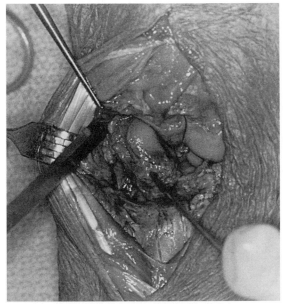

Figure 34–6. In this cadaver specimen, the thumb is to the *upper left.* A K wire has been placed in the scaphoid to use as a joystick, and the osteotome is being used to peel the capsule away from the bone. The distal pole of the scaphoid is the most difficult to remove, and often a small shell of the distal pole is left without morbidity. Care should be taken to ensure that this shell does not impinge on the radial styloid with radial deviation.

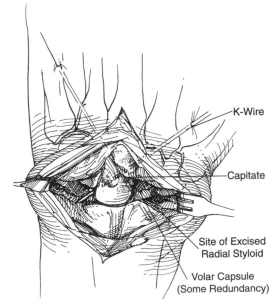

Figure 34–7. Crossed K-wire stabilization of the capitate in the lunate fossa. Note that the wires do not penetrate the articular surface. Usually the capsule is closed prior to placement of K wires in order to better assess stability.

tion of the capitate on the radius after excision of the proximal row.

Several potential errors adversely affect the outcome of this procedure. First, care must be taken to ensure that the capsular flaps are removed from bone and kept thick to allow for solid repair. If insufficient capsule remains proximally, the distal flap must be repaired through drill holes in the distal radius. During excision of the proximal row, the volar capsule, particularly the radioscaphocapitate ligament, must be protected to preserve subsequent stability of the capitate.[8] This occasionally requires that a cortical shell of distal scaphoid be left behind where it is intimate with the palmar capsular ligaments. This shell of bone, although radiographically visible, does not adversely affect the clinical outcome in any way. During excision of the proximal row, the surgeon must be careful not to damage the articular surfaces of the capitate and lunate fossa. Perhaps the two most common pitfalls are failure to recognize impingement of the trapezium on the radial styloid[5, 10] and failure to recognize significant degenerative changes that should preclude this procedure.

When intraoperative inspection reveals significant degenerative changes of the lunate fossa and/or capitate surface, one technical alternative is applicable that has received little attention in the literature. Distraction resection arthroplasty, as described by Fitzgerald and colleagues[6] can theoretically provide results similar to those of proximal row carpectomy even for these clinically more advanced cases. In their series, there was no statistically significant difference in results between proximal row carpectomy and distraction resection arthroplasty.[6]

This technique is performed through a dorsal midline incision as follows: Approach the wrist between the third and fourth extensor compartments. Take the dorsal capsule off the edge of the distal radius to create a large distally based flap. Inspect the surfaces of the capitate and lunate fossa. If the surfaces are not significantly damaged, perform a proximal row carpectomy as described previously. If, however, the surfaces show significant cartilage or bone eburnation, remove the head of the capitate and the proximal portion of the hamate squarely at the same level using a power saw. Make this cut at the level of the body of the capitate. Perform a radial styloidectomy. Then excise the lunate and triquetrum. The scaphoid is then completely or partially resected at a level distal to the capitate osteotomy.

Next, align the hand over the distal radius and distract it approximately 2 cm. Pass three or more K wires through the radius across the resection space and into the carpus to maintain distraction, neutral deviation, and slight extension. Suture the redundant dorsal capsule to the volar capsule between the capitate and the radius, and reapproximate the proximal edge of the capsular flap to the dorsal edge of the radius. Leave the K wires in place for 6 to 8 weeks, and then gradually wean the patient from the splint.

This procedure offers a viable alternative to fusion in the patient with significant degenerative changes that otherwise preclude proximal row carpectomy. The results are similar,[6] and like proximal row carpectomy, distraction resection arthroplasty avoids the requirement for prolonged immobilization and bone grafting.

In a similar fashion, the resection interposition arthroplasty described by Tillman and Thabe[18] can be used as an alternative to PRC in the presence of a badly degenerative capitate in a patient who requires motion. Likewise, this procedure is an alternative to fusion or silicone replacement arthroplasty in the rheumatoid patient.

This procedure is performed through a transverse S-shaped incision or a standard dorsal midline incision. Perform a synovectomy and/or tenosynovectomy as required. If indicated, resect the distal ulna at this point. Carry out a subperiosteal dissection, elevating the dorsal capsule off the distal edge of the radius. Retract the extensor tendons, including the abductor pollicis longus and extensor pollicis brevis, and then resect a small section of the distal radius, including the styloid. Remodel the remaining distal surface of the radius, creating a slight concavity and a small palmar shelf, then remodel the carpal joint surface in a similar fashion. If necessary, excise a portion or all of the proximal row to gain length for the capsule. Free the palmar capsule carefully from the distal surface of the radius, and suture this distally based flap of palmar capsule to the dorsal rim of the radius. This maneuver pulls the palmar flap into the radiocarpal joint as an interpositional material. Then advance the distally based dorsal capsular flap proximally on the dorsal radius.

Splint the wrist in extension postoperatively for 4 to 6 weeks, but begin immediate finger motion. Early rehabilitation is aimed at restoring motion, and later, strengthening is begun. The results reported by Tillman and Tabe[18] in a rheumatoid population were encouraging. Flexion and ulnar deviation were reliably maintained, whereas flexion and radial deviation were less predictable. They believed this latter result to be acceptable, because extension is more desirable and functional than flexion. Although this procedure has not been reported for post-traumatic arthritis, it seems a possible alternative in the patient who refuses fusion but has severe capitate or lunate fossa degeneration that precludes proximal row carpectomy.

REHABILITATION

Following proximal row carpectomy, place the extremity in a bulky compressive dressing for 10 to 12 days. At that time, remove the sutures and apply a well-molded short-arm cast, and begin finger flexion and extension exercises. At 4 weeks postoperatively, remove the cast and pins, if present. Apply a well-molded removable palmar splint, and begin a nonresistive exercise program to mobilize the wrist. Begin strengthening exercises at 6 to 8 weeks postoperatively. Maximum strength and motion may not be achieved for 6 to 12 months. Occasionally, patients complain of inability to flex or extend the fingers in the early postoperative period. This may be due to the relative lengthening of the tendons and the alteration in Blick's curve. The patient and the therapist should be made aware that this limitation is transient and will resolve in time with therapy.

OUTCOMES

In almost all reported series on proximal row carpectomy, patients have experienced a subjective sense of weakness in the operated wrist.[1, 5, 8, 10] Objective measurements, however, have revealed grip strengths that are routinely between 60 and 90 percent of normal.[1, 5, 8-10] Most major series report an average of 44° of extension, 45° of flexion, 30° of ulnar deviation, and 5° of radial deviation at the wrist.[5, 8-10] The final range of motion and maximum strength may not be achieved for up to 1 year. Almost all patients note a significant improvement in pain, and most patients are able to return to their normal preoperative avocations and occupations, regardless of the type of work.[1, 2, 8-10, 14] In general, all series report excellent overall patient satisfaction with the procedure and its outcome. On the basis of these published outcomes and our own experience, we recommend proximal row carpectomy when appropriately indicated for the treatment of wrist pain or deformity.

References

1. Crabbe WA: Excision of the proximal row of the carpus. J Bone Joint Surg 46B:708–711, 1964.
2. Culp RW, McGuigan FX, Turner MA, et al: Proximal row carpectomy: A multicenter study. J Hand Surg 18A:19–25, 1993.
3. Dohert W, Lovallo JL: Scapholunate advanced collapse pattern in calcium pyrophosphate deposition disease of the wrist. J Hand Surg 18A:1095–1098, 1993.
4. Eaton RG, Akelman E, Eaton BH: Fascial implant arthroplasty for treatment of radioscaphoid degenerative disease. J Hand Surg 14A:766–774, 1989.
5. Ferlic DC, Mack LC, Mills MF: Proximal row carpectomy: Review of rheumatoid and nonrheumatoid wrists. J Hand Surg 16A:420–424, 1991.
6. Fitzgerald JP, Peimer CA, Smith RJ: Distraction resection arthroplasty of the wrist. J Hand Surg 14A:774–781, 1989.
7. Garcia-Elias M, Cooney WP, Linscheid RL, Chao EYS: Wrist kinematics after limited intercarpal arthrodesis. J Hand Surg 14A:791–799, 1989.
8. Green DP: Proximal row carpectomy. Hand Clin 3:163–168, 1987.
9. Inglis AE: Proximal row carpectomy for diseases of the proximal row. J Bone Joint Surg 59A:460–463, 1977.
10. Jorgenson EC: Proximal-row carpectomy: An end result study of twenty-two cases. J Bone Joint Surg 51A:1104–1111, 1969.
11. Mack GR, Lichtman DM: Proximal row carpectomy. In Lichtman DM (ed): The Wrist and Its Disorders. Philadelphia, WB Saunders, 1988, pp 320–322.
12. McAuliffe JA, Dell PC, Jaffe R: Complications of intercarpal arthrodesis. J Hand Surg 14A:1121–1128, 1989.
13. McLaughlin HL, Babb OD: Carpectomy. Surg Clin North Am 31:451–461, 1951.
13a. Nelson DL, Manske PR, Pruitt DL, et al: Lunotriquetral arthrodesis. J Hand Surg 18A:1113–1120, 1993.
14. Neviaser RJ: Proximal row carpectomy for post traumatic disorders of the carpus. J Hand Surg 8:301–305, 1983.
15. Omer EG, Capen DA: Proximal row carpectomy with muscle transfers for spastic paralysis. J Hand Surg 1:197–204, 1976.
16. Stack JK: End results of excision of the carpal bones. Arch Surg 57:245–252, 1948.
17. Stamm TT: Excision of the proximal row of the carpus. Proc R Soc Med 38:74–75, 1944.
17a. Swanson AB: Flexible implant arthroplasty for arthritic disabilities of the radiocarpal joint. Orthop Clin North Am 4:383–394, 1973.
18. Tillman K, Thabe H: Technique and results of resection and interposition arthroplasty of the wrist in rheumatoid arthritis. Reconstr Surg Traumatol 18:84–91, 1981.
19. Tomaino MM, Miller RJ, Burton RI: Scapholunate advanced collapse wrist: Proximal row carpectomy or limited wrist arthrodesis with scaphoid excision? J Hand Surg 19A:134–142, 1994.
20. White JW, Stubbins SG: Carpectomy for intractable flexion deformities of the wrist. J Bone Joint Surg 26:131, 1944.

CHAPTER 35

Implant Arthroplasty in the Carpal and Radiocarpal Joints

Alfred B. Swanson, MD, and Geneviève de Groot Swanson, MD

Disabilities of the wrist occur frequently and can develop in rheumatoid arthritis or osteoarthritis or following fractures or dislocations. Involvement of individual carpal bones and of the intercarpal, radiocarpal, and distal radioulnar joints can occur singly or in combination. The ideal goal of reconstructive procedures in the wrist and carpus is to provide pain relief with reasonable stability, strength, and mobility to assist in hand adaptations. Proper evaluation of the specific problems presented, including severity of disease, patient's age, and functional requirements, is essential to selecting the best treatment from the wide range of available procedures. Treatment recommendations are discussed for the carpal bones (trapezium, scaphoid, lunate) and for the radiocarpal joint. The concepts, indications, surgical techniques, and pitfalls of implant arthroplasty in the wrist and carpus are presented in detail.

The implants for small joint arthroplasty of the extremities are the result of more than 30 years of research by the senior author and his associates.* In 1969, the silicone implants were made available following a worldwide field clinic testing, and they have since been used in numerous patients in 83 countries. Two types of silicone elastomers have been used: the conventional silicone elastomer (CSE) and a high-performance (HP) elastomer released in 1974, which was a lower tear propagation to reduce the fracture rate in hinged implants.

In 1976, a research project was initiated to develop bone-shielding (grommet) devices to protect the midsection of the silicone flexible-hinged implant from shearing forces and lacerations due to sharp bone edges.[13] A laboratory study, in vivo animal trials, and human clinical studies were conducted to evaluate ingrowth and press-fit fixation, semicircular and circumferential designs, and nine different materials (porous polyethylene, Proplast, pyrolytic carbon, stainless steel, stainless steel mesh, ion-bombarded cobalt-chromium, smooth cobalt-chromium, titanium, and glutaraldehyde-prepared bovine pericardium). The press-fit circumferential design made of titanium provided the best implant protection and bone response at the grommet-bone interface. Ma-

chine-made circumferential titanium grommets have been used for the first metatarsophalangeal joint since 1985 and for the metacarpophalangeal joints since 1987. Semicircular press-fit grommets have been used for the radiocarpal joint since 1982.

In 1985, we reported[17] that particulate synovitis and lytic bone changes can occur around some articulating silicone implants that are subjected to excessive force-loading owing to implant oversize or malalignment, uncorrected or recurring instability, and excessive activity. These reactive problems, which occurred more often around silicone scaphoid and lunate implants than around thumb basilar implants, were also seen around silicone radial head and single stem toe implants, and more rarely around flexible hinges used without grommets. A research study was initiated with the engineering and biology departments of a local university to analyze particle-induced reactions from metals, plastics, and elastomers.[4, 7, 8] Wear debris and phagocytosis are the key events in the etiology of particulate synovitis. The "cement disease" associated with total knee and hip procedures has also been recognized as a polyethylene particulate problem. After ingesting particles, the foreign-body macrophage releases osteolytic enzymes that can compromise the arthroplasty. It was shown that small particles are more likely than larger particles to induce greater inflammatory mediator release from macrophages. The participation of antigen-specific lymphocytes or antibodies in silicone particle–induced macrophage reactions has not been demonstrated to date, failing to provide evidence of immunologic stimulation by silicone elastomers.[4, 6] In 1984, in an effort to address the silicone wear problem, the senior author selected unalloyed titanium as an alternative material for silicone spacer implants on the basis of its good bone and soft tissue tolerance as seen in the grommet study.

The senior author prefers the use of conventional silicone elastomer (CSE) for trapezium implants and the use of titanium for the single stem toe, scaphoid, lunate, convex condylar, and radial head implants.*[15, 18, 20, 21, 23, 25] It should be noted that high-performance silicone elastomer, used in combination with grom-

---

*References 10, 12, 14, 16, 18, 20, 24–27.

*Wright Medical Technology, Arlington, TN.

mets, is the preferred material for flexible-hinged implants in the metacarpophalangeal, radiocarpal, and first metatarsophalangeal joints.[1-3, 5, 16, 19, 22]

CARPAL SCAPHOID AND LUNATE

Procedures for treatment of necrosis, fracture, or fracture-dislocation and subluxation of the scaphoid and the lunate have included bone grafting, local resection, carpal bone implant arthroplasty, intercarpal fusion, proximal row carpectomy, radial styloidectomy, radial shortening, ulnar lengthening, soft tissue interposition arthroplasty, and wrist implant arthroplasty or fusion.[2, 9, 24, 28] The senior author has devised a classification of lunate and scaphoid disorders to help select the appropriate treatment according to the stages of severity of disease (Tables 35–1 and 35–2). Procedures for scaphoid and lunate titanium implant arthroplasty are discussed here in detail.

Carpal Bone Implant Arthroplasty

Carpal bone implants act as articulating spacers to maintain the relationship of the adjacent carpal bones following local resection procedures while preserving wrist mobility and stability. Their use allows correction of associated intercarpal instability, thereby preventing collapse and settling of the carpus. These implants have essentially the same shapes as their anatomic counterparts, with the concavities being more pronounced to provide greater stability. Titanium implant designs were based on the clinical experience gained from use of their silicone counterparts (Fig. 35–1). Some modifications were made to accommodate the material properties of unalloyed titanium and to enhance implant stability.

Ligamentous instability and carpal collapse are frequently associated with scaphoid or lunate disease. Total removal of these bones leaves defects in the palmar ligaments that can lead to implant instability (Fig. 35–2). A subluxated carpal implant is under abnormal shear stress; if it is also subjected to excessive loading forces across the wrist joint, eventual failure of the arthroplasty results. The palmar ligaments should be preserved during carpal bone excision by leaving a small portion of the palmar part of the bone, or they should be repaired if weakened. Associated collapse patterns should be treated at the time of implant arthroplasty, by appropriate intercarpal bone fusions. Cancellous bone, preferably obtained from the ilium, is used; resected bone, if healthy, can also be used. Firm internal fixation is obtained with staples, Kirschner or threaded wires, or, preferably, a Herbert bone screw. Cysts in contiguous bones should be curetted and bone-grafted at the time of the procedure. The implants must not be oversized and should not be used if the space is inadequate. Carpal bone implant replacement is not

Table 35–1. CLASSIFICATION AND TREATMENT FOR AVASCULAR NECROSIS OF THE LUNATE

Stage	Pathologic Conditions	Treatment Options
I	Sclerosis of the lunate with Minimal symptoms Normal carpal bone relationships	Splinting and rest Revascularization procedures Ulnar and radial lengthening or shortening
II	Sclerosis of the lunate with cystic changes with Clinical symptoms Normal carpal bone relationships	Lunate implant replacement Ulnar and radial lengthening or shortening
III	Sclerosis, cysts, and fragmentation of the lunate with Scaphoradial angle: 40°–60° Carpal height collapse: 0–5 percent Carpal translation: Minimal	Lunate implant replacement with or without intercarpal fusions
IV	Sclerosis, cysts, and fragmentation of the lunate with Scaphoradial angle: <70° Carpal height collapse: 5–10 percent Carpal translation: Moderate	Lunate implant replacement and intercarpal fusions
V	Sclerosis, cysts, and fragmentation of the lunate with Scaphoradial angle: >70° Carpal height collapse: >10 percent Carpal translation: Severe Cystic changes in contiguous bones	Lunate implant replacement and intercarpal fusions Wrist arthrodesis Ulnar impingement treatment, as needed
VI	Sclerosis, cysts, and fragmentation of the lunate with Scaphoradial angle: >70° Carpal height collapse: >15 percent Carpal translation: Severe Cystic changes in contiguous bones Significant intercarpal and radiocarpal degenerative arthritic changes	Radiocarpal implant arthroplasty Wrist arthrodesis Ulnar impingement treatment, as needed

Table 35–2. CLASSIFICATION AND TREATMENT FOR PATHOLOGIC CONDITIONS OF THE SCAPHOID

Stage	Pathologic Conditions	Treatment Options
I	Acute scaphoid fractures Acute scaphoid fracture-dislocation	Immobilization Open or closed reduction
II	Non-union of the scaphoid	Bone graft Bone stimulator

III	Avascular necrosis of a fragment with
	   Carpal height collapse: 0–5 percent
	   Lunate dorsiflexion minimal (R-L* angle: 0°–10°)
		Scaphoid implant replacement

IV	Comminuted or grossly displaced fracture
	Avascular necrosis with scaphoid degenerative arthritic changes
	Subluxation of scaphoid with degenerative arthritic changes
	Non-union of scaphoid with cystic changes with
	   Carpal height collapse: 5–10 percent
	   Lunate dorsiflexion minimal to moderate (R-L angle: 10°–30°)
	   Mild degenerative arthritic changes of contiguous bones
	   (particularly between lunate and capitate)
		Scaphoid implant replacement with or without
		  intercarpal fusions

V	Stage IV pathology of the scaphoid with
	   Carpal height collapse: >10 percent
	   Lunate dorsiflexion moderate to severe (R-L angle: >30°)
	   Mild to moderate degenerative arthritic changes of
	    contiguous bones
		Scaphoid implant replacement with intercarpal fusions
		Proximal row carpectomy
		Fusion of the proximal carpus to the radius
		Hemiarthroplasty

VI	Stage IV pathology of the scaphoid or previous surgery with
	   Carpal height collapse >15 percent
	   Lunate dorsiflexion severe (R-L angle: >30°)
	   Severe intercarpal and radiocarpal degenerative arthritic
	    changes
		Radiocarpal implant arthroplasty
		Wrist arthrodesis
		Ulnar impingement treatment, as needed

*R-L angle, radiolunate angle.

indicated in cases of advanced disease; wrist implant arthroplasty or fusion is preferred.

Lunate Implant Arthroplasty

INDICATIONS

Titanium lunate implant resection arthroplasty can be indicated in the presence of avascular necrosis (Kienböck's disease), localized osteoarthritic changes, long-standing dislocations, resistance to conservative treatment, and revision procedures. The procedure is contraindicated in cases in which arthritic involve-ment is not localized to the lunate articulations, if complete relief of pain is to be expected. In long-standing dislocations or in cases of Kienböck's disease, there may be inadequate space to fit the implant. Severe carpal instability with inadequate or irretrievable ligament or bone support for stabilizing the implant precludes the use of this procedure.

SURGICAL PROCEDURE

Use a dorsal longitudinal incision across the radiocarpal area and centered at Lister's tubercle to expose the lunate bone. A transverse skin incision may be

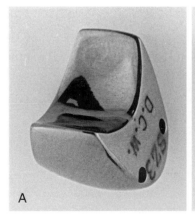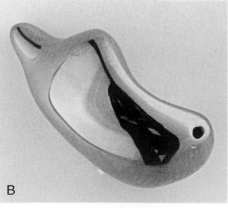

Figure 35–1. *A,* Titanium lunate implant with palmar and dorsal suture holes used for either right or left wrist. *B,* Titanium scaphoid implant with distal pole beak and suture hole in proximal pole (implant for right wrist shown).

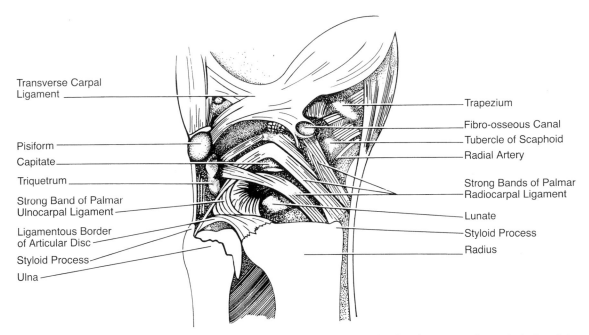

Figure 35–2. Palmar carpal ligaments. Complete excision of carpal bones (trapezium, scaphoid, or lunate) may leave "holes" or defects in palmar carpal ligaments, because they firmly attach to carpal bones. A small shell of bone should be left on the palmar capsule to preserve its continuity. (Redrawn from Swanson AB: Flexible Implant Arthroplasty in the Hand and Extremities. St Louis, CV Mosby, 1973.)

used in some of the uncomplicated cases, especially in the female. A volar approach is recommended when the lunate bone is dislocated volarly. Carefully preserve the superficial sensory branches of the radial and ulnar nerves. Incise the extensor retinaculum over the extensor pollicis longus tendon, which is mobilized for radial retraction (Fig. 35–3A). Retract the extensor carpi radials longus (ECRL) and extensor carpi radialis brevis (ECRB) tendons radially and the extensor digitorum communis tendons ulnarly. With the wrist flexed, incise the dorsocarpal ligament in a **T** shape, with the vertical extension placed over the lunate in the direction of the capitate and third metacarpal, and the horizontal extension placed over the distal radius at the insertion of the dorsal capsule (Fig. 35–3B). Then elevate the ligament close to bone.

Adequate dissection is necessary to properly identify the capitate, triquetrum, scaphoid, radius, and lunate. Take radiographs, if necessary, for further anatomic orientation. Remove the lunate piecemeal, avoiding injury to the dorsal and palmar carpal ligaments. Leave a thin, bony wafer with the palmar ligaments to assure their important continuity; their integrity must be verified and obtained to prevent palmar subluxation of the implant. If the lunate bone were totally removed, there would be a defect between the two strong bands of the palmar ulnocarpal and radiocarpal ligaments, which are attached on each side of the lunate (see Fig. 35–2). A tendon graft or a slip of the flexor carpi radialis tendon can be used if direct re-approximation of these structures is impossible.

Evaluate the associated bones for the presence of arthritic changes, loss of cartilage, surface irregulari-

ties, cystic changes, and collapse patterns. Traction and compression of the hand across the wrist joint helps reveal instability patterns, particularly vertical rotation of the scaphoid. In the presence of collapse patterns or instability of the carpus, associated limited carpal bone fusions are very important to improve the distribution of forces across the wrist joint. Rotary subluxation of the scaphoid must be corrected and the carpus stabilized, by either triscaphe or scaphocapitate fusion, using an iliac bone graft and firm internal fixation.[29] The scaphocapitate fusion is preferred when there are cystic changes in the capitate. Curette and graft pre-existing bone cysts. Because of the significant tendency for rotation of the scaphoid, we perform intercarpal bone fusions in the majority of cases.

Identify the posterior sensory branch of the interosseous nerve in its course between the distal radius and ulna. Resect about 10 mm of nerve to provide sensory denervation of part of the carpal area. Take care to avoid injury to the associated small arteries and veins.

Titanium lunate implants are made in five sizes for the right or left wrist (see Fig. 35–1A). Select an implant size that will fit comfortably into the space left by the excision of the lunate. In determining implant size, start with the smallest trial size. In long-standing dislocations of the lunate, the space can be greatly decreased, so the smallest implant should be used whenever possible. It is very important not to use an oversized implant, as doing so could result in excessive implant force-loading and displacement.

The distal surface of the lunate implant is shaped into a deep concavity that straddles the head of the

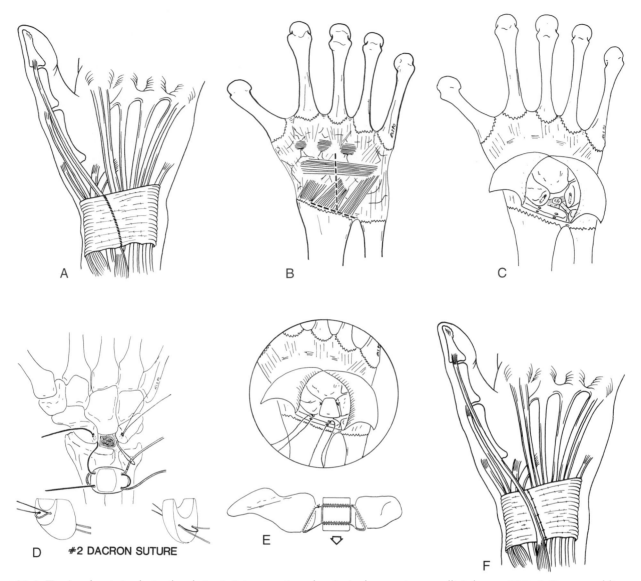

Figure 35–3. Titanium lunate implant arthroplasty. *A,* Extensor retinaculum incised over extensor pollicis longus (EPL). *B,* Dorsocarpal ligament is incised in T shape with vertical extension over lunate towards capitate. *C,* Lunate is resected, leaving small bone wafer with palmar ligaments. Small drill holes are made in palmar direction through articular surfaces of scaphoid and triquetrum. Drill holes are made in distal radius for closure of dorsocarpal ligament. *D,* With a wire loop, a #2 Dacron suture is passed through scaphoid and looped through implant palmar suture hole and then dorsal hole. Another #2 Dacron suture is similarly passed through the triquetrum and implant. Short flat implant surface articulates with the scaphoid and long flat surface with the triquetrum. *E,* As Dacron sutures are tightened, the implant becomes reduced in position. Two 2-0 Dacron sutures are passed for closure of dorsocarpal ligament. *F,* The extensor retinaculum is closed, leaving the EPL subcutaneous. (*A, B,* and *F* from Swanson AB, de Groot Swanson G, Herndon JH: Complications of arthroplasty and joint replacement at the wrist. In Epps CH Jr (ed): Complications in Orthopaedic Surgery, ed. 3. Philadelphia, JB Lippincott, 1994, pp 957–995. *C, D,* and *E* from Swanson AB, de Groot Swanson G: Implant resection arthroplasty in the treatment of Kienböck's disease. Hand Clin 9:483–491, 1993.)

capitate. The flat lateral surfaces of the implant articulate with the scaphoid (shorter surface) and triquetrum (longer surface). The proximal surface of the implant has a rounded, sloping shape that articulates with the presenting radioulnar surface. The implant has two transverse holes running laterally through its body for suture stabilization to the scaphoid and triquetral bones.

Using a 1-mm drill or a .045 Kirschner wire, make a small hole through the articular surface of the proximal pole of the scaphoid and triquetrum in a palmar

direction to pass #2 Dacron sutures to stabilize the implant, as shown in Figures 35–3*C* and *D.* Before inserting the implant, irrigate the wound thoroughly with saline solution to remove all debris. Handle the implant with blunt instruments. As the sutures are tied firmly, the implant is securely reduced into position (Fig. 35–3*E*). Verify the implant's position and stability while moving the wrist passively in all directions.

Suture the dorsocarpal ligament with 2-0 Dacron sutures passed through two small drill holes made in the dorsal distal radius before the implant was inserted (Fig. 35–3E). Secure the repair firmly with additional Dacron and Dexon sutures, inverting the knots. Suture the retinaculum over the extensor tendons, except for the extensor pollicis longus, which should be left free in the subcutaneous tissue (Fig. 35–3F). Insert multiple small drains subcutaneously, and close the skin with interrupted sutures. Apply a secure conforming dressing, including longitudinally oriented Dacron batting strips and anterior and posterior plaster splints. We prefer to use a nonelastic conforming wrapping material, such as Kling.

POSTOPERATIVE CARE

The extremity is kept elevated for 1 to 2 days, and the patient is instructed to move the shoulder and fingers. Plaster immobilization is worn for a total of 8 weeks. A long-arm thumb spica cast is applied 1 to 2 days after surgery, depending on the amount of swelling present. If a cast has been applied at surgery, it should be bivalved. Skin sutures are removed after 2 to 3 weeks through a window in the cast. At 4 weeks, a short-arm cast is applied, which is worn for another 4 weeks. The cast may be tightened or changed as needed. The rehabilitation program includes isometric gripping exercises to strengthen the extrinsic and intrinsic muscles of the hand and forearm. Use of the wrist is usually resumed at 12 weeks. Postoperative radiographs are taken to evaluate the position of the implant and bone status (Figs. 35–4 and 35–5). Postoperatively, avoidance of abusive motion is critical.

Scaphoid Implant Arthroplasty

INDICATIONS

Titanium scaphoid implant resection arthroplasty can be indicated for Preiser's disease, avascular necrosis, pseudarthroses, and arthritic involvement around the scaphoid with associated carpal instability, particularly the scapholunate advanced collapse (SLAC) wrist pattern. The titanium implant has also been used for revision of scaphoid silicone implant arthroplasties showing cystic or progressive degenerative bony changes. The procedure is not recommended in the following situations: arthritic involvement not localized to the scaphoid articulations; inadequate bone to support the implant; inadequate space to insert the implant; and severe carpal instability with inadequate or irretrievable ligament support (Fig. 35–6).

SURGICAL PROCEDURE

Make an 8- to 10-cm dorsoradial longitudinal incision across the radiocarpal joint midway between the tip of the styloid and Lister's tubercle. Carefully preserve the longitudinal veins and branches of the superficial radial nerve. Incise the extensor retinaculum over the extensor pollicis longus and retract the tendon radially. Elevate the extensor retinaculum from the third compartment radially as a flap to expose the second compartment. Mobilize the ECRL and ECRB tendons to their insertion for appropriate retraction. Protect the transverse metacarpal vessels, which are located immediately under the insertion of the wrist extensors.

The extensor tendons can be retracted radially, ulnarly, or apart from each other to expose the dorsoradial capsule of the wrist joint. Incise the dorsal capsule of the wrist in a T fashion, as shown in Figure 35–7A. With the wrist flexed, elevate the dorsal ligament from the radius by sharp dissection kept close to bone to preserve adequate tissues for re-attachment. Retracting the wrist extensor tendons radially enables identification of the scapholunate junction

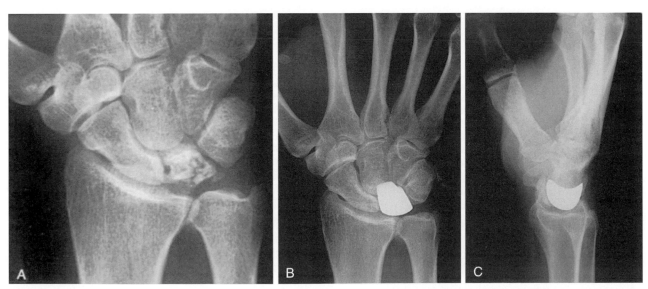

Figure 35–4. A, Preoperative radiograph of a 31-year-old heavy laborer with stage III Kienböck's disease. B and C, Radiographs taken 10 years after titanium lunate replacement shows good bone tolerance and stable implant position. The patient is pain free and works at his original job.

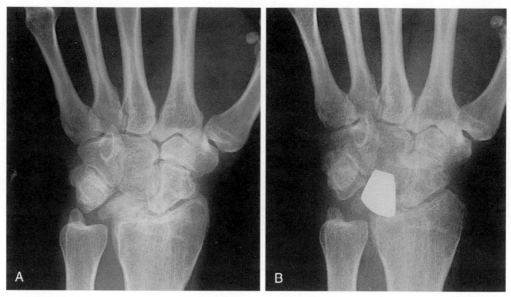

Figure 35–5. *A,* A 38-year-old boilermaker who had silicone lunate arthroplasty 15 years previously for Kienböck's disease presented with 2-year history of pain and swelling of wrist after 10 hours of heavy manual labor. This preoperative radiograph shows a lunate silicone implant, some cystic changes, scaphoid rotation, and radial styloid osteophyte. *B,* Revision procedure consisted of removal of broken lunate implant and replacement with a titanium implant; intercarpal synovectomy and fusion of scaphoid to trapezium and of hamate to capitate with iliac bone grafting; curettage and bone grafting of carpal cysts; and radial styloidectomy. Three years after revision, the patient has 30° extension, 40° flexion, and 20° radial and ulnar deviation, remains pain free, and has returned to his previous occupation.

and the capitate. Retracting the extensor tendons ulnarly allows visualization of the distal portion of the scaphoid and its articulations with the trapezoid and trapezium as well as with the radius. If necessary, intraoperative radiographs can be obtained to identify the carpal bones.

Remove the scaphoid piecemeal with a rongeur, avoiding injury to the underlying palmar ligaments and to both dorsal and palmar scapholunate ligaments. Leave a thin, bony wafer of the scaphoid in

the palmar ligament area distal to the radiocapitate ligament and extending up to the trapezium to ensure their important continuity. If the scaphoid distal pole were completely removed, a hole would be left in the palmar supporting structures through which the implant could protrude (see Fig. 35–2).

Evaluate the associated bones for the presence of arthritic changes, loss of cartilage, surface irregularities, cystic changes, and collapse patterns, as previously described for lunate implant arthroplasty. In the pres-

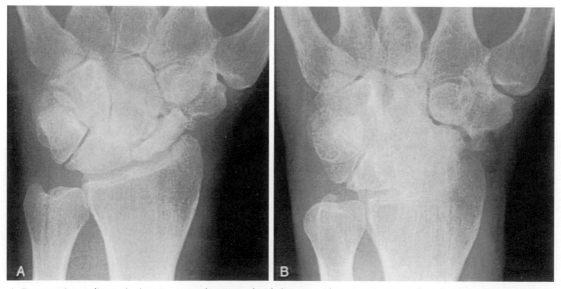

Figure 35–6. *A,* Preoperative radiograph showing a grade VI scaphoid disease with severe intercarpal and radiocarpal degenerative changes. *B,* Postoperative radiograph taken 10 years after a radiocarpal fusion.

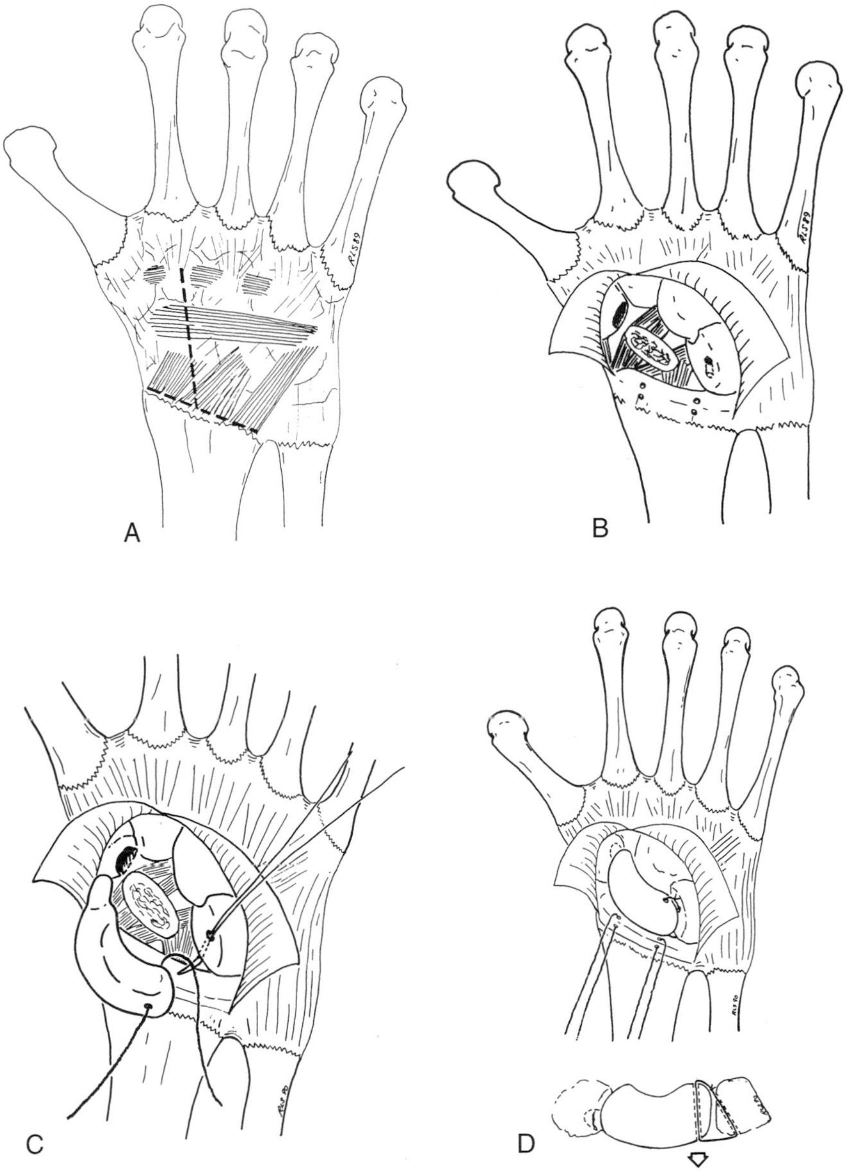

Figure 35–7. Titanium scaphoid implant arthroplasty. *A,* Dorsocarpal ligament is incised in a T shape with vertical extension over the scaphoid in the direction of the trapezoid and horizontal extension over distal radius at insertion of dorsal capsule. *B,* The scaphoid is resected, leaving a small bony wafer to preserve continuity of radiocarpal ligaments. A bony shelf is made on the undersurface of the trapezium for stabilization of the implant's distal pole. A suture hole is made through lunate for passage of fixation suture. Two drill holes are made in the distal radius to pass sutures for closure of dorsocarpal ligament. *C,* The distal pole of the implant is stabilized in the bony shelf made in the trapezium's undersurface. The proximal pole is stabilized with a #2 Dacron suture passed through the lunate and the implant suture hole. The suture is pulled through the hole in the lunate with a wire loop. *D,* As the #2 Dacron suture is tightened securely, the implant becomes reduced firmly in position. (From Swanson AB, de Groot Swanson G, Herndon JH: Complications of arthroplasty and joint replacement at the wrist. In Epps Jr CH (ed): Complications in Orthopaedic surgery, ed 3. Philadelphia, JB Lippincott, 1994, pp 957–995.)

ence of collapse patterns or instability, rotation of the lunate must be corrected and the carpus stabilized by fusion of the lunate to the capitate or to the triquetrum and hamate using an iliac bone graft and firm internal fixation. Curette and bone-graft pre-existing bone cysts. Resect approximately 1 cm of the posterior sensory branch of the posterior interosseous nerve to provide some sensory denervation of part of the carpal area, as described for lunate implant arthroplasty.

The titanium scaphoid implants are made in five sizes each for the right and left hand (see Fig. 35–1*B*). Using trial implants, determine the implant size, starting with the smallest size. It is very important not to use an oversized implant to avoid excessive implant force-loading and displacement. Handle the implant with blunt instruments.

Stabilize the distal beak of the scaphoid implant either in a bony channel prepared in the undersurface of the trapezium, or between the trapezium and trapezoid, according to individual variations in carpal anatomy (Fig. 35–7*B*). Stabilize the proximal pole by passing a #2 Dacron suture through a 1-mm drill hole made in the lunate and then through the implant suture hole (Fig. 35–7*C* and *D*). Use a wire loop to pass the suture through the hole in the lunate. Prior to inserting the implant, determine the integrity of the palmar ligaments and capsule and, if necessary, tighten them with sutures.

The methods for suturing the dorsal capsule, the extensor retinaculum, and the skin and applying the operative dressing are similar to those described for lunate implant arthroplasty.

POSTOPERATIVE CARE

The extremity is kept elevated for 1 to 2 days, and shoulder and finger movements are encouraged. A

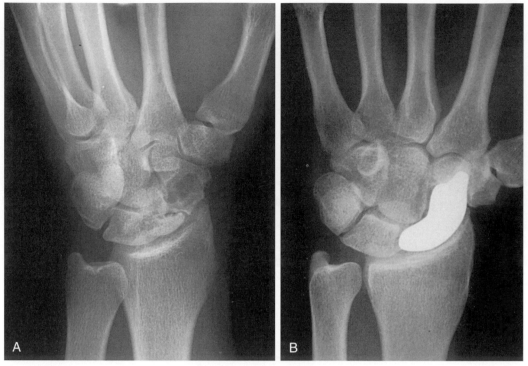

Figure 35–8. *A,* Preoperative radiograph of a 28-year-old manual laborer presenting with a painful and disabling scaphoid fracture non-union with stage IV pathology. *B,* Radiograph taken 7 years after a scaphoid titanium implant arthroplasty shows excellent bone tolerance and implant position. The patient is pain free and performs heavy manual labor and recreational activities.

long-arm thumb spica cast is applied for 4 weeks, and a short-arm thumb spica cast is used for an additional 4 weeks. If a plaster cast is applied at surgery, it should be bivalved. Postoperative care and rehabilitation are similar to those described for lunate implant arthroplasty (Figs. 35–8 to 35–11).

Pitfalls of Lunate and Scaphoid Implant Arthroplasty and Their Prevention

The risks and complications of carpal implant replacement are (1) implant rotation or subluxation, (2) progressive carpal instability or collapse with progression of disease to other carpal articulations or to the radiocarpal joint, and (3) infection, wound breakdown, or neuroma formation.

Revision procedures may be indicated for symptomatic progression of disease to other carpal articulations, for implant subluxation or fracture, or for bone cyst formation. Such procedures include synovectomy of the surrounding tissues, removal or replacement of the implant, curettage of cysts with cancellous bone grafting, selective intercarpal bone fusions, and implant arthroplasty or arthrodesis of the radiocarpal joint (see Figs. 35–5, 35–10, and 35–11). In cases of particulate synovitis, the implant should be removed, and appropriate corrective sur-

gery should be carried out. Good results have usually followed revision surgery.

The senior author has inserted 30 titanium lunates in 29 patients since 1985. The majority of patients had Kienböck's disease stages III to V. Associated limited intercarpal bone fusions, notably scaphocapitate and scaphotrapeziotrapezoid (STT) fusions, were carried out in the more advanced stages. The patients were predominantly males with an average age of 34 years. Postoperatively, patients have experienced decreased pain and improved strength and function. The vast majority of patients are completely pain free. Several experience only mild pain with very strenuous activity. There have been no cases of bone cyst formation or bone reaction to the implant. There were two revision procedures. One implant was replaced 1 year postoperatively because of subluxation incurred following acute trauma, and one wrist was fused owing to progressive ulnar translation of the proximal carpal row.

The senior author has performed 105 titanium scaphoid implant arthroplasties in the past 10 years. Postoperatively, the patients had improved hand function with decreased pain. Carpal height and congruity of the contiguous carpal bones have been well maintained. Two revisions to a wrist fusion were required because of progressive degenerative changes at the radiocarpal joint. There has been no evidence of bone or soft tissue reaction to the titanium implants to date.

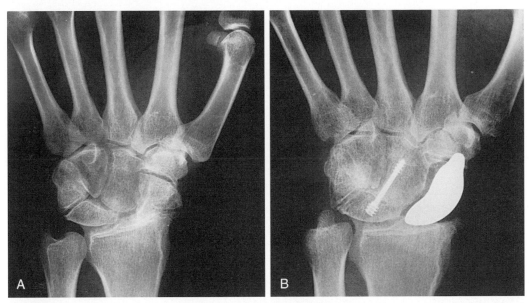

Figure 35–9. *A*, Preoperative radiograph of a scapholunate advanced collapse wrist pattern with severe osteoarthritic changes at scaphoradial articulation, and between lunate and capitate and triquetrum and hamate. The joint between the lunate and radius is preserved. *B*, Radiograph taken 7 years postoperatively, showing a titanium scaphoid implant replacement with arthrodesis between the lunate, capitate, and hamate. A Herbert screw was used to secure the lunate capitate fusion. The patient has an excellent functional result. (From Swanson AB, de Groot Swanson G, Herndon JH: Complications of arthroplasty and joint replacement at the wrist. In Epps Jr CH (ed): Complications in Orthopaedic Surgery, ed 3. Philadelphia, JB Lippincott, 1994, pp 957–995.)

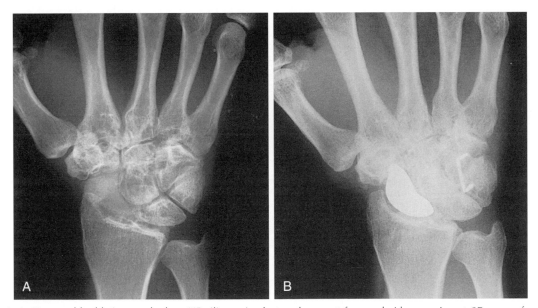

Figure 35–10. *A*, A 42-year-old athletic man had an HP silicone implant replacement for scaphoid non-union at 27 years of age. Eleven years later, he complained of having wrist pain on activity for the last year. The radiograph taken at this time demonstrated cystic changes at base of metacarpals and carpal bones. *B*, The revision surgical procedure included replacement of the silicone implant with a titanium implant, curettage of cysts and iliac bone grafting, fusion of the capitate to the lunate, and staple fixation of the hamate to the triquetrum. Five years later, the patient has a pain-free functional result. (From Swanson AB, de Groot Swanson G, Herndon JH: Complications of arthroplasty and joint replacement at the wrist. In Epps Jr CH (ed): Complications in Orthopaedic Surgery, ed 3. Philadelphia, JB Lippincott, 1994, pp 957–995.)

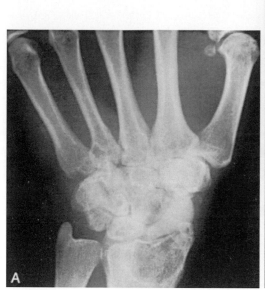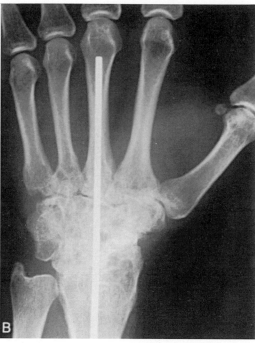

Figure 35–11. *A*, A bricklayer with stage VI disease developed cystic and degenerative changes and carpal collapse six years after scaphoid replacement with an oversized HP silicone implant. *B*, Postoperative radiograph shows revision to wrist fusion with iliac bone graft and intramedullary wire fixation. The patient has been back at work without symptoms for the past 10 years. (From Swanson AB, de Groot Swanson G, Maupin BK, et al: Scaphoid implant resection arthroplasty: Long-term results. J Arthroplasty 1:47–62, 1986, © 1986 Churchill Livingstone Inc., New York.)

The following considerations are essential for long-term good results in lunate implant arthroplasty:

1. Patient selection: In the young, active, or hard-laboring patient, associated procedures, including limited intercarpal fusion, motion restriction by soft tissue capsular reconstruction, and strict postoperative care and instructions, are indicated. Alternative nonimplant procedures such as soft tissue reconstruction or arthrodesis may be considered.

2. Identification of prior disorders: These include preoperative collapse or instability patterns, bone cysts, and arthritis of other intercarpal joints.

3. Meticulous surgical technique.

4. Stabilization of collapse deformities: An STT or scaphocapitate fusion is recommended in lunate implant arthroplasty. If there is lunate instability in a wrist requiring scaphoid implant arthroplasty, a lunocapitate or lunotriquetral fusion may be considered. Intercarpal fusions are carried out with cancellous bone grafting (preferably iliac bone) and internal fixation.

5. Presence of pre-existing subchondral bone cysts: Such cysts must be treated at the time of carpal bone implant arthroplasty by curettage and cancellous bone grafting. Failure to recognize and treat pre-existing cysts will result in their progression.

6. Implant sizing: If there is inadequate space, an implant should not be used; if used, an implant must not be oversized.

7. Stabilization of the implant: Stability is ob-

tained by capsuloligamentous reconstruction. The titanium implants have suture holes for stabilization to contiguous carpal bones.

8. Plaster cast immobilization for a minimum of 8 weeks and avoidance of excessive or abusive motion postoperatively.

We believe that lunate and scaphoid implant arthroplasties are useful procedures. Long-term good results can be achieved if the pathologic condition is well identified, the severity of disease is not too advanced, and the proper surgical indications and techniques are followed.

THUMB BASAL JOINTS

In any reconstructive surgery of the thumb, the entire ray must be considered—its balanced musculotendinous system, and the position, mobility, and stability of all three articulations. Each joint may be affected primarily or secondarily by imbalances of the other joints, as seen in the boutonnière and swan-neck deformities.

The problems that develop at the basal joints of the thumb are different in osteoarthritis and rheumatoid arthritis. Proper evaluation of the location of the arthritic involvement and of the condition and alignment of adjacent bones is essential in selecting the preferred method of treatment. The pathologic condition can involve the trapeziometacarpal joint, with or

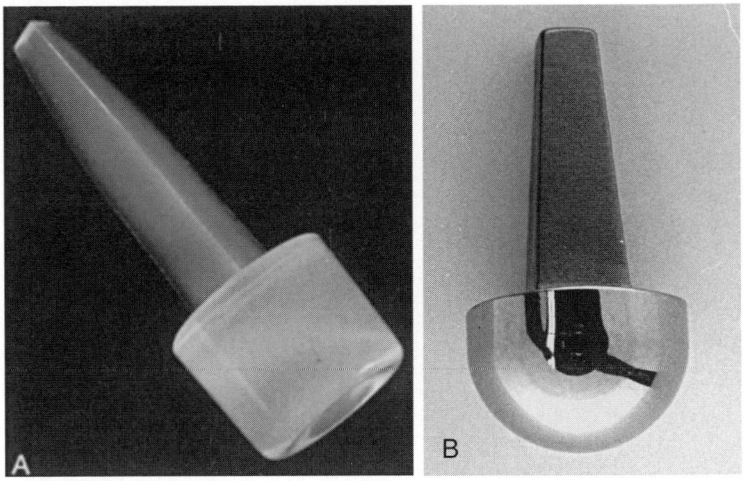

Figure 35–12. Implants for reconstruction of the thumb basal joints. *A,* Trapezium implant made of conventional silicone elastomer (CSE). *B,* Titanium convex condylar implant used with trapeziometacarpal joint arthroplasty.

without involvement of peritrapezial articulations or other carpal bone articulations; this can be present with or without resorption or displacement of adjacent carpal bones. The proper method of treatment must be selected from the following possibilities: resection arthroplasty of the trapeziometacarpal joint or of the entire trapezium with or without a titanium or a conventional silicone elastomer (CSE) condylar implant in the former or a CSE trapezium implant in the latter (Fig. 35–12).

Implant resection arthroplasty of the basal joints of the thumb helps maintain a smooth articulating joint space with improved joint stability, mobility, relief of pain, and strength. Selection of the appropriate treatment, meticulous capsuloligamentous stabilization, and correction of associated deformities of the thumb ray are essential for a good result.

Trapezium implants made of CSE are preferred in cases of pantrapezial involvement in patients with osteoarthritis. In isolated trapeziometacarpal involvement in patients with osteoarthritis, titanium convex condylar implants are recommended. In patients with rheumatoid arthritis, or with severe erosive osteoarthritis, resection arthroplasty with soft tissue interposition or fusion is preferred.

Trapezium Implant Arthroplasty

INDICATIONS

Trapezium implant resection arthroplasty is indicated in cases of degenerative or post-traumatic arthritis (e.g., following an old Bennett's fracture) with localized pain and palpable crepitation on the "grind test" (circumduction with axial compression of the thumb) and radiologic evidence of pantrapezial arthritic changes. This procedure is contraindicated when there is severe displacement, resorption, or involvement of contiguous carpal bones. Associated thumb ray deformities must be corrected.

SURGICAL PROCEDURE

Make a 7-cm longitudinal incision centered over the trapezium and parallel to the extensor pollicis brevis (EPB) tendon, as shown in Figure 35–13*A.* Expose the flexor carpi radialis (FCR) tendon at the wrist through a separate incision. Carefully identify and preserve branches of the superficial radial nerve (Fig. 35–13*B*). Small transverse veins may be ligated; however, longitudinal veins should be spared. Incise the retinaculum of the first dorsal compartment longitudinally, and carry the dissection down between the abductor pollicis longus (APL) and EPB tendons. Expose and mobilize the radial artery, protecting it by proximal retraction with a small rubber tubing; ligate the small arterial branches going into the trapeziometacarpal joint (Fig. 35–13*C*). Incise the joint capsule in a T fashion, and elevate the flaps off the underlying bone. Identify the trapezioscaphoid and trapeziometacarpal joints. Traction on the thumb allows further freeing of the dorsal capsular attachments around the trapezium. It is important to keep the dissection close to the bone to avoid injury to the artery, the underlying tendons, and the capsule.

Section the trapezium into pieces and remove it piecemeal with a bone-biting rongeur, including its ulnar distal projection, which is often seen between the first and second metacarpals. Traction on the thumb or distal retraction, with a small two-pronged rake retractor on the base of the metacarpal facilitates the exposure. Leave small flecks of bone with the underlying capsule to preserve good palmar capsuloligamentous support; this is especially true on the radial palmar aspect of the trapezium, where it attaches to the transverse carpal ligament and to the underlying thenar muscles (see Fig. 35–2). Trim osteophytes or irregularities on the distal end of the scaphoid or trapezoid. The trapezium should be positively identified to prevent removing portions of adjacent bones. We routinely perform a partial trapezoidectomy to more fully expose the scaphoid facet for proper implant seating (Fig. 35–13*C*).

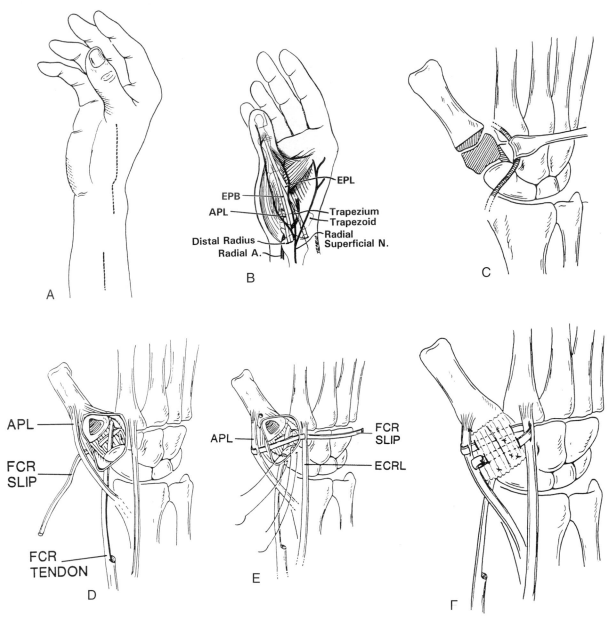

Figure 35–13. Trapezium implant arthroplasty. *A,* Incision centered over trapezium, parallel to extensor pollicis brevis tendon, has a short transverse arm over the distal wrist crease to continue proximally. The flexor carpi radialis tendon is exposed through a separate incision. *B,* Anatomic relationships of abductor pollicis longus *(APL),* extensor pollicis brevis *(EPB)* and extensor pollicis longus *(EPL)* tendons, and superficial radial nerve *(N)* and artery *(A)* at base of thumb. *C,* Radial artery branch is identified and protected. The trapezium and base of the first metacarpal are resected, and partial trapezoidectomy is performed. *D,* Flexor carpi radialis *(FCR)* tendon slip (preserving metacarpal insertion) is passed under FCR tendon and laterally through radial capsule and abductor pollicis brevis muscle. *E,* FCR tendon slip *(FCR SLIP)* is passed medially through the APL tendon and lateral capsule, across the trapeziectomy site, through the medial capsule, under the radial artery branch, and through the distal portion of the extensor carpi radialis longus *(ECRL).* 3-0 Dacron sutures are passed through capsular reflections off the scaphoid for capsular closure. *F,* The implant is inserted, and the FCR slip is folded under the dorsal capsule, looped through the APL, and sutured. Capsular reflections are sutured proximally and distally. The APL is advanced distally on the metacarpal. (*A,* and *C* through *E* from Swanson AB, de Groot Swanson G: Implant arthroplasty for the thumb basal joints. Semin Arthrop 2:91–98, 1991; *B* is from Swanson AB: Disabling arthritis at the base of the thumb—treatment by resection of the trapezium and flexible (silicone) implant arthroplasty. J Bone Joint Surg Am 54:456–471, 1972.)

Bring the base of the metacarpal up into the wound and square it off with a rongeur, leaving most of its cortical and subchondral bone intact. Osteophytes, especially on its medial portion, should be removed. Probe the intramedullary canal of the metacarpal first with a thin broach or a small curette to prevent inadvertent perforation through its side wall and consequent extrusion of the implant stem through this defect. We then use special burs with a small leader point to develop a triangular intramedullary shape, which should be no larger than necessary to receive the implant stem easily. If the canal is enlarged, insert bone chips to provide intramedullary stability of the stem.

The appropriate-sized implant should fit the trapeziectomy space, with its collar sitting properly on the metacarpal base and its base well medialized over the distal scaphoid facet to allow full and stable circumduction of the thumb. Use trial implants to select the proper size; of the five available sizes, implant sizes 2 and 3 are most commonly needed. Thoroughly irrigate the wound with saline to remove all debris before inserting the implant.

It is important to secure the implant in place over the scaphoid by reconstruction of the capsuloligamentous structures around the implant. Inspect the palmar capsule and ligaments in the depths of the wound for inadvertent tears or "holes." If present, such holes should be sutured so that there is firm support from the palmar capsule.

Expose the FCR tendon in the forearm, and dissect a 7- to 8-cm slip, developed from its radial third, distally to the fibro-osseous canal. Pull the tendon slip up into the site of the trapeziectomy, and dissect it to its insertion on the second metacarpal, which should be carefully preserved. Take care to avoid transverse lacerations of the tendon slip. Pass a small hemostat through the abductor pollicis brevis (APB) muscle to pull the tendon slip under the residual portion of the FCR tendon and then through the APB muscle (Fig. 35–13D). Pass the slip medially through the APL tendon and the lateral capsule, then across the trapeziectomy site, through the medial capsule, under the radial artery branch, and through the distal portion of the ECRL tendon (Fig. 35–13E). It is important not to pull the slip too tight, because a tight slip may tend to lift the implant from the floor of the wound; this can be prevented by placing the tendon slip under the FCR tendon and suturing it to the FCR tendon and to the palmar capsule. Retracting the radial artery proximally, place three 3-0 Dacron sutures through the preserved capsular reflection off the scaphoid to secure the closure of the capsule (Fig. 35–13E). After inserting the implant, pass the slip under the dorsal capsule, loop it through the APL tendon, and suture it as shown in Figure 35–13F. In some cases, sutures may be passed through a small drill hole made in the proximal end of the metacarpal to securely close the distal portion of the capsular repair. Repair the capsule with 3-0 Dacron sutures or other nonabsorbable material, using multiple inter-

rupted sutures and inverting the knots. Advance the APL tendon distally on the metacarpal, and tenodese the EPB tendon to the APL tendon insertion over the metacarpal to help abduction and restrict its hyperextension action on the first metacarpophalangeal joint. Loosely close the first dorsal compartment over the APL and EPB tendons, but leave the EPL tendon subcutaneous. Close the incision and drain it carefully avoiding the branches of superficial radial nerve. Apply a conforming dressing, including anterior and posterior plaster splints.

POSTOPERATIVE CARE

The extremity is kept elevated, and the drains are removed in 24 hours. Depending on the amount of soft tissue swelling, a short-arm thumb spica cast is applied and is worn for 6 weeks; sutures are removed through a window in the cast at 3 weeks. The patient then starts guarded abduction and opposition exercises while wearing a removable first web-space roll to maintain metacarpal abduction. Active flexion-adduction exercises without the first web-space roll are started 8 to 10 weeks after surgery. The use of the roll is gradually discontinued at 12 weeks (Figs. 35–14 and 35–15).

Trapeziometacarpal Implant Arthroplasty

INDICATIONS

The titanium convex condylar implant is preferred for isolated involvement of the trapeziometacarpal joint in the osteoarthritic thumb (see Fig. 35–12B). This procedure is not indicated in the presence of poor bone stock, such as seen in severe erosive osteoarthritis and in some patients with rheumatoid arthritis.

SURGICAL PROCEDURE

The surgical approach to the trapeziometacarpal joint is similar to that described for the trapezium implant. Incise the capsule in a T shape over the trapeziometacarpal joint. Resect a minimal amount of bone from the base of the metacarpal to preserve a firm bone shelf to support the implant. Then resect the articulating projection of the trapezium to the second metacarpal that can limit abduction and cause subluxation of the first metacarpal base. Using a power bur, shape the distal facet of the trapezium in a concavity slightly larger than the implant head (Fig. 35–16A). Remove enough bone to create a joint space of approximately 4 mm and to allow 45° radial abduction of the first metacarpal. Then prepare the intramedullary canal of the first metacarpal in a rectangular shape to accept the implant stem. Select the largest size implant that will provide a tight press-fit of the

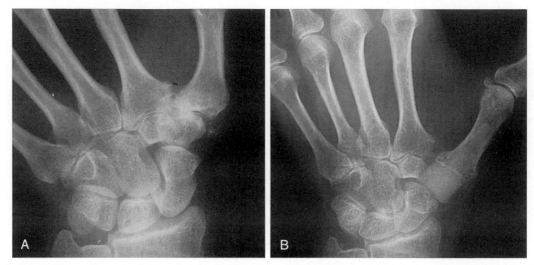

Figure 35–14. *A,* Preoperative radiograph of the wrist of a 54-year-old woman with pantrapezial degenerative arthritis and subluxation of the carpometacarpal joint. *B,* Radiograph taken 20 years postoperatively of trapezium implant (original silicone elastomer no. 372) arthroplasty showing excellent bone tolerance and an intact implant. Patient also had capsulodesis of the metacarpophalangeal joint to check hyperextension. She has pain-free thumb function with full range of motion, and she continued heavy factory work for 11 years after surgery until her retirement. (From Swanson AB, de Groot Swanson G: Implant arthroplasty for the thumb basal joints. Semin Arthrop 2:91–98, 1991.)

stem in the metacarpal. Use bone chips for intramedullary grafting if needed.

Prepare a distally based slip of the APL tendon, 8 cm long and 2 mm wide, from its medial aspect, preserving its insertion on the radial aspect of the base of the first metacarpal. Using a wire loop, pass the slip through the dorsolateral capsular reflections off the trapezium, and from inside out through a 2- to 3-mm drill hole made in the radiodorsal aspect of the metacarpal (Fig. 35–16*B*). Pass a 2-0 Dacron suture in the same drill hole to secure the capsuloliga-

mentous repair. Irrigate the wound, and insert the implant (Fig. 35–16*C*). Then pass the tendon slip through the dorsomedial capsular reflections off the trapezium. Holding the thumb in 45° abduction, pull the slip up tight and pass it through the insertion of the APL tendon (Fig. 35–16*D*). When the slip is pulled up tight, it draws the metacarpal slightly ulnarward, providing an excellent checkrein to radial subluxation of the base of the metacarpal. Advance the APL tendon distally and tenodes it to the EPB tendon over the capsular repair. Suture the end of the

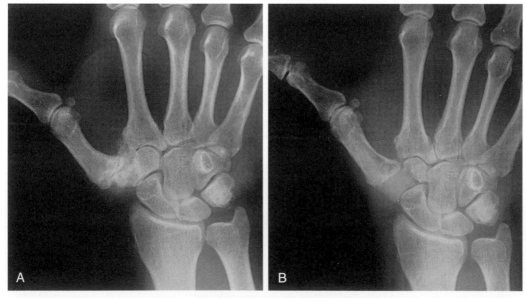

Figure 35–15. *A,* Pantrapezial degenerative arthritis with subluxation of carpometacarpal joint. *B,* Result 13 years after trapezium implant arthroplasty with the original silicone elastomer. Note partial trapezoidectomy, excellent host tolerance, and implant position. The patient is pain free and has an excellent clinical result. (From Swanson AB, de Groot Swanson G: Flexible implant resection arthroplasty in the upper extremity. In Jupiter JB (ed): Flynn's Hand Surgery, ed 4. Baltimore, Williams & Wilkins, 1991, pp 342–386.)

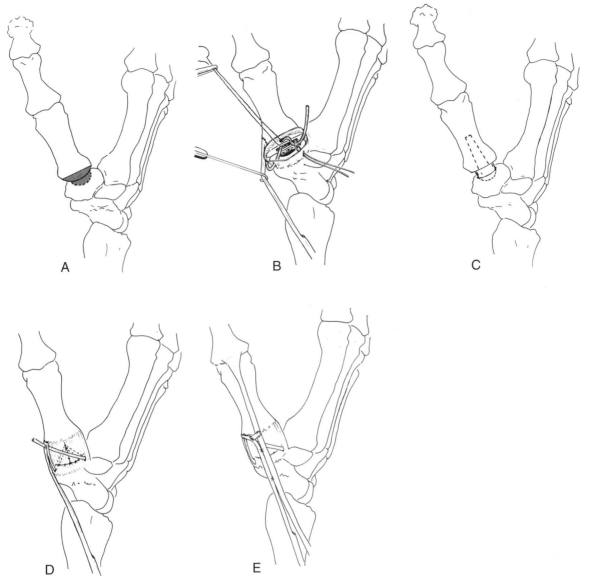

Figure 35–16. Titanium trapeziometacarpal implant arthroplasty. *A,* The base of the metacarpal is excised, a concavity is shaped in the distal facet of the trapezium, and the medullary canal is prepared in a rectangular shape. *B,* An 8-cm slip is made of the medial third of the abductor pollicis longus (APL) tendon and passed with a wire loop through the dorsolateral capsular reflections off the trapezium and pulled from inside-out through a drill hole made in the radiodorsal aspect of the metacarpal. A 2-0 Dacron suture is passed through the same hole to secure the capsuloligamentous repair. The APL slip is then passed through the dorsomedial reflections off trapezium. *C,* Snug fit of implant head in trapezial concavity. *D,* The slip is passed over the capsule through the APL tendon insertion. The capsular closure is completed with 3-0 Dexon sutures, with inversion of the knots. *E,* The APL tendon insertion is advanced distally and "tenodesed" to the extensor pollicis brevis (EPB) tendon over the capsular repair. The end of the APL slip is sutured over the EPB tendon.

APL slip over the EPB tendon (Fig. 35–16*E*). This repair helps abduct the metacarpal and prevents hyperextension of the MP joint. If a secure capsular closure can be achieved with 2-0 Dacron sutures passed through small drill holes in the base of the first metacarpal, reinforcement with a slip of APL tendon is not always necessary. However, the APL tendon insertion is always advanced distally.

Any associated deformities of the thumb ray must be corrected. The techniques for wound closure, postoperative immobilization, and therapy are similar to those described for trapezium implant arthroplasty.

Because of the narrow joint space, the usual range of motion obtained with the trapezium implant cannot be expected. Nevertheless, this technique can provide a stable, pain-free, functional thumb joint (Fig. 35–17).

SPECIAL CONSIDERATIONS

Adduction of the first metacarpal and hyperextension of the metacarpophalangeal joint promote lateral subluxation of the carpometacarpal joint and contracture of the adductor pollicis muscle, resulting in a swan-

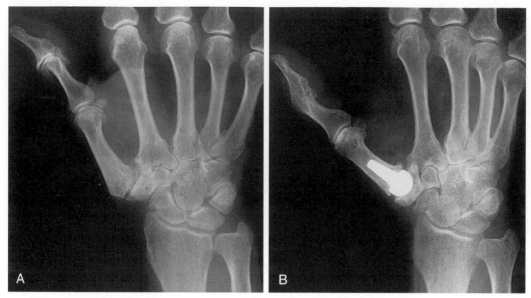

Figure 35–17. *A,* Preoperative radiograph of wrist of a 66-year-old woman with painful osteoarthritic involvement of trapeziometacarpal and interphalangeal (IP) joints. *B,* Radiograph taken 8 years postoperatively shows fusion of the IP joint and a well-seated titanium condylar implant. Note the bone deposition around the implant stem. The patient is pain free and is very pleased with her functional result.

neck collapse deformity. Correction of hyperextension at the metacarpophalangeal joint is essential to prevent subluxation of the implant.

Adduction Contracture of the First Metacarpal. If the angle of abduction between the first and second metacarpals is not at least 45°, the origin of the adductor pollicis muscle should be released from the third metacarpal through a separate palmar incision.

Hyperextension Deformity of the Metacarpophalangeal Joint. If the metacarpophalangeal joint hyperextends less than 10°, no treatment is necessary, except to apply the postoperative cast so that the metacarpal, not the proximal phalanx, is abducted. If the metacarpophalangeal joint hyperextends 10° to 20°, it is pinned in 10° flexion for 4 to 6 weeks. If

hyperextension of the joint is greater than 20° with good flexion, lateral stability, and adequate articular surfaces, a palmar capsulodesis of the metacarpophalangeal joint, as described by the senior author,[12] is indicated to preserve available flexion and to restrict the hyperextension (Fig. 35–18*A*). The metacarpophalangeal joint is fused when the ligaments and articular surfaces are inadequate. Implant arthroplasty of the metacarpophalangeal joint is not indicated in this situation.

Boutonnière Deformity. The boutonnière deformity of the thumb is usually not associated with arthritis of the basal joints of the type that would require implant arthroplasty. However, when this situation occurs, fusion of the metacarpophalangeal joint and

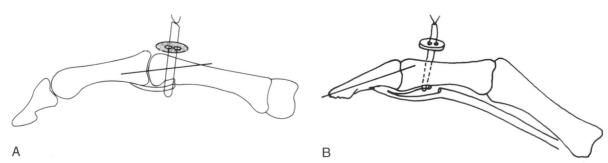

A   B

Figure 35–18. *A,* Palmar capsulodesis: The palmar aspect of the joint is exposed through lateral incision. The proximal membranous insertion of the palmar plate is incised, preserving the tendinous attachment to the sesamoid bone. Periosteum is stripped from the palmar aspect of the metacarpal neck, and two drill holes are made and converted into a small concavity with a curette. The detached proximal end of the palmar plate is drawn into the concavity with a pullout wire, and tension is adjusted to obtain 10° to 15° metacarpophalangeal (MP) joint flexion. The pullout wire is removed at 3 weeks. Kirschner wire fixation is used for 6 weeks. *B,* Flexor tenodesis of the thumb interphalangeal (IP) joint: A distally based flexor pollicis longus slip is drawn with a pullout wire into a concavity made on the palmar aspect of the neck of the proximal phalanx to obtain 10° to 15° flexion of the IP joint. The pullout wire is removed at 3 weeks. Kirschner wire fixation of distal joint is used for 6 weeks. (*A* redrawn from Swanson AB: Flexible Implant Arthroplasty in the Hand and Extremities. St Louis, CV Mosby, 1973. *B* from Swanson AB, de Groot Swanson G: Thumb disabilities in rheumatoid arthritis: In AAOS Symposium on Tendon Surgery of the Hand. St Louis, CV Mosby, 1975, p 233.)

release of the extensor pollicis longus at the distal joint may be performed at the same time as the basal joint reconstruction.

Interphalangeal Joint. A flexible hyperextension deformity of the distal interphalangeal joint with lateral stability and adequate articular surfaces can be corrected with a flexor tendon hemitenodesis (Fig. 35–18*B*). If the articular surfaces are destroyed but there is reasonably good joint stability and motion, implant arthroplasty may be considered to preserve pain-free motion. An unstable joint requires fusion.

Pitfalls of Thumb Basal Joint Implant Arthroplasty and Their Prevention

The success of thumb basal joint implant arthroplasty requires stability of the arthroplasty, proper implant medialization, a firm capsuloligamentous repair, correction of associated deformities, and adequate postoperative immobilization. The procedure is technically demanding because of the close association of the branches of the superficial radial nerve and radial artery, which must be carefully protected and preserved at surgery.

In 1989, we conducted a radiographic study of 59 trapezium implant arthroplasties that had been performed between 1965 and 1974 using the original silicone elastomer (no. 372) to specifically study the bone response.[17] After an average 187 months of follow-up, bone response was excellent in the majority of cases. There were mild cystic changes of contiguous bones in three cases and moderate changes in three cases, one of which was revised to a soft tissue interposition arthroplasty 13 years after the original procedure. This review encompassed cases from our early surgical experience, and it is of note that cystic changes occurred in cases in which the implant had not been properly medialized over the scaphoid or associated imbalance of the thumb ray, mainly hyperextension of the metacarpophalangeal joint, had not been corrected. Since 1986, we have used a conventional silicone elastomer (CSE) trapezium implant in 63 thumbs, and complications requiring a revision procedure have not occurred to date.

The senior author has performed titanium convex condylar implant arthroplasty in 130 hands since 1985.[15] Postoperatively, overall patient satisfaction was 96 percent, with good functional strength, motion, and pain relief. Bone remodeling which stabilized over the first 6 months was noted as follows: cut-end of the metacarpal accommodated the implant shape; bone deposition around the intramedullary stem; and deepening of trapezial concavity with bone deposition and apparent fibrocartilage formation around the implant head. There were no cystic or erosive changes in the carpal bones, no progressive wear or peritrapezial arthritis, nor heterotropic bone formation. The following considerations are important in reconstruction of the thumb basal joints:

1. There are definite separate indications for the use of the conventional silicone elastomer trapezium and titanium condylar implants.

2. Proper medialization of the trapezium implants on the scaphoid facet and of the condylar implants on the trapezial surface must be obtained. A partial trapezoidectomy and resection of exostoses at the base of the first metacarpal are important to ensure stable seating of the trapezium implant.

3. Firm capsuloligamentous reconstruction, with a slip of flexor carpi radialis tendon for trapezium implants or a slip of abductor pollicis longus tendon for trapeziometacarpal implants, is critical. However, if the capsule is adequate in the latter, good stability can be obtained by placing 3-0 Dacron sutures through small drill holes in the base of the first metacarpal.

4. Precise preparation of the intramedullary canal and insertion of additional bone chips around the implant stem if the canal is enlarged are essential to stability and bone remodeling.

5. Associated imbalances of the thumb ray, especially hyperextension of the metacarpophalangeal joint and adduction contracture of the first metacarpal, must be corrected at the time of basal joint reconstruction.

6. Proper immobilization is necessary.

We believe that implant reconstruction of the basal thumb joints can provide pain-free, stable mobility and improved strength. The complications are few and essentially retrievable. The recommended operative procedures are challenging and must be carefully executed to obtain rewarding results.

RADIOCARPAL JOINT

The radiocarpal, distal radioulnar, and intercarpal joints can be affected individually or in combination. Synovitis and tendon involvement are common, especially in rheumatoid arthritis. Therefore, selection of the appropriate treatment must depend on the localization and severity of involvement, instability, deformity, arthritic destruction, and the patient's requirements. The senior author has devised a classification of wrist disease based on the localization and severity of disease to assist in selection of the appropriate treatment (Table 35–3; Figs. 35–19 to 35–24).[11, 18, 19, 20, 24, 25]

Radiocarpal Joint Implant Arthroplasty

The wrist is the key joint for proper hand function, and disabilities about the wrist can result in severe functional handicaps. A stable wrist is necessary for proper transmission of forces from the forearm to the digits. However, a mobile wrist is important for positioning the hand in functional adaptations. A double-stemmed, flexible-hinged implant for the ra-

Table 35–3. CLASSIFICATION AND TREATMENT FOR WRIST ARTHRITIS

Stage	Pathologic Conditions	Treatment Options
I	Transient synovitis, pain, and weakness without instability or deformity in radiocarpal, intercarpal, and distal radioulnar joints; tendon involvement present	Physical treatment: protection, splinting, therapy Medical treatment: injection of steroids or alkylating agents or both
II	Persistent synovitis, pain, and weakness, without instability or deformity in radiocarpal, intercarpal, and distal radioulnar joints; tendon involvement present	Surgical treatment: synovectomy of tendons, joints; capsular stabilization of wrist joint and tendon rebalancing
III	Distal radioulnar deformity and destruction, with a stable radiocarpal joint	Partial or total resection of distal ulna with ligament and tendon reconstruction Shortening of ulna and reconstruction of stability with capsuloligamentous and tendon repair
IV	Arthritis limited to a stable radiocarpal joint	Fusion of proximal row carpus to the radius Radiocarpal implant arthroplasty Treatment of distal radioulnar joint as needed
V	Arthritis limited to the radiocarpal joint with ulnar translation instability	Fusion of proximal row to the radius Fusion of segment of distal ulna to the radius with osteotomy of the proximal ulnar diaphysis Radiocarpal implant arthroplasty Treatment of distal ulna as needed

VI	Subluxation of the radiocarpal joint
	Severe intercarpal and radiocarpal arthritic changes
	Destruction of the proximal carpal row
	Stiffness of the wrist
	  Tendon balance achievable
		Radiocarpal implant arthroplasty
		Wrist arthrodesis
		  Treatment of distal radioulnar joint as needed

VII	Severely unstable wrist
	Loss of bone in the carpus and distal radius
	Progressive bone destruction (multilans type)
	Great physical activity requirements of the patient
	  Tendon balance unachievable
		Wrist arthrodesis
		  Treatment of distal radioulnar joint as needed

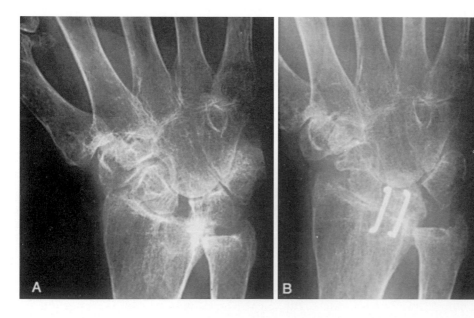

Figure 35–19. *A,* Preoperative radiograph of patient with rheumatoid arthritis, showing collapse deformity of the carpus with ulnar translation and arthritis of the radiocarpal joint (stage V). *B,* Postoperative radiograph showing relocation of the carpus with fusion of the lunate to the radius. Alternatively, the scaphoid can also be fused to the radius. Useful, pain-free mobility is achieved at the midcarpal joints.

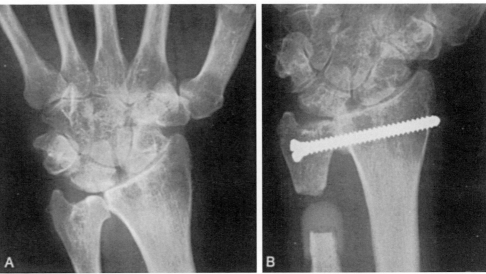

Figure 35–20. *A,* Preoperative radiograph of a patient with ulnar translation tendency and minimal arthritic changes (stage V). *B,* Postoperative result following a synovectomy and a Lauenstein (Sauvé-Kapanji) procedure. A silicone cap was used on the ulna at the pseudarthrosis level in this case.

diocarpal joint was first developed by the senior author in 1967.[12] The implant has a barrel-shaped midsection, slightly flattened on its dorsal and volar surfaces; the core of the implant contains a Dacron reinforcement to provide axial stability and resistance to rotatory torque. Since 1974, the double-stemmed, flexible-hinged implant has been made of high-performance (HP) silicone. It is available in five sizes (see Fig. 35–22). Implant design modifications have included a wider midsection and a shorter distal stem. Press-fit semicircular titanium grommets have also been developed and used since 1982 to protect the implant's midsection from shearing forces and to improve the durability of the arthroplasty.

The implant acts as a flexible hinge to help maintain an adequate joint space and alignment while support-

ing the development of a new capsuloligamentous system. Vertical and lateral movements occur through its flexible midsection and stems. The axis of motion of the wrist is at the level of the head of the capitate. In severely diseased wrists, however, radiocarpal and intercarpal articular movements have been altered. Contrary to rigid and cemented implants, the flexible hinge with its unfixed stems allows adjustments to the required axis of rotation, with little resistance, as demonstrated on cinefluorographic studies. Furthermore, this procedure is essentially retrievable; the implant is easily replaced or the wrist fused if indicated (see Fig. 35–24). Reinforcement of the capsule to restrict motion and balance of the musculotendinous system are very important to obtain good clinical results, durability, and biologic tolerance.

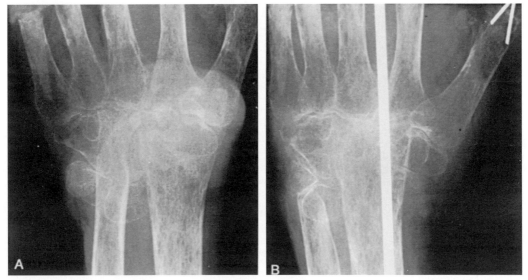

Figure 35–21. *A,* Preoperative radiograph showing severe destruction of the carpus. The patient had multiple wrist tendon ruptures, pain, and instability (stage VII). *B,* Postoperative radiograph showing wrist fusion with an intramedullary wire fixation.

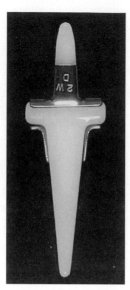

Figure 35–22. Radiocarpal flexible hinge and titanium grommets (dorsal view).

INDICATIONS

Implant resection arthroplasty of the wrist is indicated in patients with rheumatoid arthritis, osteoarthritis, and post-traumatic disabilities who have (1) instability of the wrist due to subluxation or dislocation of the radiocarpal joint, (2) severe deviation of the wrist, causing musculotendinous imbalance of the digits, (3) stiffness or fusion of the wrist in a nonfunctional position, or (4) stiffness of a wrist and a need for wrist motion for hand function.

Reconstruction of the wrist should be performed before finger joint reconstruction, unless extensor tendon ruptures are present. The distal radioulnar joint is treated as necessary. This procedure is contraindicated in patients with opened epiphyses, inadequate skin, bone, or neurovascular system, or irreparable tendon damage, and in uncooperative individuals. The authors do not recommend this method for patients who perform heavy manual labor.

SURGICAL PROCEDURE

Make a straight, longitudinal dorsal incision, taking care to preserve the superficial sensory nerves. Incise the extensor retinaculum to form a radially based flap between the first and second compartments, as shown in Figure 35–23A. Make a narrow distal retinacular flap to relocate the extensor carpi ulnaris in reconstruction of the ulnar head. Perform synovectomy of the extensor compartments, taking special care to remove only the synovium. Carefully preserve the dorsal capsuloligamentous structures for later resuture, and reflect them from the underlying radius and carpal bones as a distally based flap (Fig. 35–23B).

Part of the proximal carpal row is usually absorbed, and the remnants are displaced toward the palm on the radius. Perform a proximal row carpectomy, and square off the proximal edge of the capitate. Part of the distal scaphoid and the triquetrum can be retained in some cases. Injury to the underlying tendons and neurovascular structures should be avoided. Square off the end of the radius to fit against the distal carpal row, which should be left intact because of its importance in maintaining the stability of the metacarpals (Fig. 35–23C). Prepare the intramedullary canal of the radius with a broach, curette, or air drill to receive the proximal stem of the implant. The radiocarpal subluxation should be completely reduced. If there is a severe radiocarpal dislocation with soft tissue contracture, it is preferable to shorten the distal radius rather than to remove more of the carpal bones. Insert the distal stem of the implant through the capitate into the intramedullary canal of the third metacarpal. Precise positioning is ensured by carefully passing a wire or a very thin broach through the capitate and the base of the intramedullary canal of the third metacarpal. A Kirschner wire can be passed into the metacarpal and out through its head to verify the intramedullary orientation. Use an air drill for the final reaming procedure. The distal stem should not extend distal to the metaphysis of the third metacarpal and should be shortened as necessary.

Figure 35–23. Radiocarpal joint implant arthroplasty. *A,* The extensor retinaculum is incised to form radially based flap between the first and second compartments. The narrow distal flap is used for relocation of the extensor carpi ulnaris (ECU) tendon in reconstruction of ulnar head. *B,* Capsuloligamentous structures are elevated as a distally based flap from the underlying radius and carpal bones. *C,* The usual areas of bone resection. *D,* Before the implant is inserted, sutures are placed through the interosseous membrane and the edge of the radius to stabilize the distal ulna and sixth compartment retinaculum. *E* and *F,* Palmar capsuloligamentous structures are reefed proximally and/or distally, as required, with 2-0 Dacron sutures passed through small drill holes made in the palmar cortex of the distal radius and/or capitate. Sutures for reattachment of the dorsal capsuloligamentous flap are passed through drill holes in dorsal distal radius. *G,* The proximal stem of the implant fits into intramedullary canal of radius, and the distal stem is inserted through the capitate into the intramedullary canal of the third metacarpal, not to extend beyond proximal metaphysis. The distal grommet is placed dorsally and the proximal grommet palmarly. *H,* The capsuloligamentous flap is sutured over the implant. *I,* The retinacular flap is positioned under the extensor tendons. The proximal retinacular flap is sutured over the extensor tendons to prevent bow-stringing. The extensor pollicis longus tendon is left subcutaneous. The narrow distal flap is used as a pulley to relocate the ECU tendon over the distal ulna. (*A, B, H,* and *I* from Swanson AB & de Groot Swanson: Flexible implant arthroplasty of the radiocarpal joint. Semin Arthrop 2:78–84, 1991; *E* from Swanson AB, de Groot Swanson G, Maupin BK, et al: Flexible implant arthroplasty of the radiocarpal joint—surgical technique and long-term study. Clin Orthop 187:94–106, 1984; *F* from Swanson AB, de Groot Swanson G: Flexible implant arthroplasty in the upper extremity. In Jupiter JP (ed): Flynn's Surgery, ed 4. Baltimore, Williams & Wilkins, 1991, pp 342–386.)

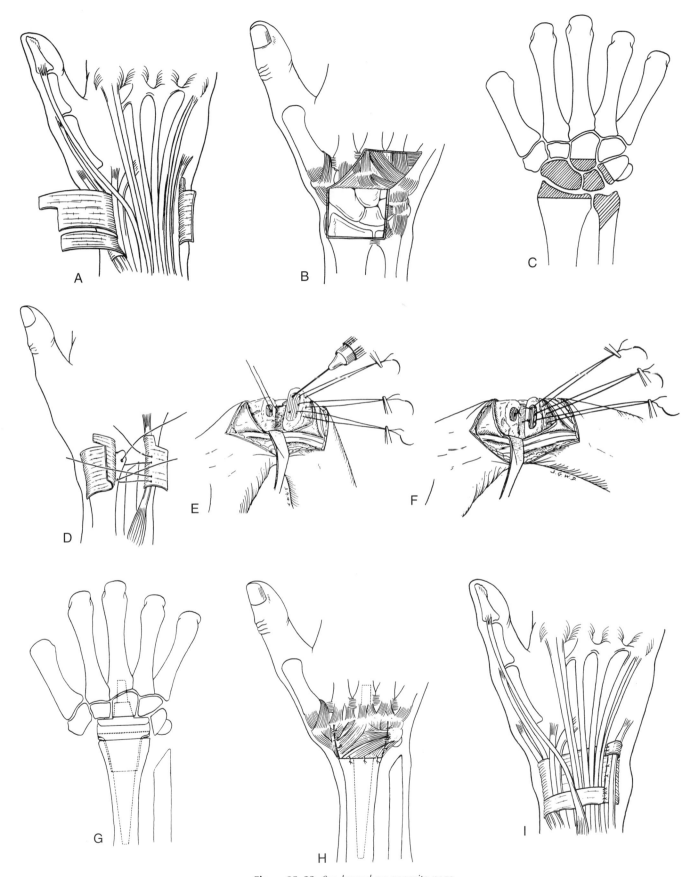

Figure 35–23. *See legend on opposite page*

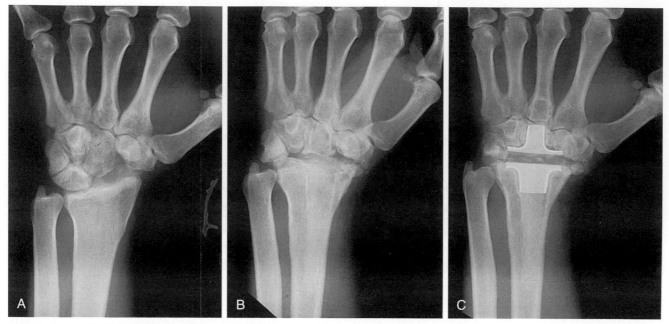

Figure 35–24. *A,* This 29-year-old man who performed heavy manual labor was referred for wrist pain 2 years after scaphoid implant arthroplasty for scaphoid non-union. The radiograph showed implant palmar rotation and cystic changes at the base of the capitate and the radial shift. *B,* Eight years after revision to radiocarpal flexible hinge and continued heavy work, the patient developed pain with motion. The radiograph showed collapse of the joint space. Separation of the implant's distal stem and minimal synovitis were noted at time of revision to a wrist flexible hinge with grommets. *C,* Radiograph taken 7 years postoperatively shows excellent bone and soft tissue tolerance with bone deposition. The patient has a pain-free 40° flexion, 20° extension, 10° radial deviation, and 5° ulnar deviation with 105-lb grip strength. He continues heavy labor and is very pleased with these functional results.

Determine the proper implant size by the fit of the proximal stem in the radius, using a sizing set. Then center the hand over the radius. Adequate bone preparation and soft tissue release allow passive motion without buckling or impingement of the implant. The bone ends should be smooth and should abut the implant's midsection. A 1.0- to 1.5-cm joint space between the radius and the carpus is usually required. Shape the distal radius and the base of the capitate to allow a precise press-fit of the appropriate size grommet. Place the distal grommet dorsally and the proximal grommet palmarly. The grommet sizes correspond to the implant sizes.

Smooth the bone ends with a diamond bur, and slightly groove them laterally to enable the slightly curvilinear grommet shoulder to seat directly on the bone ends without protruding laterally. There should be sufficient bone stock to allow a good press-fit; otherwise, the grommet could rotate. The grommets must be accurately centered over the bone ends to avoid impingement on the intramedullary canal on one side, which could cause bone resorption. Achieve final seating of the grommet with gentle pressure using a flat instrument, taking care to avoid bending or distorting the grommet. If it is too loose, try the next larger size. When necessary, a grommet size larger than the implant can be used, but never use a size smaller than the implant. With grommets in place, insert the implant sizer, and assess the joint space, flexion-extension and axial alignment.

Obliquely resect the distal ulna as needed. To stabi-lize the distal radioulnar joint, which is essential to provide wrist stability, attach the sixth dorsal compartment retinaculum to the interosseous membrane or radius (Fig. 35–23*D*).

Repair of both the palmar and the dorsal capsulo-ligamentous structures around the implant is critical. Reef the palmar ligaments proximally or distally or both, according to where they are loose (Fig. 35–23*E* and *F*). For proximal palmar reefing, pass 2-0 Dacron sutures through two small drill holes made in the palmar distal edge of the cut end of the radius. For distal palmar reefing, pass a 2-0 Dacron suture through a small drill hole made in the cut end of the capitate. Then pass 3-0 Dacron sutures for re-attachment of the dorsal carpal ligament through three small drill holes made in the dorsal cortex of the distal radius (Fig. 35–23*E* and *F*). Place all sutures prior to inserting the implant and grommets.

Thoroughly irrigate the wound with triple-antibi-otic solution, and press-fit the grommets. First, in-sert the proximal stem of the implant into the intra-medullary canal of the radius. Then, introduce the distal stem through the capitate into the intramedul-lary canal of the third metacarpal (Fig. 35–23*G*). After implant insertion and wound closure, test the repair so that approximately 20° each of extension and flexion and 10° each of ulnar and radial devia-tion are possible on passive manipulation. An exces-sive range of motion may increase the potential for implant failure and does not improve wrist function significantly. If necessary, tighten the capsule laterally with sutures passed through the radial and ulnar cortex of the radius. Adequate ligamentous repair is essential for proper function and durability of the implant.

Next, bring the previously prepared distal extensor retinaculum flap over the wrist joint under the extensor tendon and suture it in place (Fig. 35–23*H*). Evaluate the pull of the extensor tendons of the wrist joint, and shorten or transfer the tendons, as required, to obtain wrist extension without lateral deviation. The ECRL may be transferred under the ECRB to attach to the third metacarpal by a suture through the bone or may be interwoven into the distal attachment of the ECRB. Repair the extensor tendons of the digits if necessary. We often use one of the flexor superficialis muscles for tendon transfer to reconstruct ruptured extensor digitorum communis tendons. If isolated extensor tendons are ruptured, side-to-side suture can be performed. Ruptures of the extensor pollicis longus tendon can be repaired by transferring the extensor indicis proprius tendon. Suture the narrow proximal extensor retinaculum flap over the extensor tendons to prevent bow-stringing (Fig. 35–23*I*). Leave the extensor pollicis longus tendon in a subcutaneous position. Complete reconstruction of the distal radioulnar joint by using a retinacular flap from the sixth dorsal compartment to relocate the extensor carpi ulnaris tendon dorsally.

Close the wound in layers, and insert small silicone drains subcutaneously. Apply a voluminous, conforming hand dressing with a palmar splint, with the wrist in neutral position.

POSTOPERATIVE CARE

The arm is elevated for 1 to 2 days. A dorsally well-padded, short-arm cast is applied with the wrist in neutral position, and it is fitted with outriggers that hold rubber-band slings to keep the fingers in extension if the tendons have been repaired. This cast is worn for approximately 4 to 6 weeks to ensure satisfactory stability of the wrist. A dorsal window is made in the cast for wound inspection and suture removal. After cast removal, an active exercise program is begun to achieve 20° each of flexion and extension and 10° each of radial and ulnar deviation. Therapy includes strength-building exercises for forearm musculature. The patient should avoid excessive or abusive activity. Passive stretching exercises are not recommended.

Pitfalls of Wrist Flexible Implant Resection Arthroplasty and Their Prevention

Flexible implant resection arthroplasty of the wrist is a technique-intensive method that requires appropriate patient selection, operative indications, and staging; specialized instrumentation; precise bone preparation; secure capsuloligamentous reconstruction to align and restrict wrist motion; stabilization of the distal radioulnar joint; reconstruction of tendon ruptures and imbalances; and 6 weeks of postoperative immobilization, well-planned therapy, and avoidance of excessive activities. Respect for the soft tissues during surgery as well as the use of wound drainage, limb elevation, and thick dorsal padding under the cast can prevent wound healing problems and secondary infection. This radiocarpal joint treatment method is not recommended for patients who perform heavy manual labor and lifting.

The durability of wrist implant arthroplasty has been related to implant shape and material, protection of the implant-bone interface, restriction of the range of motion, surgical technique, and control of disease progression. Since 1967, we have made a number of modifications on the basis of our clinical experience and evaluation of results.

A review of 25 revision procedures for implant fracture in wrists that had been operated on without grommets disclosed fracture rates of 16 percent for no. 372 original silicone elastomer implants and of 8 percent for high-performance elastomer implants.[19] The improved tear resistance of high-performance silicone elastomer appears to play a significant role in the better durability of the implant. The common denominator in these fracture cases was an excessive arc of motion. Before revision surgery, wrists with fractured implants averaged 46° of extension to 40° of flexion, and 23° of ulnar deviation to 15° of radial deviation. This arc of motion—86° of flexion-extension and 38° of radial-ulnar deviation—was greater than the average reported in cases in the 1983 study (60° of flexion-extension and 28° of radial-ulnar deviation). Excessive motion in the vertical and lateral planes produces a circumductory motion that is destructive to the implant, even in the presence of grommets. Therefore, the capsuloligamentous reconstruction around the implant must check wrist motion to no more than 20° each of flexion and extension, and 10° each of ulnar and radial deviation. Recurrent synovitis and imbalance of the proximal and distal joints, however, eventually can compromise capsuloligamentous stability, favoring excessive mobility and implant failure.

On rare occasions, particulate synovitis was seen around the high-performance silicone flexible hinges used without grommets. We continue to use high-performance elastomer for the double-stemmed hinged implants, however, because of its excellent tear resistance. The introduction of grommets has helped to decrease further the incidence of implant fractures and particulate synovitis by improving the bone-implant interface. The hinged midsection abuts the smooth gliding surface of the titanium grommets, protecting the implant from sharp bone edges and reducing the formation of particulate debris. Favorable bone remodeling and deposition are seen at the grommet-bone interface (Figs. 35–24 and 35–25). The distal half-grommet placed dorsally and the proximal

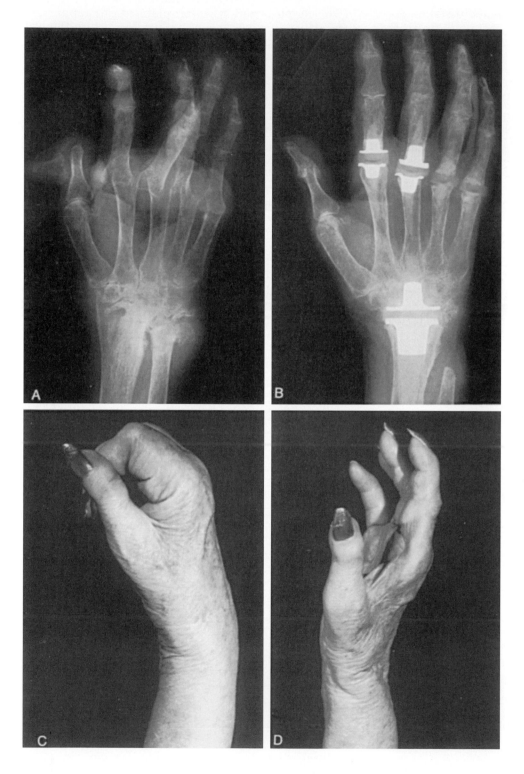

Figure 35–25. *A,* Preoperative radiograph showing severe rheumatoid arthritic involvement of the hand and wrist with complete destruction of the carpus and distal radioulnar joint (stage IV). *B,* Reconstruction of the wrist with a silicone flexible hinge implant using proximal and distal grommets. A resection of the distal ulnar was done. Note the fusion of the distal joint of the thumb and the silicone implant resection arthroplasty of the metacarpophalangeal joints of the index and middle fingers; grommets were used proximally and distally. *C* and *D,* Good correction of deformities, with a pain-free, useful range of motion.

half-grommet placed palmarly protect the implant at the areas of maximum shear forces. At the level of 170 sites where titanium grommets lined the bone, there were three (1.8 percent) stem-midsection separations. Two patients had a mutilans type of rheumatoid arthritis with severe synovitis and wrist instability and an average 150° arc of flexion-extension and 90° arc of lateral deviation. The third patient, a very active jail warden, had a wrist implant arthroplasty with grommets for advanced Kienböck's disease and continued to overuse his wrist after surgery. In all three cases, the arthroplasty was revised to a wrist fusion. Circumferential grommets have been used successfully in the metacarpophalangeal joints and great toe first metatarsophalangeal joints. Evaluation of circumferential grommets for the wrist implant is ongoing.

An important and unique factor is that this method does not require cement or significant bone resection. In cases of infection or implant failure, the implant can be removed or replaced as necessary, or the procedure can be converted to an arthrodesis by bone grafting. Flexible-hinged implant resection arthroplasty of the wrist has a useful place in the reconstruction and rehabilitation of the upper extremity.

References

1. Beckenbaugh RD: Implant arthroplasty in the rheumatoid hand and wrist: Current state of the art in the United States. J Hand Surg 8(Part 2):675–678, 1983.
2. Beckenbaugh RD, Linscheid RL: Arthroplasty in the hand and wrist. In Green DP (ed): Operative Hand Surgery, ed 3. New York, Churchill Livingstone, 1993, pp 143–187.
3. Capone RA: The titanium grommet in flexible implant arthroplasty of the radiocarpal joint: A long-term review of 44 cases. J Plast Reconstr Surg 96:667–672, 1995.
4. DeHeer DH, Owens SR, Swanson AB: The host response to silicone elastomer implants for small joint arthroplasty. J Hand Surg 20A(Part 2):S101–109, 1995.
5. Ishikawa H, Hanyu T, Murasawa A: The use of grommets for flexible hinge toe implants. Clin Orthop 316:173–179, 1995.
6. Isomäki HA, Hakulinen P, Joutsenlahti U: Excess risk of lymphomas, leukemia and myeloma in patients with rheumatoid arthritis. J Chronic Dis 31:691, 1978.
7. Kane KR, DeHeer DH, Owens SR, et al: Adsorption of collagenase to particulate titanium: A possible mechanism for collagenase localization in periprosthetic tissue. J Appl Biomater 5:353–360, 1994.
8. Kane KR, Mochel DM, DeHeer DH, et al: Influence of titanium particle size on the in vitro activation of macrophages. Contemp Orthop 28:249–261, 1994.
9. Lichtman DM, Alexander AH, Mack GR, et al: Kienböck's disease—update on silicone replacement arthroplasty. J Hand Surg 7:343–347, 1982.
10. Nalbandian RM, Swanson AB, Maupin BK: Long-term silicone implant arthroplasty—implications of animal and human autopsy findings. JAMA 250:1195–1198, 1983.
11. Sauvé-Kapandji H: Nouvelle technique de traitement chirurgical des luxations récidivantes isolées de l'extremité inférieure du cubitus. J Chir (Paris) 47:589, 1936.
12. Swanson AB: Flexible Implant Arthroplasty in the Hand and Extremities. St Louis, CV Mosby, 1973.
13. Swanson AB: A grommet bone liner for flexible implant arthroplasty. Bull Prosth Res Rehab Eng Res Devel BPR10-35 18:108–114, 1981.
14. Swanson AB: Silicone implant arthroplasty in the hand, upper extremity, and foot—25 years' experience. In Silicone in Medical Device—Conference Proceedings. US Dept of Health and Human Services Publication FDA 92-4249. Rockville, MD, US Government Printing Office, 1991, pp 233–259.
15. Swanson AB: Titanium small joint implant arthroplasty. In Proceedings of the 6th Congress of the International Federation of Societies for Surgery of the Hand, Helsinki, Finland, July 3–7, 1995. Bologna, Italy, Monduzzi Editore, 1995, pp 1173–1177.
16. Swanson AB, Bayne LG, Cracchiolo A, et al: The use of silicone implants in orthopaedic surgery. Contemp Orthop 29:363–380, 1994.
17. Swanson AB, de Groot Swanson G, Maupin BK, et al: Failed carpal bone arthroplasty: Causes and treatment. J Hand Surg 14A(Part 2):417–424, 1989.
18. Swanson AB, de Groot Swanson G: Reconstructive surgery for the rheumatoid hand. In Netter FH (illus): The CIBA Collection of Medical Illustrations, vol 8 (part 2): Musculoskeletal System. Summit, NJ, Ciba-Geigy, 1990, pp 219–232.
19. Swanson AB, de Groot Swanson G: Flexible implant arthroplasty of the radiocarpal joint. Semin Arthrop 2:78–84, 1991.
20. Swanson AB, de Groot Swanson G: Flexible implant resection arthroplasty in the upper extremity. In Jupiter JB (ed): Flynn's Hand Surgery, ed 4. Baltimore, Williams & Wilkins, 1991, pp 342–386.
21. Swanson AB, de Groot Swanson G: Implant arthroplasty for the thumb basal joints. Sem Arthrop 2:91–98, 1991.
22. Swanson AB, de Groot Swanson G, Maupin BK, et al: The use of the grommet bone liner for flexible hinge implant arthroplasty of the great toe. Foot Ankle 12:149–155, 1991.
23. Swanson AB, de Groot Swanson G: Implant resection arthroplasty in the treatment of Kienböck's disease. Hand Clin 9:483–491, 1993.
24. Swanson AB, de Groot Swanson G, Herndon JH: Complications of arthroplasty and joint replacement at the wrist. In Epps Jr CH (ed): Complications in Orthopaedic Surgery, ed 3. Philadelphia, JB Lippincott, 1994, pp 957–995.
25. Swanson AB, de Groot Swanson G: Joint reconstruction in the hand and wrist. In Harris NH, Birch R (eds): Postgraduate Textbook of Clinical Orthopaedics, ed 2. Oxford, Blackwell Scientific, 1995, pp 609–643.
26. Swanson AB, Livengood LC, Sattel AB: Local hypothermia to prolong safe tourniquet time. Clin Orthop 264:200–208, 1991.
27. Swanson AB, Poitevin LA, de Groot Swanson G, Kearney J: Bone remodeling phenomena in flexible implant arthroplasty in the metacarpophalangeal joints. (Kappa Delta Award Presentation.) Clin Orthop 205:254–267, 1986.
28. Taleisnik J: The Wrist. New York, Churchill Livingstone, 1985.
29. Watson HK, Hempton RF: Limited wrist arthrodesis. 1: The triscaphoid joint. J Hand Surg 5:320, 1980.

CHAPTER 36

Total Wrist Arthroplasty

Robert D. Beckenbaugh, MD

HISTORY AND CONCEPTS

Total wrist arthroplasty refers to the surgical resection of all or a portion of the carpus, removal of the articulating surface of the radius and usually the ulna as well, and replacement with an articulated implant. Conceptually, silicone interpositional arthroplasty accomplishes the same result and is discussed in a separate chapter.

The concept of using an articulated, nonhinged prosthesis in the wrist was simultaneously developed by Meuli[1] in Switzerland and Volz[2] in Arizona in the early 1970s. With the development of appropriate prosthetic materials and methylmethacrylate bone cement for fixation of components in total hip arthroplasties during the 1960s, these pioneers sought to apply to the wrist the principles learned from the replacement of other joints in the body.

The need for the development of a total wrist replacement became evident as a result of the limited surgical options available in the treatment of destructive wrist arthrosis. Arthrodesis can successfully relieve pain and provide stability to the wrist. However, in patients with rheumatic disease involving the elbows, the shoulder, and the hand, absence of wrist motion further accentuates the overall upper extremity disability. Some patients with noninflammatory wrist disease occasionally have careers with special needs for wrist motion, for example, some professional musicians and some mechanics working in small spaces. Synovectomy in rheumatic disease and proximal row carpectomy in traumatic disease have achieved successful relief of pain and restoration of mobility but have had variable predictability and longevity. The goals in developing a total wrist replacement are to provide a mobile, stable, painless wrist with reasonable durability. Experience has shown that the concept is viable, but problems associated with its development have been encountered.

The First Designs

Meuli[1] elected to proceed with a ball-and-socket trunnion design, whereas Volz[2] developed a dorsovolar tracking model (Fig. 36–1).

The Meuli design allowed rotation within the articulation and significant extents of motion before prosthetic impingement. The prosthesis was thus essentially unconstrained in most degrees of motion, in a biomechanical sense. As will be seen, however, in the functional mode, the distal cup firmly encompasses the ball, and if stress is applied to the hand with the wrist held motionless by soft tissue constraints (capsule or muscle), the resultant forces are transmitted to the stems as if the prosthesis were constrained.

The Volz design essentially incorporated a flexion-extension arc of motion but was a "sloppy" fit, allowing slight anteroposterior and radial ulnar translation: A moderate amount of radial ulnar deviation can occur, but only a few degrees of carpal rotation are possible. Thus, whereas the Volz design incorporates a smaller range of intrinsic motion, it is functionally less constrained than the Meuli design, owing to the loose contact fit between the proximal and the distal components.

Both designs utilized two-pronged distal compo-

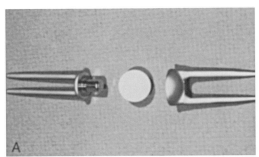
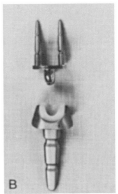

Figure 36–1. *A,* Meuli prosthesis: Trunnionated ball is added after fixation of components. Distal cupped portion is on the right. *B,* Volz prosthesis: Polyethylene bearing is press-fitted into proximal component. (*A* from Beckenbaugh RD, Linscheid RL: Total wrist arthroplasty: Preliminary report. J Hand Surg 2:337–344, 1977.)

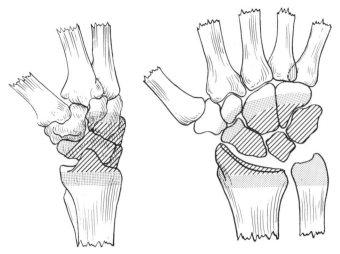

Figure 36–2. Hatched area shows the amount of bone resection needed for insertion of a Meuli prosthesis. Dotted area shows optional bone resection in patients with collapse and dislocation of carpus and ulna. (From Beckenbaugh RD, Linscheid RL: Total wrist arthroplasty: Preliminary report. J Hand Surg 2:337–344, 1977.)

nents for seating in the medullary canals of the nonmobile index and long metacarpals. The purpose of utilizing both metacarpals was to enhance fixation. In some cases, because of the fixed intermetacarpal distance, this seating was technically difficult to achieve. The process was facilitated by the Meuli device because of the ability of its stems to be bent with special instruments. The location of fixation in

the index and the long metacarpals proved to be biomechanically unsound in many patients, however, as is discussed later.

With the Meuli design, two lengths of polyethylene ball insertions were available to adjust tension as necessary. In both techniques, the distal ends of the radius and the ulna and all of the carpus except the distal portion of the distal row were resected (Fig. 36–2). Both techniques utilized methylmethacrylate cement for fixation of the prosthetic stems.

Initial reports of wrist arthroplasties with these prostheses demonstrated satisfactory motion and pain relief. Deformity was occasionally a problem.[2, 3]

Problems and Design Changes

The major early problem with total wrist arthroplasty was balance. With both prosthetic designs, a significant number of patients developed ulnar deviation deformity and contractures. Analysis of case failures and biomechanical evaluation confirmed that insertion of the distal component within the second and third metacarpals abnormally placed the prosthetic center of rotation too radially, functionally lengthening the ulnar lever arm (Fig. 36–3).[3, 4] Initially, this problem was managed in the Meuli design by bending stems or altering their placement to the third and fourth metacarpals or by tendon transfers of the extensor carpi ulnaris to the center of the wrist. Lack

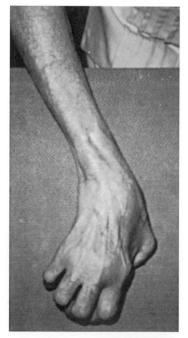

Figure 36–3. Ulnar deviation stance secondary to radial center of rotation in wrist with Meuli prosthesis. (From Beckenbaugh RD, Linscheid RL: Total wrist arthroplasty: Preliminary report. J Hand Surg 2:337–344, 1977.)

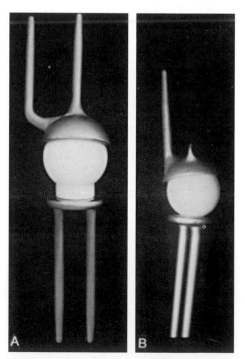

Figure 36–4. A, Offset Meuli design. Note the third metacarpal stem centered in the prosthetic cup. B, Single-stem Meuli design, lateral view. Single stem is centered over the cup and placed dorsally to enhance extension. (From Beckenbaugh RD: Total joint arthroplasty: The wrist. Mayo Clin Proc 54:513–515, 1979.)

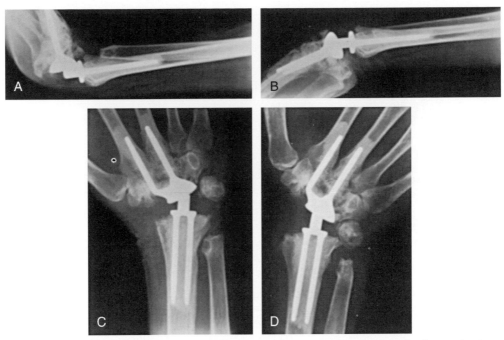

Figure 36-5. Excellent balance and movement, as seen on these motion views 1 year after Meuli offset total wrist arthroplasty.

of predictability of these measures and loosening of stems in the mobile fourth metacarpal demonstrated the need for prosthetic modification. Meuli modified his stem structure by off-setting the stems on the distal component; Volz,[1] Hamas,[4] and I[5] developed single-stemmed centered distal components with off-set dorsal volar stems to enhance dorsiflexion (Fig. 36-4). These modifications significantly reduced balance problems in total wrist arthroplasty, but the difficulty in precisely placing single-stemmed components led to persistence of problems in some cases (Figs. 36-5 and 36-6).

In addition to the problems of recurrent deformity, other causes of total wrist arthroplasty failure were eventually encountered.[6-10] Infections occurred at a rate of less than 2 percent and required prosthetic removal. Dislocations were infrequent and were managed by closed treatment, but those that were associated with deformity usually required revision surgery.[6]

By far the most significant problem of total wrist arthroplasty has related to stem fixation. Loosening of the distal component and stress shielding of the proximal component have occurred in more than 50 percent of cases in our long-term experience with the Meuli prosthesis; these changes paralleled the findings in early cemented hip designs. *Stress shielding* refers to the absorption of cortical bone adjacent to the articulating surface of the prosthesis; it has been seen with use of both the Meuli and the Volz prostheses. It occurs only in the proximal component and comes from absence of stress to the bone adjacent to the cemented proximal stem (Fig. 36-7). Stress shielding is common but rarely reaches the extreme shown in Figure 36-7. Its occurrence

implies the need for a more uniform method of fixation of the proximal stem.

Another distressing problem associated with total wrist arthroplasty has been loosening of the distal component. Unlike total joint loosening at other anatomic locations, this complication in the wrist is rarely associated with significant pain. Rather, it can result in decreasing motion, a tendency toward deformity, and eventual impingement within the carpal canal. With the Meuli design, as the distal component loosens, it tends to migrate volarly into the carpal canal. This may cause symptoms of median neuropa-

ERRORS IN SINGLE STEM

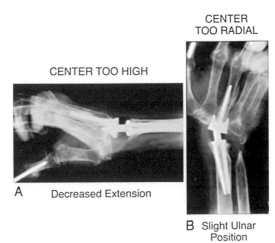

CENTER TOO HIGH

CENTER TOO RADIAL

A Decreased Extension

B Slight Ulnar Position

Figure 36-6. Malpositioned single-stem wrist arthroplasty. A, Dorsally positioned stem results in decreased dorsiflexion. B, Radially positioned stem results in increased ulnar deviation.

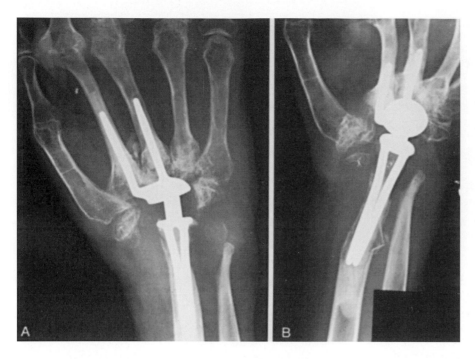

Figure 36–7. Stress shielding. *A*, Three-month postoperative view of Meuli prosthesis. Note that the proximal cortex extends to the base of the prosthesis. *B*, One year later, the distal cortex has resorbed; all fixation is proximal, and the radius has fractured. This is an extreme example of this phenomenon.

thy but more importantly may result in attritional ruptures of the flexor tendon at the edge of the prosthesis (Fig. 36–8).

The loosening rate for the Meuli prosthesis distal component has reached 50 percent in our cases. The loosening is believed to occur because of the close fit between the proximal ball and the distal cup. Functional wrist activities, such as pushing open a door, pushing up from a chair, or even moderate lifting, place great stress on the prosthetic stems. Be-

cause the wrist is flexed in position by the capsule and musculotendinous units in the dorsiflexed position, the force of the proximal stem and ball is transmitted directly and completely to the inferior portion of the cup, producing angular forces on the distal stems, and causing loosening. In the Volz design, the "sloppiness" of the fit plus the slight subluxation of the component dampens this force, and loosening occurs much less frequently.[11, 12]

The presence of this loosening phenomenon with

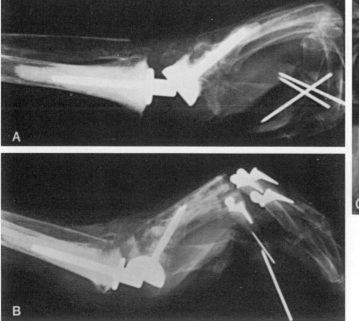

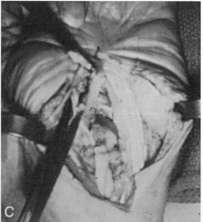

Figure 36–8. Immediate postoperative *(A)* and 6-year follow-up *(B)* radiographs. The distal cup has loosened and migrated into the carpal canal. *C*, The instrument holds the ruptured end of a flexor tendon, which is the result of attrition over the cup of the prosthesis.

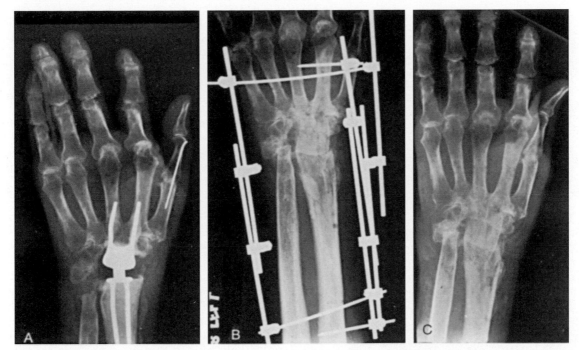

Figure 36–9. *A,* Radiograph taken 3 months after operation in a patient with infection. *B,* The prosthesis has been removed, an iliac graft has been inserted, and stabilization has been accomplished with external fixation. *C,* Three months after grafting, the arthrodesis is solid. A cast may be used in lieu of fixation. (From Cooney WP III, Beckenbaugh RD, Linscheid RL: Total wrist arthroplasty: Problems with implant failures. Clin Orthop 187:121–128, 1984.)

the ball-and-socket design has led me to believe that the design is an unsatisfactory configuration for total wrist arthroplasty. The problem is experienced less commonly with the Volz design, but with the low contact area and loose bone fit, there is greater potential in this prosthesis for wear problems and polyethylene deformity. Painless clicking and a slight sense of instability are also occasionally associated with use of the Volz prosthesis, owing to the loose fit.

Salvage

Fortunately, salvage following failed total wrist arthroplasty has always been possible. Conversion to arthrodesis may be achieved with the addition of iliac bone graft.[8, 9] Occasionally, resection arthroplasty with or without Silastic interposition is indicated. Arthrodesis is achieved by removal of the prosthesis and insertion of the bone graft in the space formerly occupied by the arthroplasty (Fig. 36–9). To remove the prosthesis, it is generally easiest to split the dorsal cortex of the radius and the metacarpals with an osteotome. The medullary canals are then opened like a book, and the component and its cement mantle are disimpacted. The cortices then close elastically, and graft insertion is permitted. As an alternative, the cement may be slowly removed with an osteotome and drills. If grafting is not performed, casting for 4 months generally results in a stable and painless wrist pseudarthrosis, although with significant shortening.

Current Considerations

As results deteriorated with the first generation of implants (Meuli and Volz), other designs were being developed in an attempt to improve durability, balance, and function. The early Meuli and Volz designs are no longer used. Meuli has developed a small-diameter, capture ball-and-socket design for use without cement and reports satisfactory early results.[13]

Four other prosthetic designs have been developed and used, all of which incorporate ellipsoidal articular designs. The Guepar prosthesis has been developed by Alnot.[10] The device has a nonmetal-backed polyethylene component proximally and is fixed with screws distally (Fig. 36–10). Early results are nonconclusive.

Clayton and Ferlic, in cooperation with Volz, have

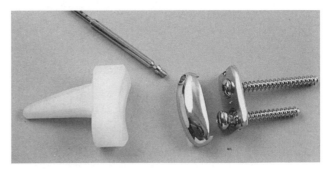

Figure 36–10. Prosthesis developed by Alnot.

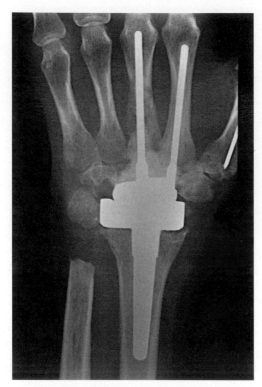

Figure 36–11. CFV prosthesis.

developed a new prosthesis designed for biologic fixation with a proximal ball and distal cup portion (Fig. 36–11). After initial success, some problem with balance and fixation has occurred, and the device is being further modified (DC Ferlic, MD, personal communication).

Menon simultaneously has developed an implant similar to the Guepar device (Fig. 36–12). The pros-

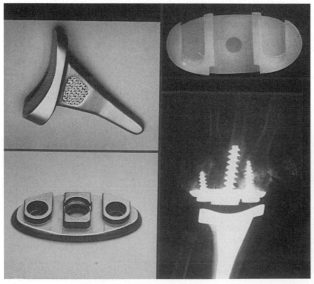

Figure 36–12. Menon prosthesis.

thesis has metal backing at the radial component and screw fixation distally. Early experience with the device has been very good.[14]

My colleagues and I have developed an ellipsoidal partially coated design with offset stems for improved centering (Figs. 36–13 and 36–14). The device is biaxial and has been utilized with success with up to 10 years of follow-up.[8, 15] Because of continuing problems with loosening, new distal components and new designs have been developed for use in patients who have bone deficiency or are undergoing revision surgery (Figs. 36–15 and 36–16).[8]

Future Considerations and Conclusions

The concept of total wrist arthroplasty has been successful. Current devices allow excellent function but poor relief of pain. The main technical problem that persists is that of loosening of the distal component. Improved stem design and prosthetic interface design will likely reduce this problem. It is anticipated that new biologic or mechanical fixation systems will need to be developed before durability can be completely ensured. Failed wrist arthroplasty can always be salvaged with arthrodesis or revision, and new designs have increased salvage with mobility. The operation remains a "higher-risk higher-reward" procedure for those patients with arthritis who wish for relief of pain and correction of deformities as well as preservation of motion.

TECHNIQUE

Perform total wrist arthroplasty through a dorsal longitudinal incision centered at the wrist. Expose the dorsal wrist capsule through an incision of the fourth dorsal compartment in a straight longitudinal manner. Then perform an extensor tenosynovectomy as necessary and retract the extensor tendons ulnarly. Open the third dorsal compartment with the scissors, and sharply elevate the retinaculum radially off the tendons of the extensor pollicis longus and the radial wrist extensors. Perform a local tenosynovectomy, remove Lister's tubercle, and retract the tendons radially or ulnarly as necessary during the procedure. After exposing the second dorsal compartment tendons, elevate the periosteum off the radial styloid region to identify and observe the first dorsal compartment tendons at the radial styloid. Subsequently, protect these tendons from damage with a retractor during resection of the distal radius.

By radially retracting the extensor tendons, expose the distal radioulnar joint. Make an incision longitudinally in the distal radioulnar joint capsule, preserving a 2-mm edge of soft tissue on the radius for later repair of the soft tissue envelope around the resected distal ulna. Then expose the ulna subperiosteally and

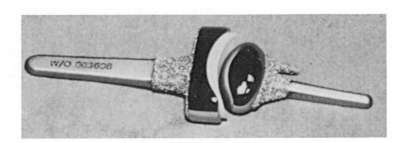

Figure 36–13. Biaxial wrist prosthesis. The radial component stem is offset radially, and the metacarpal component is curved to match the shape of the long metacarpal. The major clinical problem remains with distal component loosening, but revision surgery has been possible and successful.

resect the smallest amount necessary to allow clearing of the resected distal ulna from impingement upon the remaining sigmoid notch of the radius. Elevate the extensor carpi ulnaris and its sheath subperiosteally from the distal ulna prior to resection. At the conclusion of the procedure, snugly suture the periosteal and capsular flaps to the rim of soft tissue left on the distal radius to provide stability of the distal radioulnar joint.

Following a resection of the distal ulna, incise the capsule transversely at the radiocarpal joint from the radial styloid to the extensor carpi ulnaris. Then split the capsule longitudinally from the base of the long metacarpal proximally to the radius and elevate by sharp dissection two distally based corner flaps to expose the dorsal carpus to the carpometacarpal joints of the index, long, and ring metacarpals. Perform a local synovectomy as necessary.

Resect the distal radius with a sagittal saw perpendicular to its long axis in a fashion to allow the least amount of bone resection necessary to square off the distal end of the radius for insertion of the prosthesis. This will generally include 1 to 1.5 cm of radial styloid and 0.5 cm of sigmoid notch bone. Prior to removal of the divided distal radial bone, use the power saw to resect the capitate through its basal neck area, extending radially through the radial scaphoid joint and ulnarly through the hamate to allow excision of the entire proximal carpal row as well as the distal radius. This should leave a space of 2 to 2.5 centimeters, depending on the size of the

prosthesis to be utilized. Subperiosteally expose the proximal shaft of the long finger metacarpal, and place two Homan retractors on either side of it to allow visualization of the axis of the long metacarpal. Identify the medullary canals of the capitate and long metacarpal, and use specially prepared awls and reamers to expand them to accept the distal stem of the metacarpal component. It is necessary to prepare an additional tract in the medullary canal of the trapezoid to accept the radial stud of the distal component. Achieve as precise a fit as possible through reaming and impaction of bone and the use of power tools until the trial impactor reamers are seated snugly against the base of the distal carpal row and metacarpal. Prepare the medullary canal of the radius at the central portion with the provided awls. Use the impactor reamers to press the medullary bone of the radius. In general, the radius component is seated without the use of methylmethacrylate cement for fixation.

Perform a trial fit. If the fit is satisfactory, inject the medullary canal of the capitate and long metacarpal and the trapezoidal stub area with methylmethacrylate cement. Next, insert and compress the distal component. After setting the radial component, impact it home and articulate the joint. At this point, test the tension. It is preferable to have a tension such that one can just distract the joint on longitudinal traction of the hand. Repair the dorsal capsule to the

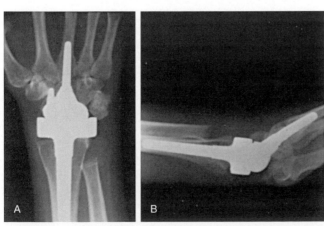

Figure 36–14. Radiographic appearance of biaxial wrist.

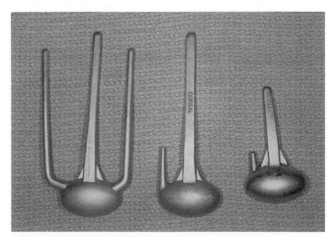

Figure 36–15. For revisions and bone deficient (methotrexate prednisone) patients, improved fixation is suggested with long single-pronged or double-pronged components.

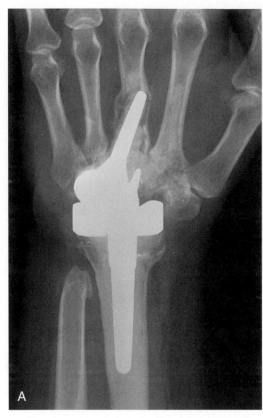
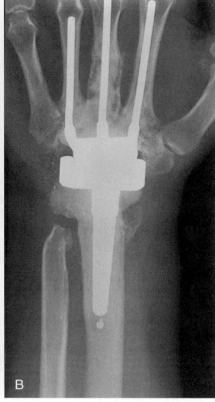

Figure 36–16. *A,* Loosening of distal component after fall and long metacarpal fracture. *B,* Radiographic appearance 4 years after revision surgery with multipronged components.

distal radius and soft tissues about the distal ulnar area of the wrist. Then repair the extensor retinaculum over the tendons of the second, third, and fourth dorsal compartments as a single layer. If there is total deficiency of the dorsal capsule, a portion of the retinaculum may be split transversely and utilized to cover the prosthesis, but in every instance, retain a portion of the retinaculum to cover the extensor tendons, to prevent dorsal bow-stringing as well as volar subluxation of the tendons during wrist flexion. Close the remainder of the wound, place a suction drain, and apply a long-arm compression dressing with the wrist in supination.

Postoperative Care

Dressings are changed at 1 to 2 days and a long-arm cast is worn for 2 weeks. After the 2-week immobilization, a short-arm cast is applied. A longer period seems necessary to stabilize the distal radioulnar joint; in my experience, however, 2 weeks of immobilization in a long-arm cast has been satisfactory clinically to allow mobilization of the elbow at this time.

If at the end of 2 weeks, the wrist is noted to be very stiff (less than 5° each of motion in dorsal and palmar flexion), active wrist motion may be started at this time. Otherwise, wrist range of motion is deferred until 4 to 8 weeks following surgery, depending on the tightness of the joint motion.[16]

The anticipated and desired range of motion is within the general parameters of 30° each of dorsal and palmar flexion and 5° each of radial and ulnar deviation. Motion in excess of these ranges may be associated with higher risks of loosening, wear, or instability. Patients should be advised to restrict activities with their hand and wrist on a "common-sense" basis. Athletic activities, such as tennis, golf, and skiing, and impact activities, such as hammering and use of vibrating tools, are not allowed.

SUMMARY AND CONCLUSIONS

Since the inception of total wrist arthroplasty in the early 1970s, much has been learned. Wrist replacement appears to be clinically viable and preferable to arthrodesis, in view of the early functional results, with outcomes of the "best" wrist arthroplasties being far superior to those of the traditional alternatives such as arthrodesis and biologic arthroplasty. Contraindications to the use of the procedure have been an unacceptable loosening rate and difficulties in achieving proper balance. The latter problem has been satisfactorily corrected with progressive design improvement, but prosthetic longevity and security of fixation have not yet been delineated. Upon failure of a total implant, a satisfactory salvage is possible; this fact provides impetus to the continued efforts to achieve a mobile, stable, and durable wrist implant.

References

1. Meuli HC: Reconstructive surgery of the wrist joint. Hand 4:88–90, 1972.
2. Volz RG: The development of a total wrist arthroplasty. Clin Orthop 116:209, 1976.
3. Beckenbaugh RD, Linscheid RL: Total wrist arthroplasty: Preliminary report. J Hand Surg 2:337–344, 1977.
4. Hamas RS: A quantitative approach to total wrist arthroplasty: Development of a "precentered" total wrist prosthesis. Orthopedics 2:245, 1979.
5. Beckenbaugh RD: Total joint arthroplasty: The wrist. Mayo Clin Proc 54:513–515, 1979.
6. Cooney WP III, Beckenbaugh RD, Linscheid RL: Total wrist arthroplasty: Problems with implant failures. Clin Orthop 187:121–128, 1984.
7. Bosco JA III, Bynum DK, Bowers WH: Long-term outcome of Volz total wrist arthroplasties. J Arthroplasty 9:25–31, 1994.
8. Rettig ME, Beckenbaugh RD: Revision total wrist arthroplasty. J Hand Surg 18A:798–804, 1993.
9. Ferlic DC, Jolly SN, Clayton ML: Salvage for failed implant arthroplasty of the wrist. J Hand Surg 17A:917–923, 1992.
10. Alnot JY: L'arthroplastie totale Guepar de poignet dans la polyarthrite rheumatoide. Acta Arth Berl 54:178, 1988.
11. Volz RG: Total wrist arthroplasty: A clinical review. Clin Orthop 187:112–120, 1984.
12. Dennis DA, Ferlic DC, Clayton ML: Volz total wrist arthroplasty in rheumatoid arthritis: A long-term review. J Hand Surg 11A:483, 1986.
13. Meuli HC, Fernandez DL: Cemented total wrist arthroplasties. J Hand Surg 20A:115–122, 1995.
14. Ferlic DC, Menon J, Meuli HC: Indications and techniques for total wrist arthroplasty. Presented at the Instructional Course Lecture on Total Wrist Arthroplasty, American Society for Surgery of the Hand 47th Annual Meeting, Phoenix, AZ, 1992.
15. Beckenbaugh RD, Brown ML: Early experience with biaxial total wrist arthroplasty. Presented at the American Society for Surgery of the Hand, Toronto, September, 1990.
16. Beckenbaugh RD: Arthroplasty of the wrist. In Morrey BF (ed): Reconstructive Surgery of the Joints, ed 2. New York, Churchill Livingstone, 1996, pp 387–409.

CHAPTER 37

Partial Wrist Fusions: Intercarpal and Radiocarpal

Paul G. Feldon, MD, Edward A. Nalebuff, MD, and
Andrew L. Terrono, MD

PARTIAL WRIST FUSION

Fusions of wrist joints have been performed for many conditions that result in painful, unstable, or arthritic intercarpal or radiocarpal joints. Complete wrist fusion is a time-honored, predictable, and reliable salvage procedure for these conditions. It provides a stable, pain-free wrist and reasonable upper extremity function, as long as forearm rotation and elbow and shoulder motion are preserved.

In many patients, however, the disease causing symptoms is confined to only one joint or several of the joints making up the wrist unit. Stabilizing the involved joints may decrease pain while preserving some wrist motion. Even significant loss of motion allows functional use of the wrist. Brumfield and Champoux[4] demonstrated that functional use of the wrist required a range of 45° (15° of palmarflexion and 30° of dorsiflexion). Palmer and associates,[41] using more sophisticated measuring techniques, demonstrated that even less range of motion was sufficient for most normal daily activities (30° of extension, 5° of flexion, 10° of radial deviation, and 15° of ulnar deviation). Thus, limited wrist fusions that preserve some wrist motion have considerable appeal in the treatment of localized problems of the wrist.[13]

Several experimental studies have described the normal kinematics of the wrist.[48, 74-76] Other studies have demonstrated the theoretic effects of various intercarpal fusions on wrist motion.

Rozing and Kauer[47] showed, in an experimental cadaver study, that fusion of the radioscaphoid or radioscapholunate joint preserved 40 percent of the flexion-extension arc. Fusion of the midcarpal joint (scaphoid-capitate-lunate) preserved 59 percent of the flexion-extension arc. Meyerdierks and colleagues[37] showed similar results. In their in vitro study, fusions that crossed the radiocarpal joint preserved approximately 45 percent of the flexion-extension arc of motion, and fusions that crossed the intercarpal rows preserved 73 percent. Fusions within a carpal row preserved 88 percent of the flexion-extension arc. A study by Gellman and coworkers[20] showed very similar preservation of motion with sim-

ulated intercarpal fusions: 41 percent preservation of flexion-extension with radioscapholunate fusion and 58 percent preservation of flexion-extension with fusion of all of the intercarpal joints.

Although limited intercarpal arthrodeses have been used for scaphoid non-unions and localized arthritides for many years, only for the past 15 years have these fusions been advocated for conditions such as carpal instability and Kienböck's disease or as an adjunct to silicone rubber implant arthroplasty of the carpus. The experiences of Watson and associates[65-73] encouraged many surgeons to begin using various combinations of intercarpal fusions for conditions affecting the wrist and particularly for wrist instabilities.

In clinical series of intercarpal fusions, most authorities have reported preserving at least a 50 percent of range of wrist motion, and some have reported considerably higher ranges.[1, 23, 27, 65, 69, 70, 72, 77] Radiolunate and radioscaphoid fusions result in greater loss of wrist motion.[33, 51, 69] Bach and colleagues[2] reported a 48° flexion-extension arc and a grip strength of 70 percent that of the other side after radius-scaphoid-lunate fusion. Tomaino and associates[58] reported an average flexion-extension arc of 70° (51 percent) and a grip strength of 68 percent of the opposite side in their combined series of intercarpal fusions. Pisano and associates[44] found an average 68° flexion-extension arc and a grip strength 74 percent that of the uninvolved side after scaphocapitate fusion. These clinical studies are remarkably consistent, both among themselves and with the motion predicted by the in vitro studies described earlier.

The success rates and predictability of limited wrist fusions in treating various wrist problems have been varied, however. Watson and associates[72] reported no significant long-term effects from various combinations of limited wrist fusions for as long as 12 years. In contrast, later literature reflects the less than optimal effectiveness and predictability of some intercarpal fusions as well as relatively high complication rates for these procedures.* It has become clear that some fusions are more effective and predictable

---

*References 9, 17, 18, 25, 27, 29, 35, 46, 59, 60.

than others. Tomaino and coworkers[58] substantiated theoretic concerns that wrist kinematics altered by intercarpal fusion will lead to arthritis at unfused or adjacent joints.[17, 19, 20, 29, 37, 38] Viegas and colleagues[64] have demonstrated that scaphoid-trapezium-trapezoid (STT) and scaphoid-capitate fusions transmitted wrist load disproportionately through the scaphoid fossa of the radius, and Garcia-Elias and associates[19] showed increased sliding motion of the lunate on the radius after the same fusions. The increased load-bearing on the radius and the greater shear on the lunate from the intercarpal fusion may place these areas at risk for early degenerative arthritis.

Few outcome studies for intercarpal fusions are available. Tomaino and coworkers[58] found a disparity between patient satisfaction and the scores obtained on wrist rating scales. They and Siegel and Ruby[51] found that patient satisfaction and ultimate outcome depended more on pain relief than on the amount of motion retained after intercarpal fusion. In their review of the literature, Siegel and Ruby[51] showed that none of the intercarpal fusions reliably provided complete pain relief, and that less than 50 percent of patients who had undergone any type of intercarpal arthrodesis had complete relief of pain.

Thus, the treatment of some wrist conditions by partial arthrodesis remains controversial. The published results of intercarpal wrist fusions have not been consistent, and the long-term results are variable.* It is accepted that limited wrist fusions in certain conditions can stabilize the wrist, relieve pain, and arrest or prevent progressive loss of carpal height. However, patients being considered for intercarpal fusion should be aware of the limitations of the procedure, of the tradeoff of wrist motion for stability and pain relief, the long period of rehabilitation necessary before the final result has been obtained, and that the long-term effects of these procedures are not well known. Proper patient selection is important when intercarpal fusion is considered for "dynamic" instabilities. These conditions are more difficult to diagnose and, in our experience, respond less predictably to intercarpal fusion than do "static" instabilities or arthritic conditions. We caution our patients with dynamic instability that more than one surgical procedure may be necessary. Static and dynamic instabilities are discussed in more detail later.

Establishing the proper diagnosis is one of the keys to success in any surgical procedure. No testing or imaging technique has supplanted careful history and physical examination in this regard. Routine radiographs with wrist positioned in neutral are mandatory. We have found that a wrist arthrogram obtained by an experienced radiologist can be very helpful. When a diagnosis cannot be established with certainty, we now recommend diagnostic arthroscopy before proceeding with an intercarpal fusion. Arthroscopy enables visualization of the articular car-

tilage, intercarpal ligaments, and articular alignment, damage to which may not be detected by imaging techniques. Unrecognized ligament injuries or osteochondral lesions may contribute to the failure of a partial wrist fusion.

COMPLICATIONS OF PARTIAL WRIST FUSION

A review of the literature on partial wrist fusions reveals relatively high rates of complications.[17, 18, 27, 29, 35, 38] The most common complications are non-union, incomplete pain relief, and progressive arthrosis at the radioscaphoid and other joints. Other reported complications are pin tract infections, osteomyelitis, avascular necrosis of the lunate, reflex sympathetic dystrophy, nerve damage, and tendon rupture.

Siegel and Ruby's review and study[51] confirm our experience that fusions with the greatest surface area (scaphoid-capitate-lunate, scaphoid-capitate-lunate-triquetrum, and total intercarpal fusion) have the lowest rates of non-union. In their review, these fusions had the lowest complications rates. Our experience over the last 12 years is similar to that of many of the other surgeons whose work has been referenced. In our own combined series of intercarpal fusions, the overall results can be characterized as "50%"—that is, 50 percent relief of pain, 50 percent range of motion, 50 percent grip strength, and a 50 percent revision rate after intercarpal fusion. Nonetheless, we have found that several of the partial wrist fusions are very effective and predictable. These are STT fusion for degenerative arthritis, radiocarpal fusions for rheumatoid disease, capitate-lunate-hamate-triquetrum (four-corner) fusions combined with scaphoid excision for isolated radioscaphoid arthritis, and lunotriquetral (LT) fusion for instability of the LT joint. Like Siegel and Ruby,[51] we have the most confidence in complete intercarpal fusions for wrist instability. In our own series of partial wrist fusions, the complete intercarpal fusion has been the most reliable procedure for providing adequate (if not complete) pain relief as well as acceptable motion.

INDICATIONS

There are several general indications for limited wrist arthrodesis.

Non-United Fractures of the Scaphoid Bone

Limited wrist arthrodeses were first described for the treatment of this condition.[54] Although scaphocapitate fusion still may be a treatment alternative in longstanding symptomatic scaphoid non-union with

---

*References 2, 3, 7, 10, 11, 15, 17, 18, 23, 25, 27, 29, 33, 35, 38, 40, 44, 46, 58, 60.

preservation of the radioscaphoid joint, bone grafting and/or electrical stimulation remain the first procedures of choice. The natural history of untreated scaphoid non-unions[21, 22, 49, 66, 67, 71] results in radioscaphoid arthritis and/or progressive carpal collapse which require treatment either by a more extensive intercarpal fusion, by scaphoid resection arthroplasty supplemented by an intercarpal fusion, or by total wrist fusion.[14, 26, 59, 62, 63]

Localized Arthritis of the Carpus

Arthritis limited to one or several of the carpal articulations can be treated by partial carpal fusion. Osteoarthritis involving the scaphoid, trapezium, and trapezoid joints is perhaps the most common condition for which intercarpal fusion should be considered. Limited arthrodesis of the involved joints is an excellent procedure, particularly if there is already some loss of wrist motion.[11, 45, 50, 77] Localized arthritis from sepsis also may be amenable to treatment by limited wrist fusion, either intercarpal or radiocarpal.

Rheumatoid Arthritis

Intercarpal and radiocarpal fusions for wrist involvement in rheumatoid arthritis are being done with increasing frequency. They are useful in arresting carpal translocation and in preserving motion when only a portion of the wrist joint has been destroyed.[3, 7, 16, 33, 39, 56, 57]

Rheumatoid arthritis has a propensity to affect mainly the radiocarpal joints and to selectively spare the midcarpal area. Therefore, reconstructive procedures may be necessary on only a limited portion of the wrist joint. Partial wrist fusion is considered in patients whose wrist radiographs show sparing of the midcarpal joints with destruction limited to the radiocarpal area (Fig. 37–1) and whose wrists are painful but are minimally deformed and retain a significant amount of mobility. Ulnar translocation of the carpus is one of the major indications for a partial wrist fusion. The extent of ulnar translocation is determined by checking the relationship of the lunate to the ulnar border of the distal radius.

Neutral-position radiographs that show less than 50 percent of the lunate articulating with the radius indicate ulnar translocation of the carpus. Contraindications to partial wrist fusion in rheumatoid arthritis include rapidly progressive disease, nonfunctioning or ruptured wrist extensor tendons, and intraoperative discovery of significant arthritic involvement of the midcarpal joints.

If the radioscaphoid joint is found to be preserved at the time of surgery, only a lunate-radius fusion is done. This corrects deformity and halts continued

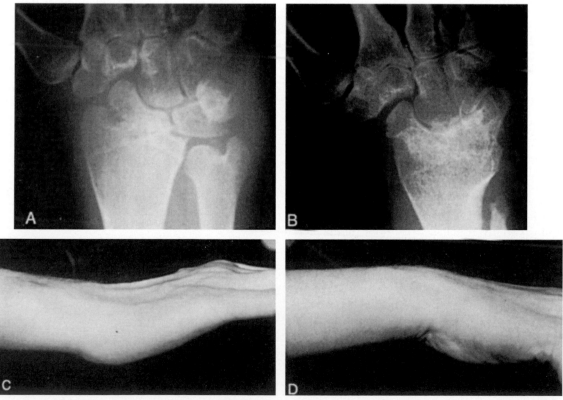

Figure 37–1. An example of limited wrist fusion. *A,* Preoperative radiograph demonstrates preserved midcarpal joints and ulnar translocation of the carpus. *B,* Postoperative radiograph demonstrates solid fusion with improved carpal alignment. *C,* Early postoperative wrist extension. *D,* Postoperative wrist flexion.

ulnar translocation of the wrist and may preserve more motion than a total radiocarpal arthrodesis. This approach has been advocated by Chamay and associates[7] and by Linsheid and Dobyns.[33] If the radioscaphoid joint is less than optimal, a radioscapholunate fusion is done to eliminate the potential for progressive disease at the radioscaphoid joint.

The surgical technique for partial wrist fusion in patients with rheumatoid arthritis varies only slightly from that described for those without it (see later). In patients with rheumatoid arthritis, the distal ulna is resected if it is unstable or if it is a source of pain, as determined preoperatively. The ulnocarpal ligaments are preserved for reconstruction. The ulnarly translocated carpus is shifted radially into more normal anatomic alignment. Local bone graft is added to the fusion site if necessary. Internal fixation with Kirschner (K) wires and/or screws is used.

Carpal Instability

The carpus is intrinsically unstable. Its stability is provided by the shape and contact of the individual carpal bones and by the intrinsic and extrinsic wrist ligaments. Loss of ligamentous support can result in varying degrees of carpal instability, which may cause symptoms of pain and clicking in the wrist and altered load transmission and which may lead to progressive degenerative arthritis of the carpus. Instability can occur at the scapholunate joint, the lunotriquetral joint, or the midcarpal joints. The diagnosis of these instabilities is straightforward in so-called static instability, in which the collapse pattern is present at all times and therefore is apparent on radiographs of the wrist. The use of intercarpal fusions in the treatment of these instability patterns has been reported by several surgeons as having reasonable functional results.*

"Dynamic" carpal instability does not occur until stress or load is applied to the wrist. Thus, provocative tests are required to demonstrate the instability. The unloaded wrist appears normal on standard radiographs. Stress views or cineradiographs may or may not show the instability pattern. Establishing an accurate diagnosis is critical in determining the appropriate treatment, particularly if intercarpal fusion is being considered. The surgeon must be certain that the fusion selected will correct the instability. Even when the diagnosis is accurate, the outcome of intercarpal fusions done for instability is not predictable. Persistent symptoms may require extension of the fusion to control symptoms.[31, 74] For these reasons, all nonoperative treatment options should be exhausted before an intercarpal fusion is considered for wrist instabilities.

---

*References 1, 10, 15, 23, 27, 28, 31, 34, 42, 43, 65, 67, 69, 70, 72.

Adjunct to Implant and Resection Arthroplasty of the Wrist

Resection arthroplasty of the scaphoid supplemented by fusion of the capitate, lunate, hamate, and triquetrum (four-corner fusion) is an established and useful procedure in treating localized radioscaphoid arthritis (scapholunate advanced collapse, or SLAC, wrist), which usually occurs as the result of scaphoid nonunion or chronic scaphoid instability.[14, 26] Although silicone rubber implant arthroplasty was popular in the 1980s, such procedures have fallen out of favor because of the limited ability of silicone rubber to bear load without deforming and because of the high incidence of particulate synovitis.[53] Partial wrist fusions done in conjunction with silicone rubber carpal implantation were advocated as a way to minimize such deformation and synovitis.[55] Nonetheless, the use of silicone carpal implants has largely been abandoned except in special cases.

Treatment of Kienböck's Disease

Partial carpal fusion is an alternative salvage procedure for advanced Kienböck's disease.[22]

Chuinard and Zeman[8] advocated the fusion of the capitate to the hamate in Kienböck's disease. They postulated that this fusion would prevent progressive proximal migration of the capitate as the avascular lunate bone collapsed. This procedure never gained wide acceptance, and its theoretic basis has been challenged.[61] Watson and colleagues[73] have advocated STT fusion for Kienböck's disease, on the basis that this fusion will provide a load-bearing column radial to the capitate-lunate axis, thereby decreasing the load borne by the lunate and preventing progressive carpal collapse. Such treatment for Kienböck's disease has the disadvantage of limiting wrist motion. Trumble and associates[61] have shown significant reduction in lunate compression during wrist loading after STT fusion but not after capitate-hamate fusion. Lichtman advocates the use of STT fusion for stage IIIB Kienböck's disease in order to treat the secondary carpal instability (see Chapter 18).

Salvage Surgery for Partial Carpal Bone Loss

Partial loss of carpal bone stock may occur from high-impact injuries such as motor vehicle accidents and gunshot wounds, following tumor resection, and as the result of avascular necrosis of bones such as the scaphoid following Preiser's disease (osteonecrosis of the scaphoid) or scaphoid fracture with proximal pole non-union.

It may be possible to salvage partial wrist function and prevent progressive carpal collapse and degenerative arthritis by performing a limited carpal fusion;

for example, fusion of the scaphoid to the capitate and excision of the distal pole of the scaphoid.[56, 65] Campbell and Koekarn[6] have described the use of inlay grafts about the wrist following bone resection in tumor surgery.

Wrist Stabilization in Neurologic Conditions

Limited wrist fusion has also been described for stabilization in cases of flail wrists following radial nerve palsy and for loss of wrist control in cerebral palsy.[50] Partial or total wrist fusion can be used in conjunction with tendon transfers to improve both function and cosmesis. Although these fusions will limit motion, they can improve the ability of a tendon transfer to provide function at a more distal site.

SPECIFIC LIMITED WRIST FUSIONS

Scaphoid-Lunate Fusion

Although scaphoid-lunate fusion would seem the most logical intercarpal fusion to consider in scapho-

lunate dissociation, it has not been advocated widely. Hastings and Silver[23] reported their experience with this procedure in 1984. Watson[65] specifically recommends against this combination, not only because it is difficult to obtain union but also because bone volume at the fusion site may be inadequate to carry the load imposed at the junction of the lunate and scaphoid during wrist use.

Satisfactory clinical results have been reported when bony union at the fusion site was obtained. However, in these series, the average non-union rate was 62.5 percent.[23, 24, 35] Persistent pain occurred in greater than 50 percent of wrists in Hom and Ruby's series,[24] even though the range of wrist motion was 94 percent and grip strength was 88 percent of those on the other side. Our results in two cases were disappointing, both patients requiring extension of their fusions to obtain union. We agree with Hom and Ruby[24] and Watson[65] that scapholunate fusion is neither a predictable nor a reliable fusion for scapholunate dissociation.

Scaphoid-Trapezium-Trapezoid Fusion

STT fusion was reported by Sutro[54] in 1946 for the treatment of a non-united scaphoid fracture and in

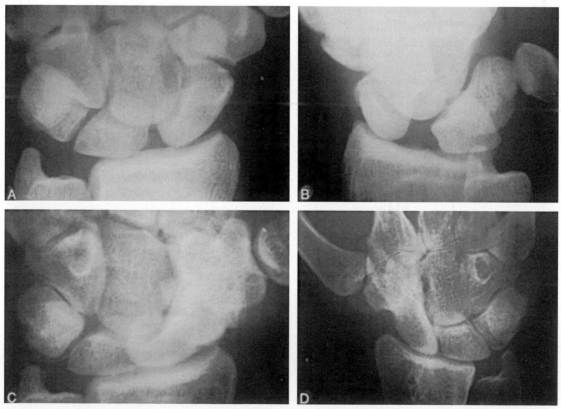

Figure 37–2. *A*, A 27-year-old firefighter with a symptomatic scapholunate dissociation that prevented him from working. *B*, The extent of the dissociation is seen on the oblique view of the wrist. *C*, Treatment by scaphoid-trapezium-trapezoid (STT) fusion stabilized the scaphoid and eliminated his pain. He was able to return to his regular work 5 months after surgery. At that time, his grip strength was 80 lb (90 percent of that of the contralateral side). Wrist flexion was 55°, extension was 55°, ulnar deviation was 28°, and radial deviation 10°. *D*, A 26-year-old secretary was treated for dynamic scaphoid instability by STT fusion. The scapoid was "over-reduced," locking it into an excessively horizontal position. Although the patient's symptoms were alleviated and she was able to return to work, radial deviation of the wrist was limited. Over-reduction of the scaphoid is one of the most common errors made during STT fusion.

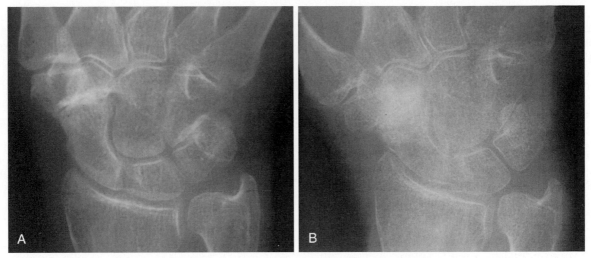

Figure 37–3. *A,* Degenerative arthritis of the scaphoid-trapezium-trapezoid in a 53-year-old woman (dominant hand). *B,* Radiographs taken 6 months after surgery show a solid STT fusion. The patient had complete relief of her preoperative wrist pain and was able to return to work as a housecleaner. Wrist extension was 35°, flexion 42°, radial deviation 10°, and ulnar deviation 26°. Grip strength was 20 lb. The wrist range of motion and grip strength after intercarpal fusion usually improve slowly up to the ninth postoperative month.

1967 by Peterson and Lipscomb[42] for rotatory subluxation of the scaphoid. It was popularized by Watson and Hempton[70] with their report in 1980. Many surgeons have reported their experience with this fusion since that time.* The kinematics of the wrist following STT fusion have been studied by Kleinman,[27] who has shown that the capitate moves with the STT fusion mass. The ulnar carpus is not affected by the fusion, because a plane of motion develops between teh scaphoid and the lunate bones. This disruption of the scapholunate link preserves the normal kinematics of the hamate and triquetrum. Wrist motion following STT fusion is therefore a combination of motion between the scaphoid and lunate bones and radiocarpal motion. Garcia-Elias and colleagues[19] showed increased sliding motion of the lunate on the radius and postulated that the resultant greater shear stress on the lunate and its adjacent ligaments could potentially affect the long-term results of STT fusion.

The indications for STT fusion include both static and dynamic scaphoid instability (Fig. 37–2) without the presence of radioscaphoid arthritis, or in localized degenerative arthritis of the STT joints. Its use in the treatment of Kienböck's disease has also been reported.[61, 73] We believe that the STT fusion is most useful in patients with degenerative arthritis of the scaphoid-trapezium joint (Fig. 37–3). In these patients, we prefer to perform the fusion through a volar approach similar to but slightly more distal than the volar approach used for scaphoid non-union, rather than using the dorsal approach described by Watson.[70] We still use the dorsal approach for STT fusions done for scaphoid instability, because it is easier to inspect the radioscaphoid joint and to align the scaphoid and lunate from the dorsal side. We adhere

to Watson's principles and technique of STT fusion (Fig. 37–4).

In the series of STT fusions with long-term follow-up reported by Siegel and Ruby,[51] the average non-union rate was 15 percent and that of persistent pain of some degree was 44 percent. The average range of motion was 67 percent and the average grip strength 77 percent of those on the other side.

Kleinman and Carroll[29] reported a 4 percent incidence of degenerative arthritis between the styloid process of the radius and the scaphoid after STT fusion. Affected patients showed response to radial styloidectomy. These researchers postulated two

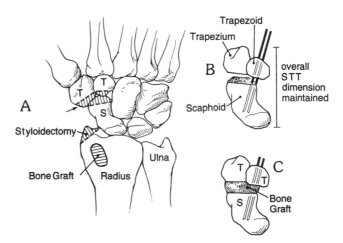

Figure 37–4. The technique of STT fusion as described by Watson.[68] *A* and *B,* The articular cartilage and subchondral bone are removed from the joint surfaces to expose cancellous bone. Care is taken to preserve the overall dimensions of the carpus. *C,* Bone graft obtained from the distal radius is packed between the prepared surfaces after the scaphoid has been stabilized with two longitudinal Kirschner wires placed across the trapezoid and scaphoid.

---

*References 10, 11, 15, 17, 18, 25, 27–29, 72, 77.

mechanisms for the degenerative changes: altered mechanics at the radius-scaphoid junction as the result of the STT fusion and incomplete reduction of the scaphoid at the time of the STT fusion.[29] Watson and Dhillon[68] noted a 35 percent incidence of painful radial styloid impingement after STT fusion, and they now advocate performing a radial styloidectomy at the time of STT fusion. For the same reason, Watson and Rao also caution against a position of excessive scaphoid extension (see Chapter 32).

Scaphoid-Capitate Fusion

With indications similar to those for STT fusion, scaphoid-capitate fusion restricts wrist motion more than the STT fusion but is easier to perform through a longitudinal, dorsal midline excision. A broad surface contact area is available for fusion, decreasing the risk of non-union. We have been satisfied with the results of this fusion in patients with scapholunate dissociation. We have used it in conjunction with placement of a lunate implant to diminish the compressive load on the implant, transmit load across the wrist, and prevent carpal collapse. However, we no longer use lunate implants. Scaphoid-capitate fusion also has been used as a salvage procedure for non-union of proximal pole fractures of the scaphoid bone with avascular necrosis of the non-united fragment.[46]

Pisano and colleagues[44] found a non-union rate of only 12 percent for scaphoid-capitate fusion. However, 41 percent of patients in their series had persistent postoperative pain. The average range of motion after fusion was 47 percent and the average grip strength was 74 percent of those on the opposite side.

Scaphoid-Capitate-Lunate Fusion

Scaphoid-capitate-lunate fusion includes the midcarpal joint and therefore can be used for midcarpal instability or for scapholunate dissociation with significant dorsiflexion instability of the lunate. Its use in late Kienböck's disease and in diffuse intercarpal arthritis with preservation of the radiocarpal joints also has been described.[22, 57] As with all midcarpal fusions, it limits wrist motion considerably.

Because of the large bone surface area available for scaphoid-capitate-lunate fusion, the average non-union rate in two separate series was low (12 percent).[23, 46] In spite of the low non-union rate, however, the rate of persistent postoperative pain was high, and the average loss of wrist motion was 50 percent in these series. The average postoperative grip strength was 60 percent of the opposite side.[26, 35, 46, 51, 63]

Capitate-Lunate Fusion

Fusion of the capitate and lunate is used for stabilization of the midcarpal joint, particularly when combined with scaphoid resection for radioscaphoid arthritis. Other indications are degenerative arthritis limited to the midcarpal joint, lunate fractures, and Kienböck's disease.[65]

In two series, the average non-union rate after capitate-lunate fusion was 29 percent; 45 percent of patients had persistent pain after the fusion. The average range of motion was 60 percent and the average grip strength was 71 percent of those on the opposite side.[51] We use the lunate-capitate-hamate-triquetrum or "four-corner" fusion (described later) for similar indications and find a lower non-union rate and improved reliability. Inclusion of the hamate and triquetrum in the fusion does not reduce the postoperative motion significantly compared with the capitate-lunate fusion alone.

Lunate-Triquetrum Fusion

Lunate-triquetrum fusion has been described for symptomatic lunotriquetral instability and/or dissociation by Alexander and Lichtman.[1] It reproduces the most common of the congenital carpal coalitions, which usually are asymptomatic.[52] Taleisnik[56, 57] has suggested this fusion for static volar collapse deformities.

In the series of lunate-triquetrum fusions reported, non-union occurred on average in 27 percent and persistent pain in 50 percent (average) of patients. The average range of motion after fusion was 83.5 percent and the average grip strength was 64.5 percent of those on the opposite side in two series.[34, 35, 40, 43, 51] Our own experience with this fusion has been improved through a modification of the surgical procedure to ensure anatomic, congruent alignment of the proximal articular surfaces of the lunate and triquetrum. The radiocarpal joint is opened to allow direct visualization of the proximal articular surfaces. The anatomic boundaries of the lunotriquetral unit are preserved by using an inlay graft, which spares the articular cartilage margins between the bones (Fig. 37–5). Careful preoperative assessment and attention to surgical detail have decreased the non-union rate and improved both the subjective satisfaction and functional outcome rates in our series. We continue to use the lunate-triquetrum fusion for instability of the triquetrum and for symptomatic tears of the lunotriquetral ligament (Fig. 37–6).

Lunate-Capitate-Hamate-Triquetrum Fusion

The lunate-capitate-hamate-triquetrum fusion, often referred to as the four-corner fusion, can be used for both midcarpal[31] and lunotriquetral[1] instabilities. It does not cause significantly more loss of wrist motion than a capitolunate fusion alone. It provides very wide surfaces for bone union and results in a stable

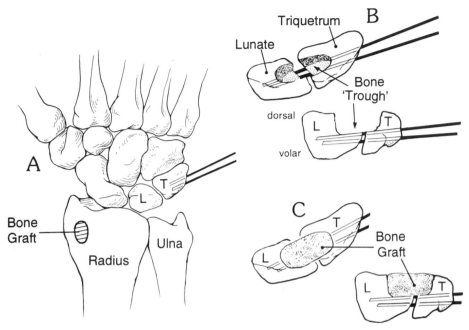

Figure 37–5. *A*, The "inlay" technique of lunotriquetral fusion: Two parallel Kirschner wires are placed across the volar aspect of the joint (see *C*) under flouroscopic control. *B*, An oval of bone is removed from the dorsal aspect of the joint. This maneuver preserves a rim of cartilage between the two bones so that the carpal dimensions and bone alignment remain normal. *C*, A corticocancellous bone graft harvested from the radius is tamped into the defect. Note that the proximal articular surfaces of the lunate and triquetrum are aligned.

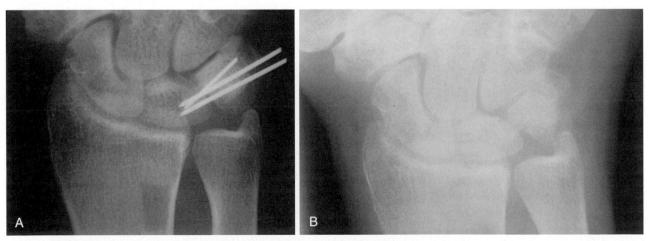

Figure 37–6. *A*, Postoperative radiograph of inlay lunotriquetral fusion showing Kirschner wires and bone graft in place. The distalmost pin was used to secure the graft. *B*, A solid fusion was obtained. At 4 months, a strut of bone bridges the joint.

carpus (Fig. 37–7). Combined with scaphoid resection, four-corner fusion has become one of the standard procedures for the treatment of localized radioscaphoid arthritis[14, 34, 59, 60, 66] (Fig. 37–8). Postoperative casting in slight ulnar deviation has decreased the problem of radial deviation deformities and loss of ulnar deviation range of motion in our patients. In the four series reported, the average union rate was low (8 percent).[35, 59, 60, 66] In the three series reporting range of motion after fusion, the average range of motion was 52 percent and the average grip strength was 71 percent of those on the opposite side.[59, 60, 66]

Triquetrum-Hamate Fusion

Fusion of the triquetrum and hamate stabilizes the midcarpal joint and has been used for midcarpal instability and for degenerative changes between the triquetrum and hamate. Documenting instability of this joint is difficult. It is one of the most mobile joints in the carpus. The dorsal stabilizing ligaments are thin, and an arthrotomy increases the laxity. Alexander and Lichtman[1] recommend pinning the joint at the time of surgery to confirm the diagnosis and ensure that the instability has been corrected prior to preparing the joint for fusion.

Complications of this procedure include persistent albeit less severe clicks after operation, as well as pain over the hamate hook, and degenerative changes of the pisotriquetral joint. K wires placed across the triquetrum-hamate joint can easily impinge the median nerve or flexor tendons at the distal end of the carpal canal. This fusion is rarely used now, having been supplanted in our and others' practices by the four-corner fusion for symptomatic midcarpal instability (Fig. 37–9).[31]

Total Intercarpal Fusion

We use a total intercarpal fusion in patients with multiple areas of intercarpal arthritis and in patients with instability not corrected by a more localized fusion. After total fusion, motion occurs only at the radiocarpal joint, resulting in significant loss of wrist motion. In our series, most wrists with total intercarpal fusions have been stable and pain free, and the patients have been able to return to work requiring strenuous use of the hands. There may be some clicking during radial and ulnar deviation as the fixed scapholunate unit slides over the ridge in the radius that separates the scaphoid fossa from the lunate fossa (Fig. 37–10). The non-union rate is low for this procedure because of the large surface areas available for fusion. Siegel and Ruby[51] have a 100 percent union rate in their series, as have we in our series. We have found the total intercarpal fusion to be one of the most predictable and reliable of the intercarpal fusions. A loss of motion of about 50 percent can be expected. Siegel and Ruby[51] report average grip strength after fusion to be 65 percent (Fig. 37–11).

Radioscaphoid Fusion

Radioscaphoid fusion can be used when there is extensive localized arthritis of the articulation between the radius and the scaphoid and in rheumatoid arthritis (Fig. 37–12). This combination allows wrist mo-

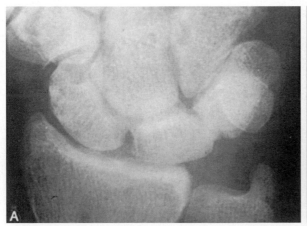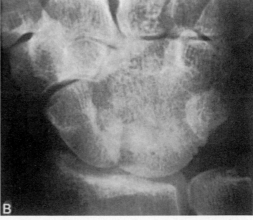

Figure 37–7. *A,* Lunotriquetral fusion in a 37-year-old firefighter who injured his wrist in a fall, after which he had signs and symptoms of triquetrum instability. Five months after surgery, his grip strength was 70 lb (64 percent of the contralateral side). Wrist flexion was 50°, wrist extension was 50°, ulnar deviation was 15°, and radial deviation was 20°. *B,* A 24-year-old woman was treated by lunate-capitate-hamate-triquetrum ("four-corner") fusion for midcarpal instability. Nine months after surgery, her grip strength was 35 lb (54 percent of the contralateral side). She had intermittent aching pain after prolonged use of the wrist. Wrist flexion was 30°, wrist extension was 50°, ulnar deviation was 10°, and radial deviation was 10°.

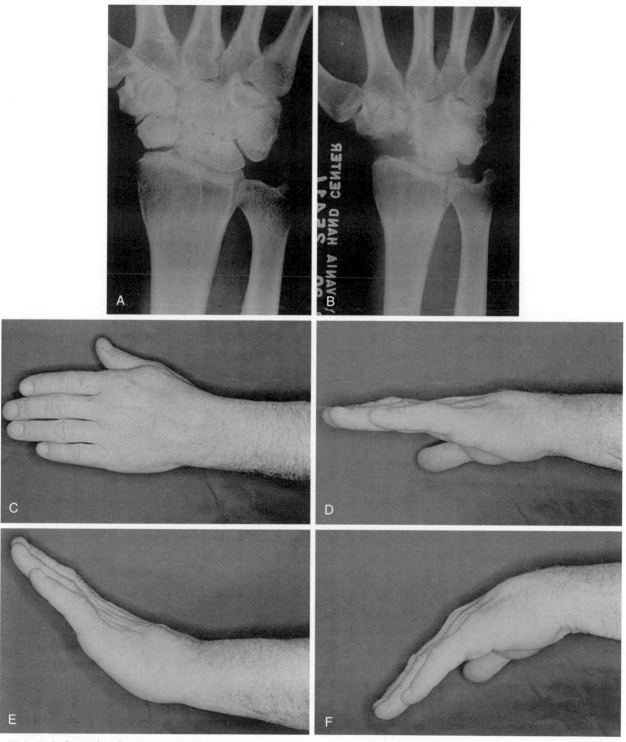

Figure 37–8. *A,* Radiographs of a 28-year-old laborer with a painful wrist and limited motion from a long-standing scaphoid non-union. *B,* The scaphoid was resected, and a "four-corner" (capitate-lunate-hamate-triquetrum) fusion performed. *C* and *D,* After fusion, the wrist is balanced at rest. *E* and *F,* Wrist extension and flexion.

Illustration continued on following page

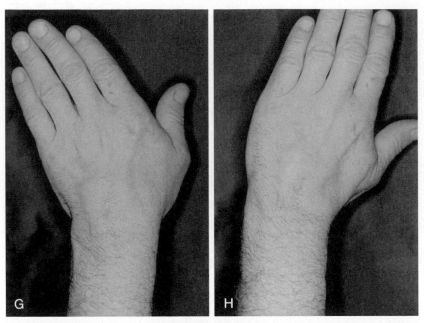

Figure 37–8 *Continued G* and *H,* Ulnar and radial deviation.

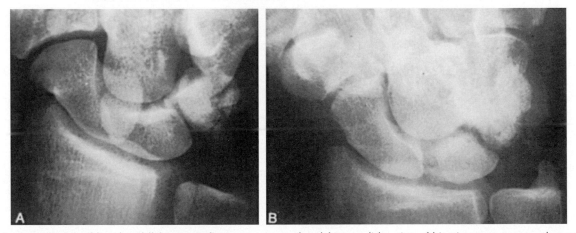

Figure 37–9. *A,* An 18-year-old student fell from a rooftop, sustaining a closed fracture dislocation of his triquetrum among other extremity and abdominal injuries. The fracture dislocation was treated by open reduction and primary triquetrum-hamate fusion. *B,* Nine months after treatment, the wrist was asymptomatic. The patient's grip strength was 85 lb (85 percent of that of the contralateral side). Wrist flexion was 56°, wrist extension was 75°, ulnar deviation was 20°, and radial deviation was 15°.

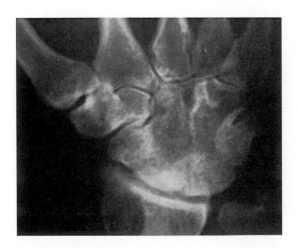

Figure 37–10. A 28-year-old man sustained a wrist injury when the bit of a large post-hole boring machine became bound in concrete, resulting in sudden rotatory stress. He underwent a pancarpal fusion for complex wrist instability. He was able to return to work as a house painter 6 months after the fusion. Grip strength was 95 lb (76 percent of that of the contralateral side). Wrist flexion was 15°, wrist extension was 40°, ulnar deviation was 10°, and radial deviation was 10°.

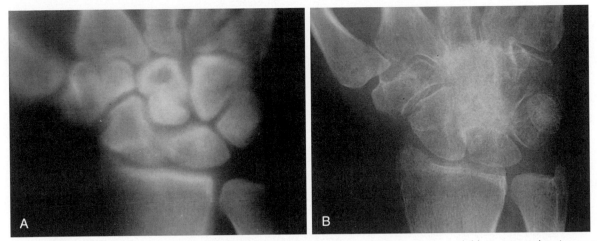

Figure 37–11. *A,* Avascular necrosis of the capitate in a 36-year-old woman who injured her wrist as a child. *B,* A complete intercarpal fusion alleviated her pain, and at 4 months, her wrist extension was 40°, wrist flexion 25°, and grip strength 35 lb (78 percent of that on the contralateral side).

tion only through the midcarpal joints and results in significant loss of motion. It can be combined with a radiolunate arthrodesis if the lunate-radius articulation is involved.

Radiolunate Fusion

Taleisnik[57] has proposed radiolunate fusion for lunate instability with either dorsal or volar instability patterns when strong grip is required. Other indications include post-traumatic degenerative disease involving the radiocarpal joints (destruction of the articular surfaces of the radius and/or proximal articular surfaces of the scaphoid and lunate bones with preservation of the midcarpal articular surfaces) and rheumatoid arthritis with localized degenerative changes of

the radiolunate articulation or ulnar translocation of the carpus[7, 40, 56, 57] (Fig. 37–13). Fusion of the proximal row or the scaphoid or lunate bones individually to the distal articular surface of the radius allows motion, albeit limited, of the wrist through the midcarpal joints. In our series, radiolunate fusion has provided a stable wrist with minimal pain but with restriction of wrist motion to approximately 33 percent of normal.

TECHNIQUE OF INTERCARPAL FUSION

Surgical Exposure

We prefer dorsal longitudinal incisions for all intercarpal fusions except for the STT fusion done for

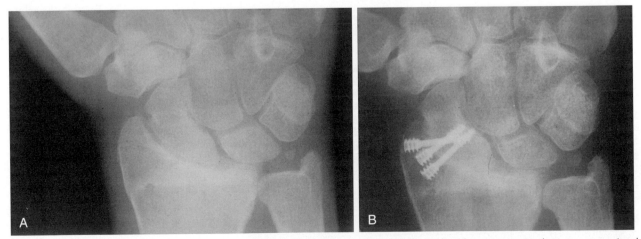

Figure 37–12. *A,* Radioscaphoid arthritis in a 30-year-old man following an intra-articular radius fracture sustained 11 years previously. *B,* Radiolunate fusion using Herbert screws for internal fixation. Five years after surgery, wrist extension is 35°, and wrist flexion is 28°. Ulnar deviation is 20°, and radial deviation is 18°. Grip strength is 80 lb (87 percent of that on the contralateral side). The patient is active athletically but complains of mild wrist pain after prolonged mountain-biking.

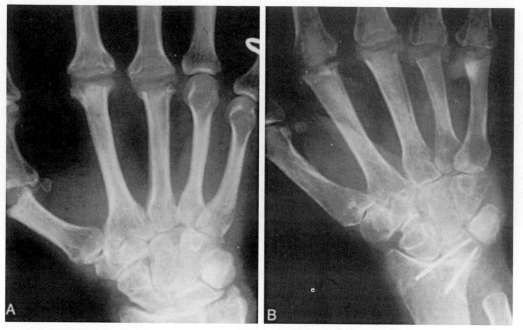

Figure 37–13. An example of radiolunate fusion. *A,* Note narrowing of the radiolunate joint with ulnar translocation. *B,* Ulnar translocation is corrected. Note preservation of the articular cartilage between the scaphoid and the radius.

osteoarthritis (described later). A slightly curved incision (convex side radialward) matches the normal slight ulnar deviation stance of the hand, although we now use a straight longitudinal incision for most of our intercarpal fusions. The incision need not be longer than 2 to 3 inches. This length provides excellent exposure of most of the carpus as well as access to the distal radius for obtaining bone graft (Fig. 37–14).

Transverse incisions may heal with a less conspicuous scar, but they limit exposure and increase the risk of damage to the superficial sensory nerves. It is difficult to extend or incorporate a transverse scar into the incision necessary for revision surgery. We

have found that meticulous wound closure and proper placement yield cosmetically acceptable longitudinal scars.

The wrist capsule can be approached between the second and third extensor compartments, between the third and fourth compartments, or through the fourth compartment. The extensor tendons must be retracted to expose the dorsal wrist capsule. One approach is to divide the retinaculum longitudinally in the midportion of the fourth compartment, and to divide the vertical septa of the retinaculum between compartments 3 through 5. This maneuver allows the extensor tendons to be retracted to either side.

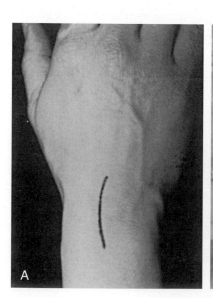
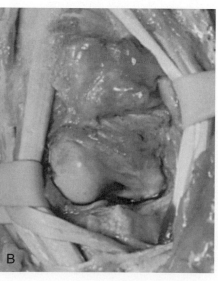

Figure 37–14. *A,* Our preferred incision for access to the wrist for intercarpal fusion (other than STT: it is difficult to reach the STT joints through this incision) and for total wrist fusion. A slight curve is used for aesthetic reasons, although a straight incision is equally effective for exposure. The incision may be moved slightly to the radial side or to the ulnar side of the midline in order to enhance exposure on one side or the other of the carpus. *B,* With a longitudinal incision, skin flaps have been retracted, the fourth dorsal compartment has been incised, retinacular flaps and extensor tendons have been retracted, and the wrist capsule has been incised to expose the carpus. The proximal pole of the scaphoid bone is seen on the left (rotated vertically), and the chronically stretched scapholunate interosseous ligament and the lunate are seen to the right of the scaphoid.

Care must be taken to identify and protect the extensor pollicis longus tendon as it crosses the second compartment tendons distal to Lister's tubercle. Alternatively, the dorsal wrist capsule may be exposed by making a longitudinal incision carried down through periosteum between the third and fourth dorsal compartments. The entire fourth retinacular compartment can be mobilized as a unit by subperiosteal dissection.[32] This step avoids exposing the individual finger extensors, preserves the restraining function of the retinaculum, and minimizes adhesions between the tendons. The capsule is exposed by retracting the extensor pollicis longus tendon radialward and the fourth compartment ulnarward. We prefer this approach because our patients have had less difficulty in regaining active finger range of motion and less pain with finger motion if the tendons within the fourth compartment were left undisturbed.

The terminal branch of the posterior interosseous nerve (radial nerve) lies in the floor of the fourth compartment. The wrist may be partially denervated by dividing this nerve as described by Buck-Gramcko[5] for rheumatoid wrist disease and by Dellon[12] for chronic wrist pain.

The capsule may be opened longitudinally or with a T or cross-shaped capsular incision, depending on how much of the carpus must be visualized. We prefer a U-shaped capsular incision based either radially or ulnarly. Such an incision allows a large flap of capsule to be placed over the midportion of the carpus following the fusion, providing a smooth bed for the extensor tendons without a longitudinal suture line while affording excellent exposure. Loose closure can be obtained by tacking back the corners of the flap.

If the patient's symptoms or clinical findings are suggestive of damage on the ulnar side of the carpus, the triangular fibrocartilage complex and/or distal radioulnar joint is exposed by mobilizing the tendons of the fifth and sixth compartments. The capsular incision can be extended or a second flap of capsule can be elevated if a fusion on the ulnar side of the wrist is to be done.

Tight closure of the capsule is not necessary and probably is not desirable. Maximum wrist motion will be obtained after intercarpal fusion if the wrist motion limits are determined by the bony constraints and not compounded by capsular fibrosis. Tight closure combined with normal scar contracture and prolonged immobilization may produce more restriction in motion than the theoretic limits imposed by any given bony fusion. Therefore, we close the capsule loosely with several absorbable sutures. The capsule should provide a smooth bed for extensor tendons but should not limit wrist motion unless a capsulodesis effect is desired for a specific reason.

Preparation of the Carpus for Fusion

Exploration of the wrist prior to fusion is critical. The presence of synovitis, capsular tears, cartilage erosion, and/or interosseous ligament damage should alert the surgeon to unsuspected intercarpal problems. Such a finding may require an alternative solution to the preoperative plan. For example, the presence of radioscaphoid arthritis precludes performing an STT fusion.

After the fusion to be performed has been selected, careful attention must be given to carpal alignment. The restoration of normal alignment may require capsular releases and/or manipulation. If the scaphoid is to be incorporated into the fusion, it should be aligned so that its proximal articular surface is reduced concentrically with the scaphoid fossa of the radius, but not over-reduced so that the bone lies too "horizontally." Reduction of the scaphoid so that the scapholunate angle is less than the normal 45° would limit radial deviation more than is necessary and may not provide concentric reduction of the proximal pole. Over-reduction of the scaphoid is probably the most common error committed during an STT fusion. However, fusing the scaphoid in too vertical a position can also lead to radioscaphoid arthritis.[27, 28, 29] The specific technique used for STT fusion as described by Watson and Hempton[70] is shown in Figure 37–4 and is described in Chapter 32.

When the lunate is to be a part of the fusion, we attempt to correct the alignment of this bone if it is volarly or dorsally tilted. A K wire introduced vertically into the body of the lunate can be used as a "handle" or "joystick" to correct rotation. It is removed after the lunate is secured with a horizontal K wire to another of the carpal bones. Concentric alignment without a step-off between the cartilage surfaces of the bones to be fused is critical to the success of all intercarpal fusions, especially a lunotriquetral fusion. Direct vision is imperative to align the proximal articular surfaces of these bones.

If the lunate is not to be fused, as in STT arthrodesis, the dorsal surface of the lunate can be decorticated to supplement lunate stability with a "capsulodesis" for mild to moderate lunate rotation. Fusion may be required to correct severe lunate rotation. Correction of lunate rotation keeps the lunate reduced concentrically in the lunate fossa of the radius and provides more normal contour of the entire articular surface of the proximal carpal row.

Watson and his coworkers[69, 70] emphasize the importance of preserving the overall dimension of the carpus, including that portion selected for fusion, when preparing the bone surfaces. It is easy to "shrink" the carpus as cartilage and subchondral bone are removed during preparation. Less commonly, the overall dimension of the carpus can be expanded by the overzealous addition of bone graft. If we are concerned about maintaining alignment or carpal dimension, we pin the carpus in the position desired for intercarpal fusion prior to removal of articular cartilage and subchondral bone. The wrist is held in neutral by an assistant. The carpal bones are reduced and fixed with one or two transversely oriented K wires. Articular cartilage and subchondral bone are removed by working around the pins that prevent the carpal bones from migrating. If the pins remain undamaged and solidly fixed, they are retained and used for final fixation of the fusion. If a pin is damaged by the osteotome or saw, it is replaced after the final pins used for internal fixation are inserted. The difficulty in working around the pins is offset by the ease in maintaining proper carpal alignment. This technique may become less useful as the surgeon gains experience with partial wrist fusion techniques.

Cartilage Removal and Bone Preparation

An osteotome, rongeurs, or a "micro" sagittal saw is used to remove articular cartilage and subchondral bone. Standard high-speed power burs should not be used, because the heat generated might cause thermal necrosis of the bone and interfere with primary bone healing. The only non-unions in one case in our series of intercarpal fusions occurred after we used burs to remove articular cartilage. We have used the Midas Rex system to prepare fusion sites without adverse effect. With this system, extreme care must be taken to protect adjacent structures and soft tissues. Removing the cartilage with other instruments before using the Midas Rex system to remove subchondral bone prevents the burs from becoming fouled.

The subchondral bone should be removed or softened by "fish-scaling" to expose cancellous bone, maximizing the potential for primary bone healing and joint fusion. Fish-scaling can be accomplished with the sagittal saw, rongeurs or osteotome, or by making multiple perforations in the subchondral plate using the sharp point of a 0.045-inch K wire driven in a high-speed drill after the articular cartilage has been removed with rongeurs or curettes.

Internal Fixation

K wires (0.045-inch diameter) are used for internal fixation. They are inserted easily and usually can be removed without undue difficulty in the office using local infiltration anesthesia. We prefer to cut the pins below the skin level. The pin ends should be palpable but should not tent the skin. If they are left too long, they may cause skin irritation or pain under the postoperative dressing or cast. If a pin erodes through the skin, we remove it as soon as possible to minimize the possibility of a pin tract infection. However, if the pins are cut too short, they may be difficult to palpate after healing has occurred, and their removal in the office may be difficult if not impossible. It is safer and less frustrating to remove such buried pins in the operating room under optimal conditions and adequate anesthesia with a C-arm image intensifier available to aid in localization of the pin.

The use of K wires for internal fixation is not without problems, including arterial puncture, nerve impingement, tendon impingement, pin breakage, and difficulty with pin removal. Smooth pins should be used to minimize soft tissue damage. Rarely, puncture of the radial artery occurs, manifested as large amounts of bright red blood escaping from the pin site. In this case, we remove the pin and apply pressure to the bleeding site. In our experience, such bleeding has stopped without permanent damage to the artery or distal circulation. Impingement of a superficial sensory nerve by a pin is manifested as intense pain in a localized area after recovery from the anesthetic. The pin should be removed as soon as possible, with care taken to protect the involved nerve from further damage. Transient paresthesias and/or numbness in the distribution of the affected nerve usually occur and resolve slowly over several weeks. Tendon impingement is signified by pain in a localized area with wrist, thumb, or finger motion. When this occurs, we remove the pin as soon as possible to avoid tendon attrition. On several occasions, steroid injection of the first dorsal compartment has been necessary for semi-acute or chronic tenosynovitis that we have attributed to scarring or bleeding from injury to the sheath by a pin. Careful pin insertion technique combined with palpation of the subcutaneous structures prior to insertion can minimize these complications. Some surgeons favor open pin insertion, because direct visualization minimizes injury to subcutaneous structures.

Before the pins are cut short, the wrist should be moved through its range of motion to make sure that the pins do not impinge the radiocarpal joint. We now use a "mini" C-arm image intensifier routinely to verify pin placement and length before cutting the pins. Pins should not be placed across the radiocarpal joint during an intercarpal fusion. Preservation of radiocarpal joint motion acts as a "safety valve" to decrease stress at the intercarpal fusion site.

Variable-pitch screws, such as the Herbert screw, or cannulated variable-pitch screws, such as the Herbert-Whipple or Acutrak screw, can be used for internal fixation of intercarpal or radiocarpal fusions. The mechanical advantage of fixation with such devices is attractive. They can be left in place after union has occurred and will not impinge tendons or other structures. However, it is commonly necessary to make a counter-incision for these screws to be inserted, adding to operative time and soft tissue trauma.

Bone Graft

The distal metaphysis of the radius provides an excellent source of bone graft for most limited carpal fusions and is a good alternative to bone from the iliac crest.[36] A corticocancellous graft can be harvested by removing a cortical window from the dorsal metaphyseal area after the periosteum has been reflected. Access to the metaphysis can be obtained by retracting the extensor tendons in the proximal portion of a longitudinal wound or through a separate transverse incision over the metaphysis. If a transverse incision is used, the interval between the tendons of the first and second compartments or between the second and third compartments is opened to expose the dorsal cortex of the radius. A cortical window is removed with osteotomes or a small sagittal saw. Cancellous bone is harvested with curettes. We usually use the cortical window as a strut at the fusion site and do not replace it. Care is taken not to penetrate the subchondral bone and articular surface of the distal radius.

If a large bone defect is present or if the distal radius has been used previously as a bone graft donor site, sufficient bone may not be available from the distal radius. In these cases, iliac bone graft should be used. If there is any question that the amount of bone available from the radius will be insufficient, permission should be obtained in advance for an iliac bone graft.

Drains

We do not use drains routinely in intercarpal fusions in young healthy patients with normal skin and subcutaneous tissue. When there has been an unusual amount of intraoperative bleeding, or if the patient may be prone to bleeding (e.g., with frequent use of nonsteroidal antiinflammatory medications just before surgery), we use either a small Penrose drain or a suction drain to avoid hematoma formation. We routinely use drains in wrist procedures on patients with rheumatoid arthritis because of the atrophic skin and minimal subcutaneous tissue over the wrist in such patients. If used, the drain should be placed in the subcutaneous space, dorsal to the repaired extensor retinaculum. The drain is removed on the first or second postoperative day.

Dressing and Postoperative Management

A bulky compressive dressing is applied with the wrist held in neutral position by a volar plaster splint that stops short of the metacarpal heads. It is our preference to leave the fingers free so that early postoperative motion can be started. Occasionally, the fingers must be supported for several days to minimize postoperative pain. Watson and Hempton[70] suggest application of a volar splint to prevent use of the hand for grip, which would add compressive load to the fusion site. We prefer to start finger motion on the first postoperative day, but we warn our patients about the potential adverse effect of strenuous grip or use of the wrist on bone healing at the fusion site. We use a sugar-tong splint for several days for comfort,

followed by a short-arm cast. A thumb spica is added if the fusion includes the radial side of the carpus. The cast is brought as proximal as possible on the forearm without causing impingement of the antecubital fossa when the elbow is flexed.

The retained K wires are removed between 6 and 8 weeks if radiographs show satisfactory progress toward bone union. External support with a short-arm or short-arm thumb spica cast is continued for 8 to 10 weeks, until there is radiographic evidence of bone union. Other surgeons recommend the use of a long-arm cast for several weeks after surgery.[57, 70] We find that it is helpful to use a removable splint for 2 to 3 weeks after the solid cast is discontinued to "wean" the patient from external support. The patient can wear the splint when in public or during activity but can use and move the wrist when in a safe environment.

Pin Removal

We use the following technique for pin removal in the office. If a pin cannot be identified definitely by palpation, we consider removing it in the operating room. For pin removal in the office, the skin is prepared with povidone-iodine solution after the desquamated epithelium has been removed and the patient has washed the hand, wrist, and forearm with soap and water. The surgeon dons sterile gloves and palpates the pin end. The skin and subcutaneous tissue overlying the pin are infiltrated with a local anesthetic such as lidocaine. The punctate bleeding from the anesthetic injection serves to mark the pin site, because the pin may not be palpable after the soft tissues have been distended by the anesthetic. A small longitudinal incision (usually 2 to 3 mm in length) is made directly over the pin end. A small sterile scissors or curved hemostat is used to mobilize soft tissues from around the pin. The end of the pin is grasped with a medium-sized needle holder that has a "diamond jaw"–type inner surface. It is easier to extract the pin when jaw of the needle holder is aligned axially with the pin. Having a recent radiograph in view aids in localizing the pin and applying the needle holder in the correct plane. When the pin end has been firmly engaged in the jaws of the needle holder, the needle holder is rotated back and forth in a 90° arc as the pin is withdrawn. This motion helps free the pin from bone. Care must be taken to avoid dividing branches of subcutaneous sensory nerves, or grasping these nerves with the needle holder as the pin is engaged. The longitudinal incisions also aid in avoiding sensory nerve damage. We leave the incisions open if they are shorter than 3 mm, and close longer incisions loosely with 5–0 or 6–0 nylon. The pin removal sites are dressed with adhesive bandages. We have had no infections from the removal of retained pins in the office in our patients.

Rehabilitation

After solid external immobilization is discontinued, we start a gentle range-of-motion program. Care must be taken by the patient and by the therapist to avoid forced wrist motion. We emphasize progressive grip strengthening rather than motion for the first several months after surgery. Wrist motion increases steadily over 6 to 9 months after surgery. Vigorous attempts to regain motion early can cause an exacerbation of wrist pain. Anti-inflammatory medication is helpful for some patients during the first few weeks of therapy.

A gradual increase in wrist motion over 9 to 12 months can be expected as new planes of motion develop around the fusion site and the wrist capsule stretches.[27, 72]

SUMMARY

Limited wrist fusion is a reasonable alternative to total wrist fusion or implant arthroplasty in static instabilities of the wrist, localized arthritis of the carpus, loss of carpal bone stock from fracture, or avascular necrosis. Intercarpal fusion is a valuable adjunct to carpal implant arthroplasty and has a role in the treatment of Kienböck's disease. Relief of symptomatic dynamic instability can be obtained with this technique, but the correct diagnosis and localization of the site of instability are critical in obtaining satisfactory results. The patient and procedure must be selected carefully, in view of studies showing that less than 50 percent of patients who had any type of intercarpal fusion had complete relief of preoperative wrist pain. Careful attention must be given to the diagnostic evaluation, selection of fusion, carpal alignment, surgical technique, and postoperative management. Unsatisfactory results may be salvaged by extension of the intercarpal fusion, conversion to a total wrist fusion, or, in some cases, proximal row carpectomy.

References

1. Alexander CE, Lichtman DM: Ulnar carpal instabilities. Orthop Clin North Am 15:307–320, 1984.
2. Bach AW, Almquist EE, Newman DM: Proximal row fusion as a solution for radiocarpal arthritis. J Hand Surg 16A:424–431, 1991.
3. Bertheussen K: Partial carpal arthrodesis as treatment of local degenerative changes in wrist joints. Acto Orthop Scand 52:629–631, 1981.
4. Brumfield RH, Champoux JA: Biomechanical study of normal functional wrist motion. Clin Orthop 187:23–25, 1984.
5. Buck-Gramcko D: Denervation of the wrist joint. J Hand Surg 2:54–61, 1977.
6. Campbell CJ, Koekarn T: Total and subtotal arthrodesis of the wrist. J Bone Joint Surg 46A:1520–1533, 1964.
7. Chamay A, Della Santa D, Vilaseca A: Radiolunate arthrodesis, factor of stability for the rheumatoid wrist. Ann Chir Main 2:5–17, 1983.
8. Chuinard RG, Zeman SC: Kienböck's disease: An analysis and rationale for treatment by capitate-hamate fusion. Orthop Trans 4:18, 1980.
9. Clendenin MB, Green DP: Arthrodesis of the wrist: Complications and their management. J Hand Surg 6:253–257, 1981.
10. Cooney WP: Intercarpal fusions. J Hand Surg 9A:601, 1984.
11. Crosby EB, Linsheid RL, Dobyns JH: Scaphotrapezial trapezoidal arthrosis. J Hand Surg 3:233–234, 1978.
12. Dellon AL: Partial dorsal wrist denervation: Resection of the distal posterior interosseous nerve. J Hand Surg 10A:527–533, 1985.
13. Douglas DP, Peimer CA, Koniuch MP: Motion of the wrist after simulated limited intercarpal arthrodesis. J Bone Joint Surg 69A:1413–1418, 1987.
14. Eaton RG, Akelman E, Eaton BH: Fascial implant arthroplasty for treatment of radioscaphoid degenerative disease. J Hand Surg 14A:766–774, 1989.
15. Eckenrode JF, Louis DS, Green TL: Scapho-trapezium-trapezoid fusion in the treatment of chronic scapholunate instability. J Hand Surg 11A:497–502, 1986.
16. Feldon PG, Millender LH, Nalebuff EA: Rheumatoid arthritis. In Green D (ed): Operative Hand Surgery, ed 3, vol II. New York, Churchill Livingstone, 1993, p 1632.
17. Fortin PT, Louis DS: Long-term follow-up of scapho-trapezio-trapezoid arthrodesis. J Hand Surg 18A:675–681, 1993.
18. Frykman EB, Ekenstam FA, Wadin K: Triscaphoid arthrodesis and its complications. J Hand Surg 13A:844–849, 1988.
19. Garcia-Elias M, Cooney WP, An KN, et al: Wrist kinematics after limited intercarpal arthrodesis. J Hand Surg 14A:791–799, 1989.
20. Gellman H, Kauffman D, Lenihan M, et al: An in vitro analysis of wrist motion: The effect of limited intercarpal arthrodesis and contributions of the radiocarpal and midcarpal joints. J Hand Surg 13A:378–383, 1988.
21. Gordon LH, King D: Partial wrist arthrodesis for old ununited fractures of the carpal navicular. Am J Surg 102:460, 1961.
22. Graner O, Lopes EI, Carvalho, BC, et al: Arthrodesis of the carpal bones in the treatment of Kienböck's disease, painful ununited fractures of the navicular and lunate bones with avascular necrosis, and old fracture-dislocations of carpal bones. J Bone Joint Surg 48A:767–774, 1966.
23. Hastings DE, Silver RL: Intercarpal arthrodesis in the management of chronic carpal instability after trauma. J Hand Surg 9A:834–840, 1984.
24. Hom S, Ruby LK: Attempted scapholunate arthrodesis for chronic scapholunate dissociation. J Hand Surg 16A:334–339, 1991.
25. Ishida O, Tsai TM: Complications and results of scapho-trapezio-trapezoid arthrodesis. Clin Orthop 287:125–130, 1993.
26. Kirschenbaum D, Schneider LH, Kirkpatrick WH, et al: Scaphoid excision and capitolunate arthrodesis for radioscaphoid arthritis. J Hand Surg 18A:780–785, 1993.
27. Kleinman WB: Long-term study of chronic scapho-lunate instability treated by scapho-trapezio-trapezoid arthrodesis. J Hand Surg 14A:429–445, 1989.
28. Kleinman WB, Steichen JB, Strickland JW: Management of chronic rotatory subluxation of the scaphoid by scapho-trapezio-trapezoid arthrodesis. J Hand Surg 7:125–136, 1982.
29. Kleinman WB, Carroll C: Scapho-trapezio-trapezoid arthrodesis for treatment of chronic static and dynamic scapholunate instability. A 10-year perspective on pitfalls and complications. J Hand Surg 15A:408–415, 1990.
30. Lichtman DM, Schneider, JR, Swafford AR, et al: Ulnar midcarpal instability—clinical and laboratory analysis. J Hand Surg 6:515–523, 1981.
31. Lichtman DM, Bruckner JD, Culp RW, Alexander CE: Palmar midcarpal instability: Results of surgical reconstruction. J Hand Surg 18:307–315, 1993.
32. Linscheid RL: Correspondence Newsletter, American Society for Surgery of the Hand, July 11, 1985.
33. Linscheid RL, Dobyns JH: Radiolunate arthrodesis. J Hand Surg 10A:821–829, 1985.
34. Maiten EC, Bora FW, Osterman AL: Lunato-triquetral instability: A cause of chronic wrist pain. J Hand Surg 13A:309, 1988.

35. McAuliffe JA, Dell PC, Jaffe R: Complications of intercarpal arthrodesis. J Hand Surg 18A:1121–1128, 1993.

36. McGrath MH, Watson HK: Late results with local bone graft donor sites in hand surgery. J Hand Surg 6:234–237, 1981.

37. Myerdierks EM, Mosher JF, Werner FW: Limited wrist arthrodesis: A laboratory study. J Hand Surg 12A:526–529, 1987.

38. Minami A, Ogino T, Minami M: Limited wrist fusions. J Hand Surg 13A:660–667, 1988.

39. Nalebuff EA, Garrod KJ: Present approach to the severely involved rheumatoid wrist. Orthop Clin North Am 15:369–380, 1984.

40. Nelson DL, Manske PR, Pruitt DL, et al: Lunotriquetral arthrodesis. J Hand Surg 18A:1113–1120, 1993.

41. Palmer AK, Werner FW, Murphy D, Glisson BS, et al: Functional wrist motion: A biomechanical study. J Hand Surg 10A:39–46, 1985.

42. Peterson HA, Lipscomb PR: Intercarpal arthrodesis. Arch Surg 95:127–134, 1967.

43. Pin PG, Young L, Gilula LA, et al: Management of chronic lunotriquetral ligament tears. J Hand Surg 14A:77–83, 1989.

44. Pisano SM, Peimer CA, Wheeler DR, et al: Scaphocapitate intercarpal arthrodesis. J Hand Surg 16A:328–333, 1991.

45. Rogers WD, Watson HK: Degenerative arthritis at the triscaphe joint. J Hand Surg 15A:232–235, 1990.

46. Rothman MB, Manske PR, Pruitt DL, et al: Scaphocapitolunate arthrodesis. J Hand Surg 18A:26–33, 1993.

47. Rozing PM, Kauer JMG: Partial arthrodesis of the wrist: investigation in cadavers. Acta Orthop 55:66–68, 1984.

48. Ruby LK, Cooney WP, Linscheid RL, et al: Relative motion of the selective carpal bones: A kinematic analysis of the normal wrist. J Hand Surg 13A:1–10, 1988.

49. Ruby LK, Stinson J, Belsky MR: The natural history of scaphoid non-union. J Bone Joint Surg 67A:428–432, 1985.

50. Schwartz S: Localized fusion at the wrist joint. J Bone Joint Surg 49A:1591–1596, 1967.

51. Siegel JM, Ruby LK: Midcarpal arthrodesis. J Hand Surg 21A:179–182, 1996.

52. Simmons BP, McKenzie WD: Symptomatic carpal coalition. J Hand Surg 10A:190–193, 1985.

53. Smith RJ, Atkinson RE, Jupiter JB: Silicone synovitis of the wrist. J Hand Surg 10A:47–60, 1985.

54. Sutro CJ: Treatment of nonunion of the carpal navicular bone. Surgery 20:536, 1946.

55. Swanson AB, Maupin BK, Swanson GD, et al: Lunate implant resection arthroplasty: Long-term results. J Hand Surg 10A:1013–1024, 1985.

56. Taleisnik J: Subtotal arthrodeses of the wrist joint. Clin Orthop 187:81–88, 1984.

57. Taleisnik J: Evaluation of the rheumatoid wrist. In The Wrist. New York, Churchill Livingstone, 1985, pp 335–363.

58. Tomaino MM, Miller RJ, Burton RI: Outcome assessment following limited wrist fusion: Objective wrist scoring versus patient satisfaction. Contemp Orthop 28:403–410, 1994.

59. Tomaino MM, Miller RJ, Cole I, et al: Scapholunate advanced collapse wrist: Proximal row carpectomy or limited wrist arthrodesis with scaphoid excision? J Hand Surg 19A:134–142, 1994.

60. Trumble T, Bour CJ, Smith RJ, et al: Intercarpal arthrodesis for static and dynamic volar intercalated segment instability. J Hand Surg 13A:384–390, 1988.

61. Trumble T, Glisson RR, Seaber, AV, et al: A biomechanical comparison of the methods for treating Kienböck's disease. J Hand Surg 11A:88–93, 1986.

62. Urbaniak JR: Arthrodesis of the hand and wrist. In Evarts CM (ed): Surgery in the Musculoskeletal System. New York, Churchill Livingstone, 1990, pp 777–782.

63. Viegas SF: Limited arthrodesis for scaphoid nonunion. J Hand Surg 19A:127–133, 1994.

64. Viegas SF, Patterson RM, Peterson PD, et al: Evaluation of the biomechanical efficacy of limited intercarpal fusions for the treatment of scapho-lunate dissociation. J Hand Surg 15A:120–128, 1990.

65. Watson HK: Limited wrist arthrodesis. Clin Orthop 149:126–136, 1980.

66. Watson HK, Ballet FL: The SLAC wrist: Scapholunate advanced collapse pattern of degenerative arthritis. J Hand Surg 9A:358–365, 1984.

67. Watson HK, Brenner LH: Degenerative disorders of the wrist. J Hand Surg 10A:1002–1006, 1985.

68. Watson HK, Dhillon HS: Intercarpal arthrodesis: In Green DP (ed): Operative Hand Surgery. New York, Churchill Livingstone, 1993, pp 113–130.

69. Watson HK, Goodman ML, Johnson TR: Limited wrist arthrodesis. Part II: Intercarpal and radiocarpal combinations. J Hand Surg 6:223–233, 1981.

70. Watson HK, Hempton RF: Limited wrist arthrodesis. Part I: The triscaphoid joint. J Hand Surg 5:320–327, 1980.

71. Watson HK, Ryu J: Degenerative disorders of the carpus. Orthop Clin North Am 15:337–353, 1984.

72. Watson KH, Ryu J, Akelman E: Limited triscaphoid arthrodesis for rotatory subluxation of the scaphoid. J Bone Joint Surg 68A:345–349, 1986.

73. Watson HK, Ryu J, DiBella A: An approach to Kienböck's disease: Triscaphe arthrodesis. J Hand Surg 10A:179–187, 1985.

74. Weber ER: Concepts governing the rotational shift of the intercalated segment of the carpus. Orthop Clin North Am 15:193–207, 1984.

75. Youm Y, Flatt AE: Kinematics of the wrist. Clin Orthop 149:21–32, 1980.

76. Youm Y, McMurtry RY, Flatt AE, et al: Kinematics of the wrist. J Bone Joint Surg 60A:423–431, 1978.

77. Zemel NP, Stark HH, Ashworth CR, et al: Operative treatment for isolated scaphotrapezial-trapezoidal arthritis. J Hand Surg 10A:436, 1985.

CHAPTER 38

Arthrodesis of the Wrist: Indications and Surgical Technique

Edward A. Nalebuff, MD, Andrew L. Terrono, MD, and Paul G. Feldon, MD

A stable, pain-free wrist is a prerequisite for normal hand function. Wrist fusion is the salvage procedure of choice for a variety of conditions, including arthritis, infection, tumor, trauma, and loss of wrist motor function, as well as for failure of other wrist procedures, such as arthroplasty and limited wrist fusion. Fortunately, the upper extremity functions well with a stable and painless wrist that does not move. As long as the forearm, elbow, and shoulder joints have relatively well-preserved function and are able to position the hand in space, patients have minimal loss. Most patients adapt rapidly to wrist fusion, particularly when the hand is pain free and aligned with the axis of the forearm.

Some patients object to or resist the recommendation of wrist fusion. The same patients are the most ardent advocates of fusion after the procedure has been performed and their pain has resolved. Then, they realize that their loss of function is not as great as they had anticipated. One young person in our practice who resisted wrist fusion for several years was so pleased with her result after fusion that she offered to organize a patients' "wrist support group." A preoperative trial of wrist immobilization in a light short-arm cast to stimulate wrist fusion may be helpful in some cases. We reassure patients that the procedure is reliable and predictable.

Flexible implant or total wrist arthroplasty is an acceptable salvage procedure in patients with inflammatory arthritis who have moderate wrist deformity, good bone stock, adequate wrist motors, and a spontaneous or surgical fusion on the other side. However, wrist arthrodesis is our procedure of choice in wrists with severe deformity, poor bone stock, poor soft tissue support, osteoarthritis, or post-traumatic arthritis.[6, 13, 27] Because of the propensity of rheumatoid disease to affect mainly the radiocarpal joints and to selectively spare the midcarpal area, partial or limited wrist fusion may be effective in selected patients (see Chapter 37).

INDICATIONS

The indications for total wrist fusion are pain (with or without loss of motion), instability, or both. These symptoms may be secondary to post-traumatic degenerative joint disease following intra-articular fracture of the radius or carpal bones; to degenerative changes from chronic loss of ligament support resulting from rheumatoid arthritis, infection, trauma, or tumor; and to loss of motor control of the wrist with wrist deformity as the result of polio or acquired hemiplegia, either flaccid or spastic.[5, 10, 22, 31]

In the patient with rheumatoid arthritis, a total wrist arthrodesis should be performed for the significantly deformed wrist with poor quality bone stock and limited soft tissue support, especially if the wrist extensor tendons have ruptured. A limited carpal fusion should not be done when radiographs show destruction of both the radiocarpal and midcarpal joints. A history of a previous wrist joint infection or the permanent need for crutch support also precludes wrist arthroplasty as a reconstructive procedure, making total wrist arthrodesis our choice in these situations.[24]

Dick[10] considers wrist fusion to be contraindicated in patients with the following conditions: (1) open epiphyseal plates, (2) quadriparesis in which wrist motion is required for the performance of tendon transfers or for modified grasp and transfer techniques, and (3) major sensory deprivation in the hand.

POSITION FOR WRIST FUSION

The position in which the wrist should be fused is controversial. The recommendations by different surgeons range from neutral to 30° of wrist extension, with 0 to 10° of ulnar deviation. To facilitate toilet and hygiene functions in patients with bilateral wrist fusion, some authorities recommend fusing one wrist in neutral or slight extension and the other wrist in neutral or palmar flexion up to 30°.[10, 31] Milford[22] prefers 10° to 20° of extension, with the third metacarpal and the radius aligned. Dick[10] prefers 15° to 20° of wrist extension, except that in patients with wrist deformity secondary to spastic hemiplegia, he uses the neutral position. For patients with bilateral wrist fusion, he suggests that the dominant wrist be fused in 20° of extension and the nondominant side in neutral extension. Haddad and Riordan[14] recommend that the wrist be fused with slight dorsiflexion and slight ulnar deviation. This position aligns the shaft of the second metacarpal with the radius.

Our preferred position for unilateral wrist fusion is 5° to 10° of extension and 5° of ulnar deviation. It is our opinion that this position provides the best compromise between function and cosmesis. For bilateral wrist fusion, the dominant wrist should be fused in the position just described, and the nondominant wrist in neutral.

INCLUSION OF CARPOMETACARPAL JOINTS IN WRIST FUSION

Haddad and Riordan[14] recommend that the second and third carpometacarpal (CMC) joints be included in the fusion to prevent the development of painful motion at these joints after wrist fusion. In our experience, such motion has occurred only in patients who perform very heavy labor, in patients who use the hand-wrist-forearm unit for repetitive or strenuous activities, and in patients with previous injuries of the carpometacarpal joints (EA Nalebuff, MD, personal communication, 1986; RK Ruby, MD, personal communication, 1986). We include the second and third carpometacarpal joints in the fusion mass in patients whose employment or avocations will stress the carpometacarpal joints. We do not routinely fuse these joints in patients who have only light or moderate use of the extremity or in those who have rheumatoid arthritis.

TECHNIQUES OF WRIST FUSION

Many techniques for wrist fusion have been described (see also Chapter 37).[1, 5, 10, 14, 19, 22, 23, 26] Most of these techniques use the dorsal approach to expose the radiocarpal joints. Articular cartilage is removed from the joints to be fused. Bone graft is added from the iliac crest, the distal radius, or other sources as needed. Most of these techniques also use internal fixation to maintain the wrist in the desired position.

Haddad and Riordan[14] described a radial approach to the wrist, a block resection of the radiocarpal, intercarpal, and second and third carpometacarpal joints, and insertion of a contoured iliac crest strut graft. This method does not disturb the extensor tendons, enter the distal radioulnar joint, or add bone bulk around the wrist, and derives some stability from the corticocancellous strut graft. Extreme care must be taken in this procedure to avoid damaging the branches of the superficial radial nerve.

Various types of internal fixation devices have been used to stabilize the wrist fusion until bone union occurs. Rods,[23] staples,[1] and compression plate[4, 15, 16, 17, 19] all have been advocated. The precontoured tapered ASIF plate has become an excellent device for the osteoarthritic and post-traumatic wrist.[15–17] The bulk on the dorsum of the wrist is significantly decreased with this plate. Therefore, there is less interference with gliding of the extensor tendons, easier closure of the dorsal soft tissue, and less pressure on the dorsal skin postoperatively. The plate often does not have to be removed.

In patients with rheumatoid arthritis, we have used Steinmann pin internal fixation almost exclu-

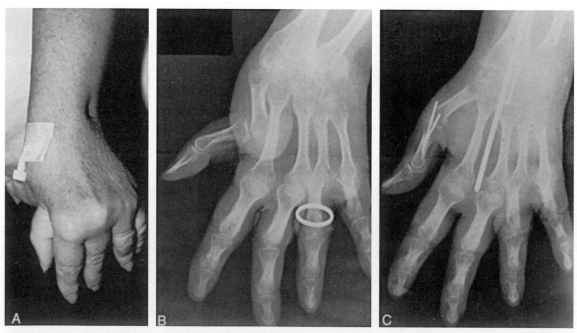

Figure 38–1. An example of total wrist fusion with intermetacarpal technique. *A*, Preoperative appearance of wrist affected with rheumatoid arthritis. Note ulnar shift of the carpus. *B*, Radiograph demonstrates severe deformity. Midcarpal joints are severely involved. *C*, Postoperative radiograph shows improved wrist alignment, with Steinmann pin fixation between the second and third metacarpals.

sively.[23, 24, 26] Several variations of this technique use intermetacarpal, intrametacarpal, and dual intermetacarpal pins.[12, 23, 24, 26, 28] The advantage of this method is its relative simplicity and speed, which allows other procedures to be performed concomitantly. The technique also allows a briefer period of postoperative immobilization (approximately 3 weeks of short-arm immobilization). In patients with osteoarthritis or post-traumatic arthritis, we prefer the dual-pin or plate fixation technique.

We use three different methods of Steinmann pin fixation for our wrist arthrodesis.[12, 23, 24, 26, 28] In the first, the intermetacarpal technique, we place a single Steinmann pin between the second and third metacarpals and drive it into the medullary canal of the radius (Fig. 38–1). In the second, the intrametacarpal technique, we place the Steinmann pin within the medullary canal of the third or, occasionally, the second metacarpal and then into the radius (Figs. 38–2 and 38–3). In the third technique (dual-pin technique), we use two intermetacarpal pins (Figs. 38–4 and 38–5). When a substantial amount of carpus remains for bone fixation distally, or if the metacarpophalangeal joint is to be preserved, either of the intermetacarpal techniques is employed. We also use the intermetacarpal techniques if the medullary canals of the metacarpals are particularly narrow, as is common in patients with juvenile rheumatoid arthritis. In this situation, the small-diameter Steinmann pin needed to enter the medullary canal of the metacarpal would fit loosely in the radius, and the fixation would not be stable.

In wrists with severe bone loss, we obtain distal stability by placing the Steinmann pin within the shaft of the third metacarpal; this is known as the intrametacarpal wrist fusion technique. The added bone fixation with the pin in this intramedullary position is mandatory in patients with the "arthritis mutilans" variant. Because of the destroyed carpus in arthritis mutilans, the attempted fusion is essentially between the radius and the bases of the metacarpals.

Approach

Carefully apply and pad a brachial tourniquet without twisting the skin. Inflate the tourniquet to 100 mmHg above systolic pressure. We often use double tourniquets, alternated hourly, to decrease the local damage and prolong safe tourniquet time.[11]

Make a straight longitudinal dorsal incision centered over the wrist joint. Use the length of the incision needed for the specific technique. Do not use zigzag or S-shaped incisions because of their increased incidence of skin necrosis. Meticulously preserve the dorsal veins and cutaneous nerves in the subcutaneous flaps. If needed, raise thick flaps by taking the dissection directly down to the extensor retinaculum. In rheumatoid arthritis, divide the midportion of the fourth compartment to perform a dorsal tenosynovectomy. If needed, divide the vertical septa of the retinaculum between compartments three through six. Take care to identify and protect the extensor pollicis longus (EPL) tendon as it crosses the second compartment distal to Lister's tubercle. Retract the tendons in Penrose drains to expose the capsule.

The terminal branch of the posterior interosseous

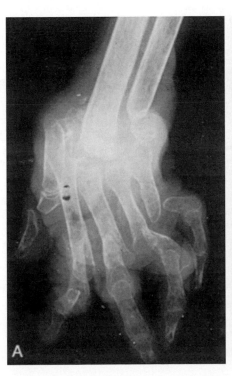
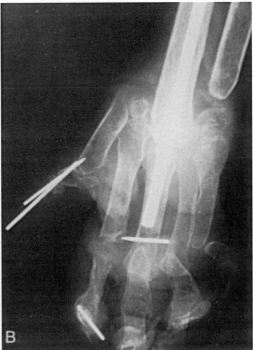

Figure 38–2. An example of total wrist fusion with intrametacarpal technique. *A,* Preoperative radiograph shows complete loss of the carpus secondary to rheumatoid arthritis. *B,* Postoperative fixation with a large Steinmann pin. A transverse Kirschner wire is used to prevent distal migration.

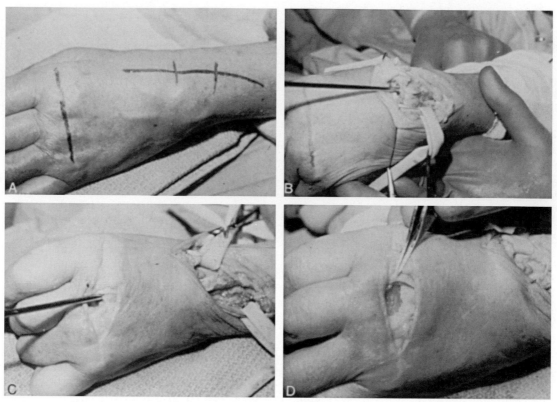

Figure 38–3. This figure demonstrates the intrametacarpal technique with metacarpophalangeal joint arthroplasty. *A,* Typical wrist incision for fusion. *B,* A Steinmann pin is inserted into the radius to predetermine length. *C,* Final insertion of the Steinmann pin via the third metacarpal head, prepared for prosthesis insertion. *D,* Note the Swanson prosthesis after Steinmann pin wrist fixation.

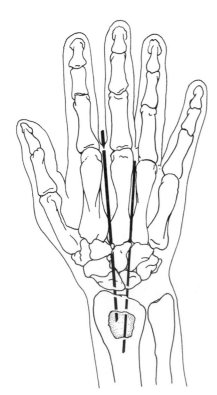

Figure 38–4. Dual-pin technique for wrist fusion. Steinmann pins are inserted through the dorsal aspects of the second and third web spaces. A dorsal window in the radius allows the pins to be driven into the radius under direct vision.

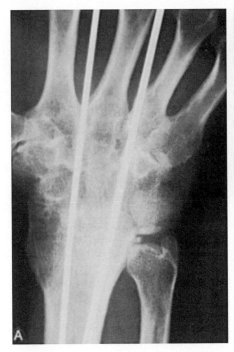
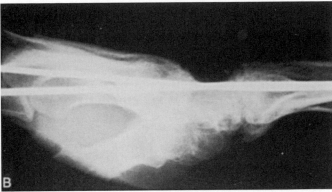

Figure 38–5. *A* and *B,* Two views of total wrist fusion using iliac crest bone graft and dual intermetacarpal rod internal fixation for post-traumatic arthritis of the wrist. Note wrist fusion position in slight dorsiflexion and slight ulnar deviation.

nerve lies in the floor of the fourth compartment. Partially denervate the wrist by dividing this nerve.[3, 9] Alternatively, when a tenosynovectomy is not needed, identify the EPL tendon distally, and open the third compartment completely.[33] Retract the EPL tendon with a Penrose drain. For radial exposure, osteotomize Lister's tubercle. This step facilitates subperiosteal exposure and provides a flat surface for a plate as well as an entrance for radial bone graft. Subperiosteal elevation of the fourth compartment completes the exposure of the radius. In Steinmann pin fixation, divide the capsule transversely and open it as a distally based flap. With plate fixation, open the capsule longitudinally.

Remove the articular cartilage from the distal radius, from the proximal and middle carpal rows, and, if necessary, from the carpometacarpal joints of the second and third metacarpals. We usually do not include the scaphotrapeziotrapezoid (STT) joint. We usually fuse the lunotriquetral and triquetrohamate joints in all patients, but not the firm articulation between the capitate and hamate if it is uninvolved in patients without rheumatoid arthritis. Expose bleeding cancellous bone using sharp osteotomes, curettes, and rongeurs. Do not use high-speed burs because of the risk of thermal bone necrosis. Remove enough bone from the proximal row to allow correction of any wrist deformity. Pack bone graft from the distal radius (Lister's tubercle), the distal ulna (if this is resected at the same time), or the iliac crest between the carpal bones. We prefer local bone graft when sufficient, especially when using a plate. Use iliac crest bone graft in a failed previous fusion, in a significant bone defect, or if other sources are not available. If needed, reconstruct the distal radioulnar joint (see Chapter 24) to allow painless forearm rotation. If there is significant ulnar impaction, removal of a portion of the proximal ulnar carpal row is an alternative to ulnar shortening (see Fig. 38–8).[32]

Intermetacarpal Steinmann Pin Technique

Prepare the bone surfaces for fusion as described. Enter the medullary canal of the radius with a pointed awl, and by hand, insert the largest size Steinmann pin possible into the medullary canal of the radius. At this time, determine the length of the pin needed (to be cut later). Remove the pin from the radius. Cut the pointed proximal end of the pin to minimize the risk of perforating the radial cortex, and attach the pin to a power drill. With the wrist in flexion, and aiming for the space between the second and third metacarpal heads, carefully drill the pin distally through the carpus. Then remove the pin from the drill and tap it through the soft tissue; to prevent injury, do not drill the pin through the soft tissue. It is critical that the pin be parallel with the third metacarpal shaft to avoid unwanted deviation of the hand when the pin is re-inserted into the radius. After the pin emerges through the skin between the metacarpal heads, withdraw it until just the tip is flush with the proximal aspect of the carpus. Carefully determine the length of the pin needed. A pin that is too short may migrate postoperatively. A pin that is too long may become impacted in the proximal portion of the radius or may perforate or split the radius. Cut the pin distally to its appropriate length.

Add bone chips to the radiocarpal space. Confirm correct alignment of the hand in relation to the forearm before finally seating the pin. Tap the pin into the radius, and countersink it approximately 2 cm proximal to the level of the metacarpophalangeal joints. Carefully tapping the pin into the radius instead of drilling it helps prevent perforation of the radial cortex by the pin. Use a bone staple or an obliquely placed Kirschner wire for additional stability, if needed. Obtain intraoperative radiographs if there is any question about the position of the pin (see Fig. 38–1).

Intramedullary Steinmann Pin Technique

In the rheumatoid patient with loss of bone stock, introduce the pin into the third metacarpal bone to augment stability. To obtain exposure and prepare the bony surfaces of the radiocarpal joint, use the techniques as previously described. As in the intermedullary technique, the Steinmann pin is hand placed into the medullary canal of the radius to determine the length needed.

Countersink the distal end of the Steinmann pin sufficiently to allow insertion of the proximal stem of a metacarpophalangeal (MP) joint implant. Consider this factor when determining the final pin length. Insert the Steinmann pin directly into the canal of the metacarpal after resecting the head. Then tap the pin into the prepared opening into the radius. Place a bone plug (metacarpal head or distal ulna) in the metacarpal canal to help prevent the rod from backing out. When the pin is fully inserted, there should be just sufficient space for the proximal stem of an MP joint implant (see Fig. 38–3).[25]

If the MP joint does not need replacement, open the dorsal articular surface of the metacarpal with a small awl, and introduce the Steinmann pin. The defect produced becomes covered with fibrocartilage (see Fig. 38–2). If the MP joint is uninvolved, insert the pin either through an opening in the distal dorsal metacarpal shaft or by using the intramedullary rod technique as advocated by Mannerfelt and Malmsten.[21] This latter technique does allow more leeway in determining wrist position, because the flexible pin is bent to provide wrist extension. However, the rod is more difficult to insert than a Steinmann pin and may not provide as rigid fixation. The dual-pin technique may be a better alternative in these cases.

Comparison of Intermetacarpal and Intrametacarpal Steinmann Pin Internal Fixation Techniques

The intrametacarpal technique is technically easier to perform than the intermetacarpal method and ensures good alignment by lining up the medullary canals of the third metacarpal and radius. With the intermetacarpal technique, use care to avoid aligning the wrist in exaggerated ulnar deviation, which can occur if the insertion of the pin is not parallel to the third metacarpal shaft. In the intramedullary technique, it may be necessary to use a smaller-diameter pin, thus reducing the fixation. With the intermetacarpal technique, late removal of the pin is often necessary but it is easy. Ordinarily, we do not remove an intramedullary pin. Both techniques of wrist fusion can correct angular deformities and lateral shift of the carpus in relation to the radius.

The intrametacarpal technique holds the wrist in neutral flexion-extension because of the rigidity of the Steinmann pin. This position is excellent for most patients with rheumatoid arthritis.[20] To vary the amount of flexion or extension of the wrist by 5° to 10° in the intermetacarpal technique, alter the direction of the Steinmann pin while driving it into the radius.

Dual-Pin Technique

The single-pin techniques previously described dictate that the wrist be positioned very close to neutral flexion-extension. The single pin, even though large in diameter, may not provide secure rotatory stability. Therefore, we have developed a modification for wrist fusion in patients both with and without rheumatoid arthritis.[12, 26, 28]

Prepare the wrist as described previously. Rather than use a single, large Steinmann pin, we use two relatively thin pins (5/64 inch to 7/64 inch in diameter). Insert the pins through the dorsal aspect of the second and third web spaces between the metacarpal bones, across the carpus, and into the medullary canal of the radius. This maneuver results in a "stacked-pin" effect in the radius, which provides rotational stability as well as anteroposterior and lateral stability without the need for supplementary internal fixation (see Figs. 38–4 and 38–5). The pins are thin enough to bend after their insertion into the radius, allowing final correction and adjustment of the wrist position. Thus, if slightly more extension is desired after the rods are in place, gently manipulate the wrist into the desired position. The use of thinner pins minimizes the potential for compression of the intrinsic muscles of the hand (interossei) by a large rod, which may result in fibrosis and secondary intrinsic contracture.

Take care to insert the pins through the dorsal portion of the web space to avoid damage to the neurovascular structures in the palm. Occasionally it is useful to make a small cortical window in the dorsal distal radius to guide the pins into the medullary canal of the radius under direct vision (see Fig. 38–4). Harvest additional cancellous bone graft from the distal radius as well. Cut the pins short beneath the skin in the web spaces.

We use the dual-pin technique in patients with

rheumatoid arthritis even when carpal bone stock is minimal. Its advantages include ease of hardware insertion and removal, stable fixation, and the ability to adjust the position of the wrist at the time of surgery in both the anteroposterior and lateral planes (see Fig. 38–5). Postoperatively, we use a short-arm cast that allows early forearm motion.

Surgical Technique for ASIF Plate Fixation

For the patient with post-traumatic arthritis or osteoarthritis and for the occasional patient with rheumatoid arthritis, ASIF plate fixation is an excellent technique.[4, 15–17]

Use the approach through the third compartment with transposition of the EPL tendon. Prepare the wrist joint as described previously, including the third and, occasionally, the second carpometacarpal (CMC) joints. Expose the third CMC joint using an osteotome to remove the overlying bone.

We use a specially designed titanium, low-contact dynamic compression plate produced by Synthes (Paoli, PA) for wrist arthrodesis (Fig. 38–6). Recessed screw heads, tapered plate edges, and a tapered distal plate width avoid dorsal prominence. Three different plates are available. Two of the plates are precontoured, one with a short bend for smaller wrists and one with a longer bend for larger wrists. The precontoured plates provide 10° of extension. The third plate is straight and is used when the other plates are not appropriate, such as when using a large corticocancellous graft. Each plate has eight holes for screws. Three 2.7-mm screws are used in the metacarpal, one 2.7-mm screw in the capitate, and four 3.5-mm screws in the radius.

Choose the appropriate plate and contour the wrist to fit it. Shave bone from the dorsal aspect of the distal radius, lunate, scaphoid, capitate, and third

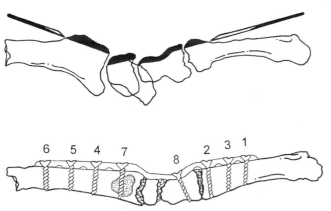

Figure 38–6. ASIF technique for wrist fusion. The dorsal aspect of the radius, carpal bones, and third carpometacarpal (CMC) joint is contoured to accept the plate. The precontoured plate is applied with the screws in the appropriate order (indicated by numbers *1* to *8*) after bone graft is placed.

metacarpal base with an osteotome until the bone fits the plate (see Fig. 38–6). With the plate temporarily positioned, make a window radial to the plate to harvest bone graft if needed. Leave the distal 1 cm of radial cancellous bone in place to avoid perforation of the distal radial surface. In cases of significant bone loss of the proximal row (Kienböck's disease or trauma), we remove the proximal row and use it for bone graft; we therefore do not use the iliac crest[2, 30] (Fig. 38–7). We always prepare the iliac crest, but the local shavings and distal radius graft are often enough.[15, 16]

Evaluate the ulnar carpus to make sure that shortening the wrist has not caused ulnar impaction. Insert bone graft, and position the plate over the third metacarpal. Mark the most distal hole, making sure that the most proximal of the three metacarpal screws will be in the metacarpal base and not the CMC joint. To see the whole shaft of the metacarpal, remove the plate and place the screw in the center of the metacarpal. Drill a 2-mm hole for the 2.7-mm screw in the center of the metacarpal directly posterior to anterior. Placement of the screw directly posterior to anterior prevents a rotational deformity. Center the two other metacarpal screws. Use standard ASIF technique to secure the plate to the metacarpal.

Align the plate over the radius. Achieve a slight amount of ulnar deviation by skewing the position of the plate. Check the most proximal hole to ensure satisfactory position of the plate over the radius. Manually compress the wrist. Eccentrically place the second-most distal radius screw. Place the remaining radial screws and the capitate screw in the appropriate order (see Fig. 38–6). A small fluoroscopy unit facilitates accurate plate and screw placement. Obtain intraoperative radiographs to confirm position and fixation (Fig. 38–8). Close the wound as described in the next section.

Closure

It is advisable to use either a suction or Penrose drain. Close the capsule loosely with an absorbable suture. Cover the distal plate using dorsal fascia and periosteum. If the third compartment was opened initially, leave the EPL tendon subcutaneous. If needed, cover the plate using the extensor carpi radialis brevis. If the fourth compartment was opened, transpose either all or half of the extensor retinaculum under the extensor tendons. Close the subcutaneous tissue and skin with interrupted suture. Apply a bulky dressing. Immobilize the limb in anterior and posterior short-arm splints for support and compression. Use a sugar tong splint if a distal radial ulnar joint procedure was done simultaneously.

POSTOPERATIVE CARE

Change the dressing and splint and remove the drain on the first postoperative day. Encourage immediate

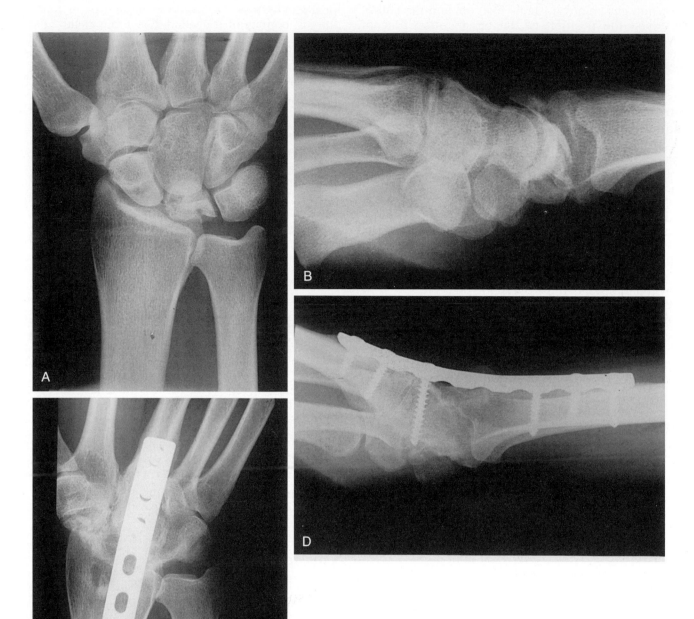

Figure 30–7. This patient is a 28-year-old heavy laborer with stage IIIB Kienböck's disease who needed a strong, painless wrist. *A* and *B*, Preoperative radiographs documenting stage IIIB Kienböck's disease. *C* and *D*, Postoperative radiographs after proximal row carpectomy and low-contact dynamic plate fixation prior to the availability of the precontoured plate. The proximal row along with distal radial bone was used as bone graft. The iliac crest was not used for bone graft.

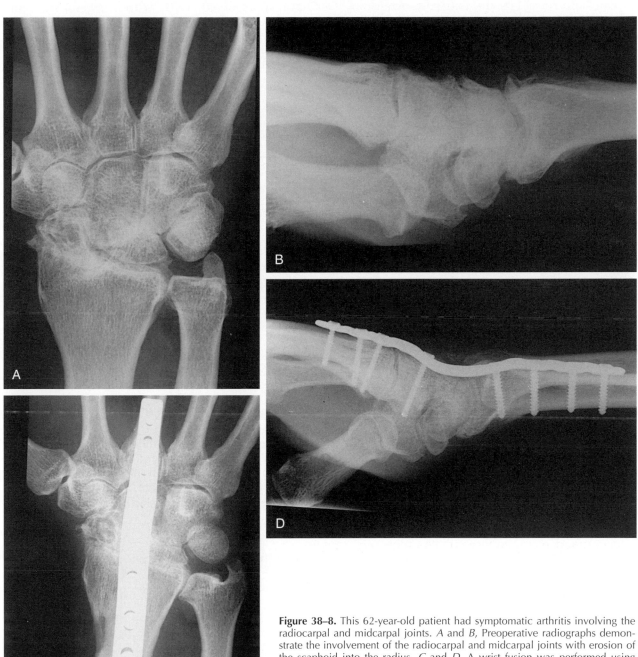

Figure 38–8. This 62-year-old patient had symptomatic arthritis involving the radiocarpal and midcarpal joints. *A* and *B*, Preoperative radiographs demonstrate the involvement of the radiocarpal and midcarpal joints with erosion of the scaphoid into the radius. *C* and *D*, A wrist fusion was performed using the precontoured ASIF plate. The triquetrum was excised to prevent ulnar impaction secondary to the scaphoid eroding into the radius and subsequent loss of height. Distal radial bone, the excised triquetrum, and the dorsal shaving were used as bone graft. The iliac crest was not used as bone graft.

finger and thumb motion to prevent stiffness and extensor tendon adhesions. Extending the MP joints with the proximal and distal interphalangeal joints flexed can help to isolate the extrinsic extensors. If the internal fixation provides satisfactory rotatory stability, apply a short-arm cast or splint for 3 weeks, after the sutures are removed. With plate fixation, simply apply a compressive garment and thermoplastic splint. Short-arm immobilization facilitates early motion of the elbow and shoulder as well as the forearm and is much easier for patients to tolerate, particularly those with rheumatoid arthritis. Preoperatively instruct patients who require crutches in the use of platform crutches, which are employed until the fusion has consolidated.

With single Steinmann pin fixation, we usually leave the pin in place. If it causes discomfort, it can be removed as early as 4 months postoperatively, after the fusion has healed. With the dual-pin technique, we usually remove the pins after bone union, between 4 and 6 months postoperatively.

We usually remove the pins using local anesthesia. We make a vertical incision in the web space and grasp the pin end with a large diamond-jaw needle holder. A Craig pin extractor can also be used. If the pins produce no symptoms, however, we leave them in place.

COMPLICATIONS OF WRIST FUSION

Many complications following wrist fusion have been reported.[7, 34] The most common complication in the series evaluated by Clendenin and Green[7] was pseudarthrosis. In post-traumatic cases, ASIF technique has been reported to have a lower rate of pseudarthrosis.[15, 18] Some complications are technique dependent. Those specific to ASIF plate technique include the need for a secondary extensor tenolysis (3.5 percent) and plate tenderness. The incidence of these complications may be decreased by the new plate design.[16]

Complications of the Steinmann pin techniques include pin migration, which causes flexor tendon impingement and/or a mechanical block to metacarpophalangeal joint flexion, and pin breakage. Other complications, regardless of technique, occur rarely but include deep wound infection, superficial skin necrosis, transient median nerve or superficial radial nerve compression, reflex sympathetic dystrophy, and fracture of the healed fusion. Carpometacarpal pain has been seen following wrist fusion, and as described previously, we recommend including the third CMC joint in the fusion when a plate is used. We include both the second and third CMC joints in young patients, especially heavy laborers, when the dual-pin technique is used.[8] Uncommon complications of iliac crest graft include hematoma, pain, and pelvic fracture.

Several of our patients have had transient sensory neuropathies of the median nerve following wrist fusion. Patients with severe flexion deformities with shortening are most susceptible. These complications have all resolved, most within several days of the procedure. We have seen no superficial skin necrosis since we began using a straight or slightly curved longitudinal skin incision. Skin necrosis occurred occasionally when we were using zigzag or S-shaped incisions, and we do not recommend such incisions for this reason. Large-diameter Steinmann pins have caused intrinsic contractures with decreased metacarpophalangeal joint motion (i.e., loss of extension) after being placed between the metacarpals in some of our patients. Smaller-diameter pins have not caused this complication.

CONCLUSION

Total wrist arthrodesis remains the single most predictable and reliable surgical procedure for treating wrist problems, regardless of their cause. Most patients tolerate wrist fusion because it is stable and painless and permits strenuous use. Most patients are able to return to their regular occupations, even though some modifications in the use of the extremity may be necessary. However, mechanics and others who must position their hands in tight or cramped spaces (i.e., behind engines) have difficulty. Sports activities that require wrist motion also are more difficult. Many patients have been able to modify the use of their arms after wrist fusion so that they are still able to enjoy their chosen sports and avocations. According to American Medical Association's *Guides to the Evaluation of Permanent Impairment*, total wrist fusion in "neutral" position results in a 30 percent loss of upper extremity function.[35] Total wrist fusion is an excellent option in the surgical treatment of wrist disease.

References

1. Benkeddache Y, Gottesman H, Fourrier P: Multiple stapling for wrist arthrodesis in the nonrheumatoid patient. J Hand Surg 9A:256–260, 1984.
2. Bolano LE, Green DP: Wrist arthrodesis in post-traumatic arthritis: A comparison of two methods. J Hand Surg 18A:786–791, 1993.
3. Buck-Gramcko D: Denervation of the wrist joint. J Hand Surg 2:54–61, 1977.
4. Buck-Gramcko D, Lohman H: Compression arthrodesis of the wrist. In Tubiana R (ed): The Hand. Philadelphia, WB Saunders Co. 1985, vol. 2, pp 723–729.
5. Campbell CJ, Koekarn T: Total and subtotal arthrodesis of the wrist. J Bone Joint Surg 46A:1520–1533, 1964.
6. Carroll RE, Dick HM: Arthrodesis of the wrist for rheumatoid arthritis. J Bone Joint Surg 53A:1365–1369, 1971.
7. Clendenin MB, Green DP: Arthrodesis of the wrist—complications and their management. J Hand Surg 6:253–257, 1981.
8. Dass G, Feldon P: Carpometacarpal pain after wrist fusion. Presented at the 1993 Annual Meeting of the American Society for Surgery of the Hand, Kansas City, Missouri.
9. Dellon AL: Partial wrist denervation; resection of the distal posterior interosseous nerve. J Hand Surg 10A:527–533, 1985.

10. Dick HM: Wrist and intercarpal arthrodesis. In Green DP (ed): Operative Hand Surgery. New York, Churchill Livingstone, 1982.
11. Dreyfuss UY, Smith RJ: Sensory changes with prolonged double-cuff tourniquet time in hand surgery. J Hand Surg 13A: 736–740, 1988.
12. Feldon PG, Millender LH, Nalebuff EA: Rheumatoid arthritis in the hand and wrist. In Green D (ed): Operative Hand Surgery. New York, Churchill Livingstone, 1993, pp 1587–1690.
13. Flatt, AE: Care of the Arthritic Hand, ed 4. St Louis, CV Mosby, 1983.
14. Haddad RJ, Riordan DC: Arthrodesis of the wrist. J Bone Joint Surg 49A:950–954, 1967.
15. Hastings H: Arthrodesis of the osteoarthritic wrist. In Gelberman RH (ed): Master Techniques in Orthopaedic Surgery: The Wrist. New York, Raven Press, 1994, pp 345–360.
16. Hastings H: Total wrist arthrodesis for post-traumatic conditions. The Indiana Hand Center Newsletter 1:1–15, 1993.
17. Hastings H, Weiss APC: Wrist arthrodesis for posttraumatic arthritis: A prospective study of plate and local bone graft application. Presented at the 1993 Annual Meeting of the American Society for Surgery of the Hand, Kansas City, Missouri.
18. Hannington KR, Strickland JW, Wiedeman GP, et al: Arthrodesis for post-traumatic arthritis of the wrist: Reliability and function. Paper presented at the 1987 Annual Meeting of the American Society for Surgery of the Hand, San Antonio, Texas.
19. Larsson S: Compression arthrodesis of the wrist. Clin Orthop 99:146–153, 1974.
20. Linscheid RL, Dobyns JH: Rheumatoid arthritis of the wrist. Orthop Clin North Am 2:649–665, 1971.
21. Mannerfelt L, Malmsten M: Arthrodesis of the wrist in rheumatoid arthritis; a technique without external fixation. Scand J Plas Reconstr Surg 5:124–130, 1971.
22. Milford L: The Hand. St Louis, CV Mosby, 1982.
23. Millender LH, Nalebuff EA: Arthrodesis of the rheumatoid wrist: An evaluation of sixty patients and a description of a different surgical technique. J Bone Joint Surg 55A:1026–1034, 1973.
24. Millender LH, Nalebuff EA: Arthrodesis of the rheumatoid wrist. J Bone Joint Surg 55A:1026–1034, 1973.
25. Millender LH, Phillips C: Combined wrist arthrodesis and metacarpal joint arthroplasty in rheumatoid arthritis. Orthopedics 1:43–48, 1978.
26. Millender LH, Terrono AL, Feldon PG: Arthrodesis of the rheumatoid wrist. In Gelberman RH (ed): Master Techniques in Orthopaedic Surgery: The Wrist. New York, Raven Press, 1994, pp 287–300.
27. Nalebuff EA, Garrod KJ: Present approach to the severely involved rheumatoid wrist. Orthop Clin North Am 15:369–380, 1984.
28. O'Donovan T, Feldon P, Belsky MR: Dual rod fixation for wrist fusion. Presented at the 1990 Annual Meeting of the American Society for Surgery of the Hand, Toronto.
29. Richards RR, Patterson SD, Hearn TC: A special plate for arthrodesis of the wrist: Design considerations and biomechanical testing. J Hand Surg 18A:476–483, 1993.
30. Richards RS, Roth JH: Pancarpal fusion with proximal row carpectomy. Presented at the 1993 Annual Meeting of the American Society for Surgery of the Hand, Kansas City, Missouri.
31. Taleisnik J: The Wrist. New York, Churchill Livingstone, 1985.
32. Trumble T, Easterling KJ, Smith RJ: Ulnocarpal abutment after wrist arthrodesis. J Hand Surg 13A:11–15, 1988.
33. Weil C, Ruby LK: The dorsal approach revisited. J Hand Surg 11A:911–912, 1986.
34. Zachary SV, Stern PJ: Complications following AO wrist fusion. Presented at the 1993 Annual Meeting of the American Society for Surgery of the Hand, Kansas City, Missouri.
35. American Medical Association: Guides to the Evaluation of Permanent Impairment, 4th ed. Chicago, American Medical Association, 1993.

CHAPTER 39

Amputations About the Wrist

Gary R. Pollock, MD, PharmD, Robert H. Meier, III, MD, and David M. Lichtman, MD

Next to the brain, the hand is the greatest asset to man, and to it is due the development of man's handiwork.

Sterling Bunnell, MD

There are approximately 90,000 people with upper extremity amputations in the United States; of these, 12 to 15 percent have amputations about the wrist.[14, 16] In marked contrast to amputations in the lower extremity, those in the upper extremity are mostly due to trauma, with a lesser number secondary to tumors, congenital anomalies, or peripheral vascular disorders.

The classic demographic description of an upper extremity amputee is a young, healthy male who has sustained a work-related injury to the dominant hand. The most common level, through the proximal to middle radius and ulna, accounts for 57 percent of all arm amputations.[10, 14] Outcome studies evaluating the functional return of patients either to their previous occupation or to a similar vocation are lacking. Unlike lower extremity amputees, only 50 percent of upper extremity amputees choose to wear a prosthesis.

GOALS OF AMPUTATION MANAGEMENT

A complete and thorough understanding of surgical principles is mandatory in order to achieve functional restoration of the amputated upper extremity. However, functional rehabilitation of the patient involves much more than the surgical procedure. For full rehabilitation of the amputee, nine distinct phases have been developed that identify treatment goals and objectives as well as provide a method to measure progress and to recognize problems.[12] These nine phases are:

Phase I:	Preoperative
Phase II:	Surgical reconstruction
Phase III:	Acute postoperative
Phase IV:	Preprosthetic
Phase V:	Prosthetic fabrication
Phase VI:	Prosthetic training
Phase VII:	Community integration
Phase VIII:	Vocational rehabilitation
Phase IX:	Follow-up

Each phase deals with distinctly different aspects of the rehabilitation program. Although the focus of this chapter is on amputations about the wrist, these nine phases can be applied to all levels of amputation in both upper and lower extremities.

REHABILITATION PROGRAM

Preoperative Phase

In traumatic amputations, the preoperative planning phase is usually a short and stressful period. It is desirable, however, to discuss the surgical options and goals of rehabilitation with the patient and family to the extent possible. In amputations performed for medical reasons (e.g., malignant tumors), more time is available for planning and discussion. In this case, the entire treatment team can be utilized, and consultations obtained from the physiatrist, prosthetist, and physical therapist.

The first order of business during the planning phase is selecting the appropriate level of amputation. Usually, the traumatic injury or medical condition dictates the required level. Preservation of maximum length is also desired. Under certain circumstances, however, especially in amputations about the wrist, it may be in the patient's best interest to elect a more proximal level.

During the initial evaluation, it is important to perform a complete physical examination to rule out subtle concomitant injuries. A brachial plexus injury masked by a more dramatic distal amputation can markedly affect the patient's postoperative ability to operate an upper extremity terminal device.

AMPUTATION LEVELS

General Considerations

Amputation levels about the wrist are partial hand (transmetacarpal and transcarpal), wrist disarticulation, and distal forearm (transradial). In order to select the appropriate level, the surgeon must first understand the patient's unique social and physical requirements. These are related to (1) the pathologic condition for which the amputation is being performed, (2) the status of the skin, nerves, and circulation of the distal segments, (3) the neurovascular status and residual motion of the proximal limb segments, (4) the cosmetic needs of the patient, (5) the functional needs of the patient, and (6) the status of the other arm. A thorough knowledge of the patient's general health and medical condition is also necessary. This information, combined with a thorough understanding of the contemporary applications and limitations of the upper extremity prosthesis, helps the surgeon select the most appropriate amputation level for each patient.

Transcarpal Level

Under most circumstances, a transcarpal amputation is undesirable, and we believe a wrist disarticulation is a much more preferable level, even in bilateral amputations. However, some patients with transcarpal amputations note that the transcarpal level is useful for "bimanual" activities. One advantage of the transcarpal level is retention of full forearm pronation and supination, if the distal radioulnar joint is intact. However, with a prosthesis, the bulky distal segment makes fitting a terminal device more difficult, with a less desirable cosmetic result than that of a standard transradial amputation (Fig. 39–1). Therefore, most patients, especially women, prefer a wrist disarticulation or a transradial amputation. Those patients who choose to have a transmetacarpal or transcarpal level can use an opposition post or pad for grasping objects in lieu of a terminal device. These passive prostheses do not function as precisely as a standard terminal device but do give better sensory feedback.

Wrist Disarticulation

Wrist disarticulation is an excellent amputation level (Fig. 39–2). With an intact distal radioulnar joint, most forearm pronation and most supination are retained. Residual rotation at this level is approximately 120°, with a proportional loss of rotation as the level proceeds proximally. Long distal forearm

amputations have a residual rotation of 100° to 120°; mid-forearm amputations, 60° to 100°; and short-forearm amputations, 0 to 60°.[9] However, even with preservation of all forearm rotation, only 50 percent can be utilized by the prosthesis. The length of residual forearm in a wrist disarticulation also improves the mechanical level arm for controlling the terminal device.

The principal disadvantage of this level of amputation is the relatively long and bulky prosthetic wrist unit required (see Fig. 39–9B). For this reason, most women, particularly those with slim wrists, prefer a more proximal level of amputation.

Distal Forearm Level

Distal forearm (transradial) amputations allow for considerable residual limb pronation and supination; but as previously discussed, rotation is lost as the level proceeds proximally. If less than 50 percent of the forearm length remains, residual limb pronation and supination are lost with use of a prosthesis. The principal advantage of a transradial amputation is that it permits a myofascial closure, which provides a good soft tissue envelope and a more cylindrical contour of the terminal stump. The bone is transfixed in the soft tissues, preventing unwanted movement. The residual muscles remain at their resting length, improving kinesthetic feedback, which is important to prosthetic training. In addition, the use of a standard wrist unit is cosmetically acceptable. Overall, this level of amputation is very successful at meeting the functional and cosmetic needs of most patients (Fig. 39–3).

Bilateral Upper Limb Amputation

Bilateral upper limb amputation is unquestionably a catastrophic injury. Preservation of length is of the utmost importance, and the longer residual extremity usually becomes dominant. Most cases should be referred to specialized centers that are capable of offering the patient with bilateral upper extremity ampu-

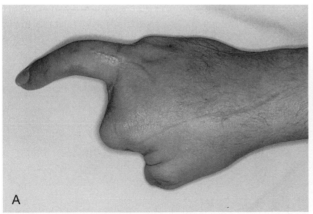
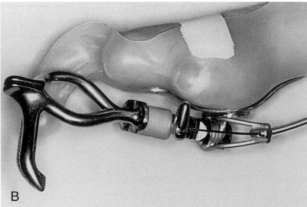

Figure 39–1. *A,* Transmetacarpal amputee with a single sensate digit. *B,* This illustration demonstrates how difficult the terminal device is to fit.

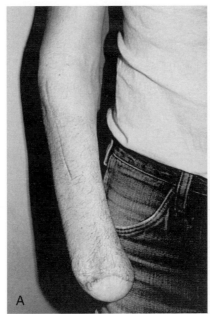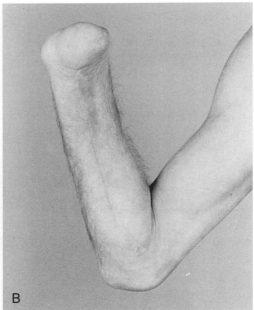

Figure 39–2. Wrist disarticulation, dorsal view *(A)* and palmar view *(B)*.

tation a comprehensive and complete rehabilitation program.

Surgical Reconstruction Phase: Surgical Techniques

The goal of amputation surgery is to create a terminal stump that is maximally efficient and functionally receptive to a prosthesis. The skin and subcutaneous tissues must provide adequate soft tissue coverage and remain pliable. The overlying skin should be sensate, but not overly sensitive. Secondary procedures, including split-thickness skin grafts and free or rotational pedicle flaps, may be required to achieve these goals.

TRANSCARPAL AMPUTATION

Fashion the skin flaps with a long palmar flap and a short dorsal flap in a ratio of 2:1. Dissect the flaps proximally, exposing the soft tissues to the level of the proposed amputation. Pull the digital flexor and extensor tendons distally, transect them, and allow them to retract into the forearm. Dissect and remove the wrist flexors and extensors from their insertion sites. At this time, if passive terminal stump flexion and extension are desired, some surgeons re-insert the wrist flexors and extensors into the carpus in line with their normal position. We see little advantage to this modification under most circumstances, and it only increases the already bulky nature of the distal terminal stump.

With gentle traction, pull distally and ligate the median and ulnar nerves along with the branches of the sensory radial nerve. Allow them to retract into the soft tissues proximally. Doubly ligate the ulnar

and radial arteries at a point proximal to the amputation level. Transect the exposed bone, and contour all sharp edges. The level of amputation through the carpus should preserve as much of the distal and proximal carpal rows as possible.

Obtain hemostasis after releasing the tourniquet. Use interrupted sutures to close the subcutaneous tissues and skin. Insert a drain of choice to evacuate

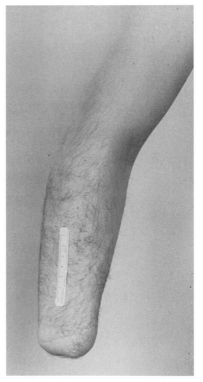

Figure 39–3. Distal forearm (transradial) amputation, dorsal view.

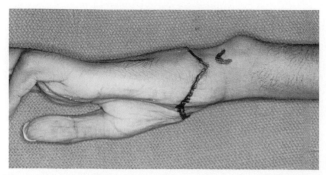

Figure 39–4. Wrist disarticulation showing the long palmar and short dorsal flaps from the ulnar side.

any residual hematoma. Apply a rigid plaster pressure dressing.

WRIST DISARTICULATION

Fashion the skin flaps with a long palmar flap and a short dorsal flap in a ratio of 2:1. Begin the incision 1 to 2 cm distal to both the radial and ulnar styloid processes and carry it volarly and dorsally in a fishmouth fashion (Fig. 39–4). Reflect the soft tissues and skin flaps together proximally to the radiocarpal joint. Identify the digital and wrist flexor and extensor tendons, pull them distally, transect them, and allow them to retract into the forearm.

With gentle traction, pull distally and ligate the median, ulnar, radial sensory, and posterior interosseous nerves. Allow them to retract into the soft tissues proximally. Doubly ligate the ulnar, radial, anterior interosseous, and posterior interosseous arteries at a point proximal to the radiocarpal joint. Incise the wrist ligaments and joint capsule circumferentially to complete the disarticulation. Resect the radial and ulnar styloid processes, and contour the bone to a smooth round terminal stump (Fig. 39–5). The major benefit of this amputation level is forearm rotation, which depends on preservation of a functioning dis-

tal radioulnar joint and triangular fibrocartilage complex. Therefore, take care not to resect too much ulnar styloid.

Obtain hemostasis after releasing the tourniquet. Use interrupted sutures to close the subcutaneous tissues and skin (Fig. 39–6). Insert a drain of choice to evacuate any residual hematoma. Apply a rigid plaster pressure dressing.

DISTAL FOREARM (TRANSRADIAL) AMPUTATION

Maximum length should always be preserved with distal forearm amputations. Fashion palmar and dorsal skin flaps of equal lengths. Design the flap length to measure approximately half the diameter of the forearm at the chosen level. Dissect the soft tissues and skin flaps proximally to the level of the bone amputation. Remove a minimum of 2 cm of distal radius and ulna to accommodate the prosthetic wrist unit. Transect the tendons and muscle bellies transversely on the volar and dorsal aspects of the forearm at the level of the bone amputation. With gentle traction, pull distally and ligate the median, ulnar, radial sensory, and posterior interosseous nerves; allow them to retract into the soft tissues proximally. Doubly ligate the radial, ulnar, anterior interosseous, and posterior interosseous arteries at a point proximal to the amputation level. Transect the radius and ulna, leaving the radius approximately 1 to 2 cm longer. Contour and smooth with a rasp any rough bone edges.

All transradial amputations should have a myofascial closure.[5] Fashion the closure utilizing a long volar flap of flexor digitorum superficialis muscle pulled distally around the end of the bones and sutured to the deep dorsal fascia. Obtain hemostasis after releasing the tourniquet. Use interrupted sutures to close the deep fascia, subcutaneous tissues, and skin. Insert a drain of choice to evacuate any residual hematoma. Apply a rigid plaster pressure dressing.

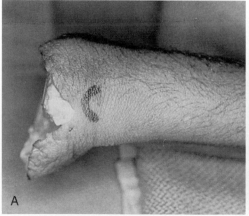
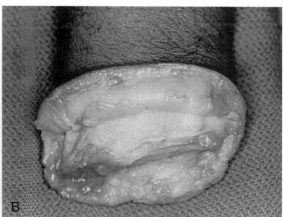

Figure 39–5. Rounded terminal stump after resection of the radial and ulnar styloid processes with palmar and dorsal skin flaps. *A,* Lateral view. *B,* Top view.

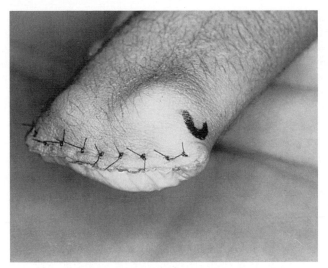

Figure 39–6. Interrupted suture closure of the terminal stump.

Under special circumstances, in which either the radius or the ulna is considerably longer, a one-bone forearm may be created if there is adequate soft tissue coverage. This procedure allows preservation of length without compromising prosthetic function.

KRUKENBERG'S PROCEDURE

The Krukenberg procedure converts a forearm stump into radial and ulnar rays to provide a pincer-like grasp motored by the pronator teres muscle. Sensibility and prehension are provided at the terminal segment. The most agreed-upon indication for this procedure is a sight-impaired person with bilateral upper extremity amputations. It is sometimes favored over a mechanical prosthesis by children with congenital bilateral amputations, for whom the radial and ulnar pincer hand usually becomes dominant. In a bilateral amputee, the procedure is usually performed on the patient's dominant side. This procedure is more widely used in Europe and developing countries, where prosthetic restoration is less utilized or may not be provided. The surgical technique is well described by Swanson[19] and Nathan and Trung.[15]

ACUTE POSTOPERATIVE PHASE

The acute postoperative phase of the rehabilitation program begins with skin closure and ends when the wound is healed and the sutures are removed. The goals for this phase include promotion of wound healing, control of incisional and phantom pain, and maintenance of the physical condition and residual motion of proximal limb segments. In most instances, patients also begin a postoperative therapy program designed to help them change hand dominance, if necessary, and learn to adapt to changes in body image. Patient education and instruction in the uses of the available prosthetic components are initiated, along with identifying sources of prosthetic funding.

In the immediately postoperative period, the surgical dressing plays a critical role in obtaining good wound healing and pain control. In all cases, a pressure dressing should be utilized, either an elastic wrap applied from distal to proximal or a rigid plaster dressing. The actual shaping and shrinking of the limb will be initiated in the next phase of the rehabilitation program. The advantages of a rigid plaster dressing over an elastic wrap in the acute postoperative period are that (1) control of edema is better, (2) incisional and phantom pain is better reduced, (3) wound healing is improved, and (4) a body-powered hook or functional hand can be attached for early prosthetic training.

Postoperative pain control is best achieved with intravenous patient-controlled analgesia or with an indwelling continuous nerve block followed by oral analgesics. Phantom pain, when severe, can be devastating for an amputee. It is stronger and of longer duration in the upper extremity than in the lower extremity. Approximately 5 to 10 percent of all amputees are estimated to experience severe progressive phantom pain.[18]

The remaining body segments provide substitute function for those lost to an amputation and are also utilized to power upper extremity prostheses. Therefore, active range-of-motion and strengthening exercises for the shoulder girdle, elbow, and residual forearm should be initiated immediately. The goal is to enlarge muscle mass to facilitate socket suspension, increase electromyographic (EMG) signals useful in myoelectric training, and maintain limb mobility and stability. Emphasis should be placed on movement by the scapula and shoulder. These segments are critical to the operation and function of the standard terminal device.

The scapular stabilizers are the levator scapula, serratus anterior, and trapezius muscles. The proximal muscles that assist in shoulder mobility are the pectoralis major and latissimus dorsi. The muscles that act on the glenohumeral joint are the deltoid, biceps, and triceps. Bilateral scapular motion in all planes is important for the amputee who will use a body-powered prosthesis. Biscapular protraction and glenohumeral flexion are important for maximum cable excursion to provide terminal device activation. Because the proximal limb segments are so vital to the terminal device, the residual limb evaluation that began in the preoperative phase must continue throughout the restoration process.

A change in hand dominance, if necessary, along with training in one-handed activities allows the patient to become more confident and feel a sense of accomplishment. Adaptive equipment may also be introduced at this time. As patients are introduced to the various prosthetic options available and begin to understand their use, they begin to recognize the potential for functional return of the extremity. Emotional support from the family and psychologic counseling are very important to help the amputee adjust and cope with the loss. In today's medical environ-

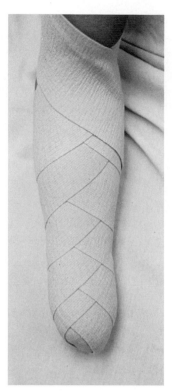

Figure 39–7. "Figure-eight" elastic wrap used to shape and shrink the residual limb.

ment, funding for prosthetic restoration is critical, because without external sources of funding, prosthetic restoration is economically prohibitive for most patients.

Preprosthetic Phase

The preprosthetic phase of the rehabilitation program prepares the residual limb for prosthetic fitting. This task should be accomplished in the shortest time possible, varying from 3 to 6 weeks. The goals are shaping and shrinking, desensitization, continued strengthening and mobility, and independence in activities of daily living.

Once the sutures are removed, the patient begins to shape and shrink the residual limb. This task is accomplished with an elastic wrap or pressure garment. Approximately 50 percent of the total shrinkage occurs during this phase. The elastic wrap is applied in a figure-eight, distal-to-proximal fashion and worn at all times except during bathing (Fig. 39–7). The wrap should be removed and re-applied every 4 hours to conform to the dynamic changes of the limb and should never be removed for more than 20 minutes at a time. Desensitization procedures can begin on the incision and terminal stump.

Use of a rigid plaster dressing immediately after surgery greatly reduces the need for continuous monitoring and rewrapping of the terminal stump during this period. The only dressing change required is for

suture removal, followed by application of a similar rigid plaster dressing. With an attached terminal device, prosthetic training can also begin earlier in the rehabilitation process. This early training greatly enhances the patient's appreciation and understanding of the various terminal devices available.

Prosthetic Fabrication Phase

Next comes the actual prescription for and fabrication of the prosthesis. This phase requires active participation by the patient and is a team effort on the part of the surgeon, physiatrist, prosthetist, and therapist. The choice of prosthetic components depends on the amputee's functional and cosmetic requirements. An orientation to realistic patient expectations will assist in determining which component designs will best meet these needs. For unilateral amputation, usually only one prosthesis is sufficient; however, patients with bilateral amputation should have a spare prosthesis in case of loss or breakage of the prostheses being worn daily.

PROSTHETIC COMPONENTS: TERMINAL DEVICE AND WRIST UNIT

The terminal device is the most important component for the upper extremity amputee. Because the device provides minimal sensory feedback, vision is essential for proper control.

The choices for the terminal device are a cosmetic (passive) hand, (Fig. 39–8), a cable-driven (body-powered) hand or hook (Fig. 39–9), and an electric hand or hook (Fig. 39–10). An electric hand or hook can be controlled either myoelectrically or by a switch. The most commonly prescribed terminal device in the U. S. is a body-powered cable-driven hook. It is the most accepted and most widely used device because it is lightweight, inexpensive, and the most durable. Also available are a variety of special terminal devices for sporting activities, such as bowling,

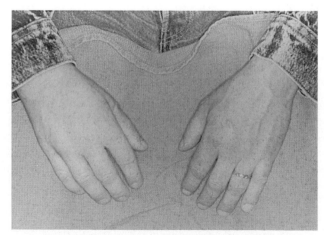

Figure 39–8. Cosmetic (passive) right hand prosthesis.

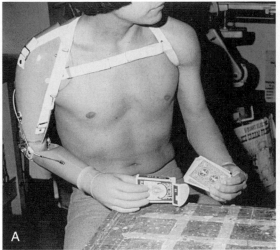
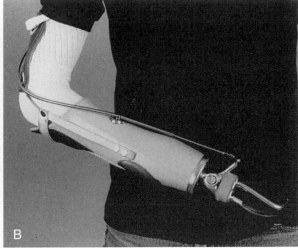

Figure 39–9. Cable-driven (body-powered) hand prostheses. *A* This prosthesis is being used by an above-elbow amputee. *B,* This prosthesis is being used by a wrist-disarticulation amputee. Note the size and position of the wrist unit.

baseball, and basketball, as well as tools for specialized work functions.

The wrist unit links the terminal device to the prosthetic forearm, providing flexion, extension, supination, and pronation. No contemporary wrist units currently provide wrist motion in all planes simultaneously. Also, wrist units cannot reproduce ulnar or radial deviation. A wrist flexion unit can improve function by placing the terminal device through three positions of passive flexion: neutral, 25° of flexion, and 50° of flexion (Fig. 39–11). At least one wrist flexion unit is preferred on the dominant side in patients with bilateral upper extremity amputation. The body-powered and myoelectric prostheses have

a wrist rotator available for pronation and supination, which is very helpful for such patients. For the active heavy duty user, a locking, quick-change wrist unit permits securing of the terminal device into a desired position of supination or pronation and also allows quick and easy changing of different functional components.

Most wrist units are aluminum constructs with adjustable nylon bushings, and they move with constant friction. A minimum of 6 cm is required to cosmetically accommodate a constant-friction wrist unit. This length requirement significantly affects the cosmetic appearance of both wrist disarticulations and distal transradial amputations.

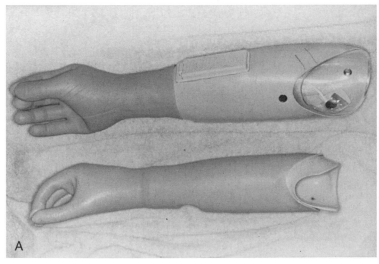
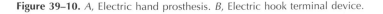
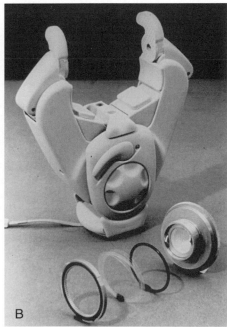

Figure 39–10. *A,* Electric hand prosthesis. *B,* Electric hook terminal device.

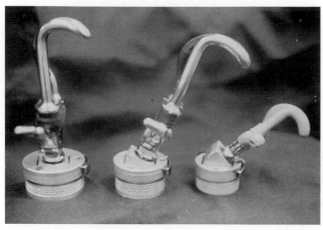

Figure 39–11. A wrist flexion unit. This device links the terminal device (shown) to the prosthetic forearm for passive flexion.

COSMESIS VERSUS FUNCTION

When choosing an upper limb prosthesis, the patient must decide whether the prosthesis is to be used for cosmetic or functional purposes. When the outward appearance or cosmesis of a prosthesis is more important, a cosmetic hand should be selected that utilizes a cosmetic glove. Some factors limiting the use of a cosmetic hand are that (1) cosmetic hands have fewer functional capabilities, (2) a cosmetic glove must match the appearance (skin color and texture) of the other hand, (3) cosmetic gloves are sensitive to sunlight, temperature, dyes, and chemicals, and (4) cosmetic gloves are less durable than a metal hook and may be torn or cut easily. Overall, the cosmetic glove design is functionally and structurally inferior to the durable metal hook design. Many patients, especially women in socially oriented vocations, select a cosmetic hand as their primary prosthesis. Others choose this cosmetic feature for social activities only, and their primary prosthesis is a metal hook used for all other activities. When only the function component of a prosthesis is important to the amputee, a hook is the best option. It is durable and can be used for a wide variety of vocational and recreational activities.

HAND VERSUS HOOK

Selection of a hand or hook depends on the patient's needs. As previously discussed, this decision can be influenced by the choice between cosmesis and function as well as the inherent limitations of each type of terminal device as applied to its expected uses. A hand suffices when nonstrenuous activities are performed. The passive cosmetic hand is lightweight and can provide excellent cosmetic restoration. The myoelectric hand is the most costly but provides pinch force. It also requires less harnessing and strapping, making it easier to apply. Hooks are preferred for vocations requiring manual dexterity. Hooks also perform very well in situations requiring

strenuous activity. Some amputees prefer both a hand and a hook for their interchangeability. The hand or hook either is voluntarily cable opened and springs closed or is voluntarily cable closed and springs open. Most amputees choose a voluntary-opening type hook. The hand or hook can be activated by a body-powered harness and cable system or a myoelectric/electric system.

BODY POWERED VERSUS MYOELECTRIC

After the choices between cosmesis and function and between hand and hook have been made, the decision between a body-powered system and a myoelectric/electric system must be addressed.

In 1812, Ballif introduced the principle of hand operation by shoulder and arm movement.[1] The current design for limb prosthesis came from the research and development of artificial limbs that began after World War II. The standard upper limb prosthesis is body powered. Shoulder and arm movements operate the terminal device through a shoulder harness-and-cable system (Fig. 39–12). This arrangement consists of a flexible elbow hinge with triceps pad as it crosses the elbow and a figure-eight harness with axillary loop for proximal control. A Bowden single-cable system is used to control the terminal device. Body-powered prostheses are preferred by approximately 90 percent of upper extremity amputees. They are relatively inexpensive, functional, and reliable, and they have some sensory proprioceptive feedback from the shoulder harness-and-cable control system.[14]

The use of myoelectric prostheses began in the early 1950s. The design is self-contained and is more cosmetically appealing than the standard prosthesis. Contraction of residual limb muscles is used to activate the terminal device, which opens or closes an electric hand or hook and can produce supination, pronation, and/or rotation of an electric wrist unit. Although myoelectric units are generally heavier and require higher suspension forces, they require less harnessing and strapping and are, therefore, more comfortable than the standard body-powered design. However, they are more complex and have more moving parts, so they have high maintenance requirements and are subject to occasional breakdowns. The cost of a myoelectric unit is also significantly greater than that of a body-powered hand or hook. Another potential disadvantage is that myoelectric units are battery operated, requiring a daily battery charge.

The myoelectric prosthesis is favored when greater grip strength and pinch force is required or when the desired functions or tasks cannot be achieved by a body-powered system. Some patients prefer to own a myoelectric prosthesis in addition to a body-powered design.

HYBRID SYSTEMS

Combination (hybrid) systems are tailored to the patient's needs and used primarily for amputations

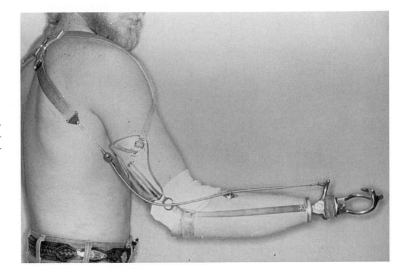

Figure 39–12. A shoulder harness and cable system for operating the terminal device of a standard body-powered prosthesis. This prosthesis is being used by a distal forearm (transradial) amputee.

about the elbow. They usually consist of either a cable-driven elbow unit coupled with an electric terminal device or an electric elbow unit coupled with a cable-driven terminal device.

PROSTHETIC PRESCRIPTION

The prescription for a prosthetic limb must take into consideration all the patient variables that ultimately affect the outcome of functional restoration. These variables may change as the rehabilitation program evolves. The entire management team must be aware of these changes and prepared to alter the prosthetic prescription as the need arises.

A typical prescription for a body-powered prosthesis, written for a patient with a unilateral wrist disarticulation, has the following features:

1. Figure-eight harness with axillary loop.
2. Bowden single-control cable.
3. Flexible elbow hinge with triceps pad.
4. Trimline distal socket with minimum length.
5. Constant-friction wrist unit or locking quick-change friction unit for the active heavy duty user.
6. Terminal device, cable-driven hand or cable-driven hook.

Prosthetic Training Phase

The sixth phase of the rehabilitation program is prosthetic training, which incorporates the prosthetic wearing and use patterns into the patient's day-to-day activities. Bimanual activities are initiated, and vocational and recreational activities are explored. The patient's emotional responses to the prosthesis and the amputation itself must be followed very closely during this phase. The amputee usually becomes acutely aware of the shortcomings of prosthetic function, cosmesis, and comfort.

Upper extremity human limb substitutes are designed to reproduce the complex activities performed by the hand and wrist. The proportionate prosthetic "gain," or restoration of function, is smaller for the hand and wrist than for any other amputation level.[9] The patient with a unilateral upper extremity amputation can perform approximately 90 percent of the activities of daily living without using a prosthesis.[8] Therefore, even minimal problems can directly result in a patient's choosing to not wear a prosthesis. In contrast, approximately 90 percent of below-knee amputees choose to wear a prosthesis.[20] This reality emphasizes the need for quality, comprehensive prosthetic training for the upper extremity amputee.

Community Integration Phase

During the community integration phase, the emphasis is taken off the prosthesis and put on returning the patient to the community. Careful assessment of the patient's ability to engage in occupational and leisure activities is essential to understanding his or her functional outcome. The patient's ability to make decisions and resume the pre-injury role with family and community are closely observed and encouraged.

Vocational Rehabilitation Phase

Patients with unilateral arm amputation should be expected to continue in gainful employment but may require further education or retraining in order to achieve their vocational goals. Patients with bilateral arm amputation commonly return to work following intense prosthetic training and vocational rehabilitation. However, the potential for an upper extremity amputee is practically limitless, given the resources available for rehabilitation.

Follow-up Phase

The follow-up phase, which measures the ultimate success of the prosthetic rehabilitation program, is a life-long process. Emphasis on appropriate use, care, and maintenance of the prosthesis, ensuring of prosthetic comfort, and sustained community and family support of the upper extremity amputee are all aspects of the follow-up phase.

SUMMARY

One of the most challenging decisions in the care of massive upper extremity injuries is whether salvage of the traumatized digit or hand is feasible or advisable. The functional capacity of the patient must not be sacrificed in an attempt to salvage marginal tissue. A dysvascular, insensate hand is far less functional than an appropriate prosthesis. Therefore, surgical judgment must be based on a thorough evaluation of the individual case. The decision-making process for any amputation must focus on the individual's rehabilitation requirements, taking into consideration the physiologic, psychologic, vocational, and avocational needs.

True functional restoration of a hand with a prosthesis is a major undertaking. The prognosis is affected by the level of amputation, as well as the quality of the terminal stump, of the prosthetic fit, and of prosthetic education and training. The goals of amputation management, as described for each of the nine phases, can be achieved by incorporating the methodology described for amputations about the wrist.

References

1. American Academy of Orthopaedic Surgeons: Historical development of artificial limbs. In Orthopaedic Appliance Atlas, Vol 2: Artificial Limbs. Ann Arbor, MI, JW Edwards, 1960, pp 1–22.
2. American Academy of Orthopaedic Surgeons: Wrist disarticulation and transradial amputation. In Atlas of Limb Prosthetics: Surgical, Prosthetic, and Rehabilitation Principles. St Louis, Mosby–Year Book, Inc., 1992, pp 237–240.
3. Baumgartner RF: The surgery of arm and forearm amputations. Orthop Clin North Am 12:805–817, 1981.
4. Bennet JB, Alexander CB: Amputation levels and surgical techniques. In Comprehensive Management of the Upper-Limb Amputee. New York, Springer-Verlag, 1989, pp 1–10.
5. Bohne WHO: Atlas of Amputation Surgery. New York, Thieme, 1987.
6. Burgess EM: Amputation. In The Elbow and its Disorders. Philadelphia, WB Saunders, 1993, pp 740–749.
7. Esquenazi A, Leonard JA, Meier RH, et al: Prosthetics. Arch Phys Med Rehabil 70 (Suppl):207, 1989.
8. Flatt AE: The Role of reconstructive surgery. In The Care of Congenital Hand Anomalies. St Louis, Quality Medical Publishing, 1994, pp 11–14.
9. Klopsteg PE, Wilson PD: The biomechanics of the normal and of the amputated upper extremity. In Human Limbs and Their Substitutes. New York, McGraw-Hill, 1954, pp 169–221.
10. LeBlanc MA: Patient populations and other estimates of prosthetics and orthotics in the USA. Orthot Prosthet 27:38–44, 1973.
11. Louis DS: Amputations. In Operative Hand Surgery. New York, Churchill Livingstone, 1993, pp 53–98.
12. Meier RH: Upper limb amputee rehabilitation. In Esquenazi A (ed): Prosthetics: State of the Art Reviews. Philadelphia, Hanley and Belfus, 1994.
13. Milford LW, Jobe MT: Amputations. In Crenshaw AH (ed): Campbell's Operative Orthopaedics, 8th ed, St Louis, Mosby–Year Book, 1992, pp 3201–3232.
14. Muilenburg AL, LeBlanc MA: Body-powered upper-limb components. In Crenshaw AH, Meier RH III (eds): Comprehensive Management of the Upper-Limb Amputee. New York, Springer-Verlag, 1989, pp 28–38.
15. Nathan PA, Trung NB: The Krukenberg operation: A modified technique avoiding skin grafts. J Hand Surg 2:127–130, 1977.
16. Pillet J, Mackin EJ: Aesthetic hand prosthesis: Its psychologic and functional potential. In Rehabilitation of the Hand: Surgery and Therapy. St. Louis, Mosby–Year Book, 1995, pp 1253–1263.
17. Sears HH: Approaches to prescription of body-powered and myoelectric prostheses. Phys Med Rehab Clin North Am. 2:361–371, 1991.
18. Shenaq SM, Meier RH, Brotzman B: The painful residual limb: Treatment strategies. In Crenshaw AH, Meier RH III (eds): Comprehensive Management of the Upper-Limb Amputee. New York, Springer-Verlag, 1989, pp 72–77.
19. Swanson AB: The Krukenberg procedure in the juvenile amputee. J Bone Joint Surg 46A:1540, 1964.
20. Tooms RE: Amputations of lower extremity. In Crenshaw AH (ed): Campbell's Operative Orthopaedics, 8th ed, St Louis, Mosby–Year Book, Inc., 1992, pp 689–702.
21. Tooms RE: Amputations of upper extremity. In Crenshaw AH (ed): Campbell's Operative Orthopaedics. St. Louis, Mosby–Year Book, 1992, pp 711–721.
22. Tooms RE: Amputation surgery in the upper extremity. Orthop Clin North Am 3:383, 1972.

PART IX
Wrist Therapy and Rehabilitation

CHAPTER 40

Assessment

Emily Jeter, OTR/L, Gregory G. Degnan, MD, and
David M. Lichtman, MD

THE CURRENT ROLE OF THE HAND THERAPIST IN CONSERVATIVE TREATMENT OF WRIST DISORDERS

"The disorientation and confusion brought on by the premature arrival of the future, can be fatal to those not prepared for it."[1] Bionics, biosensors, virtual reality, digitally controlled machines, and other technology will forever change the job of the hand therapist. Computer software programs will dramatically change the evaluation and treatment of our patients. Algorithms based on computer-generated data will allow for timely, appropriate, and cost-effective treatment, with results reported objectively in the form of percentage of probability.

These technologic advances will unquestionably assist the therapist and surgeon in patient evaluation and the formulation of a treatment plan. It is vital, however, that we do not lose sight of the fact that no amount of technology can replace the clinical experience and judgment of a well-trained surgeon or therapist. Likewise, no amount of machinery or technologic data can replace the benefit of hands-on treatment from an empathetic therapist. The power of the healing hands can never be overlooked or lost in the shuffle of the paperwork produced by our technology. Further, it is essential that the hand surgeon not be so overwhelmed by the technologic data produced in the therapy department as to overlook the need for continued communication with therapists and his or her own need to perform hands-on examination and history-taking.

Initial Evaluation

We believe that the therapist's initial evaluation of a patient sets the stage for subsequent outcome. We focus on several specific areas during this interview and examination. First, we establish the specific involved structures and the exact extent of the injuries or disease process. Second, we evaluate the needs of the patient. These include occupational and avocational needs. We then assess the rehabilitative potential of the patient. This is a purely subjective but critical evaluation. It is based on the perceived cognitive abilities, cooperation, and desires of the patient. The occupational needs of the patient and their rehabilitation potential are often key determinants of the final treatment plan. Next we establish a treatment plan that includes short-term and long-term goals. Finally, and perhaps most importantly, we interact with patients as individuals, addressing their concerns and providing the information they need to be active participants in their care.[2]

General History and Patient-Specific History

An accurate history is the first essential step in the examination and evaluation of the wrist. The therapist records the patient's age, hand dominance, occupation, and avocations. After obtaining the background data, we document the patient-specific history. We record the exact mechanism of injury, as well as the time and date of the injury, and any prior treatment. Prior surgical procedures, infections, medications, and previous therapy are also noted.

We believe strongly that it is also important, during this interview process, to assess the impact that the injury or disease process has upon the patient's family, economic, and social life. The effects include changes in activity levels and changes in patterns of work and/or play. We also make a point to discuss openly any negative impact that the problem may have on the patient's body image.

Physical Examination

When performing our hands-on physical evaluation of the wrist, we focus on two broad areas. First, we define the injury and anatomic lesion as accurately as possible. Second, we evaluate the remaining function of the extremity to determine the degree of disability that the patient may experience in work or activities of everyday life.[3]

The physical examination performed by the therapist should be similar, in most regards, to that performed by the hand surgeon. It is vital to perform a good general examination as well as specific provocative tests in order to obtain a baseline and gauge subsequent progress throughout the course of therapy. A detailed description of the examination is covered in Chapter 6; we will, therefore, focus on those areas of the examination that are often specific to the therapist.

Tissue tension testing is crucial in defining a patient's baseline condition and in monitoring progress. It is also often useful when one is attempting to decide whether further therapy is indicated or surgical intervention is required. We perform specific hands-on testing of active range of motion for all joints individually as well as during synchronized motion, documenting any pain or crepitus associated with this motion.

We then assess passive range of motion, again testing each joint individually as well as during synchronized motion. When reaching the endpoint of a specific range, the therapist should note and document the "feel" of that endpoint. A rigid, sudden endpoint indicates a bony block or rigid joint contracture, whereas a softer, "bouncier" endpoint implies scarring or contracture that will respond to different measures.

Diagnostic Examination

Hand therapists have in their armamentarium a battery of diagnostic tests that, owing to logistics and time constraints, are not readily available in the surgeon's office setting. We believe that as part of the initial evaluation and treatment plan, it is important to establish baseline values in the areas where the focus of the therapy will be concentrated. These areas include sensation, prehensile pattern, pinch strength, grip strength, volumetrics, and functional capacity in a simulated work environment.

When measuring sensibility the hand therapist should remember that the stimulus provided by the therapist is interpreted by the patient, resulting in test information that is vulnerable to bias regardless of what stimulus is used. Two-point discrimination is the most commonly used method of assessing sensibility in the hand. A number of studies, however, have shown several problems with this method. Bell and Buford[4] demonstrated that even experienced hand therapists and surgeons applied different forces in their one-point and two-point testing sessions that exceeded the resolution or sensitivity threshold for normal sensation. Additionally, they found that interrater reliability was poor.

We prefer the Semmes-Weinstein monofilament discrimination test to assess the threshold of stimulus necessary for the perception of light touch to deep pressure. This test assesses the ability to detect a punctate stimulus. This is the initial and most simple level of sensation in the hand. The test is unique in that it allows the examiner to reliably and consistently control the amount of force applied. The monofilaments are handheld probes consisting of nylon monofilaments inset at right angles to lucite rods. The probes are of equal length with increasing diameters. In the large, 20-filament set, each monofilament is marked with a number, ranging from 1.65 to 6.65. The number represents the logarithm of 10 times the force in milligrams required to bow the monofilament (log 10 Fmg).

We use the Bell-Krotoski testing procedure to test the fingertip pulps with the patient's hand fully supported and vision occluded. Testing should be demonstrated on an area of intact sensibility. The patient is asked to give a verbal response when he or she feels the filament.

The monofilament is applied perpendicular to the palmar skin of the fingertip until it bows (Fig. 40–1). Filaments marked 2.44 through 4.08 are applied three times to the test area, whereas filaments 4.17 through 6.65 are applied only once per trial in a given area. Testing usually begins with filament 2.44 or 2.83, which is considered the normal range of values. If

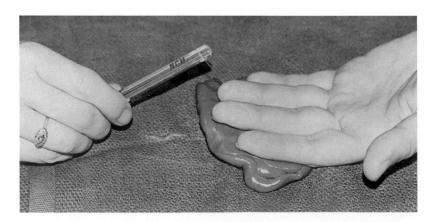

Figure 40–1. Semmes Sensory Test application: The dorsal aspect of the hand is placed in putty to provide a constant and even stimulus to the back of the fingers. The monofilament collapses under a given force, which is determined by the filament's diameter and length. This controls the magnitude of the applied pressure.

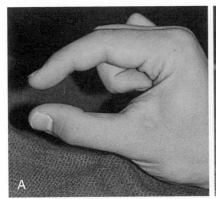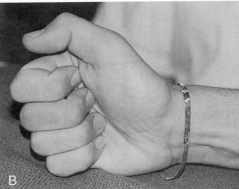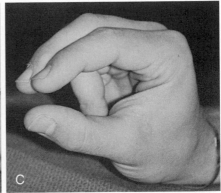

Figure 40–2. Prehension patterns: *A,* tip; *B,* lateral; and *C,* three-jaw chuck.

the patient can accurately identify the touch of either of these filaments, sensibility is normal in the area being tested, and testing can be discontinued. If the patient cannot identify the touch of these filaments, the therapist should progressively apply each next larger monofilament until touch pressure can be identified for all fingertips.[5]

In prehensile use, the hand is considered to have two parts, the thumb and the rest of the digits. Most activity combines thumb and index finger prehension. Three patterns of prehension occur most commonly: tip, lateral, and three-jaw (or palmar pinch) (Fig. 40–2). Prehensile pattern may be determined using the Moberg prehension test (Fig. 40–3). This test assesses the patient's willingness and ability to perform fine motor tasks using the thumb and index finger. Pinch strength may be measured by using a pinch gauge or pinchmeter (Fig. 40–4). The average result of three trials is recorded.[6]

A patient's ability to function is also related to muscle strength. Hand grip strength has been an indi-

cator for determining strength since 1880. Bechtol, in 1954, produced a grip dynamometer with adjustable hand spacings that measured hand grip force in pounds.[6] The Jamar dynamometer has been shown to be a reliable test instrument when standard positioning of subjects is used and the instruments are well calibrated[7] (Fig. 40–5). In our practice, we prefer measuring grip strength in kilogram force at all five positions of testing. Normal adult values for the five consecutive grip positions consistently produce a bell-shaped curve. The first, fifth, and fourth positions should be the weakest, with the strongest values occurring at the third and second handles. We use this normal grip curve to help us identify patients for whom motivation is questionable. Murray[8] has described a clinical correlation between "flat" curves and patients who were found to have "significant personality problems."

The mechanical dynamometer may be too gross to measure the grasp in the weak hand, and in these cases, we use a sphygmomanometer to record grips of lesser power. The blood pressure cuff is rolled to a 5-cm diameter and inflated to 50 mm Hg. The pa-

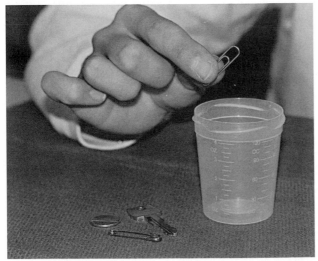

Figure 40–3. Moberg pick-up test. This test determines the patient's willingness and ability to use the thumb and index finger for normal fine-motor tasks.

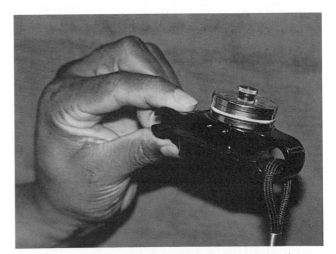

Figure 40–4. The pinch gauge is used to provide reliable and accurate measurements of pinch strength.

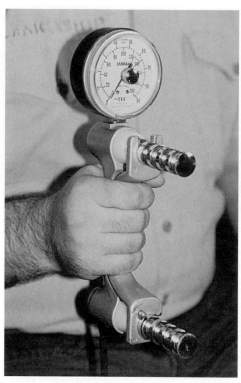

Figure 40–5. Jamar dynamometer: This device provides an accurate measure of grip strength and can also be used to assess the compliance and cooperation of the patient. (Courtesy of Asimow Engineering, Los Angeles, CA.)

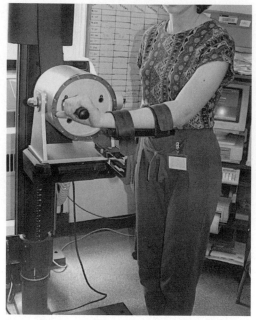

Figure 40–7. Baltimore Therapeutic Equipment Company Work Simulator (BTE). (Courtesy of Baltimore Therapeutic Equipment Co., Baltimore, MD.)

tient then squeezes the cuff, and we record the increase above 50 mm Hg.[9]

Currently, there are no normal standards for hand volume or circumference. Swelling must be considered relative to the uninvolved extremity and relative to change over time in response to activity or treatment. We measure edema using water displacement or circumferential measurements (Fig. 40–6). Several volumeters are commercially available, and the evaluator should know the reliability of the instrument being used prior to testing.

We obtain volumetric measurements with a volumeter as follows: The patient submerges one hand at a time into the container until the web space between the third and fourth digits rests on a dowel within the container. The displaced water flows out of a spout on the side of the container and is then measured in a graduated cylinder.[10]

In the hand rehabilitation setting, it is not usually feasible or space efficient to have many different machines or tools from industry available. We use work simulators, such as the Baltimore Therapeutic Equipment Company Work Simulator (BTE), to assist us in providing the information needed to make determinations regarding patient progress in therapy and return-to-work status (Fig. 40–7). We use the BTE to test patients' ability to perform the physical demands

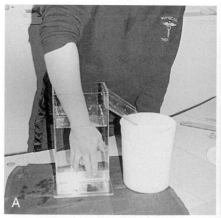
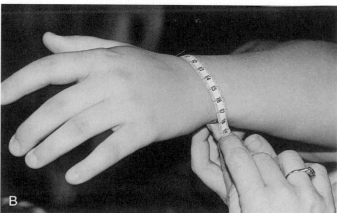

Figure 40–6. Techniques for measuring edema. *A*, Volumeter; *B*, circumferential measurement.

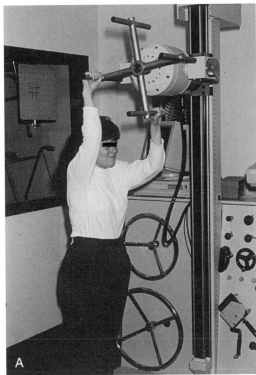

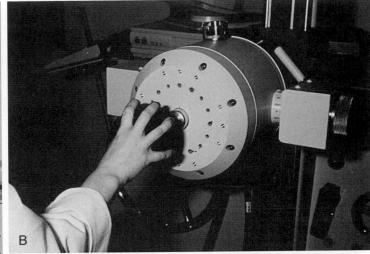

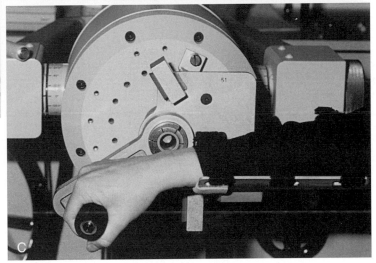

Figure 40–8. Variations in height *(A)*, shaft angle *(B)*, and patient position *(C)* available with the BTE Work Simulator. (Courtesy of Lido Work Simulation Systems, Loredan Biomedical, Inc., West Sacramento, CA.)

of their jobs or avocational activities. This machine is a mechanical device with attachments designed to simulate the upper-extremity motions utilized during job tasks. The tool attachments are selected to match the patient's job, and the machine quantifies the patient's ability to perform the necessary tasks.

The BTE has a calibrated braking system into which each of the tools is placed, providing the resistance against which the patient works. The patient must apply force in excess of the resistance to move the tool attachment. The machine calculates the work output by multiplying the force applied by the distance that the tool attachment was moved. Additionally, the machine measures the patient's endurance (power output) by dividing the work produced by the time required. We instruct the patient to exert maximum effort for 2 minutes, with both the dominant and the nondominant hand. The values for work and endurance are calculated for each hand, and the two are compared. The results are interpreted by comparing the injured and uninjured sides.

We use all 19 attachments for exercise and simulation of specific job tasks included with the BTE to simulate a wide variety of job tasks. Specific exercise use of the work simulator can include pinch and grip strengthening, supination and pronation, radial and ulnar deviation, wrist flexion and extension, palmar and fingertip desensitization, finger flexion and extension, elbow flexion and extension, internal and external shoulder rotation, and shoulder flexion and extension. Variations in height, shaft angle, and patient position create a wide range of possible uses for each attachment and exercise mode[11] (Fig. 40–8).

REASSESSMENT AND PREOPERATIVE ASSESSMENT TREATMENT PLANNING FOR THE SURGICAL CANDIDATE

The initial evaluation of the patient is critical, because it provides the baseline data against which the patient's progress is measured. If a data point is not obtained prior to initiation of treatment, neither the surgeon nor the therapist will be able to truly measure the patient's total progress. We believe that one of the keys to therapy is periodic reassessment and plotting of the data points to accurately assess the efficacy of any given treatment plan and to guide those plans accordingly. Therefore, at appropriate post-injury or postoperative intervals, we reassess the patient with specific attention to joint range of motion, soft tissue equilibrium, motor testing, grip and pinch strength, sensory status, and hand volume. Additionally, we periodically obtain objective data on functional capabilities through the use of work simulators. These periodic post-injury or postoperative assessments are essential in coordinating and altering the long-range therapy plan.

We believe that preoperative evaluation by the hand therapist can be extremely useful. This is particularly true for the rheumatoid patient and any patient whose postoperative therapy will require frequent patient-therapist interaction and a complex rehabilitative protocol. The hand therapist's preoperative evaluation can help the surgeon predetermine which patients are good rehabilitative candidates. The determination may, in some cases, alter the ultimate surgical decision. For example, the patient with a degenerative scapholunate advanced collapse deformity (SLAC wrist) who demonstrates poor rehabilitative potential would be far better served by an arthrodesis, whereas a good candidate for rehabilitation might benefit more from a proximal row carpectomy.

Additionally, the patient who is aware preoperatively of what will be expected postoperatively finds it easier to arrange his or her work and home life to ensure compliance. Finally, a preoperative hand therapist's assessment facilitates formulation of a long-term treatment plan that is in keeping with the goals and desires of the referring surgeon. The ultimate goals are to align the patient's expectations with the treatment team's abilities and to ensure maximum functional outcome.

References

1. Waylett-Rendall J: Hand therapy of the future—a profession for the 21st century. J Hand Ther 5(A):182, 1992.
2. Kasdan AS, McElwain NP: Return-to-work programs following occupational hand injuries. Occup Med State Aut Rev 4:539–545, 1989.
3. Magee DJ: Orthopedic Physical Assessment. Philadelphia, WB Saunders, 1987.
4. Bell-Krotoski J, Buford WI: The force/time relationship of clinically used sensory testing instruments. J Hand Therapy 1:76, 1988.
5. Tan AM: Sensibility testing. In Stanley BG, Tribuzi SM (eds): Concepts in Hand Rehabilitation. Philadelphia, FA Davis, 1992.
6. Totten PA, Flinn-Wagner S: Functional Evaluation of the Hand. In Stanley BG, Tribuzi SM (eds): Concepts in Hand Rehabilitation. Philadelphia, FA Davis, 1992.
7. Fess EE: A method for checking Jamar dynamometer calibration. J Hand Ther 1:28, 1987.
8. Murray J: The patient with the injured hand (presidential address). J Hand Surg 7:543, 1982.
9. Swanson AB, Swanson GG, Goran-Hagert G: Evaluation of hand impairment. In Hunter JM, Schneider LH, Mackin EJ, Callahan AD (eds): Rehabilitation of the Hand, ed 3. Baltimore, CV Mosby, 1990.
10. Nicholson B: Clinical Evaluation. In Stanley BG, Tribuzi SM (eds): Concepts In Hand Rehabilitation. Philadelphia, FA Davis, 1992.
11. Pendergraft KJ, Cooper JK, Clark GL: The BTE Work Simulator. In Hunter JM, Schneider LH, Mackin EJ, Callahan AD (eds): Rehabilitation of the Hand, ed 3. Baltimore, CV Mosby, 1990.
12. Schultz-Johnson K: Work hardening: A mandate for hand therapy. Hand Clin 7:597–610, 1991.

CHAPTER 41

Conservative Rehabilitation

Emily Jeter, OTR/L, Gregory G. Degnan, MD,
and David M. Lichtman, MD

GENERAL PRINCIPLES

Evaluation is the cornerstone of sound clinical decision-making. The clinician's evaluative skill is dependent on an in-depth understanding of structural and functional anatomy, the effects of injury and disease on tissue, and concepts of wound healing. The integrity of the entire treatment process hinges on our ability to evaluate and assess patient signs and symptoms carefully and to use that assessment as the basis for care.[1] Baseline assessment and continued re-evaluation are crucial in determining if whether conservative management has failed and when surgery should be considered.

A great variation exists in the type and severity of wrist injuries requiring some form of rehabilitation. Despite these variations, certain general principles of rehabilitation apply universally to all hand and wrist injuries. The key to a successful therapy program is adaptation of those principles to the specific injury. Good communication between the physician and the therapist facilitates the incorporation of these principles into the rehabilitation plan.

We apply these general principles in the same sequence for all injuries. Our rehabilitation protocol is divided into specific phases. The five treatment phases are as follows: phase I, edema inflammation control; phase II, development of a favorable soft tissue environment; phase III, range of motion (ROM); phase IV, strengthening (isometric, isotonic, isokinetic); and phase V, work hardening/conditioning (Table 41–1).

Phases I, II, and III overlap significantly in terms of the techniques and modalities used and of the timing of application of these modalities. In phase I, we utilize such modalities as ice, supported elevation, retrograde massage, Coban wraps, and compression garments to control the swelling. Incorporating range of motion (phase III) at this point, when feasible, also helps control the edema, because motion is critical to moving fluid out of the hand (Fig. 41–1). We emphasize to the patient that "wiggling" the fingers is not adequate to milk the edema out of the hand. Forceful, active motion sufficient to compress the dorsal veins provides adequate pressure to propel the fluid out of the hand. We rarely use heat at this stage of treatment, because the resultant increased blood flow to the area contributes to local inflammation and persistent edema. Control of the local inflammation is essential to prevent persistence or reaccumulation

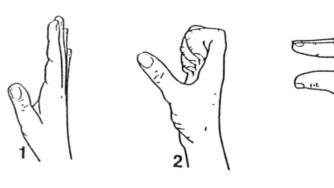
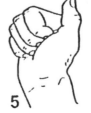

Figure 41–1. Range-of-motion exercises: Specific instructions are given to the patient to ensure that in exercises 2, 4, and 5, the patient supplies sufficient force to "milk" the fluid out of the hand.

Table 41–1. REHABILITATION PROGRAM FOR CONSERVATIVE TREATMENT OF WRIST DISORDERS*

Phase I: Edema Control

Ice application
Supported elevation
Compression garments
Iontophoresis
Coban wraps
Retrograde massage
Range-of-motion exercises
Electrical stimulation

Phase II: Development of Favorable Soft Tissue Environment

Scar massage
Whirlpool
Moist heat pack
Elastomer application
Ultrasound/iontophoresis
Paraffin

Phase III: Range of Motion

Tendon gliding exercises
Fluidotherapy
Dynamic splinting
Continuous passive motion devices
BTE/LIDO

Phase IV: Strengthening (Isometric, Isotonic, Isokinetic Exercises)

Theraputty
BTE/LIDO
Hand grippers
Free weights

Phase V: Work Hardening/Conditioning

BTE/LIDO
Ergonomic/adaptive equipment
Simulated vocational/avocational activities

*BTE/LIDO = Work simulation systems.

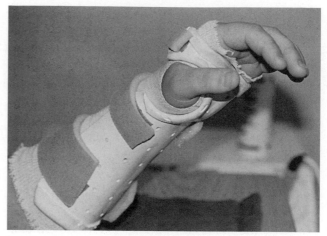

Figure 41–2. Wrist immobilization splint that allows motion of unaffected joints.

if we are to return the hand to its normal level of function. The mainstays of our treatment regimen during this phase are scar massage, stretching, iontophoresis, and the various modalities that provide heat to the soft tissues.

Scar massage is the mainstay of treatment in the early part of phase II, because it aids in desensitizing the wound and helps break up the adhesions between the skin and underlying structures (Fig. 41–4). It is also convenient because the patient can perform this activity at home. The next focus during this phase is the stretching of the soft tissues, joints, and musculotendinous units. We facilitate this manual passive

of edema. Nonsteroidal anti-inflammatory drugs (NSAIDs) may be indicated at this stage. We use splinting to rest the affected parts and decrease local inflammation. Splints vary for the different conditions, but all provide immobilization of the affected part while allowing motion of the unaffected parts (Fig. 41–2). Another useful adjunct in phases II and III is iontophoresis, the induction of topically applied medication into tissue by the application of low-voltage direct galvanic current (Fig. 41–3). It is effective in the treatment of inflammatory disorders and scar formation. Iontophoresis can induce dexamethasone or other steroid into soft tissue.[2]

In phase II of the rehabilitation program, we attempt to restore a favorable soft tissue environment. The inevitable consequences of injury and edema in the hand are scarring and stiffness. After we have brought the acute inflammation of injury or disease under control, we are left with the scarring which is the inevitable result of inflammation and edema. The extent of scarring, fibrosis, and stiffness is directly related to the duration and severity of the swelling and immobilization. It is essential to restore normal motion to the joints and suppleness to the soft tissues

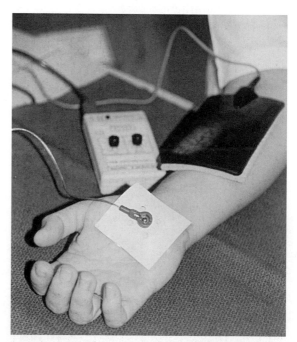

Figure 41–3. Iontophoresis: The induction of topically applied ions into tissue by application of low-voltage direct galvanic current. This modality is useful in the control of edema and inflammation.

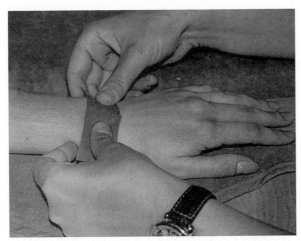

Figure 41–4. Scar massage using Dycem (nonslip material) for scar tissue mobilization. This is one of the mainstays of treatment during phase II in the development of a favorable soft tissue environment.

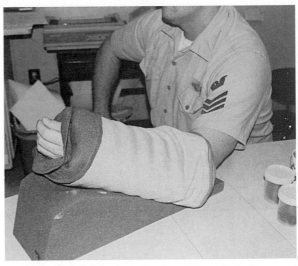

Figure 41–5. Moist heat pack application. This method of heat application is inexpensive and convenient, although patients should be cautioned that its inappropriate use can lead to thermal injury.

stretching through the use of heat modalities. After inflammation is under control, heat becomes an essential adjunct to the remainder of the therapy regimen, until normal function returns. Heat assists in restoration of soft tissue equilibrium by (1) increasing blood flow to the local area, (2) aiding in the resolution of inflammatory infiltrates, (3) helping reduce spasm, (4) assisting with pain relief and thereby facilitating cooperation with therapy, and (5) increasing the extensibility of the collagen in the soft tissue and decreasing joint stiffness.

Heat may be transferred to the tissue via three different pathways: conduction, convection, and conversion. Conduction is the transfer of heat between two objects; examples are the hot packs and paraffin baths we use prior to initiating therapy, to loosen the joints and heat up the soft tissues. Hot packs are the most commonly used form of heat because they are inexpensive, convenient, and easy to apply (Fig. 41–5). We have found them to be very effective, but we caution patients that hot packs may be dangerous. The average temperature of the hydrocollators far exceeds the temperature necessary for thermal injury. It is crucial that the packs be used with eight to ten layers of towels to protect the skin and help maintain the heat of the pack. We apply a hot pack for approximately 20 minutes and then initiate therapy. It takes the body anywhere from 30 to 45 minutes to decrease the temperature of the soft tissues within 1 cm of the skin. This provides a sufficiently long "window of opportunity" to work on passive stretch. Heat must be used with great caution, however, in patients with poor circulation or altered sensation.

When dealing with joint contractures, we prefer paraffin treatments to hot packs (Fig. 41–6). We have found that the paraffin is well tolerated by patients and allows better passive stretch, perhaps because it makes total contact and provides circumferential soft tissue heating.

Convection, the second mode of heat transfer, occurs via transfer of heat between a moving medium and a static surface. Examples of convection are whirlpool and fluidotherapy. We generally limit the use of whirlpool in this phase to those patients who have wounds requiring mechanical débridement (Fig. 41–7). The standard accepted temperature range for whirlpool (37.8–40°C) is below the reported therapeutic range for soft tissue (41–45°C).

Fluidotherapy involves convection heating using heated dry particles of corn husk (Fig. 41–8). Temperatures for this modality range from 43.3°C to 48.8°C, and treatments last for 20 minutes. We prefer this modality because it also reduces hypersensitivity of the hand. In fact, we occasionally use fluidotherapy at lower temperatures to decrease sensitivity even in the presence of edema.

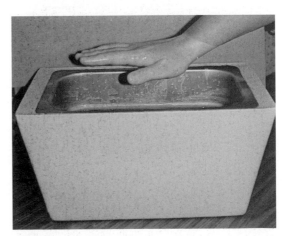

Figure 41–6. Paraffin application. Because this is a total-contact heat source, it allows excellent passive stretch and is well tolerated by patients.

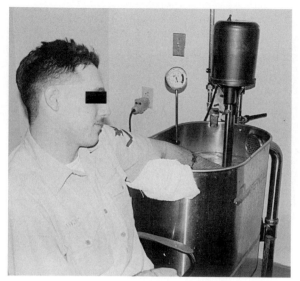

Figure 41–7. Hand whirlpool for mechanical débridement.

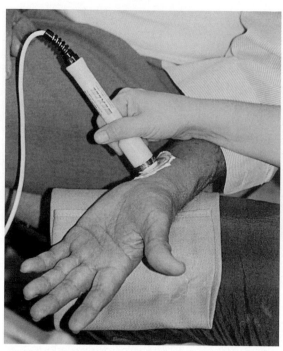

Figure 41–9. Application of phonophoresis. This modality provides heat to deep tissues by converting nonthermal energy into heat in the deep tissue layers. (Courtesy of EXCEL.)

Finally, heat can be transferred by conversion, which involves the penetration of nonthermal energy into deep tissue and its conversion to heat. Ultrasound and phonoporesis belong to this category of heating modalities (Fig. 41–9). They are particularly useful when deep tissues are involved and require

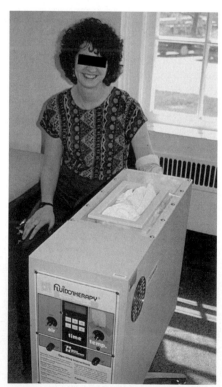

Figure 41–8. Fluidotherapy for assisting active range of motion: A method of providing heat by convection, this modality also helps diminish hypersensitivity of the hand. (Courtesy of Fluidotherapy: Henley Inc., Sugarland, TX.)

heat treatment without overheating the overlying superficial tissues. We use conversion for treatment of scar tissue but find it particularly useful for deep scar adherent to overlying incisions and scar that is restricting tendon gliding. It should be noted, however, that ultrasound may delay tendon healing, and we therefore do not recommend its use before 8 weeks following tendon repair.

Phase III of the rehabilitation program focuses on restoration of normal motion. This phase really overlaps with the first two phases, because it is extremely important to begin range of motion as early as possible. After we have achieved soft tissue equilibrium, however, our main focus is on aggressive range of motion. Active, active-assisted, and aggressive range-of-motion exercises become the mainstays of treatment. We also use splinting during this phase to provide static or dynamic stretch and improve motion (Fig. 41–10).

When the patient achieves a comfortable, functional range of motion, we shift our focus to phase IV, strengthening. The performance of specific "putty" exercises of increasing resistance is usually the first step (Fig. 41–11), and the patient progresses to spring-loaded grippers as tolerated. Light weights are initiated as tolerated and we then encourage the patient to incorporate heavy functional activities into the daily routine. We utilize periodic Jamar grip measurements to monitor the patient's progress and to determine when to advance to the next phase.

Most patients do not require phase V rehabilitation; they are able to maximize their motion and strength

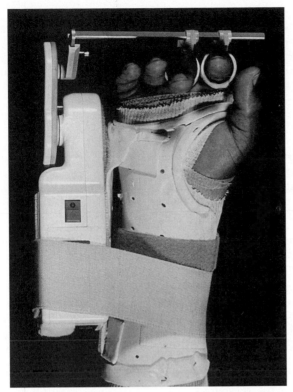

Figure 41–10. Splinting with a dynamic continuous passive motion (CPM) component to provide dynamic stretch to improve motion. (Courtesy of Continuous Passive Motion, Kinetic Continuous Passive Motion, Smith & Nephew, Germantown, WI.)

lator for the daily therapy of such patients as well as for their evaluations (see Chapter 40).

SYNDROMES OF WRIST OVERUSE

Overuse is defined as a level of repetitive microtrauma sufficient to overwhelm the tissues' ability to adapt. Microtrauma indicates damage at the microscopic or molecular level and can be produced by either a tension or a shear load. A one-time, excessive stress may cause microtrauma, but it usually results from repetitive loading episodes at a force or elongation level well within the physiologic range. Poor technique and improper equipment are additional factors that contribute to the development of overuse syndromes.[3] Our goals of treatment in phases I and II are to address the acute inflammatory condition and to prevent any further generation of fibrous adhesions or scarring due to chronic inflammation. We instruct the patient to avoid aggravating activities, with education for restructuring any inciting occupational or recreational activities. During this phase of treatment, we institute a program of rest, ice, splinting, and NSAIDs. If these measures fail, the patient is usually referred back to the surgeon for consideration of steroid injection. Once the acute inflammation is controlled, we progress to some form of heat treatment and begin phase III to restore range of motion with stretching and active range-of-motion exercises. Finally, the patient begins a strengthening program to prevent recurrences. A change in technique or equipment is often necessary for a return to work or athletic activity.

de QUERVAIN'S DISEASE

With stenosing tenosynovitis of the abductor pollicis longus (APL) and extensor pollicis brevis (EPB), we perform an initial evaluation of pain, edema, and range of motion to obtain baseline information in order to gauge progress with treatment. We usually

without formal work hardening. There is, however, a subset of patients who do require work hardening to return them to their work environment. These include, patients whose pathology and/or treatment has left them with significant loss of motion or strength, and patients whose job-related activities predispose them to recurrence of their symptoms. When dealing with these patients, we are aggressive about beginning work simulation during the late stages of strengthening. We commonly use the BTE work simu-

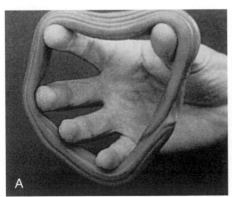
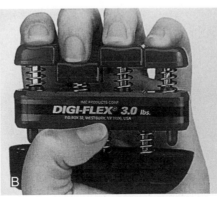
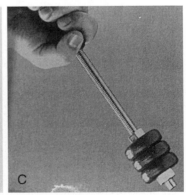

Figure 41–11. Hand strengthening devices: *A,* resistive putty; *B,* spring-loaded hand gripper; *C,* free weight. (Courtesy of Mac Products Corp., Westbury, NY.)

defer the measurement of strength until the pain has diminished to a tolerable level. Pain with palpation is recorded along with a subjective report of activities that cause pain. We document the presence of the Finkelstein's test and pain with active radial deviation of the wrist (see Chapter 6).

We visually assess swelling over the first dorsal compartment and measure edema by water displacement using either a Volumeter or circumferential measurements at the wrist, thumb, proximal phalanx, and interphalangeal (IP) joints.

We routinely perform goniometric measurements of thumb active and passive ranges of motion, including flexion and extension of the thumb metacarpophalangeal (MP) and IP joints. We note limitation of active range of motion secondary to pain, measure opposition of the thumb to the digits, evaluate the web space, measure wrist range of motion, and assess digital flexion. Range-of-motion measurements of the involved hand should be compared with those in the normal hand.[4]

In the inflammatory phase, we initially manage the patient with rest. We place the thumb in a thumb gauntlet splint, long opponens splint (Fig. 41–12), or thumb spica splint. The short-arm splint holds the wrist in 15° extension, the thumb palmarly abducted, and the MP joint in 10° of flexion. We then test for pain with IP flexion and resisted IP extension. If these maneuvers cause pain, we include the IP joint in the splint in an extended position. Immobilization is discontinued at the IP joint when the patient does not have pain with this motion.

Initially, we instruct the patient to wear the splint both day and night and to remove it only for hygiene or exercise purposes. Exercises include three-times-daily gentle, active range of motion of the thumb and wrist out of the splint. Active exercises of the nonimmobilized joints are encouraged, including tendon gliding exercises of the fingers.

We control inflammation through noninvasive techniques, such as ice massage for 3 minutes or application of a cold pack over the inflamed tendons

for 10 minutes three to four times daily. We reduce pain and inflammation by providing six to eight treatments of iontophoresis, followed by 10 to 15 minutes of cryotherapy. If we are unable to calm the inflammation with these modalities, we refer the patient back to the surgeon for possible corticosteroid injection.

We advance the patients through the acute phase depending on the response to treatment. Patients gradually wean themselves from the splint as the exercise schedule progresses. Various strengthening activities are implemented during the therapy program, with our goals to include strengthening of grip and pinch and increasing the patient's ability to perform job tasks.

INTERSECTION SYNDROME

Intersection syndrome describes an inflammatory condition located at the crossing point of the first dorsal compartment muscles (APL and EPB) and the radial wrist extensors: extensor carpi radialis longus (ECRL) and extensor carpi radialis brevis (ECRB). Pain and swelling are noted 4 to 6 cm proximal to the radial carpal joint on the dorsal surface of the forearm. In severe cases, palpable crepitus is observed with wrist or thumb motion.

Intersection syndrome is generally attributed to repetitive extension and flexion of the wrist or to direct trauma. Finkelstein's test elicits pain at the intersection site. The most difficult entity to differentiate from an early intersection syndrome is de Quervain's disease. These two entities can be differentiated by their unique locations of pain and swelling. Nonoperative measures, such as rest, splinting in 15° to 20° wrist extension, NSAIDs, and ice, may be tried initially.

We recommend at least 6 weeks of conservative treatment, to include splinting in a long opponens or thumb spica splint, anti-inflammatory agents, six to eight treatments of iontophoresis, and a corticosteroid injection, if necessary. After a successful course of treatment, it is important to slowly rehabilitate the patient. Wrist curls are an important preconditioning exercise but should be performed only if they do not induce pain.[2]

EXTENSOR CARPI ULNARIS TENOSYNOVITIS/SUBLUXATION

The sixth dorsal compartment is a common site of upper extremity stenosing tenosynovitis. Extensor carpi ulnaris (ECU) tendinitis is one of many pathologic entities that produce pain and swelling along the dorsal ulnar aspect of the wrist, so the diagnosis may be overlooked.[3] This site is one of the most common areas of rheumatoid tenosynovitis, which in this case produces subluxation of the ECU from the compartment. Forearm hypersupination and forced

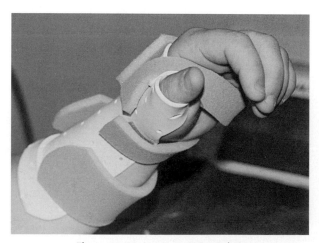

Figure 41–12. Long opponens splint.

ulnar wrist deviation can also produce ECU subluxation.

Pain, tenderness, and swelling at the dorsal ulnar aspect of the wrist may be present. If subluxation of the tendon is occurring, the patient notes a recurrent "snapping" over the wrist that can be reproduced by active forearm supination with ulnar deviation. If subluxation is the cause of the tenosynovitis and the history suggests that subluxation is acute, we recommend splinting of the wrist for 6 weeks with the wrist in slight dorsiflexion (Fig. 41–13).

During the inflammatory phase of ECU tenosynovitis, rest and splinting are the mainstays of treatment using a volar wrist "cock-up" splint with slight ulnar deviation to take stress off of the ECU tendon. Massage and ice are useful to diminish the inflammation and swelling. Iontophoresis is the next step if there is response to these measures. If necessary, this step is followed by corticosteroid injection into the ECU sheath.

When the inflammation and edema are under control, we move to phase III, range of motion. Once active range of motion is symmetric with the unaffected extremity, we can progress to phase IV, strengthening. In the strengthening phase, we emphasize resisted wrist extension and heavy grip with the wrist in the extended position.

DEGENERATIVE JOINT DISEASE OF THE WRIST

Degenerative arthritis of the wrist occurs in very specific patterns. The sequence and progression of these patterns is consistent. The most common pattern is the SLAC wrist (scapholunate advanced collapse) deformity (SLAC wrist), and the second most common is triscaphe arthritis, followed by distal radioulnar joint degenerative joint disease (DJD) and combination patterns. On the basis of the pathomechanics of the degenerative process, we have incorporated the following concepts into the phase-specific treatment program to manage DJD of the wrist.

During phase I, evaluating and controlling inflammation is our primary treatment concern. Modalities and techniques of treatment that we rely on include rest, ice application, and supportive splinting of the wrist, usually in neutral or slight extension.

In phase II, we consider the status of all the tissues in the hand, including tendon, muscle, and nerve. The destructive process often goes beyond the joint capsule to affect soft tissues. Therefore, we seek to preserve the integrity of these tissues and to maintain their function using a combination of deep heat modalities and range of motion.

We also recommend focusing on joint systems rather than isolated joints. Structures of the hand are interdependent in providing the stability and mobility necessary for function. Forces act across multiple joints, with changes at one joint (whether by disease or therapeutic intervention) altering the forces acting on the adjacent joints. Therefore, treatment cannot be isolated to an individual joint and should address joint systems. Modalities and techniques of treatment that we recommend include proper positioning through splinting, range-of-motion, progressive resistive exercises, and ergonomics/adaptive equipment.[5]

CONSERVATIVE TREATMENT OF THE CARPOMETACARPAL JOINT

The configuration of the ligaments and the saddle shape of the carpometacarpal (CMC) joint allow rotation and the four other motions of flexion/extension and abduction/adduction. The trapezium sits palmar to the other carpals, thus allowing the thumb to move in an arc around the fingers. Because of this large range of motion and the accompanying normal joint mobility, this joint most commonly requires stabilizing rather than dynamic splinting.

The common deforming force, particularly as seen in osteoarthritis or rheumatoid arthritis, is the strong pull of the adductor pollicis muscle, which originates palmarly on the third metacarpal and inserts on the

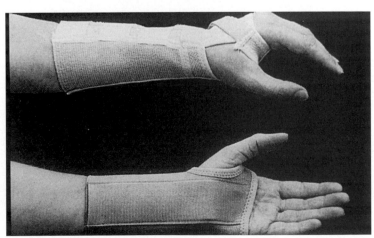

Figure 41–13. Wrist immobilization splint. Many off-the-shelf variations are available. They can also easily be custom molded from appropriate materials by the therapist.

first metacarpal and extensor hood mechanism. The other short intrinsics of the thumb that originate on the carpals and insert primarily on the distal aspect of the first metacarpal provide a deforming force to flex the first metacarpal. Insertion of the long adductor muscles into the metacarpal base aggravates the deformity. With strong intrinsic muscles and frequent powerful pinching and flexion movements, the dorsal aspect of the CMC joint is stressed, allowing the first metacarpal to sublux dorsally and radially in relationship to the trapezium. This also, with time, allows the metacarpophalangeal (MP) joint to become lax and develop a hyperextension deformity.

Any splint fitted to stabilize dorsoradial subluxation of the CMC joint must apply a stabilizing extension force to the palmar and ulnar aspects of the distal end of the metacarpal while providing counterpressure to the dorsoradial aspect of the base of the metacarpal. Stabilizing this joint in relationship to the other metacarpals is mandatory to support the CMC joint during pinching. Additionally, we ensure that the splint prevents hyperextension at the MP joint. It is also critical to assess the hand for the presence of a first web space contracture. This deformity often is present and requires a web space splint to stretch the soft tissues (Fig. 41–14).

We put our patients in a full-time splinting program for 1 month. If during that time the symptoms improve, we then attempt to wean them. If they do not improve, or if we are unable to wean them from full-time splint wear, we recommend steroid injection.

Patients may experience functional limitations with various aspects of the activities of daily living. These limitations often vary and may change from day to day in the same patient. Such problems may be the result of pain, deformity, loss of range of motion, fatigue, or decreased muscle strength. Some patients may require the use of adaptive equipment to function independently. In some cases, the need for equipment may be only temporary, to help the patient through a flare-up and to protect the joint.

For patients who show response to conservative management, we stress that the underlying disease has not changed, and we therefore advocate the use of joint protection techniques to prevent recurrence of symptoms. Joint protection techniques are methods of performing daily activities with a minimal amount of stress to the joints to reduce pain, preserve joint structures, and conserve physical energy. These techniques consider the implications of the disease process and integrate them with the person's lifestyle. Basic principles of joint protection are as follows:

1. Respect pain.
2. Maintain muscle strength and range of motion.
3. Balance work and rest.
4. Avoid deforming positions/prolonged positioning.
5. Use stronger and larger joints when possible.
6. Use necessary adaptive equipment.
7. Conserve energy.

CONSERVATIVE TREATMENT OF THE RHEUMATOID WRIST

The wrist, the key joint for proper function of the hand, may be affected by rheumatoid arthritis. As with other inflammatory diseases, treatment can be divided into three stages according to disease stage:

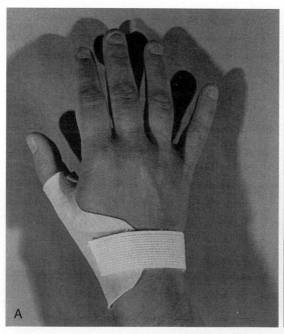
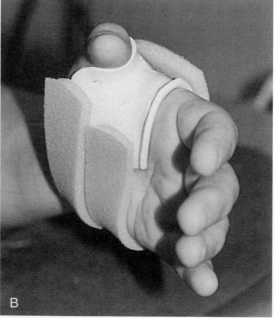

Figure 41–14. *A,* Short opponens splint for immobilization of the carpometacarpal joint. *B,* Web spacer splint for first web space stretch.

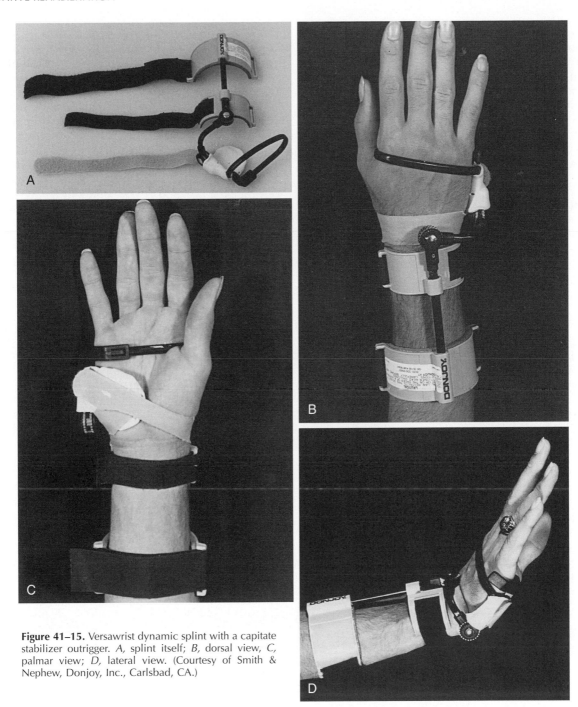

Figure 41–15. Versawrist dynamic splint with a capitate stabilizer outrigger. *A,* splint itself; *B,* dorsal view, *C,* palmar view; *D,* lateral view. (Courtesy of Smith & Nephew, Donjoy, Inc., Carlsbad, CA.)

the acute stage, the subacute stage, and the chronic stage. The goals of treatment are similar in each stage, that is, to decrease pain and swelling, maintain joint mobility, and prevent or minimize joint deformity.[5]

The rehabilitative approach to the rheumatoid patient has an inherent paradox. The emphasis of the rehabilitation protocol swings in a pendulum fashion from an emphasis on rest and splinting to an emphasis on more strenuous exercise, depending on the stage of the rheumatoid disease. It is important that the rehabilitation team have a heightened awareness

of what phase of disease the patient is in and that they educate the patient to be aware of these phases and adjust their own therapy accordingly.

In the acute inflammatory phase of the disease, we use resting wrist splints, maintaining a balanced neutral position to provide rest and support while counteracting the deforming forces that usually result in radial collapse of the wrist. We continue with gentle range-of-motion exercises to maintain joint mobility.

As the acute inflammation subsides, we gradually

increase exercise and activities as tolerated by the patient. Joint protection principles are introduced at this time.

In the chronic stage, emphasis is put on joint protection, activities of daily living, and exercises to increase strength and endurance. Resting splints, for either the whole hand or the wrist, are used to reduce inflammation, to rest and support weakened structures, to properly position joints, to minimize joint deformity, and to improve function.

MIDCARPAL INSTABILITY: SPLINTING

The common physical manifestation of midcarpal instability is a painful, palpable wrist clunk when moving from radial to ulnar deviation. This is produced as the proximal row snaps from flexion to extension as the palmarly subluxed capitate head seats itself back into the lunate fossa. We have designed an orthosis that can reduce the VISI (volar intercalated segmental instability) deformity or palmar subluxation of the capitate prior to initiation of motion. When successful, use of this orthosis prevents the abnormal snapping of the capitate and thus prevents the painful synovitis that accompanies this abnormal motion. The splint is a modification of a commercially available splint that allows wrist motion in the flexion/extension plane.[6] We add an outrigger to apply a palmar-to-dorsal stabilizing force to the pisiform, which reduces the proximal row VISI deformity and prevents palmar subluxation of the capitate (Fig. 41–15).

The splint is applied and worn for all activities for 4 to 6 weeks in an effort to reduce the synovitis. If we are able to eliminate the synovitis, avoidance of aggravating activities may be all that is necessary to prevent recurrence of symptoms.

DYNAMIC STABILIZATION THROUGH RETRAINING

Palmar midcarpal instability may be an exaggerated laxity of normal carpal support ligaments. As in the shoulder and knee, secondary restraints, primarily musculotendinous, can provide added support when needed. Our clinical experience has shown that balanced activation of wrist extensors and flexors tightens the wrist unit, rebalances midcarpal joint forces, and corrects the VISI sag of palmar midcarpal instability. If the patient can be trained to fire these muscles prior to initiating ulnar deviation, then the clunk can be eliminated. More investigative work is required to determine whether muscle strengthening, motor reeducation, and biofeedback techniques will be practical in treating this condition.

CONCLUSION

The basic principles described in this chapter apply to nearly all hand and wrist injuries and disorders. The key to a good, successful therapy program is tailoring the program to the individual patient according to the patient's needs, abilities, and response to the modalities as they are applied. It is essential to understand the purpose and mechanism of each of the therapeutic modalities used, to ensure that they are not applied in a haphazard fashion but rather are applied during the specific phase of treatment that will maximally benefit the patient. Good communication among the surgeon, therapist, and patient is crucial in achieving the ideal therapy plan.

References

1. Nicholson B: Clinical Evaluation. In Stanley BG, Tribuzi SM (eds) Concepts: Concepts in Hand Rehabilitation. Philadelphia, FA Davis, 1992.
2. Harris PR: Iontophoresis: Clinical research in musculoskeletal inflammatory conditions. J Orthop Sports Phys Ther 4:109–112, 1982.
3. Kiefhaber TR, Stern PJ: Upper extremity tendinitis and overuse syndromes in the athlete. Clin Sports Med 11:39–43, 1992.
4. Baxter-Petralia P, Penney V: Cumulative trauma. In Stanley BG, Tribuzi SM (eds): Concepts in Hand Rehabilitation. Philadelphia, FA Davis, 1992.
5. Marx H: Rheumatoid arthritis. In Stanley BG, Tribuzi SM (eds): Concepts in Hand Rehabilitation. Philadelphia, FA Davis, 1992.
6. Lichtman DM, Schneider JR, Swafford AR, et al: Ulnar midcarpal instability. Clinical and laboratory analysis. J Hand Surg 6:515–523, 1981.

CHAPTER 42

Postoperative Wrist Rehabilitation

Emily Jeter, OTR/L, Gregory G. Degnan, MD,
and David M. Lichtman, MD

PHASES OF POSTOPERATIVE WRIST REHABILITATION

Healing and rehabilitation after wrist surgery follow a predictable sequence of events that can be influenced by the surgeon and therapist. Rehabilitation of the wrist is based on a sound knowledge of the biology of wound healing, how this knowledge relates to tissues of the wrist, and how healing can be optimized to achieve the best functional result after injury.[1] A team approach is essential to achieving optimal results. The therapy of the educated patient, performed under the guidance of the therapist and surgeon, ensures that gliding planes and soft tissue equilibrium are restored and tissues are strengthened through an individually designed and supervised therapy program that follows phase-specific treatment goals. We select therapeutic modalities and treatment techniques on the basis of a knowledge of their actions and of the wound healing process in the wrist (see Table 41–1).

Initially, we focus our treatment in phase I, the inflammatory phase of postoperative wrist healing, on edema control. Prevention of a prolonged inflammatory response is essential in minimizing edema, soft tissue and periarticular tightness, decreased motion, and the potential for permanent loss of function. During this phase, we incorporate procedure-specific splint immobilization to rest tissues traumatized by either surgery or injury. Therapeutic motion is encouraged; however, if started too early and without control, it will only aggravate the trauma, perpetuating the inflammatory response.

In phase II, we continue our focus on preventive management through the development of a favorable soft tissue environment. This approach minimizes scar tissue formation and results in less need for prolonged management in the maturation phase. Our clinical management in these phases, which overlap, consists of: (1) wound care and dressings to provide an optimal environment for healing, (2) edema control measures, such as Coban wrapping, retrograde massage, intermittent compression, and icing, (3) active and passive motion, focusing on tendon glide and controlled passive stretch, and (4) splinting, for immobilization purposes.

In phase III, range of motion, and phase IV, strengthening, we continue to overlap with the previous phases and focus on the maturation of scar tissue with heat modalities (paraffin or moist heat), scar mobilization using massage and compression, and splinting using low-load and long-duration approaches. Active, active-assisted, and passive range-of-motion exercises to increase total active range of motion at the wrist are emphasized, and as range of motion improves, isometric, isokinetic, and isotonic strengthening are added to the program.

Finally, in phase V, work hardening/conditioning, we focus on the use of work-oriented tasks as the ultimate treatment tool to restore range of motion, strength, and coordination. In work hardening, the patient works with activities that simulate the resistance, repetition, duration, and biomechanics of the occupation to which he or she hopes to return. The use of the Baltimore Therapeutic Evaluator (BTE), or work familiar tasks (e.g., filing, lifting) are structured and graded to progressively increase stamina (energy at top speed), endurance (necessary for prolonged activity), physical tolerances, productivity, and, ultimately, confidence. Equilibrium must be restored to the injured tissues, and the tissues must withstand a high level of physical stress without inflammation before a patient may participate in a work hardening/conditioning program. A clinic program consisting of high resistance and maximum repetition exercise does not qualify as work hardening.[2] In a true work hardening/conditioning program the patient performs tasks using the same muscle groups, range of motion, repetitions, and duration that would be necessary for performance of his or her particular job. Ideally, the rehabilitation program is performed using the pre-injury job tasks at the job site, with the therapist monitoring the results.

This general approach to the postoperative patient closely parallels our conservative therapeutic approach to the patient with an injured wrist described in Chapter 41. Specific surgical procedures demand specific postoperative regimens but the general treatment rationale remains the same for all injured and postoperative patients. The treatment for postoperative patients is described here according to the surgical procedure.

PROXIMAL ROW CARPECTOMY

The majority of candidates for a proximal row carpectomy (PRC) have a severely disabled painful wrist

709

with a limited arc of motion and decreased grip strength. Our treatment goals are to decrease wrist pain, increase and maintain range of motion at the wrist to 50% to 70% of normal, and increase and maintain grip strength to 50% to 80% of normal.[3] Despite Jamar grip strength measurements, which may reveal grip strength of 70% to 80% of that in the unaffected side, patients may complain of subjective weakness or instability when performing heavy gripping activities. For patients with this complaint, we provide a stabilizing wrist splint, such as an elastic wrist support strap, for any activities involving heavy grip (Fig. 42–1).

Therapists and surgeons should be aware and should warn all their patients that some patients undergoing carpectomy note an inability to flex the fingers in the immediate postoperative period. This inability is secondary to an alteration of the Blick's curve for the musculotendinous unit due to shortening of the wrist. It will resolve, and with continued therapy for active range of motion and strengthening, the muscles will readjust and function normally.

Postoperatively, we place the patient's wrist in a bulky dressing with a volar wrist/forearm plaster splint for 10 to 14 days. In this early postoperative period, we focus on edema control using elevation, retrograde massage, active tendon gliding exercises, and cryotherapy as indicated. At 10 to 14 days, we remove the sutures, put the patient in a short-arm cast, and give instructions for continued digital range of motion and edema management. The cast is removed 1 to 2 weeks later, and we begin active and gentle passive range-of-motion therapy under a therapist's supervision. At this point, we also encourage use of the extremity for activities of daily living. For the next 6 to 8 weeks, we continue splint protection for heavy activities and sleeping. We use a lightweight removable orthosis. During this period, we increase the passive range-of-motion and stretching exercises and start the patient on a progressive resistive strengthening program. Depending on the patient's hand dominance and nature of work, we return the patient to sedentary work 2 to 3 weeks postoperatively; to light duty at 6 to 8 weeks; and to

manual labor as soon as adequate strength is demonstrated, usually 6 to 12 months.[4]

LIMITED INTERCARPAL FUSION

Limited intercarpal fusion, or intercarpal arthrodesis, is currently popular for the treatment of carpal instabilities and, when combined with scaphoid excision, is also popular for the treatment of scapholunate advanced collapse (SLAC) or scaphoid non-union advanced collapse (SNAC) wrist. This is the procedure of choice when the patient's job requires some wrist mobility and the radiocarpal joint is relatively free of arthritic involvement. The procedure is often considered in the same patients for whom a proximal row carpectomy is contemplated. Preoperative therapy evaluation can often help the surgeon decide which procedure is more appropriate for the individual patient. Patients who are not good rehabilitative candidates are probably better served by intercarpal fusion, because the end result of proximal row carpectomy is very dependent on patient cooperation with postoperative therapy. Patients who have preexisting small joint degenerative joint disease (DJD) or who would otherwise not tolerate prolonged immobilization would be better served by proximal row carpectomy.

With a limited intercarpal fusion, our treatment goals are to ensure fusion by protecting the wrist until the graft has incorporated, to maintain range of motion of the unaffected small joints of the hand, to ensure gliding of the extensor tendons.

Our postoperative protocol for limited intercarpal fusions includes immediate postoperative casting with emphasis on control of finger and hand edema and maintenance of active and passive range of motion of the digits of the hand. Elevation, Coban wrapping of the fingers, and aggressive range of motion of the finger joints are the focus in the first 2 to 4 weeks postoperatively. Casting is continued until radiographic fusion is evident, usually at 8 to 10 weeks. At this point, the Kirschner wire fixation and cast are removed, and we focus our attention on the wrist. As soon as the cast is removed, we begin an active and active-assisted wrist range-of-motion program. In a few weeks, passive stretch is initiated. This is facilitated by the use of heat modalities prior to any stretching of the capsular or ligamentous tissues. As pain diminishes, we begin a strengthening program, starting with pure gripping such as of putty and progressing as tolerated to exercises requiring wrist motion as well as grip strength. Aggressive strengthening is begun at this point with the expectation that maximum motion and grip strength will not be achieved for 6 months to a year following limited intercarpal arthrodesis. Finally, when the patient appears to have reached a plateau in the range-of-motion and strengthening program, we start them on a work hardening/

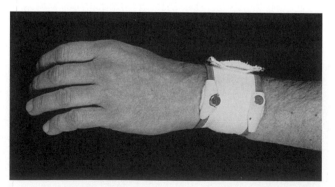

Figure 42–1. Elastic wrist support strap, useful in assisting stability when performing heavy activities. It can also be used to keep the ulna in a reduced position.

conditioning program; this usually occurs between 4 and 6 months postoperatively.

TOTAL WRIST FUSION

Wrist arthrodesis gives up motion for stability and pain relief. It often is performed as salvage surgery for other procedure failures and in heavy laborers with advanced radiocarpal instability or arthritis. We recommend fusing the dominant hand in 10° of extension and 5° of ulnar deviation to best facilitate functional activities. The average time for bony fusion varies from 8 to 12 weeks. Another 12 weeks of phase-specific rehabilitation is usually necessary to reach maximum benefit.

Our rehabilitation program for wrist fusion is similar to that discussed for limited intercarpal fusion, except that there is greater emphasis on extensor tendon gliding and small joint (digit) mobility. The dissection for this surgical procedure is greater than that for most intercarpal fusions, and the potential for postoperative scarring is therefore greater. We occasionally use a thermoplastic splint for protection of the fusion following cast removal and begin an aggressive strengthening program at that time.[5] Rigid dorsal plate fixation enables early cast removal and commencement of soft tissue therapy.

SWANSON WRIST ARTHROPLASTY

In the rheumatoid patient with good bone stock, reasonable preoperative motion, and a well-balanced wrist, silicone wrist arthroplasty is a viable salvage option that provides good pain relief and still allows for some limited motion of the wrist. Preoperatively, we explain to the patient that the goals of flexion and extension are 30° in either direction to avoid breakage of the implant.

As with all postoperative rehabilitation, we must ensure that edema control and maintaining motion at the unoperated joints is an integral part of the rehabilitation protocol. Postoperatively, we splint the wrist in neutral in a bulky compressive dressing for 3 weeks. During this time, we focus our efforts on edema control and range of motion of the metacarpophalangeal (MP) and proximal interphalangeal (PIP) joints. At 3 weeks postoperatively, we remove the bulky dressing and fit the patient with a static immobilization splint. The wrist is held in 15° of extension, and the splint is worn between exercise sessions and at night (Fig. 42–2). Active and gentle, passive range-of-motion exercises are initiated for the wrist and digits six to eight times daily for 10 to 15 minutes. Occasionally, we find it necessary to incorporate dynamic splinting of the digits to increase composite flexion or active extension (Fig. 42–3).

At 6 weeks postoperatively, we institute a program of passive range of motion, emphasizing flexion and extension. We instruct the patient to avoid radial and

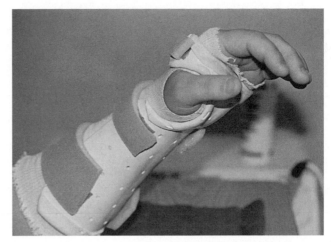

Figure 42–2. Static wrist support splint with the wrist position at 15° dorsiflexion.

ulnar deviation to protect the implant. Splinting is discontinued when the wrist is stable and the patient is asymptomatic. Splinting may be necessary for 8 to 10 weeks. At 8 weeks, the patient begins supervised, gentle, progressive strengthening of the wrist and hand, using graded resistive putty or free weights. At 12 weeks, we allow the patient to gradually resume normal activities.[7] A light supportive splint is used indefinitely for support during heavy activities.

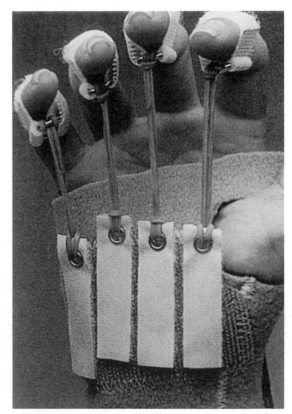

Figure 42–3. Dynamic outrigger splint to increase finger range of motion.

CARPOMETACARPAL ARTHROPLASTY (LIGAMENT RECONSTRUCTION TENDON ARTHROPLASTY TECHNIQUE)

Our long-term treatment goals following carpometacarpal (CMC) arthroplasty are to provide a pain-free joint, to increase range of motion, and to increase strength and functional use of the hand. Immediately postoperatively, we place the patient in a bulky thumb spica splint for 2 weeks. The interphalangeal joint is left free, and range of motion is encouraged at this joint. At 2 weeks, the bulky postoperative dressing and sutures are removed, and edema control measures are initiated. We fit the patient with a thumb spica cast or splint with the interphalangeal (IP) joint left free for range of motion (Fig. 42–4). The cast or splint is worn continuously until we initiate active and active-assisted motion of the MP joint at 4 weeks. This is performed by the patient or therapist holding the CMC joint in abduction.

At 6 to 8 weeks, the CMC joint pin, if used, is removed, and active motion of the CMC joint is begun. We emphasize abduction, extension, and opposition to each fingertip.[8] Aggressive soft tissue desensitization for the scar over the harvested flexor carpi radialis may be necessary. Scar massage and desensitization techniques to address the problem of irritation and neuritis of the superficial radial sensory nerve may also be required. Splinting is continued between exercise sessions and at night for patient comfort. If necessary, at 7 weeks, we initiate dynamic splinting to increase MP and IP joint motion if the CMC joint is well stabilized, and these joints have not responded to therapy. At 8 to 10 weeks, we discontinue the static splint if the joint is stable and the patient is asymptomatic. We begin gentle strengthening, including grip and pinch. At 10 to 12 weeks, normal use of the hand may be resumed without

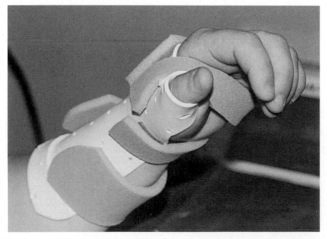

Figure 42–4. Long opponens splint for carpometacarpal and metacarpophalangeal joint stabilization.

restrictions, provided that the joint is stable and the patient is asymptomatic.[8]

PROCEDURES FOR RHEUMATOID ARTHRITIS

Wrist Synovectomy

Postsynovectomy patients with rheumatoid arthritis have specific therapy demands, in that there is a distressing tendency for the operated joints to stiffen. Therefore, in most cases, we initiate early aggressive range of motion of the joints that have undergone synovectomy. Maintenance of the range of motion of the adjacent joints also is emphasized. In the rheumatoid wrist, a certain amount of postoperative stiffness is often desirable, to add stability. It is therefore important for the patient, surgeon, and therapist to have a common understanding of the goals of surgery. In order to achieve desired motion, we use the normal postoperative mobilization techniques, with one exception. We use heat sparingly and with great care in patients with rheumatoid arthritis, because their skin tends to be thin and easily damaged. It does not tolerate the standard modalities of the heat packs prior to range-of-motion exercises.

Postoperatively, we apply a bulky dressing and splint the wrist in neutral. If distal radioulnar joint (DRUJ) stabilization was performed, the forearm is held in supination with a sugar-tong splint. Forearm supination is maintained for approximately 3 weeks (Fig. 42–5). At this time, we remove the splint and start both forearm and wrist motion.

The length of postoperative splinting depends on the amount of wrist ligament laxity present preoperatively and the extent of ligament disruption found at the time of surgery. The greater the laxity, the longer the wrist is splinted postoperatively. Splinting for 4 to 6 weeks may be necessary to allow enough capsular healing to provide stability. The range of motion after wrist synovectomy is 30° to 40° of flexion and extension.[10] If other procedures are performed (e.g., tendon transfers or repair), the postoperative therapy must be modified accordingly.

Darrach Procedure

Our postoperative treatment for the Darrach procedure in patients with rheumatoid arthritis requires specific, individualized attention, because it is usually only one of several procedures performed simultaneously. Concomitant procedures often include reconstruction of ruptured extensor tendons, extensor tenosynovectomy, and wrist synovectomy. The therapy for the Darrach procedure itself must be incorporated into the overall program, so that it does not interfere with the rehabilitation or healing process for the other procedures performed. Generally, we initiate active range-of-motion exercises at 3 to 5 days

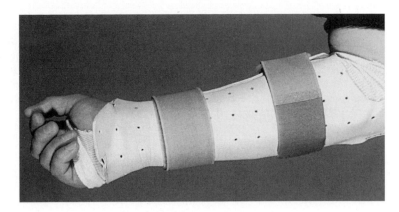

Figure 42–5. Sugar-tong forearm supination splint with the wrist support in neutral.

postoperatively, when the bulky dressing is removed. If the surgical area for the Darrach procedure is painful, exercises are initially minimized. When the Darrach procedure is performed in conjunction with a procedure to stabilize the DRUJ, the following protocol is utilized: for the first 3 weeks postoperatively, the arm remains in a bulky compressive dressing with the elbow flexed at 90° and the forearm supinated. (To aid in patient comfort, we may remove the bulky dressing at 2 weeks and fit the patient with a long-arm splint in the same position.) Three weeks postoperatively, a wrist immobilization splint is fabricated and applied in 15° of dorsiflexion for the patient to wear between exercise sessions and at night for comfort. Active and passive range-of-motion exercises are initiated for the wrist and forearm on an hourly basis. It is important to note that patients may have some discomfort along the area of the distal ulna as they attempt forearm rotation. This discomfort generally diminishes by 6 weeks postoperatively.

Some patients have mild residual dorsal subluxation of the distal ulna and find it much more comfortable to have a distal ulna strap applied approximately 2 inches proximal to the distal ulna to help keep the distal ulna reduced. At 6 weeks, the wrist immobilization splint may be discontinued, as long as the patient has no pain. Gentle strengthening is initiated.[7]

POSTOPERATIVE REHABILITATION FOLLOWING EXTERNAL FIXATION OF DISTAL RADIUS FRACTURES

External fixation presents its own set of problems for the therapist. Our immediate postoperative treatment is designed to maximize motion of the small joints and prevent pin tract infections. At 2 to 3 days postoperatively, we remove the bulky compressive dressing and begin daily pin care with hydrogen peroxide to minimize the risk of pin tract infection. A light compressive dressing may be applied with even compression around the pins. Active and gentle passive forearm range-of-motion exercises are initiated unless otherwise advised by the surgeon. We apply passive forearm rotation proximal to the fracture site and

within the patient's comfort level. We focus heavily, at this point, on active range of motion of the metacarpophalangeal joints and proximal interphalangeal joints. The index finger often presents a challenge, because the metacarpal pin can bind the extensor to this finger. The patient is also reminded that elbow and shoulder motion are important. Along these lines, we discourage the use of slings except in the immediate postoperative period.

Mobilization of the fingers and (later) the wrist is greatly facilitated by avoidance of over-distraction by the external fixation. If extrinsic tightness is noted early, the surgeon should consider decreasing the force of distraction.

Depending on fracture stability and consolidation, the external fixator is generally removed at 6 weeks. We immediately initiate active range-of-motion exercises to the wrist and forearm. These are performed for 10 minutes each hour. A wrist immobilization splint may be prescribed between exercise sessions and at night for protection. As soon as it is tolerated by the patient, we initiate strengthening with Theraputty and hand exercisers.

At 8 to 10 weeks, when the fracture is clinically and radiographically healed, we begin passive range-of-motion exercises. Occasionally, we use dynamic splinting to provide a constant resistive force in a patient who has a rubbery end point to the motion but is not progressing with standard techniques. Progressive resistive exercises are incorporated at this point.[7]

Scar massage and desensitization may be required in some patients following external fixation.

OPEN REDUCTION AND INTERNAL FIXATION OF SCAPHOID FRACTURES

Open reduction and internal fixation of scaphoid fractures and non-unions can often provide a stable construct amenable to early motion. This is especially true when the compression screws developed by Herbert and Herbert/Whipple have been used. Good communication between the surgeon and therapist can lead to early mobilization and return to function, even before complete fracture healing occurs.

Following stable fixation of a scaphoid fracture (e.g., utilizing a Herbert screw), range of motion may begin 7 to 14 days postoperatively. The postoperative dressing and splint are removed, and the patient is fitted with a long opponens splint, which will provide adequate stabilization during the early phases of rehabilitation. In the early rehabilitative period, we concentrate on healing soft tissues in an optimal environment to maximize range of motion. We pay particular attention to wrist extension, because we have found it consistently to be the motion most commonly lost after the volar surgical approach to the scaphoid is employed. If a dorsal approach has been used in the fixation of a proximal pole fracture, more emphasis is placed on wrist flexion.

We start aggressive active motion in the early postoperative period. As soft tissue healing becomes complete at 3 to 4 weeks, active-assisted range of motion is added. As fracture healing progresses, we shift the emphasis to strengthening and passive stretch if required.

CONCLUSION

It is important to realize that surgery is a controlled form of injury and that most wrist injuries require some form of rehabilitation. Although great variation exists in the type and complexity of wrist procedures, the general principles of rehabilitation are the same. Mobilization of the stiff wrist cannot be started until the injured tissues have healed enough to provide some stability. If the type of immobilization used is properly applied and active exercises are performed during the healing phase, joint stiffness proximal and distal to the wrist should not be a problem. After healing of the bony and soft tissue structures of the wrist is complete, the focus shifts to the wrist joint itself, with the long-term goals to maximize range of motion and strength.

References

1. Smith KL: Wound Healing. In Stanley BG, Tribuzi, SM (eds): Concepts in Hand Rehabilitation. Philadelphia, FA Davis, 1992.
2. Schultz-Johnson K: Work hardening: A mandate for hand therapy. Hand Clin 7:597–610, 1991.
3. Aiello B: Proximal row carpectomy. In Clark GL (ed): Hand Rehabilitation, A Practical Guide. New York, Churchill Livingstone, 1993, p 311.
4. Van Heest AE, Hous, JH: Proximal Row Carpectomy. In Gelberman RH: The Wrist. New York, Raven Press, 1994.
5. Stanley BG: Therapeutic exercise: Mobility in the hand. In Stanley BG, Tribuzi SM (eds): Concepts in Hand Rehabilitation. Philadelphia, FA Davis, 1992.
6. Swanson AB, de Groot Swanson G: Treatment Considerations and Resource Materials for Flexible Implant Arthroplasty. Grand Rapids, MI, Blodgett Memorial Medical Center, 1987.
7. Cannon NM (ed): Diagnosis and Treatment Manual for Physicians & Therapists. Indianapolis, The Hand Rehabilitation Center of Indiana, P.C., 1991.
8. Gorman RJ: The carpometacarpal joint arthroplasty. In Clark GL (ed): Hand Rehabilitation, A Practical Guide. New York, Churchill Livingstone, 1993.
9. Nalebuff EA, Garrod KJ: Present approach to the severely involved rheumatoid wrist. Orthop Clin North Am 15:369–380, 1984.
10. Feldon P, Millender LH, Nalebuff EA: Rheumatoid arthritis in the hand and wrist. In Green DP (ed): Operative Hand Surgery, Vol 2. New York, Churchill Livingstone, 1993.
11. Cooney WP, Linscheid RL, Dobyns JH: Scaphoid fractures: Problems associated with nonunion and avascular necrosis. Orthop Clin North Am 15:381–391, 1984.

Index

Note: Page numbers in *italics* refer to illustrations; page numbers followed
by (t) refer to tables.